Preface

Musculoskeletal surgery is one of the great success stories of medicine today. Our understanding of how bone and soft tissues grow and heal is increasing dramatically year by year. New biomaterials, which are coming much closer to providing strong long-lasting substitutes for the body's own tissues, are being created for use when natural healing is not possible. The result is that we can now treat more conditions than ever before, and produce excellent functional results where previously patients were doomed to be crippled for life.

Trauma and orthopedic surgery deals with pain, deformity, and loss of function in the musculoskeletal system. Many of the conditions that we manage are preventable. Indeed, poliomyelitis has now been eradicated in most countries of the world. The workload from the sequelae of this terrible disease will disappear in our lifetime. However, trauma, whether on the roads, in the workplace, or as a result of war, is proving much more difficult to prevent. Although its incidence is dropping in the developed world, the increase in the range and severity of treatable trauma has meant that the surgical workload has continued to increase beyond all recognition. As people live longer, osteoarthritis has become a major health problem, condemning many of the elderly to years of pain, and the frustration and cost of loss of independence. Joint replacement, first of the hip and then of other major joints in the body, now allows us to transform these people back into outgoing independent members of society, who can once again live a full and pain-free life. In the three volumes of this book we have attempted to show the full depth and breadth of this rapidly moving subject, presenting the basic science on which these new developments are based as well as the actual techniques and the indications for them.

A disquieting trend has been the widening gulf between the way in which musculoskeletal surgery is practised in the developed countries of the world. This makes no sense. If a particular treatment is used because it is the best and most cost-effective in one developed country, it is likely that this will also be the case in another. Many of the differences in treatment between countries appear to be the result of ignorance, and not of a genuine difference in needs. This book is specifically designed to address this problem. By involving leading authorities from internationally recognized centers in the United States, Europe, and elsewhere, it brings together the most authoritative opinions from wherever they can be found. It is designed to provide the information on which best practice can be based.

For some time now there has been no book covering the whole field of musculoskeletal trauma and orthopedics, although there are many excellent books covering specialist areas within the field. We have attempted to fill this gap with a textbook taking in research, theory, and decision-making skills, as well as the principles of operative techniques. The subject is enormous. Although we have tried to be comprehensive, there may be some omissions, and the editors welcome readers' comments and suggestions as to how we can improve the book in future.

The book is organized to serve as an easily accessible yet comprehensive source of information. It is divided into five major sections covering fundamental science, adult orthopedics, trauma, pediatric orthopedics, and pediatric trauma. Each section has been designed to allow the reader to find answers to specific questions while still providing chapters that can be read as independent units. The content is extensively referenced, highly illustrated, and punctuated with summary boxes throughout.

We would like to think that this book should be on the shelf of every practising orthopedic surgeon, whether in training or not. It should also be available in every medical library as a reference work, for primary care doctors, and for those involved in developing policy for health care in the future. Wherever it is, it should soon be well thumbed. It is designed to be cosmopolitan, comprehensive, and clear to read. If we have succeeded, it will be pulled from its shelf on a daily basis to settle a lingering doubt about a fact or an opinion, or indeed to spur the reader to do further research into yet another area of clinical practice where not all is as simple as might appear at first glance.

The Editors
Oxford and Iowa City
February 2002

Oxford Textbook of
Orthopedics and
Trauma

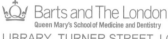

Project Editor	Roberta Nichols
Indexer	Jill Halliday
Production Controller	Gill Watts
Development Manager	Kate Martin
Design Manager	Claire Walker
Text Designer	Jonathan Coleclough
Illustrations	by Technical Graphics Department, Oxford University Press
Publisher	Richard Marley

Section Editors

The foot
C.L. Saltzman, Professor, Department of Orthopaedic Surgery and Biomedical Engineering, University of Iowa, Iowa City, USA

Paediatrics
M.J. Bell, Consultant Orthopaedic Surgeon, Sheffield Children's Hospital, Sheffield

Tumors
F.H. Sim, Professor of Orthopedics, Mayo Medical School, Rochester, USA

Volume 1

Oxford Textbook of
Orthopedics and Trauma

Edited by

Christopher Bulstrode
Professor of Trauma and Orthopaedics, University of Oxford

Joseph Buckwalter
Department of Orthopedic Surgery, University of Iowa, Iowa City, USA

Andrew Carr
Nuffield Professor of Orthopaedic Surgery, Nuffield Orthopaedic Centre, Oxford

Larry Marsh
Department of Orthopedic Surgery, University of Iowa Hospital, Iowa City, USA

Jeremy Fairbank
Consultant Orthopaedic Surgeon, Nuffield Orthopaedic Centre, Oxford

James Wilson-MacDonald
Consultant Orthopaedic Surgeon, John Radcliffe Hospital, Oxford

and

Gavin Bowden
Nuffield Orthopaedic Centre, Oxford

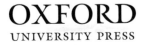

OXFORD
UNIVERSITY PRESS

OXFORD

UNIVERSITY PRESS

Great Clarendon Street, Oxford OX2 6DP

Oxford University Press is a department of the University of Oxford.
It furthers the University's objective of excellence in research, scholarship,
and education by publishing worldwide in

Oxford New York

Auckland Bangkok Buenos Aires Cape Town Chennai
Dar es Salaam Delhi Hong Kong Istanbul Karachi Kolkata
Kuala Lumpur Madrid Melbourne Mexico City Mumbai
Nairobi São Paulo Shanghai Taipei Tokyo Toronto
with an associated company in Berlin

Oxford is a registered trade mark of Oxford University Press
in the UK and in certain other countries

Published in the United States
by Oxford University Press Inc., New York

© Oxford University Press, 2002

The moral rights of the author have been asserted

Database right Oxford University Press (maker)

First edition published 2002

A catalogue record for this title is available from the British Library

Library of Congress Cataloging in Publication Data
(Data available)

ISBN 0 19 262681 7

10 9 8 7 6 5 4 3 2 1

Typeset in Minion
by Wyvern 21 Ltd, Bristol
Printed in Great Britain
on acid free paper by
Butler & Tanner Ltd, Frome, Somerset

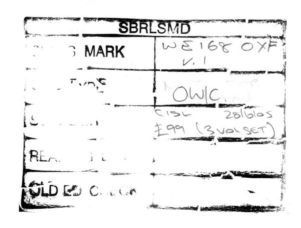

Contents

Index [1]

Volume 2

Part 2 Adult orthopedics

Index [1]

Volume 3

Part 3 Trauma

Part 4 Pediatric orthopedics

Part 5 Pediatric trauma

Index [1]

List of Contributors

Seref Aktas Associate Professor in Orthopaedic Surgery, Trakya University Faculty of Medicine, Edirne, Turkey

Patricia E. Allen Consultant Orthopaedic Surgeon, Bristol Children's Hospital, Bristol, UK

A. Amendola Associate Professor, Orthopedic Surgery, University of Western Ontario, London, Ontario, Canada

Howard S. An Morton International Professor of Orthopaedic Surgery, Rush Medical College, Rush-Presbyterian-St.Luke's Medical Center, Chicago, Illinois, USA

Robert B. Anderson Miller Orthopaedic Clinic Faculty, Carolinas Medical Center, Charlotte, North Carolina, USA

Paul A. Anderson Clinical Associate Professor, Orthopedic Surgery, University of Washington, Seattle, Washington, USA

Carola A.S. Arndt Associate Professor of Pediatrics, Mayo Medical School; Consultant, Department of Pediatrics and Adolescent Medicine, Division of Pediatric Hematology/Oncology, Mayo Clinic, Rochester, Minnesota, USA

Roger M. Atkins Consultant Orthopaedic Surgeon and Reader in Orthopaedic Surgery, Bristol Royal Infirmary, Bristol, UK

Bridget L. Atkins Consultant Microbiologist, Oxford Radcliffe Hospitals; Honorary Consultant Physician, Bone Infection Unit, Nuffield Orthopaedic Centre, Oxford, UK

Terry S. Axelrod Division of Orthopaedic Surgery, Sunnybrook Health Science Centre, Toronto, Canada

David C. Ayers Director of Joint Replacement Surgery, SUNY Upstate Medical University, Syracuse, New York, USA

L.C. Bainbridge Consultant Hand Surgeon, Pulvertaft Hand Clinic, Derby, UK

Gordon Bannister Consultant Orthopaedic Surgeon, North Bristol NHS Trust, UK

R. Barbieri Assistant Professor, Department of Orthopaedics, New Jersey Medical School, Newark, New Jersey, USA

Aires A.B. Barros D'Sa Consultant Vascular Surgeon, Royal Victoria Hospital, Belfast; Honorary Lecturer in Surgery, The Queen's University of Belfast, UK

D. Beaman Attending Physician, Legacy Emmanuel Hospital, Portland, Oregon, USA

James H. Beaty Professor, University of Tennessee-Campbell Clinic Department of Orthopaedic Surgery; Chief-of-Staff, Campbell Clinic, Memphis, Tennessee, USA

Fred F. Behrens Professor and Chairman, Department of Orthopaedics, New Jersey Medical School, Newark, New Jersey, USA

George C. Bennet Consultant Orthopaedic Surgeon, Royal Hospital for Sick Children, Glasgow, UK

G. Bentley Professor and Director of Orthopaedics, Institute of Orthopaedics, University College London, UK

Anthony R. Berendt Consultant Physician-in-Charge, Bone Infection Unit, Nuffield Orthopaedic Centre, Oxford, UK

Richard A. Berger Department of Orthopaedics, New Jersey Medical School, Newark, New Jersey, USA

J. Sybil Biermann Department of Orthopaedic Oncology, University of Michigan, Ann Arbor, Michigan, USA

William F. Blair Steindler Orthopaedic Clinic, Iowa City, Iowa, USA

G.W. Blunn Professor, Centre for Biomedical Engineering, Institute of Orthopaedic and Musculoskeletal Science, University College London; Royal National Orthopaedic Hospital Trust, Stanmore, UK

Earl R. Bogoch Professor, Department of Surgery, University of Toronto, Canada

Henry H. Bohlman Department of Orthopaedics and Rehabilitation, Oregon Health Sciences University, Portland, Oregon, USA

D. Glynn Bolitho Associate Professor, Division of Plastic Surgery, University of California, San Diego, California, USA

S.R. Bollen Consultant Orthopaedic Surgeon, Bradford Royal Infirmary, Bradford, UK

A. Bonomo Shoulder Fellow, Nuffield Orthopaedic Centre, Oxford, UK

Norbert Boos Associate Professor, Chief of Spine Surgery, Orthopedic University Hospital Balgrist, Zürich, Switzerland

O.M. Böstman Consultant Orthopaedic Surgeon, Department of Orthopaedic and Trauma Surgery, University Hospital, Helsinki, Finland

Robert B. Bourne Professor of Adult Reconstructive Surgery, University of Western Ontario, London, Ontario, Canada

Martin I. Boyer Division of Orthopaedic Surgery, Sunnybrook Health Science Centre, Toronto, Canada

Anthony Bradlow Consultant Rheumatologist, Royal Berkshire and Battle Hospitals NHS Trust, Reading, UK

Michael E. Brage Assistant Professor of Orthopaedic Surgery, University of California, San Diego, California, USA

Richard A. Brand Professor, Department of Orthopedic Surgery, University of Iowa, Iowa City, Iowa, USA

Eric A. Brandser Associate Professor, Director Musculoskeletal Imaging, University of Iowa, Iowa City, Iowa, USA

T.R.W. Briggs Consultant Orthopaedic Surgeon, Royal National Orthopaedic Hospital Trust, Stanmore, UK

Jeffrey T. Brodie Fellow, Division of Foot and Ankle Surgery, Department of Orthopaedic Surgery, Mayo Clinic Scottsdale, Arizona, USA

Nigel S. Broughton Consultant Orthopaedic Surgeon, Frankston Hospital, Frankston, Victoria, Australia

Joseph A. Buckwalter Professor and Chair, Department of Orthopaedics, University of Iowa, Iowa City, Iowa, USA

Christopher Bulstrode Clinical Reader and Honorary Consultant, Nuffield Department of Orthopaedic Surgery, John Radcliffe Hospital, Oxford, UK

Peter Burge Consultant Hand Surgeon, Nuffield Orthopaedic Centre, Oxford, UK

Chris Caddy Consultant Plastic Surgeon, Northern General Hospital, Sheffield, UK

Jason H. Calhoun Professor and Chairman, Department of Orthopedics and Rehabilitation, University of Texas Medical Branch, Galveston,Texas, USA

Margaret Callan Medical Research Council Senior Fellow and Honorary Consultant Rheumatologist, John Radcliffe Hospital, Oxford, UK

Douglas A. Campbell Consultant Hand Surgeon, St James' University Hospital, Leeds, UK

Andrew Carr Consultant Orthopaedic Surgeon, Nuffield Orthopaedic Centre, Oxford, UK

James B. Carr Associate Professor of Orthopedic Surgery, Medical College of Virginia, Richmond, Virginia, USA

Maurizio A. Catagni Chief of the Ilizarov Unit, Department of Orthopaedics, Lecco General Hospital, Italy

Fabio Catani Assistant Professor of Orthopaedic Surgery, University of Bologna, Istituti Ortopedici Rizzoli, Bologna, Italy

A. Catterall Emeritus Consultant Orthopaedic Surgeon, Royal National Orthopaedic Hospital, Stanmore, Middlesex, UK

F. Cavina Pratesi Resident, Policlinico G.B. Rossi, University of Verona, Italy

Jens R. Chapman Associate Professor of Orthopaedic and Neurological Surgery, Harborview Medical Center, University of Washington School of Medicine, Seattle, Washington, USA

Edward Y. Cheng Associate Professor, Department of Orthopaedic Surgery, University of Minnesota, Minneapolis, Minnesota, USA

Jai Chitnavis Specialist Registrar in Orthopaedics, Nuffield Orthopaedic Centre, Oxford, UK

Peter Choong Professor of Orthopaedics, University of Melbourne; Professor and Director of Orthopaedics, St Vincent's Hospital and Peter MacCallum Cancer Institute, Melbourne, Australia

James Christie Consultant Trauma Surgeon, Edinburgh Orthopaedic Trauma Unit, Edinburgh, UK

Richard J. Claridge Assistant Professor of Orthopaedics, Mayo Clinic Scottsdale, Arizona, USA

Charles R. Clark Professor of Orthopaedic Surgery and Biomedical Engineering, University of Iowa, Iowa City, Iowa, USA

N.M.P. Clarke Consultant Orthopaedic Surgeon and University Reader in Orthopaedics, Southampton General Hospital, Southampton, UK

Jonathan Clasper Consultant Orthopaedic Surgeon, Frimley Park Hospital, Frimley, UK

Andrew S. Cole Consultant Trauma and Orthopaedic Surgeon, Southampton University Hospital, Southampton, UK

V.B. Conboy Consultant Orthopaedic Surgeon, Torbay Hospital, Torquay, UK

John Connolly Academic Chairman, Department of Orthopaedic Surgery, Orlando Regional Medical Center, Orlando; Clinical Professor, Department of Orthopaedic Surgery and Rehabilitation, University of Miami School of Medicine, Miami, Florida, USA

Paul H. Cooke Consultant Orthopaedic Surgeon, Foot and Ankle Surgery Service, Nuffield Orthopaedic Centre, Oxford, UK

Ian Corry Consultant Orthopaedic Surgeon, Royal Victoria Hospital, Belfast, UK

Kathryn E. Cramer Associate Professor of Orthopaedics, Wayne State University, Detroit, Michigan, USA

Alvin H. Crawford Professor of Pediatrics and Orthopedic Surgery, Director of Pediatric Orthopedic Surgery, Cincinnatti Children's Hospital Medical Center, Cincinatti, Ohio, USA

R. Crawford Director of Orthopaedics, Mater Hospital, Brisbane, Australia

Michael W. Cripps Medical School, Southwestern University, Dallas, Texas, USA

H. Alan Crockard The National Hospital for Neurology and Neurosurgery, London, UK

David J. Dandy Consultant Orthopaedic Surgeon, Addenbrooke's Hospital, Cambridge, UK

Károly M. Dávid Consultant Neurosurgeon, Department of Neurosurgery, Oldchurch Hospital, Romford, UK

Dennis J. Davin Assistant Clinical Professor, Oregon Health Sciences Center, Portland; Clinical Attending, Providence Medical Center, Portland, Oregon, USA

T.R.C. Davis Consultant Hand Surgeon, Queen's Medical Centre, Nottingham; Special Professor in Trauma and Orthopaedic Surgery, University of Nottingham, UK

W. Hodges Davis Director, Fellowship Program, Carolinas Medical Center and Miller Orthopaedic Clinic, Charlotte, North Carolina, USA

Jill Dawson Research Fellow, Department of Public Health and Primary Care, University of Oxford, UK

Thomas A. DeCoster Professor of Orthopaedic Surgery, University of New Mexico, Albuquerque, New Mexico, USA

R. Dehne Department of Pediatric Orthopedics, Children's Hospital, New Orleans, Louisiana, USA

J.M. de Leeuw Cambridge Hip and Knee Unit, BUPA Cambridge Lea Hospital, Cambridge, UK

Robert W. Demetrius Senior Resident in Dermatology, Mayo Clinic and Mayo Foundation, Rochester, Minnesota, USA

S.D. Deo Specialist Registrar, Orthopaedics and Trauma, Nuffield Orthopaedic Centre, Oxford, UK

R.N. de Steiger Consultant Orthopaedic Surgeon, Department of Surgery, Royal Melbourne Hospital, Melbourne, Victoria, Australia

J. Dheenadhayalan Consultant Orthopaedic Surgeon, Ganga Medical Centre and Hospitals, Coimbatore, India

Joseph Dias Consultant Orthopaedic Surgeon, University Hospitals of Leicester, UK

Robert A. Dickson Professor of Orthopaedic Surgery, University of Leeds; Director, University of Leeds Centre for Spinal Research; Consultant Orthopaedic Spinal Surgeon, St James's University Hospital, Leeds, UK

James H. Dobyns Emeritus Professor, Department of Orthopedic Surgery, Mayo Graduate School of Medicine, Rochester, Minnesota, USA

John P. Dormans Chief of Orthopaedic Surgery, Children's Hospital of Philadelphia; Professor of Orthopaedic Surgery, University of Pennsylvania School of Medicine, Philadelphia, Pennsylvania, USA

Frank E. Dowling Consultant Orthopaedic Surgeon, Our Lady's Hospital for Sick Children, Dublin, Ireland

Darren Drosdewech Assistant Professor, Orthopedic Surgery, University of Western Ontario, London, Ontario, Canada

J. Dubousset Professor of Paediatric Orthopaedics, Université René Descartes, Paris; Hôpital Saint-Vincent-de-Paul, Paris, France

D.G. Dujon Northern General Hospital, Sheffield, UK

Paul J. Duwelius Adjuvant Associate Professor of Orthopaedics, Oregon Health Sciences University, Portland; Clinical Attending, St Vincent Hospital, Portland, Oregon, USA

J. Dvorak Professor of Neurology, University of Zürich; Chairman, Department of Neurology, Schulthess Klinik, Zürich, Switzerland

Deborah M. Eastwood Consultant Orthopaedic Surgeon, Royal National Orthopaedic Hospital, London, UK

A.J. Edge Consultant Surgeon, Trauma and Orthopaedics, Worthing and Southlands NHS Trust Hospitals, Worthing, UK

Sally E. Edmonds Consultant Rheumatologist, Nuffield Orthopaedic Centre, Oxford, UK

Georges Y. El-Khoury Professor of Radiology and Orthopedics, Vice-Chair Department of Radiology, University of Iowa, Iowa City, Iowa

David Elliott Consultant Hand and Plastic Surgeon, St Andrew's Centre for Plastic Surgery, Chelmsford, UK

James Elliott Consultant Orthopaedic Surgeon, Musgrave Park Hospital, Belfast, UK

Mark E. Emerton Consultant Orthopaedic Surgeon, Leeds General Infirmary, Leeds, UK

Roger Emery Consultant Orthopaedic Surgeon, St Mary's Hospital, London, UK

David M. Evans Consultant Hand Surgeon, The Hand Clinic, Oakley Green, Windsor, UK

Jeremy Fairbank Consultant Orthopaedic and Spine Surgeon, Nuffield Orthopaedic Centre, Oxford, UK

Gordon Findlay Consultant Neurosurgeon, Walton Centre for Neurology and Neurosurgery, Liverpool, UK

Ray Fitzpatrick Professor of Public Health and Primary Care, University of Oxford, UK

J.A. Fixsen Consultant Orthopaedic Surgeon (Retired), Great Ormond Street Hospital for Sick Children, London, UK

A.S. Floyd Consultant Orthopaedic Surgeon, Milton Keynes General Hospital, Milton Keynes, UK

John M. Flynn Assistant Orthopaedic Surgeon, Children's Hospital of Philadelphia; Assistant Professor of Orthopaedic Surgery, University of Pennsylvania School of Medicine, Philadelphia, Pennsylvania, USA

Julian R. Flynn Consultant Orthopaedic and Trauma Surgeon, Milton Keynes General Hospital, Milton Keynes, UK

Christian Foglar Baylor College of Medicine, Houston, Texas, USA

R. Forster Hand Surgeon, Port St Lucie, Florida, USA

Deborah A. Frassica Assistant Professor of Radiation Oncology, Johns Hopkins University, Baltimore, Maryland, USA

Frank J. Frassica Professor of Orthopaedics and Oncology, Johns Hopkins University, Baltimore, Maryland, USA

Helen Frost Research Fellow, Queen Margaret University College, Edinburgh, UK

Evanthia C. Galanis Senior Associate Consultant, Division of Medical Oncology, Mayo Clinic and Mayo Foundation; Assistant Professor of Oncology, Mayo Medical School, Rochester, Minnesota, USA

C.S.B. Galasko Professor of Orthopaedic Surgery, University of Manchester; Consultant Orthopaedic Surgeon, Salford Royal Hospitals NHS Trust; Consultant Orthopaedic Surgeon, Royal Manchester Children's Hospital NHS Trust, Manchester, UK

B. Gardner Consultant Surgeon in Spinal Injuries, National Spinal Injuries Centre, Stoke Mandeville Hospital, Aylesbury, UK

Martin Gargan Consultant Trauma and Orthopaedic Surgeon, University Department of Orthopaedic Surgery, Bristol Royal Infirmary, Bristol, UK

Kevin L. Garvin Professor and Chairman, Department of Orthopaedic Surgery and Rehabilitation, University of Nebraska Medical Center, Omaha, Nebraska, USA

Mark C. Gebhardt Frederick W. Jane Associate Professor of Orthopedic Surgery, Harvard Medical School, Cambridge, Massachusetts; Associate Orthopaedic Surgeon, Massachusetts General Hospital and Children's Hospital, Boston, Massachusetts, USA

Gregory M. Georgiadis Associate Professor, Department of Orthopaedic Surgery, Medical College of Ohio, Toledo, Ohio, USA

E.J. Ghadiali Consultant Neuropsychologist, Walton Centre for Neurology and Neurosurgery, Liverpool, UK

Paul Giangrande Consultant Haematologist, Oxford Radcliffe Hospitals NHS Trust, Oxford, UK

C.L.M.H. Gibbons Consultant Orthopaedic Surgeon, Nuffield Orthopaedic Centre, Oxford, UK

Grey Giddens Consultant Surgeon, Royal United Hospital, Bath, UK

Henk Giele Consultant Plastic, Reconstruction, and Hand Surgeon, and Florey Lecturer in Clinical Medicine, Radcliffe Infirmary, Oxford, UK

Thomas J. Gill Massachusetts General Hospital, Harvard Medical School, Boston, Massachusetts, USA

W.J. Gillespie Professor and Dean, Dunedin School of Medicine, University of Otago, New Zealand

Jan Gillquist Professor Emeritus of Sports Medicine, Faculty of Health Sciences, Linköping University, Sweden

Steven Gitelis Professor and Associate Chairman, Department of Orthopaedic Surgery, Rush Medical College, Chicago, Illinois, USA

Nicholas Goddard Consultant Orthopaedic Surgeon, Royal Free Hospital, London, UK

Caroline J. Goldberg Research Fellow, Children's Research Centre, Our Lady's Hospital for Sick Children, Dublin, Ireland

Charles C. Greenough Consultant Orthopaedic Surgeon, Middlesbrough General Hospital, Middlesbrough, UK

Michael Grevitt Consultant Spinal Surgeon, Queen's Medical Centre, University Hospital, Nottingham, UK

Franz Grill Head, Paediatric Orthopaedic Department, Orthopaedic Hospital, Speising, Vienna, Austria

A.O. Grobbelaar Consultant Plastic Surgeon, Mount Vernon Hospital, Northwood, Middlesex, UK

R. Gundle Consultant Orthopaedic Surgeon, Nuffield Orthopaedic Centre, Oxford, UK

Andrew P. Gutow Department of Orthopaedics, Emory University School of Medicine, Atlanta, Georgia, USA

R. Handley Trauma Unit, Critical Care Centre, John Radcliffe Hospital, Oxford, UK

Michael E. Hantes Orthopaedic Surgeon, Ioannina, Greece

Robert A. Hart Assistant Professor, Department of Orthopaedics, Oregon Health Sciences University, Portland, Oregon, USA

Edward J. Harvey Department of Orthopaedic Surgery, McGill University, Montreal General Hospital, Montreal, Quebec, Canada

A. Hashemi-Nejad Consultant Orthopaedic Surgeon, Royal National Orthopaedic Hospital, Stanmore, UK

Michael Hejna Instructor, Department of Orthopaedic Surgery, Rush Medical College, Chicago, Illinois, USA

T.E.J. Hems Consultant Hand and Orthopaedic Surgeon, Victoria Infirmary, Glasgow; Honorary Clinical Senior Lecturer, University of Glasgow, UK

Ralph Hertel Director of the Shoulder and Elbow Service, Department of Orthopaedic Surgery, Inselspital, University of Bern, Switzerland

A.J. Heywood Consultant Plastic Surgeon, Stoke Mandeville Hospital, Aylesbury, UK

Susan Hicks Chartered Physiotherapist, Royal Berkshire and Battle Hospitals NHS Trust, Reading, UK

J.L. Hobby Research Fellow, Orthopaedic Research Unit and Department of Radiology, University of Cambridge, UK

Mark Hoffer Lowman Professor of Children's Orthopaedics, University of Southern California, Los Angeles, California, USA

Brian Holdsworth Consultant Orthopaedic Surgeon, Queen's Medical Centre, University Hospital, Nottingham, UK

James B. Holmes Michigan Orthopedic Center, Ypsilanti, Michigan, USA

Gavin M. Holt Lecturer and Honorary Specialist Registrar, University of Sheffield, UK

Jon D. Hop Consulting Orthopedic Surgeon, Holland, Michigan, USA

Francis J. Hornicek Assistant Professor of Orthopaedic Surgery, Harvard Medical School, Cambridge, Massachusetts; Assistant Orthopaedic Surgeon, Massachusetts General Hospital and Children's Hospital, Boston, Massachusetts, USA

G.E.D. Howell Consultant Orthopaedic and Trauma Surgeon, The Royal Hospital Haslar, Gosport, UK

M.J.S. Hubbard Consultant Orthopaedic Surgeon, The Knee Clinic, Robert Jones and Agnes Hunt Orthopaedic Hospital, Oswestry, UK

Susan M. Huson Consultant Clinical Geneticist, Oxford Radcliffe Hospitals, Oxford, UK

Imran Ilyas Consultant Orthopaedic Surgeon, King Faisal Specialist Hospital and Research Centre, Riyadh, Saudi Arabia

John N. Insall Chief, Adult Knee Reconstruction, Beth Israel Medical Center; Clinical Professor of Orthopedics, Albert Einstein Medical College, New York, USA

Mark Jackson Consultant Senior Lecturer, Trauma and Orthopaedic Surgery, University Department of Orthopaedic Surgery, Bristol Royal Infirmary, Bristol, UK

J.R. Jenner Consultant in Rheumatology and Rehabilitation, Addenbrooke's NHS Trust, Cambridge, UK

James O. Johnston Professor of Clinical Orthopaedics, University of California, San Francisco, California, USA

Benjamin Joseph Professor of Orthopaedics, Head of Paediatric Orthopaedic Service, Kasturba Medical College, Manipal, Karnataka, India

Gregoris Kambouroglou Consultant Trauma Surgeon, John Radcliffe Hospital, Oxford, UK

John J. Kamp Certified Prosthetist Orthotist, American Prosthetics, Davenport, Iowa, USA

Johan Kärrholm Professor of Orthopaedics, Sahlgrenska University Hospital, University of Göteborg, Sweden

Scott S. Kelley Assistant Professor of Orthopaedics, School of Medicine, University of North Carolina at Chapel Hill, North Carolina, USA

John Kenwright Nuffield Professor of Orthopaedic Surgery, University of Oxford; Consultant Orthopaedic Surgeon, Nuffield Orthopaedic Centre, Oxford, UK

Shahid Khan Specialist Registrar in Orthopaedics and Trauma, Bristol Royal Infirmary, Bristol, UK

Todd A. Kile Chair, Division of Foot and Ankle Surgery, Department of Orthopaedic Surgery, Mayo Clinic Scottsdale, Arizona, USA

G.J.W. King Associate Professor, Hand and Upper Limb Centre, University of Western Ontario, London, Ontario, Canada

Jenö Kiss Asistant Professor of Orthopaedic Surgery, Department of Orthopaedics, Semmelweiss University, Budapest, Hungary

Kaj Klaue Universität Bern, Klinik für Orthopädische Chirurgie, Inselspital, Bern, Switzerland

Mark A. Konodi Senior Literature Analyst, Harborview Medical Center, University of Washington School of Medicine, Seattle, Washington, USA

Paul F. Lachiewicz School of Medicine, University of North Carolina at Chapel Hill, North Carolina, USA

Om Lahoti Consultant Orthopaedic Surgeon, University Hospital, Lewisham, London, UK

Simon Lambert Consultant Surgeon, Royal National Orthopaedic Hospital, Stanmore, and Royal Free Hospital, London, UK

E.E.G. (Charles) Lautenbach Founder and Consultant, Bone Sepsis Unit, Johannesburg Hospital, South Africa

F. Lavini First Assistant, Policlinico G.B. Rossi, University of Verona, Italy

L. Scott Levin Chief, Division of Plastic, Reconstructive, Maxillofacial and Reconstructive Surgery; Associate Professor of Plastic and Orthopaedic Surgery, Duke University Medical Center, Durham, North Carolina, USA

A. Levy Clinical Assistant Professor, Department of Orthopaedics, New Jersey Medical School, Newark, New Jersey, USA

Steven A. Lietman Assistant Professor of Orthopaedic Surgery, Johns Hopkins University, Baltimore, Maryland, USA

Ronald W. Lindsey Baylor College of Medicine, Houston, Texas, USA

Benjamin A. Lipsky Professor of Medicine, University of Washington School of Medicine, Seattle, Washington, USA

René Louis Professor of Orthopaedic and Chief, Department of Orthopaedic and Joint Surgery, Hôpital de la Conception, Marseilles, France

John A. McCulloch Professor of Orthopaedics, Northeastern Ohio Universities College of Medicine, Rootstown, Ohio, USA

Douglas J. McDonald Professor of Orthopedics, Department of Orthopedic Surgery, St Louis University Health Sciences Center, St Louis, Missouri, USA

I.S.H. McNab Nuffield Orthopaedic Centre, Oxford, UK

E. McNally Consultant Musculoskeletal Radiologist, Nuffield Orthopaedic Centre, Oxford; Honorary Senior Lecturer, University of Oxford, UK

Martin A. McNally Consultant in Limb Reconstruction Surgery, Nuffield Orthopaedic Centre, Oxford; Honorary Senior Lecturer in Orthopaedics, University of Oxford, UK

Malcolm Macnicol Consultant Orthopaedic Surgeon and Senior Orthopaedic Lecturer, Royal Hospital for Sick Children and Princess Margaret Rose Orthopaedic Hospital, Edinburgh, UK

Henry McQuay Clinical Reader in Pain Relief, University of Oxford, UK

Margaret M. McQueen Consultant Orthopaedic Surgeon, The Royal Infirmary of Edinburgh, UK

A.C. Macey Consultant Orthopaedic Surgeon, Sligo General Hospital, Sligo, Ireland

John H. Mader Attending Physician, Reid Memorial Hospital, Richmond, Indiana, USA

Jon T. Mader Professor, Department of Internal Medicine and Department of Orthopedics and Rehabilitation; Chief, Section of Surgical Infectious Disease, University of Texas Medical Branch, Galveston, Texas, USA

D. Mahalick Department of Neurosurgery, Director of Neuropsychological Services, New Jersey Medical School, Newark, New Jersey, USA

Rajesh Malhotra Associate Professor of Orthopaedic Surgery, All India Institute of Medical Sciences, New Delhi, India

J. L. Marsh Professor of Orthopedic Surgery, University of Iowa, Iowa City, Iowa, USA

James Martin Department of Orthopaedic Surgery, University of Iowa Hospitals and Clinics, Iowa City, Iowa, USA

Theodore Miclau Baylor College of Medicine, Houston, Texas, USA

Kerry R. Mills Professor of Clinical Neurophysiology, King's College London, UK

Sohail K. Mirza Assistant Professor, Director of Spinal Research Unit, Harborview Medical Center, University of Washington School of Medicine, Seattle, Washington, USA

R. Mitchell Consultant Radiologist, Royal National Orthopaedic Hospital Trust, Stanmore, UK

John A. Miyano Department of Orthopaedics, University of Washington School of Medicine, Seattle, Washington, USA

Berton R. Moed Professor of Orthopaedic Surgery, Wayne State University, Detroit; Chief, Department of Orthopaedic Surgery, Detroit Receiving Hospital, Detroit, Michigan, USA

Jennifer Klaber Moffett Deputy Director, Institute of Rehabilitation, University of Hull, UK

David A.F. Morgan Associate Professor of Orthopaedic Surgery, Holy Spirit Hospital, Brisbane, Australia

T.R. Morley Consultant Spinal Surgeon, Royal National Orthopaedic Hospital, Stanmore, UK

W.A. Morrison Professor of Surgery, St Vincent's Hospital, University of Melbourne, Australia

J. Dougall Morrison Consultant in Rehabilitation, Prosthetic Service, Nuffield Orthopaedic Centre, Oxford, UK

Robert C. Mulholland Special Professor in Orthopaedic and Accident Surgery, University of Nottingham, UK

Peter M. Murray Associate Professor of Orthopedic Surgery, Mayo Graduate School of Medicine, Rochester, Minnesota; Senior Associate Consultant, Mayo Clinic, Jacksonville, Florida, USA

D. Murray Consultant Orthopaedic Surgeon, Nuffield Orthopaedic Centre, Oxford, UK

Sydney Nade Department of Surgery, University of Sydney Westmead Hospital, Sydney, Australia

Antonio G. Nascimento Consultant, Section of Surgical Pathology, Mayo Clinic and Mayo Foundation; Associate Professor of Pathology, Mayo Medical School, Rochester, Minnesota, USA

Ian W. Nelson Consultant Orthopaedic Surgeon, North Bristol NHS Trust, Bristol, UK

Kenneth J. Noonan Associate Professor, Department of Orthopaedics, University of Wisconsin, Madison, Wisconsin, USA

Olarewaju J.O. Oladipo Clinical Fellow, Department of Orthopedic Surgery, Boston City Hospital, Boston, Massachusetts, USA

Christopher W. Oliver Consultant Trauma Surgeon, Edinburgh Orthopaedic Trauma Unit, Edinburgh, UK

Steven A. Olson Associate Professor of Orthopaedic Surgery, Duke University Medical Center, Durham, North Carolina, USA

David M. Oster Denver Orthopaedic Specialists, Denver, Colorado, USA

Clark C. Otley Assistant Professor of Dermatology, Mayo Clinic and Mayo Foundation, Rochester, Minnesota, USA

John Owen St Vincent's Hospital, Melbourne, Australia

Hans H. Paessler Medical Director, ATOS-Clinic; Orthopaedic Surgeon, Heidelberg, Germany

J. Panayiotis Consultant, Department of Orthopedics, Athens University Medical School, Athens, Greece

Martyn J. Parker Orthopaedic Research Fellow, Peterborough District Hospital, Peterborough, UK

K. Parsch Orthopaedic Clinic, Olga Hospital, Stuttgart, Germany

S. Patel Moore Orthopedic Clinic, Columbia, South Carolina, USA

Leo Pinczewski Consultant Orthopaedic Surgeon, Mater Misericordiae Hospital, Australian Institute of Musculo-Skeletal Research, Sydney, Australia

Tony Pohl Director of Trauma, Department of Orthopaedics and Trauma, Royal Adelaide Hospital, Adelaide, Australia

Richard Porter Formerly Professor of Orthopaedic Surgery, University of Aberdeen, UK

Martyn L. Porter Consultant Orthopaedic Surgeon, Wrightington Hospital, Wigan, UK

Charles T. Price Surgeon in Chief, Nemours Foundation, Orlando, Florida, USA

Douglas J. Pritchard Professor of Orthopedic Surgery, Mayo Foundation, Rochester, Minnesota, USA

Laura Prokuski Assistant Professor, Department of Surgery, University of Wisconsin, Madison, Wisconsin, USA

Gerardine Quaghebeur Consultant Neuroradiologist, Radcliffe Infirmary, Oxford, UK

S. Rajasekaran Head of Department of Orthopaedics and Spine Surgery, Ganga Medical Centre and Hospitals, Coimbatore, India

L. Renzi Brevio First Assistant, Policlinico G.B. Rossi, University of Verona, Italy

Paul Rhys Davies Centre for Spinal Studies and Surgery, University Hospital, Queen's Medical Centre, Nottingham, UK

W.J. Ribbans Consultant Orthopaedic Surgeon, Northampton General Hospital NHS Trust, Northampton, UK

Peter Richards Consultant Paediatric Neurosurgeon, Radcliffe Infirmary, Oxford, UK

Horst Rieger Department of Trauma and Hand Surgery, Westfälische Wilhelms-Universität, Münster, Germany

Barry L. Riemer Director, Orthopaedic Fracture Division; Professor, Department of Orthopaedic Surgery, Allegheny University of the Health Sciences, Pittsburgh, Pennsylvania, USA

Robert A. Robinson Professor, Department of Pathology, University of Iowa College of Medicine, Iowa City, Iowa, USA

Michael G. Rock Professor, Orthopedic Surgery, Mayo Clinic and Mayo Foundation, Rochester, Minnesota, USA

Randall K. Roenigk Professor of Dermatology, Mayo Clinic and Mayo Foundation, Rochester, Minnesota, USA

Aaron G. Rosenberg Department of Orthopaedics, New Jersey Medical School, Newark, New Jersey, USA

L. Rosenbloom Consultant Paediatric Neurologist, Alder Hey Children's Hospital, Liverpool, UK

N.D. Rossiter Nuffield Orthopaedic Centre, Oxford, UK

Pietro Ruggieri Assistant Professor, Rizzoli Orthopaedic Institute, Bologna, Italy

L.A. Rymaszewski Stobb Hill Hospital, Glasgow, UK

Diva R. Salomao Consultant, Section of Anatomic Pathology, Mayo Clinic and Mayo Foundation; Assistant Professor of Pathology, Mayo Medical School, Rochester, Minnesota, USA

Angela Sandall Chartered Physiotherapist, Royal Berkshire and Battle Hospitals NHS Trust, Reading, UK

Ann Sandison Consultant Histopathologist, Royal National Orthopaedic Hospital Trust, Stanmore, UK

T. Sarkhel Specialist Registrar in Orthopaedics, SW Thames Training Programme, UK

G. Schippinger Associate Professor of Traumatology, Medical School, University of Graz, Austria

Dietrich Schlenzka Associate Professor, ORTON Orthopaedic Hospital, Invalid Foundation, Helsinki, Finland

J. Schwappach Swedish Medical Center, Englewood, Colorado, USA

Giles R. Scuderi Associate Chief, Adult Knee Reconstruction, Beth Israel Medical Center; Assistant Clinical Professor of Orthopedics, Albert Einstein Medical College, New York, USA

F.J. Seibert Consultant Trauma Surgeon, Medical School, University of Graz, Austria

C.A. Shackleton Pain Relief Unit, Churchill Hospital, Oxford, UK

T.K. Shanmugasundaram Emeritus Professor of Orthopaedic Surgery, Madras Medical College, Chennai, India

Ajoy Prasad Shetty Consultant Orthopaedic Surgeon, Ganga Medical Centre and Hospitals, Coimbatore, India

Konsei Shino Professor of Orthopaedics and Rehabilitation, Osaka Prefecture College of Health Sciences; Clinical Associate Professor, Department of Orthopaedic Surgery, Osaka University Medical School, Osaka, Japan

Evelyn Shortall Research Fellow, Department of Public Health and Primary Care, University of Oxford, UK

Donald G. Shurr Certified Prosthetist Orthotist, University of Iowa, Iowa City, Iowa, USA

Franklin H. Sim Consultant, Department of Orthopedics, Mayo Clinic and Mayo Foundation; Professor of Orthopedics, Mayo Medical School, Rochester, Minnesota, USA

Joseph F. Slade III Assistant Professor, Section of Hand and Extremity Surgery, Department of Orthopaedics and Rehabilitation, Yale University School of Medicine, New Haven, Connecticut, USA

Matthew S. Slater Chief Resident, Cardiothoracic Surgery, Oregon Health Sciences University, Portland, Oregon, USA

P.J. Smith Consultant in Plastic and Hand Surgery, Great Ormond Street Hospital for Sick Children, London, UK

Roger Smith Consultant Physician, Nuffield Orthopaedic Centre, Oxford, UK

David H. Sochart Consultant Orthopaedic Surgeon, Manchester Arthroplasty Unit, North Manchester General Hospital, Manchester, UK

Mark J. Spoonamore Center for Orthopaedic Spinal Surgery, USC University Hospital, Los Angeles, California, USA

Carl L. Stanitski Professor of Orthopedic Surgery, Medical University of South Carolina, Charleston, South Carolina, USA

David Stanley Consultant in Orthopaedics and Trauma Surgery, Northern General Hospital NHS Trust, Sheffield, UK

J.K. Stanley Consultant in Upper Limb Surgery, Wrightington Hospital, Wigan, UK

J. Stothard Consultant Hand and Upper Limb Surgeon, Middlesbrough General Hospital, Middlesbrough, UK

Michael D. Sussman Former Chief of Staff, Shriners Hospital for Children; Clinical Professor of Orthopedic Surgery, Oregon Health Sciences University, Portland, Oregon, USA

K. Swan Professor of Surgery, Department of Surgery, New Jersey Medical School, Newark, New Jersey, USA

Darren R. Swenson Research Assistant, University of New Mexico, Albuquerque, New Mexico, USA

M.F. Swiontkowski Professor and Chair, Department of Orthopaedic Surgery, University of Minnesota, Minneapolis, Minnesota, USA

R. Szyszkowitz Professor of Traumatology, Medical School, University of Graz, Austria

Shawn Tavares Consultant Orthopaedic Surgeon, Royal Berkshire Hospital, Reading, UK

B.A. Taylor Department of Spinal Surgery, Royal National Orthopaedic Hospital, Stanmore, UK

David Tearse Department of Orthopaedic Surgery, University of Iowa College of Medicine, Iowa City, Iowa, USA

D. Temperley Consultant Radiologist, Wrightington Hospital, Wigan, UK

H.T. Temple Associate Professor of Orthopaedic Oncology, University of Florida, Gainesville, Florida, USA

David C. Templeman Wayzata Orthopaedics, Wayzata, Minnesota, USA

Alexander Templeton Professor of Pathology, Rush Medical College, Chicago, Illinois, USA

D.D. Theile Plastic Surgeon, Princess Alexandra Hospital, Brisbane, Queensland, Australia

T.N. Theologis Consultant Orthopaedic Surgeon, Nuffield Orthopaedic Centre, Oxford; Honorary Senior Clinical Lecturer, University of Oxford, UK

Michael Thomas Consultant Orthopaedic Surgeon, Heatherwood and Wexham Park Hospitals Trust, East Berkshire, UK

P.B.M. Thomas Senior Lecturer in Orthopaedics and Honorary Consultant, Keele University Medical School, Stoke-on-Trent, UK

Karl-Göran Thorngren Professor of Orthopedic Surgery, Lund University Hospital, Lund, Sweden

I.A. Trail Consultant in Upper Limb Surgery, Wrightington Hospital, Wigan, UK

Thomas E. Trumble Chief of Hand and Microvascular Surgery, Department of Orthopaedic Surgery and Sports Medicine, University of Washington School of Medicine, Seattle, Washington, USA

Donald D. Trunkey Professor of Surgery, Department of Surgery, Oregon Health Sciences University, Portland, Oregon, USA

S.K. Tucker Department of Spinal Surgery, Royal National Orthopaedic Hospital, Stanmore, UK

B.C. Twaddle Consultant Orthopaedic Surgeon, Auckland Hospital, Auckland, New Zealand

R.N. Villar Cambridge Hip and Knee Unit, BUPA Cambridge Lea Hospital, Cambridge, UK

Richard Vlasak Section of Orthopedic Oncology, Department of Orthopedic Surgery, Watson Clinic, Lakeland, Florida, USA

Don Wallace Milton Keynes General Hospital, Milton Keynes, UK

William C. Warner Jr Associate Professor, University of Tennessee - Campbell Clinic Department of Orthopedic Surgery, Memphis, Tennessee, USA

David Warwick Consultant Orthopaedic Surgeon, Southampton University Hospitals, Southampton, UK

J. Tracy Watson Professor of Orthopaedic Surgery, Wayne State University, Detroit; Vice-Chief, Department of Orthopaedic Surgery, Detroit Receiving Hospital, Detroit, Michigan, USA

John K. Webb Director, Centre for Spinal Studies and Surgery, University Hospital, Queen's Medical Centre, Nottingham, UK

Jonathan Webb Consultant Orthopaedic Surgeon, Southmead Hospital, Bristol, UK

Kristy Weber Assistant Professor of Orthopaedic Oncology, University of Texas MD Anderson Cancer Center, Houston, Texas, USA

John H. Wedge Surgeon-in-Chief, The Hospital for Sick Children, Toronto; Professor and Chairman, Department of Surgery, University of Toronto, Canada

Lars Weidenhielm Associate Professor, Department of Orthopaedics, Karolinska Institute, Stockholm, Sweden

Arnold-Peter C. Weiss Professor of Orthopaedics, Brown University School of Medicine, Providence, Rhode Island, USA

George P. Whitelaw Jr Associate Professor, Department of Orthopedics, Boston University, Boston, Massachusetts, USA

Keith Willett Nuffield Orthopaedic Centre, Oxford, UK

John R. Williams Consultant Trauma and Orthopaedic Surgeon, Newcastle upon Tyne NHS Hospitals Trust, Newcastle upon Tyne, UK

T. Williams Orthopedic Surgeon, Wisconsin, USA

Lyn Williamson Consultant Rheumatologist, Princess Margaret Hospital, Swindon, UK

J.S. Williamson Plastic and Hand Surgery Consultant, Kelowna General Hospital; Clinical Instructor, Division of Plastic Surgery, University of British Columbia, Kelowna, British Columbia, Canada

*Stig Willner Formerly Assistant Professor, Department of Orthopaedics, University Hospital, Malmö, Sweden

James Wilson-MacDonald Consultant Orthopaedic Surgeon, Nuffield Orthopaedic Centre, Oxford, UK

Ian G. Winson Consultant Orthopaedic Surgeon, Avon Orthopaedic Centre, Bristol, UK

David Woods Consultant Orthopaedic Surgeon, Princess Margaret Hospital, Swindon, UK

Paul Wordsworth Clinical Reader in Rheumatology, University of Oxford, UK

Peter Worlock Consultant Trauma Surgeon, John Radcliffe Hospital, Oxford, UK

Yoshaki Yamano Professor of Orthopaedic Surgery, Osaka City University Medical School, Osaka, Japan

A.B. Zavatsky Lecturer in Engineering Science, University of Oxford, UK

*It is with great regret that we must report the death of Stig Willner during the preparation of this textbook.

1
Fundamentals

1.1 Principles of epidemiology and research methodology

Christopher Bulstrode

Introduction

An epidemiological perspective on orthopedics

Orthopedic surgery is much more than the technical skill of being able to operate. It involves complex problem solving when deciding what the options are, and communication skills in explaining these to the patient. This requires an understanding of the evidence on which these decisions are based. The study of how this evidence is collected and analysed is basic epidemiology.

At the interface between orthopedic surgeons and health-care planners (whether governments or insurance companies) a further level of understanding of epidemiology is needed. Here there is a constructive tension between health-care providers and those who pay for this care. If left unchecked the energy and inventiveness of orthopedic surgeons could rapidly bankrupt even the best resourced health-care service. Health-care planners see it as one of their duties to try to balance the demands of orthopedic surgeons with equally powerful demands from other services. They rely on epidemiology research to provide them with the hard information on which rational decisions can be based. If we in orthopedics understand this language then we can engage in a constructive debate on how and where rationing should be applied.

The rationale behind epidemiology

Epidemiology tries to ask questions about the causes of conditions and about the rationale for treatment (Table 1). The situation is complicated in the orthopedic specialty by the fact that orthopedic surgeons do not usually cure disease, but merely alleviate symptoms. Their interventions may also cause further health-care problems. For example, the treatment of fractured neck of femur secondary to osteoporosis in an elderly patient treats the complications of the underlying condition, not the condition itself. Once the fracture has been fixed the patient may then go on to develop a bed sore. From osteoporosis to bed sore is a short pathosociological step. Similarly, in osteoarthritis of the hip a total hip replacement does not cure the arthritis, it just replaces the joint with an artificial joint which has a short life compared with the natural one. This has led to a veritable epidemic of patients needing revisions. An even more difficult problem to manage is the fact that a significant proportion of patients seeing an orthopedic surgeon (especially back surgeons) may be exaggerating or even inventing some of their symptoms, 'somatizing' their dissatisfaction with their lives. Conventional orthopedic surgery does not necessarily have appropriate models for dealing with this kind of problem, and patients may receive an operation when it is the last thing that they need, even if they are quite literally 'asking for it'.

Table 1 The orthopedic epidemiological perspective

Category	Presenting	Common orthopedic intervention	Epidemiological questions
Simple orthopedics	Pain from ecchondroma	Removal	How many ecchondromas cause no symptoms at all and can be left alone?
Elderly osteoporotic	Fractures	Fix fracture	How important is osteoporosis in causing fractures? Is it increasing in an ageing population?
Elderly arthritic	Pain in joints disability	Replace joints	How much resource do we need to put into joint replacement? What factors would reduce the need for revisions?
Psychiatric or emotionally disturbed	Backache etc.	Exclude organic diagnosis	What proportion of patients could be better managed elsewhere? How can we identify them?
Poliomyelitis	Loss of function	Tendon transfer fusions	How well is immunization working? Can the disease be eradicated?
Trauma	Broken bones	Fix fractures	What proportion of trauma is avoidable? At what social and financial cost?

Some conditions are largely preventable. If society chose to change its priorities and invest more in education and prevention, some branches of orthopedics would almost disappear. Two examples from opposite poles of medicine and the world are trauma (especially civilian gun-shot wounds) and poliomyelitis, where immunization now holds a real possibility of eradicating this dreadful disease altogether. Epidemiology is the understanding of how conditions and their treatment fit into the broader perspective of society in general.

In this chapter we describe the main principles of the subject and explain why, in the age of 'evidence-based medicine', this is important for an orthopedic surgeon.

The patterns of demand for orthopedic services are likely to change radically over the next few decades in response to the attention that each society pays to immunization, and prevention, and not just to the amount of money society decides to spend on orthopedics. These changes need to be anticipated for a cost-effective service.

Box 1 Definition of orthopedic epidemiology

1. Study of the occurrence of musculoskeletal problems and the factors which influence this
2. Study of the social and economic importance of musculoskeletal disorders
3. The value (therapeutic and economic) of screening, prevention, investigation, and treatment of musculoskeletal disorders

What can orthopedic epidemiology do?

Epidemiology is concerned with studying groups of people to obtain the information necessary to plan, implement, and evaluate service (Table 2). This could be for prevention, control, or treatment of diseases. Orthopedic surgeons are, in the main, concerned with diagnosis and treatment of the individual patient. Epidemiology provides information gathered from large numbers of patients on which a rational care plan for an individual patient can be based. Epidemiological techniques can also help orthopedic surgeons to interpret published literature critically, so that they can function more effectively.

Problems with epidemiology

Basing the care plan of a patient on a published series of 1000 cases is likely to be more reliable than basing it on the last two or three cases that you can remember in your own practice, or even on what you were taught as a trainee. Nevertheless, epidemiology, like every branch of science, is open to misinterpretation. Some of the most common of these pitfalls will be described in this chapter so that you are aware of them, and more importantly so that you do not fall into them when publishing your own studies.

Definition of disease: what is disease?

It is surprising how often we are not clear about the definition of the disease. For intra-articular disorders of the knee for example, there have been a proliferation of new diagnoses over the last 20 years—based on pathology of synovium, cartilage, ligaments, etc. Prior to the widespread use of knee arthroscopy, the majority of these would have received the diagnosis of 'internal derangement of knee' (**IDK**, which was also interpreted by many to mean 'I don't know!'). Now there is a proliferation of 'new' conditions, some of which will indeed exist and may even be treatable, whereas others will merely be normal variants which have nothing whatsoever to do with the patient's symptoms and which are best left alone.

The same is happening at present, with a proliferation of new imaging techniques such as MRI where natural variability may be interpreted as pathology if large studies of 'normal' subjects are not carried out. Comparisons between different time periods and between different observers can also create problems if there are no explicit and agreed operational criteria. An example of this in plain radiography is the definition of loosening of the hip. Gruen's lines, which were becoming a standard method by which loosening could be defined and classified after total hip replacement, have been shown to have such a large interobserver error that it is doubtful whether one individual's progress can be studied using this system, never mind comparisons made between groups.

Trials

Trials are the staple diet of epidemiologists but come in many different forms, each of which has its strengths and weaknesses.

Audit (Fig. 1)

This is probably the most basic form of scientific study. It is merely a decision by an individual or group to measure what is happening

Table 2 Epidemiology

For orthopedic surgeons the skills allow:	For the service, it gathers information necessary to:	For health care the information can be used to:
Critical interpretation of the scientific literature	Plan	Prevent
Rational decision making on individual patients	Implement	Control
Understanding of health-care needs	Evaluate	Treat

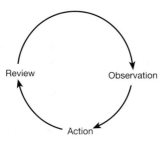

Fig. 1. The audit loop.

with their work practice. Some say that audit is not 'real' science, but science involves three stages:

- observation and identification of patterns
- formation of hypothesis
- experimentation to test hypothesis.

Audit shares the first and most important stage of the scientific process (observation). It differs from conventional scientific research in that the hypothesis formed from observation is not formally tested by experimentation. It just leads directly to a change in practice. For example, it may be noticed that there has been an increase in the number of postoperative wound infections since trauma operations (out of hours) started to share an operating room with general surgical emergencies. A decision might be made to use only the orthopedic operating room for trauma emergencies.

Box 2 Advantages and disadvantages of audit

- Currently the way that most clinical practice changes
- Relies heavily on the loop observe/change/review
- Can be used to identify problems
- Is not so good at finding logical solutions

The results in the change in practice are then observed, and provided that the outcome is an apparent reduction in infection there may be further fine tuning in practice to try to improve outcome further. For example, it may then be found that operations performed after 10 p.m. appear to have a higher infection rate than those performed earlier in the day. It may then be decided to stop all operations except absolute emergencies after 10 pm. The problem is that the change in outcome may be the result of biological variability, or may be due to some other factor which changed at the same time. In this case the higher infection rate when general and trauma share an operating room may actually have been a chance finding (despite our preconceived feelings about this). This is an example of biological variability or noise. The higher infection rate after 10 p.m. could actually be a result of the fact that only serious cases are dealt with late at night anyway and they have a higher infection rate. This is an example of a confounding factor (something that affects the outcome of a study but is not being directly measured in that study and so may confuse the results). It is not a good idea to rely too

heavily on 'audit' when trying to understand how things work. Despite this, audit performed consciously or unconsciously is probably the way in which most change in clinical practice takes place.

The retrospective study

A retrospective study is a review of clinical work that has already been performed. It is usually undertaken with a preconceived idea, such as: 'I would like to show that my new technique gives better results than what was being done before'. It is one of the easiest studies to perform but has fundamental weaknesses. It differs from audit in that the researcher usually has strong preconceived ideas about the outcome, which is often the motivation for performing the study in the first place. These ideas are likely to introduce bias into the results so the results must be treated cautiously. Most important is the fact that, like audit, it is not possible from a retrospective study to say that a treatment or investigation is better or worse than any other. The nature of a retrospective study simply does not allow this interpretation of the results. Despite this, such conclusions are common in the published literature.

Box 3 Advantages and disadvantages of the retrospective study

- Subject to bias
- Can be used to identify research questions
- Can assess the likely size of a problem for power analysis
- Cannot be used to determine which treatment is best

Retrospective studies do have a most important role to play in studying the natural history of a problem or condition and in generating hypotheses which can then be tested using a formal trial. It should be the first phase of any scientific study, providing the raw materials for the human mind's favourite pastime—searching for patterns. It is these patterns which are the grist for the mill of hypothesis formation. But a retrospective study can go no further than this. Testing the hypothesis needs more rigorous types of trial, which will be described below.

Prospective studies

A study of the natural history of an intervention can be more directed than a simple retrospective study. It can be decided in advance that patients receiving a given operation are to be followed (a prospective study). The group of patients being studied is known as a cohort. In orthopedics it is usual to accumulate cases over a period of time. This poses problems with follow-up, because at any given time each patient will have been followed for a different length of time. The technique of correcting for this so that it appears (for analysis at least) that every patient received their operation at the same time is known as survivorship analysis, and is especially important when studying the longevity of joint replacements.

Unfortunately this technique, like many other statistical manipulations, is open to abuse by the naive and by those who are statistically sophisticated but who have chosen to be 'economical with the truth'.

Box 4 **Prospective study methods**

- Decide in advance what you are going to study
- Follow the patients according to a protocol
- Cohorts may need a survivorship analysis to allow for entry at different times

The most common sources of problems are where significant numbers of patients are lost to follow-up, and it is then assumed that their outcome is the same as those who continue to be followed. A second common problem is to end up with very small numbers followed for long periods and to assume that the figures relating to these small numbers have the same reliability as the early years of follow-up where large numbers still remained in the study.

Randomized controlled trials

The randomized controlled trial (Fig. 2) is the gold standard of scientific studies in clinical medicine, because if performed properly it offers a test of a hypothesis which is as sure as anything can be in clinical medicine (a field of science dogged by variability).

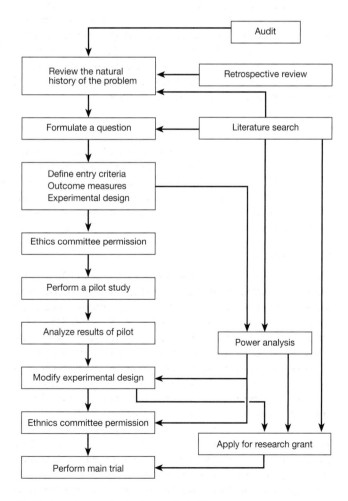

Fig. 2. Steps in a randomized controlled trial.

It is called a trial because there is an agreed protocol (way of handling the patients etc.). It is controlled because one group of patients who enter the trial do not receive the intervention being studied. They provide a baseline of what would have happened if the treatment being studied had not been performed. It is randomized because the decision as to whether an individual who has entered the trial should go into the control groups or another group is decided by random allocation. If allocation is not random it is possible that the trial organizers may consciously or even unconsciously allocate patients to influence the results of the trial. The best randomized controlled trials are blinded or even double blinded. Blinding of the trial means that the patients do not know which arm of the trial they are in. Double blinded means that the researchers do not know either, until after the experiment is finished and the results have been analysed. Only then is the code broken. The purpose of blinding is to make sure that even if patients or researchers have strong views about the value of the treatment, there is no way that they can influence the results as they do not know which group the patients are in. In medicine, blinding is relatively easy because patients can be given the tablets or placebos (tablets dressed up to look like the real thing, but containing no active ingredients). In surgery the equivalent would be a sham operation (where the anesthetic would be given, the incision made, the operating area exposed, but no active procedure performed). It may be ethical to do this in animal experimentation but it is certainly not ethical in humans, and so it is almost impossible to have controlled experiments in surgery and equally difficult to have blinded ones.

Box 5 **The randomized controlled trial**

- Can be used to determine which treatment is best
- Are designed to prevent bias
- Are very difficult to design and run well

Preparation for a randomized controlled trial

Literature search
Before starting a randomized controlled trial the natural history of the condition under study needs to be understood. A literature search may produce papers on the condition under study which will give useful information on the natural history of the condition and its treatment. They may also provide outcome measures which if used in the present trial might make the results comparable with other studies.

Pilot studies
These provide an opportunity to test out the trial methodology and to modify it before committing too many resources. If there is no previous literature on the condition, the pilot may provide information on the value of various outcome measures, so that the best can be picked for the main study.

Power analysis
This calculation allows the experimenter to determine how many patients need to be involved if there is to be a reasonable chance of getting a meaningful answer to the question being asked. It also pre-

vents the design of a larger trial than necessary (a very expensive undertaking). The following pieces of information are some of those which are required for its calculation.

1. **The probable difference that the treatment will make** If the expected difference is large (e.g. 80 per cent reduction in pain) then clearly not many patients will be needed before a difference will be detectable statistically. If the difference is only 1 per cent, then many more patients will be needed before it is shown up reliably.

2. **The variability of results** If the patients in the study have a very variable outcome anyway, a small improvement will be much more difficult to detect than if all the patients behave in exactly the same way.

3. **The level of significance** If absolute certainty about a result is necessary (the treatment is felt to be good but can have dire side-effects), then the level of significance required to demonstrate that the treatment has a real effect may be much more stringent than otherwise. In this case significance at the 1 per cent level ($p < 0.01$) might be required rather than the more usual 5 per cent level ($p < 0.05$).

4. **The level of reliability of the trial** Just as statistics can apparently suggest that things are significantly different when they are not, a trial which is too small may fail to show a difference which exists and is important. If it is vital that even a small difference is found, then a much larger trial is needed than if it is simply felt that only large differences would affect clinical practice. Obtaining the right numbers for a trial is important. If too few patients are involved the treatment may indeed make a difference, but the numbers will be so small that statistically the difference does not shown up through the noise.

Box 6 Information needed for a power analysis

- Difference expected
- Variability
- Significance level
- Reliability required

Entry criteria

If the conditions for entry into a study are very closely defined, a very homogenous group of patients will be admitted to the study. The variability in outcome will be reduced and, as we have seen from the power analysis section above, this improves the chances of a significant difference being detected. However, these same strict entry criteria will also reduce the number of patients entering the trial. The entry criteria are therefore a compromise and should be based on a group which is regarded as a clinical entity, rather than on statistical requirements.

Ethics committee permission

Trials require independent review by a group of people appointed to represent the interests of the patients. The role of an ethics committee is to encourage high-quality research with constructive criticism while defending the interests of the public who may be asked to take part.

Consent

Patients should be allowed to decide whether they wish to take part in a trial or not and therefore need to be fully informed. In order to do this the researcher should be able to say quite honestly that he or she genuinely does not know which arm of the trial offers the best treatment. This is sometimes very difficult because the stimulus to perform a trial may come from a strong wish to prove a personal belief that a given technique is valuable.

Outcome measures

Outcome measures need to be relatively common so that they can be measured. They also need to be clinically relevant, and to be recognized reliably. An example of this is the study of thrombo-prophylaxis after total hip replacement where the major reliable and clinically relevant outcome measure is death rate. However, death after total hip replacement is so rare (probably around 0.1–0.4 per cent) that huge numbers would be needed for even a major effect on death rate to be detectable. Deep vein thrombosis is common after total hip replacement and therefore it is an attractive 'surrogate' outcome in thrombo-prophylaxis studies. Very small numbers of patients are needed to demonstrate even a small effect on deep vein thrombosis rates. Unfortunately deep vein thromboses below the knee are probably not clinically relevant as they do not appear to be associated with increased death rate. This makes deep vein thrombosis rate a statistically attractive but clinically poor outcome measure in this research. It also provides an example of where statistical significance may differ from clinical significance.

Bias

There are various ways in which the outcome of a trial can be distorted accidentally or even deliberately by the researcher. Bias is a 'systematic deviation of an observation from the true clinical state'. In other words, it is not random, producing a scatter of results (variability); rather, it is a skew in one direction which distorts the results. Some of the more common types are described below.

Selection bias

The choice of patients for a trial can have a profound effect on the conclusions reached. A condition studied in a tertiary referral centre is likely to be much more severe than the same disease studied in a general practice. This leads to quite different conclusions being drawn on the most appropriate management for what might superficially seem to be the same patients. In a specialist knee injury clinic, it may be felt appropriate for most patients to have either MRI or an arthroscopy. In a general practice or open-access sports injury clinic the most appropriate primary intervention may be physiotherapy without the need for sophisticated investigation.

If a randomized controlled trial is not used, bias can occur in several other ways. Researchers may choose to study only those patients who are more likely to have the outcome they wish to demonstrate. If they believe their treatment does good, then they may choose patients who they know for other reasons are going to do well whether they receive treatment or not. An example of this is in reconstruction of the anterior cruciate ligament. To obtain good results, young highly motivated individuals with no other instability should be chosen for treatment as they are likely to do well anyway. Another common strategy is to say that an operation must be done early if a good result is to be obtained. This comment is found in the literature on pelvic osteotomies for acetabular dysplasia. Patients may indeed do better if they are operated on early, but you are also choosing a group of patients in whom it is quite possible that some will do well anyway whether they receive surgery or not. Any trial that draws this conclusion must be robust to this criticism if it is to be trusted.

Box 7 Bias: definition, causes, and cure

- Systematic deviation of an observation from the true clinical state
- Selection (e.g. choose only patients who will do well)
- Hawthorne effect—the trial itself affects the results
- Outcome measures (e.g. choose clinically irrelevant outcome measures)

Treatment bias: the Hawthorne effect

Anything which is studied intensively is likely to have a different outcome by virtue of the fact that awareness of clinicians and patients alike is heightened. On the whole, phenomena that are studied do better than those that are not, and the effect can be quite profound. The quality of teaching that a pupil receives, and indeed his or her behavior in class, is quite different when a school inspector is 'sitting in' than when a routine class is taking place.

This effect can be used by the naive or indeed unscrupulous researcher to conclude that a highly significant effect is caused by the treatment when in fact it is a result of observation only.

Outcome bias

The outcome measures used can profoundly affect the conclusions that can be drawn from a trial especially if the outcomes are only chosen after the trial has been completed. Outcome measures should be chosen for their clinical importance before the trial starts to prevent this bias.

Publication bias

Negative results are common and tend to be uninteresting. Therefore they tend not to be written up, and if they are, they are not accepted for publication. There are three problems with this. Firstly it may lull someone else into believing that the study has not been done and therefore the work is unwittingly repeated (probably a waste of time). Secondly, by the simple laws of chance, repetition of a study many times will eventually produce results showing a statistically significant difference which is probably spurious. This study will be the only one published because it shows a positive result, and so the literature will be biased. An epidemiologist approaching a meta-analysis (collecting together all the studies for analysis) would only find the tip of the iceberg (the published studies), which we already know may be biased. The result may be a further biased conclusion.

Conclusion

The important principle to remember is that facts and findings in themselves mean very little. Account must be taken of the context from which *they* were taken and the environment in which *you* are working before you can draw conclusions and apply them to your practice. The skills of epidemiology are in being able to understand how trials are performed and being able to spot the pitfalls between believing that something is true and showing how true it really is.

Further reading

Hulley, S.B. and Cummings, S.R. (1988). *Designing clinical research.* Williams and Wilkins, Baltimore, MD.

Praemer, A., Furner, S., and Rice, D.P. (1992). *Musculo-skeletal conditions in the United States.* American Academy of Orthopedic Surgeons, Rosemont, IL.

Rose, G. and Barker, D.J.P. (1981). *Epidemiology for the uninitiated.* British Medical Association, London.

1.2 Measurement

1.2.1 Classification and outcome measures

A. C. Macey

The problem with classifications— either a feast or a famine

Technological and biological advances have opened up a vast range of treatments for musculoskeletal pathology and injuries. The vogue for evidence-based interventions has also created a major problem in orthopedics, where outcomes are complex to measure.

There is no excuse for the huge range of indices (rating scales) which have appeared in orthopedics. There are now more than 225 for locomotor disease alone (Feinstein 1987). Most of these have been invented and then used without being checked for observer variability, accuracy, or relevance.

The diversity of treatments available, the problem of definable relevant outcomes, and the reliance of research on indices which have not been validated create major problems when trying to classify, code, store, and then retrieve information on progress in orthopedics.

Aims of classification

The aim of orthopedic and trauma surgeons is to restore function and prevent or relieve pain, deformity, and disability in both the short and the long term. The rationale for the development of the systems of nomenclature, classification, and coding is to ensure the following:

(1) accurate diagnosis and grading of injury or pathology;

(2) selection of the appropriate treatment;

(3) confirmation that the treatment has been effective.

An additional benefit is the ability to describe the natural history of a condition. This is the information which provides the raw material on which research questions can be based.

Finally, any profession concerned with maintaining good standards will be measuring, classifying, and collating the results of its work.

Steps in classification of outcome

1. Defining terms—this includes naming of parts, and agreeing terminology relating to actions taken. This will also include defining what constitutes normal and what is abnormal.

2. Diagnosis—use of the defined terms above to describe the pattern which makes a diagnosis.

3. Determining the natural history—recording only by observation what happens if no active intervention is undertaken.

4. Grading—setting a scale to the severity of the pathology.

A secondary problem is reporting the progress of a preselected group of patients, many of whom have already undergone non-operative treatment. Describing the subsequent clinical course of such patients as the natural history of the problem under review is misleading.

Outcome results

Once the four steps above have been completed it may be possible to analyze results logically in order to:

(1) define normality;

(2) determine appropriate treatment;

(3) define the optimum timing of interventions.

Defining normality

Normality needs to be defined and must be seen in the perspective of the quote:

> Life is a disease: and the only difference between one man and another is the stage of the disease at which he lives. (George Bernard Shaw, *Back to Methuselah*, 1921)

It needs to be defined in the following terms:

(1) the natural history of this patient;

(2) the natural history of this disease;

(3) the natural history of this patient with this disease;

(4) the natural history of this patient with this disease at this time.

The measurement of treatment in the absence of this knowledge is empirical. Symptoms may improve despite or because of the treatment.

Despite the logic of this, studies of the natural history of many diseases are limited, and so there are few yardsticks against which to judge the effectiveness or otherwise of any therapeutic intervention. This work will assess the benefit of treatments against the natural history in terms of success in prevention of pain, deformity and disability, and restoration of function in the short and long term.

Classification of classifiers

There are two types of classifiers.

1. **Splitters** subdivide as far as possible, forever seeking minor differences which can be used to create a new category.

2. **Lumpers** do the opposite—they base their classifications on overarching general principles.

Everyone concerned with classification tends to fall somewhere on the spectrum between splitters and lumpers. Splitters have the advantage that the groups that they create are homogeneous. However, their classifications are complex and tend to be unworkable. Lumpers have the advantage that their classifications are simple, but each group may contain such variability that study of it as a single group becomes meaningless.

Most accepted classifications have originated from large retrospective surveys. Their very size may make them the 'gold standard'. In fact, these classifications have frequently not been validated and may only reflect the splitter or lumper mentality of the author and the bias in the method of collection of material.

Principles of a classification

There is a basic set of requirements for a good classification.

1. **Clinical usefulness**—the classification should be needed to solve, and indeed help to solve, a clinical problem.

2. **Simplicity**—it should be as simple as possible.

3. **Reproducibility**—as far as possible the same condition of the same severity should fall into the same category however often it is reclassified and whoever does that classification (inter- and intra-observer reproducibility).

4. **Appropriate divisions**—there should be categories for all known types (grades) of condition, and there should be clear criteria which separate one grade from another.

5. **Face validity**—the scale should seem to be based on common sense.

6. **Ease of use**—this should follow on from the principles listed above.

Classification in clinical trials

Nothing ruins good results like good follow-up. (Goodfellow 1991, 1995)

Observational studies

Most reports of outcome in orthopedics are observational studies, performed by someone who has a preconceived notion of what they want to find. Whilst these can give useful indications of outcome, in most cases they are open to so much bias as to be worthless. Bias is the distortion of results in one direction. All observational studies are subject to bias (conscious or unconscious) as a result of the preconceptions of the observer. Bias should always be acknowledged and discussed in an observational study.

Randomized controlled trials

The gold standard of studies is the randomized controlled trial. These have proved difficult to perform in orthopedics. They require large numbers of patients whose diagnosis and severity grading is relatively similar (narrow entry criteria). The inclusion and exclusion criteria should also be clear and relevant to the clinical question being asked. They also require a clear research question, and clear clinically relevant outcome measures. The diversity of clinical problems and difficulties in offering equivalent and comparable treatment programs

Table 1 Ten recommendations to improve future studies in musculoskeletal surgery

1	Conduct prospective randomized trials comparing carefully selected patients treated conservatively versus surgically
2	Administer reliable and valid measures before treatment starts and at standardized follow-up times (e.g. 6 months, 1 year, 5 years, 10 years)
3	Outcome measures completed by patient or by an independent observer, not by the patient's surgeon
4	Report all inclusion and exclusion criteria for selecting patients for the study
5	Report information for all patients entered into the study and reasons for all losses to follow-up
6	Report preoperative clinical signs and symptoms
7	Report details of surgical procedures
8	Report all surgical complications or lack thereof and subsequent operations during the follow-up interval
9	Retain individual patient data to allow potential meta-analysis with other studies
10	Use appropriate statistical techniques to determine whether changes in pain and disability after surgery is statistically significant

make it difficult to recruit patients and maintain the interest of the investigators over the many years needed to complete a major trial. Classification is an essential element in designing trials. The classification should be able to handle the spectrum of disorders which cover the zone of uncertainty in management options. A simple set of recommendations to improve future studies in musculoskeletal surgery is described by Labelle and Guibert (1992) (Table 1).

Relationship of classification to need

Classification is needed by three main groups: clinicians, hospital managers and accountants, and lawyers.

Clinicians

Clinicians need classification for audit and research, and to measure the outcome of their work. They also need classification for reimbursement in systems that offer a fee for service.

In order to achieve this they need the following:

(1) agreed terminology;

(2) precise nomenclature;

(3) a method of coding;

(4) information storage and retrieval systems.

Each classification will tend to be strong in some areas and weak in others. For example, classifications relating to remuneration tend to be sensitive to degree of difficulty and time involved in managing the patient. However, they lack clinical specificity.

It is important to be aware that the group with most financial interest and resources in classification are insurers concerned with reimbursement. Their systems of classification are ill-suited to the needs of audit, research, or outcome measure.

Nomenclature classification and coding systems in use

In **uniaxial systems** only one dimension of variable is used (such as diagnosis).

The **International Classification of Disease (ICD)** was developed mainly for the use of the World Health Organization in global epidemiologic studies. Extra digits have been added by clinicians, in particular the American Academy of Orthopedic Surgery (1988), to make the classification more user friendly. Despite this, the lack of an axis to allow separate coding of elements such as the anatomic site means that the classification continues to be of little value in orthopedic and trauma surgery.

The **Read Codes** (Read and Benson 1986) are far more extensive than the ICD but suffer from the same problem of not being site based.

The system used by the **Office of Population Censuses and Surveys** (OPCS 1975) is not comprehensive and fails to code anatomic sites separately.

Diagnosis-related groups were developed in the United States to classify patients by diagnosis or procedure into groups which should in theory consume the same resources (and therefore should attract the same fee). **Health-care-related groups** are the National Health Service equivalent of diagnosis-related groups. Both systems are valueless for audit research or outcome measure.

Multiaxial systems use several axes to describe and code diagnoses. They are inevitably more complex, but have face validity and clinical relevance.

The **Systematized Nomenclature of Medicine (SNOMED)** comprises seven main axes: topology, disease, occupation, morphology, etiology, function, and procedure. The main disadvantage of this system is that it lacks a simple user interface for orthopedics and trauma.

The **AO (Arbeitsgemeinschaft Osteosynthesefragen) classification of fractures** uses 'pattern recognition' similar to that applied in a real clinical situation. Fractures are then coded by number. The classification has been carefully researched but is cumbersome in practice and is unlikely to be universally used in everyday clinical practice.

Stages of classification
Description, diagnosis, and consistency

This stage is usually first done in free text. The problem-orientated medical record approach of Weed (1971) uses the Subjective–Objective Assessment Plan (**SOAP**) format described in Table 2.

Codes and their construction

The next stage is to translate the natural language text into an alphanumeric code. A basic test of a robust code is that it will play back the precise natural description when used in reverse.

For the musculoskeletal system the code will need to be multiaxial with the site as a separate axis.

Translation from natural language to code

Automated systems to perform this task remain a major challenge in all but the simplest diagnostic areas as they require sensitivity and robustness to context, grammar, and individual variability in the use of language.

Relevance of measurements

Measurements are only relevant if they are important in determining an outcome and are reproducible, i.e. the same result is obtained

Table 2 Subjective–Objective Assessment Plan (SOAP) modified for orthopedics

Findings	Description
Patient and problem	
Subjective	
Objective	
Radiography	
Tests	
Assessment	
Plan	

each time a measurement is made regardless of who makes it. A measurement should also be sensitive, i.e. it should give a different reading if a real change has taken place.

The use of radiographs as an outcome measure

Radiographs suffer from some major problems. The first is that they are merely projected shadows, and are therefore a two-dimensional representation of a three-dimensional problem. This means that slight changes in the orientation of the patient (rotation, or even distance from the film) can have a profound effect on the measurement made. A second problem is the definition of fracture union. The inter-observer variability in the interpretation of this outcome makes it very suspect for any clinical trial.

Allowance for growth

A rapidly changing subject such as orthopedics and trauma surgery requires a classification system that is robust to rapid changes in practice and to overall expansion of the subject. Any classification based on spurious premises may have superficial credibility initially, but will rapidly show its weaknesses when it is challenged by the advances in the specialty.

Tools for patient management, audit, outcome, and research: specific classification systems for trauma and orthopedics

> It is one thing to have a fancy classification; it is another to make it work. (MacNab and McCullough 1994)

Although classification and coding of the individual patient presents considerable problems, a further aim is to group similar patients together in order to enable comparisons within patient groups and between them, for example the same pathology and grade treated differently. Three specific areas of classification are of interest:

(1) fracture classifications;

(2) orthopedic classifications;

(3) classifications relating to the whole patient.

Fracture classifications

Fracture classifications are tools with the following six purposes (Burstein 1993). Fracture classification should:

(1) assist choice of treatment for each fracture;

(2) suggest a method of treatment;

(3) provide a reasonable estimation of outcome;

(4) provide the same results every time the same patient data are reviewed (intra-observer reliability);

(5) provide the same results regardless of the user (inter-observer reliability);

(6) have a proven workability prior to general use.

Validation of a classification, including demonstrating that it does actually work in a real clinical situation, is mandatory before a classification is used for research or audit purposes. The fact that most classifications of fractures have either not been validated or have demonstrated poor intra- and inter-observer reliability diminishes the value of much of the research currently in the literature.

Orthopedic classifications

These classifications suffer from similar problems as trauma classifications, but with one added problem—the long-term follow-up of a subset of patients who have undergone nonoperative treatment is frequently described as the natural history of that condition. The problem remains that for all but the most common conditions it is extremely difficult to gather a large series which is not a subset and in which no treatment has been instituted. Without a clear description of the 'natural history' a description of the outcome of a treatment is meaningless.

Classifications relating to the whole patient

These are especially important in trauma, where high-energy injury may result in multiple injuries and where the time elapsing between the occurrence of the injury and the institution of appropriate treatment is crucial. Considerable work has been done on defining a minimum set of criteria needed for evaluating injury severity indices.

The Triage Revised Trauma Score is now the most widespread (dynamic) triage instrument (Champion et al.1989). It has been shown that a Triage Revised Trauma Score 11 of less identifies 97.2 per cent of the fatally injured patients. However, when assessing the validity of a triage score it is essential to know both its sensitivity and specificity. In the case of trauma, sensitivity is defined as the ability of the component to identify patients at risk (in this case an Injury Severity Score greater than 15) and specificity is the ability of a component to identify a patient not at risk (an Injury Severity Score less than 15).

These criteria reveal the limitations of using physiological scores alone as triage systems; a Triage Revised Trauma Score of less than 11 has a sensitivity of only 59 per cent and a specificity of 82 per cent. A CRAMS (circulation, respiration, abdomen, motor, speech) score of less than 6 has a sensitivity of 83 per cent and a specificity of only 48 per cent.

Summary

The issue of classification is the key to the advance of any clinical specialty. It should be recognized that classifications may serve different masters, and that classifications for remuneration will bear no relation to classifications for outcome measurement. Multiaxial classifications in orthopedics and trauma offer major advantages over uniaxial classifications. Before a classification is used to measure outcome it needs to be validated and then tested in the workplace. Then, and only then, can it be used as a proper scientific tool.

References

American Academy of Orthopedic Surgeons (1988). *Orthopedic ICD-9-CM.* American Academy of Orthopedic Surgeons, Rosemont, IL.

Burstein, A. (1993). Fracture classification systems: do they work and are they useful? (Editorial). *Journal of Bone and Joint Surgery, American Volume,* **75A**, 1743–4.

Champion, H.R., Sacco, W.J., Copes, W.S., Gann, D.S., Gennarelli, T.A., and Flanagan, M.E. (1989). A revision of the trauma score. *Journal of Trauma*, **29**, 623–9.

Feinstein, A. (1987). *Clinimetrics*. Yale University Press, New Haven, CT.

Goodfellow, J. (1991). Science and audit (editorial). *Journal of Bone and Joint Surgery, British Volume*, **73B**, 3–5.

Goodfellow, J. (1995). Outcomes and incomes. *EFORT Bulletin*, **3**, 3–5.

Labelle, H. and Guibert, R. (1992). Lack of scientific evidence for the treatment of lateral epicondylitis of the elbow. An attempted meta-analysis. *Journal of Bone and Joint Surgery, British Volume*, **74B**, 646–51.

MacNab, I. and McCullough, J. (1994). *Neck ache and shoulder pain*. Williams and Wilkins, Baltimore, MD.

OPCS (1975). *Classification of surgical operations*. Office of Population Censuses and Surveys, London.

Read, J. and Benson, T. (1986). Computer coding—comprehensive coding. *British Journal of Healthcare Computing*, **3**, 22–5.

Weed, L. (1971). *Medical records, medical education and patient care*. Case Western Reserve University, Cleveland, OH.

1.2.2   Statistics

Christopher Bulstrode

What are statistics and why do we need to use them?

Statistics are simply the methods we use for handling data obtained from observation and experiments. They are not as difficult as they look and mainly involve common sense, not a masters degree in pure mathematics.

We use them because orthopedics is a biological subject. Biological subjects are not completely deterministic. In other words if you do the same thing twice you might get a slightly different answer each time. Statistics is all about trying to work out whether that difference probably occurred by chance, or whether something has changed between the two occasions.

Biological variability You go to a golf driving range and drive 200 balls instead of attending postgraduate training. The first drive goes only 120 yards but the last goes an extraordinary 180 yards. Statistics may allow you to get an idea whether that last drive was simply a fluke or whether your ability to drive has improved considerably more that your orthopedic knowledge that afternoon.

The null hypothesis

A common start point for your test is the supposition that the difference you have observed is merely chance. Starting from this very gloomy point of view (the null hypothesis), you can then use a statistical test to work out how likely this difference really was to have taken place by chance.

Probability—the *p* value

If you calculate that the possibility of the difference occurring by chance is 50 per cent, it would be unwise to put much reliance on the importance of the difference observed. You may then have to abandon your hypothesis for the moment, or you may decide to design a larger or more elegant experiment to test your hypothesis. Obviously the more times you can repeat the experiment, the more results there are for the statistical test to 'see' real change in amongst the 'noise' of a biological system.

p < 0.05 (*p* < 5 per cent)

In biological systems the usual level at which notice is taken is 1 in 20. If you calculate from a statistical test that the difference you have observed could have occurred by chance only once in 20 times or less ($p < 0.05$) then the observation is said to be significant at the 5 per cent level. This is a standard level agreed by most biological scientists as being a threshold for a difference observed probably being due to a real underlying difference and not just chance. It does not mean that you have proved anything; it just says it is unlikely to have occurred by chance.

p < 0.001 (*p* < 0.1 per cent)—very highly significant results

Beware significance levels of less than 0.001 (0.1 per cent). In orthopedics it is unusual to be able to repeat an experiment often enough to obtain even 5 per cent significance. A significance of 1 per cent may mean that what you are testing is blindingly obvious (in which case there was no need to perform statistics) or that something has gone wrong in the way the experiment has been designed or analysed, and this result is spurious.

Testing the obvious After 4 weeks of going to the golf range, there seems little point in changing what are clearly becoming the habits of a lifetime, and so you continue going to the range every Friday for the rest of the year. You then persuade the statistics department to run your year's scorecard, claiming that it is an experiment in leg-lengthening that you have performed where the yards you have driven are in fact millimeters of diaphyseal lengthening. The improvement over the year comes back as 1 yard (millimeter) per week with $p < 0.01$. It was pretty obvious really, and you did not need to apply statistics to rationalize dropping out of the postgraduate training program.

Power analysis

Power analysis is a simple technique for working out how many subjects that you are likely to need in an experiment to have a reasonable chance of showing statistical significance, assuming that there really is a difference. Statisticians have computer programs for calculating this number, and will just need you to describe the experiment to them, so that they can make the calculation. Some of the questions they may ask you are as follows.

1. How great is the **variability** in observations anyway? You can imagine that if the variability is large then more subjects will be needed to show a difference between two groups than if the variability is small.

2. What kind of **difference** are you expecting to find? If you are only expecting a slight difference at best, then large numbers will be needed. If you are expecting a very large difference (unusual

in most comparisons of treatment), then far fewer patients will be needed in the study.

3. What level of **significance** will satisfy you that there is a real difference? If it is vital that you are sure that there is a difference, then a *p* level of less than 0.001 might be necessary. You will need far more patients to achieve this than if you are prepared to accept a *p* value of 0.05.

4. What **type** of data are you gathering? If the data are simple 'yes' or 'no' answers, you may need more patients than if you can measure seven or eight categories reliably.

Power analysis To calculate how many postgraduate sessions you would have to miss before you could demonstrate a statistical improvement in your standard of golf, you would need to take the following information to the statistician.

- How far you normally drive a ball and what the variability is. You might say that in 20 consecutive drives the mean was 150 yards and the range was 80 to 180 yards.

- How much you expect to improve per session. Here, you might be looking at 1 yard per session.

- What probability level you are prepared to accept. Being a reasonable person, you would probably accept $p < 0.05$.

- Can you really give all the figures in yards, or are you simply going to have to say, 'Beyond the tree half-way down the fairway'.

Type II error

If you recruit too few patients in a study you may find no apparent difference when there really is one. This is called a type II error, and causes great confusion in the orthopedic literature. If a study shows no difference between groups, this does not necessarily mean that there is no difference. It just means that any difference was too small to be detected by that trial's design and size.

Type I error

That leads on to what a type I error is, which I hope had been worrying you ever since we mentioned a type II error. A type I error is the decision that there is a real difference when actually there is not. Obviously, the higher you set the *p* value (the more likely you are to reject the null hypothesis), the more likely you will be to commit a type I error. In orthopedics it is so hard to obtain large numbers of subjects that it is difficult to obtain *p* values that are very certain, such as 0.001. The compromise that has been reached is $p < 0.05$.

The randomized controlled trial

This is really the gold standard of scientific research, and is the most elegant and powerful way of testing a hypothesis. Unfortunately, randomized controlled trials are also very difficult to perform, especially in the surgical sciences. A randomized controlled trial tests a null hypothesis (e.g. there is no difference between the incidence of pulmonary embolus after total hip replacement whether or not low-molecular-weight heparin is used). Subjects are allocated to the different arms of the study purely by chance (randomization). Any

significant differences observed between the outcomes of the two groups should serve to disprove the null hypothesis and should not be caused by any other factor such as the fact that one group are mainly patients with rheumatoid arthritis (which seems to protect against pulmonary embolus, and the other group mainly have osteoarthritis).

Experimental design You and several of your colleagues who have now joined you decide that driving at a golf range is very boring on a Friday afternoon, and it would be more interesting to play 18 holes with one of the professors who is a member of the Very Royal and Ancient Golf Club. Only three of you can play with him, and of course you make sure that you lose each week to keep Professor X happy. Nevertheless an argument has broken out as to who should play at the VRAGC and who should go to the driving range. In a flash of inspiration you decide to resolve what is likely to prove a most divisive argument by setting up a randomized controlled trial to see whether you improve more by playing with Professor X at the VRAGC or by going to the golf range. Three of you are randomly allocated to play with Professor X and three go to the driving range. Your null hypothesis is that your improved handicaps by the end of the year will be the same in each group and that no more of the group who play with Professor X will have got consultant jobs than those who go to the driving range. The statistician smells a rat and refuses to perform a power analysis on such paltry numbers despite the fact that you bring him your handicaps and tell him that you expect the driving-range group to drop their handicaps by two and the group who play with Professor X to deteriorate by one point. You are looking for significance at the 5 per cent level.

Control group

If one arm of the trial is 'no treatment', this is called the control group. It is usual to try to treat the control group in the same way as the treatment group apart from the actual treatment being tested. In medical trials, tablets given that look identical to the treatment tablet but that contain no active ingredient are called **placebo**. In surgery a mock operation (usually only performed in animal experiments) is called the **sham**.

Confounding factors and bias

Confounding factors are other variables in a trial that may have a profound effect on the outcome and invalidate the results. In a randomized controlled trial the randomization process should block this effect out by allocating subjects with these confounding factors equally to each group.

However, in small clinical trials it is very easy for factors to produce a systematic deviation in the results unless a careful look-out is kept for them. This is a **bias** and can ruin the results of study. If the study is biased towards the null hypothesis, then a type II error will be more likely to occur (no difference will be found when there was one). If the bias increases the difference between the groups then a type I error may occur (the null hypothesis is falsely disproved). The only solution is to identify factors that might do this (common examples are age and gender), and then to make sure that appropriate action is taken to minimize their effects.

Confounding factors The three who are not going to the driving range are so bored that they have volunteered to do Professor X's outpatient clinic together on Wednesday afternoon while he is away doing paperwork. Each week they rush through the clinic, and then sneak off to the local golf course. Professor X is enormously grateful. This is a confounding factor. Not only may it be responsible for any improvement in their handicap, but it may also result in their being preferred for the next three senior resident posts over their colleagues who thought they were in clover. The outcome of this study may be more influenced by a factor not included in the hypothesis (the Wednesday afternoon) than the difference being tested.

Stratification or minimization

A computer program exists which allows for a modified form of randomization while ensuring that the major confounding factors do not distort the groupings by chance (Evans 1987).

Blinding

There is a danger that if patients know which treatment they are receiving, particularly when a placebo is being used in one arm, that they will consciously or subconsciously modify their response according to whether they have received the treatment under test or not. This would invalidate the results of the trial and is a form of **bias**. The simple solution is not to allow patients to know whether they are receiving the treatment or placebo. This is very difficult in surgery where obviously it is not possible or ethical to perform a **sham** operation for the control arm.

There is also a danger that the observer is such a fervent believer in his or her hypothesis that he or she might again consciously or unconsciously modify the results to bring about a favorable result. If the observer also does not know to which group the patient belongs (treatment or control), then this bias is avoided. This is known as **double blinding**, and the **double-blinded randomized controlled trial** is the most rigorous of scientific tools used to gather evidence for efficacious practice (Sackett *et al.* 1991).

Blinding and relevance A golf handicap is awarded by a player submitting his or her own card. Therefore it is subject to bias, as the person filling it in may be economical with the truth. A better evaluation in this case would be for a golf professional to go round with each group before and after the year and assess progress. This would be an independent assessment. If the professional had no idea which group was which, then this would constitute a blinded independent assessment. If the arrangements for you to go round the golf course were made by Professor X to help him decide who should have the senior resident posts and he did not tell you why he had arranged this, then this would be a double-blinded assessment. Neither you nor the professional would be able to bias the results because you would not know what the professional was doing, and the professional would not know either. The important thing about blinding is that whoever is blinded should not know how the data might be altered to affect the outcome of the trial. However, it would not be a very good way of deciding on senior resident posts. Although it would be scientifically rigorous, it would actually be methodologically flawed because the outcome would be of very doubtful significance.

Different kinds of data

Data can take different forms which require different methods for analysis. Some examples are given below.

Nominal data

Nominal data can be assigned to different classes, but each category is no larger or better than the others—it is just different. An example would be a dome osteotomy rather than a wedge osteotomy for arthritis of the knee. They are different but cannot be put into an order.

Ordinal data

The next grade up is where the data can be ranked but not in any mathematical way. For example, to be able to walk with a stick after surgery is better than requiring crutches. Being on crutches is better than being confined to a wheelchair. Here, the outcomes can be ranked but cannot be given values which can be added and subtracted—they can only be ranked.

Interval data

Interval data are one grade stronger. For example, the range of movement of a joint in degrees can be regarded as interval data: 60° of movement is approximately twice as good as 30°.

Normally distributed data

This is a special class of interval data where we know that the numbers have been collected from a population that has a symmetrical bell-shaped distribution. Many biological variables such as height are normally distributed, and this allows very specific statistics called parametric statistics to be used in analysing the data.

On the whole in clinical orthopedics, data are not normally distributed, or if they are, we have no way of being sure. As a working rule therefore, use non-parametric statistics for the analysis of your data. It is simpler to use and easier to understand, but perhaps sometimes not as powerful as parametric statistics. One advantage is that the books describing the tests are short and simple.

Data analysis
Mean

The mean is the middle or average of a data set. If the data are normally distributed (a symmetrical bell-shaped curve), then it bisects the bell. However, if the data are very skewed the mean can be 'meaningless'.

The mean is meaningless You are now a very keen golfer and decide to share your joy in this wonderful sport with a fellow professional. You take out an anesthesiology resident to introduce him to the delights of golf and the great outdoors. He is eager but has never hit a golf ball in his life. You decide to apply your new found skills in statistics to start measuring his skills in golf. By sheer luck, his first hit goes 80 yards. After that he digs four consecutive divots, moving the ball less than 6 inches each time. Finally he breaks a new driver on the fifth drive by hitting the ground. While trying to console him over the fact that he has just broken your newest club, you cheer him with the news that his mean driving distance is 16 yards ($80 + 0 + 0 + 0 + 0$ divided by 5). This is patently rubbish. All you can say is that his best hit was 80 yards, and after that the less said the better.

The standard deviation

The standard deviation (**SD**) describes how widely the data are spread around the middle point, i.e. the mean (Fig. 1). If every reading obtained in a normally distributed data set is almost the same, the SD is very small (Fig. 1, curve B). If they are widely separated, then it is large (Fig. 1, curve A).

Standard deviation The curves in Fig. 1 might represent your burgeoning relationship with this anesthesiologist. He is making progress in leaps and bounds, but has reached that stage where his performance can be good, but tends to be erratic. Some drives are really quite good (but not as good as yours). Others are still frankly awful (curve A). Your drives, however, are long, hard, and very consistent. The mean distance is high and there is very little variability. The SD is low (curve B).

Confidence interval

When you are reporting a result based on several observations it is helpful for the reader to have some idea of how much reliance they can put on it. This will depend on how scattered the data are (the SD) and on how many data points have been collected. If there are very few data points, then the mean calculated from those few data points may be out by a long way. The confidence interval (**CI**) merely gives a range in which it is 95 per cent certain that the true mean lies.

Confidence interval You want to know on average how often you can hole a putt from 10 yards. Initially you do 10 putts and hole three.

You could just say 'I can hole 30 per cent of the time at 10 yards'. But intuitively how sure would you be that the answer was not 20 per cent or 40 per cent. Not very, I suspect! If, however, you did 100 putts and holed 38 you could say with some certainty that you can hole nearly 40 per cent of the time. The CI is the certainty you have in the answer. The 95 per cent CI for the answer from the 10 putts was ± 25 per cent. The answer from the 100 putts had a CI of ± 5 per cent. This second answer is more attractive both because it is better and because it is more reliable.

Range

In data that are not normally distributed it is simply better to give just the range, which in Fig. 2 would be very large. It is written as the difference between the highest and lowest readings in brackets after the mode, or can be written simply as the highest and lowest values.

Median

The median is the line that has equal numbers of results above and below it. If the data are very skewed, it may be more useful than the mean because it is not distorted by outlying points. For example, the median striking distance for your partner's first attempt at golf would 3 inches (remember that the mean was 16 yards) because two strikes drove the ball less than 2 inches, one drove it 3 inches, one 6 inches, and one 80 yards. In this case the median gives a better idea of the situation than the mean.

Mode

To counteract the problem of the median and mean being offset by skewed data, the mode is a line through the most common category (the peak of the bump). When data are very skewed, this can give a better description of where the center of all the points may lie (see Fig. 2).

Importance of range Figure 2 shows the relationship a couple of months later. Your partner is settling but is still a little erratic. The most likely distance (the mode) that he will drive is 100 yards. However, his average driving distance (the mean) is 86 yards. If you were

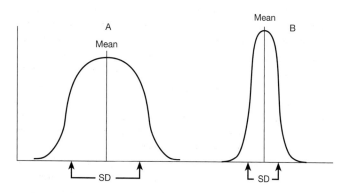

Fig. 1. The bell-shaped curves of a normal distribution. Curve A has a low mean but a high SD. Curve B has a higher mean but a lower SD.

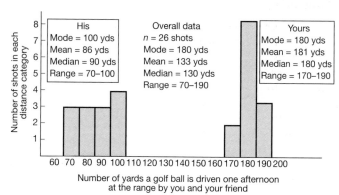

Fig. 2. Bimodal data that are not normally distributed. There are many ways of describing them.

a gambling man and wanted to wager on how far he could drive, you would be wise to bet that he could not drive more than 90 yards (the median) as his chances of driving further than that are less than 50 per cent. But note that for the overall picture of the afternoon's driving, the mean, mode, and median tell you nothing at all. The most useful piece of information might be the range.

Sensitivity and specificity

Sensitivity

One of the other problems with scientific studies in clinical medicine is the reliability of the tests being used. Some tests pick up all patients with a particular condition and no others. These tests are rare. It is important when using a test to know how reliable it is in picking up what you are trying to study. Sensitivity and specificity are the two measures most commonly used. Sensitivity is a measure of how sure you can be that a patient does not have a condition if the test is negative. A very sensitive test is useful when the treatment is cheap and harmless and the consequences of failing to make the diagnosis are dire. For example, if a child with a supracondylar fracture has pain on extending the fingers after the plaster has been applied, it is best to assume that a compartment syndrome is starting and release the plaster forthwith. You may be overreacting, but it best to be on the safe side. If he or she does not have pain on extension it is very unlikely that a compartment syndrome is developing, and so both you and the child can sleep in peace. The test is sensitive.

> **Sensitivity** An example of a test with low sensitivity is being caught speeding. The police only catch a very small proportion of people speeding. If you based your estimate of the number of people speeding on the number of prosecutions brought by the police, you would grossly underestimate the incidence of the problem. This is low sensitivity.
>
> Conversely, the fire alarms at our hospital are very sensitive indeed. There have been some fires in the past and the alarms have worked perfectly on every occasion. The alarms have a very high sensitivity—they pick up every single fire. The penalty is that they sometimes go off unnecessarily.

Specificity

Specificity is a measure of how reliable a test is when it is positive. A very specific test only reports positive if the condition really is present. This is very important in medicine because most patients and many doctors think that if a test is positive then the disease is present. Most tests are actually not very specific.

> **Trade-off between sensitivity and specificity** Although the number of prosecutions brought for speeding is a low-sensitivity test for the amount of speeding going on, it is very rare indeed that the police bring a prosecution when in fact the driver was not speeding. Therefore this test has a high specificity.
>
> However, the hospital fire alarms have a very low specificity, despite their high sensitivity, as they are always going off for no apparent reason.

Spins and snouts

A simple way of remembering which is which is 'spins and snouts'. Sp IN is short for Specificity = IN. If a specific test is positive (IN) then it likely that the patient has the condition. Therefore a specific test is useful when it is positive. Conversely, Sn OUT is short for Sensitivity = OUT. If a sensitive test is negative, then you can be very sure that you have excluded the condition.

Survivorship analysis

Survivorship analysis is a specific technique used for studying the lifetime of something which is eventually going to wear out or fail. It was originally designed for evaluating treatments being used for cancer patients where relapse or death may occur at some time in the future, but is now routinely used in orthopedics for studying the longevity of joint replacements. However, it does have limitations, and if these are not recognized, very misleading results can be presented (Murray *et al.* 1993).

The ideal test of a new joint replacement would be to put in a couple of hundred of the new design within a few weeks and then follow them as a group over the years. This is what is called a cohort study. Clearly, this may be possible in some branches of medicine, but not in joint replacement where several years may elapse before the first hundred have been put in. By that time some of the first patients who received the joint may have died, or the implant may already have failed in one or two. The method for getting round this when analysing the results is to lay out results with the first column being the result for each patient in the first year after they had received their implant irrespective of the actual year when that was. At each patient's subsequent year, you can calculate how many patients are still in the study (the number at risk of failure), how many have died, how many have been lost, and how many implants have failed. Thus, for each year after the operation you have a number for that year that failed, which you can compare with the number in that year who were still in the trial (the number at risk). Convention allows you to assume that patients who die during the study are successes up until their deaths and then simply disappear from the study without ever being counted as failures. Patients lost to follow-up are more difficult because it may be assumed that they have gone elsewhere for treatment to save embarrassment. Limited studies performed indicate that this is not necessarily true, but nevertheless it has now been suggested that that the number of failures should be calculated twice, once counting lost to follow-up as successes until their disappearance (like deaths), and once counting each patient lost as a failure. When these figures have been calculated a cumulative total failure rate year by year can be worked out by adding on the proportion failing each year to the proportion already failed from previous years. This survivorship curve should give a reasonable idea of how well an implant is standing up over the years.

However, there are problems. If revision is used as the failure point of an implant, the number that actually fail may be grossly underestimated. This is because revisions may not be performed for many reasons (no time, no expertise, no equipment, no money, patient too ill, patient too frightened, etc.). If revision operations are even delayed, never mind avoided completely, the success rate recorded may bear no relation to the truth. The other problem is that however long a study is continued joint replacement is basically an operation for the elderly who do not live long. You may find that even after 20 years of gathering patients there are very few data points beyond 10 years, simply because most patients have died within 10 years of surgery. The result is that the tail of the survivorship curve may only be based on very few patients, and therefore the chance of a failure is very low especially as by then most of them are too old to tolerate a revision. Therefore we have recommended that a survivorship curve should include a second curve which plots the worst scenario, counting all patients lost to follow-up as failures. We have also suggested that the number of patients included in each year's analysis should also be written on the curve to show how much reliance can be put on the data. Obviously if there are only five or six patients left at risk then not much reliance can be put on the data. In fact if there are fewer than 30 patients, the survivorship curve from that point on must be regarded with considerable caution. Finally, it is probably worth plotting a separate curve based on an outcome that does not depend on the health or courage of the patient, and in this case the onset of moderate continuous pain probably fills that bill. A failure rate of around 1 or 2 per cent per annum in one of our studies converts to a failure rate of over 5 per cent per annum when onset of moderate pain is plotted.

Further reading

Pocock, S.J. (1983). *Clinical trials: a practical approach.* Wiley, Chichester.

Pynsent, P.B., Fairbank, J.C.T., and Carr, A.J. (1993). *Outcome measures in orthopaedics.* Butterworth Heinemann, Oxford.

Siegel, S. and Castellan, N.J., Jr (1988). *Nonparametric statistics for the behavioral sciences* (2nd edn). McGraw-Hill, New York.

References

Evans, S. (1987). *Computer program for stratification in randomised controlled trials.* London Hospital Medical College, London.

Murray, D., Carr, A., and Bulstrode, C. (1993). Survival analysis of joint replacement. *Journal of Bone and Joint Surgery, British Volume,* **75B**, 697–704.

Sackett, D., Haynes, R.B., Guyatt, G.H., and Tugwell, P. (1991). *Clinical epidemiology* (2nd edn). Little, Brown, Boston, MA.

1.3 Principles of diagnosis and management

Aaron G. Rosenberg and Richard A. Berger

Introduction

One of the greatest appeals of orthopedics is the intellectual challenge of solving an endless variety of musculoskeletal problems. This chapter examines how to solve these problems by analyzing the process of reasoning and decision-making in orthopedics as it relates to the problems of formulating a diagnosis and then making treatment recommendation.

Medical care is often considered an art. This viewpoint stems in part from the intrinsic uncertainty in medical care combined with the overwhelming complexity inherent in treating patients who can present with a dizzying array of symptoms and unique combinations of disorders. Physicians must frequently choose a treatment before the exact diagnosis is known. Even when the diagnosis is known, the treatment outcome is often uncertain and multiple treatments may offer significantly different risks, benefits, and costs. Although physicians have always lived with and managed uncertainty, the inability or unwillingness to analyze and understand how decision-making is carried out under this uncertainty has led to the mistaken conclusion that medical decision-making is an art. Unfortunately, considering medical thinking as an art makes thinking about medical reasoning difficult and may make it impossible to study, refine, and teach.

Deductive reasoning has helped physicians in new and unfamiliar situations, but deductive reasoning by itself is of little use when essential facts are missing. Decision-making in the face of uncertainty, common to all medical situations, has been increasingly the subject of study. The recent findings of substantial regional variations in surgical and medical procedures, the drive to control costs by standardizing treatments (allowing only 'proven care' modalities), and the increase in costs of, and reliance on, high-tech diagnostic modalities (coupled with the increasing presence and reliance on computers) has led to the evolution of medical decision-making as a science unto itself. To understand decisions under uncertainty, we must first analyze the decision-making process in general.

The differential diagnosis

A patient usually seeks medical advice to treat a symptom. This presenting symptom is expressed as a chief complaint. Although the patient may or may not want to know the reason for the symptom, the patient wants the symptom eliminated quickly and painlessly. The physician must either find the cause of the problem or at least rule out the possibility of a serious and treatable disease. This task, faced by physicians daily, is often difficult since there are many possible causes of a particular symptom. There are many logical strategies for approaching this problem.

Box 1 Differential diagnosis

- Identifying the cause of the problem
- Excluding stenosis or treatable disease

Formulating a differential diagnosis is usually the initial step in solving a patient's problem and consists of compiling a list of possible or probable causes of the patient's chief complaint. These alternative diagnoses must be evaluated before finally settling on a final diagnosis. This systematic review acts as a safeguard against a premature and incorrect diagnosis. The differential diagnosis pervades all specialties and subspecialties in all fields of medicine. It is a skill that all physicians must learn and strive to master.

Methods of formulating a differential diagnosis

In medical training, students are initially, and perhaps mistakenly, taught to segregate data gathering and diagnosis testing. They are instructed to obtain all relevant data before starting to include or exclude disease processes. This method of gathering all information and then developing a conclusion is an example of inductive logic: reasoning from particular facts to a general conclusion. While this method is valuable, it is time consuming and inefficient. Deductive logic—reasoning from a general principle to specific facts—is more representative of the logic used by more experienced physicians. Yet pure deductive logic, as a strategy for formulating a differential diagnosis, is also inefficient.

Both inductive and deductive logic represent unrealistic extremes of the actual methodology physicians use to think and reason clinically. Studies of clinical problem solving show that physicians form diagnostic hypotheses on the basis of minimal clinical findings and that these hypotheses create an environment to gather additional, specific data. This process is an iterative approach between inductive and deductive reasoning. This iterative logic process has been called the hypothetico-deductive method (Fig. 1). By this process, diagnoses are either confirmed or eliminated. Diagnoses that survive are then made progressively more specific.

The emphasis in the iterative approach is on assessing information

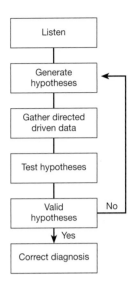

Fig. 1. Flowchart of the hypothetico-deductive method. In this iterative logic process, diagnoses are either confirmed or eliminated. Diagnoses that survive are then made progressively more specific.

as it is encountered in the evaluation of the patient. The clinical information is accumulated and interpreted as it presents or is accumulated. This ability to develop a relevant fact finding strategy is the essence of a thorough yet efficient diagnostician.

The human mind has a limited working memory. The physician can consider only a few hypotheses at once. The physician begins an evaluation of a hypothesis by matching the patient's findings with the internal representation, or model of the disease process. In this way a causation is usually inferred by logical deduction. This process assumes a good understanding of the pathophysiology of the disease. In other cases, the diagnosis is associative. In this method the physician matches the clinical findings, the progression, and the predisposing factors associated with a disease to their patient's findings. The physician then inquires about the typical features of the disease and is able to eliminate or support diagnoses from the patient's response.

The cognitive process that physicians use to confirm or discard hypotheses has been proposed in several models. In the algorithmic model, the physician follows an internal flow sheet with branching logic as the test diagnoses. In the Bayesian model, physicians change their belief in a diagnosis with each new item of information. Finally, in the linear model, findings are assigned a positive weight if true and a negative weight if false. The decision to keep or reject a diagnosis is formulated by summing these diagnostic values.

Data collection

A good diagnostician observes the patient closely before conversation is even initiated. They start to draw tentative conclusions immediately. As soon as the chief complaint is identified, the skilled physician uses the patient's age and gender to identify the main diagnostic possibilities. These first impressions then serve to determine the first line of questioning. Each subsequent answer refines the diagnosis, either confirming or refuting a hypothesis, and in turn, generating another relevant question.

Unfortunately, the skill of history taking is often the least perfected and the most neglected. Although we often blame the patient, there are probably many more poor history takers than poor historians. Too often evaluation consists of an inadequate history, where only a few questions are asked in a cursory manner. Then a large number of expensive tests are ordered, with the hopes of finding the answer via technology. Of course in some cases these results may be inaccurate, inappropriate, or poorly interpreted, and ultimately misleading. This 'shotgun approach' wastes time and money and in today's environment of cost containment is unacceptable. An important observation that has been reported is that consultants or 'experts' who are asked to solve a particular diagnostic dilemma usually do so by asking additional questions and finding something that was overlooked on the original examination, rather than by ordering additional tests.

Nowhere in the practice of medicine are interpersonal skills needed more than in taking a history. When patients give reasons why they change physicians, over half do so because of cold and impersonal interactions. Most perceive this rushed attitude as the most significant criticism. This information means that the time used for a proper history is not only good medicine but good customer relations.

Studies have shown that initial hypotheses are formed early in the interview and that the correct hypothesis can frequently be reached within 2 min of the history. The initial hypotheses are confirmed or excluded by the hypothetico-deductive method (Fig. 1). To use it, the interview must be highly directed and hypothesis driven. This method is efficient, and allows a high volume of low-value information to be skipped. However, it is highly dependent on the physician's knowledge base, template matching, and case-building skills.

The method does have pitfalls. When a physician begins to believe in a diagnostic hypothesis, conflicting data are sometimes ignored or misinterpreted. Newly acquired information may be used to confirm an existing hypothesis when it should be disregarded, used to reject the hypothesis, or used as the basis for a new hypothesis. The physician may exaggerate the importance of a finding to fit the diagnosis. It is important to recognize and avoid this mental inertia.

Physicians use their experience to estimate the likelihood that a hypothesis is true. Experience is valuable, however the likelihood that an illness is present should be based on known probability. Furthermore, the hypothesis to test first should be based on both the probability of a disease and the importance of treating it.

The physical examination can be hypothesis driven also. A screening and branching approach is most useful. A simple screening examination is done and abnormalities noted are further examined in more detail. Furthermore, the examination should be focused on proving or disproving a diagnosis on the differential list. This method, while efficient, is somewhat risky in that it is incomplete. This is particularly true in musculoskeletal medicine, where the physician is frequently working with a very specific anatomic region which is the source of the patient's complaint. The screening and branching examination should not be used when the hypothesized disease may have serious consequences if untreated. This is the disease that 'cannot be missed'.

Pathognomonic findings, when present or absent, are also useful, but unfortunately very rare. Also, a mistaken pathognomonic finding will prematurely terminate a diagnostic search. Therefore, it can be argued that pathognomonic finding not be considered as such, only as strong evidence to help prove or disprove a hypothesis.

Another common diagnostic mistake is to reassure oneself when making a diagnosis or differentiating between diagnoses when it does not matter to the patient or to the treatment. When our 'need to know' is the sole reason for pursuing a diagnosis, time and money are wasted. Furthermore, instead of looking for data to reassure, we should be searching for evidence to disprove our theory. Searching to disprove a theory is more effective at strengthening the theory when we are unable to disprove it.

On occasion, hypotheses will be slow to come to mind. This is often the case when the chief complaint is vague or when the physician does not know what diseases may be causing the patient's complaint. When this occurs, it is often useful to think of disease categories rather than specific diseases. It is useful to think of anatomy first and then broad etiology. When all else fails a good review of systems can be helpful.

There are several good rules to reduce the list of active hypotheses. Start by ranking the remaining active hypotheses and list evidence for each. Rank the active hypothesis from most to least likely on paper. Combine diagnoses with the same consequences in a cluster. If the treatment and outcomes are the same, than treating these diagnoses as different may not be useful. Lastly, consider parsimony, that a patient's complaint is likely to be caused by only one process and not by multiple processes occurring simultaneously. This rule comes from probability theory (as will be discussed later): the probability of multiple processes occurring is the product of these multiple probabilities. Most often this combined probability is lower than the probability of the presence of a single less common disease.

It should be remembered at each step in this process, from chief complaint and history to the physical examination, and finally paraclinical studies, that the possible list of diagnosis be reduced at each step. In this way the process remains efficient. Only tests that are necessary and will change your diagnosis are ordered. This saves time and especially money. Tests ordered in a 'shotgun approach' are not only expensive, but, as discussed later, without a pretest suspicion are often useless and confounding, and may even be harmful.

Orthopedic diagnosis

The initial problem to be solved in most orthopedic diagnoses is determining the anatomic source of the patients complaints. Concurrently, one must determine whether the problems are systemic or local. This phenomenon is encountered when the patient has more than a single region to which a complaint is offered. That is, when the patient has multiarticular or several regions of complaint, are they related or separate? In general it is more appropriate in a text on orthopedic surgery to discuss the patient with a single joint or anatomic complaint, and a rheumatologic text to discuss the patient with multiarticular complaints and the potential for systemic illness affecting the musculoskeletal system.

Box 2 Problems of localization

- Patient's description may not match anatomy
- Referred pain
- Pain radiation

The process of diagnosing a patient's musculoskeletal complaint usually begins by localization of the disease process through on understanding the patient's complaints as it relates to his or her perception of anatomy. For example, patients have little understanding, in general, of the anatomic terms used for pain location, and will complain of 'hip pain' when the pain is experienced in the buttock, or will refer to 'wrist pain' when the actual symptom is in the hand. A thorough understanding of where the patient is experiencing their symptoms is essential to defining the anatomic source of the patient's complaint. It is consequently essential to understand the propensity of musculoskeletal pain to be experienced in specific referral patterns. For example, in children (and some adults) hip-joint pathology is frequently experienced primarily (and occasionally exclusively) as knee pain. Low back inflammation is experienced as pain in the buttock. Actual hip-joint pathology is almost exclusively felt in the groin, but frequently patients with buttock and back complaints will present with complaints of 'hip' pain.

Additional important information is gained by determining the severity, frequency, and quality of the symptoms. Radiation of pain along specific pathways is common in the musculoskeletal system. In particular, those events that precipitate or alleviate the symptoms are essential in formulating a differential diagnosis. For example, continuous pain, rest pain, and night pain are more likely due to inflammatory or tumorous conditions, while pain related to activity is more likely due to mechanical or degenerative conditions. Important additional information is gained by asking the patient how the particular symptoms in question affect the patient's lifestyle, e.g. walking distance or time, self-care needs related to use of the region in question, or, for athletic patients, their ability to compete or perform specific maneuvers. While much of this information is not essential to making the diagnosis *per se*, severity of symptoms may be very influential in determining the next appropriate step in making the diagnosis or how the potential treatment choices compare in terms of potential improvement versus risks.

Decision analysis

The science of decision analysis has constructed models that allow investigation, study, and improvement of decision-making methods. Through these models, and the study of them, decision analysis can be better incorporated in clinical orthopedics. This section is designed to give an overview of fundamental methods and rules to allow the implementation of decision analysis in clinical practice. Furthermore, these fundamentals may allow for more efficient teaching and development of standards of care.

In these theoretical models, all diagnoses are logical conclusions from sound facts. In real practice, they are not. Medical decisions are estimates of probability.

The act of making a diagnosis is, in effect, making a decision that the patient has a particular disease process on the differential diagnosis list. Various standards of evidence can be used to determine whether or not the patient does indeed have the pathophysiologic process in question. In point of fact, the presence or absence of disease is often not a certainty, but a probability. The term 'gold standard' is frequently invoked to describe the finding (whether it be physical finding or the result of a particular laboratory investigation) that is considered the hallmark of the disease in question. For example, in microbiologic terms, the identification of a specific pathognomonic

Table 1 The 2 × 2 contingency table

	Disease present	Disease absent
Test positive	True positive	False positive
Test negative	False negative	True negative

Table 2 Example of a 2 × 2 contingency table

	Herniated lumbar disk present (10)	Herniated lumbar disk absent (90)
Positive MRI results	True-positive MRI (9)	False-positive MRI (27)
Negative MRI results	False-negative MRI (1)	True-negative MRI (63)

organism by culture is considered the gold standard in diagnosis. The finding of a specific histopathologic pattern in a bone tumor biopsy or the findings of specific bone necrosis and creeping substitution patterns in a femoral head specimen, 'classic' for osteonecrosis, can be considered such gold standards. In general the visual microscopic findings of the pathologic examination of tissue are the clearest examples of 'standards' available in the diagnosis of disease. Functional diagnoses such as reduced blood flow in coronary artery disease, or functional rotatory instability in the anterior cruciate deficient knee, will have 'standards' of diagnosis that are not based on histopathologic findings. Indeed, tests of various kinds have been devised to determine whether or not disease is actually present. The findings of these tests (whether they be physical examination, radiologic, serum chemistry, angiographic, etc.) represent attempts to determine whether or not the pathologic condition being considered is actually present. These tests can be considered to be associated with the specific disease process, as determined by comparison to a gold standard through various statistically determined elements. In discussing the diagnostic accuracy of such tests it is important to understand the fundamental elements which relate the findings of the test to the actual presence or absence of disease. These are sensitivity, specificity, prevalence, and predictive value. The basic tool to understand these variables is the 2 × 2 contingency table (Table 1).

The sensitivity of a test is its ability to detect a disease when that disease is actually present. Using a proportion, it is the percentage of the patients with a disease who have a positive test. Using the 2 × 2 contingency table,

$$\text{sensitivity} = \frac{\text{true positive}}{\text{disease present}}$$

where

$$\text{disease present} = \text{true positive} + \text{false negative}.$$

Conversely, the specificity of a test is the test's ability to accurately detect disease-free patients. Using a proportion, it is the percentage of the patients without a disease who have a negative test. Using the 2 × 2 contingency table,

$$\text{sensitivity} = \frac{\text{true negative}}{\text{disease absent}}$$

where

$$\text{disease absent} = \text{true negative} + \text{false positive}.$$

Sensitivity and specificity are characteristics of the test. They remain constant as long as the test is performed in the standard manner, without preselecting or subselecting some parameters related to the test.

The false-positive rate of a test is the test's error in not detecting disease-free patients when they are disease free. Using a proportion, it is the percentage of the patients without the disease who have a positive test. Using the 2 × 2 contingency table,

$$\text{false-positive rate} = \frac{\text{false positive}}{\text{disease absent}}$$

False-positive rate can also be calculated as 1 − specificity.

The prevalence of a disease is the proportion of patients in a given population who actually have the disease, before the results of a test are known. Prevalence is occasionally referred to as the prior probability.

Conversely, if the prevalence, the sensitivity, and specificity of a test are known, then the 2 × 2 contingency table can be completed using these three proportions. The prevalence identifies the probability a patient will be in the first column (disease present) while the remainder will be in the second column (disease absent). Sensitivity (also referred as true-positive rate) identifies the probability that if the patient is in the first column, the result of the test will be positive. Finally, the false-positive rate (1 − specificity) gives the probability that if the patient is in the second column (disease absent), the test results will be positive.

For example, start with 100 patients. If the prevalence of a herniated lumbar disk is 10 per cent and the sensitivity of MRI of the spine is 90 per cent with a specificity of 70 per cent, complete the 2 × 2 contingency table (Table 2). Ten (10 per cent) of the 100 patients will have a herniated lumbar disk (column 1), and 90 will not (column 2). Of the 10 patients in column 1 that have a herniated lumbar disk, nine (90 per cent) will have a true-positive test, leaving one with a false-negative test. Of the 90 patients without a herniated lumbar disk in column 2, 63 (70 per cent) will have a true-negative result and therefore 27 (30 per cent) will have a false-negative result.

Clinically, the most helpful probability from this table is the predictive value of a positive test. The predictive value of a positive test is the probability that a patient has the disease if the test is positive. It is the proportion of the patients with a positive test who have the disease. This information is most useful because we usually order a test to see if a patient has a disease. Using the 2 × 2 contingency table,

$$\text{positive predictive value} = \frac{\text{true positive}}{\text{test positive}}$$

where

$$\text{test positive} = \text{true positive} + \text{false positive}.$$

In the above example the positive predictive value of the test is 9/(27 + 9) or 25 per cent. In other words, the pretest probability that a patient in this group had a herniated lumbar disk was 10 per cent without any test information. The post-test probability that a patient in this group has a herniated lumbar disk has increased to only 25 per cent with a positive MRI. While the numbers in this example have been chosen to allow an easy calculation, they are reasonable estimates for an MRI of the spine in cases of herniated lumbar disk. Therefore, why is the MRI of the spine so ineffective in this example? The answer lies in the prevalence. This 10 per cent prevalence may be accurate for a patient in an orthopedic office who presents with

Table 3 Recalculated 2×2 contingency table

	Herniated lumbar disk present (70)	Herniated lumbar disk absent (30)
Positive MRI results	True-positive MRI (63)	False-positive MRI (9)
Negative MRI results	False-negative MRI (7)	True-negative MRI (21)

back pain without any other information. If the positive predictive value of an MRI is only 25 per cent, would you recommend an MRI as a routine examination for this group? Would a positive MRI result in any way alter your treatment of this patient? The answer to both is no. However, this would result in an enormous waste of valuable MRI time and money.

Using the same example of an MRI of the spine, now assume that a proper history and physical were done first to select the patients who are more likely to have a herniated lumbar disk. Let us further assume that the prevalence of a herniated lumbar disk in this pre-screened group is 70 per cent. The sensitivity (90 per cent) and specificity (70 per cent) of MRI are unchanged. Table 3 shows a recalculation of the 2×2 contingency table.

In this second example the positive predictive value of the test is $63/(63 + 9)$ or 88 per cent. In other words the probability that a patient has a herniated lumbar disk, which was 70 per cent without any test information, has increased to 88 per cent with a positive MRI of the spine. There are three important points about this example. First, the value of a good history and physical is again illustrated. Second, the positive predictive value is a function of the prevalence of the disease. The higher the prevalence the better the test is at detecting disease. Lastly, as the positive predictive value of this test is now 88 per cent, would you now recommend an MRI for this prescreened group? Would this positive result in any way alter your treatment of this patient? The answer to both questions is now yes. The answer to these questions has changed because the prevalence changed. The test, with its sensitivity and specificity, has not changed; only the prevalence of the disease has changed.

In addition to probability, the chance of an event occurring can also be expressed as an odds ratio or 'odds'. The odds of an event happening are the probability an event will happen divided by the probability it will not. Thus

$$\text{odds} = \frac{\text{probability}}{1 - \text{probability}}.$$

For example, if the prevalence is 0.50 (50 per cent), the prevalence odds are 0.50/0.50 or 1:1. As in the last example, the post-test probability of 25 per cent converted to odds becomes 0.25/0.75 or 1:3.

We can define a test's true-positive ratio, or likelihood ratio, as true-positive rate divided by false-positive rate. From the example above, the MRI has a sensitivity (true positive) of 90 per cent, a specificity (true negative) of 70 per cent, and a false-positive rate of 30 per cent. Therefore the likelihood ratio (ratio of true-positive rate to false-positive rate) is 0.90/0.30 or 3:1. The likelihood ratio, like sensitivity and specificity, is specific to the test and does not change. This intrinsic characteristic is useful, as described by Bayes' theorem.

Bayes' theorem uses the likelihood ratio to link the prevalence to the positive predictive value. In other words, the odds of the disease being present following a positive test (positive predictive value) are equal to the likelihood ratio multiplied by the odds of the disease

before the test was done (prevalence). Mathematically, Bayes' theorem can be expressed as

$$\text{positive predictive value} = \text{likelihood ratio} \times \text{prevalence}.$$

Therefore the likelihood ratio measures the discriminating power of the test. The higher the ratio, the more discriminating is the test. For example, as shown in the MRI example, with a sensitivity of 90 per cent and a specificity of 70 per cent, the likelihood ratio is 3:1. In other words, whatever the odds of the diseases was before the test, the odds following a positive test is three times greater. From the first example above, a prevalence of 10 per cent gives odds of 1:9. With a likelihood ratio of 3, the post-test odds are (3×1) to 9, or 1:3. This is the same result as calculated before; a 1:3 odds is 25 per cent (exactly the result achieved above).

Taking a different example, if the sensitivity was 70 per cent and the specificity was 90 per cent, the likelihood ratio would be 0.70/0.10 or seven times more likely to be true with a positive result. Therefore the likelihood of the disease being present increases more with a greater specificity than with a greater sensitivity. (Compare this with the prior example, where with a sensitivity of 90 per cent and a specificity of 70 per cent, the likelihood ratio was 3.)

In discussing sensitivity and specificity, it is important to understand the meaning of normal and abnormal values when the test has continuous variables. The cutoff point for a 'normal' test result is frequently determined at two standard deviations from the mean of a normal population sample. While this includes 95 per cent of the 'normal' population, it automatically results in 2.5 per cent of the normal population having abnormally high values and 2.5 per cent of the normal population having abnormally low values.

Ideally, a result could be distinguished such that no patient with the disease in question had a normal result and, conversely, no patient who was free of the disease had an abnormal result. This would represent a sensitivity of 100 per cent and a specificity of 100 per cent. Unfortunately, this does not occur, as there is always some degree of overlap between the normal and the abnormal populations. Therefore the optimal cutoff between an abnormal and a normal test result is not a fixed characteristic of the test but a value chosen by the interaction of several factors, such as the consequences of having the disease, the prevalence of the disease, and issues relating to factors such as treatment effect, risks, costs, etc.

The overlap between normal and abnormal implies a trade-off between the true-positive rate (sensitivity) and the false-positive rate $(1 - \text{specificity})$. If you change the cutoff of the normal to improve one, the other becomes worse. This trade-off is always true for continuous test results when there is a distribution overlap. In short, the sensitivity and specificity are inversely related by this cutoff value. Therefore without changing the test, as the sensitivity is increased, the specificity is decreased and the converse is also true. Therefore the likelihood ratio (sensitivity/$(1 - \text{specificity})$) is also affected by the selection of cutoff value. The best cutoff also depends on the required outcome—whether a high true-positive rate or a low false-positive rate is wanted. This involves trade-offs.

In order to resolve the trade-off, a decision must be made. This intrinsically implies a preference of one action or one outcome over another. Usually this decision process involves weighing the advantages and disadvantages of the different outcomes. The decision may be difficult and involve weighing multiple advantages and disadvantages, with clear outcomes. This is called decision under certainty. The choice then indicates a preference for one outcome over another. For example, you are going out to dinner and you must choose between your favorite Italian restaurant and your favorite French restaurant. The decision is dependent on your preference between two actions where the outcome of either choice is known.

Unfortunately, most medical decisions are more complex. The outcomes of the choice are not known with certainty at the time the decision must be made. Whether the outcome is cure, complication, or death, it is unknown at the time of the decision. When at least one of the possible outcomes is unknown, the process is called decision under uncertainty. Decision under uncertainty not only involves trade-offs between advantages and disadvantages, but must also include the probability that they will or will not occur. Therefore the preference is not the advantage of one choice over another, but for the expectation that a net advantage will occur.

To aid in the more complex process of decision under uncertainty, a model of representative decisions, a decision tree, is commonly used. This model has four parts: an option, an outcome, a probability of the outcome, and a worth or utility of the outcome (Fig. 2).

A decision tree starts at a decision point which is represented by a decision node (square box in Fig. 2). At the decision node there are several paths which represent the different options, the minimum is two. A decision tree should include any reasonable option. In most medical decisions (decision under uncertainty), one or more of the options lead to an uncertain outcome. Therefore, each option branches at a chance node (circle) to the possible or likely outcomes. The outcomes should be mutually exclusive. The outcome set generally includes continued disease, cure, complications with temporary or permanent disability, and death. Furthermore, each option has a set of outcomes (Fig. 2).

For example, in evaluating a patient with avascular necrosis of the right hip who presents with left hip pain with normal radiographs. You now must decide whether to get an MRI of the left hip. Let us only consider whether the patient has avascular necrosis of the left hip as the outcome. A simplified decision tree is shown (Fig. 3).

Once again, this is decision under uncertainty, and therefore which

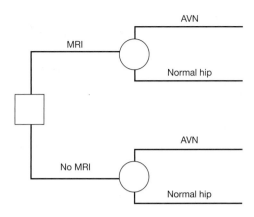

Fig. 3. Example of a simple decision tree in evaluating a patient with avascular necrosis (AVN) of the right hip who presents with left hip pain with normal radiographs. The decision as to whether to obtain an MRI of the left hip is the square node. For simplicity we only consider whether the patient has avascular necrosis of the left hip as the outcome.

actual outcome will occur is not known. Because of this uncertainty, we must estimate the probability that the outcome will occur. This may be done objectively or subjectively. It is import to remember that the probability of an outcome is based on the assumption that the option is taken.

While estimating probabilities is difficult in medicine, it is not impossible. The best estimates are objective estimates based on similar experiences, either in large published trials or in a clinician's own experience. The medical literature is full of such reports on many subjects. Clinical judgment is necessary to choose which report is most appropriate to base the probabilities of an individual outcome. Without objective data, subjective estimates must be made. Even when making subjective estimates, it is important to be objective.

The combined probabilities of all the outcome for an option should sum to 1.0. This is true since the point in the tree should include all possible outcomes that may result from that option. As shown in Fig. 4,

$$\text{probability 1} + \text{probability 2} = 1.0.$$

The final step to a simple decision tree is to assign a worth to an outcome. The worth or usefulness of an outcome to a particular person is described as a utility. The utility of an outcome is not a set value for every patient but must be modified for each patient based on their biases and preferences. In the decision tree, each outcome has a utility assigned as if the option and the outcome had resulted. The utility is assigned a value from zero to 100 per cent. The completed decision tree is shown in Fig. 5.

The decision trees drawn thus far have been examples of simple trade-offs. In this form, two or more therapies are compared (e.g. medical versus surgical treatments). Another common decision tree type is called the prophylactic trade-off, where simple observation is compared with therapy. If the patient is simply observed, either no complication will occur (the status quo) or the case will develop a complication. For example when treating a patient with a nonunion of a scaphoid fracture, you can elect to treat the nonunion or only observe it. If you observe it, it may never become a clinical problem or it may cause disabling pain and lead to a wrist fusion. The prophy-

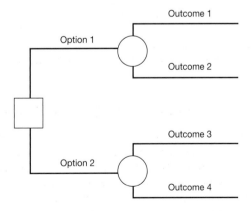

Fig. 2. A simple decision tree. A decision tree starts at a decision point which is represented by a decision node (square). At the decision node there are several paths which represent the different options; the minimum is two. In decision under uncertainty, one or more of the options lead to an uncertain outcome. Therefore, each option branches at a chance node (circle) to the possible or likely outcomes. The outcomes should be mutually exclusive.

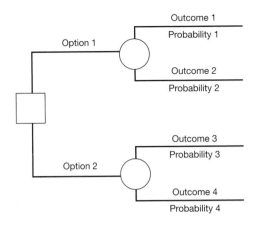

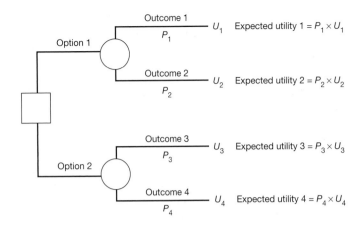

Fig. 4. A simple decision tree including the probability of an outcome occurring. It is important to remember that the probability of an outcome is based on the assumption that the option is taken. The combined probabilities of all the outcomes for an option should sum to 1.0. This is true since the point in the tree should include all possible outcomes that may result from that option. As shown, probability 1 + probability 2 = 1.0.

Fig. 6. Analyzing a decision tree using expected utility. Each outcome has an expected utility. The expected utility of an outcome is expressed as the probability of the outcome multiplied by the utility of the outcome. Thus the expected utility of an option is the sum of all the expected utilities of the outcomes for that option. For example, the expected utility of option 1 is the expected utility of outcome 1 plus outcome 2. This then can be compared with the expected utility of option 2. Whichever option has the better expected utility is considered the better option.

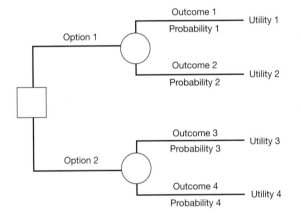

Fig. 5. A completed simple decision tree. The final step to a simple decision tree is to assign a worth or utility to an outcome. In the decision tree, each outcome has a probability and utility assigned as if the option and the outcome had resulted. The utility is assigned a value from zero to 100 per cent.

To analyze a decision tree, a method called expected utility is used, where the expected utility of a given option is represented by its utility as well as by a probability. The expected utility of an outcome is expressed as the probability of the outcome multiplied by the utility of the outcome. Therefore each outcome has an expected utility, and the expected utility of an option is the sum of all of the expected utilities which are expected of the outcome for that decision. This is shown on our decision tree (Fig. 6). In this example, the expected utility of option 1 is the expected utility of outcome 1 + outcome 2. This then can be compared with the expected utility of option 2. Whichever option had the better expected utility is considered the better option.

The decision tree is a good tool for evaluating possible outcomes, but it is very sensitive to the user's input as to utilities and probabilities. Which options and outcomes to include is based on clinical knowledge and is the crucial difference between an excellent decision-making aid and a useless waste of time. This is discussed in more detail below with regard to a specific orthopedic problem.

lactic trade-off decision tree involves time. As in the scaphoid fracture, if treatment is chosen the outcome is known now; however, if observation is chosen the outcome will be known in the future. Therefore, in time-dependent trade-offs, the trade-off is complicated by features of an immediate versus a delayed outcome. Furthermore, the best outcome may be dependent on the time frame evaluated in the decision. For example, an analysis of the results of cemented femoral stems in total hip arthroplasty at 2-year follow-up may demonstrate that prosthesis type and technique are unimportant. Therefore cost may dominate the clinical issue of prosthesis selection with no emphasis on surgical technique. Conversely, at 10- to 20-year follow-up, prosthesis type and technique may strongly influence the end result. This concept of time and cost is becoming increasingly important as insurance companies are using such data to constrain costs.

Maximum expected utility analysis

Regardless of the specific methodology used in making a therapeutic choice, the decision to proceed with a specific therapeutic intervention involves weighing or comparing the probable benefits to be achieved from the intervention against the possible risks involved. Furthermore, the risks and benefits of alternative therapies must be considered. All this is done against the backdrop of an understanding of the natural history of the disease process one is considering treating.

There is little difficulty in making treatment decisions where the natural history is well known, the consequences of treatment well described, and the likelihood of successful intervention are high compared with the risks of intervention and/or the risks of allowing the natural history of the disease process to go unchecked. In many of the conditions that are encountered in orthopedic practice these factors are well described, and it is relatively easy for the surgeon and patient to weigh out the various risks and benefits of a particular intervention in the specific clinical setting in which the patient presents. Typical examples would be the elderly patient with degenerative arthritis of the hip unresponsive to conservative measures with increasing pain and decreasing function. Total hip replacement is in most cases a rather easily made choice for this type of patient (see below on algorithms). Other typical such 'easy' examples in the appropriate patient might include carpal tunnel release, internal fixation of an intertrochanteric fracture, and arthroscopic debridement for persistent meniscal symptoms.

However, many surgical decisions are not so straightforward. In many cases multiple factors must be considered in the surgical decision; the underlying health and potential longevity of the patient, willingness to undergo surgical procedures, expected outcome, and risks of a particular intervention based on the specific anatomic and pathologic setting encountered in the individual patient. As an example, consider the issue of total knee arthroplasty reimplantation following removal of a previously placed knee which had become infected. Factors that must be considered in such a setting would include the conditions of the soft tissues (including the periarticular skin and capsular tissues), viability and integrity of the extensor mechanism, the underlying bone stock, and the neurovascular integrity of the limb. In addition, variables related to the patient's general health and functional requirements must be considered.

Decision-making in these cases can be far from straightforward. In some cases, reimplantation may be a technically easier surgical operation than arthrodesis, and in certain cases heroic attempts at infection eradication combined with bone stock and extensor mechanism reconstruction may be warranted. However, in some settings the best alternative may be to leave a chronically infected pseudarthrosis without further surgical intervention. While many of these types of complex decisions are made by the experienced surgeon on the basis of intuition, alternative, more formal methods of decision analysis may be helpful.

A basic technique for decision-making in this complex setting is a modified form of what is known as maximized expected utility analysis. Maximizing the utility of a decision simply means making a decision in such a way as to reap the maximal benefit. This technique requires the decision-maker to list the potential benefits of any intervention and assign to each benefit both a probability for its occurrence and a specific assignment of numerical ranking to the expected utility or benefit. A similar process is carried out for all of the potential risks involved with that particular decision.

In business decision-making, such utilities are mainly economic factors and can be measured in dollars, but in medical decision-making, where factors such as pain and quality of life must be taken into account, the assignment of 'utilities' is more complex. An important assumption in this method are that utilities (or outcomes) can be expressed using a common scale. This has not been realistically accomplished for many medical (or orthopedic) utilities. For example, there is no formal way to assign comparable utility weight to knee range of motion, pain-free weight-bearing, or joint stability. Similarly, it is hard to quantify on a similar scale the absence of pain, or the inability to sleep because of persistent pain. Nonetheless, an approximation of this technique (termed subjective analysis because

of the lack of specificity or objectivity to either the probability assigned or to the specific utility value itself) may be quite useful.

For any given procedure each potential benefit of the procedure can be assigned a utility factor. These can then be listed, with each utility assigned a probability. One can then sum the product of each utility factor by its probability, yielding a number representing the expected benefit of a particular intervention. The number derived from a similar sum of risk rankings multiplied by their individual probabilities can then be subtracted from the number calculated for the potential benefits of the procedure. Thus, for a given procedure with potential benefits listed as 1, 2, 3, ..., x, and risks 1, 2, 3, ..., y

$$
\begin{aligned}
\text{expected utility} = & [(\text{benefit of utility } 1 \times \text{probability of utility } 1) + \\
& (\text{benefit of utility } 2 \times \text{probability of utility } 2) \ldots \\
& + (\text{benefit of utility } x \times \text{probability of utility } x)] - \\
& [(\text{risk of utility } 1 \times \text{probability of risk } 1) + (\text{risk of} \\
& \text{utility } 2 \times \text{probability of risk } 2) \ldots + (\text{risk of utility} \\
& y \times \text{probability of risk } y)].
\end{aligned}
$$

The resulting sum can then be compared with comparable figures generated from a similar consideration of alternative procedures. In order to make complex decisions using this technique the surgeon must accurately asses multiple patient-related factors as noted above, but must also adequately judge his or her own skills, experiences, and resources as regards any particular procedure. As a minimal requirement for treating or counseling patients in these complex settings, a thorough understanding of the literature on indications, contraindications, and the expected results of various interventions is mandatory.

Thus, again as an example, the starting point for the surgeon who treats the failed total knee arthroplasty should be familiarity with the indications, contraindications, and techniques of reimplantation as well as the alternatives to reimplantation including resection arthroplasty, arthrodesis, and amputation. As mentioned previously, the risk and benefit 'utilities' are subjective at this point in time, and there is little or no specific data on the probabilities of these occurrences in specific unusual or complex settings. Nonetheless, such an analysis, even on an informal basis, can assist the surgeon in both the complex decision-making process and may also aid in communicating with the patient all of the potential risks and benefits involved in complex clinical settings as regards specific interventions.

Just as the surgeon must decide which outcomes and options to include in a decision tree based on clinical judgment, published data on similar cases, and the likelihood of occurrence, a patient should be informed of not only your recommendations, but how the decision was reached. The options and outcomes in the decision tree can and should be discussed with a patient. In this manner, the decision tree is a good tool to discuss the advantages and disadvantages of various options with the patient. This is commonly known as a discussion of risks and benefits. It is important to note that the risks of treatment is a sum of all the risks. This can be thought of in terms of medical and surgical risks. The medical risks relate to the patient's underlying general health status and specific comorbid factors which pose a risk to the patients health from pursuing the therapeutic regimen under consideration. Specific surgical risks include the specific factors that render a particular case more likely to suffer a specific complication or decrease the likelihood of an expected outcome. These risks are frequently due to specific anatomic or disease-specific variations such as proximal femoral deformity in the patient requiring a total hip arthroplasty or diabetes in a patient with as displaced ankle fracture. These factors are usually synonymous with 'comorbid' factors which are known to affect outcome. This sum of risks must be contrasted with the benefit side of the risk–benefit ratio. The benefit of a treatment can be seen as the difference between the likely outcome compared with the patient's current status. Thus, if we compare two patients: one, a patient seeking treatment for complaints of hip pain, which is present only with strenuous and prolonged physical activity, but is otherwise asymptomatic, and another, who has lost the ability to ambulate at all or to sleep without painful interruptions, both with a diagnosis of hip osteoarthritis, the benefit from the intervention will be smaller or less in the first individual than it will be in the second, more handicapped individual, who may be returned to almost normal musculoskeletal health status by performance of a total hip replacement. Of course formal comparisons of current status and expected future status should be assessed in a rigorous fashion, with the use of appropriate outcomes instruments and tools.

When a rational patient does not agree with the surgeon's recommendations, either the perceived probabilities or the utility of the outcomes that the surgeon has assigned differ from the patients. Probabilities usually differ because the surgeon's probabilities are, or should be, more soundly based on experience and science, whereas the patient's may be solely based on emotion. When this occurs, reviewing the facts and pertinent data may be useful in helping the patient make the best choice. Conversely, when utilities differ, it is because the surgeon's assumptions differ from the patient's preferences. In this situation the orthopedist must listen more closely to the patient in order to understand the patient's perceptions and wishes so as to incorporate these in the decision analysis.

The measurement of utilities is far from straightforward. Utility may be measured by reflecting on what an individual will give up and not give up to obtain an outcome. This method of measuring a person's preference incorporates all aspects of this preference in a global fashion. It is expressed as an arbitrary unit, ranging from zero to 100 per cent. Positive units are expressed as gains and negative units as losses. The expected utility is then what is projected from the decision. This analysis must include tangible and intangible considerations.

To illustrate this example, consider the opportunity to buy a lottery ticket. There are 1000 tickets being sold. Only one ticket will be chosen for a million dollar grand prize. Would you buy such a ticket, a 1 in 1000 chance to win a million dollars, for $1000.00? What is the most you would pay?

The discrepancy between the mathematical value of the ticket, $1000, and what you would sell it for, illustrates the need to include the psychological perceptions of worth into the decision analysis. A person who is a gambler would likely pay much more for this chance than a person who dislikes risks. Furthermore, a millionaire may be more willing to assume the financial risks than a person whose entire savings are $1000. Thus, preferences may be biased by many factors. Some of the most common surgical decision biases should be understood by the surgeon so that in practice they may be avoided or at least accounted for.

Aversion to risk is an important bias. As illustrated above, under most circumstances most people choose the known entity over a mathematical equivalent of gambling. Although some people are risk takers, more people are apprehensive about uncertainty and will avoid risk even if there is a cost associated with this aversion.

Anchoring or mental inertia is perhaps the strongest factor in decision bias. People tend to work from an established position. The fact that a surgeon will be most influenced by the outcome of the last similar case treated is an example of this. For example, a surgeon be more likely to treat a pilon fracture conservatively if the last pilon fracture he or she treated became infected and resulted in a below-knee amputation.

Regret is a strong psychological factor in avoiding a particular outcome of decision. In this bias, the decision-maker tends to avoid decisions that can cause harm, even if low probability. For example, a surgeon may be more likely to treat a pilon fracture conservatively, even though the surgeon may believe that operative treatment would result in a better outcome because operative treatment has a low but finite risk of a below-knee amputation.

Framing is another process that can skew a decision. Would you rather undergo a resection for osteosarcoma that has an 85 per cent survival rate or a resection that has a 15 per cent mortality rate. While these are obviously statistically identical, yet most would prefer the positive outlook rather than the negative one.

Inconsistency, over time or by example, can influence decisions. A suboptimal reduction obtained as an emergency procedure at 2 a.m. may be termed acceptable, when the same result at 10 a.m. may have been revised. In another example, a surgeon decides to operate on an elderly patient with a tibia fracture to allow early mobilization but places the patient in a long leg cast to protect the fixation thereby immobilizing the patient and achieving little or no benefit from the procedure.

Intrinsic in the utility analysis is the point of indifference. For example, would you take a medication that immediately cured you of a cold in 1 day if there were no side-effects? Would you take the same medication if 50 per cent of patients who took it developed anaphylactic shock? Most likely you would answer yes to the first question but no to the second. At what point would the risk be equal to the benefit? In other words at which point does one encounter indifference between accepting the risk of treatment versus enduring the symptoms. That would be the point of indifference. This measure can then be used as the utility.

Utility can be calculated and employed for individual patients, in which individual preference should be considered. When used to develop protocols, it is often inappropriate to consider individual preferences. Instead, approximation should be used. Unfortunately, approximations are too often used for decisions about individual preferences and the preferences of the individual patient are ignored. Furthermore, the utility is intended to be that of the patient and not the surgeon, hospital, or society. However, there may be trade-offs when the surgeons life is at risk, such as may occur in operating on patients with AIDS or active hepatitis.

As discussed above, people tend to be averse to risk and uncertainty, and will perceive a known outcome to be very different from a theoretically equal outcome that is uncertain. Furthermore, people will accept a lesser known result if it involves less uncertainty. In cases with uncertainty, risk aversion usually dominates the decision process. Although most decisions in medicine involve uncertainty, it is often useful to eliminate this uncertainty in the initial analysis.

A useful first step is to create a rank order of all outcomes. This will allow identification of which outcomes are better and which are worse. It also identifies which can be balanced by trade-offs. A simple way to assess ranking is to create a scale of zero to 100, with the worst outcome as zero, the best as 100, and the others graded relative to these. Alternatively, a visual analogy scale can be useful with the best and worst outcomes on the two ends of the scale and the other outcomes on this scale noted in between. While there is a tendency to anchor about the midpoint for middle outcomes, the relative ranking can still aid in trade-offs.

Other outcomes lend themselves to time trade-offs. This is common with an ongoing or chronic state when compared with a healthy state. For example, assume that your average life expectancy was 50 years and the utility of being healthy with both legs was 100. How would you rate the utility of your life with a below-knee amputation? One way to asses this utility would be to compare your full life expectancy with a below-knee amputation to a shorter life expectancy with both legs. For example, would you rather live for 50 years with a below-knee amputation or live for 49 years with both legs? If you choose 49 years with both legs, then would you rather live 50 years with a below-knee amputation or live 48 years with both legs? This questioning continues to 47 years, 46 years, etc. until the option of the amputation is chosen. At that point the utility for a below-knee amputation (for you) would be the years in good health that would be equal to 50 years of an amputation divided by 50 years.

One of the simplest way of assessing uncertainty is to use the standard gamble. In this method the patient chooses between two alternatives. For example, consider a patient with cancer who believes his remaining 5 years of life *without intervention* to be equal to that of undergoing a surgical procedure that, if successful, would allow him to live 20 years but also has a 50 per cent mortality rate. Then the next 5 years has 50 per cent of the utility (not 25 per cent) of the next 20 years for that patient. The patent is presumable giving up 5 years of potential life to avoid surgery and the risk of immediate death. Conversely, the patient may be placing a higher value on the next 5 years of his life than on the later 15 years.

In general there are no right or wrong answers to utility assessments, only preferences. While formal utility analysis is time consuming and not routinely practical, it can be useful in difficult cases and clearly forces the surgeon to think about potential treatment options and outcomes in a more rigorous manner. This process also helps model rational decision-making.

Without doing a formal utility assessment, we can use these principles clinically to understand our patients' attitudes about an outcome. We can deduce the relative ranks of these outcomes and propose trade-offs of known best and worst outcomes.

Clinical intuition

Experienced clinicians make most medical decisions rapidly, confident that the correct diagnosis or procedure was selected. These decisions, whether diagnostic or therapeutic, are made by relying on knowledge, experience, and judgment. They rarely consider Bayes' theorem, decision analysis, prediction rules, or algorithms. Therefore the argument that most medical thinking is intuitive may be expressed. Indeed, speedy thinking, confidence, and not relying on formal rules are characteristics of intuition.

It may be argued that making everyday clinical decisions is intuitive and that the size of this component is related to experience. Fur-

ther, although clinicians are capable of formally analyzing a clinical situation, they usually do not, unless it is required. Finally, the steps taken in rapid and intuitive decision-making may be an unconscious act. This fact sets limits on what can be learned about the process of analysis.

Darwin, in *The Origin of Species*, pointed out that habits or dispositions acquired early in life may become so entrenched that we forget that they are learned and erroneously regard them as instinctive. Therefore, intuition may be little more than rapid and automatic learned behavior. If this is true, clinical intuition may be little more than clinical habits that are gradually incorporated by the lengthy training process of medicine. Through repetition, feedback, and integration, this process is learned. Clinical intuition is highly prized by physicians and especially surgeons who have to make rapid decisions intraoperatively that cannot be encumbered by doubt. Nevertheless, a fairly substantial body of literature on judgment and decision-making has raised questions about the limitations and ultimate usefulness of intuition.

Some doubt on the usefulness of intuition has centered about conflicts or discrepancies between results arrived at by intuition and those reached by a more formal thought process. Intuition rarely considers uncertainty of outcomes, issues of risk, trade-offs, and imperfect evidence. Intuition departs from principles of decision-making at each point in the process: problem structuring, probability estimation, reaching a diagnosis, utility assessment, and final decision selection. These departures from the mathematical principles of decision-making are called heuristics and biases. Some of the biases such as aversion, regret, anchoring, and inconsistency have been discussed.

We are even biased to considering individuals versus groups. A recent study found that both lay people and physicians make different decisions when considering the patient as an individual rather than considering a patient as part of a group of identical patients. Although it seems reasonable that clinicians might employ a different approach to the two schemes, this is inconsistent with expected utility analysis. This willingness to save an individual life versus statistical lives is repeated in health-care debts and in clinical practice. This may be why individuals in society may be unwilling to pay for alcohol withdrawal programs but are willing to pay for liver transplants when the liver disease is secondary to alcoholic cirrhosis. This intrinsic tension between the individual approach and the group approach has now been magnified by cost concerns in health care. Hospital administrators and managed care officers may come to different conclusions about health-care choices because they are looking at statistical rather than individual lives. Conversely, given the same information, clinicians may come to different decisions based on their focus on individual cases. This may cause the clinicians to view these administrators as heartless and the administrators to view the clinicians as wasteful. Resolution of this conflict is, of course, beyond the scope of this chapter.

Developing treatment plans

The development of a treatment plan is dependent on many factors. These factors interact in either a simple straightforward way, or alternatively, in a complex fashion, depending on the parameters of disease encountered and the specific parameters of the patient's medical, psychologic, and social milieu. Perhaps most important in the process of developing a treatment plan is the confidence which the physician has in the diagnosis. With a firm diagnostic impression in hand, it is easier to contemplate the natural history of the disease process encountered. This information can then be compared with the clinician's understanding of the interventional consequences of various treatment modalities. On the other hand, diagnostic uncertainty can make such reasoning much more complex. While many diagnoses can be made by the history and physical examination of the patient, the use of ancillary diagnostic studies as discussed above are usually performed to either define or confirm the diagnosis.

Even in the case when a diagnosis is readily available, the decision-making process to employ surgical intervention may be difficult. An interesting method of exploring those issues, specifically related to the decision-making process regarding therapeutic intervention, is to look specifically at those thought processes involved in a specific, common therapeutic intervention. In this manner, the diagnostic intervention of total hip arthroplasty will be used to explore the type of thinking and decision processes that may be required in order to reach a decision regarding surgical intervention.

The terms 'indications' and 'contraindications', while carrying the ring of specificity, actually represent the end points of a complex decision-making process which must be carried out by the medical practitioner in conjunction with the patient. Any medical decision-making requires consideration of the potential risks and benefits of a particular intervention. This type of risk–benefit calculation is relatively uncomplicated for many diagnostic interventions, but there is clearly more at stake in most therapeutic interventions, particularly surgical ones.

The concept of indications can be defined as those situations where an individual patient will benefit from the intervention in such a way, and with sufficient likelihood, to warrant the specific risks involved in the intervention. Contraindications would connote the opposite: the risks involved, and/or the likelihood of the interventions failure to achieve the desired results, outweigh the expected benefit of the intervention. Determining whether or not a given procedure is indicated or contraindicated involves the careful evaluation of the patients complaints, pathology, and overall health status; the weighing of multiple probabilities for various positive and adverse outcomes (many of which are at best based on less than adequate data); and finally some type of judgment as to whether the final balance of risks and benefits is appropriate for the individual patient under consideration. An important consideration in the performance of any elective surgical procedure is the relative risk of perioperative events which carry with it significant morbidity or mortality. Total hip arthroplasty as initially practiced, and before the risk of thromboembolic disease was well understood, carried with it a reported mortality risk from pulmonary embolism alone, of up to 3 per cent. While this incidence has been substantially reduced, as have the initial rates of infection and other serious postsurgical morbidities, the surgeon contemplating elective surgical intervention must essentially compare the potential long-term benefits of pain reduction and improved function versus the short-term risks of death and other complications which may potentially occur following this elective surgery.

A simple example of one of the trade-offs which must be evaluated is in the setting of pharmacologic intervention for deep vein thrombosis prophylaxis, where the benefits of thrombosis and embolism reduction may be accompanied by an increased risk of serious bleeding complications. This type of 'apples and oranges' comparison of both short- and long-term risks and potential complications with the expected short- and long-term benefits of a specific intervention is common in reconstructive surgical practice, and keeps much of surgical decision-making in the realm of heuristic rather than algorithmic problem solving.

While total hip arthroplasty is the operation of choice for severe arthritic hip disease in the vast majority of patients, it is clear that in several settings other options may be more appropriate. Decision-making in this setting is dependent on many factors in addition to the underlying pathology, including the patient's age and activity demands. There are several factors (or assumptions) regarding hip arthroplasty as an interventional choice which must be kept in mind when evaluating an individual for this type of surgery.

The first assumption is that the arthroplasty is a time-limited operation. In general, arthroplasty service life can be tied to issues related to fixation longevity, component wear and the biologic effects thereof, or material failure. While multiple clinical series demonstrate relatively high component survival with a variety of fixation methods and component designs, even in relatively young and presumably active patients, it is difficult to imagine a total hip implant outliving a young adult with a normal lifespan. Thus, age becomes an important factor in the decision to proceed with total hip arthroplasty. Assuming no excessive comorbidities, and the presence of symptoms due to hip-joint pathology amenable to arthroplasty, the older patient is actually a better candidate for arthroplasty, in that the operation and implant will most likely outlive the patient. The younger individual may well require multiple surgeries over their lifetime, with increased risk and deteriorating function a potential concomitant of multiple surgeries. While it is difficult to say at what age a surgeon should strive to find reasonable alternatives to total hip arthroplasty, the pediatric and young adult patient clearly deserves an attempt at alternative treatment, such as arthrodesis or osteotomy, if such treatment will relieve symptoms sufficiently to postpone arthroplasty and not make subsequent treatment exceedingly complex.

Another assumption is that conservative treatment should be attempted prior to proceeding with arthroplasty. This may include the use of assistive devices for ambulation, weight loss, systemic or local medications, physiotherapy, and activity modification. A concerted effort at nonsurgical therapy may be more reasonable in the younger patient than in the elderly where prolonged attempts at conservative therapies can be both time consuming, and are rarely as effective in relieving symptoms and improving function as total hip arthroplasty.

In some settings, the symptoms, physical findings, and radiographic changes are severe enough to warrant consideration of total hip arthroplasty even if the patient has had no prior conservative treatment. However, in most cases, particularly in the younger patient, it may be wiser to demonstrate to the patient that conservative or nonsurgical treatment will not relieve symptoms or improve function prior to recommending more aggressive treatment with more substantial potential risks and complications. This may also depend on the patient's attitude toward surgical intervention.

The level of patient activity and symptom severity are other important factors to consider in determining whether arthroplasty is indicated. While pain is the most common complaint prior to surgical intervention, in many cases symptoms are activity related. In the patient whose symptoms are clearly amenable to activity modification, and in whom total hip arthroplasty is not an ideal operation due to age, comorbidities, or other factors, the surgeon should opt for conservative treatment. An obvious and clear-cut example would be a young athlete whose hip pain only limits his or her athletic activity. Total hip arthroplasty would not be expected to hold up to the rigors of athletic competition, so that such activity would be contraindicated following such surgery. If the individual has little or no symptoms with activity modification, then activity limitation would be a more reasonable course than proceeding with total hip arthroplasty, due to the potential serious long-term consequences of arthroplasty and the relatively small benefit obtained, as the patient must abandon competitive athletic competition in either case.

Thus, behavior modification may play a significant role in the treatment of hip disease. In attempting to understand a patient's pain pattern, the clinician must decide whether a patient has realistically modified their activity to accommodate their damaged joint. If the patient is unwilling to alter his or her lifestyle to accommodate their degenerative joint, then the likelihood is that this patient will not alter his or her lifestyle to extend the life of a prosthetic joint. For example, as noted above, a patient unwilling to give up sports or other activities which contact stress joints and which cause substantial discomfort, is probably not having enough pain to warrant intervention. On the other hand, it seems unreasonable to ask a patient to modify their lifestyle to the point of complete inactivity. Thus, limitation in functional capacity is another important factor in determining the appropriateness of total hip arthroplasty, and understanding the patient's requirements for activity of daily living is essential in this determination. A patient's ability to perform his or her job, do household tasks, and maintain personal hygiene can be used as measures of the effect of hip function on the patient's lifestyle. Walking tolerance, defined as the length of time or distance one can walk without rest, can be an important benchmark in assessing the severity of disease and limitation of function. In general, if a patient cannot perform activities of daily living despite conservative treatment, his or her hip function has decreased to the point where intervention may be indicated.

Decision-making in the clinical setting of the young patient is usually far from straightforward, but often requires consideration of multiple factors prior to recommending total hip arthroplasty. Other factors that influence the results of, and longevity of, the total hip arthroplasty would include weight and expected activity levels. Clearly the 18-year-old patient with severe multiarticular systemic inflammatory arthritis and persistent adduction contracture interfering with hygiene and impeding any attempts at ambulation would be expected to stress a total hip arthroplasty significantly less than a 30-year-old former professional football player who is 6 feet 6 inches tall, weighs 270 pounds, and suffers from isolated post-traumatic arthritis of the hip.

While radiographs are extremely helpful in deciding for whom total hip arthroplasty is appropriate, the mere existence of moderate to severe degenerative changes radiographically is not an indication for surgery.

Radiographs are but one small piece of the equation. Many patients function very well with severe radiographic changes. Likewise patients with only moderate changes can be significantly disabled. Therefore the decision to operate must be a clinical and not a radiographic one. The decision to perform surgery imminently

because a radiographic picture is sure to deteriorate is also not an appropriate stance. One must be wary of the patient with only mild radiographic changes, reasonable range of motion, and noncharacteristic hip pain. Chances of relieving this type of pain with total hip arthroplasty are remote.

In those patients with severe pain and severe radiographic changes, this conflict does not exist. Nor does it exist in the opposite situation, in those patients with severe pain and normal radiographs. In such a setting further evaluative studies of the hip may be indicated, and a search for reasons for pain in this setting may need to be focused elsewhere.

While there are few absolute contraindications to total hip arthroplasty, active, local, or systemic infection is one contraindication that most clinicians would agree on. Relative contraindications include morbid obesity, neurologic dysfunction, and remote local infection. While in each of these conditions there may be a higher failure rate, substantial reduction in pain and improvement in function may overshadow the potential risks in these populations.

The presence of substantial comorbidities may preclude the use of surgical intervention in all but the most incapacitated of patients. Certainly the risks of perioperative mortality following surgical intervention must be carefully weighed against the expected functional improvement and pain relief that can be expected to be obtained with any type of surgical intervention

Another confounding factor may center on specific anatomic abnormalities of soft tissue or bone which would place the patient at substantial increased risk from the surgical procedure itself. For example, an elderly patient with an ancient femoral neck fracture malunion, with substantial shortening and rotational deformity, with concomitant severe atherosclerotic femoral vessels may be at substantially increased risk, with the lengthening and rotational release needed for hip arthroplasty, of femoral artery thrombosis. Again, the risks of surgery must be balanced with the patients symptoms.

In those patients less than 40 years old the stakes regarding surgical intervention go up dramatically. With life expectancy stretching into the seventh and eighth decades in modern society, a prosthetic hip placed in one of these patients cannot, in most cases, be expected to last 40 years. Even in the best circumstances, these patients can count on at least one revision during their lifetime. Unfortunately, the well-publicized success of total hip arthroplasty has colored the patient's perception of nonprosthetic options in treating hip disease. Where hip fusion may be the most appropriate treatment for a manual laborer with a limited education, this option is frequently not accepted by the patient. If an appropriate osteotomy can extend the life of the natural hip, it should be given serious consideration. In this setting decision-making may be at its most complex because the expected lifespan of the patient is great. It is always necessary for the surgeon who is contemplating total hip arthroplasty in the younger patient to be familiar with the indications for alternative hip salvage procedures so that total hip arthroplasty is not the only option entertained in this patient population. While familiarity with the specific operative techniques involved in hip salvage is not necessary for all surgeons who treat arthritis of the hip, the surgeon must be able to select out and appropriately refer those younger patients who may benefit substantially from alternative treatments which will reduce pain, improve functional capability, and still allow for total hip arthroplasty at a later date.

A patient occasionally enters into this process with unrealistic expectations. These expectations must be tempered by the surgeon's experience, understanding of the patients psychologic make-up, and the surgeon's communications skills. A patient must understand that hip arthroplasty is not a panacea for multiple physical problems. This procedure affects but one joint. While an improved gait pattern may help an aching back to some degree, it will not have a major impact on other musculoskeletal disorders the patient may have. The patient must also understand the functional limitations that may still exist following hip arthroplasty. Normal range of motion may not be restored after years of contracture. Positions may have to be avoided to prevent instability. These concepts should be discussed preoperatively with the patient.

Finally, it is important to discuss the responsibility the patient must assume for their prosthetic hip. The patient must understand that this implant is a walking device designed to relieve pain. It is not a device for impact-loading sports or heavy manual labor. By assuming responsibility for their actions, the patient must realize that if they abuse their hip in this regard, they may realize the consequences through diminished longevity of the hip and subsequent need for revision surgery.

The above discussion of some of the issues related to decision-making regarding total hip arthroplasty amply indicate that this process can vary from simple to complex. In clinical decision-making it is the job of the surgeon to assess all of the patient-related factors involved in the clinical decision and to communicate this understanding to the patient. Of course such communication must be tempered by an understanding of the patient's psychologic make-up and intellectual capabilities. This informing of the patient may be a time-consuming and difficult undertaking in several settings. In cases where the surgeon does not have good data on outcomes and risks in specific conditions or in specific anatomic variations, it may be difficult to assess the real benefits or risks of surgery. Nonetheless, time spent in this exercise will reward the surgeon with patients who fully understand the goals of surgery and are better able to co-operate with their own recovery and have a greater understanding of the goals of surgery. This tends to make for a happier patient population and a more satisfying surgical practice.

Treatment recommendations—without a diagnosis

A preliminary or tentative diagnosis is usually required before making treatment or further diagnostic recommendations. However, the inability to make a 'definitive diagnosis' does not preclude treatment! Indeed, one can say that in many cases of musculoskeletal complaint, no final 'histopathologic' diagnosis is ever reached, and yet the clinician may be able to make substantial contributions to the patients recovery by appropriate therapeutic recommendations.

In many cases of 'low back pain', no clear anatomic structure is identified as diseased, no specific disease is diagnosed, and yet appropriate medication and supportive therapy can reduce the time to symptom resolution. In many cases of vague periarticular pain complaints, no definitive diagnosis is reached and yet with specific therapeutic recommendations such as physical therapy modalities, rest, exercise, and appropriate anti-inflammatory medication, the patient's symptoms resolve. The decision or need to aggressively pursue a

definitive diagnosis is based on several factors, including the severity of symptoms, the response to initial nonspecific therapies, and the degree of patient satisfaction with their progress despite the lack of a firm diagnosis. Finally, an additional factor of importance is the risk of 'missing' a diagnosis with serious potential long-term implications if appropriate treatment is not initiated.

Formal treatment recommendations

There is abundant evidence that large variations exist in the rate at which many surgical procedures are performed in different geographic locations which have very similar population demographics. Such studies can be traced back to Glover in the United Kingdom, who demonstrated widely varying tonsillectomy rate amongst various counties with similar population demographics. This phenomenon was re-demonstrated by Wennberg and Gittelsohn (1973) in a landmark study of surgery rates in the state of Vermont. Since that time others have shown that marked variation in the rates of common surgical procedures can be demonstrated both within and between different health-care systems and countries (Rutkow 1982; Wennberg and Gittelsohn 1982; Rutkow and Starfield 1984; Wennberg *et al.* 1989). Given that these analyses review populations that are quite similar demographically, there is little room but to conclude that not all of these rates can be correct or appropriate. This evidence strongly implicates the existence of significant under- and/or overutilization of multiple surgical procedures in different geographic areas. These findings, along with significant social and economic pressures on the medical profession, have led to the development of what has been termed the 'Third Revolution' in medicine—the outcomes movement (Relman 1988). This represents an attempt to apply more rigorous scientific methodology to the question of indications and contraindications for specific interventions. In addition, these data are useful in answering the questions of whether or not specific interventions have 'value' equal to their cost on a system-wide basis, and whether or not certain cost-cutting measures have an adverse effect on the population under consideration.

In particular, outcomes methodology has come to be represented by four basic and differing areas of emphasis in health-care research:

(1) the review of large databases such as governmental medical databases and national or local registries;

(2) the systematic scientific appraisal of extant literature including the use of appropriate statistical methods to combine multiple studies—'meta-analysis';

(3) the use of improved study methods to provide data more likely to yield both validity and applicability to specific populations along with better control of potential bias via methods such as randomization and the more rigorous recording of comorbid factors;

(4) the use of expanded end-point parameters of evaluation, including patient-based assessments of outcome as well as the use of rating tools or instruments that have been proven to be sensitive, reliable, and valid.

Outcomes research represents part of a continuum. Medical decisions have traditionally been made by physicians armed with medical knowledge and applied for the patient's benefit through a process of communication, negotiation, and subsequent application. However, it is also clear that there are several influences on physician decision-making that are not directly related to medical knowledge. These include administrative, social, and financial pressures and constraints (Schwartz and Griffin 1986; Plous 1993; United States Congress 1994). Because these may vary more widely than the basic components of the medical knowledge database, they may explain some of the widespread practice variations noted. However, substantial evidence exists that practice styles and decisions are most strongly influenced by varying interpretations of extant data combined with previous educational influences (Kassirer 1991; Riegelman 1991; Plous 1993).

In an attempt to bring medical and surgical practice in alignment with scientific principles related to evidence analysis, there has been a growing movement to produce formalized statements recommending specific decisions in medical practice. These range from recommendations for diagnostic imaging in various conditions (produced by the American College of Radiology) to specific treatment protocols for multiple disease states (by the American College of Physicians, The Agency for Health Care Policy and Research, and others.) Indeed the list of organizations developing formal clinical policies (ranging from specific algorithmic approaches to clinical problems to text-based policy recommendations for diagnostic interventions) spans the spectrum from Federal to academic to private agencies, and now includes third party indemnity payers.

While there is much to recommend the use of formal guidelines for the treatment of common conditions (Norton 1986) there are students of medical decision-making who claim that the algorithmic thinking process which guidelines represent are not consonant with the thought processes of clinical experts (Abernathy 1995).

These clinical 'statements' go under different names, clinical algorithms, practice parameters, clinical care guidelines, and clinical policies, depending somewhat on their formatting, the process undertaken to produce them, and their overall scope. The development of these statements can be undertaken in various ways and there are explicit methodological concerns with their production (McCormick 1994):

(1) the way in which guidelines topics are selected for production;

(2) the characteristics of the methods used to select guideline development panel members;

(3) the scope and perspective of the guideline;

(4) the methods used to extract appropriate evidence from literature sources, experts, the public, and other sources;

(5) the group processes and methods used to analyze evidence and produce agreement on recommendations;

(6) the extent of linkage between the recommendations and the evidence acquired;

(7) the degree to which the above-mentioned methodologies are explicit, documented, and available for review.

The importance of choosing appropriate topics for guideline development cannot be overemphasized. The criteria used to determine the selection of topics should be explicit. They include public health impact, the cost of the intervention evaluated, the availability of evidence, the extent of variation in clinical practice as regards the subject under consideration, and the need to evaluate appropriate usage of new technologies. Most often the process for selecting topics is based on survey, nomination, or hierarchical ranking. Frequently the nom-

inative processes discussed above are applied in a *post hoc* fashion to justify the topic reached by less formal methods.

A particular difficulty in producing guidelines is avoiding selection bias in the development of panels considering guideline related evidence. This relates to factors of panelist orientation such as academic versus community-based practice, surgical versus nonsurgical, physician versus other health-care professionals, and health-care provider versus consumer biases.

An important first step in the guideline development process relates to establishing the audience for the guideline. While in many cases, guideline development has focused on producing documents for primary care physicians, more current development efforts have included consumers, specialty physicians, and ancillary health-care professionals. Physician acceptance of a particular set of guidelines may depend on the composition of these panels and/or sponsoring bodies.

Perhaps of greatest importance in evaluating the utility of a guideline is the type of evidence available for analysis. Important questions to ask in the evaluation of any evidence derived in the treatment of patients by study include the following.

- With randomization as the gold standard, how were patients assigned to treatment groups?
- Were all patients enrolled in the study accounted for by completion?
- Were patients analyzed in the group to which they were assigned?
- Which participants, patients, observers, and health-care workers, if any, were blinded?
- Were groups similar at the start of the study?
- Aside from the variable of the treatment in question, what covariables were monitored?
- Were the groups treated similarly?
- How precise is the measurement of the treatment effect, and how large is it?

Several grading systems for analyzing evidence have been developed. The United States Preventive Service Task Force Strength of Recommendations are typical; these are relatively subjective, with type A being 'good evidence to support performing the preventive service', type B being 'fair evidence', C representing 'poor evidence', and D and E representing fair and good evidence to *discontinue* the service (Guyatt *et al.* 1995). More specific evidence-weighing criteria have been developed by other organizations.

Specific evidence criteria for grading include study homogeneity or heterogeneity, randomization, confidence intervals of the results, and the numbers needed to treat in order avoid one unwanted outcome. The number needed to treat (**NTT**) is derived from a calculation of the risk of disease if untreated (U) and the risk if treated (T). The absolute risk reduction is $U - T$ and the NNT is the reciprocal $1/(U - T)$. This reflects the number of patients that would require treatment in order to see one additional patient benefit from the treatment in question as opposed to the alternate treatment or no treatment in the case of a placebo.

The grading of the relative value of these parameters in any given study or group of studies is reflected in the grades of recommendation of the Evidence-Based Medicine Working Group (1992).

A1 Randomized controlled trials, no heterogeneity, confidence intervals (**CI**) all on one side of the threshold of the NNT.

A2 Randomized controlled trials, no heterogeneity, CIs overlap threshold NNT.

B1 Randomized controlled trials, heterogeneity, CIs all on one side of threshold NNT.

B2 Randomized controlled trials, heterogeneity, CIs overlap threshold NNT.

C1 Observational studies, CIs all on one side of threshold NNT.

C2 Observational studies, CIs overlap threshold NNT.

A slightly more complex rating system is used by the American College of Chest Physicians in evaluating thromboembolic prophylactic intervention (Cook *et al.* 1995).

Level I Randomized trials or meta-analyses in which the lower limit of the CI for the treatment effect exceeds the minimally clinically important benefit.

Level II Randomized trials or meta-analyses in which the CI for the treatment effect overlaps the minimally clinically important benefit.

Level III Nonrandomized concurrent cohort comparisons between contemporaneous patients who did and did not receive treatment.

Level IV Nonrandomized historic cohort comparisons between patients who received specific agents and former patients (from the same institution or from the literature) who did not.

Level V Case series without controls.

The AHCPR guidelines on the management of acute low back pain provide insight into one method for providing guideline-type data without specifying particular treatment recommendations or modalities specifically. This method, rather than recommending any specific treatment modality, or the timing of such interventions, offers the practitioner a review of treatment effectiveness through a formal grading process. In this method the evidence for any given treatment modality is rated based on its specific efficacy as determined from the best quality studies available in the peer reviewed literature.

The last 15 years have seen a large increase in the effort to summarize and grade levels of evidence for medical interventions. While there has been considerable progress in this field, there are still a number of methodological limitations, and further work is in progress. Unfortunately much of the current evidence for treatment effects in orthopedic research is weak. That is to say that while there have been tremendous strides in the past several decades in many areas of orthopedic treatment, there has not been as comprehensive an effort to determine when intervention and what intervention is specifically appropriate in various treatment settings. Indeed much of the orthopedic literature on treatment provides evidence which would receive the lowest grades, level V or grade C2, according to the evidence weighing schemes noted above.

Despite the relative lack of high-quality data, the drive to reduce costs and standardize treatment indications have led some third-party payers and many managed care organizations to establish basic guidelines for many interventions. Specifically, one large North American health insurer has recently established a complex protocol to evaluate whether or not a patient has had sufficient conservative therapy to warrant arthroscopic intervention for a number of knee conditions including anterior cruciate and posterior cruciate ligament insufficiency, meniscal tears, and osteochondritis desiccans.

As larger numbers of administrative and other organizations develop guidelines it would seem reasonable to review the attributes of a 'good' guideline (US Congress 1994).

Validity: the guideline, when followed, should lead to the health and cost outcomes projected for them.

Soundness: the recommendations must be based on good evidence.

Reliability: given the same evidence and methods, a similar group of development experts should arrive at similar guidelines. Given similar circumstances and patients, the guidelines should result in similar treatment plans, that is their application should be interpreted and applied consistently.

Applicability: the guidelines should be applicable to well-defined populations which should be explicitly delineated in the guideline.

Flexibility: exceptions or 'outliers' should be identified and patient preferences should be identified and considered in the guideline.

Comprehensiveness: the guidelines should include all likely clinical alternatives or indications for the use of an intervention.

Specificity: detailed descriptions of the indications for interventions along with a description of when inadequate information is present to form an opinion.

Ease of use: the guidelines should be concise, unambiguous and in a format that renders them easy to use by the clinician.

Scheduled review: guidelines should include a statement indicating when they were prepared and when they will be reviewed.

Documentation: the guidelines should explicitly and meticulously report on the procedures followed in developing the guideline, including: the participants involved, the evidence accumulation and evidence-weighing methods used, the assumptions, rationales, and analytic methods employed.

As can be seen from this impressive list of factors, a 'good' guideline can be extremely difficult, as well as expensive, to produce. In addition there is little documentation that guidelines are effective in doing what they claim to do. Unfortunately, there is little evidence that any guidelines have been widely adopted or made a significant difference in the care of patients. Sophisticated research is required to document a guidelines efficacy, and to date little such research has been done outside of the arena of cost cutting, generally in the managed care environment. However, there is evidence that the use of clinical guidelines or parameters can be effective in accomplishing a multitude of objectives.

Institution of guidelines can provide equivalent care at lower cost as documented in guiding physician choices regarding nonsteroidal anti-inflammatory medication prescribing in a managed care setting (Jones 1996). The use of algorithmic guidelines has been shown to be more effective than prose summaries of appropriate clinical behavior in teaching the management of complex clinical problems (Margolis 1989). Additional evidence for the effectiveness of guideline use in an orthopedic setting has been the development of rules for obtaining radiographs for the evaluation of injured patients (Fig. 7). Such rules, in the form of guidelines, have been established for making the decision to obtain radiographs in the emergency

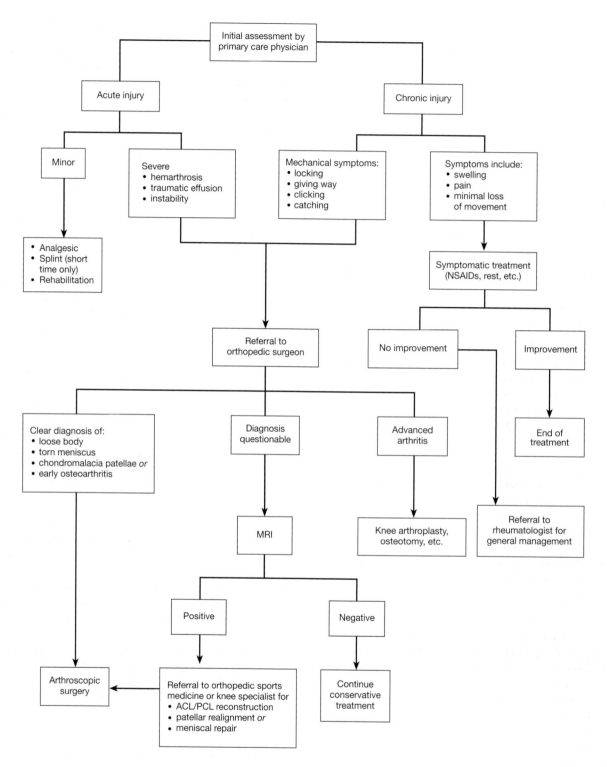

Fig. 7. Algorithm for the diagnosis and treatment of knee pain. ACL, anterior cruciate ligament; PCL, posterior cruciate ligament. (Reproduced from Jackson (1996).)

department setting. Such decision rules for acute knee injuries have been independently confirmed as providing a high degree of confidence that no fracture is present, that is 100 per cent sensitivity (95 per cent CI, 0–4 per cent) (Stiell *et al.* 1996).

Concerns about guidelines

Complaints often raised regarding guidelines include the following.

1. They represent a form of 'cook-book' medicine.

2. They reduce physician autonomy.

3. They inhibit expert physicians from employing their experience and judgment in ways that may improve outcomes for the individual patient.

4. They represent compromises in patient care where ambiguous or conflicting data exist.

5. They stifle the creative and experimental urge to improve on care methodologies.

6. By establishing specific guidelines, a formal method for injuring physicians is brought into the medical malpractice arena.

It should be clear that guidelines are not complete guides to the practice of medicine. It is rare for clinical situations to present in such a fashion that no independent thinking will be required of the clinician. Many of the clinical conditions encountered will not fit neatly into guideline parameters and so will require additional thought and evaluation beyond what the guideline can offer in the majority of clinical situations. The complaints that are enumerated above can be best evaluated on an individual basis.

Claim 1 is valid in the sense that a guideline purports to specifically define the parameters regarding diagnostic and treatment decision-making, much in the same way that cook books define the specific ingredients, their order and method of combination as well as their specific heating or cooling needs to the practitioner attempting to recreate specific type of food. The analogy to a cook book is perfectly apt. For the neophyte chef, such a document is essential to producing high-quality food! An attempt to individualize patient care via methods such as documented by the Evidence-Based Medicine Working Group (1992) represents the pinnacle of medical thinking. However, the use of such detailed analysis for every case encountered would reduce the physician to managing a single case over long periods of time and resynthesizing data analysis which may have been more appropriately done by others. Both the recipe and the guideline work as a teaching tool for conveying accurate information. Even for the expert it may well represent a specific framework around which to adapt the situation encountered regarding alteration in parameters which are not specifically addressed in the guideline or the recipe.

Claim 2 also carries a fair degree of validity. The development of guideline specifics will tend to constrain physician behavior in favor of the recommendations specified by the guideline. However, the counter-claim is equally valid; given high-quality guideline development, the synthesis of evidence should establish appropriate and inappropriate treatment choices such that any reasonable physician would deduce the specific recommendations from independent appraisal of the evidence. It is the quality of the evidence that constrains physician behavior and so reduces autonomy, not the formal evidence analysis process.

With regard to **Claim 3**, the more expert the physician the more much of any guidelines recommendations will be second nature to him or her. One may readily argue that an 'expert' physician is such because of an increased sensitivity to the parameters that render each case an individual with a disease rather an individual example of the same disease, and an expanded knowledge of the evidence available regarding diagnostic and therapeutic options for the individual patient. As previously stated, a practice guideline is not a rigid set of rules dictating physician behavior but rather a set of guideposts guiding the clinician in the general direction that such an 'expert' would head on his or her own. Expert physicians will continue to seek the individual parameters in any given patient encounter that will either lead to following the guideline or establishing the basis on which the guidelines are not appropriate in any given case. This is the case of the so-called outlier mentioned above.

Claim 4 is highly dependent on the nature of the guideline development process. In areas where ambiguous or conflicting data exist, it is unlikely that specific or firm guidelines can be developed. The purpose of guideline development is to evaluate extant data so as to establish where good data exist and also where the quality of data in a given clinical situation is poor, such that future research efforts can be directed to improving the quality of data available for decision-making in that specific clinical situation.

Claim 5 is of little validity. In almost all medical settings, any attempt to engage in creative or experimental alterations in care must be approved by an investigational review board to determine the validity of new treatment or diagnostic methodologies. These new treatments must be contrasted with standard tactics currently employed by physicians. Thus, any attempt to employ and study new strategies for intervention must have some background treatment against which comparison can be made. Guidelines exist as and can provide such background.

With regard to **Claim 6**, there is a distinct possibility that physicians who violate established guidelines will be held accountable to those guidelines as 'standards of medical care'. However, is the current situation any better, where no formal standards of care exist? What standards are currently employed in the medicolegal setting? Much has been written about this issue, and further discussion remains in the realm of medicolegal and sociological issues beyond the scope of this discussion (McIntyre 1995; National Health Lawyers Association 1995).

While in each of these claims there are components of truth, and consequently reasons for concern, the bulk of evidence has led most health policy experts to the conclusion that the time has arrived for an attempt to codify much of what has been informal in medicine for decades. The explosion of medical information, the wide variation in procedure rates identified in demographically similar areas, and attempts to rein in health-care costs have all resulted in increased interest in providing more formal directions for medical decision-making.

Conclusion

The principles of diagnosis and management enumerated above, as well as the discussion of developments in the field of formal guidelines, represent the tip of an iceberg of information regarding the underpinnings of modern medical and surgical practice. Principles of decision-making, logic, psychology, and all of the clinician's evaluation skills interact in this arena. The full complexity of these issues, as well as the interaction of the philosophical, psychologic, economic, and scientific principles which guide medical decision-making, have been summarized in detail in several excellent monographs which are recommended to the interested reader.

Further reading

Abernathy, C.M. and Hamm, R.M. (1995). *Surgical intuition. What it is and how to get it.* Hanley and Belfus, Philadelphia, PA.

Eddy, D.M. (1996). *Clinical decision making. from theory to practice.* Jones and Bartlett, Sudbury, MA.

Kassirer, J.P. and Kopelman, R.I. (1991). *Learning clinical reasoning.* Williams and Wilkins, Baltimore, MD.

McCormick, K.A., Moore, S.R., and Siegel, R.A. (1994). *Clinical practice guideline development. methodology perspectives.* AHCPR Publication No. 95–0009. United States Department of Health and Human Services, Public Health Service, Agency for Health Care Policy and Research.

National Health Lawyers Association (1995). *Colloquium report on legal issues related to clinical practice guidelines.* National Health Lawyers Association.

Plous, S. (1993). *The psychology of judgment and decision making.* McGraw-Hill, New York.

Riegelman, R.K. (1991). *Minimizing medical mistakes—the art of medical decision making.* Little, Brown, Boston, MA.

Schwartz, S. and Griffin, T. (1986). *Medical thinking—the psychology of medical judgment and decision making.* Springer-Verlag, New York.

Sox, K.C., Blatt, M.A., Higgins, M.C., and Marten, K.I. (1988). *Medical decision making.* Butterworth Heinemann, Boston, MA.

United States Congress (1994). *Office of Technology Assessment. Identifying health technologies that work: searching for evidence.* OTA-H-608. US Government Printing Office, Washington, DC.

References

Abernathy, C.M. and Hamm, R.M. (1995). *Surgical intuition. What it is and how to get it.* Hanley and Belfus, Philadelphia, PA

Cook, D.J., Guyatt, G.H., Laupacis, A., Sackett, D.L., and Goldberg, R.J. (1995). Clinical recommendations using levels of evidence for antithrombotic agents. Fourth ACCP Consensus Conference on Antithrombotic Therapy. *Chest*, **108** (Supplement), 227S–30S.

Evidence-Based Medicine Working Group (1992). Evidence based medicine. a new approach to teaching the practice of medicine. *Journal of the American Medical Association*, **268**(17), 2420–5.

Guyatt, G.H., Sackett, D.L., Sinclair, J.C., Hayward, R., Cook, D.J., and Cook, R, for the Evidence Based Medicine Working Group (1995). User's guides

to the medical literature IX. A method for grading health care recommendations. *Journal of the American Medical Association*, **274**(22), 1800–4.

Jackson, R.W. (1996). The painful knee: arthroscopy of MR imaging. *Journal of the American Academy of Orthopedic Surgeons*, **4**, 97.

Jones, D.L., Kroenke, K., Landry, F.J., Tomich, D.J., and Ferrel, R.J. (1996). Cost savings using a stepped care prescribing protocol for nonsteroidal anti-inflammatory drugs. *Journal of the American Medical Association*, **275**(12), 926–30.

Kassirer, J.P. and Kopelman, R.I. (1991). *Learning clinical reasoning.* Williams and Wilkins, Baltimore, MD.

McCormick, K.A., Moore, S.R., and Siegel, R.A. (1994). *Clinical practice guideline development. methodology perspectives.* AHCPR Publication No. 95–0009. United States Department of Health and Human Services, Public Health Service, Agency for Health Care Policy and Research.

McIntyre, K.M. (1995). Medicolegal implications of consensus statements. Fourth ACCP Consensus Conference on Antithrombotic Therapy. *Chest* **108** (Supplement), 502S–5S.

Margolis, C.Z., Cook, C.D., Barak, N., Adler, A., and Geertsma, A. (1989). Clinical algorithms teach pediatric decision making more effectively than prose. *Medical Care*, **27**, 576–92.

National Health Lawyers Association (1995). *Colloquium report on legal issues related to clinical practice guidelines.* National Health Lawyers Association.

Norton, L.W. and Eiseman, B. (1986). *Surgical decision making.* W.B. Saunders, Philadelphia, PA.

Plous, S. (1993). *The psychology of judgment and decision making.* McGraw-Hill, New York.

Relman, A.S. (1988). Assessment and accountability-the third revolution in health care. *New England Journal of Medicine*, **319**, 1220–2.

Riegelman, R.K. (1991). *Minimizing medical mistakes—the art of medical decision making.* Little, Brown, Boston, MA.

Rutkow, I.M. (1982). Unnecessary surgery: What is it? *Surgical Clinics of North America*, **62**, 613–25.

Rutkow, I.M. and Starfield, B.H. (1984). Surgical decision making and operative rates. *Archives of Surgery*, **119**, 899–905.

Schwartz, S. and Griffin, T. (1986). *Medical thinking—the psychology of medical judgment and decision making.* Springer-Verlag, New York.

Stiell, I.G., Greenberg, G.H., Wells, G.A., *et al.* (1996). Prospective validation of a decision rule for the use of radiography in acute knee injuries. *Journal of the American Medical Association*, **275**, 611–15.

United States Congress (1994). *Office of Technology Assessment. Identifying health technologies that work: searching for evidence.* OTA-H-608. US Government Printing Office, Washington, DC.

Wennberg, J. and Gittelsohn, A. (1973) Small area variations in health care delivery. *Science*, **182**, 1102–8.

Wennberg, J. and Gittelsohn, A. (1982). Variations in medical care in small areas. *Scientific American*, **246**, 120–34.

Wennberg, J.E., Freeman, J.L., Shelton, R.M., and Bubolz, T.A. (1989). Hospital use and mortality among Medicare beneficiaries in Boston and New Haven. *New England Journal of Medicine*, **321**, 1168–73.

1.4 Genetic disorders of the skeleton

Andrew Carr

Introduction

Over recent years dramatic advances have occurred in our understanding of the molecular basis of genetic disorders of the skeleton. Specific genetic mutations have been identified and this has led to a greater understanding of the biology of bone, muscle, and cartilage. In addition to these genetic advances, considerable improvement has also occurred in the treatment and management of individuals and families with these disorders. In the field of orthopedic surgery this has included increasing use of joint replacement surgery and operations to correct bone deformity and to lengthen limbs. On the horizon are medical treatments for these conditions and the next 10 to 20 years are certain to reveal considerable further change in this field.

Much progress has been made since the early pioneering days of Sir Thomas Fairbank in classifying and understanding genetic disorders of the skeleton. His work was taken on by Ruth Wynne-Davies, Christine Hall, and Graham Apley who together produced an atlas of skeletal dysplasias (Wynne-Davies *et al.* 1986). Others, notably Spranger (1988), have also made significant contributions to the classification and understanding of genetic disorders of the musculo-skeletal system.

This chapter aims to outline both clinical and genetic classifications of inherited disorders of the skeleton. It will also review issues relating to the antenatal diagnosis of these conditions and how this may be of importance to orthopedic surgeons.

Principles of classification

The concept of grouping skeletal dysplasias has existed in some form for over 50 years. Spranger (1988) proposed the idea of families of skeletal dysplasias. He felt that these were pathogenetically related, and suggested that it would be useful to classify them within groups. It is illuminating to see how dysplasia classifications have evolved over time. Table 1 illustrates the general classifications of dysplasias that have been used in this chapter. This system of subdividing by phenotype is rapidly becoming superceded by classifications based on new knowledge of the underlying genetic mutations responsible for the disorder.

Outlined in Table 2 is an up-to-date list of skeletal dysplasias with their gene mutations if known. Over the past 20 years there have been regular meetings of international working groups on skeletal dysplasias which have classified as many as 24 major groups and it is interesting to review these groups now in the light of new genetic knowledge. Of particular interest are examples such as the achondroplasia family which includes thanatophoric dysplasia which is lethal and hypochondroplasia which may be difficult to distinguish from normal; these disorders have similar features of vastly different severity and are due to mutations in the same gene.

Many of the skeletal dysplasias arise as a result of genes coding for constituents of the matrix of bone or cartilage. Figures 1, 2, and 3 illustrate schematically the major constituents of bone and cartilage and their proposed interactions. This chapter describes the clinical and radiological features of genetic disorders of the skeleton. Surgical treatments are also discussed for each of the conditions and are summarized in Table 3.

Epiphyseal disorders
Multiple epiphyseal dysplasia
Clinical features

This condition is characterized by shortness of stature and irregular epiphyseal growth involving most joints but occasionally only one pair. It is associated with premature degenerative arthritis. There is occasional minor vertebral involvement in the lower dorsal region mainly in childhood. It is one of the most common skeletal dysplasias with a variable phenotype and a prevalence of approximately 10 per million. The condition usually presents with short stature but there may also be pain and stiffness of affected joints. There are often joint contractures and occasionally scoliosis and ankle valgus. It has been subdivided into the Ribbins type with normal wrists and hands and the more severe Fairbank type where the wrists and hands are short and stubby. There is considerable overlap between the Fairbank type and pseudoachondroplasia (Briggs *et al.* 1994, 1995; Muragaki *et al.* 1996).

Radiographic features

The skull is generally normal and the spine shows occasional irregularity of endplates in the lower thoracic region. The major problem is with the limb epiphyses where joints are usually involved symmetrically. The ossification centers are late and become fragmented, and there is sometimes associated abnormality of the metaphyses. The hips are commonly involved with flat epiphyses and femoral head subluxation. In severe cases, joints become involved with degenerative arthritis very early in life. Radiographs of the hands and wrists

Table 1 Classfication of skeletal dysplasias based on phenotype

(i) Epiphyseal dysplasia
Multiple epiphyseal dysplasia, hereditary arthro-ophthalmopathy (Stickler), chondrodysplasia punctata
  (Conradi), severe rhizomolic, milder forms
(ii) Spondyloepiphyseal dysplasias
Congenita and tarda, autosomal dominant and recessive, X-linked recessive
(iii) Predominantly metaphyseal dysplasias
  Metaphyseal chondrodysplasias (MCD)
  Types: Schmid, McKusick, Jansen, Peña, with malabsorption and neutropenia, others (see also
    hypophosphatasia, rickets, included with metabolic bone disease (ix))
Spondylometaphyseal dysplasias—types Kozlowski, Sutcliffe
(iv) Short limbs/normal trunk
Achondroplasia, hypochondroplasia, dyschondrosteosis Robinow, Werner, acromesomelia,
  acrodysostosis
(v) Short limbs and trunk (may or may not be disproportionate)
Pseudoachondroplasia, diastrophic dysplasia, metatropic dwarfism, Kniest, Ellis–van Creveld, Jeune
(vi) Lethal forms of short-limb dwarfism
Thanatophoric, achondrogenesis, short rib/polydactyly syndromes, campomelic dwarfism
(vii) Increased limb length
Marfan, congenital contractural arachnodactyly, homocystinuria
(viii) Storage disorders
Mucopolysaccharide disorders, mucolipidoses, mannosidosis, sialidoses
(ix) Metabolic bone disease
Hypo- and hyperphosphatasia, hypophosphatemic rickets, pseudohypoparathyroidism
(x) Decreased bone density
Osteogenesis imperfecta group, idiopathic juvenile osteoporosis, Hajdu–Cheney (osteolysis)
(xi) Increased bone density (sclerosing bone dysplasias)
Osteoporosis, pycnodysostosis, Pyle's craniometaphyseal dysplasia, frontometaphyseal dysplasia,
  osteodysplasty (Melnick–Needles), Engelmann's craniodiaphyseal dysplasia, osteopathia striata,
  osteopoikilosis
(xii) Tumor-like disorders (bony or fibrous)
Diaphyseal aclasis, Ollier's, Maffucci's, dysplasia epiphysealis hemimelica, myositis ossificans progressive,
  polyostotic fibrous dysplasia (including Albright), melorheostosis, neurofibromatosis
(xiii) Ehlers–Danlos syndrome
(xiv) Alkaptonuria
(xv) Hemophilia
(xvi) Malformation syndromes
Apert's, Crouzon, cleidocranial, craniocarpotarsal, Cornelia de Lange, Larsen's, nail–patella, Ollier's,
  Trevor's
(xvii) Neuromuscular disorders
Duchenne and Becker muscular dystrophy, myotonic dystrophy, Charcot–Marie–Tooth, spinal
  muscular atrophy, neurofibromatosis
(xviii) Common disorders of the skeleton
Osteoarthritis, osteoporosis, rheumatoid arthritis, Dupuytren's disease, scoliosis, developmental
  dysplasia of the hip, club foot

may reveal evidence of cone-shaped epiphyses with occasional premature fusion. In the more severe forms the metacarpals and phalanges are short (Fig. 4).

Genetics

Two mutations have been identified in multiple epiphyseal dysplasia. The first is on chromosome 19p and causes a defect in the cartilage oligomeric matrix protein. The second defect is on chromosome 1p and is a type IX collagen defect.

Treatment

The most common problem requiring orthopedic treatment is hip arthritis. Hip replacement is often necessary at a young age. Tech-

nically this is a problem because of varus deformity of the femoral neck. Occasionally realignment osteotomies are performed. Great care must be taken with these because of the possibility of bringing forward the onset of osteoarthritis.

Valgus deformity of the knee may also occur and this may require correction with supracondylar femoral osteotomy. On occasions, limb-length discrepancy occurs and then an epiphyseodesis may be necessary.

Hereditary arthro-ophthalmopathy (Stickler's syndrome)

This has a spectrum of presentations and is split into two main subgroups. Stickler's syndrome with ocular involvement and Stickler's

Table 2 The mapping of skeletal dysplasias: alphabetic listing of the mapped skeletal dysplasias

Disorder	Location	Title
Achondrogenesis Ib, 600972	5q31–q34	Diastrophic dysplasia sulfate transporter
Achondrogenesis–hypochondrogenesis, type II	12q13.11–q13.2	Collagen, type II, α_1 polypeptide
Achondroplasia, 100800	4p16.3	Fibroblast growth factor receptor 3
?Acrocallosal syndrome	12p13.3–p11.2	Areocallosal syndrome
?Acrofacial dysostosis, Nager type	9q34	Acrofacial dysostosis, Nager type
Aneurysm, familial 100070	2q31	Collagen, type III, α_1 polypeptide
Apert syndrome, 101200	10q26	Fibroblast growth factor receptor 2 (bacteria-expressed kinase)
Aspartylglucosaminuria	4q32–q33	Aspartylglucosaminidase
Atelosteogenesis II, 256050	5q31–q34	Diastrophic dysplasia sulfate transporter
Bardet–Biedl syndrome 1	11q13	Bardet–Biedl syndrome 1
Bardet–Biedl syndrome 2	16q21	Bardet–Biedl syndrome 2
Bardet–Biedl syndrome 3	3p13–p12	Bardet–Biedl syndrome 3
Bardet–Biedl syndrome 4	15q22.3–q33	Bardet–Biedl syndrome 4
Campodelic dysplasia with autosomal sex, sex reversal	17q24.3–q35.1	Campomelic dysplasia 1 (sex reversal, autosomal, 1)
Cartilage–hair hypoplasia	9p13	Cartilage–hair hypoplasia
Chondrocalcinosis with early-onset osteoarthritis	8q	Chondrocalcinosis 1 (calcium pyrophosphate-deposition disease, early-onset osteoarthritis
?Chondrodysplasia punctata, rhizomelic	4p16–p14	Chondrodysplasia punctata, rhizomelic
Chondrodysplasia punctata, X-linked dominant	Xq28	Chondrodysplasia punctata 2, X-linked dominant (Happle syndrome)
Chondrodysplasia punctata, X-linked recessive, 302940	Xp22.3	Arylsulfatase E
Cleidocranial dysplasia	6p21	Cleidocranial dysplasia
Contractural arachnodactyly, congenital	5q23–q31	Fibrillin 2
?Craniofrontonasal dysplasia	Xpter–p22.22	Craniofrontonasal dysplasia
Craniosynostosis, Adelaide type	4p16	Craniosynostosis, Adelaide type
Craniosynostosis, type 1	7p21.3–p21.2	Craniosynostosis, type I
Craniosynostosis, type 2	5q34–q35	msh (*Drosophila*) homeo box homolog 2
Crouzon craniofacial dysostosis 123500	10q26	Fibroblast growth factor receptor 2 (bacteria-expressed kinase)
Diastrophic dysplasia	5q31–q34	Diastrophic dysplasia sulfate transporter
Ehlers–Danlos syndrome, type II	9q34.2–q34.3	Ehlers–Danlos syndrome, type II
?Ehlers–Danlos syndrome, type II, one form 1300010	9q34.2–q34.3	Collagen V, α_1 polypeptide
Ehlers–Danlos syndrome, type III	2q31	Collagen, type III α_1 polypeptide
Ehlers–Danlos syndrome, type IV	2q31	Collagen, type ill, α_1 polypeptide
Ehlers–Danlos syndrome, type VIIA1, 130060	17q21.31–q22.05	Collagen, α_1 polypeptide
Ehlers–Danlos syndrome, type VIIA2, 130060	7q22.1	Collagen, type I, α_2 polypeptide
Ellis–van Creveld syndrome	4p16	Ellis–van Creveld syndrome
Epiphyseal dysplasia, multiple 2	1p32	Epiphyseal dysplasia, multipe 2
Epiphyseal dysplasia, multiple 1	19p13.1	Cartilage oligomeric matric protein
Exostoses, multiple, type 1	8q24.11–q24.13	Exostoses (multiple) 1
Exostoses, multiple, type 2	11p12–p11	Exostoses (multiple) 2
Exostoses, multiple, type 3	19p	Exostoses (multiple) 3]
Familial expansile osteolysis	18q21.1–q22	Familial expansile osteolysis
?Fibrodysplasia ossificans progressiva	20p12	Bone morphogenetic protein 2
Fibromuscular dysplasia of arteries, 135580	2q31	Collagen, type III, α_1 polypeptide
Fucosidosis	1p34	Fucosidase, α-L-1, tissue
GM1-gangliosidosis	3p21.33	Galactosidase, β_1
?Goldenhar syndrome	7p	Goldenhar syndrome
Greig cephalopolysyndactyly syndrome, 175700	7p13	GLI-Kruppel family members GL13 (oncogene GL13)
Hemolytic anemia due to ADA excess	20113.11	Adenosine deaminase
Hereditary hemorrhagic telangiectasia, type II	12q	Osler–Rendu–Weber syndrome 2
Holoprosencephaly, type 3	7q36	Holoprosencephaly 3
?Holoprosencephaly 1	18pter–q11	Holoprosencephaly 1, alobar, 236100
?Holoprosencephaly 4	14q11.1–q13	Holoprosencephaly 4, semilobar
Holt–Oram syndrome	12q21.3–q22	Holt–Oram syndrome
Homocystinuria, B_6-responsive and nonresponsive types	21q22.3	Cystathionine β-synthase
Homocystinura due to MTHFR deficiency	1p36.3	Methylenetetrahydrofalate reductase
Hypercalcemia, hypocalciuric, type I	3q21–q24	Hypocalciuric hypercalcemia 1 (parathyroid Ca^{2+}-sensing receptor)
Hypocalcemia, autosomal dominant	3q21–q24	Hypocalciuric hypercalcemia 1 (parathyroid Ca^{2+}- sensing receptor)
Hypochondrodysplasia 14600	4p16.3	Fibroblast growth factor receptor 3
?Hypophosphatasia, adult, 146300	1p36.1–p34	Alkaline phosphatase, liver/bone/kidney
Hypophosphatasia, infantile, 241500	1p36.1–p34	Alkaline phosphatase, liver/bone/kidney
Hypophosphatemia, hereditary	Xp22.2–p22.1	Hypophosphatemia, vitamin D-resistant rickets
Jackson–Weiss syndrome, 123150	10q26	Fibroblast growth factor receptor 2 (bacteria-expressed kinase)

Table 2 *Continued.*

Disorder	Location	Title
?Klippel–Feil syndrome	5q11.2	Klippel–Feil syndrome
Kniest dysplasia	12q13.11–q13.2	Collagen, type II, α_1 polypeptide
Langer–Giedion syndrome	8q24.11–q24.1	Langer–Giedion syndrome chromosome region
Larsen syndrome, autosomal dominant	3p21.1–p14.1	Larsen syndrome 1 (autosomal dominant)
Mannosidosis, α_1	19cen–q12	Mannosidase, α B, lysosomal
Marfan syndrome, 54700	15q21.1	Fibrillin 1
Maroteaux–Lamy syndrome, several forms	5q11–q13	Arylsulfatase B
McCune–Albright polyostotic fibrous dysplasia 174800	20q13.2	Guanine nucleotide-binding protein (G protein), α-stimulating activity polypeptide 1
Metaphyseal chondrodysplasia, Murk–Jansen type, 156400	3p22–21.1	Parathyroid hormone receptor
Metaphyseal chondrodysplasia, Schmid type	6q21–q22.3	Collagen type X, α_1 polypeptide
Mucolipidosis II	4q21–q23	UDP-N-acetylglucosamine-lysosomal-enzyme N-acetyglucosamine phospotransferase
Mucolipidosis III	4q21–q23	UDP-N-acetyglucosamine-lysosomal-enzyme N-acetyglucosamine phosphotransferase
Mucopolysaccharidosis Ih	4p16.3	Iduronidase, α-L-1
Mucopolysaccharidosis Ih/s	4p16.3	Iduronidase, α-L-1
Mucopolysaccharidosis II	Xq28	Iduronate 2-sulfatase (Hunter syndrome)
Mucopolysaccharidosis IVA	16q24.3	Galactosamine (N-acetyl)-6-sulfate sulfatase
Mucopolysaccharidosis IVB	3p21.33	Galactosidase, β_1
Mucopolysaccharidosis VII	7q21.11	Glucuronidase, β_1
Nail–patella syndrome	9q34.1	Nail–patella syndrome
Neonatal hyperparathyroidism, 239200	3q21–q24	Hypocalciuric hypercalcemia 1 (parathyroid Ca^{2+}- sensing receptor)
OSMED syndrome, 215150	6p21.3	Collagen XI, polypeptide
Osteoarthrosis, precocious	12q13.11–q13.2	Collagen, type II, α_1 polypeptide
Osteogenesis imperfecta, 4 clinical forms, 166200, 166210, 259420, 166220	17q21.31–q22.05	Collagen I, α_1 polypeptide
Osteogenesis imperfecta, 4 clinical forms, 166200, 166210, 259420, 166220	7q22.1	Collagen, type I, α_2 polypeptide
?Osteopetrosis, 259700	1p21–p13	Colony-stimulating factor 1 (macrophage)
Osteoporosis, idiopathic, 166710	17q21.31–q22.05	Collagen I, α_1 polypeptide
Otopalatodigital syndrome, type I	Xq28	Otopalatodigital syndrome, type I
Pfeiffer syndrome, 101600	10q26	Fibroblast growth factor receptor 2 (bacteria-expressed kinase)
Pfeiffer syndrome, 101600	8p11.2–p11.1	Fibroblast growth factor receptor 1 (fms-related tyrosine kinase 2)
Pituitary ACTH-secreting adenoma	20q13.2	Guanine nucleotide-binding protein (G protein), α-stimulating activity polypeptide 1
Pseudoachondroplasia, 177170	19p13.1	Cartilage oligomeric matrix protein
Pseudohypoparathyroidism, type Ia, 103580	20q13.2	Guanine nucleotide-binding protein (G protein), α-stimulating activity polypeptide 1
Pycnodysostosis	1q21	Pyknodysostosis (pycnodysostosis)
Renal tubular acidosis–osteopetrosis syndrome	8q22	Carbonic anhydraseII
Rubenstein–Taybi syndrome, 180849	16p13.3	CREB binding protein
Russell–Silver syndrome	17q25	Russell–Silver syndrome
Saethre–Chotzen syndrome	7p21	Acrocephalosyndactyly 3 (Saethre–Chotzen syndrome)
Sanfilippo syndrome, type B	17q21	N-acetylglucosaminidase, α_1
?Sanfilippo syndrome, type C	Chr.14	Mucopolysaccharidosis, type IIIC
Sanfilippo syndrome, type D	12q14	N-acetylglucosamine-6-sulfatase
SED congenita	12q13.11–q13.2	Collagen, type II, α_1 polypeptide
Severe combined immunodeficiency due to ADA deficiency	20q13.11	Adenosine deaminase
SMED Strudwick type	12q13.11–q13.2	Collagen type II, α_1 polypeptide
Somatotrophinoma	20q13.2	Guanine nucleotide-binding protein (G protein), α-stimulating activity polypeptide 1
Split hand/foot malformation, type 2	Xq26	Split hand/foot malformation, type (ectrodactyly) 2
Split hand/foot malformation, type 1	7q21.2–q21.3	Split hand/foot malformation, type 1
Spondyloepiphyseal dysplasia tarda	Xp22.2–p22.1	Spondyloepiphyseal dysplasia, late
Stickler syndrome, type I	12q13.11–q13.2	Collagen, type II, α_1 polypeptide
Stickler syndrome, type II, 184840	6p21.3	Collagen XI, α_2 polypeptide
Symphalangism, proximal	17q21–q22	Symphalangism 1 (proximal)
Syndactyly, type II	2q31	Syndactyly type II (synpolydactyly)
Thanatophoric dwarfism, 187600	4p16.3	Fibroblast growth factor receptor 3
Treacher–Collins mandibulofacial dysostosis	5q32–q33.1	Treacher–Collins–Franceschetti syndrome 1
Trichorhinophalangeal syndrome, type I	8q24.12	Trichorhinophalangeal syndrome, type I
Triphalangeal thumb–polysyndactyly syndrome	7q36	Triphalangeal thumb–polysyndactyly syndrome
Wagner syndrome, type II	12q13.11–q13.2	Collagen, type II, α_1 polypeptide

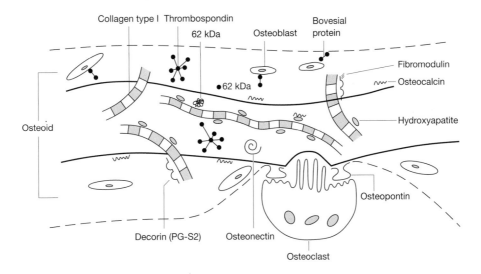

Fig. 1. Schematic illustration of bone matrix constituents and their proposed interactions.

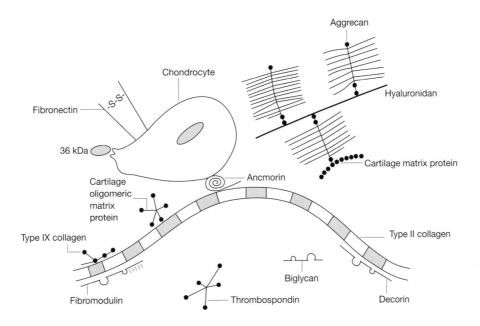

Fig. 2. Schematic illustration of cartilage matrix constituents and their proposed interactions.

syndrome without ocular involvement. There is usually enlargement of joints with eipiphyseal changes. Its frequency is low (approximately 0.1 to 0.3 per million) (Winterpacht *et al.* 1993).

Clinical features

The clinical features include a high degree of myopia with a characteristic facial appearance of flat nasal bridge and turned up nose.

Intelligence is usually normal. Occasionally short stature is present and there is sometimes associated cleft palate and hearing loss. Retinal detachment may occur.

Radiographic features

The skull has a normal vault but with small facial bones. Spinal changes include a mild irregular platyspondyly with anterior wedging

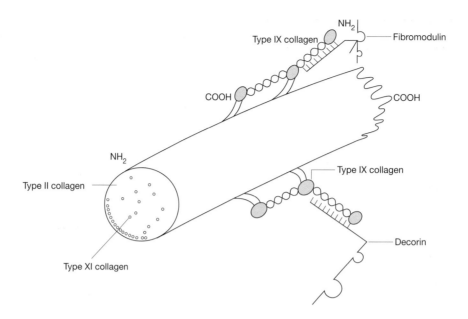

Fig. 3. Schematic representation of the type II collagen and its interactions in the extracellular cartilage matrix. Most type IX collagen molecules are covalently linked onto the surface of type II collagen. Decorin and fibromodulin interact with the cationic component of type IX collagen. Type XI collagen lies within the type II collagen bundle.

similar to Scheuermann's disease. In the long bones a characteristic appearances of a dumb-bell shape of long bone with enlarged epiphyses and metaphyses (Fig. 5).

Genetics

The ocular form of Stickler's syndrome has been mapped to chromosome 12q and the type II collagen gene. The non-ocular form of Stickler's syndrome has been mapped to chromosome 6p and the type XI collagen gene.

Treatment

Ophthalmic problems may occur and these require treatment by ophthalmic surgeons. Occasionally early onset osteoarthritis is a feature and joint replacement surgery may be necessary.

Chondrodysplasia calcificans punctata (Conradi disease)

Clinical features

This interesting disorder is characterized by stippling of the epiphyses and also by extraepiphyseal calcification. Stippling occurs only in the early years and disappears thereafter. The phenotype range is great, from a severe rhizomelic form often stillborn or perinatal lethal to a milder disorder with limb shortening. Its frequency is low at approximately 1.7 per million.

The facial appearance is of a flat face and depressed bridge of nose; the hair is often sparse and thin. Mental retardation is common in the severe forms. There are often vertebral anomalies and congenital scoliosis. Contractures of joints occur and there are associated anomalies include congenital cataracts, skin lesions, and congenital heart lesions.

Radiographic features

There is a punctate stippling of the epiphyses with calcification outside the epiphyses. This calcification is often found around the vertebral column and pelvis and disappears by 3 to 5 years. The spine demonstrates congenital vertebral anomalies with scoliosis. In the long bones there is proximal limb shortening and metaphyseal cupping and splaying (Fig. 6).

Genetics

X-linked forms have been described; X-linked dominant is localized to chromosome Xq and an X-linked progressive form localized to chromosome Xp. The rhizomelic form of chondrodysplasia punctata has been localized to chromosome 4p.

Treatment

This condition is associated with atlantoaxial instability and fusion may be necessary. Because of congenital abnormalities of the spine, spinal deformity may occur and on occasions be rapidly progressive. These may require early surgical fusion and correction. Flexion deformities may occur in the hip and knee but very rarely require surgical release.

Spondyloepiphyseal dysplasia

Clinical features

This has been separated into two main forms, congenita and tarda. In the congenita form, subgroups have been described with and without severe coxa vara. In spondyloepiphyseal dysplasia congenita, short stature with disproportionately short trunk and gross joint damage is described. The prevalence is rare, approximately 1 to 2 per million. Flat facial features are described. There are associated anomalies of

Table 3 Orthopedic surgery in inherited disorders of the skeleton

	Spine	Hips	Knees	Femur/tibia	Ankle/foot	Upper limb	Hand
Multiple epiphyseal dysplasia		Osteotomy Joint replacement	Osteotomy Joint replacement				
Stickler		Osteotomy Joint replacement	Osteotomy Joint replacement	Osteotomy			
Spondyloepiphyseal dysplasia tarda							
Spondyloepiphyseal dysplasia congenita	Atlantoaxial fusion Deformity correction	Osteotomy Joint replacement	Osteotomy Joint replacement	Corrective osteotomy	Hind foot correction fusion		
Conradi syndrome	Atlantoaxial fusion Corrective deformity	Release of hip contractures		Corrective osteotomy	Hind foot correction fusion		
Metaphyseal dysplasia	Atlantoaxial fusion	Corrective osteotomy	Corrective osteotomy				
Ellis–van Creveld syndrome				Corrective osteotomy			Polydactyly Syndactyly
Storage disorders	Atlantoaxial fusion	Osteotomy Correction of flexion contractures Joint replacement					
Marfan's syndrome	Spinal deformity correction Dural cyst						
Hemocystinurea	Spinal deformity correction						
Achondroplasia	Spinal stenosis		Correction genuvarum	Limb lengthening			
Pseudo-achondroplasia	Scoliosis correction	Osteotomy Joint replacement	Osteotomy Joint replacement				Wrist fusion
Gaucher's disease		Joint replacement					
Ochronosis (alkaptonuria)		Joint replacement	Joint replacement			Joint replacement	
Hemophilia		Syno-vectomy Arthrodesis Joint replacement	Synovectomy Arthrodesis Joint replacement				
Osteogenesis imperfecta	Spinal deformity		Telescopic rods Fractures	Fractures	Fractures	Telescopic rods	
Multiple hereditary exostoses			Removal Osteo-chondromas Corrective osteotomy Bone lengthening Tumors			Removal Osteo-chondromas Corrective osteotomy Bone lengthening Tumors	
Craniosynostoses	Craniofacial surgery						
Nail–patella syndrome			Patella stabilization			Radial head excision	
Ollier's disease (enchondromatosis)			Corrective osteotomy Lengthening			Corrective osteotomy Lengthening	
Muscular dystrophy	Spinal deformity						

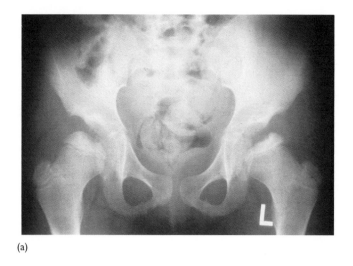

(a)

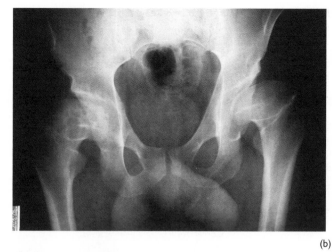

(b)

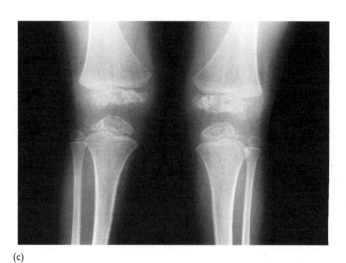

(c)

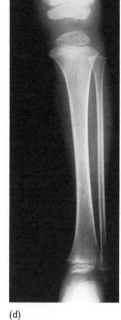

(d)

Fig. 4. Multiple epiphyseal dysplasia.
(a) Anteroposterior radiograph of the pelvis showing abnormality of both femoral capital epiphyses. (b) Anteroposterior radiograph of pelvis demonstrating flattened femoral heads with shallow acetabulae. There is early degenerative change particularly in the right hip, and both femoral heads are uncovered. (c) Anteroposterior radiographs of immature knees demonstrating small and irregular epiphyses. (d) Anteroposterior radiograph of tibia demonstrating small and irregular epiphyses.

cleft palate and club-foot. Deformities are also present particularly scoliosis and kyphoscoliosis with deformities of the knees, hips, and feet.

In spondyloepiphyseal dysplasia tarda, the prevalence is greater, approximately 3 to 4 per million, and much more normal stature is achieved. Generally the abnormalities of the epiphyses and spine are less severe than described in spondyloepiphyseal dysplasia congenita.

A very rare form has been described with a progressive arthropathy and it is unclear whether or not this condition is a true skeletal dysplasia.

Radiographic features

The radiographic features include gross abnormalities of the spine with odontoid dysplasia and loss of vertebral height. Occasionally, instability at the upper end of the cervical spine occurs and requires surgical stabilization. Limb epiphyses and metaphyses are abnormal with severe fragmentation of the epiphyses usually most marked at the proximal end of the femur (Fig. 7).

Genetics

Genetically the disorder has been localized to an abnormality of the type II collagen gene on chromosone 12q, and it is notable that in the congenita form myopia is often present (Murray *et al.* 1989; Anderson *et al.* 1990).

Treatment

The odontoid is often hypoplastic and this predisposes to atlantoaxial

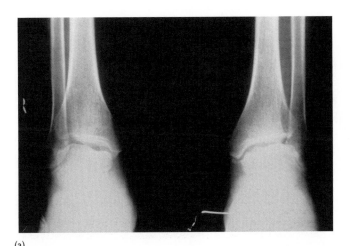

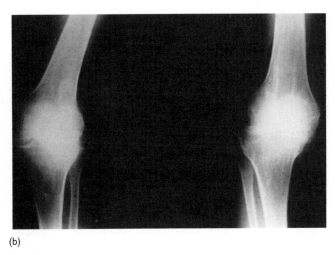

(a)

(b)

Fig. 5. Stickler's syndrome demonstrating early onset of osteoarthritis in (a) the ankle joints and (b) the knee joints.

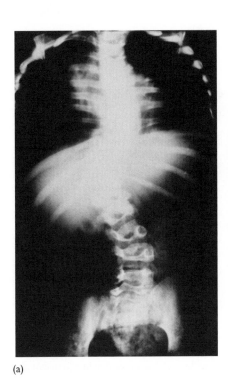

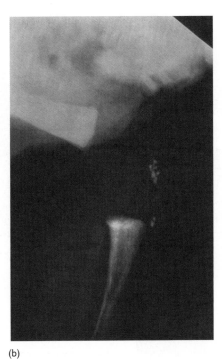

(a)

(b)

Fig. 6. Conradi syndrome. (a) Anteroposterior radiograph of spine with congenital vertebral anomalies in the mid-thoracic region and scoliosis. (b) Lateral radiograph of the knee demonstrating typical stippled calcification.

instability. Symptoms of myelopathy may occur, and if there is significant symptomatic instability then an atlantoaxial fusion is required.

Severe progressive varus deformity of the femoral neck is often encountered, and subtrochanteric valgus osteotomy may help to reduce this deformity. If this osteotomy is performed, an extension of the distal femur in conjunction with valgus osteotomy may decrease the flexion deformity of the hip and improve the lumbar lordosis which is present. Early onset of osteoarthritis is often encountered, and joint replacement surgery may be necessary.

In some cases severe genu valgum may be present, and supracondylar femoral osteotomy and realignment may be necessary.

Metaphyseal disorders

Metaphyseal dysplasia

Clinical features

A number of metaphyseal dysplasias have been described of which the most common is type Schmid. This affects predominantly the

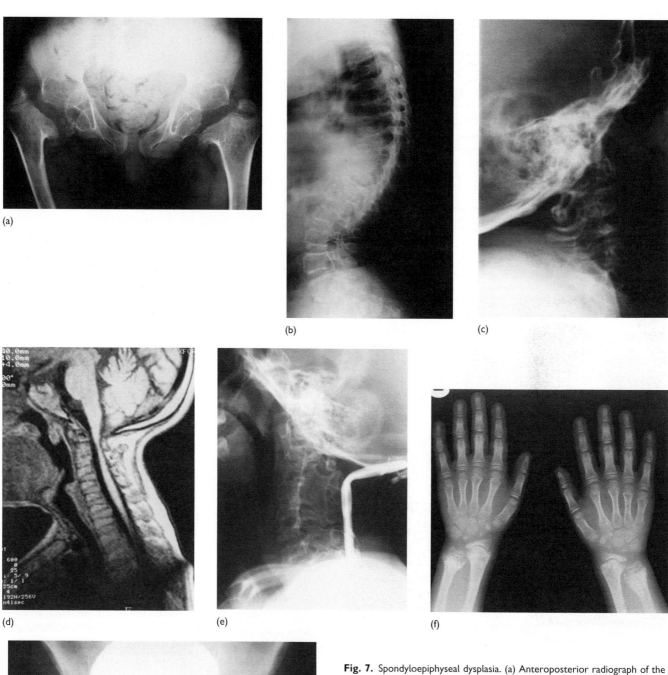

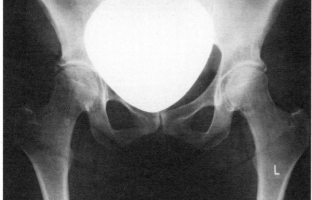

Fig. 7. Spondyloepiphyseal dysplasia. (a) Anteroposterior radiograph of the pelvis in spondyloepiphyseal dysplasia congenita, demonstrating grossly disorganized hip joints with marked coxa vara. (b) Lateral radiograph of the thoracolumbar in spondyloepiphyseal dysplasia congenita with marked platispondyly and increased lumbar lordosis. (c) Lateral radiograph of the upper cervical spine in spondyloepiphyseal dysplasia congenita demonstrating platispondyly and instability at the atlantoaxial level. (d) Magnetic resonance imaging scan of the cervical spine in spondyloepiphyseal dysplasia congenita with narrowing of the spinal canal in the upper cervical level. This patient required decompression and fusion. (e) Lateral radiograph of the upper cervical spine in spondyloepiphyseal dysplasia congenita following fusion. (f) Anteroposterior radiographs of the hands in spondyloepiphyseal dysplasia congenita with marked epiphyseal changes, particularly in the distal radius and ulnar. (g) Anteroposterior radiographs of the pelvis in spondyloepiphyseal dysplasia tarda with mild early onset osteoarthritis.

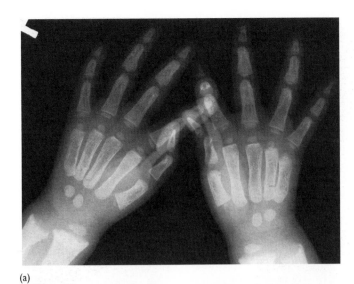

(a)

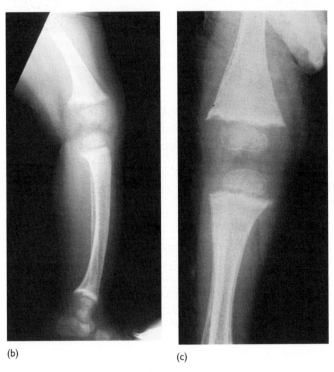

(b)　　　　　　　　(c)

Fig. 8. Metaphyseal chondrodysplasia type Schmid. (a) Anteroposterior radiographs of the hands, showing characteristic metaphyseal abnormality with flaring of the metaphyseal region. (b) Lateral radiograph of the leg, showing metaphyseal flaring but normal epiphyses. (c) This condition may be confused with nutritional rickets, which is demonstrated here with normal epiphyses and metaphyseal flaring.

upper femur and also presents with some shortness of stature. The prevalence is around 5 per million population. The condition usually presents with an abnormality of gait in childhood with lumbar lordosis. The range of severity is wide. There is often bowing of the femora and tibia (Fig. 8). The genetic abnormality is a mutation of type X collagen. The gene for type X collagen is on chromosome 6q (Dharmavaram *et al.* 1994).

Other forms of metaphyseal dysplasia also exist, including type

Jansen which is extremely rare and has a prevalence of under 0.1 per million. The metaphyses have a striking appearance of a bulbous expanded area and are irregularly mottled. Retarded growth and short stature have been reported and deafness and joint contracture are reported in association. The genetic mutation for this form of metaphyseal dysplasia has been described on chromosome 3p and appears to be an abnormality of a parathyroid hormone receptor.

Other forms of metaphyseal chondrodysplasia associated with malabsorption and neutropenia have been described. Type Peña metaphyseal dysplasia is characterized by marked dwarfing with irregular metaphyseal ossification. Some forms of metaphyseal chondrodysplasia are associated with brachydactyly and retinitis pigmentosa.

Treatment

Atlantoaxial instability occurs, and flexion and extension radiographs of the neck may be necessary to diagnose this. If the instability is significant then fusion may be necessary. In the McKusick pattern of metaphyseal chondrodysplasia, subtrochanteric valgus osteotomy is sometimes necessary. The genu varum deformity seen in this condition rarely requires surgical treatment.

Spondylometaphyseal dysplasia

A variety of forms of spondylometaphyseal dysplasia have been described, including Kozlowski and Sutcliffe types. They are very uncommon with a prevalence of less than 1 per million. The radiological features are principally those of irregular metaphyses. The spine is often involved with platyspondyly and irregularity of the endplates. Stature is usually short although intelligence is normal. One form of spondylometaphyseal dysplasia has been described as being linked to chromosome Xp (Fig. 9).

Short limbs and normal trunk
Achondroplasia

Achondroplasia is the most common form of dwarfism, and is characterized by short limbs, bulging forehead, low nasal bridge, and a lumbar lordosis. The inheritance is autosomal dominant and the prevalence is approximate 3 per million. Many individuals have limitation of elbow extension, a lumbar kyphosis in infancy, and a persistent lumbar kyphosis after 10 years of age in 20 per cent of cases. There is an occasional scoliosis and occasional genu varum. Sometimes the long fibula will disrupt ankle movement.

Radiographic features

The radiographic appearances include small facial bones with occasional hydrocephalus. There is often a short base of skull. In the spine there are short pedicles throughout the length of the spine. The interpedicular distances narrow progressively from L1 to L5. The iliac wings are often squared and the acetabular roof horizontal. The upper femoral metaphyses is splayed. Other metaphyses may also be splayed. Characteristically the hands have a starfish or trident appearance (Fig. 10).

Genetics

The genetic mutation has now been described as an abnormality of the fibroblast growth factor receptor 3 gene. This gene is located on

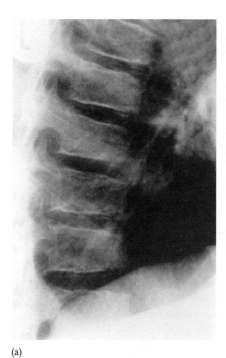

(a)

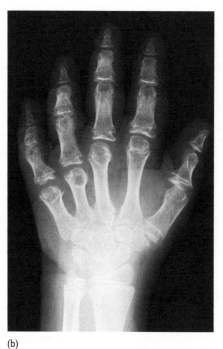

(b)

Fig. 9. Spondylometaphyseal dysplasia. (a) Anteroposterior radiograph of the lumbar spine showing flattened and irregular vertebrae. (b) Anteroposterior radiograph of the hand. The bones are short and the epiphyses abnormal.

chromosome 4p (Shiang *et al.* 1994; Bellus *et al.* 1995; Muenke and Schell 1995).

The fascinating feature of the mutation causing achondroplasia is that it is always at the same nucleotide position (nucleotide 1138). The mutation causes a single amino acid change from arginine to glycine in the transmembrane portion of the cell-surface receptor. The fibroblast growth factor is expressed in all pre-bone and cartilage, and diffusely in the central nervous system. The remarkable consistency of the phenotype in achondroplasia matches well with the very specific point mutation which always seems to cause the disorder. No other autosomal dominant condition has such consistency of phenotype and genetic mutation. The other interesting feature about achondroplasia is that it is strongly related to paternal age. The higher the paternal age the greater the risk of having an achondroplastic child. It is possible that the basis of the mutation is associated with aging sperm formation.

The function of fibroblast growth factor receptor is now under increasing investigation by biologists because of its profound importance in the development of the skeleton. It appears that the normal function of the receptor is to inhibit chondrocyte proliferation in the proliferation zone of the epiphysis. Fibroblast growth factor receptor 3 appears to regulate bone growth by limiting ossification. Another interesting feature of this mutation is that it appears to cause a turning-on of the receptor; this is known as a gain of function mutation. Obviously if some mechanism could be devised to reverse this gain of function, then there is a possibility of treatment of the condition.

Treatment

Some achondroplastics develop hydrocephalus requiring drainage. During childhood there are occasional respiratory problems due to poor development of the nasal sinuses. Some patients also develop symptoms of spinal stenosis which can be significant in some cases.

Genu varum may occur in patients with achondroplasia but they rarely require surgical treatment. Limb-lengthening procedures are now being performed in a number of cases to try and improve adult final height. This type of surgery has considerable implications in terms of possible complications. Adequate counseling of the patient and his or her family is required before undertaking such surgery.

Hypochondroplasia

This condition is difficult to distinguish from achondroplasia, except that the facial appearance is generally normal. The prevalence is approximately 3 per million and is similar to achondroplasia. Radiographic appearances are of a lumbar lordosis with slight decrease in facial bone size. On pelvic radiographs there are large capital femoral epiphyses and trochanters. Some forms of hypochondroplasia have been linked to the fibroblast growth factor receptor 3 gene located on chromosome 4p.

Dyschondrosteosis

This condition often presents with a Madelung type deformity of the distal ulnar with dorsal dislocation of the distal forearm bones. It is characterized by disproportionate growth between the radius and ulna and tibia and fibula, leading to disruptions of the ankle, knee, or wrist joints. Its prevalence is approximately 3 per million and the genetics is unknown.

Mesomelic dysplasia

This is described in a number of types including the Werner type. It is extremely rare and is characterized by absent or dysplastic tibiae with intact fibulae, five-fingered hands, and occasional preaxial polydactyly. It is sometimes associated with congenital heart defects. The genetics is unknown.

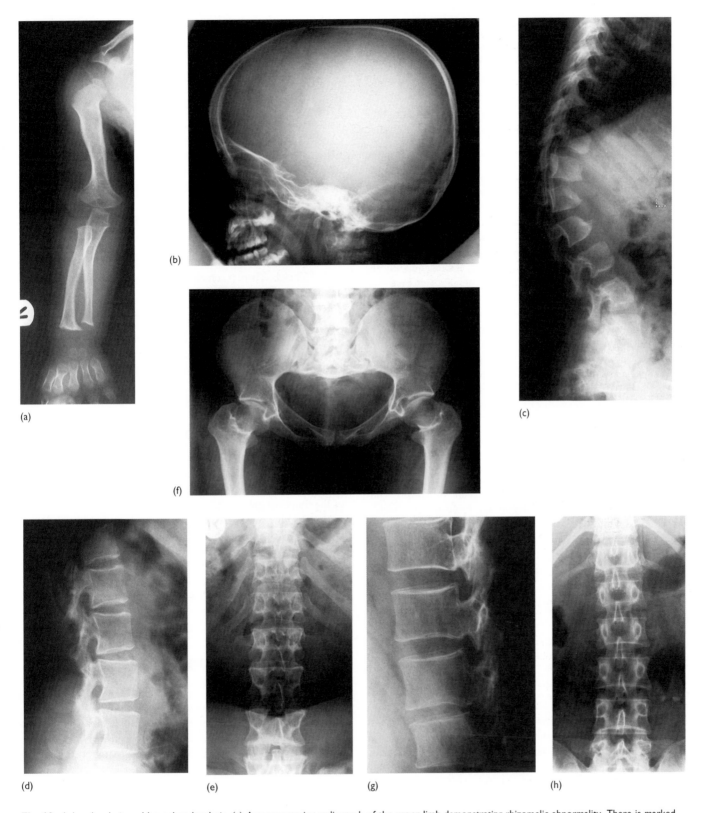

Fig. 10. Achondroplasia and hypochondroplasia. (a) Anteroposterior radiograph of the upper limb demonstrating rhizomelic abnormality. There is marked shortness of the limb which is particularly short in its upper segment. (b) Lateral radiograph of the skull with frontal bossing. (c) Lateral radiograph of the thoracolumbar spine with wedging of the L1 vertebrae. Short pedicles are also present. (d) Lateral radiograph of the lumbar spine demonstrating square vertebral bodies with very short pedicles. (e) Anteroposterior radiograph of the lumbar spine demonstrating progressive narrowing of the intrapedicular distance between L1 and L5. (f) Anteroposterior radiograph of the pelvis. The iliac wings of the pelvis are square with horizontal acetabular roofs. The greater sciatic notch is narrowed. (g) Lateral radiographs of the lumbar spine in hypochondroplasia showing less marked pedicular shortening. (h) Anteroposterior radiographs of the lumbar spine in hypochondroplasia showing no narrowing of the interpedicular distance between L1 and L5.

Acromesomelic dysplasia

Acromesomelic dwarfism is also described and is due predominantly to shortening of the forearm and leg with marked brachydactyly. It is extremely rare and the genetics is unknown.

Short limbs and trunk

Pseudoachondroplasia

Traditionally pseudoachondroplasia is classified in the short limbs and trunk group although it now seems genetically much more suitable to link it with multiple epiphyseal dysplasia. The condition is characterized by a short-limb dwarfism which is sometimes very pronounced. Premature osteoarthritis is common. The prevalence is approximately 4 per million. Clinically the hands are short. Deformities occur due to osteoarthritis of the joints. Radiographically the spine presents with variable deformities of the vertebrae and platyspondyly. The long bones are short with flared metaphyses. The predominant abnormalities are in the epiphyses which are small, irregular, and fragmented. Genetically the condition is now linked to an abnormality of the cartilage oligomeric matrix protein which is located on chromosome 19p (Fig. 11) (Briggs *et al.* 1995).

Orthopedic treatment is usually restricted to joint replacement surgery for severe disease of the hips. Occasionally other joints may be very symptomatic in which case fusion is a surgical option.

Diastrophic dysplasia

This extremely rare condition has features of short-limb dwarfism with joint contractures. Intelligence is normal, the final adult height is between 79 cm and 140 cm, and there are progressive contractures of all joints. Radiographically the spine presents with a dysplastic odontoid and variably irregular vertebral bodies. In the pelvis and hip there is flaring of the iliac wings, and the capital epiphysis is often late in appearing and may be deformed. Radiographs of the hand reveal irregular long metacarpals with bizarre ossification. An unusual feature is shortening of the first metacarpal which is sometimes placed very proximally. The condition is given the name 'hitchhiker's thumb'. Genetically the condition is interesting and has been linked to a sulfate transporter gene located on chromosome 5q.

Kniest dysplasia

This presents with abnormal facial appearance with depressed nasal bridge. There is associated deafness and myopia and marked short stature. The condition is extremely rare with a prevalence of under 0.1 per million. There is often scoliosis and joint contractures.

Radiographically the spine shows irregular platyspondyly with scoliosis and kyphosis. The long bones have broad metaphyses and irregular epiphyses. Genetically the condition is linked to the type II collagen gene on chromosome 12q.

Dyggve–Melchior–Clausen disease

This is a form of short-trunk dwarfism with mental retardation. Characteristically the spine has platyspondyly with notching on the lateral view. In some respects it is similar to Morquio's disease with sternal protrusion, scoliosis, and malalignment. The prevalence is extremely rare and the genetics is unknown.

Chondroectodermal dysplasia (Ellis–van Creveld syndrome)

This form of short-limb dwarfism is associated with abnormal hair, teeth, and nails. There is sometimes a postaxial polydactyly. Congenital heart disease is also associated. The frequency is rare and the genetics is unknown.

Hand deformities may require surgical correction including polydactyly and syndactyly. Progressive deformities of the knee, usually genu vagum, often require surgical correction with a supracondylar osteotomy of the femur. This osteotomy sometimes has to be repeated.

Lethal forms of short-limb dwarfism

There are a number of forms of lethal short-limb dwarfism. Death is usually from respiratory failure shortly after birth. The most common forms are thanatophoric dwarfism which is due to mutation of the fibroblast growth factor receptor 3 gene located on chromosome 4p. Other forms are associated with short-limbed polydactyly syndromes, the cause of which is unknown. Finally, achondrogenesis types 1 and II may occur. Achondrogenesis type I is due to an abnormality of the sulfate transport gene located on chromosome 5q and achondrogenesis type II, sometimes known as hypochondrogenesis, is due to a mutation of type II collagen gene located on chromosome 12q.

Increased limb length

Marfan's syndrome

The frequency of this condition is approximately 2 per million. However, a significantly larger number of people present with what is described as a Marfanoid habitus. The prevalence of this condition is between 15 and 20 per million. The clinical characteristics are dis-

Fig. 11. Pseudoachondroplasia. (a) Anteroposterior radiograph of the pelvis with marked destructive change in the hip joint and coxa vara. (b) Lateral radiograph of the lumbar spine with notching of the vertebral enplates and some platispondyly. (c) Anteroposterior radiograph of the knees with significant irregularity of the epiphyses which are small. There is also some abnormality of the metaphyses. (d) Anteroposterior radiograph of the shoulder with grossly disorganized proximal humerus and abnormality of the glenohumeral joint. (e) Anteroposterior radiograph of the hand showing short fingers and metacarpals with abnormality of the epiphyses. (f) Anteroposterior radiograph of the feet showing short toes and metatarsals with early degenerative change. (g) Anteroposterior radiographs of the pelvis in childhood showing an irregular and small capital epiphysis. (h) Anteroposterior radiographs of the femur in a milder form of the condition.

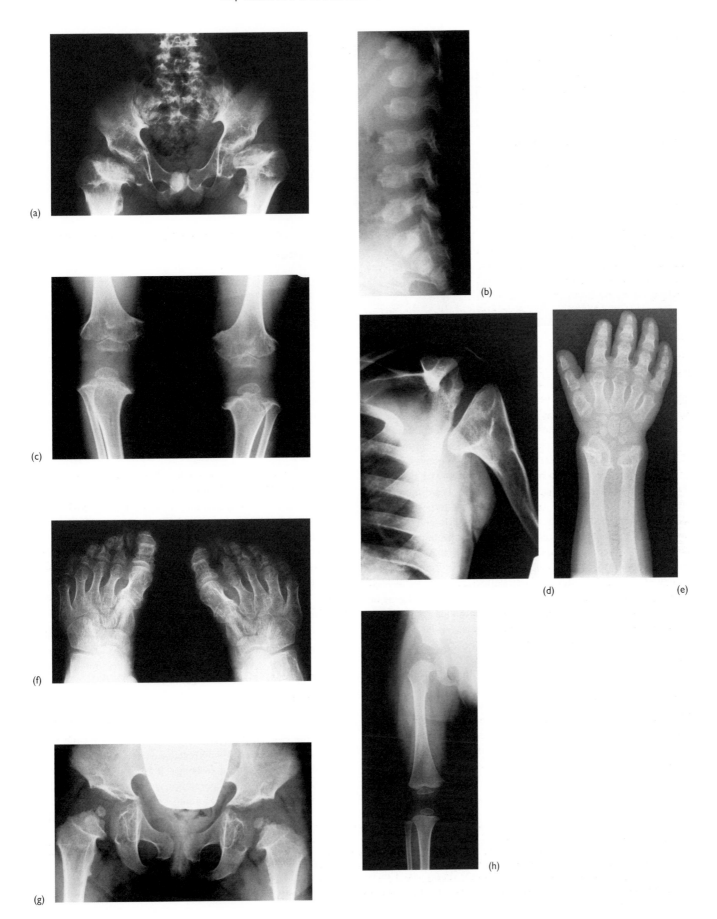

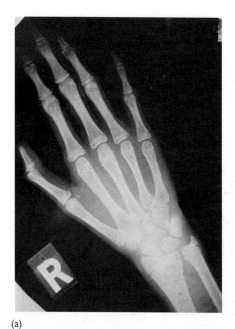

(a)

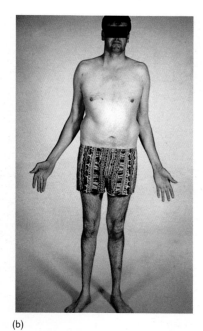

(b)

Fig. 12. Marfan's syndrome. (a) Anteroposterior radiograph of the hand with gross elongation of the phalanges and metacarpals. This is arachnodactyly. (b) Marfan's syndrome.

proportionately long limbs. There is generalized joint laxity and often associated scoliosis and herniae. Because there are no precise features in Marfan's syndrome a diagnosis requires the presence of three hard criteria (subluxed lens, aortic dilatation, and scoliosis or chest deformity). Alternatively a clear family history of Marfan's syndrome and two of these criteria are required. This system was devised by Pyeritz. In the classical Marfan's syndrome there is a dislocation of lens and aortic aneurysm. Less commonly, short sightedness, detached retina, cataract, high arch palate, and dislocation of joints may occur. Contractures of the hand are not uncommon and may form part of a separate condition known as contractural arachnodactyly. Congenital contractural arachnodactyly is also dominantly inherited with disproportionate body stature. The genetics of Marfan's syndrome has revealed an abnormality of the fibrilin I gene on chromosome 15q. Congenital contractural arachnodactyly is due to a mutation of the fibrilin II gene on chromosome 5q (Fig. 12) (Dietz *et al.* 1991; Tsipouras *et al.* 1992).

Commonly Marfan patients are managed in multidisciplinary clinics. Surgical correction may be necessary for scoliotic deformity. The main problem is with management of cardiovascular pathology. If the aortic root exceeds 4 cm in diameter then treatment with β-blockers is often advocated. If the aortic root becomes greater than 6 cm in diameter than an aortic graft replacement is indicated. Pregnancy can produce catastrophic cardiovascular problems in patients with Marfan's syndrome.

Homocystinuria

This also features body disproportion. Often mental retardation occurs with lens dislocation. There is sometimes joint laxity, arachnodactyly, and pectus excavatum. Genetically this condition is due to a mutation of the gene for cystathionine β-synthase. This is located on chromosome 21q. A second form of homocystinuria is

due to a mutation on chromosome 1p and is known to be a problem with the gene for methyl-methylenetetrahydrofolate reductase.

Storage diseases

There are two broad groups of storage diseases. Those involving the mucolipids and those involving the mucopolysaccharides. Genetically these have been grouped into mucolipidoses I and II which are due to enzyme defects localized to chromosome 4q. The mucopolysaccharidoses have been grouped into at least seven different types. These have been described as being related to enzyme deficiencies of idioronidase galactosamine and galactosidase. Various chromosomal allocations have been found and these are shown in Table 2.

Treatment

Generally surgical treatment in the storage diseases is aimed at attempting to keep the patient mobile and out of a wheelchair. This usually requires correction of joint contractures but on occasion spinal fusion is required for spinal instability.

Morquio syndrome

Unlike the Hunter and Hurler syndromes and their close relatives Scheie syndrome and Sanfilippo syndrome, this condition can be distinguished clinically at an early age. It is characterized by normal intelligence. The clinical appearance is of prominent maxilla and broad mouth. Those with Morquio syndrome are usually of short stature with a disproportionately short trunk. Deformities include a genu valgum and marked joint laxity. Radiologically the spine shows platyspondyly with an absent or dysplastic odontoid peg (Fig. 13). On chest radiographs the characteristic feature is of a marked manubriosternal angle which may be almost 90°. Radiographs of the wrists and hands are similar to those in Hurler syndrome with pointed

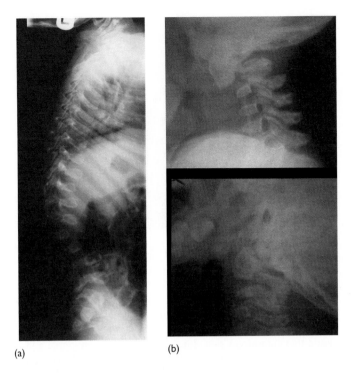

(a)

(b)

Fig. 13. Morquio syndrome. (a) Lateral thoracolumbar spine demonstrating platispondyly with a centrally protruding tongue from the anterior surface. (b) Flexion and extension views of the cervical spine demonstrating odontoid hypoplasia and atlantoaxial instability.

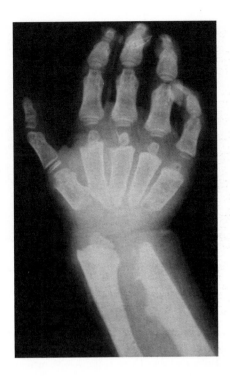

Fig. 14. Hurler syndrome. Anteroposterior radiograph of the hand, showing lack of diaphyseal modeling with disordered growth, particularly at the metaphyses. The mid-metacarpals have the feature of a pointed base in the second to fifth bones.

proximal ends to the metacarpals. However, in Morquio syndrome the small bones of the hands are well modeled.

Hurler syndrome

This storage disorder is sometimes known as gargoylism. It is characterized by short stature which is proportionate. There is a progressive mental retardation with hepatomegaly and splenomegaly. The joints are generally stiff and develop degenerative changes. The facial appearance may be normal at birth but progresses to increasing protrusion of the tongue with a large head and frontal bossing. There is often disordered breathing as the airways become progressively blocked. There may be chronic upper airways infection and deafness. Initially intelligence appears normal but mental retardation progresses. Corneal opacities are sometimes present and skeletally there is deformity of the spine with kyphosis and coxa valga. Radiographically the skull shows enlargement with thick base of skull and orbital roofs. The sella turcica is J-shaped, and evidence of hydrocephalus may be present. The vertebrae become hooked, being deficient in their anterior and superior parts. The clavicles are often broad at the medial end and ribs are paddle shaped. Pelvic radiographs show flared iliac bones with sloping acetabulae. The long bones often have lack of diaphyseal modeling and appear thick. Radiographs of the wrists and hands show pointed ends to the proximal ends of the metacarpals particularly numbers 2 to 5. Sadly, this

is a progressive disorder with death often occurring by the end of 10 to 15 years (Fig. 14).

Hunter syndrome

This is similar in onset and appearance to Hurler syndrome but is generally less severe. All the patients are male. There is a slightly longer lifespan and the radiological appearances are less marked.

The mucolipidoses

This is a group of storage diseases which present with course facial appearance and skeletal features similar to the mucopolysaccharidosis. However, in the long bones the distinguishing feature is periosteal bone formation associated with lack of modeling of the diaphysis.

Gaucher's disease

This is a disease resulting from an accumulation of glucocerebroside in organs and tissues throughout the body. Characteristically it forms in storage cells known as Gaucher's cells. This is the most common of the glycolipid storage diseases and there are three clinical types: type I, the adult non-neuronopathic chronic form; type II, the infantile neuronopathic acute form; type III, the juvenile neuronopathic subacute form. The clinical features of these three forms are as follows.

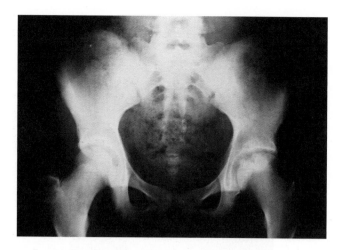

Fig. 15. Gaucher's disease showing osteoarthritis at the hip joints.

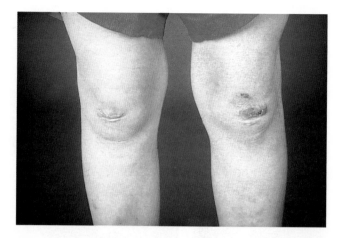

Fig. 16. Ehlers–Danlos syndrome type I showing abnormal scarring of the skin on the anterior aspect of the knee.

Type I

Type I shows organomegaly, hematological disorders secondary to hypersplenism, and bone lesions attributable to the medullury infiltration by Gaucher's cells. There is no involvement of the central nervous system.

Type II

There is early involvement of the brain and cranial nerves. The disease is fatal by 2 years of age.

Type III

There is involvement of visceral organs bone and central nervous system. Neurological symptoms are less severe and appear later. The transmission is thought to be autosomal recessive and is common in Ashkenazi Jews. Frequently ischemic necrosis occurs and there is evidence of femoral head collapse and secondary osteoarthritis (Fig. 15). Surgery is sometimes necessary to replace the hip joint for severe pain.

Ehlers–Danlos syndrome

Ehlers–Danlos syndrome is a large and somewhat heterogenous group of heritable disorders which affect tissues such as ligaments, skin, joints, blood vessels, and other internal organs. The condition is now classified into 10 different forms.

Ehlers–Danlos syndrome types I, II, and III

These forms of Ehlers–Danlos syndrome are described together because they differ only in their severity. The main features are marked joint laxity with occasional aortic and valve rupture. In the milder form (type III) the only feature is generalized hypermobility. The genetics is autosomal dominant and has recently been linked to the type V collagen located on chromosome 9q (Fig. 16).

Ehlers–Danlos syndrome type IV

This is a dreadful and life-threatening disease. It manifests with a tendency to bruising and bleeding with extreme fragility of blood vessels. The basic defect in this form of Ehlers–Danlos syndrome is an absence of type III collagen. The affected individuals have hyperelastic thin translucent skin. Joint hypermobility is minimal and is limited to the small joints. The skin covering hands and feet is often finely wrinkled. This makes the individuals look older and the condition is sometimes known as acrogeria. Unfortunately the hallmark of this type of Ehlers–Danlos syndrome is life-threatening internal bleeding from ruptures of vessels or bowel. The genetic mutation has now been localized to type III collagen which is present on chromosome 2q.

Ehlers–Danlos syndrome type V

This form of Ehlers–Danlos syndrome is extremely rare, and only two families and eight members have ever been described. It appears to X linked. All patients have the features of extensible skin but only mild tissue fragility. In may not be a separate entity.

Ehlers–Danlos syndrome type VI

This condition is due to a marked deficiency of lysyl hydroxylase. This is an enzyme involved in cross-linking of collagen. The clinical features are of generalized hypertonia. Kyphoscoliosis is often present at birth and they have a Marfanoid habitus. Osteoporosis is common but there does not appear to be a tendency to fractures. Ocular fragility sometimes leads to retinal detachment. It is inherited as an autosomal recessive trait in common with most enzyme defects.

Ehlers–Danlos syndrome type VII

This form of Ehlers–Danlos syndrome involves ligaments and joint capsules. Congenital hip dislocation at birth is common; other joints may also be dislocated including shoulders, wrists, and knees. It is an autosomal dominant condition and appears to be due to mutations in the genes for type I collagen located on chromosomes 17q and 7q (Fig. 17) (Carr *et al.* 1994).

Ehlers–Danlos syndrome type VIII

Ehlers–Danlos type VIII is a rare dominantly inherited disorder of unknown cause. Joint laxity is mild to moderate, hyperextensibility

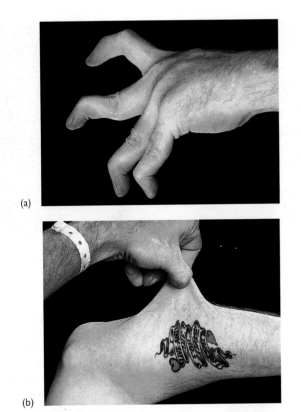

(a)

(b)

Fig. 17. Ehlers–Danlos syndrome type VII. (a) Marked joint hypermobility is present. (b) The excessive laxity of the skin is demonstrated.

is mild or absent, and fragility of the skin is mild to severe. There is no evidence of involvement of viscera. The patients have a Marfanoid habitus, and minor trauma produces bruising. Dental disease is common, with caries occurring. These characteristic features of the teeth cause it to be known as the periodontal form of Ehlers–Danlos syndrome.

Ehlers–Danlos syndrome type IX

This is sometimes known as the occipital horn syndrome. The features are a loose skin which is not easily bruisable. It is felt that this should be excluded from the Ehlers–Danlos syndrome group and should be reclassified as a disorder of copper transport.

Ehlers–Danlos syndrome type X

This is a relatively new description and is illustrated by one family only. The features are of joint hypermobility and a thin but non-velvety skin. Mitral valve prolapse occurs and the aortic root is at the upper limit of normal. As yet the biochemical and genetic bases for the disorder is not known. However, a defect in fibronectin has been suggested.

Alkaptonuria

Alkpatonuria was first recognized in 1859 by Boedeker. He remarked that the color of a patient's urine turned dark on exposure to the air. The condition was further described in 1866 by Virchow when it was associated with the pigmentation of connective tissue in a 67-year-old man. The chemical structure of alkpton was not established until 1891 by Wolkow and Baumann. It was thereafter known as homogentisic acid because of its relationship to gentisic acid.

The inheritance of alkaptonuria was first described in 1902 by Garrod who was the Professor of Medicine in Oxford. This disease marks a milestone in the understanding of human diseases and was the first condition known to be behaving as a Mendelian trait in human. The recessive character of the disease was confirmed in all the families they observed. Interestingly the localization of the homogentisic acid oxidase gene has only recently been described on chromosome 3q (Fernandez-Canon *et al.* 1996).

Clinical features

Alkaptonuria is characterized by pigmentation of the cartilage of the ear and the cornea of the eye. Deposition of the ochronotic pigment also occurs in articular cartilage. One of the characteristic features of alkaptonuria is early onset of arthritis. Wafer-thin calcification is often seen in the intervertebral discs on lateral spinal radiographs. Because of the early onset of osteoarthritis, joint replacement may be necessary. The small joints of the hands, feet, wrists, and ankles are rarely affected. The most severe involvement is in hips, knees, shoulders, and elbows (Fig. 18).

The precise relationship between deposition of the pigment and degenerative changes is not known. Histologically the ochronotic pigment involvement in cartilage is within collagen bundles which lose striation, swell, and then fracture.

Hemophilia

Hemophilia as a term was first attributed to Schonlein in 1818. It was probably first referred to in a dissertation by his pupil Hopf. The disease was well recognized by the Jews and religious writers of the fifth century AD because of the complications of circumcision in babies with hemophilia. The term hemophilia is from the Greek 'love of blood'.

It was the appearance and transmission of hemophilia within the royal families of Europe during the nineteenth and twentieth centuries that promoted much research in this area. The Tsarevich Alexis's severe hemophilia resulted in him having severe joint disease early in life. The disease is recognized as being a deficiency of factor VIII (hemophilia A) or factor IX (hemophilia B). Early therapeutic treatment with factor VIII acquired from blood donation was unfortunately complicated by high incidence of HIV-1 infection in hemophiliacs treated with these blood products between 1980 and 1995. Recently developed synthetic factors and better donor screening has essentially eradicated this problem.

Hemophilia has an incidence of 10 per 100 000 male births and its distribution is uniform around the world. Hemophilia is inherited as a sex-linked recessive disorder.

Clinical features

One of the major clinical features of hemophilia is widespread hemorrhage occurring either spontaneously or with minor trauma. Hemorrhaging may be intracerebral but is more commonly into the musculoskeletal system either into muscles or joints. Frequent hemarthrosis is the cause of early joint degeneration. The onset of the disorder and the frequency of bleeds depends on the severity of the

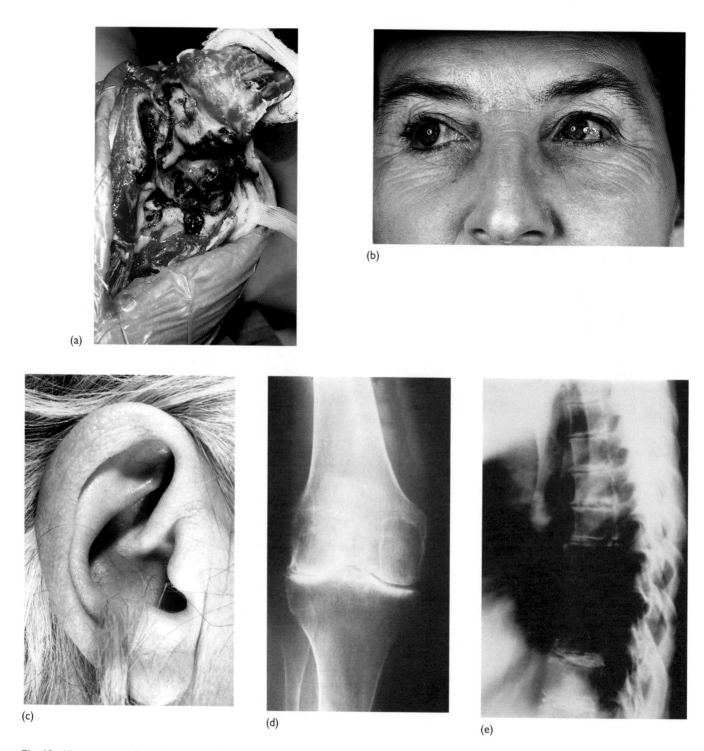

Fig. 18. Alkpatonuria. (a) Black pigmentation is present in the synovium and articular surface of the joint predisposing to early-onset osteoarthritis. (b) The sclera of the eye is blackened. (c) The cartilage of the pinna of the ear is also black. (d) Early osteoarthritis of joints is common. (e) The condition is characterized by calcification of the intervertebral discs.

factor deficiency. Levels of less than 5 per cent of factor VIII are associated with severe and recurrent bleeding. Factor VIII levels of greater than 20 per cent are much less frequently associated with bleeding problems.

Management

Hemophilia centers have been established to provide multi-disciplinary expertise for the management of hemophiliac problems. Early treatment of an acute hemarthrosis is essential if damage is to be limited. Use of synthetic factor VIII or factor IX is now routinely advocated and self-administration is possible. Because of the severity of bleeding in some patients, surgery is sometimes necessary either in the form of synovectomy or joint replacement. Occasionally nerve entrapment occurs as a result of the synovitis. For further information see Chapter 1.8.

Metabolic bone disease

A number of disorders of the skeleton arise from metabolic defects. These are discussed in greater detail in a separate section of the book. Some of these conditions will be outlined in this chapter.

Hypophosphatasia

This is a condition associated with a low alkaline phosphatase which results in poor mineralization of bone and metaphyseal defects. The frequency is not known but the condition is rare. Clinically the children often have normal stature, but with failure of bone formation short stature appears. A severe congenital form is known to be lethal and the children are often stillborn. Those that do survive have failure to thrive and often have pathologic fractures. The deformities of the bones are generally similar to those of rickets with bending of bone and metaphyseal changes. The condition is known to be due to a mutation of the alkaline phosphatase gene on chromosome 1p.

Idiopathic hyperphosphatasia

This is probably an autosomal recessive condition and is characterized by high levels of alkaline phosphatase. Clinically the children have thick and fragile bones often with patchy sclerosis. Survival is very rare. Children who do survive into infancy often have paralysis of cranial nerves due to encroachment of the cranial exit foraminae. The long bones demonstrate osteoporosis with very poor differentiation between the medulla and cortex.

Hypophosphatemic rickets (vitamin D resistant)

This interesting X-linked dominant condition is rare. Stature is often short but intelligence normal. Children usually present with limb deformity and short stature. Radiographs reveal wide epiphyseal plates which are difficult to distinguish from nutritional rickets. The metaphyses may be cupped. Looser zones are present in some bones. It should be distinguished from nutritional rickets and osteomalacia. Treatment is possible with the use of 1α-hydroxycholecalciferol and an oral phosphate. The gene for hypophosphatemia has now been localized to chromosome Xp.

Pseudohypoparathyroidsm

This is genetically now linked to a binding protein called the G protein. The chromosomal allocation is to 20q. It is a very rare condition and associated with short metacarpals and mental retardation.

Table 4 Sillence classification of osteogenesis imperfecta

Type I	Autosomal dominant	Mild form
		Mild to moderate bone fragility
		No deformity
		Blue sclerae
		Early hearing loss, easy bruising
		Mild to moderate short stature
		1A. No dentinogenesis imperfecta
		1B. Dentinogenesis imperfecta present
Type II	Autosomal dominant or recessive	Perinatal lethal or severe
		Fragility of all connective tissue
		Intrauterine fractures
		Intrauterine growth retardation
		Soft large skull
		Micromelia, beaded ribs, long bones
		Short and deformed
Type III	Autosomal recessive	Progressive deforming
		Severe bone fragility
		In utero fractures
		Severe osteoporosis
		Macrocephaly triangular facies
		Fractures with deformity and bowing
		White sclerae
		Extreme short stature, scoliosis
Type IV	Autosomal dominant	More severe than type I
		Long-bone bowing
		Light sclerae
		Moderate short stature
		Moderate joint laxity
		Type IV A. No dentinogenesis imperfecta
		Type IV B. Dentinogenesis imperfecta

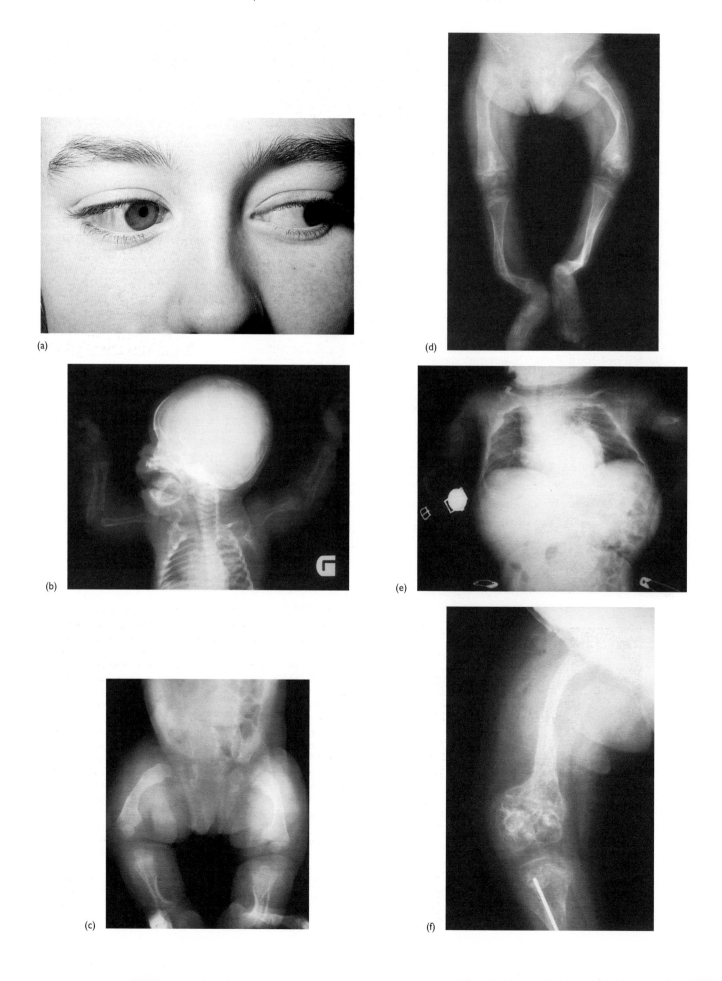

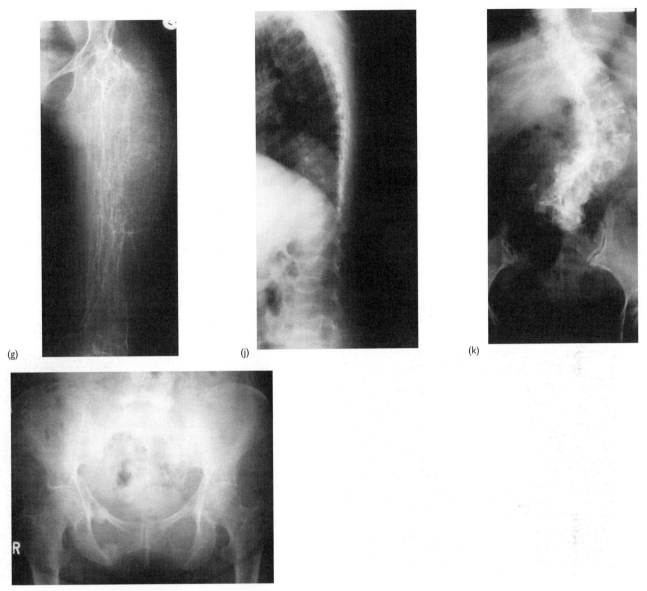

(g)

(j)

(k)

(h)

(i)

Fig. 19. Osteogenesis imperfecta. (a) The blue sclera are characteristic of type I osteogenesis imperfecta. (b) Perinatal lethal or severe. Radiograph showing a baby with severe osteogenesis imperfecta showing a lateral view of the skull with wormian bones. (c) Anteroposterior radiographs of the legs of a baby with severe osteogenesis imperfecta showing fractures and deformity of femora and tibiae. (d) Progressive deforming osteogenesis imperfecta with severe deformity of the tibia. (e) Anteroposterior radiograph of the torso in severe osteogenesis imperfecta with considerable deformity of the chest associated with severe scoliosis. The humeri are grossly deformed and shortened. (f) Severe osteogenesis imperfecta with a transverse fracture of the mid-femur. The distal femur is bulbous and deformed. This appearance is sometimes known as popcorn bone. (g) Osteogenesis imperfecta is sometimes complicated by formation of callus around bones. This is known as hyperplastic callus and is shown here in a radiograph of the femur. (h) In more mild forms of osteogenesis imperfecta fractures may be present of the superior and inferior pubic ramai as shown here. (i) In mild forms of osteogenesis imperfecta (type I) the characteristic features maybe those of generalized osteoporosis and a metaphyseal buckle fracture as shown here in the distal tibia. (j) This lateral radiograph of the thoracolumbar spine shows osteoporosis of the vertebral bodies. The bodies have collapsed. The vertebral discs are still well preserved and have an excessive convexity where they have indented the surrounding vertebral bodies. (k) Because of the gross osteoporosis, a scoliotic deformity may appear as demonstrated here in the lumbar spine.

Radiograpically, ectopic calcification sometimes occurs in subcutaneous tissues.

Conditions of decreased bone density

Osteogenesis imperfecta

This relatively common condition has a frequency of approximately 1 in 20 000 births (Byers 1993). The classification of the condition is shown in Table 4 and is a modification of the system described by Sillence. The condition is characterized by major bone fragility and fractures. The phenotype varies according to the different clinical type but all forms of the condition are due to mutations of one of the two genes for type I collagen. These are localized to chromosomes 17q and 7q. Biochemically the most common feature is a complete loss of proteinaceous material within bone. This is due to so-called null alleles. A mutation causing a null allele leads to the loss of 50 per cent of the type I collagen protein. However, some mutations lead to the production of faulty protein and therefore produce connective tissue with abnormal proteins within it. The phenotype of this type of mutation is often much worse than a simple deletion.

However, even within families with the same mutation the phenotype can vary considerably. Mutations in the gene for the α_1 chain are generally more severe than mutations in the gene for the α_2 chain. This is probably because the roles of the α_1 and α_2 chains are not identical and because the ratio of α_1 collagen to α_2 collagen collagen is 2:1. Mosaicism has also been described in cases of osteogeneses imperfecta when not all the cells of an individual are producing abnormal collagen. This can further affect the phenotype (Fig. 19).

The condition is also associated with dentinogenesis imperfecta. Dentine contains type I collagen and some types of osteogenesis imperfecta are associated with grossly abnormal teeth formation. One of the great problems with osteogenesis imperfecta is in the milder forms (particularly type IV) where repeated fractures in childhood can sometimes be put down to child abuse or neglect rather than the true underlying condition. This has produced many difficult clinical and legal problems. Some authors would contend that any type of fracture can occur in osteogenesis imperfecta; however, others state certain patterns of fracture, particularly metaphyseal chip fractures, are diagnostic of child abuse. Occasionally biochemical studies can help where abnormal proteins can be shown in tissues therefore confirming the diagnosis of osteogenesis imperfecta. Unfortunately, not all individuals with osteogenesis imperfecta can be detected with biochemical tests. Some families have also asked for antenatal diagnosis of osteogenesis imperfecta. This is sometimes possible where the specific mutation in a particular family is known. It requires the use of chorionic villous biopsies and ultrasound studies of fetuses. Unfortunately, it is not appropriate for sporadic and new cases, and even in families where the mutation is known, the technique can sometimes fail.

Treatment

Surgical correction of spinal deformities is fraught with complications although on occasions it is necessary if respiratory and cardiac complications are present. The poor bone density produces significant risk of failure of any surgical implants used to correct deformity.

In the progressive deforming form of osteogenesis imperfecta, telescoping rods have been popularized by Bailey and Dubow. The surgical technique involves multiple osteotomies of the long bone, usually the femur, and the insertion of a rod which extends during growth. This form of surgical treatment has produced a reduction in deformity and in the number of fractures in some children.

Indications for rodding are recurrent fractures, progressive deformity, and loss of function. The surgery is sometimes complicated by pulmonary hyperpyrexia, and the anesthetist should avoid muscle relaxants.

Idiopathic juvenile osteoporosis

This is an extremely rare condition which has features of osteoporosis in childhood and usually associated with remission in late teenage years. The features are those of thin and fragile bones particularly the thoracic vertebrae.

Sclerosing bone dysplasias

Osteopetrosis

This condition features bone fragility and increased bone density. There is poor modeling of bone, and occasionally osteoarthritis may develop. It is rare but probably has a prevalence of around 1 per million. Radiographs reveal a thickened skull, vault, and base, with obstructive foramina and sometimes hydrocephalus. The long bones have expanded metaphases and there is a poor distinction between cortex and medulla. The spinal radiographs also show marked increased density of the vertebral bodies. Genetically it is possible that a mutation for a macrophage colony-stimulating factor on chromosome 1p may be involved (Fig. 20).

Pycnodysostosis

This condition also appears to be due to a mutation on chromosome 1q and is characterized by short stature, osteosclerosis, and increase bone fragility. There may also be hyperplastic clavicles and dysplastic terminal phalanges. The prevalence is under 1 per million.

Craniometaphyseal dysplasia

This is a very rare condition and is similar in some ways to Pyle's disease. Its features are of metaphyseal expansion with cortical thinning, and skull radiographs show abnormal thickening of the vault and facial bones which may be severe in some cases.

Engelmann's disease (progressive diaphyseal dysplasia)

This rare condition is associated with weakness and hypertonia. There is some diaphyseal thickening of bones and sometimes sclerosis of the skull. It usually presents in infancy with failure to thrive. The genetic defect is not known.

Osteopathia striata

This is the only condition where linear striaton of bones occurs. It is very rare and the biochemical defect is not known.

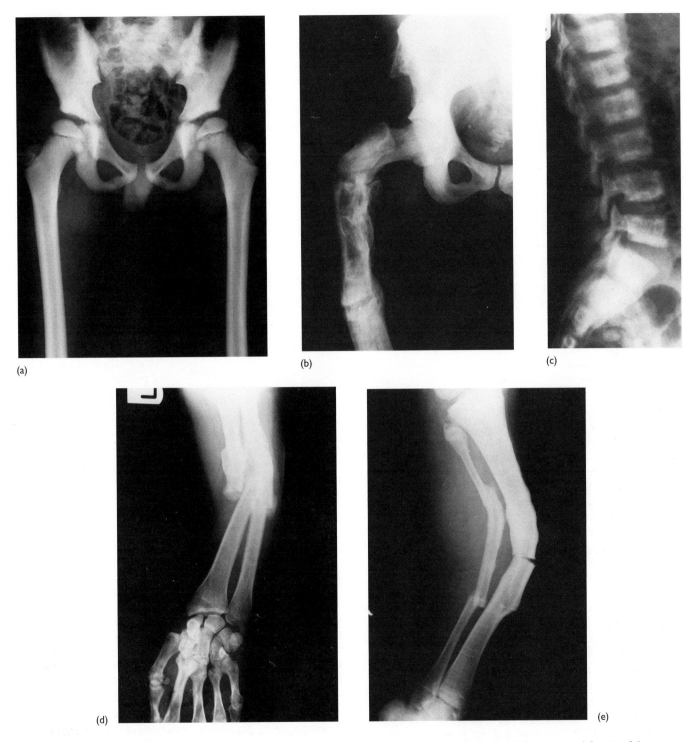

Fig. 20. Osteopetrosis. (a) Osteopetrosis affecting the pelvis and upper femora. (b) Osteopetrosis with fractures and characteristic deformity of the proximal femur. (c) Osteopetrosis affecting the lumbar spine. (d) Osteopetrosis of the forearm with fractures of the radius and ulnar. (e) Osteopetrosis of the leg with typical transverse fractures of the tibia and fibula with consequent deformity. Lines of growth arrest can also be seen.

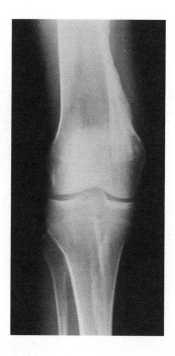

Fig. 21. Melorheostosis.

Osteopoikilosis

This condition has the characteristic appearance of stippling of the ends of long bones rather than diaphyses. It is extremely rare and the underlying cause is not known.

Melorheostosis

This unusual condition which is usually unilateral is associated with irregular masses of sclerotic bone apparently stuck to the surface of bone shafts. This may cause some interference with joint movement. The biochemical and genetic defect is not known (Fig. 21).

Tumor-like bone dysplasias

Diaphyseal aclasis (multiple hereditary exostosis)

This is the most common genetic disorder of bone with a prevalence of probably 10 per million. It is an autosomal dominant condition and recently the genetic mutation has been described in some of these cases. Localizations have been made to chromosomes 8q, 11p, and 19p. The gene has been cloned on chromosome 8q and may be a form of tumor suppressor gene. Presenting features are with bony lumps which are often noted at birth but may occur during childhood. The ribs and scapulae and pectoral and pelvic girdles are frequently the site of exostoses which may be large and may cause blocks to movement. The cartilage-capped exostoses also appear on the long bones (Fig. 22). The true extent and size of the lesions may not be evident on plain radiographs, and ultrasound or magnetic resonance imaging (MRI) of the cartilage cap will reveal their full

size. The exostoses usually stop growing at skeletal maturity; any exostosis that continues to grow or one where the cartilage cap is greater than 2 to 3 mm in size beyond the end of skeletal maturity should be regarded with some suspicion. Exostoses that are located more proximally are also suspicious. There are reports of conversion to chondrosarcoma although the true prevalence of this is not known. Exostoses of the radius and ulna commonly produce problems with rotation of the forearm.

Trichorhinophalangeal syndrome

This is characterized by sparse hair with a characteristic facial appearance with wide mouth and long nose. Exostoses occasionally occur and it has a prevalence of 5 to 10 per million. The genetic mutation is probably linked to the exostosis gene on chromosome 8q.

Malformation syndromes
Apert's syndrome

This condition forms one of the craniosynostoses which are usually distinguished by features of congenital limb anomalies and inheritance. Apert's syndrome occurs in approximately 0.5 per million births. There is abnormal fusion or early fusion of the coronal suture of the skull. Limb anomalies include distal joining of the digits particularly the second to the fourth digits. The thumb metacarpal is usually normal but there may be only one phalanx and it may be trapezoid in shape. The feet show some deformities. Genetically this condition has now been linked to an abnormality of the fibroblast growth factor receptor 2 gene located on chromosome 10q.

Crouzon syndrome

Crouzon syndrome is a similar craniosynostosis and has been linked to the same gene as Apert's syndrome. Features are those of limb abnormalities and early fusion of the skull sutures.

Cleidocranial dysplasia

This unusual condition is characterized by an abnormal facial appearance with bulging frontal bone and parietal ridges. There may be disordered eruption of teeth and the clavicles are absent (Fig. 23). This allows the shoulders to droop and to be excessively mobile. Wormian bones are present on skull radiographs and there may be failure of fusion of the mandibular epiphyses. The spinal radiograph reveals retarded ossification of vertebrae. Although the clavicles are usually absent, pseudarthrosis may sometimes occur with persistence of some parts of the clavicle. Very rarely a pseudarthrosis of the femur occurs. Interestingly the congenital pseudarthrosis of the clavicle is almost always on the right side. Genetic mutation for this condition has been localized to chromosome 6p.

Craniocarpotarsal dysplasia

This is sometimes known as the Freeman–Sheldon syndrome or whistling face syndrome. The features are of a characteristic small mouth as though the child was whistling. Intelligence is normal. There are sometimes hand and foot abnormalities with ulnar devi-

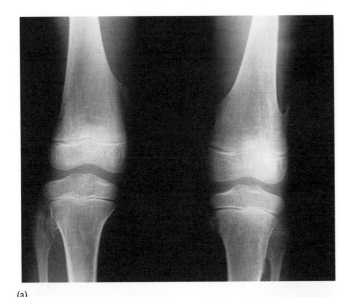

(a)

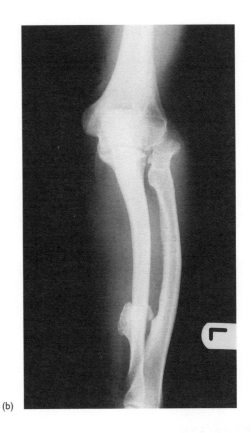

(b)

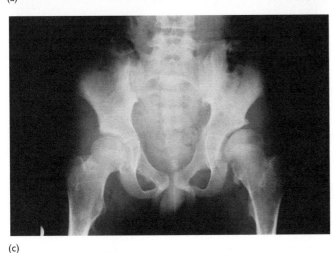

(c)

Fig. 22. Diaphyseal aclasis. (a) Osteochondromas are present in both the distal femur and proximal tibia. (b) Diaphyseal aclasis of the forearm with osteochondromas of both radius and ulnar. Osteochondroma in this region cause considerable problems with forearm rotation and function of the hand and upper limb. (c) Exostoses have occurred round the proximal femora.

ation of the hand. Occasionally congenital dislocation of the hip and scoliosis are associated. It should be differentiated from arthrogryposis. The genetic defect is not known.

Cornelia de Lange syndrome

This condition has a characteristic facial appearance with low hair line and the eyebrows meeting in the middle, with a small nose. There is mental retardation and the skeletal deformities include short metacarpals and syndactyl. The biochemistry and genetic defects are not known.

Larsen's syndrome

This is a very rare condition with a prevalence of less than 1 per million. There are multiple congenital dislocations usually of the hips and knees. The facial appearance is with a depressed nasal bridge and bulging forehead. The genetic mutation is now known to be on chromosome 3p.

Nail–patella syndrome

This rare condition has been linked to a locus determining ABO blood groups. The mutation is now known to be on chromosome 9q. Clinically it is characterized by abnormal nail development and growth. There are also often small high-riding patellae and congenital dislocation of the radial head. An additional feature is on pelvic radiograph where an iliac horn projects from the middle of the iliac wings. Occasionally renal dysfunction and proteinurea may be present (Fig. 24).

Enchondromatosis (Ollier's disease)

This condition is characterized by multiple lesions of cartilage usually occurring within the metaphyseal region of long bones. No distinct genetic pattern is known.

Clinical features

The enchondromatosis usually becomes evident in early childhood and presents with swelling of the limb bones or occasionally the

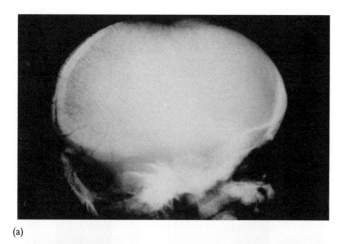

(a)

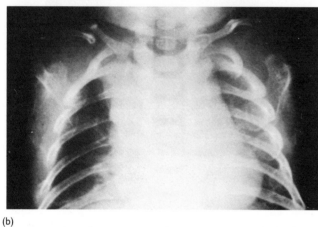

(b)

Fig. 23. Cleidocranial dysplasia. (a) Characteristic appearance of the skull with bulging fontanels and wormian bones. (b) The clavicles may be absent. The clavicles may have hypoplasia of their lateral ends.

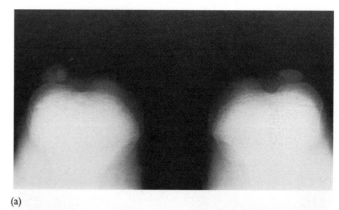

(a)

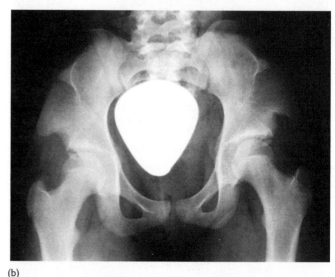

(b)

Fig. 24. Nail–patella syndrome. (a) Skyline views of the knee demonstrate small, high-riding patellae which lie over the lateral femoral condyle. (b) There are characteristic horns on the ileum.

trunk (Fig. 25). If the lesions are large and close to joints then joint deformity may occur. There is a risk of secondary chondrosarcoma. This risk is increased if they are associated with multiple soft-tissue hemangiomas. This association is known as the Maffucci syndrome.

Radiographic features

The radiographic feature is of a radiolucent lesion in the metaphyses of the long bones. There are occasional irregular areas of calcification and streaking within these lesions.

Treatment

Occasionally osteotomy is required for angular deformities; limb-length discrepancy may also require treatment with surgery. Large lesions occurring in the peripheral bones particularly the hands may require curettage and bone grafting.

Dysplasia epiphysealias hemimelica (Trevor's disease)

The clinical features of this condition usually become recognizable during childhood and present with deformity usually affecting one

limb. Most common sites are the tarsus, distal femur, and proximal tibia. The lesion is similar to an exostosis occurring on one side of the epiphyses. The complaint is not usually of pain but of deformity and limited movement.

Radiologic features

Radiologically a multicentered opacity develops adjacent to the epiphysis and may cause some widening of the metaphyses.

Treatment

Excision of the lesion is advised if it interferes with joint movement and if it is producing deformity. Leg-length discrepancy may occur as a result of the lesion and its excision. This may require further treatment.

Neuromuscular disorders
Duchenne and Becker muscular dystrophy

These have normally been considered as separate conditions. However, in 1987 the gene dystrophin was discovered and it was realized

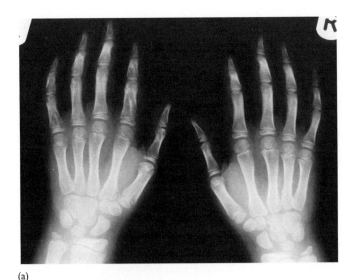

(a)

(b)

Fig. 25. Ollier's disease. (a) Enchondromas are present in the phalanges. (b) Enchondromas are present in the femur and this bone has required corrective osteotomy.

that both conditions result from mutations of this gene (Monaco and Kunkel 1988; Hoffman and Kunkel 1989).

Clinical features

Duchenne muscular dystrophy is the more severe form and usually presents in early childhood with abnormalities of gait including toe walking. The natural history of the disease is one of progressive weakness and delay in achieving normal milestones.

Becker muscular dystrophy produces a much milder phenotype with proximal weakness occurring in childhood and in early adolescence. A diagnosis can be made by finding high levels of creatinine kinase on serum analysis. Sometimes female carriers of this X-linked condition can have some symptoms with limb girdle weakness and elevated creatinine kinase levels. Scoliotic deformity may be present, and cardiac muscle abnormalities are sometimes a cause of symptoms.

Genetics

The dystrophies are due to abnormalities of the dystrophin gene located on the X chromosome. This gene is the largest human gene yet identified, and many different mutations of the gene have been found. Diagnosis of the condition can usually be made clinically and by finding high creatinine kinase levels. Muscle biopsies are sometimes useful.

Treatment

At present there is no successful treatment for the condition although surgery for spinal stabilization is sometimes indicated. There is great excitement at present because of the possibility of gene therapy for this condition, allowing cure of the disease.

Myotonic dystrophy

Myotonic dystrophy presents with a variety of phenotypes and significant spread of severity. Most severe forms present soon after birth with hypotonia and weakness. Often they are unable to breathe and feed themselves. The incidence of the severe form is much greater if the mother has myotonia than if the father has the condition. There is mental retardation.

Milder forms of myotonic dystrophy produce very few symptoms and may present only with cataracts. Presentation in childhood is usually with wasting of the temporalis muscle and the typical long narrow face. Cardiac conduction defects are sometimes present and patients may have diabetes and infertility. Mental retardation is common.

Genetics

The abnormalities are due to mutation in the gene myotonin. The abnormality within the gene is multiple copies of a three-base repeat segment of the gene known as a CTG repeat.

The more severely affected individuals with myotonic dystrophy have the greater number of repeats within the gene. This condition demonstrates an interesting genetic phenomenon known as anticipation. This involves worsening of the clinical picture with each generation. It appears that when the gene moves from one generation to another more of these trinucleotide repeats appear within the gene, producing a much more severe disease. The phenomenon occurs in a number of other human diseases.

Hereditary motor and sensory neuropathies (Charcot–Marie–Tooth disease)

The Charcot–Marie–Tooth diseases have been classified into types I and type II. Type I is the most common inherited neuromuscular disorder and is autosomal dominant. Its features are of a progressive distal muscle wasting and weakness. Reflexes are absent and there are deformities of the feet, most usually cavus and varus deformity. Electrophysiologic studies reveal slow nerve conduction. The phenotype varies but the disease is usually evident in childhood. Cases often present to orthopedic surgeons in late childhood or teenage years.

Genetics

A number of mutations have been identified to account for this disorder located on chromosomes 17 and the X chromosome. The most common mutation is found on chromosome 17p and is now classified as type IA hereditary, motor, and sensory neuropathy. This gene codes for a myelin protein gene and it seems likely that myelin is strongly implicated in this disease. The second mutation is now identified as the type IB neuropathy and is located on chromosome 1. It also codes for a myelin protein and is very rare. A third location, type IC, is suggested although the precise chromosomal location is not yet known. Three X-linked loci have also been identified.

The gene for type 2 Charcot–Marie–Tooth disease which is known to be associated with axonal degeneration has not yet been identified.

Spinal muscular atrophy

This condition has been separated into three different forms. The first, Werdnig–Hoffmann, has generalized muscle weakness and hypotonia. Premature death is common and the patients are never able to walk. The second form is Kugelberg–Welander. This is by far the mildest form and is not usually evident until 2 or 3 years of age. There is also an intermediate form where there are delayed motor milestones and usually an inability to walk.

Genetics

These three conditions appear to perform part of a continuum and have now been mapped to genetic mutations on chromosome 5. It appears that mutations arise in a gene called the survival motor neurone. It is possible that a nearby gene, which is involved in controlling programed cell death, is also influenced by these mutations. Individuals with this type of neuropathy may demonstrate a failure to inhibit cell death during development of the nervous system thus developing their neuropathy.

Clinical problems

Individuals with spinal muscular atrophy may present to orthopedic surgeons with spinal deformity and instability of the hips.

Neurofibromatosis

Neurofibromatosis is an extremely common single-gene autosomal dominant disorder. Most individuals with the mutation will demonstrate an abnormal phenotype. It is classically split into two types. Type 1 is common with a prevalence of 1 in 3500 births. Half of these will be due to new mutations. Type II is much less common and is due to mutations on chromosome 22. It occurs in 1 in 50 000 births.

Clinical features

Clinical features of type 1 include the classical *café-au-lait* spots, neurofibromatosis, abnormal bone formation, and congenital pseudarthrosis of the tibia. Scoliotic deformity may also occur and sometimes requires surgical treatment. Congenital pseudarthrosis of the tibia may also require surgical treatment, although it is often difficult to achieve bony union because of the presence of neurofibroma tissue in the tibia (Collins *et al.* 1989).

In the second form there are a very few orthopedic complications. The main abnormality is neuromatous development in the acoustic nerve.

Common disorders of the skeleton

One of the most exciting advances that has occured in the last 5 to 10 years has been the move from genetic analysis of rare single-gene disorders to an analysis of much more common genetic disorders of humans. These are known as multifactorial or complex traits. The inheritance of these conditions is inevitably much more complicated than that of single-gene disorders (McKusick and Amberger 1993; Lander and Schork 1994; McKusick 1994). There is often an interaction of environmental and genetic influences in the development of the phenotype. Often more than one gene is involved. Nevertheless, an understanding of the genetic basis of common disorders of the skeleton may lead to a significantly improved understanding of the pathologic basis of the condition and may provide new insights into possible treatments with either drug or surgical therapy. Another possibility on the far horizon is the use of gene therapy to treat some of these conditions.

Osteoarthritis

Osteoarthritis is a debilitating disease which is caused by the degeneration of articular cartilage. Its etiology can clearly be affected by the environment. There is also a strong genetic component to the disease. One way of demonstrating that a trait is genetic is to investigate for familial clustering. The estimated relative risk for siblings of patients with severe disease who have undergone total hip or total knee replacement due to osteoarthritic damage has been calculated as approximately three. That is to say that a sibling of somebody with a hip or knee replacement is three times as likely to require the operation as a control matched for age and sex from the general population.

A more classical method of demonstrating the genetic component of a complex disease trait is to examine twins. Comparison between the phenotypic concordance of monozygotic twins who share all their genes and dizygotic twins who share on average 50 per cent of their genetic loci gives an estimate of heritability. Such a study involving female twins has demonstrated a raised concordance in monozygotic twins and an estimated heritability of up to 70 per cent for osteoarthritis of multiple joints. This relative risk and twin data demonstrates strong genetic factors predisposing to osteoarthritis. It is, however, clear that the model of inheritance of osteoarthritis does not follow the classical Mendelian pattern. This places osteoarthritis in the polygenetic and multifactorial class of human disease where more than one gene and a combination of genetic and environmental factors give rise to the disease. The precise basis of many monogenic diseases of the skeleton has now been unraveled and these often involve mutations in genes coding for proteins of the extracellular matrix. Several of these genetic disorders are associated with the early onset of osteoarthritis. Understanding the genetic basis of osteoarthritis may well help with diagnosis and treatment in the future.

Osteoporosis

Osteoporosis is a disease characterized by low bone mineral density. Low bone density appears to affect around 22 per cent of women aged over 50. Osteoporosis has a significant affect on public health and results in approximately 60 000 hip fractures a year in the United Kingdom. Ninety per cent of these fractures are in people aged over 50, and 80 per cent of them are in women. The disease consumes increasing annual resources which were estimated at £750 million in 1994 in the United Kingdom. The World Health Organization definition of osteoporosis is a bone mineral density that lies more than 2.5 standard deviations below the young adult mean. It is more common in women and in the elderly and may be associated with other conditions, for example steroids, anorexia, alcohol intake, smoking, thyrotoxicosis, and malabsorption.

Early genetic work suggests a strong heritable component to bone mineral density in adults. Studies of identical and non-identical twins demonstrate an estimated genetic component of bone mineral density of between 60 and 80 per cent in both men and women. More recent studies demonstrate reduced bone mass in daughters of women with osteoporosis. This strong genetic determinant of peak adult bone mass clearly contributes to bone strength. Environmental factors and other influences such as dietary calcium intake and physical activity are important in the disease. Some early genetic linkage studies have suggested a role for the vitamin D receptor in some forms of osteoporosis. Whether this genetic abnormality is present in all of the more common forms of osteoporosis is as yet uncertain. A number of single-gene disorders are characterized by low bone density, the most important of which is osteogenesis imperfecta. This condition is known to be due to mutations in the genes coding for type 1 collagen protein.

Rheumatoid arthritis

Rheumatoid arthritis is another common disease of the skeleton associated with dramatic synovial changes and joint destruction. Relative risk and twin studies have been performed in this condition. These suggest that there is significant genetic predisposition to the disease. It is known that there is a strong link between rheumatoid arthritis and the HLA locus on chromosome 6. Whether or not any other genes outside of this region are responsible for the disease is unknown. Currently a number of groups around the world are investigating families with rheumatoid arthritis to try and determine the genetic basis for the condition.

Dupuytren's disease

Dupuytren's disease is a common condition in which proliferation of fibroblasts in the palmar and digital fascia leads to contracture of the fingers. At present the treatment is surgical and no other treatment is known to alter the progress of the disease. The prevalence is about 10 per cent in males over 65 years in northern European countries but it is very low in Asia and Africa. There is a strong genetic predisposition to Dupuytren's disease but exogenous factors may initiate the disorders in susceptible individuals.

The observation that many sufferers of Dupuytren's disease have affected relatives was made in 1838 by Goyran and confirmed by many later authors. Identical Dupuytren's disease has been found in identical twins. Strong evidence of autosomal dominant inheritance of Dupuytrens's disease was obtained by Ling who examined 832 first-degree relatives of 50 patients with Dupuytren's disease. Eight out of 50 reported a family history, but on careful examination 34 out of 50 were found to have affected relatives. After correcting for late age of onset and population prevalence, the frequency of affective individuals among first-, second-, and third-degree relatives accorded closely with predictions for a dominant mode of inheritance. There are many tissues in which the proliferation of fibroblasts leads to disease (sclerosis, pulmonary fibrosis, limited joint mobility of diabetes, wound healing, hypertrophic and keloid scarring, retinal fibrosis, and Peyroni's disease). In each case, exogenous factors, tissue-specific factors and genetic susceptibility may combine to influence the development of disease. Identification of the mutant locus or loci responsible for Dupuytren's disease may allow research into non-surgical methods of treatment.

Scoliosis

The etiology of adolescent idiopathic scoliosis remains unknown. It has been recognized for many years that there is a familial basis for the condition. The most persuasive of this evidence is from a number of twin studies. These studies suggest a heritability of 70 to 90 per cent. Indeed in some pedigrees the condition appears to behave much like a single-gene disorder. Attempts to link the disease to collagen gene markers have failed. Scoliosis is seen in Marfan's syndrome but there is no evidence to suggest that girls with idiopathic scoliosis have abnormalities of the fibrilin gene. It is probable that the gene or genes involved in adolescent idiopathic scoliosis control growth factors or proteins related to the central nervous system. Identifying the genetic mutations in idiopathic scoliosis may provide improved screening techniques and may also lead to improved treatment of the disease. Other orthopedic and muscular skeletal diseases in which a genetic base is known include development dysplasia of the hip and club-foot.

Prenatal diagnosis

A number of different methods are now available for prenatal diagnosis of genetic conditions affecting the skeleton. The first of these is the use of ultrasound. This may reveal severe skeletal abnormalities such as severe osteogenesis imperfecta by 15 to 17 weeks gestation. Ultrasound is capable of measuring the length of limbs and can also detect abnormalities of the heart, kidneys, and cranium. Unfortunately, the sensitivity and specificity of ultrasound is such that sometimes a precise diagnosis is not possible. Nevertheless, as ultrasound technology becomes more sophisticated this technique will increasingly be used to identify skeletal abnormalities *in utero*. Table 5 outlines the timing of pre- and postnatal diagnosis in their various diagnostic groups.

Alternatively, genetic tests can be used to investigate for some conditions. This requires there to be a family history of the condition. The techniques employed include the use of linked markers in dominant families, the identification of specific mutations characterized in previously affected members, and the analysis of genetic products synthesized from biopsies or from chorionic villus fibroblasts.

The precise technique used will depend very much on the information available in the family; it will also depend on the gestational age

Table 5 Possibility of prenatal diagnosis for different clinical diagnostic groups

	Prenatal diagnosis		Clinical diagnosis in neonatal period early infancy	Clinical diagnosis 2 years +
	11+ weeks gestation: chorionic villus sampling for DNA testing unless otherwise noted (*only* when known family cases)	16+ weeks gestation: ultrasound (some more secure at 24+ weeks) (for congenital malformations and short limbs)		
(i) Epiphyseal dysplasia Multiple epiphyseal dysplasia, hereditary arthro-ophthalmopathy (Stickler), chondrodysplasia punctata (Conradi), severe rhizomolic, milder forms	Conradi (rhizomelic) Stickler	Conradi (rhizomelic) Stickler	Conradi (rhizomelic) Stickler	Conradi (mild) Stickler (mild)
(ii) Spondyloepiphyseal dysplasias (SED) Congenita tarda, autosomal dominant and recessive, X-linked recessive	SED congenita	SED congenita	SED congenita	SED tarda
(iii) Predominantly metaphyseal dysplasias Metaphyseal chondrodysplasias (MCD) Types: Schmid, McKusick, Jansen, Peña Spondylometaphyseal dysplasias (SMP): Types Kozlowski, Sutcliffe	MCD Schmid, Jansen	MCD with neutropenia (from fetal blood)	MCD Jansen MCD with neutropenia	All other MCD and SMP
(iv) Short limbs/normal trunk Achondroplasia, hypochondroplasia, dyschondrosteosis Robinow, Werner, acromesomelia, acrodysostosis	Achondroplasia	Achondroplasia (also from amniocentesis for fetal cells)	Achondroplasia Acromesomelia	Hypochondroplasia Dyschondrosteosis Acrodysostosis
(v) Short limbs and trunk (may or may not be disproportionate) Pseudoachondroplasia, diastrophic dysplasia, metatropic dwarfism, Kniest, Ellis–van Creveld, Jeune	Pseudoachondroplasia Diastrophic Kniest	Ellis–van Creveld Jeune Diastrophic Metatropic Kniest	Ellis–van Creveld Jeune Diastrophic Metatropic Kniest	Pseudoachondroplasia
(vi) Lethal forms of short-limb dwarfism Thanatophoric, achondrogenesis, short-rib/polydactyly syndromes, campomelic dwarfism.	Thanatophoric, achondrogenesis (gonadal mosaics), short-rib polydactyly syndromes (by ultrasound 12+ weeks) Campomelic	All thanatophoric (also from amniocentesis)	All	—
(vii) Increased limb length Marfan, congenital contractural arachnodactyly, homocystinuria	Marfan Homocystinuria	Marfan: severe neonatal form	Marfan (neonatal) Congenital contractural arachnodactyly	Marfan Homocystinuria
(viii) Storage disorders Mucopolysaccharide (MPS) disorders, mucolipidoses (MLS), mannosidosis, sialidoses	MPS, MLS		MLS	MPS (perhaps earlier)
(ix) Metabolic bone disease Hypo- and hyperphosphatasia, hypophosphatemic rickets, pseudohypoparathyroidism	Hypophosphatasia(also by ultrasound 12+ weeks)	Hypophosphatasia	Hypophosphatasia	Hypophosphatasia Rickets Pseudohypoparathyroidism
(x) Decreased bone density Osteogenesis imperfecta group, idiopathic juvenile osteoporosis, Hajdu–Cheney (osteolysis)	Osteogenesis imperfecta (all) (types IIa and IIc also by ultrasound 12+ weeks)	Osteogenesis imperfecta (type I, some type III at 24+ weeks)	Osteogenesis imperfecta	Mild osteogenesis imperfecta Juvenile osteoporosis Hadju–Cheney
(xi) Increased bone density (sclerosing bone dysplasias) Osteoporosis, pycnodysostosis, Pyle's craniometaphyseal dysplasia, frontometaphyseal dysplasia, osteodysplasty (Melnick–Needles), Engelmann's craniodiaphyseal dysplasia, osteopathia striata, osteopoikilosis	Osteopetrosis (with carbonic hydrase deficiency)	Osteopetrosis Melnick–Needles Pycnodysostosis (family cases 24+ weeks)	Severe osteopetrosis Pycnodysostosis Severe craniometaphyseal Craniodiaphyseal Severe Melnick–Needles	All others
(xii) Tumor-like disorders (bony or fibrous) Diaphyseal aclasis, Ollier's, Maffucci's, dysplasia epiphysealis hemimelica, myositis ossificans progressiva, polyostotic fibrous dysplasia (including Albright), melorheostosis, neurofibromatosis	Neurofibromatosis Diaphyseal aclasis		Myositis ossificans Polyostotic fibrous dysplasia Melorheostosis Neurofibromatosis	All others

of the baby when prenatal diagnosis is requested. Some conditions can be detected from amniotic fluid cells but unfortunately this is not possible in conditions such as osteogenesis imperfecta because some of the cells synthesize collagen fibrils that are of a form that it is impossible to analyze on electrophoresis gels.

Molecular biology

Remarkable changes have occurred in the last 10 to 20 years in our understanding of the molecular and cellular basis of disease. This has produced an exciting new relationship between basic scientists and clinical scientists who are now collaborating in projects to understand the basis of common diseases and to determine how new knowledge may produce more effective treatments for these diseases. This section will outline some of the basic science principles involved in this work.

Structure and function of human genes

Genes are responsible for the manufacture of proteins which consist of peptide chains folded into three-dimensional structures. These proteins are essential for the normal function of tissues and are the basis of enzymes or structural tissues such as ligaments and cartilage. The precise role that the protein has is determined by its shape which is in itself dictated by the sequence of amino acids that form part of the peptide chain. This sequence of amino acids is determined by a particular section of DNA. In order to produce a protein the DNA is first transcribed into messenger RNA and this messenger RNA template is then translated into a protein.

DNA is comprised of chains of nucleotides which are wrapped around each other in a helical pattern. There are four bases—adenine, guanine, cytosine, and thymine. These bases are linked to each other by a backbone of deoxyribose molecules linked by phosphates. The variable part of the chain is therefore the nucleotide base. These nucleotides form a code which is in the form of triplets and is non-overlapping. Each triplet of bases codes for a particular amino acid. In order to replicate DNA, the DNA strands have to separate and then, through the action of enzymes, a mirror of the DNA chain is made.

The DNA is located on chromosomes of which there are 46 in the human and two sex chromosomes X and Y. Each of these chromosomes contains a large number of genes. Not all DNA codes for genes much of it is redundant material. Indeed, within a particular gene there may be further redundant sections known as exons. The parts of the gene which code for messenger RNA are known as introns. At the ends of genes are initiation and termination sequences which are usually coded AGG, or TAA, TAG, or TGA. Somewhat downstream from the start sequence, further conserved sections of DNA are almost invariably found. These appear to be involved with the regulation of transcription of messenger RNA. Figures 26 and 27 show the process of transcription and translation of DNA to messenger RNA and to a protein chain.

The tools of DNA technology

The process of splitting and rejoining of DNA is central to many of the new methodologies used in DNA research. If the DNA strands are heated and cooled then they will dissociate and reassociate. It is

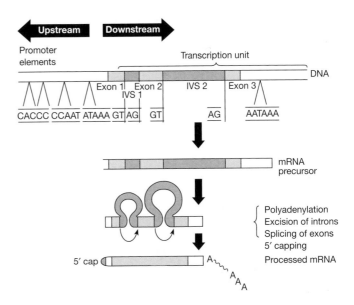

Fig. 26. Transcription. The process of transcription of DNA. Messenger RNA (mRNA) is synthesized on its DNA template. The primary transcription unit is large and comprises the entire gene unit, both introns (coding) and exons (noncoding). This mRNA precursor is then modified to produce mRNA.

possible to replicate sections of DNA using a process of heating and cooling and generate complimentary sequences which can be radio-labeled and used as gene probes. An enzyme called a reverse transcriptase can be used to synthesize a DNA copy from any messenger RNA isolated from human cells. This is known as complementary DNA.

Once a gene probe has been manufactured and is known to be complimentary to an area of particular interest such as a particular gene, then it is possible to investigate individuals or populations using gene mapping. Gene mapping requires the cellular DNA to be cut into sections so that it can be spread out on an electrophoresis gel. The process of cutting cellular DNA is accomplished using restriction endocucleases. These are enzymes that occur naturally mainly in bacteria and that cleave DNA at particular sites. Figure 28 demonstrates the process of restriction enzyme mapping which is known as Southern blotting.

Another important tool that is used in DNA research is the process of gene cloning using gene libraries. This requires a piece of DNA to be inserted into bacterial plasmids or bacterial phages. Plasmids are closed circular DNA molecules which replicate themselves within bacteria. So by inserting a gene of interest into a plasmid in a bacterium, the bacterium's DNA production machinery can be used to produce many copies of the gene. In order to produce a gene library of the whole genome, genes must be inserted into some form of vector. It has been found that one of the best vectors is the yeast artificial chromosome (**YAC**). By storing all the fragmented genes within these artificial vectors a permanent source of gene material is available. In order to access a particular part of the library a radio-labeled gene is used in a technique called colony hybridization. This radiolabeled gene probe will attach itself on a filter to the complimentary part of the library. This part of the yeast colony can then be removed and used in subsequent experiments and studies. Now that

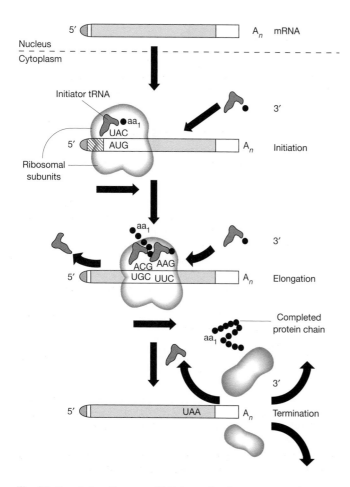

Fig. 27. Translation. Messenger RNA is translated into a protein chain by acting as a template. Amino acids are brought to the mRNA by transfer RNA (tRNA). Each triplet of basis of the mRNA corresponds to a particular tRNA and a particular amino acid. By this process the protein chain is manufactured.

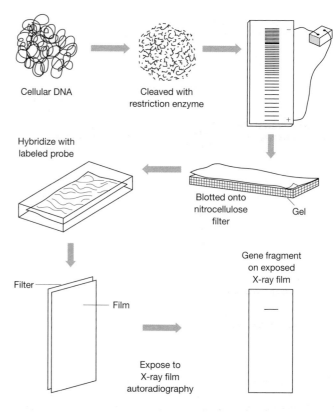

Fig. 28. Southern blotting. This is the process by which cellular DNA is cleaved into fragments by enzymes. The fragments are separated by an electrophoresis transferred onto filtered paper, hybridized with a radiolabeled gene probe, and then exposed on radiograph film. The process allows particular genes to be identified.

genes have been isolated using cloning methods, this has opened up a variety of possibilities for determining the basis of single gene and even common disorders. In order to determine exactly where the mutation is, the process of gene sequencing has to be followed.

One particular technique that has made an enormous difference to speed of experimentation has been the use of the polymerase chain reaction. This amplifies any short sequence of DNA many many times in a short period of time. The principle of the polymerase chain reaction is shown in Fig. 29.

Identification of genetic mutations in human disease

A variety of methods have been used to identify the specific mutations responsible for single-gene disorders in humans. This is obviously an extremely complex task bearing in mind that the human genome comprises somewhere around 3×10^9 to 3.5×10^9 base pairs. Contained within this mass of DNA are some 50 000 to 200 000 important genes. Despite this daunting mass of genetic information contained within each human cell, recombinant DNA technology

and the new genetics has allowed us to discover the genetic mutations responsible for a number of single-gene disorders. This type of experimental work usually begins with searching for markers for genes and by tracking these genes through families. This type of genetic analysis is known as linkage analysis. One form of genetic marker relies upon variable cutting sites for bacterial enzymes. If these cutting sites occur in DNA that does not code for proteins then it has been found that some people will have the cutting site and some people will not. Obviously, if a cutting site is absent, this will produce a longer fragment of DNA which will travel less far on an electrophoresis gel. This allows geneticists to distinguish one individual from another and in particular one genetic region from another. It is therefore possible using these restriction site markers to track regions of the genome through families to see whether or not a particular region is consistently linked to a disease within a family. Once a particular region of the human genome has been linked to a disease the next stage of experimentation is known as physical mapping and this requires a much more detailed analysis of this region of DNA on a particular chromosome. When the gene has been identified, the process of sequencing the gene to identify all the bases within it is begun. Once the sequence of the normal gene has been determined the next step is to define where the mutation is with individuals with an abnormal gene. Such techniques have produced remarkable success, particularly over the last 10 to 15 years.

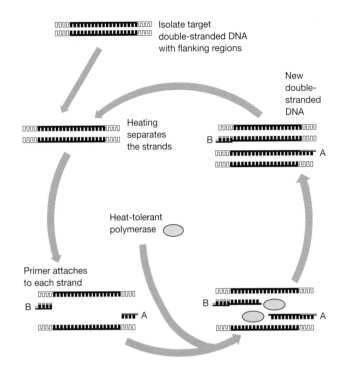

Fig. 29. The polymerase chain reaction. Certain DNA sequences can be amplified many times using a process whereby double-stranded DNA is heated and separated and bound to primers. The primers then initiate the formation of two new chains complimentary to the originals. Each time the process is repeated the amount of DNA is doubled.

Clinical applications of the new DNA technologies

Discovering the genetic defects of single-gene disorders has produced a number of possible clinical applications. These begin with diagnostic tests particularly of use in antenatal screening for severe disorders. Knowledge of the precise mutation also makes possible treatment with either drugs or vaccines and even in some cases the possibility of genetic therapy itself. Trials are already beginning in gene therapy for diseases such as cystic fibrosis.

Perhaps one of the most exciting developments occurring at the present time is the search for the genetic basis for common genetic diseases. Many diseases of the skeleton have some genetic basis including osteoarthritis, osteoporosis, and rheumatoid arthritis. Other diseases also have some genetic pattern including congenital dislocation of the hip, scoliosis, Dupuytren's disease, and club-foot. If the genetic component of these diseases can be identified then this leads to a variety of exciting possibilities. These would include the ability to understand in greater detail the environmental influences which act together with the genetic susceptibility to produce the disease. This may allow certain individuals with a particularly strong genetic predisposition to be advised about what risk factors to avoid. The other possibility is that some form of therapeutic agent may be designed to treat the disease. The possibility of treating early osteoarthritis or early osteoporosis with a drug is enticing. If this was only to reduce the severity of the diseases then this would have enormous consequences to the suffering of people and also to the costs of treating people with the diseases in their endstage.

References

Anderson, I.G.R., Marion, R.W., Upholt, W.B., and Tsipouras P. (1990). Spondyloepiphyseal dysplasia congenita: genetic linkage to type ii collagen (COL2A1). *American Journal of Human Genetics*, **46**, 896–901.

Bellus, G., Mcintosh, I., Smith, E.A., *et al.* (1995). A recurrent mutation in the tyrosine kinase doman of fibroblast growth factor receptor 3 cause hypochondroplasia. *Nature Genetics*, **10**, 357–9.

Briggs, M., Choi, H., Warman, M.I., *et al.* (1994). Genetic mapping of a locus for multiple epiphyseal dysplasia (Edm2) to a region chromosome 1 containing a type IX collagen gene. *American Journal of Human Genetics*, **55**, 678–84.

Briggs, M., Hoffman, S.M., King, L.M., *et al.* (1995). Pseudoachondroplasia and multiple epiphyseal dysplasia due to mutations in the cartilage oligomeric matrix protein gene. *Nature Genetics*, **10**, 330–6.

Byers, P. (1993). Osteogenesis imperfecta. In *Connective tissue and its heritable disorders: molecular, genetic and medical aspects* (ed. P.M. Royce and B. Steinmann), pp. 317–50. Wiley-Liss, New York.

Carr, A., Cole, W.G., Chiodo, A., Hockey, A., and Chow, C.W. (1994). The clinical features of Ehlers Danlos syndrome type VIIB resulting from a base substitution at the splice acceptor site of intron 5 of the COL1A2 gene. *Journal of Medical Genetics*, **31**, 306–11.

Collins, F., Ponder, B.A., Seizinger, B.R., and Epstein, C.R. (1989). The Von Recklinghausen neurofibromatosis region on chromosome 17—genetic and physical maps come into focus. *American Journal of Human Genetics*, **44**, 1–5.

Dharmavaram, R., Elberson, M.A., Peng, M., Kirson, L.A., Kelley, T.E., and Jimenez, S.A. (1994). Identification of a mutation in type X collagen in a family with schmid metaphyseal chondrodysplasia. *Human Molecular Genetics*, **3**, 507–9.

Dietz, H., Cutting, G.R., Pyeritz, R.E., *et al.* (1991). Marian syndrome caused by a recurrent de novo missense mutation in the fibrillin gene. *Nature*, **352**, 337–9.

Fernandez-Canon, J., Grandino, B., Bertran-Valero Debernabe, D., *et al.* (1996). The molecular basis of alkaptonuria. *Nature Genetics*, **14**, 19–24.

Hoffman, E. and Kunkel, L.M. (1989). Dystrophin abnormalities in Duchenne/Becker muscular dystrophy. *Neuron*, **2**, 1019–29.

Lander, E. and Schork, N.K. (1994). Genetic dissection of complex traits. *Science*, **265**, 2037–48.

McKusick, V. (1994). *Mendelian inheritance in man: catalogs of autosomal dominant, autosomal recessive and X-linked phenotypes*, p. 11. Johns Hopkins University Press, Baltimore, MD.

McKusick, V. and Amberger, J.S. (1993). The morbid anatomy of the human genome: chromosomal location of mutations causing disease. *Journal of Medical Genetics*, **30**, 1–26.

Monaco, A. and Kunkel, L.M. (1988). Cloning of the Duchenne/Becker muscular dystrophy focus. *Advances In Human Genetics*, **17**, 61–98.

Muenke, M. and Schell, U. (1995). Fibroblast-growth-factor receptor mutations in human skeletal disorders. *Trends in Genetics*, **11**, 308–13.

Muragaki, Y., Mariman, E.C., Van Beersum, S.E., *et al.* (1996). A mutation in the gene encoding the alpha 2 chain of the fibril-associated collagen IX, COL9A2, causes multiple epiphyseal dysplasia (MED2). *Nature Genetics*, **12**, 103–5.

Murray, L., Bautista, J., James, P.I., and Rimoin, D.I. (1989). Type II collagen defects in the chondrodysplasias I. Spondyloepiphyseal dysplasias. *American Journal of Human Genetics*, **45**, 5–15.

Shiang, R., Thompson, L.M., Zhu, Y.Z., *et al.* (1994). Mutations in the transmembrane domain of FGFR3 cause the most common genetic form of dwarfism, achondroplasia. *Cell*, **78**, 335–42.

Spranger, J. (1988). Bone dysplasia 'families'. *Pathology and Immunopathology Research*, **7**, 76–80.

Tsipouras, P., Del Mastro, R., Sarfarazi, M., *et al.* and The International Marfan Syndrome Collaborative Study (1992). Genetic linkage of the Marfan syndrome, ectopia lentis, and congenital contractural arachnodactyly to the fibrillin genes on chromosomes 15 and 5. *New England Journal of Medicine*, **326**, 905–9.

Winterpacht, A., Hilbert, M., Schwarze, U., Mundlos, S., Spranger, J., and Zabel, B.U. (1993). Kniest and Sticklers dysplasia phenotypes caused by collagen type II gene (COL2A1) defect. *Nature Genetics*, **3**, 323–6.

Wynne-Davies, R., Hall, C., and Apley, G.A. (1986). *An atlas of skeletal dysplasias*. Churchill Livingstone, Edinburgh.

Appendix 1

Clinical diagnostic groups	Prenatal diagnosis		Clinical diagnosis in neonatal period/early infancy	Clinical diagnosis 2 years+
	By ultrasound examination[a]	By genetic (G) / biochemical (B) testing[b]		
(i) *Predominantly epiphyseal dysplasias* Multiple epiphyseal dysplasia, hereditary arthro-ophthalmopathy (Stickler), chrondrodysplasia punctata (Conradi), severe rhizomelic, milder forms	Conradi (rhizomelic) have stippled epiphyses (18+ weeks)	Conradi B Stickler G*	Conradi (rhizomelic), Stickler	Conradi (mild) Stickler (mild)
(ii) *Spondyloepiphyseal dysplasias (SED)* Congenita: classical type, others with distal involvement, e.g. brachydactyly Tarda: autosomal dominant and recessive, X-linked recessive	SED congemta (18+ weeks)	SED congenita G*	SED congenita	SED tarda

(iii) *Predominantly metaphyseal dysplasias*
Metaphyseal chondrodysplasias (MCD)
    Types: Schmid, McKusick, Jansen, Peña, with malabsorption and neutropenia, others
    (see also hypophosphatasia, rickets, included with metabolic bone disease (ix))
Spondylometaphyseal dysplasias (SMP)
    Types Kozlowski, Sutcliffe
		MCD with neutropenia G*
		MCD Schmid G*
		MCD Jansen G*
			MCD Jansen
			MCD with neutropenia
				All other MCD and SMP

(iv) *Short limbs/normal trunk* Achondroplasia, hypochondroplasia, dyschondrosteosis Robinow, Werner, acromesomelia, acrodysostosis, others	Achondroplasia (20+ weeks)	Achondroplasia G	Achondroplasia Acromesomelia	Hypochondroplasia Dyschondrosteosis Acrodysostosis
(v) *Short limbs and trunk* (may or may not be disproportionate) Pseudoachondroplasia, diastrophic dysplasia, metatropic dwarfism, Kniest, Ellis–van Creveld, Jeune, others (see also storage disorders (viii))	Pseudoachondroplasia (20+ weeks) Diastrophic (16+ weeks) Kniest (18+ weeks) Metatropic (18+ weeks) Ellis–van Creveld (Jeune) (20+ weeks)	Pseudoachondroplasia G* Diastrophic G* Kniest G*	Ellis–van Creveld, Jeune Diastrophic Metatrophic Kniest	Pseudoachondroplasia
(vi) *Lethal forms of short-limbed dwarfism* Thanatophoric, achondrogenesis, short rib/polydactyly syndromes, campomelic dwarfism, others (see also hypophosphatasia (ix) and osteogenesis imperfecta (x))	Thanatophoric (16+ weeks) All others Achondrogenesis (16+ weeks) Campomelic (16+ weeks) Short-rib syndromes (16+ weeks)	Thantophoric G Achondrogenesis G* Campomelic G*	All	—
(vii) *Increased limb length* Marfan, congenital contractural arachnodactyly, homocystinuria		Marfan G* Homocystinuria B	Marfan (neonatal) Congenital contractural arachnodactyly	Marfan Homocystinuria
(viii) *Storage disorders* Mucopolysaccharide disorders (MPS), mucolipidoses (MLS), mannosidosis, sialidoses		MPS, MLS B	MLS	MPS
(ix) *Metabolic bone disease* Hypo- and hyperphosphatasia, hypophosphatemic rickets, pseudohypoparathyroidism, others (see also metaphyseal disorders, (iii))	Hypophosphatasia (16+ weeks)	Hypophosphatasia B, G*	Hypophosphatasia	Hypophosphatemic rickets Pseudohypoparathyroidism
(x) *Decreased bone density* Osteogenesis imperfecta (OI) group, idiopathic juvenile osteoporosis, Hajdu–Cheney (osteolysis), others (also membrane bone disorder – cleidocranial dysostosis)	OI type II A, B, C (16+ weeks) OI type III (24+ weeks)	OI G*	OI Cleidocranial	Mild OI Juvenile osteoporosis Hajdu–Cheney Cleidocranial
(xi) *Increased bone density (sclerosing bone dysplasias)* Osteoporosis, pycnodysostosis, Pyle's craniometaphyseal dysplasia, frontometaphyseal dysplasia, osteodysplasty (Melnick–Needles), Engelmann, craniodiaphyseal dysplasia, osteopathia striata, and osteopoikilosis	Osteopetrosis (20+ weeks) Pycnodysostosis (20+ weeks)	Osteopetrosis (carbonic anhydrase deficiency type only) B, G*	Severe osteopetrosis Pycnodysostosis Severe craniometaphyseal Craniodiaphyseal Severe Melnick–Needles	All others
(xii) *Tumor-like disorders (bony or fibrous)* Diaphyseal aclasis, Ollier, Maffucci, dysplasia epiphysealis hemimelica, myositis ossificans progressive, polyostotic fibrous dysplasia (including Albright), melorheostosis, neurofibromatosis		Neurofibromatosis G*	Myositis ossificans Polyostotic fibrous dysplasia Melorheostosis Neurofibromatosis	

[a] Specialist scanning required to establish correct diagnosis.
[b] G*, genetic testing not available except for known familial mutations.
Reproduced with permission of the Skeletal Dysplasia Group.

Appendix 2 The non-lethal skeletal dysplasias

Diagnostic groups[a]	Under 2 years ▼	2 years and over ▲	Increased	Reduced: Trunk	Reduced: Limbs	Rhizomelic	Mesomelic	Skull/Cranium: Size	Density	Suture fusion (Early ▲ / Late ▼ / Wormian W)	Facial bones	Mandible	Spine: Scoliosis / kyphosis	Persistent ovoid	Platyspondyly	Odontoid dysplasia	Other
(i) Multiple epiphys. dys.		▲			(+)										(T.11, 12)		
Hered. arthro. ophth.	▼	▲									▼	(▼)	(+)		+		
Chondro. punctata (severe & mild forms)	▼	▲			+	(+)	(+)				(▼)		+	+			Corona clefts
(Conradi)					(Asym.)												
(ii) Spondyloepiphys. congenita	▼			+	+	(+)					(▼)		(+)	+	+	+	
Tarda – X-linked		▲		+									(+)		+		Post vert. lump
– Dom. rec.		▲		+									(+)		+		
– Progressive arth.		▲		(+)									(+)		+		
(iii) Metaphys. dys. – Schmid		▲			Lower								(+)				
– McKusick	(▼)	▲			+				(▲)				(+)			(+)	
– Jansen	▼			+	+			▼	▲	(▲)	+						
– with malabsorp., neutropen.		▲															
Spondylometaphyseal dys.		▲		+									(+)		+		
(iv) Achondroplasia	▼				+	+		▲			▼		T-L kyphos				Pedicles ▼
Hypochondroplasia		▲			+	+		(▲)			(▼)						
Dyschondrosteosis		▲			+		+										
Acromesomelia	▼	▲			+		+				(▼)		(+)		(+)		Pedicles ▼
Acrodysostosis		▲			(+)		(+)	(▲)			(▼)						Pedicles ▼
(v) Pseudochondroplasia		▲		+	+								+	(+) (Triangular)	(+)		
Diastrophic dysplasia	▼			+	+								+		(+)	+	Pedicles (▼)
Metatropic dysplasia	▼			+	+								+		++	(+)	
Kniest disease	▼			+	+						▼		+		(+)	(+)	Coronal clefts
Dyggve–Melchior–Clausen		▲		+	+			(▼)							+	(+)	
Chondro. ecto. (Ellis–van Creveld)	▼			(+)	+		+				Teeth ▼						
Asphyx. thor. dys. (Jeune)	▼	▲		(+)	+												
(viii) Storage diseases																	
MPS – Hurler	▼	▲		+	+			▲	▲	Sag. ▲			Condyles ▼ (T-L kyphos)	+	Hooked	(+)	
– Hunter		▲		+	+			(▲)	(▲)				T-L kyphos	+	Hooked	(+)	
– Scheie		▲															
– Sanfilippo		▲							(▲)					+			
– Mannosidosis		▲						▲					(T-L kyphos)				
– Maroteaux–Lamy		▲		+	+			(▲)	(▲)	Sag. ▲			Condyles ▼ T-L kyphos	+	Hooked	(+)	
– Morquio		▲		+	+								T-L kyphos	+	Early hooked / Later tongued	++	
MLS – GM, gangliodidiosis type 1	▼	▲						▲	▲	▲			Condyles ▼ T-L kyphos	+	Hooked		
(ix) Metabolic bone disease																	
Hypophosphatasia	▼	▲		(+)	(+)				▲								
Hyperphosphatasia		▲		(+)	(+)			▲	▲								
Hypophosphatemic rickets		▲			+			(▲)	(▲)	(▲)			(+)				
Pseudo-hypoparathyroid		▲		(+)	(+)			Ectopic cal.									Pedicles ▼
(x) Decreased bone density																	
Osteogen. imperfecta	▼	▲		(+)	(+)			▲	(Platybasia) ▼	W ▼	▼	(Teeth)	(+)		Biconcave (+)		
Idiopath. juv. osteoporosis		▲		(+)											(+)		
Osteolysis (Hajdu–Cheney)		▲							(Platybasia) ▼	W ▼							
(Cleidocranial dys.)		▲		(+)	(+)			▲	(▼)	W ▼			(+)				Fusion delayed
(xi) Sclerosing bone dysplasias																	
Osteopetrosis – severe	▼			+	+				▲[b]				Infection				Sandwich
– mild		(▲)							(▲)								
Pycnodysostosis	▼	▲		+	+				▲	W ▼	▼	▼ Infection					
Craniometaphyseal	▼							▲	▲[b]			▲ Teeth					
Pyle's metaphyseal dys.		▲	(+)														
Frontometaphyseal		▲		(+)	(+)			Frontal ▲	▲						(▼)	Segmental anomalies	
Melnick–Needles		▲	(+)						▲						(▼)	(+)	
Engelmann		(▲)	(+)					▲	▲								
Craniodiaphyseal	▼			(+)	(+)			▲	▲[b]			▲	▲				
Osteopathia striata		(▲)							▲[b]								

(xii) Tumor-like disorders

Diaphyseal aclasis, Ollier, Maffucci, dysplasia epiphysealis hemimelica, fibrodysplasia (myositis) ossificans progressiva, polyostotic fibrous dysplasia, melorheostosis: nearly always diagnosed over the age of 2 years; all are asymmetric with shortening and/or malalignment confined to the affected part, with patchy sclerosis. Malignant change is rare, except in Maffucci.

---

[a] 'Lethal dwarfs' and 'increased limb length' omitted.   [b] Wherever skull base is involved there may be cranial nerve compression.   ▲▼ Increase / decrease over normal.

Principal radiologic features — Thorax (Cage, Ribs, Clavicle); Pelvis — Ilium (Wings, Base), Acetab. (Under-developed ▼ / Protrusio ▲); Limbs (Epiphysis, Metaphysis, Diaphysis), Deformity (Coxa vara, Malalignment), Wrist / Hands; Ossification (Advanced ▲ / Delayed ▼). Principal associated anomalies or complications. Further investigations: Radiology (R), Hemotology (H), Biochemistry (B), Genetic (G).

Cage	Ribs	Clavicle	Wings	Base	Acetab.	Epiphysis	Metaphysis	Diaphysis	Coxa vara	Malalignment	Wrist / Hands	Ossification	Principal associated anomalies or complications	Further investigations
					(▼) (▲)	+	(+)		(+)	+	(+)	▼		(G)
						+	(+) Infancy dumb-bell						Cleft palate, myopia, hearing ▼	(G)
						(+)	(Cupped)		(+)	Punctate calcif.			Cataract, heart, skin lesions	B
Carinatum			▼			+(less distally)	+		++			▼ (Hip)	Cleft palate, myopia	R (Cl.2)
						+								
						+					(MC ▼)	▲		
						+			Contracture	+ ('Rheumatoid')				
							+		+					B (? rickets)
	▲Ant.						+				▼		Blood ▼, Hair▼	B,H
						▲	++		(+)	+	+		Hearing ▼, Fractures	B
	Infant ▼						+		+		▼		Cyclical neutropenia	B,H
				▲			+		(+)					
(▼)	(▼)		▼	Spur			+		(+)	Tib / fib	+		Spinal stenosis	G
						(+)				Tib / fib	(+)			G
									+	Disl. ulna ('Madelung')				
			▼				+		+		▼			
			▼								▼	▲ Hands		(G)
Post-cupping			▼	▼		++	++		+		▼ 1st MC	▼ (Hips)	(Gross joint laxity)	(G)
			(▲)	▼		+	+		(+)	Contracture	▼ 1st MC	▲ ▼	Cleft palate	R,(Cl.2)G
▼	▼		▼			(+)	Dumb-bell	▼		+		▼		(G)
▼	▼					(+)	▲		(+)			▲	Cleft palate, myopia, hearing	
Carinatum				Lace like		(+)	+					▼	(Mental retard.)	
▼(improves later)	▼		(▼)	Spike					(+)	Fusion capi/ham Post-ax. poly.		(▲) Infant	Heart, hair ▼	(G)
▼(improves later)	▼		(▼)	Spike			(+)			(Post-ax. poly.)		(▲) Infant	(Nephritis)	
All may:	Med. ▲	▲	▼	▼		+	(+)	▲	(C. valga)	Hip dislocation contractures	MC 2-5 pointed bases		(Mental retard.)	B,G
	Med. (▲)	▲	▼	▼		+	(+)		(C. valga)	Contracture	As Hurler		(Mental retard.)	B,G
										Contracture	Contracture			B,(G)
Ant. ▲		(▲)	(▼)	(▼)						Contracture			(Mental retard.)	B
Post. ▼		(▲)	(▼)	(▼)									(Mental retard.)	B,(G)
	Med. ▲	▲	▼	▼		+	+	▲	(C. valga)	Contracture	As Hurler			B,(G)
Carinatum	Med. ▲	▲	▼	▼		+	+		(C. valga)	G. valgum ++	As Hurler but well modeled	▲ Hip-early ▼ Hip-late	Joint laxity, atlantoaxial instability	R,(Cl.2),B,(G)
(G)	Med. (▲)	▲	▼	▼		+			(C. valga)		As Hurler		Periosteal cloaking	
							+	(+)		+		▼	Fractures	B,(G)
▲ Dense 'rosary'					▲	▲			+	+	Modeling		Fractures	B
					(▲)		Cupped		(+)	+		▼ Prem. fusion	Fractures	B,(G)
											MC 3, 4, 5 ▼		Hypocalcemia	B,(G)
(Beaded)				(Trefoil)	▲					+		▼	Fractures (blue sclerae) (deafness)	(G)
												▼	Fractures	
▼	Thin				(▲)				+	T.P. ▼		▼	Fractures	
			▼	(Pubic symph. wide)						T.P. ▼		▼	(Pseudarthroses)	
(▲)	(▲)		Arcuate bands		▲	▲					'Bone-in-bone'		Fractures, pancytopenia	(G)
(▲)	(▲)		Arcuate bands										(Fractures)	(B)
+	▼		▼							T.P. ▼			Fractures	
(▲)	▲						▲	(Early) ▲			Modeling ▼		Fractures	
			Med. ▲				▲				Modeling ▼			
	▼ Constrict.		Grooved ▼				▼			Wavy	Modeling ▼		Cosmetic only	
	▼ Constrict.		Grooved ▼		▲		▼	Constric.		Wavy	T.P. ▼			
(▲)	▲							▲			Modeling ▼		Pain, muscle weakness	
▲	▲							▲						
							Striations							

Appendix 3 Skeletal dysplasias presenting at birth[a]

Diagnosis[b]		Always lethal[c]	Limbs Short	Bent/ angulated	Dislocation	Femur / tibia / fibula	Poly- dactyly	Skull Ossification	Ribs Short	Beaded/ fractured	Spine Platy- spondyly	Some absent ossification	Pelvis 'Trident' 'Spiky'	Bone density ▲ ▼ + fracture	Genetic 'abnorm.' identified
Achondroplasia	– hetero.		Rhizo.						+				+		+
	– homo.	+	Rhizo.						+				+		+
Thanatophoric	I	+	++	+					++		++		+		+
	II	+	+	+				Clover leaf	+		+		+		+
(Thanatophoric variants)															
Achondrogenesis	I	+	++					▼	+	+		+			+
	II	+	++						+			+			+
Hypochondrogenesis		+	+						+		+	+			+
Spondyloepiphyseal dysplasia congenita			(Rhizo.)						+		+				+
Osteogenesis imperfecta	IIA	+	+	+				▼	+	+			▼+		+
	IIB	+	+	+					+				▼+		+
	IIC	+	+	+				▼	+				▼+		+
	III		(+)	(+)					+				▼+		+
Hypophosphatasia	Lethal	+	+			Fib. ▼		▼	+	+		+	▼+		+
	Surviving			+											+
Campomelic		+		+	+	Fib. ▼									+
Kyphomelic			Rhizo.	+											
Diastrophic			+		+						(+)				
			(1st MC ++)								(Scoliosis)				
Metatropic			+			Dumb-bell			+		++				
Kniest			+			Dumb-bell					(+)				
Fibrochondrogenesis		+	+			Dumb-bell			++		++				
Chondrodysplasia punctata			Rhizo. (+)											Stippled ectopic calcification ▲+	+
Osteopetrosis								▲						▲+	+
Pycnodysostosis								▲						▲+	+
Short-rib syndromes															
I Saldino–Noonan		+	+				+		++				+		
II Majewski		+	Meso.			Oval tibia	+		++						
III Verma–Naumoff		+	+				+		++				+		
Beemer		+	Meso.				(+)		++						
Asphyxiating thoracic (Jeune)			(+)				(+)		++				+		
Ellis–van Creveld			Meso.				+		++				+		
Atelosteogenesis	I	+	Rhizo.	+	+	Fib. ▼			+		+				
	II	+	Rhizo.		+	Fib. ▼									
	III		Rhizo.		+	(Fib. ▼)									
Boomerang / de la Chappelle		+	+	+		Fib. ▼			+		+	(+)	(+)		
Opsismodysplasia			+						+		+	+	+		
Schneckenbecken		+	+			Dumb-bell			+			+	+		
Dyssegmental dysplasia	I		+	+					+						
	II	+	+	+					+						

Reproduced with permission of the Skeletal Dysplasia Group.

[a] All these findings should easily be observed by the nonspecialist.

[b] Grouped according to main radiographic features and (approximately) in descending order of frequency.

[c] Short limbs can be identified on ultrasound by 20 weeks gestation in the lethal conditions and a few nonlethal conditions.

() The findings may be present but mild, or absent.

▼ Reduced, short, hypoplastic, or absent.

▲ Increased, dense.

Tissues should be stored from all these severe skeletal dysplasias to enable confirmatory genetic testing and/or prenatal diagnosis. Cryopreserved fibroblasts are suggested.

1.5 The musculoskeletal system: structure and function

Christopher Bulstrode

Cells and matrix

Higher animals are made up of cells and matrix—the material surrounding the cells. The cells determine to a large degree the active functions of the tissue such as muscle. The matrix determines the mechanical properties of the tissue. Tissues such as bone whose main function is support (a mechanical property) have a high ratio of matrix to cells. Tissues such as muscles (functional) are mainly cellular.

The function of the matrix

The matrix serves two main mechanical functions in the human body. It may prevent tissues being torn apart (tension) or it may stop tissues collapsing (compression). Tensile forces predominate in tissues like tendons and ligaments, while compressive forces are more often found in bones and the interverbral disk. In other tissues, such as articular cartilage, there may be a blend of compression and shearing forces. The structure of the matrix of each tissue is adapted to cope with the stresses it encounters.

Substances in the matrix

The main constituent of the matrix is water which is held in equilibrium with the intracellular water by the osmotic pressure of the salts it contains. Where the matrix needs to resist compression, large feather-shaped molecules with a molecular weight of several million daltons which are intensely hydrophilic (they attract water) hold the matrix together (Fig. 1).

These molecules are proteoglycans, long chains of hyaluronic acid with multiple negatively charged side-arms made up of sulfated disaccharides. If proteoglycans and water were the only constituents of the matrix it would swell into an amorphous jelly. To make a strong structure such as articular cartilage which can keep its shape and resist shearing forces one further component is required—collagen (Fig. 2).

Collagen is a long triple-helix polymer which resists stretching although it can be compressed easily. Collagen is laid down in bundles, layers, or even mats wherever distraction forces may be significant (Fig. 3). It is equivalent to the reinforcing steel rods found in concrete skyscrapers or the carbon strands found in carbon fiber. The combination of an incompressible matrix (proteoglycans and water) and an unstretchable net of collagen creates a composite struc-

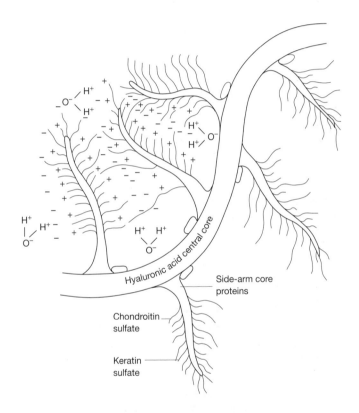

Fig. 1. Proteoglycans—long feathery molecules covered in negative charges which are highly attractive to water molecules (hydrophilic) and create the turgor pressure in the matrix.

ture whose strength and mechanical properties far exceed those of its individual components. This is the characteristic of a good composite material. Depending on the arrangement of the collagen fibers the matrix can specifically resist compression (articular cartilage), tension (the annulus of the intervertebral disk), and distraction (ligaments). However, in order to resist bending, one further component is required in the composite. That substance is hydroxyapatite—a rigid crystal of calcium and phosphate (a form of ceramic)—which converts a strong but flexible matrix into the rigid and unyielding structure of bone. The hydroxyapatite crystal is weak in tension but very strong in compression. When mixed into a composite it resists bending. The crystals are only 25 μm long but are laid down in layers,

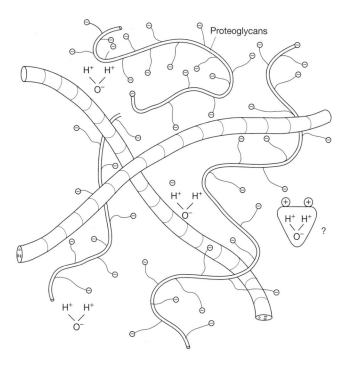

Fig. 2. Matrix consisting of hydrophilic proteoglycans, water, and collagen creating a tense structure which can resist multidirectional compression.

creating bone, which for its weight is one of the strongest composite materials known.

Bone

Bone is a dynamic composite material. It is continuously being resorbed and laid down. Its structure at the microscopic and macroscopic level is specifically designed to cope with and respond to loading. In contrast with invertebrates who shed and regrow their exoskeleton throughout their lives, mammalian bone is an internal skeleton and grows steadily up to adulthood. After this it remains active, continuously being removed and replaced by new bone. This appears to serve two important functions. Firstly, it allows the skeleton to remodel in response to changes in demand and loading. Secondly, it prevents fatigue fractures developing under repetitive loading, a problem that invertebrates avoid by regularly shedding their skeleton and growing a new one.

The composite consists mainly of collagen (strong in distraction) and hydroxyapatite (strong in compression). This results in a material which is also strong in torsion and bending. Macroscopically the structure of bone is designed to give maximum strength with minimum weight. Although human bones are not filled with air, as is the case with many bird bones, the center of the bone (where loads are least) tends to be a lightweight web of trabecular bone (a scaffolding structure) while the cortex (where is strength to resist torsion and bending is most needed) is solid bone.

The central portion of long bones (the diaphysis) is mainly concerned with resisting compression and resisting bending and torsion. Therefore the shape approximates to a thin-walled tube (like a bicycle frame) (Fig. 4). Muscles, tendons, and ligaments are bound firmly

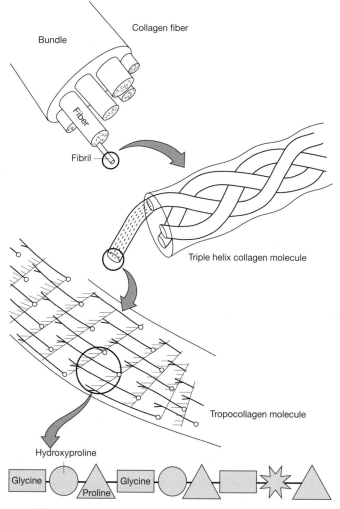

Fig. 3. Collagen—a triple helix of strands made from tropocollagen molecules. Each type of collagen has a characteristic repeating pattern of amino acids usually involving glycine, hydroxyproline, and proline. Collagen is very strong in tension.

to the bone structure by fiber anchors buried deep into the cortex of the bone. These collagen anchors are cemented to the bone with hydroxyapatite (Fig. 5).

In the bone under these areas of external load, the trabecular pattern is modified to cope with these forces. Under a relatively flat load-bearing articular surface the trabeculae are arranged in sweeping arches, strikingly similar to the patterns seen in the roofs of medieval cathedrals (Fig. 6). The similarity is no mere chance. Both are load-bearing structures using the minimum of material (and hence weight) to support the maximum amount of load. Trabeculae are also needed where there are tension forces, not just compression. The proximal end of the femur has large compressive forces on the medial side and distractive forces on the lateral side where the abductor muscle inserts. Trabecular patterns designed to cope with compression fan out from the calcar up to the articular surface of the femoral head. On the lateral side, a second set of trabeculae at right angle to

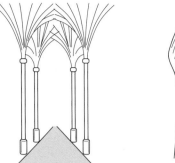

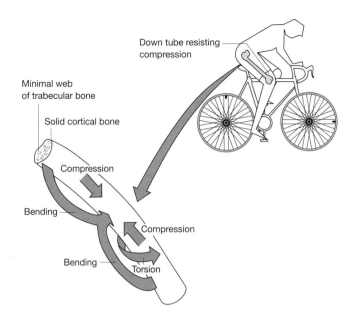

Fig. 4. Bone, like the tubing in the frame of a bicycle, is hollow and designed to be light yet resist bending, compression, and torsion forces.

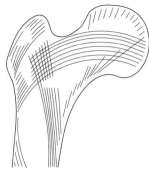

Fig. 6. The design of the ceiling arches in a medieval church mirrors the trabecular pattern of bone because each serves a similar function.

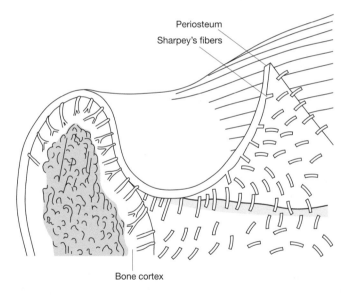

Fig. 5. External structures are bound to the bone by collagenous Sharpey's fibers embedded in hydroxyapatite.

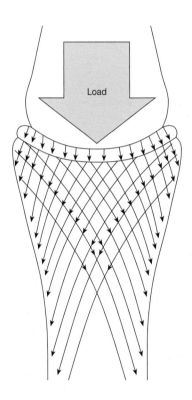

Fig. 7. The trabecular pattern of the neck of the femur is designed to provide maximum strength in the calcar where compression is greatest, and through the top of the femoral neck where tension forces will be largest.

the first arch up and across from the lateral cortex to counter the tension forces (Fig. 7). The line of the trabeculae appears to be partly determined genetically (the genome contains information on how the body should be laid out, the so-called 'genetic *anlage*') but is also modified by the loads passing through the bone. After a fracture or osteotomy, the load passing through bone will change in magnitude and direction. The trabecular patterns are modified in response to this over the subsequent months and years. This response is known as Wolff's law and stated in simple terms says that bone responds to

changes in the magnitude and direction of load by remodeling the shape and thickness of the cortex and of the trabecular pattern inside.

In osteoporosis there is a general reduction in bone mass. Thick trabeculae become thinner, thinner trabeculae may disappear altogether. The radiographic result is a coarsening of the main trabecular pattern. The reason for this paradox is that the main trabeculae may become slightly thinner in osteoporosis but do not disappear, but the small cross-trabeculae disappear and allow the main trabecu-

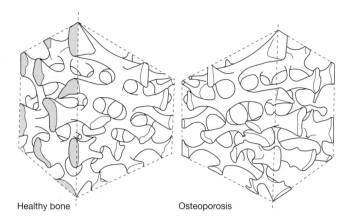

Healthy bone   Osteoporosis

Fig. 8. In osteoporosis there is generalized loss of bone. The thick longitudinal stress-bearing trabeculae become thinner, and thin cross-bridging trabeculae disappear altogether. On radiography the loss of the cross-bridges enhances the definition of the longitudinal trabeculae, making the bone look stronger not weaker.

lae to stand out even more clearly than before, making the bone look stronger rather than weaker on radiographs (Fig. 8).

Embryology of the musculoskeletal system

The differentiation and organization of the embryo starts with the formation of the notochord during gastrulation. It is only at this stage that ectoderm cells become programed to form neural tissue. The signal to start forming the notochord seems to come from a layer of dorsal mesoderm in contact with the ectoderm, which induces the ectoderm to infold and form the neural tube. The limb buds start to form shortly after this. They are produced by rapid division of mesoderm cells (the progress zone) which bulge out as a result of their fast growth. The thin layer of ectoderm lying over the end of the limb bud, called the apical epidermal ridge, seems to stimulate proliferation of the mesoderm beneath. Removal of this apical epidermal ridge at an early stage prevents limb formation altogether. Removal of the apical epidermal ridge late on in limb-bud formation results in normal proximal limb development but absent digits and other

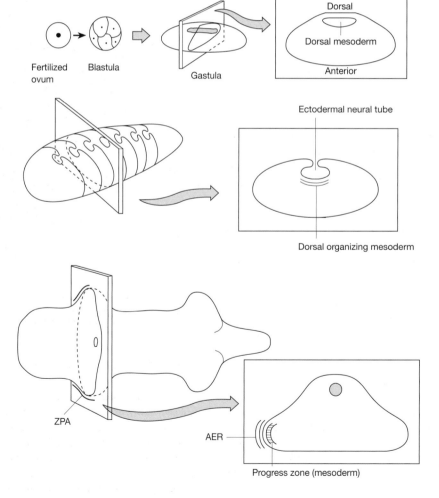

Fig. 9. Formation of the neural tube, followed by limb buds stimulated by the apical ectodermal ridge (AER). Orientation of the limb is controlled by the zone of polarizing activity (ZPA).

distal structures. The apical epidermal ridge seems to control the longitudinal growth of the limb.

The anteroposterior differentiation of the limb is controlled by an area of mesenchyme along the posterior margin of the limb bud known as the zone of polarizing activity. The apical epidermal ridge, the underlying mesenchymal progress zone, and the zone of polarizing activity all work together to produce the normal limb. Cells left behind from the progress zone at any early stage are destined to become part of the proximal limb. Those which leave the progress zone later make up the distal part of the limb (Fig. 9).

The gene controlling the ability of one group of cells to initiate differentiation in another goes by the splendid name of 'sonic hedgehog' and it is this gene which is implicated in the activity of the apical ectodermal ridge cells in the zone of polarizing activity, and indeed the mesenchymal cells which induce the notochord. Activation of this gene in responsive cells seems to be mediated by retinoic acid. The signal sent out by the cells in which 'sonic hedgehog' is active appears to be fibroblast growth factors 2 and 4, and possibly bone morphogenetic protein 2. Downstream cells activated by these signals exhibit activity from the so-called Hoxa and Hoxd genes which appear to control the more detailed organization of the limb and give individual cells a positional address.

Formation of bone

The first clue to the formation of bone is an area of mesenchyme where cells are slightly more densely packed. These cells start to lay down a matrix consisting of a high proportion of collagen type II. The cells round the periphery of this condensation flatten to form a perichondrium. Bone morphogenetic protein 2 is implicated in the early stages of the formation of this cartilage *anlage* (model of the bone); later, tumor growth factor β_2 appears to take over this function. Several other molecules in this family of growth differentiation factors have now been identified, but it is still not clear to what extent the concentration of given growth differentiation factors and a cell's knowledge of its 'positional address' determine its potential for differentiation and organ formation.

The cells within the cartilage model of a bone are larger and set further apart than those at the ends. It is in this central area that the cartilage matrix becomes calcified and the cells die. The cells in the putative periosteum around this area start to lay down osteoid which is converted to bone. The calcified cartilage matrix is now invaded by new blood vessels and cells apparently derived from the walls of these vessels start to lay down osteoid which converts to bone. This method of laying down bone within a cartilage *anlage* is known as endochondral ossification and occurs almost everywhere in the human body apart from the skull and the clavicle (Fig. 10).

Osteocytes become incarcerated in rings of bone laid down around blood vessels, creating a pattern of interlinking rings with a Haversian canal running down the center (Fig. 11).

The ossification of the bone spreads out from the ossification centers, each of which forms at a characteristic age and can be used to age skeletons by radiography. The last areas to ossify are the epiphyseal plates, where longitudinal growth of the bone will continue until adulthood (Fig. 12).

The diameter of bones also increases during growth through bone laid down under the periosteum. At the same time, bone remodeling

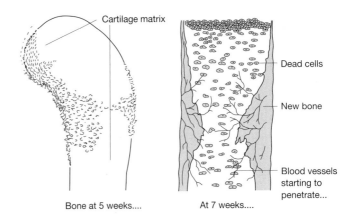

Fig. 10. Formation of bone at 10 weeks from a condensation of mesenchyme. This is followed by the formation of a cartilage model (*anlage*). The cartilage cells then die (apoptosis) and bone is laid down in place of the cartilage.

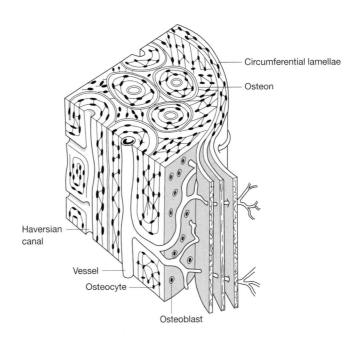

Fig. 11. Osteocytes become incarcerated in rings of bone laid down around blood vessels, creating a pattern of interlinking rings with a Haversian canal running down the center.

may take place on the inner side of the cortex enlarging the diameter of the medulla in proportion the dimensions of the rest of the bone.

In the cortical bone, ossification continues in rings around each blood vessel. The osteoblasts laying down the bone become incarcerated within the bone and are left dormant as osteocytes. These cells are connected by thin cytoplasmic processes, and may be important in calcium homeostasis, as well as possibly sending signals about the load being experienced in the area, which could induce bone remodeling. Each layer of bone laid down around the vessel has the collagen arranged at a certain orientation. The next layer will have its collagen at a different orientation, creating a layered effect which

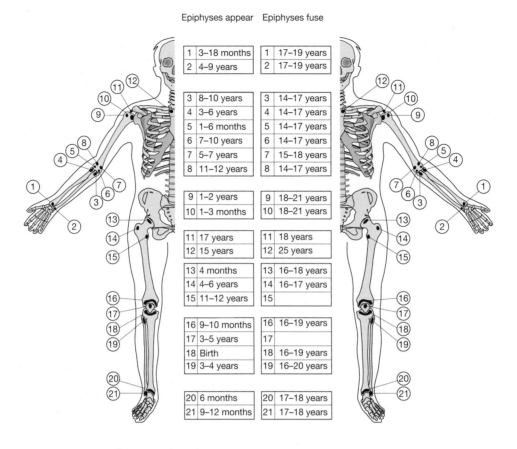

Fig. 12. Atlas of bone age. On the right side of the skeleton are the ages when centers of ossification first appear. On the left are the ages when the plates close. Sophisticated atlases can be used to calculate the age of a patient from the appropriate plain radiographs.

is exceptionally strong (the same principle as is used in plywood). In the center of these sets of concentric rings the blood vessels flow in the Haversian canal (Fig. 11).

Wherever bone is being laid down, fat and active osteoblasts will be visible coating its surface. Beneath them will be a thin layer of osteoid which has not yet been mineralized. Normally it is about 10 μm thick; each layer takes about 10 days to mineralize. An unusually thick layer of osteoid suggests that there may be a problem with bone mineralization such that it cannot keep pace with osteoblast activity (osteomalacia).

Where bone is quiescent, the bone surfaces will be smooth and lined with thin inactive osteocytes. There will be no layer of osteoid visible.

In the adult there is a dynamic equilibrium between osteoclastic activity (resorbing bone) and osteoblastic activity (new bone being laid down) (Fig. 13).

Osteoclasts are large multicellular structures with a large volume of cytoplasm (possible highly specialized macrophages). They are frequently found working in groups when they form a cutting cone in the bone (a tunnel which is drilled into old bone). In the cavity created, osteoblasts line the walls of the cavity and lay down new bone to replace that which was resorbed (Fig. 14). Osteoclasts are enzymatically very active. They appear to absorb bone by sealing off

an area of bone, and then moving into very close contact with that bone. The cytoplasm in close contact becomes highly indented, creating what is known as a brush border. There are large numbers of mitochondria and lysosomal inclusion bodies. The pH under the brush border becomes very low (acidic) and the bone is decalcified. The osteoid is absorbed and collagen is removed with collagenase. There is a close link between the activity of the osteoclasts and of the osteoblasts, maintaining a constant mass of healthy bone and keeping the plasma levels of calcium and phosphate at the correct level. This linkage is probably mediated by cytokines which pass between the two cell types, osteoclasts (removing bone) and osteoblasts (rebuilding). If osteoclastic activity outstrips osteoblastic activity, a progressive reduction in bone mass occurs. This is known as osteoporosis. If this is rapid then plasma calcium and phosphate may rise (as in myeloma and other bone-lysing tumors). Excessive activity by the osteoblasts increases bone mass and removes calcium and phosphate from the plasma.

Blood supply to bone

The blood supply to the center of the bone originally enters at the zones of ossification. There is usually one in the shaft (diaphysis) of the bone and at least one to each end (epiphysis). As the bone elong-

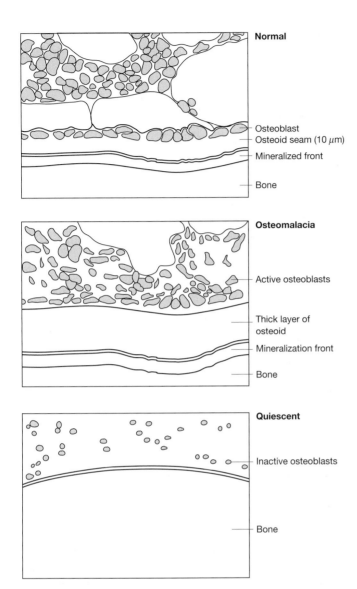

Fig. 13. Bone is normally in dynamic equilibrium, with old bone being removed and new bone constantly being laid down. Mature bone has a thin layer of osteoid on its surface, where mineralization of newly laid down osteoid has not yet occurred. In conditions where there is insufficient calcium, the layer of osteoid will be thickened because mineralization cannot keep up with the deposition of new osteoid. In elderly patients, bone activity may be reduced and the layer of osteoid may become very thin.

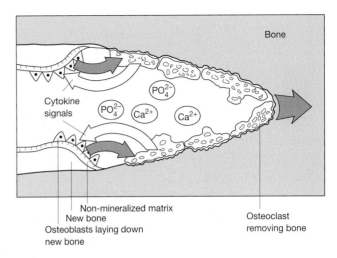

Fig. 14. A cutting cone in mature bone. Osteoclasts are cutting into old bone, resorbing as they go. Behind them, osteoblasts are laying down new bone communicating via cytokines.

in a capillary net in the bone immediately beneath the articular cartilage (the subchondral bone). However, the main supply of oxygen and nutrients to the articular cartilage is by diffusion through the synovial fluid and not from the subchondral vessels (Fig. 15).

Nerve supply to bone

Little is known about the nerve supply to bone. The periosteum is well innervated, but the only nerves entering the bone marrow appear to be unmyelinated sympathetic fibers which travel in the walls of the nutrient vessels, and disperse with them. It is these fibers that presumably mediate the deep aching which comes from bone when there is raised intraosseous pressure, as occurs in osteoarthritis and avascular necrosis.

Bone growth and the epiphyseal plate

Bone normally forms within a cartilage *anlage* (model). The longitudinal growth of bone at the epiphyseal plate is no exception. Growth plates consist of a series of histologic layers which merely represent the stages that bone goes through when it is produced. The epiphyseal plate actually moves forward and, like a comet, leaves a trail behind it which in this case is the final stages of bone formation. At the front of the epiphyseal plate (the comet's head) there are relatively undifferentiated and quiescent reserve cells, ready to be activated and move the epiphyseal plate forward. This is the reserve cell layer. In this quiet area, the epiphyseal artery supplies nutrients to the growing epiphyseal plate. Immediately behind the resting cell layer are cells which are rapidly dividing and separating, driving the resting layer and the epiphysis forward.

This layer creates the cells needed to produce the matrix of the epiphyseal plate. This is known as the proliferative layer. Cells are budded off into the tail of the comet, staying behind and maturing as the proliferative layer continues forward. The cells grow larger and

ates at the epiphyseal plates the nutrient artery entry point tends to become oblique but has a consistent anatomic entry point for each bone. A secondary but equally important blood supply forms in the periosteum, supplying the outer surface of the bone and linking with the vessels from the nutrient artery by collaterals. There may be a circumferential ring of vessels around the epiphyseal plate supplying both the epiphysis and the diaphysis, but blood vessels do not cross the epiphyseal plate itself during growth, or even in adulthood when activity in the growth plate has ceased. The articular cartilage of the joint itself has no blood supply, but the epiphyseal vessels terminate

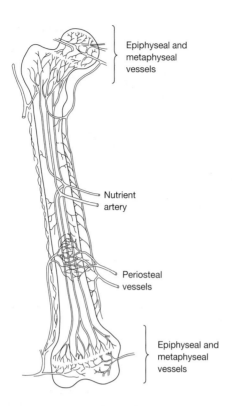

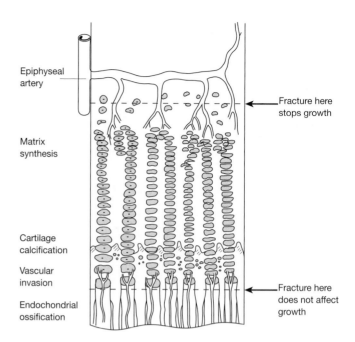

Fig. 16. Articular cartilage. The layers of collagen are oriented to resist the forces to which they are subjected. The surface layer is horizontal to resist shearing forces. The deeper layers are vertical to provide struts for the hydrostatic pressure which serves as a shock absorber.

Fig. 15. (a) Blood supply of an adult long bone: nutrient arteries enter the diaphysis obliquely (because of growth), and periosteal vessels surround the bone; epiphyseal vessels supply the subchondral bone (and the epiphyseal plate until growth is completed). (b) The layers of the epiphyseal growth plate: a fracture through the layer of calcification (the common site—Salter–Harris 2) does not harm growth; a fracture through the reserve layer (the rarer Salter–Harris 4 and 5) is more likely to affect growth by damaging the blood supply to the growth plate.

Joints

Embryology

Joints initially appear in the embryo as condensations of mesenchyme. At around 8 weeks there appears to be a line along which cell death occurs. A cleft is created which develops into the joint. In the typical diarthrodial joint the cells around the cleft contribute to the synovium and articular cartilage.

Healing and longevity

Articular cartilage receives its oxygen and nutrients through the synovium and is relatively acellular, consisting mainly of a highly complex arrangement of collagen. It therefore has very limited powers of healing, although it can mount a healing response. Therefore joint surfaces should be able to sustain many millions of loading cycles without wearing out, and should have low friction and resist shearing forces as well as simple compression.

Anatomy in relation to function

The collagen fibers in the articular cartilage are arranged on the surface as a mat to resist shearing. Deeper down they are vertical. This assists in the load-bearing function of the cartilage because there is a high concentration of proteoglycans between the collagen fibers which draw in water and create the turgor pressure of the cartilage. This pressure constrained by the vertical collagen fibers converts articular cartilage into a hydroelastic suspension system which cushions and spreads load across its joint surface. The indentation of the outer layer of articular cartilage as a load moves across it squeezes

start producing matrix. Columns of cells are produced; those closest to the proliferative layer are still small and young, and those further back are larger and older (hypertrophied) and surrounded by the cartilage matrix that they have produced. This zone is the hypertrophic zone.

Finally, even further from the advancing front it can be seen that the hypertrophied cells are now starting to die (apoptosis) and the cartilage matrix is starting to calcify. This layer (the calcification layer) is an environment ideal for laying down new bone. New blood vessels from the nutrient artery of the metaphysis grow into the back of this zone and from their walls cells appear which remove the calcified cartilage and start to lay down new endochondral bone.

Scanning from the distal side of the epiphyseal plate to the proximal is equivalent to traveling through time, demonstrating in sequence each phase of new bone formation. From the orientation of the epiphyseal plate it can be seen that any fracture of the proximal side is in effect a simple fracture of new bone which can heal normally. Injury to the distal part of the epiphysis (the head of the comet) cuts of the blood supply to the cells about to create the next phase of the plate and effectively stops the plate's forward movement (Fig. 16).

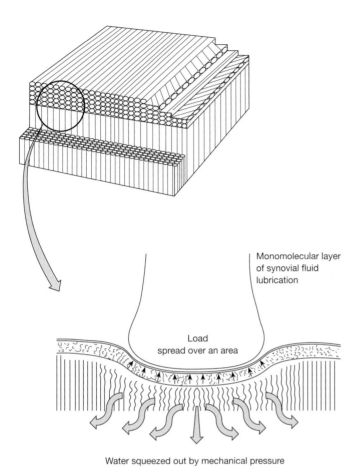

Monomolecular layer
of synovial fluid
lubrication

Load
spread over an area

Water squeezed out by mechanical pressure

Fig. 17. The structure of the intervertebral disk in relation to function. Sheets of collagen laid in oblique sheets (like plywood) allow some movement but resist expansion. The central nucleus pulposus has a high concentration of proteoglycans which create a hydrostatic pressure which resists compression and acts as a shock absorber.

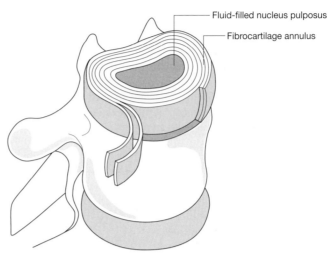

Fluid-filled nucleus pulposus
Fibrocartilage annulus

Fig. 18. The intervertebral disk is designed like a pneumatic tire in cross-section. The fluid-rich nucleus pulposus resists compression. The tough fibrocartilage annulus is the tire casing, allowing small amounts of movement but creating (with the nucleus pulposus) a compressible shock absorber.

out synovial fluid lying within the articular cartilage This creates a fluid lubrication layer between the articular cartilage surfaces. This goes a long way to explain why articular surfaces have such a very low coefficient of friction *in vivo* (Fig. 17).

The synovial membrane

The synovial membrane consists of a thin layer of lining cells lying on a subintimal layer of fat and fibrous tissue. The intimal cells or synoviocytes consist mainly of two classes of cells. One group appears to be mainly synthetic and probably produce hyaluronate for the synovial fluid as well as nutrients for the cartilage cells. The second group are macrophage type cells and probably clear away and detritus created by the movement of the joint.

Fibrocartilage

Fibrocartilage is a special form of cartilage where the matrix is mainly collagen. It is very strong in tension, but alone does not have the shock-absorbing or lubricating qualities of articular cartilage. It is found for example in the annulus of the intervertebral disk, where

in combination with the proteoglycan rich nucleus pulposus it provides a very strong load-bearing joint with a limited range of movement in all planes. The spine is a fundamental load-bearing structure in the human body but must nevertheless allow some movement between each vertebral body while resisting forces producing slip of one vertebra on another. This function is served by an incompressible central fluid-filled sac (the nucleus pulposus) surrounded by several layers of finrocartilage (the annulus). The collagen fibers of each layer are set obliquely and at the opposite angle to the layers each side. The laminated gaiter effect allows limited movement, including torsion, but is able to strongly resist excessive movement and load (Fig. 18).

Calcium and phosphate homeostasis

The skeleton is also involved in the vital homeostasis of calcium and phosphate. Both ions are important in physiology. Calcium is needed for neuromuscular conduction especially in the myocardium. It is also important for clotting. Phosphate has an equally important role in acting as one of the ions needed to buffer the pH of the body fluids.

Homeostasis of these ions can be influenced in four main ways.

1. The intake may be disturbed (usually because of poor diet—dietary rickets). In fact calcium can also be secreted into the bowel, and the amount taken up is controlled by the hormonal state and not just the dietary availability.

2. The regulation of levels in the body may be affected by disorders in the homeostatic mechanisms (inappropriate levels of parathyroid hormone, calcitonin, or vitamin D).

3. The kidneys may be unable to resorb calcium and/or phosphate so they are lost from the body (renal rickets). Large amounts of calcium and phosphate pass out into the proximal renal tubule

in the glomerular filtrate. Most is then reabsorbed from the tubules. This mechanism is under hormonal control.

4. The bone may be destroyed and ions released by the destructive process (myeloma and other bone tumors). There is a continuous exchange of calcium and phosphate between the plasma and bone, but only some of the bone salts appear to be available for rapid release, the rest can only be mobilized slowly when needed. This mechanism is also under hormonal control.

Any disease process may affect more than one of these four causes of dysfunction, so that the final result in terms of whether the serum calcium is raised or reduced and whether the phosphate is affected in the same way or not depends on the actual disease and the body's response to it. However, if both calcium and phosphate are raised, their solubility product may be exceeded in which cases calcium phosphate may be deposited spontaneously in the tissues. The complexities of calcium and phosphate metabolism are discussed in Chapter 2.7.1.

Further reading

Johnson, R.L., Riddle, R.D., and Tabin, C.J. (1994). Mechanism of limb patterning. *Current Opinion in Genetics and Development*, 4, 535–42.

Tickle, C. (1994). On making a skeleton. *Nature*, **368**, 587–8.

1.6 Tumors

1.6.1 Endoprosthetic replacement of skeletal malignancies

T. R. W. Briggs and G. W. Blunn

Introduction

The primary goal of the bone tumor surgeon is the survival of the patient. This involves complete removal of the malignancy, which will involve removal of a segment of bone and additionally often removal of soft tissues associated with the tumor. The success of this technique has greatly increased since the introduction of neoadjuvant chemotherapy. A second goal of the bone tumor surgeon should be the preservation of limb function (Cannon 1997). Springfield *et al.* (1988) reported that survival rate as well as recurrence were similar between amputation and limb salvage operations in patients with osteosarcoma. There are various techniques available to the surgeon for limb salvage.

Amputation versus reconstruction in the management of osteosarcoma

These include the use of autografts, allografts, prosthetic implants, and modified amputations such as rotationplasty. Thus, a comparison of the survival of patients with bone tumors around the knee joint which had been treated using amputation or by limb salvage surgery showed that the local recurrence of disease in both groups was around 10 per cent. It has been shown that the use of endoprosthetic replacements in the distal femur for the treatment of osteosarcoma provides no greater risk in terms of patient survival than amputation (Simon *et al.* 1986; Rougraff *et al.* 1994). In addition a comparison of the functional results between above-knee amputation and limb salvage using endoprostheses indicate that limb salvage has

Box 1

- Survival rates are similar
- Function better with reconstruction
- Growing children may require multiple operations for reconstruction
- If prognosis is limited an endoprosthesis may give better quality of life

better functional results and is more energy efficient than amputation (Otis *et al.* 1985). The energy expenditure during gait and functional results are best after limb salvage where knee joint function is restored when compared with knee arthrodesis and rotationplasty. The only time when limb salvage techniques can be questioned is when young patients are involved and where preservation of limb length would require multiple operations (Sugarbaker *et al.* 1982). Extendible prostheses used to treat young growing patients with bone tumors are generally temporary as the implant will need to be revised at least once during the patient's life (Schindler *et al.* 1998). Conversely, it can be argued that where the prognosis for the survival of the patient is limited, then considering the time scale, the use of an endoprosthesis provides the fastest and most functional outcome.

Comparison between different methods of limb salvage is often difficult, as patient populations between studies are highly variable. Problems associated with the use of large allografts are different from the problems associated with the use of large prosthetic implants. For example, in a series of 870 massive frozen allografts used for the treatment of segmental defects there was a 10 per cent infection rate within the first year and a risk of fracture of 19 per cent within the first 3 years. However, after this period 75 per cent of the grafts became stable and were considered to be successful. An additional complication with osteoarticular allografts is that after approximately 6 years osteoarthritis is a problem and a high percentage of patients require total joint replacements. Rotationplasty was first used as a limb salvage technique for the treatment of osteosarcoma in the distal femur by Kotz and Salzer (1982). Although this technique produces good functional results (Hanlon and Krazbich 1999) the use of an external prosthetic device is required and the cosmetic appearance of the reconstruction is sometimes not acceptable. Other promising reconstructive techniques that have recently been developed utilize living bone to replace the excised tumor. One technique involves the use of vascularized fibula autograft (Han *et al.* 1992; Usui *et al.* 1996) and the other utilizes distraction osteogenesis (Said and El-Sherif 1995; Tsuchiya *et al.* 1997). Whilst the advantages of both techniques are clear the major disadvantage is that marginal excision is required in most cases where the tumor is subarticular in position and involvement of the joint cannot be treated. Another problem is that in patients with malignant disease where the prognosis is poor, the time taken for distraction followed by a period of remodeling may be excessive. In comparison the main problems associated with endoprosthetic replacements are infection and fixation of the implant to the bone.

In the United Kingdom limb salvage operations in supraregional bone tumor centers involving the use of endoprosthetic replacements have been used extensively since the 1970s and more generally since the 1980s. Modern neoadjuvant chemotherapy and improved histo-pathological diagnosis have improved the survival rate of patients with osteosarcoma to 60 per cent at 5 years (Rougraff *et al.* 1994). Functional results of bone tumor patients treated with endo-prosthetic replacement are superior to those treated by massive allog-rafts. In addition it has been shown that endoprosthetic reconstruc-tion is cost-effective when compared with amputation (Grimer *et al.* 1997).

Growing implants

An important development in the design of massive endoprosthetic replacements was made in 1976 with the use of extendible (growing) implant (Scales *et al.* 1987). A large number of bone tumors occur in adolescent patients where resection of the tumor involves removal of the epiphyseal growth plate. These implants consist of an actively growing part which replaces the excised area of bone and a passively growing part which fixes the implant into the unaffected bone on the opposing side of the joint (Figs 1 and 2). The actively growing part, which replaces the epiphyseal growth plate, has a telescopic shaft, which is extended by turning a worm-wheel screw mechanism using a hexagonal driver inserted through a small incision. In order to keep pace with growth of the contralateral limb, active extension of the shaft is performed periodically (usually when the leg-length discrep-ancy becomes greater that 5 to 10 mm). In a series of 12 patients with custom-made extendible distal femoral replacements the mean lengthening over 8 years was 5.2 cm which on average was carried out over six operations (Schindler *et al.* 1997). In most other studies lengthening between 1 and 2 cm was accomplished at each extension.

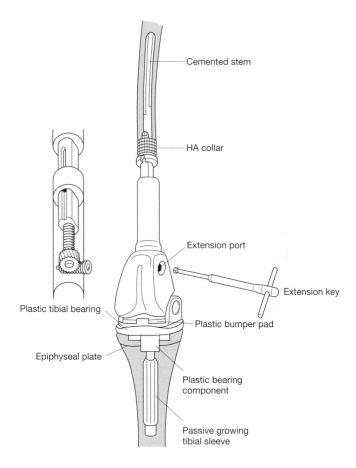

Fig. 2. Schematic diagram showing extendable prostheses.

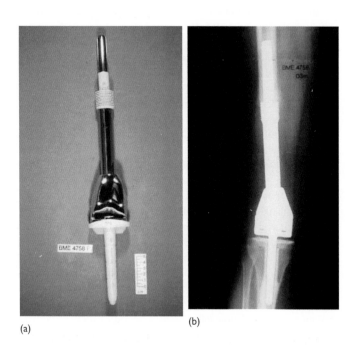

(a)   (b)

Fig. 1. (a) Photograph of a distal femoral replacement with rotating-hinge knee joint, hydroxyapatite-coated collar, and intramedullary stem partly coated with hydroxyapatite. This implant was used to replace an osteosarcoma of the distal femur. (b) Radiograph taken 3 months postoperatively showing the distal femoral replacement *in situ.*

In these studies lengthening was carried out over a number of opera-tions, usually between six and twelve (Schiller *et al.* 1995; Schindler *et al.* 1997). The failure rate for these extendible implants is high with aseptic loosening given as the main reason for revision which may be between 66 and 83 per cent as in a series that was followed up for more than 5 years (Kenan *et al.* 1991; Schiller *et al.* 1995; Schindler *et al.* 1997). Implants used in these patients must therefore be regarded as temporary devices which at some stage, after the patient has finished growing will be replaced by another implant.

The passively growing implant consists of a plateau that is seated on the epiphysis and a stem that penetrates the growth plate (Inglis *et al.* 1992) but does not prevent growth (Cool *et al.* 1997). This stem is polished so that it slides within the intrameduallary cavity as the epiphyseal plate grows. Over the last decade the design of the extending mechanism in bone tumor implants used in the two supra-regional bone tumour centers in the United Kingdom has been changed. The original worm drive was replaced with a system whereby a series of ball bearings were forced into the implant and push apart the telescopic shaft. This system was in turn replaced by a design that was extended by a series of different sized collars of varying sizes. Apart from aseptic loosening infection the other major complication of massive implants in children was infection with rates up to 40 per cent (Schiller *et al.* 1995). The increase in the rate of infection is due to the additional intermittent surgical interventions required to extend the implant. Several major orthopedic companies

Box 2 Complications of growing implants

- Infection due to multiple operations (up to 40 per cent)
- Aseptic loosening (60 to 80 per cent)

have since developed growing implants that are all based on a worm drive or Jacobs chuck mechanism (Eckardt *et al.* 1991*b*, 1993; Kotz *et al.* 1991*b*; Lewis *et al.* 1991). Additionally, a number of experimental designs are investigating the use of growing implants that can be extended noninvasively (Verkerke *et al.* 1991).

Survival and fixation of massive implants

Survival of massive endoprosthetic replacements is generally not as successful as conventional joint replacements. In reported series mechanical failure due to fatigue fracture can account for up to 10 per cent of implant-related failures (Eckardt *et al.* 1991*a*). Infection of primary massive endoprostheses appears to be higher than with conventional arthroplasty but is comparable to other reconstructive techniques (Malawar and Chou 1995). Infection appears to be site dependent and for distal femoral replacements can be as high as 7.5 per cent (Bradish *et al.* 1987), rising to over 20 per cent for some proximal tibial replacements (Grimer *et al.* 1991). However, provided infection is avoided and that implants are strong enough to withstand mechanical failure the main problem associated with failure of the implant is aseptic loosening (Unwin *et al.* 1993*a*; Wirganowicz *et al.* 1999). The survival rate depends not only on the site of the implant but also on the age of the patient and on the amount of bone remaining after excision of the tumor. The survival rate for distal femoral, proximal femoral, and proximal tibial replacements is different.

Causes of failure of massive implants

Proximal femurs are more successful in terms of aseptic loosening than distal femurs or proximal tibias. Figure 3 shows the survival rate for distal femoral replacements in patients under 20 years, between 20 and 60 years, and over 60 years of age. At 120 months the survival rate for patients under 20 years of age with distal femoral replacements is below 45 per cent, whereas for older patients the survival rate is over 65 per cent. Another factor that can significantly influence survival of distal femoral replacements is the amount of bone resected during removal of the tumor (Fig. 4). Distal femurs where a small amount of bone was removed had a greater survival rate than implants where larger amounts of bone were removed. The

Box 3

- Fatigue fracture—10 per cent
- Infection in distal femur—7.5 per cent
- Infection in proximal tibia—20 per cent
- Aseptic loosening—40 to 70 per cent

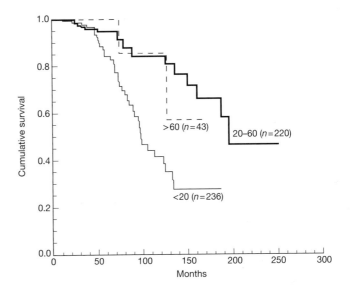

Fig. 3. The effects of age on the survival of distal femoral prostheses.

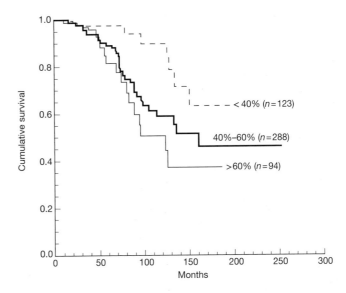

Fig. 4. The effects of the level of resection on the survival of distal femoral prostheses.

reason for this is due to the offset loading which induces greater bending moments the more proximal the intramedullary stem is positioned in the femur (Fig. 5). When age and the amount of bone are both taken into account, patients with distal femoral replacements under the age of 20 years with over 60 per cent of the femur resected had the poorest outcome (Unwin *et al.* 1996).

Factors influencing survival of massive implants

Loosening in massive endoprosthetic implants follows a sequence of events which begins with the osteolysis of the bone adjacent to the shoulder of the implant and a reduction of bone density adjacent to the shoulder (Blunn *et al.* 1991*a*; Ward *et al.* 1997). This osteolysis

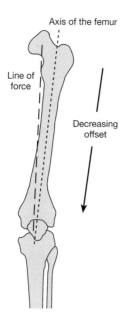

Fig. 5. Schematic diagram showing the effect of the position of the stem in the femur on the offset line of force. The more distal the stem is positioned (i.e. the less bone resected) the more the offset force is reduced and the bending moment on the stem is reduced.

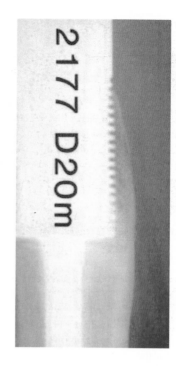

Fig. 6. Radiograph showing bony ingrowth into a hydroxyapatite-coated grooved collar on a distal femoral replacement.

Box 4

- Site—proximal femur better than distal
- Length—long implants fare badly
- Age of patient—younger patients do less well

progresses along the periprosthetic bone implant interface resulting in the development of an extension of radiolucent lines towards the tip of the stem. Using telemetry, Taylor *et al.* (1997) have compared the forces at the stem tip with those passing through the shaft of the implant showing that with time more load is transferred through the stem tip compared with load transfer at the shoulder of the implant. This uncoupling of load from the shoulder of the implant happens quickly. Taylor *et al.* (1997) showed that over a 23-month period the ratio of the mean tip force to the shaft force steadily increased from 25 to 63 per cent. Histological observations of bone remodeling around these implants is consistent with this progressive transfer of load to the stem tip. Histological data of retrieval specimens showed that changes in the distribution of load are accompanied by the formation of a fibrous tissue membrane under the shoulder with increased bone porosity and reduced bone diameter which indicates disuse osteoporosis.

Other authors have indicated that loosening may be associated with wear-debris-induced osteolysis (Ward *et al.* 1997).

In order to combat loosening in patients with massive endoprosthetic replacements the fixation of implants has been augmented using collars around the shaft that allow bone to integrate with the implant. This makes use of reactive bone formation that grows from the transaction site over the shaft of the implant to form a bony bridge. These collars are constructed from sintered porous titanium beads (Chao and Sim 1985; Gottsauner-Wolf *et al.* 1991; Ward *et al.* 1993) and can be augmented with bone graft. Although bone ingrowth into the collars occurs in some cases the use of an hydroxyapatite coating provides more reliable results. In our Institution a comparison of hydroxyapatite collars with porous collars has shown that in cases without graft augmentation the incidence of bone integration occurred in over 70 per cent of cases with hydroxyapatite in the distal femur compared with no ingrowth recorded in porous collars (Fig. 6). In addition, the size of the radiolucent lines around the intramedullary stem could be inversely correlated with the amount of bone ingrowth into the hydroxyapatite collar (Cobb *et al.* 1991; Unwin *et al.* 1993b). Bony bridging is believed to reduce loosening by acting as a 'purse string' which seals the bone–implant interface (Ward *et al.* 1997), preventing the migration of wear particles. Osseointegration of the bony bridge may also lead to the preservation of load transfer at the shoulder of the implant. In addition to reducing the number of radiolucent lines around the intramedullary cemented stem, ingrowth into the hydroxyapatite collar was also a major factor in the survival of distal femurs. A study of 402 patients with fixed-hinge knee joints was compared with rotating hinge designs with and without hydroxyapatite collars (Unwin *et al.* 1999). This study showed that probability of surviving aseptic loosening was 92 per cent in the fixed-hinged group and 100 per cent in the rotating hinges with hydroxyapatite collars at 5 years duration. In addition the number of radiolucent lines around distal femurs with rotating hinges alone was reduced when compared with fixed hinges. However, the number of radiolucent lines was reduced even further when a combination of a rotating hinge with a hydroxyapatite-coated collar was used.

For young patients with massive endoprostheses fixed using intramedullary cemented stems, growth of the skeleton may be an import-

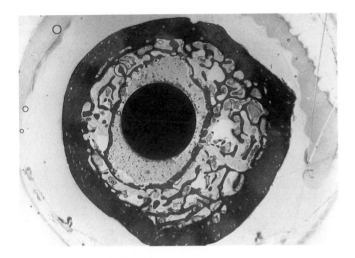

Fig. 7. Transverse histological section through an intramedullary stem of a distal femoral replacement in the diaphyseal region of the femur in a 16-year-old patient. This shows the formation of a neocortex, a region of cancellous bone, and outer denser cortical bone. When the implant was inserted (at age 12) the cement was located against dense cortical bone.

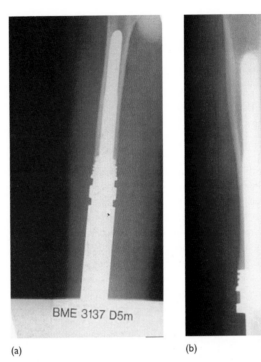

(a)　　　　　　　　(b)

Fig. 8. (a) Radiograph taken 5 months postoperatively showing uncemented intramedullary stem. (b) Radiograph of the patient shown in (a) taken 2 years postoperatively showing remodeling due to stress protection resulting in loss of bone on the periosteal surface.

ant factor in aseptic loosening. In all patients with securely fixed intramedullary stems located in the diaphysis bone, remodeling results in the formation of a neocortex surrounding the cement. For young patients the formation of this neocortex is more important because of centrifugal bone growth resulting in an increase in the girth (Fig. 7). In a normal bone this results in an increase in diameter of the intramedullary cavity. Therefore as growth proceeds, bony support for the neocortex which holds the stem in place may be reduced (Blunn and Wait 1991; Blunn *et al.* 1991*b*).

A development which appears to reduce loosening substantially, particularly in young patients with distal femur and proximal tibial replacements, is the use of uncemented intramedullary stems. This type of fixation has been used successfully in designs such as the Kotz modular femoral and tibial reconstruction and in its modified form as the Howmedica modular resection device. These designs have intramedullary stems with porous ingrowth areas. The implants are stabilized by extracortical plates that are attached using screws. Compared with cemented stems the incidence of aseptic loosening of these designs is reduced but other complications occur such as fracture of stems and screws which attach the extracortical plate to the bone and resorption of bone under the shoulder of the implant (Capanna *et al.* 1994; Morris *et al.* 1995).

Methods for reducing aseptic loosening

In our center, where appropriate, implants are anchored to the bone using an uncemented stem that is partly coated with hydroxyapatite.

Box 5

- Bone ingrowth collars
- Hydroxyapatite coating of implants
- Partial coating to reduce stress protection

Indications for the use of these implants include the age of the patient and the amount of bone resection. Fixing these uncemented designs in a widely divergent intramedullary canal is not possible. Initially stems were fully hydroxyapatite coated. The implants where the stem was fully hydroxyapatite coated appeared to be associated with periosteal cortical bone remodeling, particularly under the shoulder, leading to loss of the bone. This remodeling occurs quickly and could be seen after only 6 months. Using finite element analysis it has been shown that this bone loss is due to stress protection. This bone loss stabilizes, and in active patients bone re-forms in this region with time (Fig. 8). Histology of two cases that have been retrieved as a result of amputation, due to recurrence of the disease, shows that even where cortical remodeling occurs leading to wasting, bone is adherent to the surface of the hydroxyapatite.

Pelvic replacements

Local resection of the periacetabular region of the pelvis has become an established alternative to hindquarter amputation in the management of primary bone tumors around the pelvis. In tumors of the pelvis a long latency period in clinical symptoms is often involved, which is why muscle, ischial and femoral nerves, and iliac or femoral vessels are involved. Extensive resections are also involved. Surgery is complicated and blood loss, orientation, nerve damage, and wound closure are complications associated with removal of the tumor (Allan *et al.* 1995). Reconstruction after tumor removal involves options that include arthrodesis, allografts, a saddle type of femoral prostheses or a hemipelvis reconstruction with a total hip replacement. Endoprosthetic reconstruction with a saddle implant involves inserting a modular femoral stem with a saddle-shaped proximal part that articulates against a notch in the iliac remnants after major acetabular bone loss (Aboulafia *et al.* 1991). The saddle–bone articulation allows for flexion and abduction. An additional bearing below the saddle allows rotational movement. In the United Kingdom prior to 1990 hemipelvis reconstruction with an endoprosthesis usually involved a two-stage procedure. The implant was designed around a mould of the resected specimen. This involved considerable delay between the resection and reconstruction and involved double the surgical risk to the patient. A one-stage reconstruction is now used where CT scans are used to make a model of the pelvis using rapid prototype techniques. This type of approach is used in other centers in Japan (Shinjo *et al.* 1991), Europe (Kotz *et al.* 1991*a*), and in the United States.

Having decided on the resection level, an implant is made from a block of titanium alloy that fits onto the bone. The bone model is used for surgical planning and for checking the fit of the implant. The implant has flanges which fit over the anterior and posterior aspect of the ilium and two divergent pins which can be cemented in place. The largest pin is fixed within the iliopubic bar and the

other pin is located into the medullary space of the ilium. A cup is cemented into the implant and a femoral component is inserted (Fig. 9). Patients treated by these techniques are thankfully few in number and major centers often report on a small number of cases. However, reports of these techniques have shown complications associated with wound healing, dislocation of the hip, and nerve palsy.

A novel approach that requires the use of endoprostheses for the treatment of periacetabular bone tumors is the use of a homolateral proximal femoral autograft. In these cases the proximal femur is swung through 180° to fill in the pelvic defect. The acetabular cup is implanted into the cancellous bone of the greater trochanter and this articulates with a massive proximal femoral replacement that replaces the proximal femur. This technique was developed by Puget *et al.* (1991) and results seem to be more reliable than those with hemipelvic implants.

Soft-tissue complications

Problems associated with soft tissues involve coverage of the implant and attachment of muscles to the implant. These problems are associated with reattachment of specific muscle groups to the implant such that the functional outcome of the reconstruction can be improved and with wound healing such that infection is avoided. Complications associated with proximal tibial and distal femoral replacements include the problem of soft-tissue coverage and these replacements are most often associated with soft-tissue problems. Tumors around the knee frequently extend into the surrounding soft tissues. The removal of these tissues in combination with the effects of chemotherapy makes management of the soft tissues important in

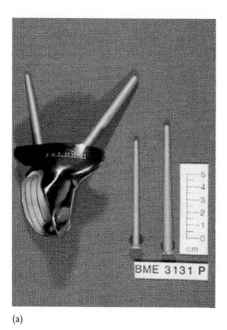

(a)

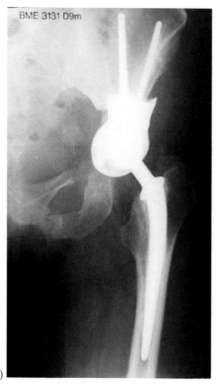

(b)

Fig. 9. (a) Photograph of a hemipelvic replacement. (b) Radiograph of patient with hemipelvic and hip joint replacement.

limb salvage. A solution has been to use gastrocnemius rotation flaps (Malawer and McHale 1989) and tissue transfer with a myocutaneous free flap and the latissimus dorsi as the donor muscle (Horowitz *et al.* 1991).

Tumor surgery of the proximal tibia is associated with reconstruction of the extensor mechanism. Previously this involved the use of a Terylene mesh that was sown into the patellar tendon and passed through the shaft of the implant in the region of the tibial tuberosity. This artificial tendon rubbed on the titanium alloy shaft and generated wear debris. In some cases the tissue overlying the prosthesis in the shin region was discolored and darkly stained. A fluid-filled sac could be detected which when aspirated produced a sterile black fluid containing titanium debris. In addition the tendon also caused local inflammation and a sinus developed which at first was aseptic but which soon became infected. These complications are now prevented by the use of gastrocnemius rotational flaps to the front of the tibia and the attachment of the patellar tendon to this transferred muscle. For example, in a study of 151 patients with proximal tibial replacements over a 20-year period the rate of infection was reduced from 36 to 12 per cent by reconstructing with a rotational gastrocnemius flap (Grimer *et al.* 1999).

Fixation of tendons to metallic implants can improve the function and stability of endoprosthetic replacements (Gottsauner-Wolf *et al.* 1994; Markel *et al.* 1995). Devices used for the incorporation of the tendon into the implant usually involve a clamp to secure the tendon into a titanium mesh that is used to incorporate the bone. In animal experiments it has been shown that use of autogenous tendon and bone block results in fixation of physiological strength through bone ingrowth into the titanium mesh (Gottsauner-Wolf *et al.* 1994). The techniques used for reattachment depend on the margins of the tumor and often where there is involvement of soft tissues tendon attachment is difficult simply because there is little tendon left after surgery. Attachment of the patellar tendon to the implant is advantageous because the power that the quadriceps develops can be transferred directly to the implant. This has been attempted by clamping the patellar tendon to the implant. Often this involves lengthening the tendon by downward transfer of a piece of patellar bone and tendon. This turned down piece of tendon remains attached to the main tendon body (Cannon 1997).

Another complication associated with the soft tissues occurs in replacement of the proximal humerus. Owing to resection of soft tissues during surgery patients have limited abduction movement of the shoulder and in addition where a hemiarthroplasty is used the humeral head often migrates out of the glenoid during movement. This superior subluxation of the humeral head can be controlled by using a captive glenoid component which is screwed into the scapula. Another method is to encourage fibrosis around the head by using a Terylene mesh that is attached to the edges of the resected rotator cuff or the glenoid labrum and to the shaft of the proximal humeral replacement (Ayoub *et al.* 1999).

Revision of massive endoprostheses

As bone tumors occur in relatively young patients, combined with the use of chemotherapy to prevent secondary lesions occurring, patients can be expected to outlive their implant. In addition, as massive implants generally are not as successful as those for total joint arthroplasty then the proportion of primary implants requiring a revision procedure is high. Therefore the success of long-term limb salvage using endoprostheses after tumor resection generally depends on the prosthetic longevity and on the management of prosthetic failures. The options for revision of primary massive endoprostheses include amputation, arthrodeses, the use of vascularized fibula allografts, and the use of a revision implant. Of these options revision using another massive implant is the most common. For example in a study from the Mayo Clinic over a period of 10 years, 208 primary implants were for limb salvage inpatients with tumors. In this series, reoperations were required in 52 patients and of these, 35 were prosthetic revisions. Of these 35 patients 12 needed a third operation (Shin *et al.* 1999). The chance and frequency of a revision operation increased as patients survived longer. Revision of these implants with another endoprosthesis is associated with a number of difficulties not encountered in primary implants. Bone loss associated with infection or aseptic loosening may reduce the bone stock available. Endosteal lysis associated with debris or infection may reduce the strength and quality of bone so that the eroded area has to be bypassed to ensure good fixation. In these situations a number of options are available which include the use of extracortical plates with or without intramedullary stems, stems anchored with a lag screw which passes into the femoral neck, and the use of Wagner-type cutting flutes which anchor the implant in viable bone.

Functional outcomes

The need for a standardized system for measuring the function of various limb salvage and ablative procedures led to the development of an internationally recognized system (Enneking *et al.* 1993) which is called the Musculoskeletal Tumour Society Rating Scales. This system assesses the function of the reconstruction after surgical treatment of musculoskeletal tumors in the lower limb by assigning numerical (0–5) values for pain, function, emotional acceptance, walking ability, use of supports, and gait. In the upper limb gait, walking supports, and walking ability are replaced by hand positioning, manual dexterity, and lifting ability. Other schemes have been used to measure the functional outcome, namely the Toronto Extremity Salvage Score (Davis *et al.* 1999) and the Short Form 36. The Short Form 36 represent patients perceptions of their mental and physical health whilst the Toronto Extremity Salvage Score measures physical function. These schemes have recently been compared with the Musculoskeletal Tumour Society Rating. The main difference between these schemes is that the clinician completes the Musculo-skeletal Tumour Society Rating Scales.

Future of endoprosthetic replacement

Over the last 20 years limb salvage has become more widely used. This has been due to the use of neoadjuvant chemotherapy which has made limb-sparing surgery possible. The use of endoprosthetic replacement has proved sucessful and is probably the most frequently used technique for the preservation of the limb after tumor surgery. However, other techniques are being developed such as the use of distraction osteogenesis and vascularized grafts which may replace the use of massive replacements for certain indications such as diaphyseal replacements. However, extra-articular resections and removal of most tumors with safe margins usually require joint replacements. At the moment the only alternative to the use of a joint replacement is the use of massive allografts. Allografts are associated with problems such as incorporation into the host bone, infection, and osteoarthritis of the joint. However, the use of composite endoprosthetic replacements with living autografts may be a way of preserving host bone and avoiding complications associated with aseptic loosening of the fixation.

Tissue engineering techniques which involve growth of bone cells in the laboratory, prior to their use in the body are a new and exciting avenue but again these techniques would have to be used in conjunction with a reinforcing implant as initial strength is important.

Whatever the future holds the expertise of specialist surgeons, bioengineers, and biologists will be required to advance the field of limb salvage.

References

Aboulafla, A., Faulks, C., Li, W., Buch, R., Matthews, J., and Malawer, M. (1991). Reconstruction using the saddle prosthesis following excision of malignant periacetabular tumors. In *Complications of limb salvage: prevention, management and outcome* (ed. K.L.B. Brown), p. 223. ISOLS, Montreal.

Allan, G., Bell, R.S., Davis, A., and Langer, F. (1995). Complex acetabular reconstruction for metastatic tumor. *Journal of Arthroplasty*, **10**, 301–6.

Bacci, G., Springfield, D., Capanna, R., Picci, P., Bertoni, F., and Campanacci, M. (1985). Adjuvent chemotherapy for malignant fibrous histiocytoma in the femur and tibia. *Journal of Bone and Joint Surgery, American Volume*, **67A**, 620–5.

Blunn, G.W. and Wait, M.E. (1991). Remodelling of bone around intramedullary stems in growing patients. *Journal of Orthopedic Research*, **9**, 809–19.

Blunn, G.W., Hua, J., Wait, M.E., and Walker, P.S. (1991a). Correlation of stress distribution with bony remodelling in retrieved femora with proximal femoral replacements. In *Complications of limb salvage: prevention, management and outcome* (ed. K.L.B. Brown), pp. 445–50. ISOLS, Montreal.

Blunn, G.W., Wait, M.E., and Scales, J.T. (1991b). Remodelling of bone around massive prostheses used in growing patients. In *Limb salvage—major reconstructions in oncologic and nontumoral conditions* (ed. F. Langlais and B. Tomeno), pp. 601–8. Springer-Verlag, Berlin.

Bradish, C.F., Kemp, H.B.S., Scales, J.T., and Wilson, J.N. (1987). Distal femoral replacement by custom-made prostheses. *Journal of Bone and Joint Surgery, British Volume*, **69B**, 276–84.

Cannon, S.R. (1997). Massive prostheses for malignant bone tumours of the limbs. *Journal of Bone and Joint Surgery, British Volume*, **79B**, 497–506.

Capanna, R., Morris, H.G., Campanacci, D., Del Ben, M., and Campanacci, M. (1994). Modular uncemented prosthetic reconstruction after resection of tumours of the distal femur. *Journal of Bone and Joint Surgery, British Volume*, **76B**, 178–86.

Chao, E.Y. and Sim, F.H. (1985). Modular prosthetic system for segmental bone and joint replacement after tumor resection. *Orthopedics*, **8**, 641–51.

Cobb, J.P., Unwin, P.S., Walker, P.S., and Blunn, G.W. (1991). Extracortical bone bridging to enhance fixation. In *Complications of limb salvage: prevention, management and outcome* (ed. K.L.B. Brown), pp. 409–411. ISOLS, Montreal.

Cool, W.P., Carter, S.R., Grimer, R.J., Tillman, R.M., and Walker, P.S. (1997). Growth after extendible endoprosthetic replacement of the distal femur. *Journal of Bone and Joint Surgery, British Volume*, **79B**, 938–42.

Davis, A.M., Bell, R.S., Badley, E.M., Yoshida, K., and Williams, J. (1999). 1. Evaluating functional outcome in patients with lower extremity sarcoma. *Clinical Orthopaedics and Related Research*, **358**, 90–100.

Eckardt, J.J., Eilber, F.R., Rosen, G., *et al.* (1991a). Endoprosthetic replacement for stage IIB osteosarcoma. *Clinical Orthopaedics and Related Research*, **270**, 202–13.

Eckardt, J.J., Eilber, F.R., Rosen, G., Kabo, J.M., Safran, M., and Mirra, J.M. (1991b). Expandable endoprostheses for the skeletally immature: the initial UCLA experience. In *Limb salvage—major reconstructions in oncologic and nontumoral conditions* (ed. F. Langlais and B. Tomeno), pp. 585–90. Springer-Verlag, Berlin.

Eckardt, J.J., Safran, M.R., Eilber, F.R., Rosen, G., and Kabo, J.M. (1993). Expandable endoprosthetic reconstruction of the skeletally immature after malignant bone tumor resection. *Clinical Orthopaedics and Related Research*, **297**, 188–202.

Enneking, W.F., Dunham, W., Gebhardt, M.C., Malawar, M., and Pritchard, D.J. (1993). A system for the functional evaluation of reconstructive procedures after surgical treatment of tumors of the musculoskeletal system. *Clinical Orthopaedics and Related Research*, **286**, 241–6.

Gottsauner-Wolf, F., Rock, M.G., Pritchard, D.J., Sim, F.H., and Chao, E.Y.S. (1991). Extracortical bone bridging for endoprosthetic shaft anchorage in segmental bone/joint defect replacement. In *Complications of limb salvage: prevention, management and outcome* (ed. K.L.B. Brown), pp. 439–41. ISOLS, Montreal.

Gottsauner-Wolf, F., Egger, E.L., Schultz, F.M., Simm, F.H., and Chao, E.Y.S. (1994). Tendons attached to prostheses by tendon–bone block fixation: an experimental study in dogs. *Journal of Orthopedic Research*, **12**, 814–21.

Grimer, R.J., Carter, S.R., and Sneath, R.S. (1991). Endoprosthetic replacements of the proximal tibia. In *Limb salvage—major reconstructions in oncologic and nontumoral conditions* (ed. F. Langlais and B. Tomeno), pp. 285–92. Springer-Verlag, Berlin.

Grimer, R.J., Carter, S.R., and Pynsent, P.B. (1997). The cost-effectiveness of limb salvage for bone tumours. *Journal of Bone and Joint Surgery, British Volume*, **79B**, 558–61.

Grimer, R.J., Carter, S.R., Tillman, R.M., *et al.* (1999). Endoprosthetic replacement of the proximal tibia. *Journal of Bone and Joint Surgery, British Volume*, **81B**, 488–94.

Han, C.-S., Wood, M.B., Bishop, A.T., and Cooney, W.P. (1992). Vascularized bone transfer. *Journal of Bone and Joint Surgery, American Volume*, **74A**, 1441–9.

Hanlon, M. and Krajbich, J. (1999). 1. Rotationplasty in skeletally immature patients. *Clinical Orthopaedics and Related Research*, **385**, 75–82.

Horowitz, S.M., Lane, J.M., Otis, J.C., and Healey, J.H. (1991). Prosthetic arthroplasty of the knee after resection of a sarcoma in the proximal end of the tibia. A report of sixteen cases. *Journal of Bone and Joint Surgery, American Volume*, **73A**, 286–93.

Inglis, A.E., Jr, Walker, P.S., Sneath, R.S., Grimer, R., and Scales, J.T. (1992). Uncemented intramedullary fixation of implants using polyethylene sleeves: a roentgenographic study. *Clinical Orthopaedics and Related Research*, **284**, 208–14.

Kenan, S., Bloom, N., and Lewis, M.M. (1991). Limb-sparing surgery in skeletally immature patients with osteosarcoma. The use of an expendable prosthesis. *Clinical Orthopaedics and Related Research*, **270**, 223–30.

Kotz, R. and Salzer, M. (1982). Rotation-plasty for childhood osteosarcoma of the distal part of the femur. *Journal of Bone and Joint Surgery, American Volume*, **64A**, 959–69.

Kotz, R., Kutschera, H.P., and Windhager, R. (1991*a*). Early experience with implantation of pelvic prostheses designed by CAD. In *Complications of limb salvage: prevention, management and outcome* (ed. K.L.B. Brown), p. 211. ISOLS, Montreal.

Kotz, R., Schiller, C., Windhager, R., and Ritschl, P. (1991*b*). Endoprostheses in children—first results. In *Limb salvage—major reconstructions in oncologic and nontumoral conditions* (ed. F. Langlais and B. Tomeno), pp. 591–9. Springer-Verlag, Berlin.

Lewis, M.M., Kenan, S., and Bloom, N. (1991). The expandable adjustable prosthesis: an alternative to amputation in growing children with malignant tumors of the extremities. In *Limb salvage—major reconstructions in oncologic and nontumoral conditions* (ed. F. Langlais and B. Tomeno), pp. 579–84. Springer-Verlag, Berlin.

Malawer, M. and Chou, L. (1995). Prosthetic survival and clinical results with use of large segment replacements in treatment of high-grade bone sarcomas. *Journal of Bone and Joint Surgery, American Volume*, **77A**, 1154–65.

Malawer, M. and McHale, K. (1989). Limb sparing surgery for high grade malignant tumors of the proximal tibia. Surgical technique and method of extensor mechanism reconstruction. *Clinical Orthopaedics and Related Research*, **239**, 231–48.

Markel, M.D., Wood, S.A., Bogdanske, J.J., *et al.* (1995). Comparison of healing of allograft/endoprosthetic composites with three types of gluteus medius attachment. *Journal of Orthopedic Research*, **13**, 105–14.

Morris, H.G., Capanna, R., Del Ben, M., and Campanacci, D. (1995). Prosthetic reconstruction of the proximal femur after resection for bone tumors. *Journal of Arthroplasty*, **10**, 293–9.

Otis, J.C., Lane, J.M., and Kroll, M.A. (1985). Energy cost during gait in osteosarcoma patients after resection and knee replacement and after above-the-knee amputation. *Journal of Bone and Joint Surgery, American Volume*, **67A**, 606–11.

Puget, J., Tricoire, J.L., Colombier, J.A., Chiron, P., and Utheza, G. (1991). Limb salvage in large periacetabular tumoural defects. In *Complications of limb salvage: prevention, management and outcome* (ed. K.L.B. Brown), p. 215. ISOLS, Montreal.

Rougraff, B.T., Simon, M.A., Kneisl, J.S., Greenberg, D.B., and Mankin, H.J. (1994). Limb salvage compared with amputation for osteosarcoma of the distal end of the femur. A long-term oncological, functional, and quality-of-life study. *Journal of Bone and Joint Surgery, American Volume*, **76A**, 649–56.

Said, G.Z. and El Sherif, E.K. (1995). Resection-shortening-distraction for malignant bone tumours: a report of two cases. *Journal of Bone and Joint Surgery, British Volume*, **77B**, 185–8.

Scales, J.T., Sneath, R.S., and Wright, K.W.J. (1987). Design and clinical use of extending prostheses. In *Limb salvage in musculoskeletal oncology* (ed. W.E. Enneking), pp. 52–61. Churchill Livingstone, New York.

Schiller, C., Windhanger, R., Fellinger, E.J., Salzer-Kuntschik, M., Kaider, A., and Kotz, R. (1995). Extendable tumour endoprostheses for the leg in children. *Journal of Bone and Joint Surgery, British Volume*, **7B**, 608–14.

Schindler, O.S., Cannon, S.R., Briggs, T.W.R., and Blunn, G.W. (1997). Stanmore custom-made extendible distal femoral replacements. Clinical experience in children with primary malignant bone tumours. *Journal of Bone and Joint Surgery, British Volume*, **79B**, 927–37.

Schindler, O.S., Cannon, S.R., Briggs, T.W.R., Blunn, G.W., Grimer, R.J., and Walker, P.S. (1998). Use of extendable total femoral replacements in children with malignant bone tumors. *Clinical Orthopaedics and Related Research*, **357**, 157–70.

Shin, D.S., Weber, K.L., Chao, E.Y.S., An, K.N., and Sim, F.H. (1999). Re-operation for failed prosthetic replacement used for limb salvage. *Clinical Orthopaedics and Related Research*, **358**, 53–63.

Shinjo, K., Asai, T., Saito, S., *et al.* (1991). Dacron fabric enveloped alumina ceramic pelvic prostheses for cementless reconstruction of periacetabular tumor defects. In *Complications of limb salvage: prevention, management and outcome* (ed. K.L.B. Brown), p. 235. ISOLS, Montreal.

Simon, M.A., Aschliman, M.A., Thomas, N., and Mankin, H.J. (1986). Limb-salvage treatment versus amputation for osteosarcoma of the distal end of the femur. *Journal of Bone and Joint Surgery, American Volume*, **68A**, 1331–7.

Springfield, D.S., Schimdt, R., Graham-Pole, J., Marcus, R.B., Spanier, S.S., and Enneking, W.F. (1988). Surgical treatment for osteosarcoma. *Journal of Bone and Joint Surgery, American Volume*, **70A**, 1124.

Sugarbaker, P.H., Barofsky, I., Rosenberg, S.A., and Gianola, F.J. (1982). Quality of life assessment of patients in extremity sarcoma clinical trials. *Surgery*, **91**, 17–23.

Taylor, S.J.G., Perry, J.S., Meswania, J.M., Donaldson, N., Walker, P.S., and Cannon, S.R. (1997). Telemetry of forces from proximal femoral replacements and relevance to fixation. *Journal of Biomechanics*, **30**, 225–34.

Tsuchiya, H., Tomita, K., Minematsu, K., Mori, Y., Asada, N., and Kitano, S. (1997). Limb salvage using distraction osteogenesis. A classification of the technique. *Journal of Bone and Joint Surgery, British Volume*, **79B**, 403–11.

Unwin, P.S., Cobb, J.P., and Walker, P.S. (1993*a*). Distal femoral arthroplasty using custom-made prostheses: the first 218 cases. *Journal of Arthroplasty*, **8**, 259–68.

Unwin, P.S., Blunn, G., Cannon, S.R., *et al.* (1993*b*). The effectiveness of hydroxyapatite coated and porous beaded collars for bony bridging in bone tumour: Stanmore massive endoprotheses. In *Limb salvage—current trends* (ed. S.K. Tan *et al.*), pp. 459–66. ISOLS, Singapore.

Unwin, P.S., Walker, P.S., and Blunn, G.W. (1995). A radiographic and retrieval study, comparing porous collared and hydroxyapatite coated segmental femoral replacements. *Transactions of the Orthopedics Research Society*, **20**, 747.

Unwin, P.S., Cannon, S.R., Grimer, R.J., Kemp, H.B.S., Sneath, R.S., and Walker, P.S. (1996). Aseptic loosening in cemented custom-made prosthetic replacements for bone tumours of the lower limb. *Journal of Bone and Joint Surgery, British Volume*, **78B**, 5–13.

Unwin, P.S., Walker, P.S., Briggs, T.W., *et al.* (1999). Rotating hinged, hydroxyapatite coated versus fixed hinged, uncoated distal femoral replacements. A study of 402 cases. *Proceedings of the 10th International Symposium on Limb Salvage, Cairns, Australia*.

Usui, M., Ishii, S., Naito, T., Wada, T., Yamawaki, S., and Isu, K. (1996). Limb-saving surgery in osteosarcoma by vascularised fibular graft. *Journal of Orthopedic Science*, **1**, 4–10.

Verkerke, G.J., van den Kroonenberg, H.H., Grootenboer, H.J., *et al.* (1991) *In vitro* and *in vivo* experiments of a lengthening element for a modular femur endoprosthetic system. In *Limb salvage—major reconstructions in oncologic and nontumoral conditions* (ed. F. Langlais and B. Tomeno), pp. 609–12. Springer-Verlag, Berlin.

Ward, W.G., Johnston, K.S., Dorey, F.J., and Eckardt, J.J. (1993). Extramedullary porous coating to prevent diaphyseal osteolysis and radiolucent lines around proximal tibial replacements: a preliminary report. *Journal of Bone and Joint Surgery, American Volume*, **75A**, 976–87.

Ward, W.G., Johnston, K.S., Dorey, F.J., and Eckardt, J.J. (1997). Loosening of massive proximal femoral cemented endoprostheses. *Journal of Arthroplasty*, **12**, 741–50.

Wirganowicz, P.Z., Eckardt, J.J., Dorey, F.J., Eilber, F.R., and Kabo, J.M. (1999). Etiology and results of tumor endoprosthesis revision surgery in 64 patients. *Clinical Orthopaedics and Related Research*, **358**, 64–74.

1.6.2 Biopsy for suspicion of tumor

T. W. R. Briggs, R. Mitchell, and Ann Sandison

Bone and soft-tissue tumors are rare and constitute less than 1 per cent of all malignancies. Such tumors should, when possible, be treated at specialized tertiary centers where there is a dedicated multidisciplinary team of medical, nursing, and counseling services to manage these often difficult problems.

A poorly performed biopsy at a non-specialist center is reported to be the major cause of error and failure of limb salvage in two review articles (Mankin *et al.* 1996; Springfield and Rosenberg 1996). Our experience supports the view of Simon and Biermann (1991) that whilst biopsy itself demands relatively few technical skills, the decisions related to the performance of the biopsy require considerable thought and experience. Histological characterization of a potential bone or soft-tissue tumor has a major impact on both the decision-making process and subsequent pathway of management, whether that be by primarily surgical treatment or by a combination of other therapies including chemotherapy or radiotherapy.

Radiology

Plain film imaging remains the cornerstone of radiological classification of bone tumors. Cross-sectional imaging with CT, MRI, and SPECT is used to amend benign/aggressive/malignant levels of confidence and to provide further information regarding management (Table 1). This is particularly true for intramedullary spread, extent of the subperiosteal extraosseous mass, or the likely presence of breakthrough of the periosteum and contamination of soft-tissue planes. Establishing radiologically the probability of malignancy at the presentation stage is essential to good management, as a percutaneous biopsy probe can then be used which is compatible with the planned surgical access, allowing the biopsy tract to be excised at the time of surgery. Close collaboration between surgeon and radiologist and a knowledge of each other's working practices are essential.

CT imaging is particularly valuable in spinal and pelvic lesions, where information from plain film analysis can be limited. With contrast supplementation it can, in conjunction with MRI, provide

Table 1 Comparison of MRI and CT in descending order of importance

Features best shown on MRI
Marrow signal change
Extraosseous mass
Cortical destruction
Matrix characterization

Features best shown on CT
Detail of bone destruction
Matrix characterization
Extraosseous mass
Marrow signal change

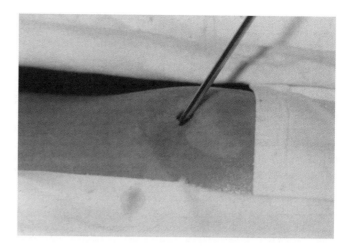

Fig. 1. Jamshidi needle biopsy of a proximal tibia.

detailed identification of the integrity of adjunct neurovascular structures.

Percutaneous biopsy is now standard practice. Given the increase in the use of CT and ultrasound for accurate needle placement, biopsy is now primarily a radiologist-led procedure.

Role of percutaneous needle diagnosis

Percutaneous needle biopsy of suspected bone tumors is well established, with a reported accuracy of 78 to 97 per cent (Ayala and Zornosa 1983; El-Khoury *et al.* 1983; Stoker *et al.* 1991; Fraser-Hill and Renfrew 1992). In our unit most cases are initially histologically classified on percutaneous biopsy (Fig. 1). A diagnostic accuracy of 95 to 97 per cent, irrespective of the image guidance system used, is obtainable (D.R. Remedios and R. Mitchell 1998, unpublished work; Saifuddin *et al.* 2000).

Selection of specific biopsy techniques

This is ideally planned on an individual basis with all the assessment imaging to hand. Attempts have been made at other centers to pro-

Box 1 Percutaneous biopsy for suspicion of tumor

- Needs careful planning
- Gives as good a diagnostic yield as open biopsy
- Minimizes morbidity

Box 2 Guidance systems for percutaneous biopsy

- Ultrasound—ideal for superficial soft-tissue lesions
- CT—best for deep lesion
- MRI—not always available

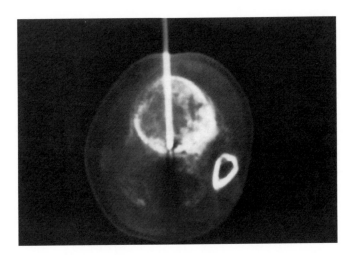

Fig. 2. Axial scan of CT-guided biopsy of osteosarcoma of tibia.

vide an algorithm for selection (Logan *et al.* 1996). Fluoroscopy has been the most accessible guidance system, but it has been superseded by CT or ultrasound. In other centers specialist biopsy-designed MRI is available.

CT guidance is used primarily for bone-based pathology and for deep soft-tissue tumors that are beyond the focus of a standard ultrasound probe (Fig. 2). Ultrasound is suitable for superficial soft-tissue lesions and for bone-based pathology such as osteosarcomas which commonly have a large extraosseous 'soft-tissue' component at the time of presentation (Saifuddin *et al.* 1998). It has the added advantage of minimal tumor disturbance, but depends on the confidence of the histopathologist to make the diagnosis from such partially representative samples. Areas of tissue necrosis which are unhelpful to the final diagnosis may also be available if the biopsy is guided by ultrasound. Careful selection is required to maintain accuracy of diagnosis (Saifuddin *et al.* 2000). The avoidance of critical anatomical structures within the biopsy field will affect the choice of guidance system and both CT and ultrasound play a role. Targeting of the specific lesion in a vertebrae or the pelvis is considerably more accurate with CT than with either ultrasound or biplane fluoroscopy. CT also allows biopsy of smaller lesions with confidence and the final position of the needle can be reliably recorded. This is important for retrospective confirmation of needle position in non-diagnostic pathology reports.

The site and method of approach must provide samples that are adequate for diagnosis and deliver them with the minimum amount of morbidity. Two attempts at percutaneous biopsy are justified. Lesions such as aneurysmal bone cysts and necrotic soft-tissue tumors are the common sources of our negative biopsies. Percutaneous biopsy yield compares well with open biopsy and is more cost-effective (Fraser-Hill *et al.* 1992; Skrzynski *et al.* 1996). The more accurate targeting from cross-section imaging outperforms the standard fluoroscopic guidance system available in theater. In experienced hands percutaneous biopsy can be performed quickly, with less patient morbidity, and at a fraction of the cost of open surgical biopsies.

High diagnostic yield percutaneous biopsies can only be obtained if the histopathologist can deal with such relatively small needle

samples and achieve a diagnosis with a high level of confidence. It is important that the imaging is discussed with the pathologist whenever a histology request is made. This is an essential collaborative stage where two specialties must be acutely aware of each other's needs.

Patient preparation and tissue handling

Informed consent for outpatient percutaneous biopsy is obtained at the referral/assessment outpatient appointment. This is usually done by the specialist bone tumor consultant supported by a nurse counselor. All patients are given a date for biopsy; in our unit we aim to perform all imaging and subsequent biopsy within 7 to 10 working days of the clinical appointment, scheduling times reflected by the level of anesthesia required, either local anesthetic alone or local anesthetic plus intravenous sedation, or in the younger patient, especially children, general anesthesia requiring an anesthetist to be present.

Needle systems

Several needle systems have been devised for biopsies of the musculoskeletal system. In our unit we routinely use two needle types.

Jamshidi needle

This cutting needle with a tapered end (aiding tissue retention) and a disposable trocar is used for lesions that are predominantly osteoblastic and centrally sited within bone, often for predominantly lytic or mixed intraosseous lesions that have an intact surrounding rim or cortex. It is unsuitable for soft-tissue biopsy work. The Jamshidi needle is available in two lengths and three gauges (8, 11, and 13). The smaller needle gauge is used for pediatric work. The central trocar is used to aid dense cortical penetration or to obtain a surface hole.

This device is a one-part instrument and has to be pulled out in its entirety to obtain a specimen, making reintroduction difficult in unsuccessful first passes. These needles are disposable and of good ergonomic robust design, and therefore are used almost exclusively for bone biopsies.

Trucut or Temno (preloaded) needles

These are predominantly used for soft-tissue extraosseous soft-tissue specimens, or when cortical bone destruction allows access to the medulla. Sizes used vary from 11 to 14 gauge and produce a slice of tissue. Hemorrhagic lesions may fail to produce a satisfactory core, but direction under ultrasound or CT guidance improves the diagnostic yield. Multiple specimens can be provided for the pathologist.

Box 3 Advantages and disadvantages of biopsy needles

- Jamshidi needle—ideal for bone lesions; difficult to introduce
- Trucut—best for soft-tissue lesions; hemorrhagic lesions produce poor specimens

With all specimens care is taken to reduce tissue crush and slides may be prepared by the operator but we prefer to deliver our specimens fresh and unfixed to the histopathology department. In cases of potential infective diagnoses additional samples must be sent for microbiology examination.

Technique

Full aseptic conditions are observed in all cases, and the appropriate method of anesthesia, depending on the age of the patient, is selected. Younger patients and those with Ewing's sarcoma and osteosarcoma, which account for a significant number of our cases, require general anesthesia.

Having chosen the radiological technique that complements the percutaneous biopsy, a small stab incision is made with a 15 blade at the site of entry of the needle and the selected needle type inserted. Care must be taken in cases of suspected malignant but contained lesions not to take the needle beyond the point of natural tissue hold-up. For example, with a subperiosteal osteosarcoma contamination of the medulla from the biopsy must be avoided. In tumors close to joints it is imperative that the biopsy is located in such a way that the joint cavity is not contaminated by needle placement.

Technical problems

Cylindrical bones can provide problems of needle slippage. The trocar should be used to provide a focal pit in the bone. Drills may be needed for extremely sclerotic lesions. Combinations of needles can also be used. An 11-gauge Jamshidi needle can be used to provide an access track to pathology suitable for Trucut sampling. A 14-gauge soft-tissue needle can then be fed along the track of the bone tunnel (White *et al.* 1996).

In the investigation of local recurrent disease the presence of prosthetic metalwork precludes the use of MRI-guided biopsy, and ultrasound or CT become the methods of choice.

Patient aftercare

There are usually no problems. Mild analgesia must be provided and directed to coincide with the wearing off of local anesthetic. Occasionally hemostasis can be a problem with extremely vascular tumors such as aneurysmal bone cysts or telangiectatic malignant lesions. In our experience this requires a combination of firm local pressure and admission for a few hours observation.

Histopathology perspective

The clinical differentiation between benign and malignant conditions may be difficult and whilst excisional biopsy of a benign lesion is acceptable, this is not the case with malignant lesions. Bone and soft-tissue tumors may undergo a wide variety of secondary changes,

Box 4 Delivery of specimens

- Avoid crush
- Deliver fresh and unfixed if possible
- Send specimens for microbiology also if infection suspected

including necrosis, fibrosis, and active bone formation, so that lesional tissue may be obscured. Inappropriate sampling compromises the opportunity for adequate local control and limb salvage surgery (Skrzynski *et al.* 1996; Serpe and Pitcher 1998).

The aim of the biopsy is to provide sufficient material to enable the pathologist to make an accurate tissue diagnosis knowing that ancillary studies, such as immunohistochemistry, cytogenetic, and molecular techniques, may also be required. In specialist centers needle biopsy (Fig. 3) has been proven to be just as accurate as open biopsy (Stoker *et al.* 1991; Mankin *et al.* 1996), with less morbidity and more convenience to the patient, as well as being more cost-effective (Skrzynski *et al.* 1996). To achieve diagnostic accuracy with such small tissue samples, full and accurate clinical information is essential to the pathologist, as are specialist laboratory techniques.

Handling the specimen

In our unit the biopsy material is sent dry and unfixed to the pathologist, which allows imprint preparation to be made to ensure that lesional tissue is present in a sample. The imprints may be quickly stained with hematoxylin and eosin or with alkaline phosphatase. Performance of these stains takes between 10 and 30 min. Assessment of the biopsy by imprint is routinely used as it quickly confirms the presence of lesional tissue and usually shows whether a tumor is benign or malignant. In a large proportion of cases a diagnosis can be made. An imprint preparation can also indicate a failed biopsy, allowing immediate rebiopsy which reduces the anxiety for the patient. A positive alkaline phosphatase stain combined with classical radiology may allow a diagnosis of osteosarcoma to be made on imprint cytology. The level of sterility of our samples allows tissue to be cultured for cytogenetic analysis or development of cell lines if sufficient material is available. Between one and three cores (Fig. 4) of tissue are routinely taken, and some tissue may be used for ultra-structural analysis as well as tissue culture. Some of the tissue cores may be snap frozen for tumor banking and/or DNA and RNA analysis.

Special stains may be performed on imprint preparation; for example, periodic acid–Schiff stain may help to distinguish between

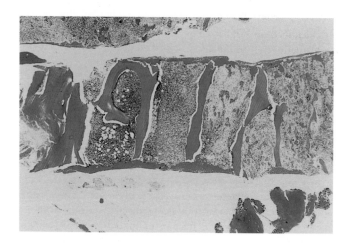

Fig. 3. Needle core biopsy of osteosarcoma of distal femur stained with hematoxylin and eosin.

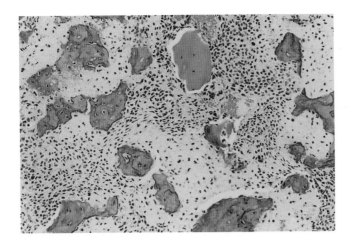

Fig. 4. Needle core biopsy of osteosarcoma of distal femur demonstrates tumor cells, tumor bone, and residual normal lamellar bone.

rhabdomyosarcoma, Ewing's sarcoma, and lymphoma when the lesion is a malignant round cell tumor. A positive alkaline phosphatase stain in such a tumor would indicate a small cell osteosarcoma. Immunohistochemical staining is possible on imprint preparations using alkaline phosphatase–antialkaline phosphatase techniques, such as those routinely applied to cytological preparations from fine-needle aspiration. This method is used only in exceptional circumstances in our unit as more reliable immunostaining is obtained on formalin-fixed paraffin-embedded tissue.

Soft-tissue tumors are most likely to need immunohistochemistry to achieve diagnosis. However, primary bone tumors, including the malignant round cell tumors such as lymphoma, Ewing's sarcoma, and rhabdomyosarcoma, and the spindle cell sarcomas, for example leiomyosarcoma and malignant fibrocytoma, also require a panel of histochemical stains to be performed.

Specific chromosome translocations have been associated with soft-tissue sarcomas, and examples are listed in Table 2.

These translocations can be detected using conventional cytogenetics, interphase cytogenetics, or molecular techniques, including fluorescent *in situ* hybridization (FISH and M-FISH) (Squire and Perlikowski 1998). Specific chromosome translocations have not been identified in primary bone sarcomas, apart from Ewing's sarcoma/peripheral primitive neuroectodermal tumor, but these tumors are difficult to analyze because they are relatively few in number and show complex changes.

Table 2 Examples of chromosome translocations associated with soft-tissue sarcomas

Ewing's sarcoma/PPNET	t11;22 (q24;q12)
Desmoplastic round cell tumor	t11;22 (q13;q12)
Synovial sarcoma	tX;18 (p11.1;q11.2)
Clear cell sarcoma	t12;22 (q13;q12)
Myxoid liposarcoma	t12;16 (q13;p11)
Extraskeletal myxoid chondrosarcoma	t9;22 (q22;q12)

PPNET, peripheral primitive neuroectodermal tumor.

Conclusion

Needle biopsy of bone soft-tissue tumors is both safe and accurate when performed in a specialist center. Radiologists are best placed to perform most biopsies as they have a number of imaging modalities at their disposal, enabling them to take the most appropriate tissue sample. The main disadvantage to pathologists is the small amount of tissue available, but with careful planning and appropriate handling of the specimen, combined with meticulous clinical information and diagnostic expertise, needle biopsy is not a barrier to application of modern diagnostic techniques or to research.

References

Ayala, R.G. and Zornosa, A. (1983). Primary bone tumors: percutaneous needle biopsy. *Radiology*, **149**, 675–9.

El-Khoury, G.Y., Terepka, M.D., Mickelson, M.R., Rainville, C.T., and Zaleski, M.S. (1983). Fine needle aspiration biopsy of bone. *Journal of Bone and Joint Surgery, American Volume*, **65**, 522–5.

Fraser-Hill, M.A. and Renfrew, D.L. (1992). Percutaneous needle biopsy of musculo-skeletal lesions. Effective accuracy and diagnostic utility. *American Journal of Radiology*, **158**, 809–12.

Fraser-Hill, M.A., Renfrew, D.L., and Hilsenrath, P.E. (1992). Percutaneous needle biopsy of musculo-skeletal lesions–cost effectiveness. *American Journal of Radiology*, **158**, 813–19.

Logan, P.M., Connell, D.G., O'Connell, J.X., Munk, P.L., and Janzen, D.L. (1996). Image guided percutaneous biopsy of muskulo-skeletal tumours. *American Journal of Radiology*, **166**, 137–41.

Mankin, H.J., Mankin, C.J., and Simon, M.A. (1996). The hazards of the biopsy; revisited. *Journal of Bone and Joint Surgery, American Volume*, **78**, 656–63.

Saifuddin, A., Burnett, S.T.D., and Mitchell, R. (1998). Pictorial review: ultrasonography of primary bone tumours. *Clinical Radiology*, **53**, 239–46.

Saifuddin, A., Mitchell, R., Burnett, S., Sandison, A., and Pringle, J. (2000). Ultrasound guided needle biopsy of primary bone tumours. *Journal of Bone and Joint Surgery, British Volume*, **82**, 50–4.

Serpe, J.W. and Pitcher, M.E. (1998). Preoperative core biopsy of soft tissue tumours facilitates their surgical management. *Australian and New Zealand Journal of Surgery*, **68**, 345–9.

Simon, M.A. and Biermann, J.S. (1991). Biopsy of bone and soft tissue lesions. *Journal of Bone and Joint Surgery, American Volume*, **75**, 616–21.

Skrzynski, M.C., Biermann, J.S., Montagu, A., and Simon, M.A. (1996). Diagnostic accuracy and change savings of outpatient core needle biopsy compared with open biopsy of muskulo-skeletal tumours. *Journal of Bone and Joint Surgery, American Volume*, **78**, 644–9.

Springfield, D.S. and Rosenberg, A. (1996). Biopsy: complicated and risky (editorial). *Journal of Bone and Joint Surgery, American Volume*, **78**, 639–43.

Squire, J.A. and Perlikowski, S. (1998). Molecular cytogenetics in modern pathology. In *Progress in Pathology*, Vol. 4 (ed. R. Kirkham and N.D.R. Lemoir). Churchill Livingstone, Edinburgh.

Stoker, D.J., Cobb, J.P., and Pringle, J.A.S. (1991). Needle biopsy of musculo-skeletal lesions. A review of 208 procedures. *Journal of Bone and Joint Surgery, British Volume*, **73**, 498–500.

White, L.M., Schweitzer, M.E., and Deely, D.M. (1996). Co-axial percutaneous needle biopsy of osteolytic lesions with intact cortical bone *American Journal of Radiology*, **166**, 143–4.

1.6.3   Overview of musculoskeletal tumors

1.6.3.1 Musculoskeletal tumors and lesions that resemble tumors

Joseph A. Buckwalter and Kristy Weber

Musculoskeletal tumors, and some lesions that resemble tumors, present exceptionally difficult diagnostic and treatment problems. These lesions vary greatly in anatomic location, tissue origin and composition, clinical presentation, response to treatment, and natural history. They may appear in any region of the musculoskeletal system, consist of or involve almost any tissue including bone, cartilage, fibrous tissue, bone marrow, lymphoid tissue, nerve, blood vessel, and lymphatic vessel, and arise in patients of any age. They may destroy normal tissue and cause dramatic signs and symptoms including intolerable pain, massive swelling, severe disability, and pathologic fracture or they may have little effect on normal tissues and remain asymptomatic. They vary in natural history from lesions that spontaneously regress to those that rapidly spread and lead to death despite early diagnosis and aggressive treatment. Despite their diversity, many benign and malignant neoplasms and lesions that resemble neoplasms have similar clinical presentations and appearances on imaging studies.

Box 1

- Difficult diagnostic and treatment problems
- Appear in any region of the musculoskeletal system. Consist of or involve almost any tissue including bone, cartilage, fibrous tissue, bone marrow, lymphoid tissue, nerve, blood vessel, and lymphatic vessel. Arise in patients of any age
- May present with pain, diffuse swelling, a discrete mass, neurologic or vascular compromise, pathologic fracture, or as an incidental finding on physical examination or imaging studies
- Common benign lesions of the musculoskeletal system can resemble malignant lesions
- Appropriate staging studies are a critical part of optimal treatment
- Biopsies must be carefully planned and performed to provide a definitive diagnosis and allow for the best treatment
- Current treatment offers the possibility of cure for many patients with primary malignancies of bone and soft tissue, and improved quality and duration of life for others and for patients with metastatic disease
- Definitive care of a patient with a malignant bone or soft-tissue tumor requires a multidisciplinary approach that includes experienced radiologists, pathologists, medical oncologists, radiation oncologists, and surgeons

Clinical presentation

Patients commonly become aware of the presence of a bone or soft-tissue tumor or lesion that resembles a tumor because of pain. In some individuals the pain is associated with a firm mass or poorly defined swelling. Loss of musculoskeletal function due to weakness, sensory, or vascular deficits, decreased range of motion, or pathologic fracture occurs in some patients with tumors. Less frequently, physicians discover asymptomatic bone and soft-tissue lesions during a physical examination or an imaging study performed for other reasons.

Pain

Pain is often the first symptom of a growing benign or malignant neoplasm, but the type and pattern of pain varies. Bone and soft-tissue tumors can cause symptoms that range from excruciating, sharply localized pain to mild vague discomfort. However, not all tumors cause pain, and some neoplasms reach large size or metastasize before the patient experiences significant discomfort. Patients commonly describe the pain associated with an enlarging bone or soft-tissue tumor as a deep aching that interferes with normal activities, makes it difficult to go to sleep, and awakens them from sleep. Often, rest does not relieve the pain. Occasionally the pain may be referred to a location distant to the tumor. A tumor involving the hip or soft tissues near the hip may cause pain extending down the thigh to the knee or pain localized to the knee; a tumor of the cervical spine may cause pain radiating down the arm; and, neoplasms of the lumbar spine or pelvis may cause discomfort in the buttock, thigh, or leg. Because of this referred pain, the physician may perform an extensive examination and evaluation of a site distant from the tumor. For example, it is not unusual for a patient with a lesion of the mid or proximal femur to complain of knee pain, and therefore have extensive studies of their knee before radiographs of the proximal femur reveal the presence of the lesion responsible for their symptoms. Some non-neoplastic lesions of the musculoskeletal system, including osteomyelitis, Paget's disease, and bone necrosis due to bone infarction can cause pain similar to the pain caused by a growing benign or malignant neoplasm. Unlike the pain caused by most growing neoplasms, musculoskeletal pain caused by stress fractures or soft-tissue strains generally increases or occurs with activity and decreases or disappears with rest.

Swelling or a mass

Many soft-tissue and some bone neoplasms cause diffuse swelling or firm, discrete masses. Others produce only a slight increase in overall limb circumference, while still others do not cause a detectable mass or swelling. Infrequently, the reaction of normal tissues to a neoplasm near or involving a synovial joint causes a joint effusion. Bleeding within a tumor can cause a sudden increase in size and pain. There may be erythema, vascular dilatation, and increased warmth in the skin over the neoplasm, and tumors can erode through the skin. When neoplasms cause a firm tender erythematous mass, they can easily be mistaken for abscesses. Tumors confined to bone cannot be palpated and deep soft-tissue tumors may produce little or no increase in limb circumference. This is a particular problem with deep soft-tissue tumors of the thigh, hip, and shoulder. These lesions can reach substantial size without producing a palpable mass, particularly in obese or muscular patients. Intrapelvic, intra-abdominal, and intrathoracic neoplasms originating in musculoskeletal tissues may also grow to large size before they cause signs or symptoms. For these reasons, lack of a palpable mass or measurable swelling does not eliminate the possibility of a musculoskeletal neoplasm, and the presence of a well-defined mass does not necessarily indicate the presence of a neoplasm since some non-neoplastic lesions including soft-tissue hematomas, traumatic neuromas, and infections can produce masses.

Loss of function

Most patients with musculoskeletal tumors detect the presence of the tumor because of pain, swelling, or both; but, occasional patients present with an initial complaint of loss of function. This may result from neurologic deficit, pathologic fracture, joint contracture, or restriction of joint motion due to the tumor. Neurologic deficits may be subtle. A patient with a slowly growing soft-tissue sarcoma of the posterior thigh may develop gradual sciatic nerve compression causing weakness of the calf muscles. Alternatively, the neurologic deficits may be severe and occur acutely. For example, rapid enlargement of a primary or metastatic spinal lesion may cause sudden compression of the spinal cord or nerve roots. Physicians should suspect the presence of a neoplasm in any patient who sustains a fracture following minor trauma. Some of these patients will report that they had pain at the site of the fracture before the injury. Plain radiographs will often show some irregularity of the bone near the fracture site, but occasionally these irregularities are difficult to identify or the neoplasm may have caused a diffuse decrease in bone density rather than a localized abnormality. Therefore, even without obvious radiographic evidence of a lesion, patients who sustain a fracture following trauma that would not be sufficient to fracture a normal bone should be carefully evaluated for the presence of a neoplasm.

Incidental discovery

Evaluations performed for other reasons occasionally reveal a previously unsuspected neoplasm. During the course of a routine physical examination, a physician may detect a soft-tissue or bone mass, subtle neurologic deficit, or slight increase in limb circumference. Plain radiographs, CT scans, MRI studies, or bone scans ordered to evaluate an acute injury, infection, or chronic musculoskeletal disorder may show unexpected abnormalities such as bone destruction, new bone formation, soft-tissue swelling, or increased uptake of radioactive tracer that suggest the presence of a bone or soft-tissue neoplasm.

Initial evaluation

Patients who have symptoms, signs, or incidental findings that suggest the presence of a bone or soft-tissue tumor should have an initial evaluation that includes a detailed history and physical examination. Plain radiographs should be performed even when a soft-tissue tumor is suspected rather than a bone neoplasm. They may show soft-tissue calcification or bone involvement. Bone scans can be helpful in demonstrating the extent of skeletal involvement, but a negative bone scan does not eliminate the possibility of a bone tumor. In

particular, myeloma and metastatic renal cell carcinoma may not cause easily detectable abnormalities on a bone scan. These tumors cause bony destruction without appreciable reactive bone formation. CT scans are helpful in evaluating the extent of cortical bone destruction and new bone formation. They can also assist in the evaluation of some soft-tissue lesions, but MRI is currently the best method of evaluating soft-tissue tumors as well as the extent of bone marrow involvement. The role of PET scans in the initial evaluation of suspected bone and soft-tissue tumors is not yet clear. After imaging studies have been performed to identify and define the lesion, staging studies should be done to evaluate the degree of local extension and the possibility of metastatic spread.

Deciding if and how a biopsy should be performed is a critical part of the definitive care of patients with suspected bone and soft-tissue neoplasms. Lack of careful planning and performance of a biopsy can yield nondiagnostic tissue and compromise future treatment. For these reasons, biopsies should be performed by individuals with experience in the treatment of bone and soft-tissue neoplasms and when possible they should be performed by the individuals who will be providing the future surgical treatment of the patients.

Classification of musculoskeletal tumors and lesions that resemble tumors

Lesions that can resemble bone and soft-tissue neoplasms

Musculoskeletal disorders that can resemble neoplasms occur more frequently than neoplasms (Table 1). The symptoms, signs, and imaging studies of some injuries, infections, metabolic bone diseases, developmental disorders, and diseases of unknown etiology may closely resemble neoplasms. For example, stress fractures can mimic bone-forming neoplasms, and osteomyelitis and Ewing's sarcoma are often difficult to distinguish based on the history, physical findings, and plain radiographs. Aneurysmal bone cysts can destroy segments of the skeleton and have the appearance of an aggressive neoplasm on plain radiographs. Ganglia, hematomas, abscesses, and myositis ossificans cause soft-tissue masses that can resemble soft-tissue sarcomas. In some instances these benign lesions can be distinguished from malignant tumors by physical examination and imaging studies, but in others a biopsy may be necessary.

Benign bone and soft-tissue neoplasms

Benign neoplasms of bone and soft tissue (Table 2) occur more commonly than malignant neoplasms. The behavior of benign neoplasms varies considerably. Some enlarge to a certain size, usually during skeletal growth, and then remain unchanged indefinitely, thus they might be considered developmental disorders rather than neoplasms.

Lesions that follow this pattern include osteochondromas, enchondromas, and some lymphangiomas and hemangiomas. Other lesions including giant cell tumors of tendon sheath, elastofibromas, and pigmented villonodular synovitis may behave like inflammatory or reactive disorders, but some lesions like giant cell tumors of bone, desmoid tumors, and osteoblastomas aggressively invade and destroy

Table 1 Lesions that can resemble bone and soft-tissue neoplasms

Lesions that can resemble bone neoplasms	Lesions that can resemble soft-tissue neoplasms
Stress fractures	Hematomas
Osteomyelitis	Ganglia
Metabolic bone disease (osteoporosis, osteomalacia, hyperparathyroidism)	Myositis ossificans
Simple/unicameral bone cysts	Nodular fasciitis
Aneurysmal bone cysts	Abscesses
Fibrous cortical defects/nonossifying fibromas	Traumatic neuromas
Bone islands	Aneurysms
Fibrous dysplasia	
Bone necrosis	
Paget's disease	

Table 2 Benign bone and soft-tissue neoplasms

Benign bone neoplasms	Benign soft-tissue neoplasms
Osteoid osteoma	Lipoma
Osteoma	Hemangioma
Osteoblastoma	Lymphangioma
Giant cell tumor of bone	Glomus tumor
Chondromyxoid fibroma	Neurofibroma and neurilemmoma
Osteochondroma	Extra-abdominal desmoid tumor
Enchondroma	Elastofibroma
Periosteal chondroma	Giant cell tumor of tendon sheath
Hemangioma	Pigmented vilonodular synovitis
Chondroblastoma	Synovial chondromatosis
Langerhans' cell histiocytosis	Intramuscular myxoma

normal tissue. Because of the differences in their behavior, benign neoplasms require different treatments. Many osteochondromas and enchondromas can be left untreated; but others, including giant cell tumors, desmoid tumors, and osteoblastomas, almost always require surgical resection. Some of these lesions may be capable of metastasizing despite their benign histologic appearance; in particular, rare patients with giant cell tumors and chondroblastomas have developed lung lesions with the histologic appearance of the primary bone neoplasm. Although Langerhans' cell histiocytosis is listed among the benign neoplasms, it is not certain that it is a neoplasm

and this disorder varies from a disseminated fatal illness in infants to a benign localized bone lesion in adults.

Primary malignant bone and soft-tissue neoplasms

Primary malignant musculoskeletal neoplasms (Table 3) occur less frequently than benign lesions and, unlike benign neoplasms, they frequently cause disseminated disease and death. Some malignant neoplasms develop in or near previously existing benign lesions

Table 3 Malignant bone and soft-tissue neoplasms

Primary malignant bone tumors	Primary malignant soft-tissue tumors
Adamantinoma	Liposarcoma
Osteosarcoma	Malignant fibrous histiocytoma
Chondrosarcoma	Fibrosarcoma
Ewing's sarcoma	Leiomyosarcoma
Malignant vascular tumors of bone	Synovial cell sarcoma
Myeloma	Neurofibrosarcoma
Lymphoma	Malignant vascular tumors
Fibrosarcoma	Rhabdomyosarcoma
Malignant fibrous histiocytoma	Epitheloid sarcoma
Chordoma	Clear cell sarcoma
	Skin tumors (melanomas, basal cell carcinomas and squamous cell carcinomas)

including osteochondromas (especially in patients with hereditary multiple exostoses), enchondromas (especially in patients with Ollier's disease and Maffucci's syndrome), fibrous dysplasia (especially in patients with polyostotic fibrous dysplasia), chronic draining osteomyelitis, bone infarcts, Paget's disease, and neurofibromas (especially in patients with neurofibromatosis). In some instances, the development of a malignant neoplasm presumably results from expression of pre-existing malignant potential. This may explain the appearance of malignant neoplasms in patients with Ollier's disease and neurofibromatosis. In other lesions, development of a malignant neoplasm presumably results from an alteration in the originally normal cells near the lesion. This may explain the development of malignant lesions in patients with chronic draining osteomyelitis or bone infarcts. Although a wide variety of primary bone tumors have been identified, the vast majority of patients with primary malignancies of bone suffer from one of four types of tumor: myeloma, osteosarcoma, chondrosarcoma, or Ewing's sarcoma. Soft-tissue sarcomas occur much more frequently than primary bone tumors and include liposarcoma, malignant fibrous histiocytoma, fibrosarcoma, synovial cell sarcoma, neurofibrosarcoma, and malignant vascular tumors. The incidence of malignant bone and soft-tissue tumors varies with age. Myeloma, soft-tissue sarcoma, and chondrosarcoma rarely occur before the age of 35 but then increase in frequency with age. Osteosarcoma has a bimodal age distribution with one peak in late adolescence and another smaller peak in late adult life. Ewing's sarcoma occurs primarily in people under the age of 30. Malignant neoplasms of bone vary in their clinical presentation. For example, myelomas frequently present as bone pain without a mass or swelling and generalized weakness in elderly debilitated people, whereas osteosarcomas commonly present as sharply localized bone pain and a mass in children and adolescents without systemic symptoms. Current treatment of these neoplasms also varies from systemic chemotherapy and radiation therapy used for myeloma to combinations of systemic chemotherapy and surgery used for most osteosarcomas. In contrast to malignant bone neoplasms, malignant soft-tissue neoplasms vary less in clinical presentation and current treatment. Most of them present as a mass that sometimes, but not always, causes pain. Surgical resection, with wide margins when possible, is the primary treatment of soft-tissue sarcomas. Most patients also receive radiation of the region of the sarcoma. The role of chemotherapy in the treatment of soft-tissue sarcomas is being investigated in multiple medical centers, but thus far it is not widely used for the treatment of nonmetastatic soft-tissue sarcomas.

Metastatic disease of the musculoskeletal system

Metastatic disease of the skeleton (Table 4) occurs at least 20 times more frequently than primary malignant tumors of bone and soft tissue combined. Nearly all malignant tumors have shown the ability to metastasize to bone; but carcinomas of the breast, lung, and prostate produce more than 80 per cent of bone metastases and about half of the patients with breast, lung, or prostate cancer eventually develop bone metastases. Renal cell cancers, gastrointestinal cancers, gynecologic cancers, and thyroid cancers also commonly involve bone. Although bone metastases occur primarily in adults of middle age or older, they occasionally affect younger adults, and neuroblastomas and tumors of renal origin can metastasize in children. Soft-tissue sarcomas and primary malignancies of bone seldom metasta-

Table 4 Metastatic neoplasms

Neuroblastoma
Renal tumors of childhood
Carcinomas
Breast
Prostate
Kidney
Lung
Thyroid

size to bone. Metastatic bone lesions cause pain, and frequently will cause pathologic fractures. They occur most frequently in the vertebrae, pelvis, ribs, and proximal appendicular skeleton, and seldom occur in the hands or feet or the musculoskeletal soft tissues. Most patients with bone pain or pathologic fractures due to skeletal metastases have a known primary malignant neoplasm, but some patients present with skeletal metastases as the first indication of the primary malignancy. For this reason the possibility of metastatic carcinoma should be investigated in patients with bone lesions. In some of these patients, biopsy of the bone lesion will show a poorly differentiated metastatic carcinoma, and physical examination, imaging studies, and laboratory studies will not find the primary lesion.

Although plain radiographs often demonstrate bone destruction with areas of reactive new bone formation in patients with metastatic disease, the tumor must destroy a substantial portion of the bone before a plain radiograph will show an abnormality. For this reason, radioisotope scanning offers a more sensitive method of detecting metastatic disease, although it may not show some destructive lesions including bone lesions due to myeloma and in some instances, renal cell carcinomas. If plain radiographs and radionuclide imaging fail adequately to demonstrate the bone abnormalities in a patient with metastatic disease, CT and MRI may provide more detailed information. Although most metastases destroy bone, metastases from carcinomas of the prostate and breast can stimulate bone formation and therefore appear as regions of increased bone density.

Treatment of metastatic disease of the skeleton can help preserve musculoskeletal function and relieve or prevent pain. It includes prophylactic internal fixation of involved bones to prevent fracture and relieve pain, internal fixation of pathologic fractures, amputation when other treatments would be inadequate, radiation therapy, and for some neoplasms chemotherapy and hormonal therapy.

Summary

Lesions that resemble neoplasms, benign neoplasms, primary malignant neoplasms, and metastatic neoplasms can involve all parts of the musculoskeletal system. They vary in clinical behavior from developmental disturbances of the musculoskeletal tissues that resolve spontaneously, to benign neoplasms that left untreated will destroy bone and soft tissue, to highly malignant neoplasms that cause death despite aggressive treatment. Partially because neoplasms of bone and soft tissue occur infrequently, many physicians including orthopedists may not suspect neoplastic disease in a patient with vague discomfort, swelling, loss of musculoskeletal function, or incidentally discovered unexplained physical findings or abnormalities on imaging studies. Because common benign lesions of the musculo-skeletal system may initially resemble malignant lesions, even when a physician identifies the presence of a musculoskeletal abnormality he or she may not consider the possibility of malignant disease. Even if he or she considers the possibility of malignant disease, distinguishing neoplasms from non-neoplastic lesions can be difficult when the patient is first seen by a physician. For example, synovial sarcomas have been initially diagnosed and treated as ganglia and osteosarcomas have been initially diagnosed and treated as stress fractures. For these reasons, patients with symptoms, signs, or abnormalities on imaging studies that suggest the presence of a musculoskeletal neoplasm should have a careful initial evaluation. Based on this evaluation the physician must decide if the patient can be treated symptomatically, observed, have further laboratory and imaging studies, be referred to a center specializing in the care of musculoskeletal tumors, or have immediate treatment. Conditions that can require immediate treatment include pathologic fractures and impending pathologic fractures, neurologic deficits or impending neurologic deficits, and uncontrolled pain. Current treatment offers the possibility of cure for many patients with primary malignancies of bone and soft tissue, and improved quality and duration of life for others and for patients with metastatic disease. In most instances the definitive evaluation and biopsy of a lesion that may be malignant should be performed by an orthopedist with experience in the management of these problems. The optimal care of a patient with a malignant bone or soft-tissue tumor requires a multidisciplinary approach that includes experienced radiologists, pathologists, medical oncologists, radiation oncologists, and surgeons.

1.6.3.2 Biopsy of musculoskeletal tumors

J. Sybil Biermann

The biopsy of musculoskeletal tumors may seem an uncomplicated task. It is not. A biopsy can do harm, and needs to be done well if a reliable diagnosis is to be made from it. This requires good team work between the surgeon, radiologist, and pathologist.

Box 1

- Biopsy of potentially malignant tumors should be performed in medical centers with the resources necessary to provide definitive treatment of patients with these diseases
- Patients should have a complete evaluation before biopsy
- Biopsy techniques include fine-needle aspiration, core-needle biopsy, incisional biopsy, and excisional biopsy
- Selection of the appropriate biopsy technique and location is critical for obtaining a diagnosis and for optimal future treatment of the patient

General considerations

Biopsy is best performed in a center which specializes in the diagnosis and management of musculoskeletal tumors. There is always a temptation to biopsy a lesion so that a diagnosis can be made which will determine whether a patient needs to be referred to a large specialist center, which may be some distance away. In the case of a potentially malignant tumor, this temptation should be avoided for the following reasons:

(1) additional imaging may be required prior to biopsy;

(2) a musculoskeletal pathologist should be available when the biopsy is taken for accurate interpretation of the material retrieved;

(3) the quality of the biopsy, incision, and technique may profoundly affect the treatment and prognosis of the patient.

One of the key issues concerning the biopsy of musculoskeletal lesions is the understanding that primary malignant tumors of the musculoskeletal system usually are best managed with complete surgical removal. Frequently, surgery is used in conjunction with adjuvant chemotherapy or radiation, but the use of adjunctive therapy does not replace the necessity of complete surgical removal in an *en bloc* fashion. Not only should every attempt be made to remove primary nonmetastatic tumors completely when possible, but also contamination of the surgical field with tumor at the time of definitive resection increases the risk of tumor recurrence locally. Whether radiation is used postoperatively or not makes no difference to the need for complete surgical removal if at all possible.

The biopsy tract should be removed in its entirety at the time of resection if complete surgical excision is to be obtained. The biopsy track is considered contaminated since it is assumed to have had tumor spillage within it. Since the biopsy track must be removed with the specimen, it must be planned to lie in the line of any planned surgical incision that is required. This is most easily done if the surgeon who is doing the definitive surgery, and who is most experienced in the options for surgical approach, also plans and carries out the biopsy. Surgeons or radiologists who are less knowledgeable regarding these issues may inadvertently place the biopsy in an inappropriate site and compromise the future care of the patient. In studies performed by members of the Musculoskeletal Tumor Society, there was a 4.5 per cent rate of amputations which were necessary because of prereferral biopsy problems (Mankin *et al.* 1982, 1996).

Patients often ask whether a properly performed biopsy or the biopsy process itself could cause tumor spread. There is no clinical evidence to suggest that patients who undergo biopsy do worse than those who do not (Brostrom *et al.* 1979). However, one cannot stress strongly enough that an inappropriately performed biopsy of a musculoskeletal lesion may significantly compromise a patient's care, and can even result in the loss of limb-sparing surgical options, even when the patient is subsequently referred.

Prebiopsy staging and evaluation

Reaching a diagnosis from the biopsy material should not just rely on the histology. A thorough history and physical examination, and appropriate laboratory and radiographic staging studies need to be carried out prior to biopsy and be available to the pathologist (Simon and Biermann 1993). For the majority of bone tumors, the plain film with its report gives a likely diagnosis. The film and the report should be made available to the pathologist.

Generally, all possible investigations should be carried out before biopsy to assist in making a definitive diagnosis. For example, an older adult patient presenting with a lytic lesion of aggressive appearance may be suspected of having a primary or metastatic bone malignancy. A whole-body bone scan which shows multiple lesions will clarify the diagnosis and even reveal a lesion which would be simpler to biopsy. Or, in the case of a sclerotic lesion of bone in an adolescent, thin-cut CT scans may demonstrate a classic nidus of an osteoid osteoma which could not otherwise be seen; this may help direct the biopsy as well as assist planning of definitive management. Imaging and other investigations may make the biopsy unnecessary.

For example, a patient may be found with a serum electrophoresis consistent with multiple myeloma having presented with multiple lytic lesions of bone. In the case of a renal cell carcinoma the dangerous complications of open biopsy (torrential hemorrhage), may be avoided.

No matter how atraumatic, biopsy always entails some degree of tissue damage which, with its resultant edema, may then cause abnormalities on CT and MRI postoperatively. Thus the actual extent and nature of the underlying abnormality may be obscured if images are obtained following the biopsy. It may then be difficult to plan the margins of surgical resection in the face of poor quality imaging. Bone marrow biopsy may be considered at the time of biopsy for some malignancies; however, if whole-body bone scanning is performed following bone marrow biopsy, spurious positive results may be reported.

In cases of highly suspected bone malignancy in which preoperative chemotherapy is generally given (Ewing's sarcoma or osteosarcoma) it may be desirable to establish central venous access at the time of biopsy to expedite chemotherapy and avoid a second sedation or general anesthetic. However, this is best done following chest CT since complications related to venous access, or even a general anesthetic, may interfere with radiographic evaluation of the lung fields and misdirect further care of the patient.

Biopsy techniques

There are four ways in which the biopsy specimen may be secured. Biopsies may be obtained via fine-needle aspiration (**FNA**), core-needle biopsy, open incisional biopsy, or excisional biopsy. The advantages and disadvantages of each are discussed below, as well as recommendations as to optimum.

FNA obtains the least diagnostic material, but with the least invasiveness. Using sterile techniques, a narrow-bore needle (usually 21 to

23 gauge) is attached to a 10 to 20 cm³ syringe, and negative pressure is maintained in the syringe while the surgeon moves the needle through the lesion (Arca *et al.* 1995). Cells are detached from the neoplasm and aspirated into the barrel of the syringe. The cytopathologist, who is usually available to receive the specimen immediately, then expels the aspirated material onto a glass slide and stains the specimen. Immediate evaluation under the microscope is then possible. Passes of the needle which produced an equivocal diagnosis can be repeated in the hope of achieving a clear diagnosis.

The disadvantage of FNA is that the cells obtained have lost the tissue-architectural clues which may be important in the evaluation of a sarcoma (Hadju and Melamed 1971). Also, tumor grading cannot be established with any reasonable degree of certainty, which is a major drawback since the grade of the sarcoma may significantly affect treatment decisions. In most centers the use of FNA for musculoskeletal neoplasms is usually restricted to evaluation of local or regional nodal recurrence in patients with previously established diagnoses of malignancy. Because it is a relatively atraumatic technique, it can be quite useful in the evaluation of retroperitoneal masses under CT guidance. Its role in extremity sarcomas is less well defined, although some have reported success with routine use in the setting of very experienced surgeons, radiologists, and cytopathologists.

Although FNA is used primarily for soft-tissue lesions, it may also be used successfully in some bone lesions (Katz *et al.* 1980). FNA for bone lesions may be associated with a high rate of non-diagnostic material—29 per cent in one series.

Other problems occurring with FNA are false-positive and false-negative diagnoses.

Core-needle biopsy

Core-needle biopsy has been reported increasingly as an economical and effective technique to obtain diagnostic material, especially in soft-tissue sarcomas. These needles obtain material through hollow-tipped needles, and obtain actual tissue samples rather than cellular material retrieved via FNA. The area is prepared, using full sterile

Box 5 Problems with fine-needle aspiration

- High rate of nondiagnoses
- False positives—no architecture
- False negatives—inadequate biopsy

Box 6 Incisional biopsy

- Short longitudinal incision
- Direct sharp dissection through compartment
- No skin flaps
- Minimize hematoma
- Tourniquet well proximal to lesion

precautions and the needle is introduced percutaneously by the surgeon, based on palpation of physical landmarks and the evaluation of the previously obtained images. Less commonly, the radiologist may be directed to perform these biopsies under fluoroscopic, CT, or ultrasound guidance. However, good communication between surgeon and radiologist is necessary in these cases to ensure that the radiologist selects a biopsy site that does not interfere with further care of the patient, and which provides the best tissue for diagnosis.

Core needles (Fig. 1) can be used in the operating suite or in the outpatient clinic area under local anesthesia and the specimens processed for histopathology, special studies, or other tests. Typically, several cores are obtained at 5-mm successive passes through one entry site. This provides the maximum amount of tissue while reducing tissue trauma and contamination by tumor to a minimum.

Cores may be sent for different preparation (freezing, fixing, cytogenetics) based on a plan made by the surgeon and pathologist together. Core biopsy performed in the outpatient clinic setting can result in substantial cost savings, when compared with open biopsy in the operating suite. The diagnostic accuracy is about 80 per cent, so that both surgeon and patient must be prepared for an open biopsy if an inadequate specimen is obtained. The use of the core needle can avoid catastrophic complications of wound breakdown in an open biopsy in patients with compromised skin due to a rapidly expanding lesion in a difficult position. The amount of superficial tissue which will need to be removed with the specimen *en bloc*

should the lesion prove to be a primary malignancy is reduced to a minimum. Even partially anticoagulated patients can have a needle biopsy with minimal bleeding, provided that adequate precautions are taken. This includes taking a minimum number of cores and holding pressure on the biopsy site for several minutes after the biopsy.

Although core-needle biopsy has significantly increased in popularity because of its cost-savings potential and expediency, incisional open biopsy remains the conventional and gold standard method for securing adequate tissue at the time of biopsy.

Generally, longitudinal incisions are best in the extremities. Since the vast majority of limb structures run longitudinally, these incisions will cover the fewest number of structures, and fewer normal structures will have to be removed at the time of *en bloc* resection (Fig. 2). The incisional length should be kept to the minimum required to retrieve appropriate tissue (Fig. 3). Dissection should be carried

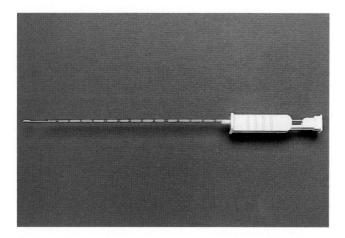

Fig. 1. Core biopsy needles such as this Trucut biopsy needle allow for percutaneous removal of a small piece of tissue. Upon introduction of the needle and extension of the inner obturator, tissue herniates into the specimen notch. After the outer cannula is advanced over the obturator, the needle can be withdrawn and the tissue emptied. Unlike cytology, core-needle biopsy permits evaluation of tissue architecture. Core-needle biopsy is especially appropriate for soft-tissue lesions and soft-tissue extensions of bone tumors.

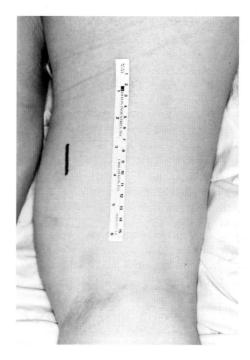

Fig. 2. Planned incision for biopsy of a 17-cm mass in the posterior thigh of a 78-year-old woman. Biopsy incisions in the limbs should be vertical and as short as possible to permit subsequent *en bloc* excision should the lesion prove malignant. Contamination of major neurovascular structures should be avoided.

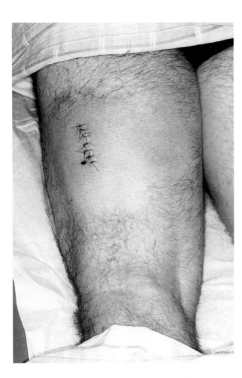

Fig. 3. Longitudinal biopsy incision created for the evaluation of a soft-tissue mass which was revealed to be a myxoid liposarcoma in a 40-year-old man. In general, closure of biopsy incisions should be performed with sutures as close to the skin edge as possible. Subcuticular closure would have been preferable in this case.

Box 7 Biopsy technique

- Methylmethaurylate to plug bone
- Close in layers
- Subcuticular to skin
- Drain tract in incision line
- Minimal tissue for frozen section to confirm

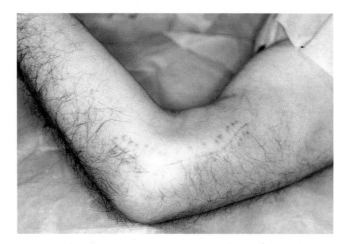

Fig. 4. Biopsy incision used for the concurrent incisional biopsy of a neurofibrosarcoma and ulnar nerve transposition in a 78-year-old man. Biopsies should not be performed in concert with other procedures, since this will extend the zone of contamination should the lesion prove malignant. Wide mattress sutures in this case have also extended the area of skin contamination. *En bloc* resection of a biopsy incision in this case would be difficult, and the treating surgeon is forced to choose between leaving potentially contaminated tissue or performing an amputation.

down directly to the area of interest. Skin flaps and blunt dissection should be avoided.

Since all portions of the biopsy wound are potentially contaminated, all hematomas at biopsy should be kept to a minimum at definitive excision and malignant cells contained. Thus any resultant hematoma must be removed with the specimen, or suboptimal excision must be accepted. Compression dressings should be applied to all biopsy sites to reduce hematoma formation, and the patient's clotting factors checked before surgery.

The use of a tourniquet has been controversial; however, it can be safely used for biopsy, provided it is placed well proximal to the lesion. Since pressure on the tumor has the capacity to embolize tumor cells, an Esmarch bandage should not be applied. The limb can be partially exsanguinated using gravity by elevation for 3 to 5 min prior to tourniquet inflation. However, the tourniquet should be deflated and hemostasis achieved prior to closure. Refractory bleeding can be controlled by use of topical hemostatic agents, cautery, and pressure in the soft tissues. Bone windows can be plugged using methylmethacrylate, which will prevent extrusion of marrow contents into the biopsy tract and beyond.

Closure of the biopsy wound should be meticulous, and in layers to reduce hematoma and tumor spillage. Since the entire wound will be excised with the specimen, every attempt to keep the closure close to the incision should be made (Fig. 4). Subcuticular skin closure is preferred over mattress sutures, or even simple sutures, since these extend the skin which will need to be resected ultimately. The drain site, including the exit point, is considered to be a part of the biopsy tract. If a drain must be used, it should exit the wound in line with the incision, as close as possible to the incision site, to reduce the amount of normal tissue that will have to be removed with the tumor.

Only as much material as is necessary to establish the diagnosis and obtain additional tests such as cytogenetics, immunohistochemistry, or electron microscopy should be obtained. A frozen section should be performed at the time of biopsy to ensure that representative material rather than reactive or normal tissue has been obtained. Once the presence of representative tissue has been established, the minimal amount of tissue required to complete planned tests should be harvested. There is no need to sample additional parts of the tumor once it has been confirmed that diagnostic tissue has been obtained. Additional tumor sampling will result in increased hematoma formation and increased chance of tumor embolization at no benefit to the patient.

Box 8 Excision biopsy

- Only for lesions less than 5–mm diameter
- Subcutaneous lesions likely to be benign

The same considerations regarding hemostasis, tourniquet use, and placement of incisions apply to open excisional biopsies. While occasionally appropriate, the open excisional biopsy is widely overutilized, particularly with soft-tissue masses, and often creates substantial difficulties for subsequent caregivers (Lawrence *et al.* 1987; Noria *et al.* 1996).

However, there are some occasions where open excisional biopsy is appropriate. In lesions that are less than 5 cm in greatest dimension and which are subcutaneous, a primary excisional biopsy is often appropriate. Fewer than 1 in 200 of these lesions is likely to turn out to be a primary malignancy, so this is a rational approach (Rydholm and Berg 1983). In the case of larger deep lesions, excisional biopsy is only appropriate when the appearance on MRI is most consistent with lipoma. Since fat has distinctive imaging characteristics relative to most other tumors, this determination can be made by evaluating multiple sequences to ascertain that the lesion always is isointense with the subcutaneous fat.

Excisional biopsy of large deep lesions which turn out to be sarcomas is one of the major pitfalls which may occur in the biopsy situation. Noria *et al.* (1996) followed patients who had had an unplanned resection of a sarcoma in this manner, and found that they ultimately had a higher local failure rate despite reoperation and sometimes chemotherapy. Also, in the postoperative setting, modalities such as MRI or CT have difficulty in establishing whether or not there is residual tumor.

Occasionally, excisional biopsy may be appropriate for an expendable bone lesion with a benign appearance. Lesions in the fibula or ribs may be particularly amenable to this. However, it should be stressed that if the lesion has the potential to be a primary malignancy of bone, excisional biopsy will be inappropriate even for a small lesion, since consideration will need to be given to wide resection and possibly preoperative chemotherapy.

Biopsy placement

The decisions of where to biopsy a lesion and what technique is most appropriate are heavily influenced by the requirement that the biopsy track will need to be excised *en bloc* should the lesion prove to be a primary malignancy (Fig. 5).

Generally, biopsy tracks should avoid neurovascular structures where possible. A common misconception is that nerves of blood vessels should be identified and retracted during the biopsy procedure. However, since all portions of the biopsy wound will subsequently be considered to be contaminated with tumor, this may result in an unnecessary neurovascular contamination. This will then result in either the neurovascular structures being resected unnecessarily, contamination of the limb at the time of limb salvage, or amputation to achieve complete tumor removal.

Biopsy sites are best placed such that dissection proceeds through a minimum of normal tissue. However, if normal tissue is between the incision and the tumor, it is best to dissect through a muscle rather than in intermuscular planes or intervals. Standard orthopedic approaches generally exploit internervous planes and intermuscular intervals. However, if tumor contamination takes place in an interval, spread of hematoma or tumor may more rapidly gain access to other parts of the limb. In contrast, if a portion of a normal muscle is split

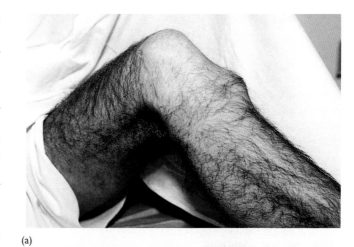

(a)

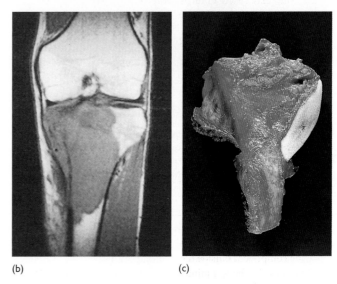

(b)   (c)

Fig. 5. (a) Clinical appearance of the lower extremity of a 21-year-old man who presented with a 2-month history of swelling and pain about the proximal leg. (b) Coronal T_1-weighted MRI showing marrow extent of the abnormality in the proximal tibia, and soft-tissue extension of the lesion out of the bone medially. The lesion proved to be a malignant fibrous histiocytoma of bone. (c) In order to ensure complete tumor removal, the anteriomedial needle biopsy tract was resected *en bloc* with the specimen at the time of tumor resection. Where possible, biopsy of the soft-tissue mass outside the bone is preferable to making a bone window. The biopsy tract is considered contaminated with tumor, and its *en bloc* removal is necessary at the time of resection of malignant tumors.

to gain access to the tumor, that muscle portion can be resected *en bloc* with the tumor.

Longitudinal incisions in the extremities allow a minimum number of structures to be violated during the performance of the biopsy. However, incisions around the limb girdles may be different, and a knowledge of both limb-sparing and amputation options is necessary for planning.

Role of the frozen section

Accurate evaluation of the musculoskeletal biopsy is best performed in the setting of good communication between the surgeon, radiologist, and pathologist. Pathologists, especially those less experienced in evaluating musculoskeletal neoplasms, may be misdirected in the absence of adequate clinical information and consequently may be less helpful. A frozen section performed at the time of open biopsy can ensure that the surgeon has obtained adequate material for diagnosis, and prevent unnecessary return trips to the operating room. Sarcomas in particular have an inherent diagnostic trap. The reactive zone around the tumor may appear markedly abnormal yet be composed only of nondiagnostic reactive host material.

If the material is sent to the center following biopsy, there may be significant limitations regarding additional tests which can be performed. This may result in an incomplete pathology evaluation or, alternatively, a need for rebiopsy. If the diagnosis of lymphoma is suspected the pathologist needs extra fresh tissue to snap freeze for additional studies which cannot be performed on fixed tissue. With the pathologist available to look at the material intraoperatively, appropriate apportioning of the biopsy specimen to fixative, freezing, cytogenetics, or other molecular studies can be arranged.

Bone biopsy

Bone biopsy can be carried out by FNA, core, or open techniques. Spine lesions are often relatively inaccessible, with the needle techniques often being the most effective. Trephine-type needles can be used to penetrate the cortex and retrieve material (Moore *et al.* 1979).

Bone should not be entered unless absolutely necessary. If there is soft-tissue component outside the bone then biopsies should be taken from that. Mostly, the less mineralized areas of the tumor result in a higher likelihood of diagnostic tissue and fewer processing problems for the pathologist. However, if a bone tumor has a soft-tissue extension or if the soft-tissue portion is inaccessible due to location, the bone can be entered. This is best achieved by the creation of a circular or oblong hole, preferably in an area where the bone is already attenuated. Square or rectangle holes have stress concentrations at the corners and are more likely to result in pathologic fracture. Use of methylmethacrylate in the biopsy hole following the completion of harvest of diagnostic material can reduce the chance of a stress fracture and help to prevent further extrusion of the tumor into the soft tissues around the biopsy site.

Every precaution should be taken to reduce the chance of pathologic fracture either at the time of biopsy or during subsequent treatment prior to resection. Fractures are associated with hematoma and presumed tumor contamination, so a pathologic fracture in a malignant bone tumor means that the surgeon needs to perform a more extensive resection. The limb should always be held carefully while the patient is anesthetized. Once the biopsy hole is made, the limb may be even more susceptible to a stress fracture. Consideration should be given to casting, splinting, or bracing the limb for postoperative protection. For lower-extremity lesions, the patient should usually remain non-weight-bearing following a bone biopsy until there is evidence that the bone strength has returned.

Further reading

Arca, M.J., Biermann, J.S., Johnson, T.M., and Chang, A.E. (1995). Biopsy techniques for skin, soft-tissue, and bone neoplasms. *Surgical Oncology Clinics of North America*, **4**, 157–74.

Techniques for the biopsy of skin, soft-tissue, and bone neoplasms are presented. Practical suggestions as well as the importance of prebiopsy staging, and multidisciplinary co-ordination are reviewed.

Lawrence, W., Jr, Donegan, W.L., Natarajan, N., Mettlin, C., Beart, R., and Winchester, D. (1987). Adult soft tissue sarcomas. A pattern of care survey of the American College of Surgeons. *Annals of Surgery*, **205**, 349–59.

A nationwide survey of soft-tissue sarcomas in the United States over two separate 2-year time periods. The overuse of excisional biopsy was demonstrated in these data. Adverse prognostic factors in this large group of patients included positive surgical margins, large tumors, and retroperitoneal or mediastinal sites.

Moore, T.M., Neyers, M.H., Patzakis, M.J., Terry, R., and Harvey, J.P. Jr (1979). Closed biopsy of musculoskeletal lesions. *Journal of Bone and Joint Surgery, American Volume*, **61A**, 375–80.

The results of 531 closed biopsies performed at a single hospital are presented. Accurate diagnosis was achieved in 66 per cent of bone lesions and 76 per cent of soft-tissue lesions.

Noria, S., Davis, A., Kandel, R., *et al.* (1996). Residual disease following unplanned excision of a soft-tissue sarcoma of an extremity. *Journal of Bone and Joint Surgery, American Volume*, **78A**, 650–5.

Patients who had had an unplanned excision of a sarcoma (excisional biopsy) prior to referral had a higher likelihood of having positive margins at definite surgery and ultimately had a higher local recurrence rate than those treated only at the referral center. Additionally, residual tumor was difficult to detect although it was present in 35 per cent of patients who had had a previous excision.

Rydholm, A. and Berg, N.O. (1983). Size, site and clinical incidence of lipoma. Factors in the differential diagnosis of lipoma and sarcoma. *Acta Othopaedica Scandinavica*, **54**, 929–93.

A review of 428 patients presenting with lipoma during 1 year in a defined population were reviewed and compared with data for soft-tissue sarcomas. Tumors larger than 5 cm located in the thigh and deep to the fascia are more likely to be sarcomas.

Simon, M.A. and Biermann, J.S. (1993). Biopsy of bone and soft-tissue lesions. *Journal of Bone and Joint Surgery, American Volume*, **75A**, 616–21.

This review of the biopsy process for musculoskeletal lesions covers the need for staging, biopsy techniques, and the importance of multidisciplinary co-operation in caring for patients with musculoskeletal tumors.

References

Arca, M.J., Biermann, J.S., Johnson, T.M., and Chang, A.E. (1995). Biopsy techniques for skin, soft-tissue, and bone neoplasms. *Surgical Oncology Clinics of North America*, **4**, 157–74.

Brostrom, L.A., Harris, M.A., Simon, M.A., Cooperman, D.R., and Nilsonne, U. (1979). The effect of biopsy on survival of patients with osteosarcoma. *Journal of Bone and Joint Surgery, British Volume*, **61B**, 209–12.

Hadju, S.L. and Melamed, M.R. (1971). Needle biopsy of primary malignant bone tumors. *Surgery, Gynaecology and Obstetrics*, **133**, 829–32.

Katz, R.L., Silva, E.G., DeSantos, L.A., and Lukeman, J.M. (1980). Diagnosis of eosinophilic granuloma of bone by cytology, histology, and electron microscopy of transcutaneous bone-aspiration biopsy. *Journal of Bone and Joint Surgery, American Volume*, **62A**, 1284–90.

Lawrence, W., Jr, Donegan, W.L., Natarajan, N., Mettlin, C., Beart, R., and Winchester, D. (1987). Adult soft tissue sarcomas. A pattern of care survey of the American College of Surgeons. *Annals of Surgery*, **205**, 349–59.

Mankin, H.J., Lange, T.A., and Spanier, S.S. (1982). The hazards of biopsy in patients with malignant primary bone and soft-tissue tumors. *Journal of Bone and Joint Surgery, American Volume*, **64A**, 1121–7.

Mankin, H.J., Mankin, C.J., and Simon, M.A. (1996). The hazards of the biopsy, revisited. *Journal of Bone and Joint Surgery, American Volume*, **78A**, 656–63.

Moore, T.M., Neyers, M.H., Patzakis, M.J., Terry, R., and Harvey, J.P. Jr (1979). Closed biopsy of musculoskeletal lesions. *Journal of Bone and Joint Surgery, American Volume*, **61A**, 375–80.

Noria, S., Davis, A., Kandel, R., *et al.* (1996). Residual disease following unplanned excision of a soft-tissue sarcoma of an extremity. *Journal of Bone and Joint Surgery, American Volume*, **78A**, 650–5.

Rydholm, A. and Berg, N.O. (1983). Size, site and clinical incidence of lipoma. Factors in the differential diagnosis of lipoma and sarcoma. *Acta Othopaedica Scandinavica*, **54**, 929–93.

Simon, M.A. and Biermann, J.S. (1993). Biopsy of bone and soft-tissue lesions. *Journal of Bone and Joint Surgery, American Volume*, **75A**, 616–21.

1.6.3.3 Staging and surgical margins in musculoskeletal tumors

Peter Choong

Introduction

Surgery has a primary role in the management of musculoskeletal tumors. The goals of surgery are firstly local control of disease and secondly preservation of function (Nelson and Thompson 1990; Rougraff 1995). While these goals are achievable by surgery alone in benign tumors, radiotherapy and chemotherapy are often combined with surgery in managing bone and soft-tissue sarcomas. Successful treatment depends upon a knowledge of the precise anatomical location of the tumor, the extent of dissemination, if any, and the anticipated biologic behavior of the tumor. Compilation of this knowledge is often referred to as staging of the tumor. Following staging, surgical margins are designed to optimize local control of disease.

Principles of staging

There are two aspects to staging musculoskeletal tumors, namely clinical and pathologic staging. Clinical staging defines the local and systemic extent of the disease which is required in the planning of appropriate measures to achieve control of tumor. Clinical staging relies on a variety of imaging studies which not only pinpoint the anatomical location of the tumor but also serve as baseline indices for post-treatment comparisons. Pathologic staging categorizes tumors according to their predicted biological behavior which may range from indolence to widespread metastasis. Pathologic staging relies on biopsy of the tumor and therefore should follow clinical staging.

Accurate staging is important for minimizing over- and under-treatment, performing meaningful analyses, and comparing clinical outcome in controlled studies of cancer treatment.

Clinical staging

Clinical staging should be performed prior to biopsy because hemorrhage, surgical artifacts, and tissue reactions may confound the results of imaging studies, particularly highly sensitive modalities such as MRI. Restaging should also be performed immediately prior to definitive surgery if preoperative adjuvant therapy has been utilized. This permits a reassessment of the tumor's relationship to adjacent structures, particularly if there has been an alteration in size. Furthermore, the resolution of bone and soft-tissue edema allows a more accurate appraisal of the intramedullary and soft-tissue tumor border. Under these circumstances, surgical margins can be planned to maximize the potential for limb-sparing surgery.

Imaging studies
Plain radiography

Plain radiography is the first investigation performed after suspicion of any musculoskeletal tumor. Conventional films are useful for demonstrating the size, site, mineralization, periosteal reaction, nature, and number of skeletal lesions. Soft-tissue tumors are less easily demonstrated unless they contain significant quantities of calcium, hemosiderin, or fat. However, the effect of soft-tissue tumors on bone (e.g. saucerization, erosion, invasion, or sclerosis) is better seen with conventional radiography than with other forms of imaging modalities. Plain radiographs are also important for planning the size requirements of prosthetic or allograft implants. Plain radiography does not allow delineation of intramedullary tumors or their extraskeletal extensions, factors which are an essential part of clinical staging. Other difficulties include identifying early skeletal destruction where 30 to 40 per cent of bone destruction is required before the lesion becomes detectable (Bassett *et al.* 1981).

Features which raise suspicion of malignancy include cortical destruction, sclerosis, periosteal new bone formation, and intramedullary or extracortical mineralization (Fig. 1).

Radionuclide scintigraphy

Scintigraphy is a valuable tool for screening the entire skeleton for bone and soft-tissue involvement (Scott and Larson 1993; Hugosson

Box 1

- Optimal treatment of musculoskeletal tumors requires accurate clinical and pathologic staging

- Clinical staging defines the local and systemic extent of the disease and is based on the history and physical examination, imaging studies, and in some instances serologic studies

- Pathologic staging categorizes tumors according to their potential for local tissue destruction and metastases and is based primarily on histologic examination of the tumor

- Surgical margins are defined as intralesional, marginal, wide, and radical

- Generally, achieving a wider surgical margin decreases the probability of local recurrence, but determining the appropriate surgical margin for a specific patient depends on a variety of factors including the clinical and pathologic stage of the disease, the effects of adjuvant therapy, and the patient's preference

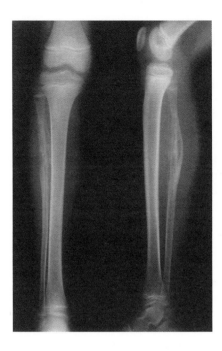

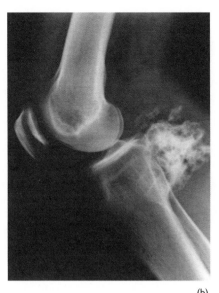

(b)

(a)

Fig. 1. (a) Ill-defined fibular lesion with permeative destruction and an aggressive periosteal reaction consistent with Ewing's sarcoma. Intramedullary extension is not clearly seen. (b) Soft-tissue mineralization erosive outline and a prominent soft-tissue shadow suggest malignant change in this osteochondroma.

et al. 1994). Bone scans are useful for determining bone involvement, the singularity or multiplicity of lesions within a specific bone (Anez *et al.* 1993), the presence of osseous metastosis (Shapeero *et al.* 1993), the response to chemotherapy therapy (Menendez *et al.* 1993) (Fig. 2), or the presence of recurrence (Hugenholtz *et al.* 1994).

Analogues of technetium-99m such as medronate methylene diphosphonate (**MDP**) or ethane-1-hydroxy-1,1-diphosphonate are the most commonly used. Recently, thallium has gained recognition as an alternative isotope for imaging bone and soft-tissue sarcoma because of its increased specificity for tumors (Menendez *et al.* 1993; Rosen *et al.* 1993; Caluser *et al.* 1994) (Fig. 3). Thallium incorporation, which is closely linked with the metabolism of the tumor, may have a role in determining the response of these tumors to chemo- or radiotherapy, the presence of local or regional (lymph node) metastases, and the presence of local recurrence which thallium scintigraphy is able to differentiate from scar (Terui *et al.* 1994) (Fig. 4). [^{67}Ga]Citrate is another isotope which may have a role in assessing soft-tissue involvement because it concentrates more readily in tumors than [^{99}Tc^m]MDP (Cogswell *et al.* 1994; Lin *et al.* 1994).

The advantages of radionuclide scanning are its high sensitivity and ability to screen the entire skeleton. Disadvantages of scintigraphy include a low specificity for differentiating tumor from fracture, infection, and inflammation and a limited ability to define of the tumor border.

The presence of tumors is usually identified by an increase in tracer uptake, a hot spot, which represents an area of repair or reaction within or around the lesion. Occasionally, tumors arise which induce destruction and very little new bone formation. These tumors are photopenic and produce cold spots which may be missed unless there is increased activity in surrounding bone or sufficient background activity in the skeleton to allow their detection. Multiple myeloma, lymphoma, metastatic renal, and thyroid carcinoma often produce cold spots (Ragsdale *et al.* 1981).

Computed tomography

CT provides better tissue contrast than plain radiographs and is the preferred examination for assessing osseous involvement by tumor (Massengill *et al.* 1995). By modulating the analysis of differences between tissue densities, bone or soft-tissue windows can be generated which permit examination of the marrow space, adjacent soft tissue and also the extraosseous extension of the tumor (Fig. 4).

The value of CT is in detecting intramedullary lesions which are not readily visible on conventional radiographs, the ability to display cross-sectional anatomy, and the ability to demonstrate early cortical and trabecular destruction (Hogeboom *et al.* 1991; Slavotinek *et al.* 1991). CT is particularly useful in areas with complex anatomy such as the pelvis, hip, and spine. High resolution CT is limited to horizontal planar images with reconstructed views in the longitudinal axis lacking the same degree of definition. Soft-tissue imaging by CT is inferior to that of MRI (Hogeboom *et al.* 1992).

Three-dimensional CT reconstruction of musculoskeletal structures is available (Fishman *et al.* 1993; Magid 1993). This technique is useful for demonstrating surface lesions such as parosteal osteosarcomas, osteochondromas, and heterotopic bone formation, and for highlighting soft-tissue masses and contrast-enhanced vasculature (Fishman *et al.* 1993). This is relevant to lesions that arise close to or impinge on adjacent joints. Manipulation of images even allows subtraction of other parts of the anatomy from the image to isolate the area of interest (Plumley *et al.* 1995). Thus, three-dimensional CT has a limited role in surgical planning (Magid 1993), although the information does not contribute to the diagnosis.

Magnetic resonance imaging

MRI is the single most valuable study in the assessment of musculoskeletal tumors (Arca *et al.* 1994; Kroon *et al.* 1994; Iwamoto *et al.* 1995; Kransdorf and Murphey 1995). This technique, which does not

pathology including fluid collections and edema (Fig. 5(b)). Spin–echo proton-density weighted images highlight cortical involvement by tumor.

Gradient–echo images are mainly used for three-dimensional or volume acquisition scanning.

The short tau inversion recovery (**STIR**) sequence is employed to suppress the signal from fat in soft tissue and marrow. Fat-suppression techniques enhance the identification of marrow and soft-tissue lesions (Fig. 5(c) and (d)).

The advantages of MRI include its ability to detect bone and soft-tissue lesions with a particular sensitivity to marrow pathology, its ability to provide accurate anatomic images in the horizontal, longitudinal, sagittal, and coronal planes, and the ability to demonstrate blood flow which can be interpreted like angiograms (Bloem *et al.* 1988; Arca *et al.* 1994; Kransdorf 1994). However, there are limitations with MRI, including lack of specificity, suboptimal imaging of bone and areas of mineralization, and sensitivity to surgical and implant artifacts (Hogeboom *et al.* 1992; Arca *et al.* 1994).

MRI should be performed prior to biopsy and commencement of neoadjuvant therapy. A subsequent MRI should be performed to restage the tumor after neoadjuvant therapy to assess response (Figs 6(a) and (b)) and to demonstrate a clearer image of the tumor border after resolution of edema (Figs 6(c) and (d)).

Angiography

Angiography is no longer routinely used for staging because much of the information is now available with MRI and CT. Nonetheless, it remains the most reliable method of demonstrating vascular anatomy, particularly if major vessels are thought to be displaced or if vascular reconstructions are anticipated during surgery. It is also important when vascular tumors are to be resected. Angiography allows preoperative embolization to be performed, and major arterial feeders can be targeted for ligation intraoperatively.

Pathologic staging

Pathologic staging of tumors is undertaken either before or after surgery. Traditionally, definitive staging has been performed postoperatively because of the availability of the whole tumor for examination. The use of preoperative adjuvant therapy such as chemotherapy or radiotherapy can influence the result if there has been massive tumor necrosis which may prevent reliable grading, histologic, immuno-histochemical, or cytogenetic examination.

For preoperative pathologic staging to be accurate, sufficient, and representative tissue must be obtained at biopsy to confirm the diagnosis and to characterize the biology of the tumor. In the majority of cases, open biopsy is the technique used to procure tissue. In Scandinavia the practice of fine-needle aspiration cytology over the last two decades has been refined to the level where information regarding the histology, grade, cytogenetics, molecular genetics, and electron microscopy are now possible from needle aspirates alone, and open biopsy is less frequently performed for musculoskeletal tumors (Åkerman *et al.* 1987; Willén *et al.* 1995).

Pathologic staging stratifies tumors according to their aggressiveness, that is, the tendency to metastasize (malignancy). Appropriate primary and adjuvant therapy can be planned to minimize local and distant recurrence by first identifying tumors with a greater or

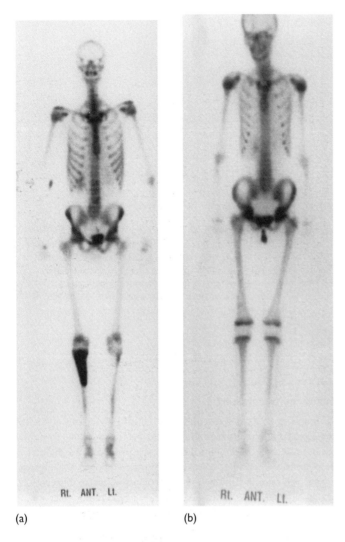

(a)   (b)

Fig. 2. Technetium isotope scan demonstrating (a) pre- and (b) post-chemotherapy appearances.

employ ionizing radiation, allows multiplanar imaging and provides the best contrast discrimination of all modalities. The availability of MRI has reduced the number of investigations required in the clinical staging of tumors (Bloem *et al.* 1988).

MRI utilizes the energy emitted by hydrogen nuclei in stimulated tissues to generate images. Radiofrequency pulses are generated and directed through areas of interest during which the pulse excites hydrogen nuclei within tissues that it crosses. Subsequent relaxation of the hydrogen nuclei is associated with the emission of a signal which is characteristic for different tissues. The acquisition of data allows accurate reconstruction of anatomy and pathology with high-resolution soft-tissue contrast.

Three main pulse sequences are employed, spin–echo, gradient–echo, and inversion recovery, and these sequences give rise to signals of different intensities that are referred to as proton-density weighted, T_1-weighted, and T_2-weighted images.

Spin–echo T_1-weighted images are excellent for demonstrating marrow pathology, soft tissues, and cortical bone (Fig. 5(a)). Spin–echo T_2-weighted images are better for demonstrating soft-tissue

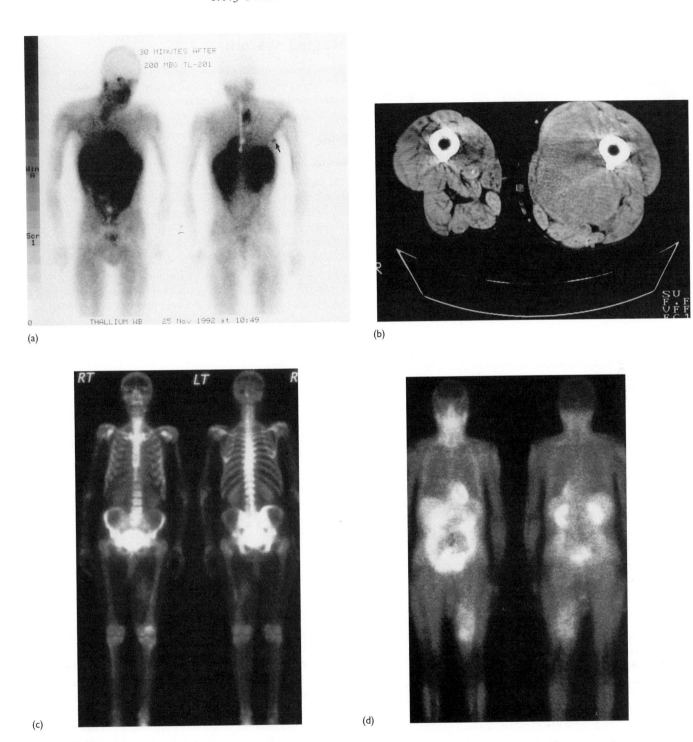

Fig. 3. (a) Concentration of thallium in thoracic vertebra and rib of previously resected vertebral osteosarcoma suggesting recurrence of tumor. (b) Malignant fibrous histiocytoma of adductor compartment of left thigh. (c) Weak uptake of technetium isotope in comparison with (d) thallium.

lesser likelihood of metastasis. This approach helps to optimize limb-sparing surgery and reduce the morbidity of treatment.

Grading is a process of categorizing malignancy using histological characteristics, and is an important feature of pathologic staging. Clear correlations exist between grade and metastasis. The grade of a tumor is determined by a combination of features including its cellularity, the degree of pleomorphism, mitotic activity, necrosis,

and its infiltrative nature. Grades range from low to high and are classified into two (Enneking 1986), three (Russell *et al.* 1977; Jensen *et al.* 1991), or four (Angervall *et al.* 1986) grade systems.

The importance of a grading system is that it selects patients according to the aggressiveness of their tumors who may be suitable candidates for more intensive therapy. However, the subjective nature of assessing many of these histologic characteristics can result

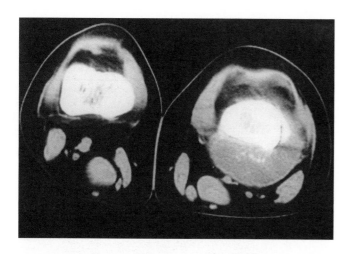

Fig. 4. CT scan demonstrating distal femoral osteosarcoma. Note mineralization within soft-tissue component of tumor.

in variations in assigning grades by different pathologists despite using the same grading system (Alvegård and Berg 1989). This is further compounded by several grading systems which employ different criteria. Uniformity in grading is essential for ensuring the reliability of this parameter as a prognostic factor, and also for analysing the responses to treatment.

The clinical implications of grade in one tumor may not always be equivalent to grading in other tumors. Some tumors may behave aggressively despite a moderate degree of pleomorphism or lack of mitoses; examples include synovial sarcoma and alveolar soft-tissue sarcoma. Other tumors such as infantile fibrosarcoma are relatively low grade despite their cellularity and prominent mitotic activity.

Histologic type or subtype can also be used as a means of establishing tumor grade. For example, parosteal osteosarcoma and low-grade central osteosarcoma are two entities which are classified as low grade and can be treated with surgery alone without risk for metastasis. In contrast, conventional osteosarcoma and dedifferentiated primary bone sarcomas are classified as high grade because of the significantly increased risk for metastasis, and for which adjuvant chemotherapy is always required. Alveolar rhabdomyosarcoma, extraskeletal Ewing's sarcoma, and synovial sarcoma are examples of high-grade tumors, whereas well-differentiated liposarcoma and myxoid liposarcoma are designated as low-grade tumors.

There is a need for more objective means of assessing grade. In this regard, discrete features such as tumor necrosis (Gustafson 1994), vascular invasion (Gustafson 1994), proliferative activity (Choong *et al.* 1994, 1995b), DNA content (Alvegård *et al.* 1990), and cytogenetic abnormalities are under investigation as potential alternatives to conventional grading.

Staging systems

Several staging systems for musculoskeletal tumors are currently in use. At present, one main system is used for bone tumors, while several are employed for soft-tissue sarcomas.

Bone

Benign

The staging of benign bone tumors reflects the local behavior of the lesion and not its tendency to recur or spread, although this tendency can be inferred from the stage if inadequate treatment is performed (Enneking 1986).

Latent tumors are those which have been present and undetected for long periods of time. These tumors are characterized by radiologic features which include a well-defined sclerotic margin that is occasionally associated with remodeling of bone. Latent benign tumors may be left if unsymptomatic or removed with curettage and cementation or bone grafting. Fibrous dysplasia and simple bone cysts are examples of latent tumors.

Active tumors are those which are often symptomatic and are characterized by a lytic or mixed lytic–sclerotic lesion that is poorly defined in part or all of its perimeter. Occasionally, the cortex surrounding these lesions is extremely thin, and the tumors present after pathologic fracture. These tumors increase in size as demonstrated by changes in serial radiographs, and the predominantly lytic character and the lack of sclerosis are hallmarks of increased activity. Most aneurysmal bone cysts and giant cell tumors are examples of active benign tumors.

Aggressive tumors are those which grow rapidly, and frequently expand the bone of origin. It is not uncommon to find a soft-tissue component associated with aggressive benign lesions and this feature may be mistaken for a more sinister lesion. The cortical thinning and expansion seen with active lesions are present to a much greater degree in aggressive benign tumors. Advanced giant cell tumors are examples of aggressive tumors.

Malignant

The staging system most commonly used for bone sarcomas is the Surgical Staging System (Table 1) proposed by the Musculoskeletal Tumour Society (**MSTS**) (Enneking 1986). The components in this staging system include tumor grade (low or high), location (intra- or extracompartmental), and distant metastasis (present or absent). The applicability of this system to both bone and soft tissues reflects a similar behavior of either tumor group irrespective of histotype. The application of this staging system to bone and soft-tissue sarcomas will be discussed together.

The characteristic of grade is primarily based upon histologic findings of increasing cellular atypia, mitotic counts, necrosis, and vascularity. The MSTS system combines clinical and radiological criteria with the histological features to classify low (G1) and high (G2) tumors.

Size of the tumor is closely linked with the behavior of the tumor (Delepine *et al.* 1990; Davis *et al.* 1994; Choong *et al.* 1995a; Fein *et al.* 1995; Singer *et al.* 1995). Large tumors (over 5 cm) are associated with a poorer survival rate than small tumors (less than 5 cm). Size

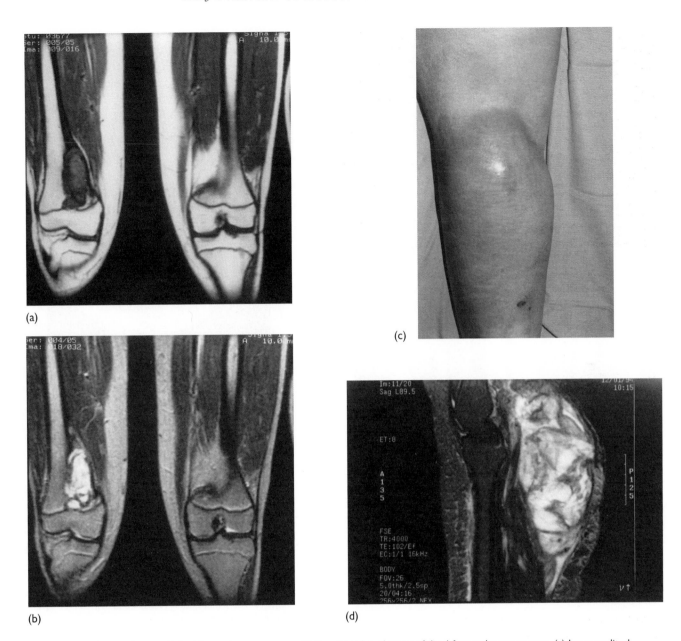

Fig. 5. (a) T_1-weighted coronal image of distal femoral osteosarcoma. (b) T_2-weighted axial image of distal fermoral osteosarcoma. (c) Large popliteal liposarcoma highlighted with (d) short tau inversion recovery (STIR) sequence on MRI.

also has major implications for local treatment because larger tumors may engage vital structures necessitating more extensive resections, reconstructions, and the use of adjuvant therapy. The MSTS system, however, employs the site (T) of the tumor rather than its size as a staging parameter. Tumors are classified into those that are intracompartmental and others which are extracompartmental because of the rationale that intracompartmental tumors that are confined by an anatomical fascia are less likely to recur than tumors which have transgressed the fascia of their compartment of origin. Intracompartmental (T1) tumors are those which are intramuscular, intraarticular, and superficial to the deep fascia. Extracompartmental (T2) lesions are those that arise in extracompartmental tissue, extend from

one compartment to another, or which are subcutaneous and engage the deep fascia. Involvement of regional nodes or distant structures (M0 to M1) are poor prognostic signs.

Enneking *et al.* (1980) evaluated 397 extremity sarcoma patients using this system and reported 5-year disease-free survival rates of 97 per cent (stage IA), 89 per cent (stage IB), 73 per cent (stage IIA), 45 per cent (stage IIB), and 8 per cent (stage III).

As a result of the restrictive definition of compartmentalization, it was difficult to discriminate between small intramedullary tumors which touched the periosteum and aggressive lesions which engaged and crossed the periosteum into the adjacent soft tissue. Spanier *et al.* (1990), refined the classification of stage IIB osteosarcomas by

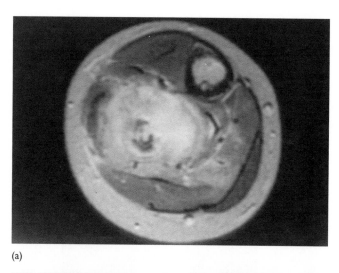

(a)

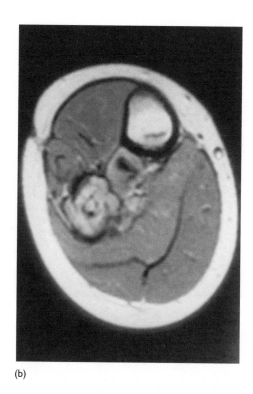

(b)

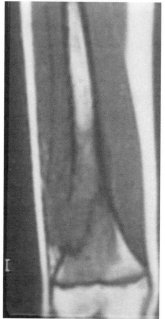

(c)

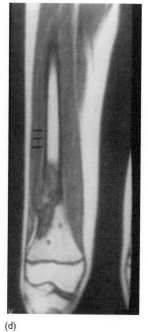

(d)

Fig. 6. MRI of lesion in Fig. 1 demonstrating marked diminution of soft-tissue component and edema between (a) pre- and (b) postchemotherapy images. (c) Pre- and (d) post-chemotherapy images from another patient demonstrating resolution of marrow edema and improved definition of tumor margins.

Table 1 Musculoskeletal Tumour Society Surgical Staging System

Stage	Grade (G)	Site (T)	Metastasis (M)
IA	Low (G1)	Intracompartmental (T1)	None (M0)
IB	Low (G1)	Extracompartmental (T2)	None (M0)
IIA	High (G2)	Intracompartmental (T1)	None (M0)
IIB	High (G2)	Extracompartmental (T2)	None (M0)
III	Any grade	Any site	Yes (M1)

Table 2 Anatomic extent of stage IIB osteosarcomas

Extent	Definition
E1	Tumor touches but does not elevate or penetrate periosteum
E2	Tumor elevates but does not penetrate periosteum
E3	Tumor penetrates into but not through periosteum
E4	Minimal periosteal extension not into a defined structure or space, seen as a nodule of 1–cm or less just outside the periosteum
E5	Tumor invades any one of the following: tendon, ligament, periarticular structures, joint, muscle, bone, space, popliteal fossa, or axilla
E6	Tumor invades two structures or more

dividing them into six subcategories based upon their local growth patterns (Table 2). Tumors that invaded two or more structures (E6) had a six times greater risk of disease recurrence than tumors that were more circumscribed. Of patients with IIB tumors, those with E6 tumors had a 38 per cent 5-year survival while those with non-E6 tumors had an 82 per cent survival. This study highlights the obser-

Table 3 American Joint Committee for Cancer Staging System

Stage	Grade (G)	Size (T) (cm)	Lymph node (N)	Metastasis (M)
IA G1T1N0M0	1	&60; 5	No	No
IB G1T2N0M0	1	> 5	No	No
IIA G2T1N0M0	2	&60; 5	No	No
IIB G2T2N0M0	2	> 5	No	No
IIIA G3T1N0M0	3	&60; 5	No	No
IIIB G3T2N0M0	3	> 5	No	No
IVA G1–3T1–2N1M0	Any grade	Any size	Yes	No
IVB G1–3T1–2N0M0	Any grade	Any size	No	Yes

vation that the local extent of tumor has an important influence over the prognosis of patients with osteosarcoma.

Soft-tissue sarcomas

American Joint Committee for Cancer Staging System

The American Joint Committee for Cancer (**AJCC**) Staging and End Results (Russell *et al.* 1977) proposed a more complex staging system for soft-tissue sarcomas based upon four parameters including histologic grade, tumor size or local invasion, nodal involvement, and metastasis (Table 3). This system was constructed with data collected from 1215 soft-tissue sarcomas treated at 13 institutions over an 8-year span. This system utilized the TNMG classification, wherein T represented tumor size or local invasion of nerves, blood vessels, or bone, N represented nodal involvement, M referred to metastasis, and G was the grade of the tumor. Tumors of the viscera were excluded. Rhabdomyosarcoma, synovial sarcoma, and certain angiosarcomas were regarded as high grade, regardless of degree of differentiation. The differences between this system and that recommended by the MSTS are an increase in the number of grades and the use of tumor size rather than compartmentalization in the AJCC model, resulting in three extra stages.

As with the MSTS system, survival inversely correlated with stage. The 5-year overall survival was 75 per cent for stage I tumors, 55 per cent for stage II tumors, 29 per cent for stage III tumors, and 7 per cent for stage IV tumors. While there are similarities between the AJCC and MSTS systems, the former has been encumbered by several factors. Firstly, the existence of nine stages is thought to be cumbersome; secondly, the addition of head, neck, and retroperitoneal tumors in up to 40 per cent of cases may be a confounding factor because treatment of these and extremity tumors are different; thirdly, node involvement and metastasis are classified separately even though both have the same prognosis and regional lymph node involvement is given a better prognosis than tumors which invade bone, nerve, or a major vessel.

The strong correlation between clinical stage and histologic grade of the tumor in the AJCC system suggests that the overall prognostic value of the AJCC system is the same as for histologic grade alone.

Lund Staging System

The main difficulty encountered with a multilevel staging system is the presence of many intermediate survival groups. The decision as to how these patients should be treated has not been satisfactorily addressed. The Lund Sarcoma Group analyzed parameters derived from a population-based series of 508 soft-tissue sarcomas (Gustafson 1994), which included the age and sex of the patient, the location of the tumor and its depth, size, and malignancy grade, the presence of tumor necrosis or vascular invasion, the DNA histogram type, the adequacy of local treatment, and local recurrence. They found that size, tumor necrosis, and vascular invasion were the most important prognostic factors for metastasis-free survival. In order to minimize the number of survival groups in their staging system, they constructed a scheme whereby all patients with only one of the three prognostic factors were grouped together, and those with more than one were isolated into a second group. The 5-year survival was 81 per cent for the former group and 32 per cent for the latter group. Identifying such widely separated good and poor survival patients allows the selection of candidates for prospective trials of chemotherapy from the latter group.

Staging of recurrent soft-tissue sarcomas

Despite adequate treatment, local recurrence occurs in 10 to 20 per cent of soft-tissue sarcoma patients. Furthermore, a large proportion of patients with soft-tissue sarcoma initially present to tertiary referral centers with local recurrence following primary surgery performed elsewhere (Serpell *et al.* 1991). The therapeutic options for these patients still remain controversial, partly because of disagreements over the role of local recurrence in the aetiology of metastasis (Collin *et al.* 1987; Gustafson *et al.* 1991; Gaynor *et al.* 1992). Rational treatment of patients with local recurrence requires the identification of survival groups to whom optimal therapy can be offered.

The growth rate (increase in size over time) of local recurrence may have prognostic implications for metastasis. Choong *et al.* (1995a) combined this parameter with histologic evidence of necrosis and devised a staging system for recurrent tumors that identified very good (90 per cent) and poor (0 per cent) 5-year metastasis-free survival groups. Patients with low growth rate indices for local recurrence could be treated with surgery alone with a small risk for metastasis, while those patients treated for local recurrence with high growth rate indices had a far greater risk of metastasis, thus targeting them as potential candidates for trials of chemotherapy.

Surgical margins

Surgery is the mainstay of treatment for musculoskeletal tumors. The high recurrence rates and the initial belief that local control was paramount for survival lead to amputation being the surgical technique of choice. Over the last decade, better imaging, improved chemotherapy, and more sophisticated radiotherapy have facilitated attempts to remove the tumor while preserving limb function and minimizing local recurrence.

The principles of surgical margins are similar for bone and soft-tissue sarcomas and are based on the pattern of growth of the tumor (Simon and Enneking 1976). Musculoskeletal tumors are surrounded by a nontumorous reactive zone containing inflammatory cells and neovascular tissue. This pseudocapsule contains microscopic extensions of tumor which may be continuous with, or satellites of, the main tumor mass. Tumors usually grow in a longitudinal fashion within their compartment of origin, respecting the naturally occurring barriers such as fascia, cortical bone, periosteum, joint capsule and synovium, and neurovascular sheaths. Extension across these barriers is a characteristic of aggressive tumors or a late phenomenon. Metastasis typically occurs to the lung and lymph node involvement is rare. Local recurrence rates correlate directly with the quality of the surgical margin and an appreciation of the characteristics of the host–tumor relationship is important in the planning of oncologic margins (Figs 7 and 8).

Definition of surgical margins

Intralesional margins imply a procedure which crosses the pseudocapsule and enters into the substance of the tumor. Often tumor tissue is removed piecemeal. Curettage is an example of intralesional surgery. Recurrence is guaranteed with intralesional margins as macroscopic evidence of tumor remains after surgery. Intralesional margins are only used in benign tumors such as bone cysts, aneurysmal bone cysts, and giant cell tumors.

Marginal margins are those in which a tumor is removed in one piece and the plane of dissection passes through the pseudocapsule or reactive zone. Excisional biopsies or tumors which are shelled out are examples of surgery with marginal margins, and microscopic residual tumor often exists. Approximately three-quarters of malignant tumors will recur after surgery with marginal margins.

Wide margins include the entire tumor and its pseudocapsule or reactive zone and a cuff of normal tissue *en bloc*. During this procedure, tumor is never seen. Surgery with wide margins does not remove all tissue from the affected compartment. Consensus has not been reached on the definition of what constitutes a cuff of normal tissue. In principle, the proximal or distal cut edge of normal muscle represents a wide margin if it is 5 cm or more from the tumor border. Removal of bone at a similar distance beyond the tumor also constitutes a wide margin. Surgical margins which include the normal fascia surrounding the muscle of an intramuscular tumor is regarded

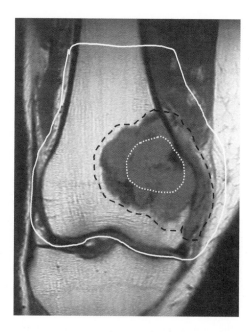

Fig. 7 Coronal MRI of distal femoral osteosarcoma with extraosseous extension of tumor. The intralesional margin (dotted line), the marginal margin (broken line), and the wide margin (full line) are indicated. A radical margin would be a resection of the entire tumor-bearing compartment, which would imply a total femoral resection.

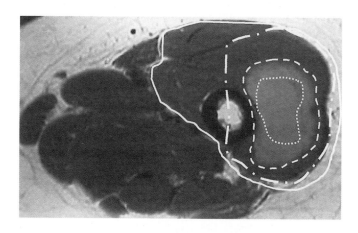

Fig. 8. Axial MRI of soft-tissue sarcoma of the thigh lying adjacent to mid-diaphysis of the femur. The intralesional margin (dotted line), the marginal margin (broken line), and the wide margin (chain line) are indicated. A radical margin (full line) would be a resection of the entire tumor-bearing compartment which would imply a total quadriceps resection including a section of femoral diaphysis.

as wide even though the absolute thickness of the muscle and fascial cuff is less than 5 cm. Synovium which covers the periosteal extension of a distal femoral tumor is regarded as an anatomic barrier and if excised *en bloc* with the tumor constitutes a wide margin.

Radical margins are achieved when the entire tumor-bearing compartment is removed *en bloc*. For bone sarcomas, radical margins include the *en bloc* removal of the bone of origin and the entire soft-tissue compartment into which the tumor has entered. For soft-tissue sarcomas, this includes anatomical fascia surrounding that compartment and bony borders when present. Radical margins are associated with the lowest risk of recurrence.

With limb-sparing surgery as the preferred technique, the majority of uncomplicated bone or soft-tissue resections aim at wide surgical margins. The use of chemotherapy has improved the rate of local control in osteosarcoma while allowing wide excisional limb-sparing surgery (Damron and Pritchard 1995; Jaffe *et al.* 1995). Similarly, radiotherapy has had a major influence on decreasing the size of surgical margins in soft-tissue sarcoma resections. Specifically, combination radiotherapy and marginal surgery has had the same results as surgery with wide margins alone, and the recurrence rates for surgery with wide margins combined with radiotherapy are similar for radical surgical margins alone (Karakousis *et al.* 1991; O'Connor *et al.* 1993). If vital neurovascular structures are adjacent to the tumor, marginal surgery may be selected and combined with adjuvant therapy. In selected tumors, such as those which are completely within a single muscle, or subcutaneous and not engaging the deep fascia, surgery with wide margins alone may be sufficient to achieve local control (Rydholm *et al.* 1991). Decisions regarding choice and combination of modalities need to be tailored to each case.

Although limb-sparing surgery is a major aim of tumor surgery, amputation is indicated if the potential for local recurrence remains high even after anticipated optimal limb-sparing procedures, if the result of limb-sparing surgery is a functionless limb, or if the morbidity associated with complex reconstruction outweigh the benefits of early rehabilitation after amputation. Amputations are also classified by the same margins (intralesional, marginal, wide, and radical) that are achieved and are subject to similar recurrence rates. Optimizing surgical margins, and thus local control of tumor, requires accurate preoperative imaging of the tumor and surrounding anatomy. Surgical planning includes the selection of an appropriate position for the biopsy site. Improperly placed biopsy incisions may prevent the possibility of limb salvage surgery (Mankin *et al.* 1982).

References

Åkerman, M., Killander, D., Rydholm, A., and Rööser, B. (1987). Aspiration of musculoskeletal tumors for cytodiagnosis and DNA analysis. *Acta Orthopaedica Scandinavica*, **58**, 523–8.

Alvegård, T.A. and Berg, N.O. (1989). Histopathology peer review of high-grade soft tissue sarcoma: the Scandinavian Sarcoma Group experience. *Journal of Clinical Oncology*, **7**, 1845–51.

Alvegård, T.A., Berg, N.O., Baldetorp, B., *et al.* (1990). Cellular DNA content and prognosis of high-grade soft tissue sarcoma: the Scandinavian Sarcoma Group experience. *Journal of Clinical Oncology*, **8**, 538–47.

Anez, L.F., Gupta, S.M., Berger, D., and Spera, J. (1993). Scintigraphic evaluation of multifocal hemangioendothelioma of bone. *Clinics in Nuclear Medicine*, **18**, 840–3.

Angervall, L., Kindblom, L.G., Rydholm, A., and Stener, B. (1986). The diagnosis and prognosis of soft tissue tumors. *Seminars in Diagnostic Pathology*, **3**, 240–58.

Arca, M.J., Sondak, V.K., and Chang, A.E. (1994). Diagnostic procedures and pretreatment evaluation of soft tissue sarcomas. *Seminars in Surgical Oncology*, **10**, 323–31.

Bassett, L.W., Gold, R.H., and Webber, M.M. (1981). Radionuclide bone imaging. *Radiologic Clinics of North America*, **19**, 675–702.

Bloem, J.L., Taminiau, A.H., Eulderink, F., Hermans, J., and Pauwels, E.K.J. (1988). Radiologic staging of primary bone sarcomas: MR imaging, scinti-

graphy, angiography, and CT correlated with pathologic examination. *Radiology*, **169**, 805–10.

Caluser, C.I., Abdel-Dayem, H.M., Macapinlac, H.A., *et al.* (1994). The value of thallium and three-phase bone scans in the evaluation of bone and soft tissue sarcomas. *European Journal of Nuclear Medicine*, **21**, 1198–205.

Choong, P.F.M., Akerman, M., Gustafson, P., *et al.* (1994). Prognostic value of Ki-67 expression in 182 soft tissue sarcomas. Proliferation—a marker of metastasis? *Acta Pathologica, Microbiologica, et Immunologica Scandinavica*, **102**, 915–24.

Choong, P.F., Gustafson, P., Willen, H., *et al.* (1995a). Prognosis following locally recurrent soft-tissue sarcoma. A staging system based on primary and recurrent tumour characteristics. *International Journal of Cancer*, **60**, 33–7.

Choong, P.F.M., Akerman, M., Rydholm, A., *et al.* (1995b). Proliferating cell nuclear antigen (PCNA) and Ki-67 expression in soft tissue sarcoma. Is prognostic importance histotype specific? *Acta Pathologica, Microbiologica, et Immunologica Scandinavica*, **103**, 797–805.

Cogswell, A., Howman, G.R., and Bergin, M. (1994). Bone and gallium scintigraphy in children with rhabdomyosarcoma: a 10-year review. *Medical Pediatric Oncology*, **22**, 15–21.

Collin, C., Godbold, J., Hajdu, S., and Brennan, M. (1987). Localized extremity soft tissue sarcoma: an analysis of factors affecting survival. *Journal of Clinical Oncology*, **5**, 601–12.

Damron, T.A. and Pritchard, D.J. (1995). Current combined treatment of high-grade osteosarcomas. *Oncology (Huntington)*, **9**, 327–43.

Davis, A.M., Bell, R.S., and Goodwin, P.J. (1994). Prognostic factors in osteosarcoma: a critical review. *Journal of Clinical Oncology*, **12**, 423–31.

Delepine, N., Delepine, G., Desbois, J.C., Cornille, H., and Mathe, G. (1990). Results of multidisciplinary limb salvage in 240 consecutive bone sarcomas. *Biomedical Pharmacotherapy*, **44**, 217–24.

Enneking, W.F. (1986). A system of staging musculoskeletal neoplasms. *Clinical Orthopaedics and Related Research*, **204**, 9–24.

Enneking, W.F., Spanier, S.S., and Goodman, M.A. (1980). A system for the surgical staging of musculoskeletal sarcoma. *Clinical Orthopaedics and Related Research*, **153**, 106–20.

Fein, D.A., Lee, W.R., Lanciano, R.M., *et al.* (1995). Management of extremity soft tissue sarcomas with limb-sparing surgery and postoperative irradiation: do total dose, overall treatment time, and the surgery–radiotherapy interval impact on local control? *International Journal of Radiation Oncology, Biology, Physics*, **32**, 969–76.

Fishman, E.K., Wyatt, S.H., Bluemke, D.A., and Urban, B.A. (1993). Spiral CT of musculoskeletal pathology: preliminary observations. *Skeletal Radiology*, **22**, 253–6.

Gaynor, J.J., Tan, C.C., Casper, E.S., *et al.* (1992). Refinement of clinicopathologic staging for localized soft tissue sarcoma of the extremity: a study of 423 adults. *Journal of Clinical Oncology*, **10**, 1317–29.

Gustafson, P. (1994). Soft tissue sarcoma. Epidemiology and prognosis in 508 patients. *Acta Orthopaedica Scandinavica*, **259** (Supplement), 1–31.

Gustafson, P., Rooser, B., and Rydholm, A. (1991). Is local recurrence of minor importance for metastases in soft tissue sarcoma? *Cancer*, **67**, 2083–6.

Hogeboom, W.R., Hoekstra, H.J., Mooyaart, E.L., Freling, N.J. and Schrafordt, K.H. (1991). MRI and CT in the preoperative evaluation of soft-tissue tumors. *Archives of Orthopaedic and Trauma Surgery*, **110**, 162–4.

Hogeboom, W.R., Hoekstra, H.J., Mooyaart, E.L., *et al.* (1992). MRI or CT in the preoperative diagnosis of bone tumours. *European Journal of Surgical Oncology*, **18**, 67–72.

Hugenholtz, E.A., Piers, D.A., Kamps, W.A., *et al.* (1994). Bone scintigraphy in nonsurgically treated Ewing's sarcoma at diagnosis and follow-up: prognostic information of the primary tumour site. *Medical and Pediatric Oncology*, **22**, 236–9.

Hugosson, C., Lindahl, S., and Rifai, A. (1994). Primary pelvic bone tumours in children and adolescents—imaging correlation. *Acta Radiologica*, **35**, 549–54.

Iwamoto, Y., Oda, Y., Tsumura, H., Doi, T., and Sugioka, Y. (1995). Three-dimensional MRI reconstructions of musculoskeletal tumors. A preliminary evaluation of two cases. *Acta Orthopaedica Scandinavica*, **66**, 80–3.

Jaffe, N., Patel, S.R., and Benjamin, R.S. (1995). Chemotherapy in osteosarcoma. Basis for application and antagonism to implementation; early controversies surrounding its implementation. *Hematology and Oncology Clinics of North America*, **9**, 825–40.

Jensen, O.M., Hogh, J., Ostgaard, S.E., Nordentoft, A.M., and Sneppen, O. (1991). Histopathological grading of soft tissue tumours. Prognostic significance in a prospective study of 278 consecutive cases. *Journal of Pathology*, **163**, 19–24.

Karakousis, C.P., Emrich, L.J., Rao, U., and Khalil, M. (1991). Limb salvage in soft tissue sarcomas with selective combination of modalities. *European Journal of Surgical Oncology*, **17**, 71–80.

Kransdorf, M.J. (1994). Magnetic resonance imaging of musculoskeletal tumors. *Orthopedics*, **17**, 1003–16.

Kransdorf, M.J. and Murphey, M.D. (1995). MR imaging of musculoskeletal tumors of the hand and wrist. *Magnetic Resonance Imaging Clinics of North America*, **3**, 327–44.

Kroon, H.M., Bloem, J.L., Holscher, H.C., van der Woude, H.J., Reijnierse, M., and Taminiau, A.H. (1994). MR imaging of edema accompanying benign and malignant bone tumors. *Skeletal Radiology*, **23**, 261–9.

Lin, W.Y., Kao, C.H., Hsu, C.Y., Liao, S.Q., Wang, S.J., and Yeh, S.H. (1994). The role of Tc-99m MDP and Ga-67 imaging in the clinical evaluation of malignant fibrous histiocytoma. *Clinics in Nuclear Medicine*, **19**, 996–1000.

Magid, D. (1993). Two-dimensional and three-dimensional computed tomographic imaging in musculoskeletal tumors. *Radiology Clinics of North America*, **31**, 425–47.

Mankin, H.J., Lange, T.A., and Spanier, S. (1982). The hazards of biopsy in patients with malignant primary bone and soft tissue tumours. *Journal of Bone and Joint Surgery, American Volume*, **64A**, 1121–7.

Massengill, A.D., Seeger, L.L., and Eckardt, J.J. (1995). The role of plain radiography, computed tomography, and magnetic resonance imaging in sarcoma evaluation. *Hematology and Oncology Clinics of North America*, **9**, 571–604.

Menendez, L.R., Fideler, B.M., and Mirra, J. (1993). Thallium-201 scanning for the evaluation of osteosarcoma and soft-tissue sarcoma. A study of the evaluation and predictability of the histological response to chemotherapy. *Journal of Bone and Joint Surgery, American Volume*, **75A**, 526–31.

Nelson, T.E. and Thompson, R.C. (1990). Management of soft-tissue tumors of the extremity and trunk. *Current Opinion in Orthopedics*, **1**, 409–15.

O'Connor, M.I., Pritchard, D.J., and Gunderson, L.L. (1993). Integration of limb-sparing surgery, brachytherapy, and external-beam irradiation in the treatment of soft-tissue sarcomas. *Clinical Orthopaedics and Related Research*, **289**, 73–80.

Plumley, D.A., Grosfeld, J.L., Kopecky, K.K., Buckwalter, K.A., and Vaughan, W.G. (1995). The role of spiral (helical) computerized tomography with three-dimensional reconstruction in pediatric solid tumors. *Journal of Pediatric Surgery*, **30**, 317–21.

Ragsdale, B.D., Madewell, J.E., and Sweet, D.E. (1981). Radiologic and pathologic analysis of solitary bone lesions. Part II: Periosteal reactions. *Radiology Clinics of North America*, **19**, 749–83.

Rosen, G., Loren, G.J., Brien, E.W., et al. (1993). Serial thallium-201 scintigraphy in osteosarcoma: correlation with tumour necrosis after preoperative chemotherapy. *Clinical Orthopaedics and Related Research*, **293**, 302–6.

Rougraff, B.T. (1995). Surgical management of osteosarcoma. *Current Opinion in Orthopaedics*, **6**, 69–72.

Russell, W.O., Cohen, J., Enzinger, F., et al. (1977). A clinical and pathological staging system for soft tissue sarcomas. *Cancer*, **40**, 1562–70.

Rydholm, A., Gustafson, P., Rooser, B., et al. (1991). Limb-sparing surgery without radiotherapy based on anatomic location of soft tissue sarcoma. *Journal of Clinical Oncology*, **9**, 1757–65.

Scott, A.M. and Larson, S.M. (1993). Tumour imaging and therapy. *Radiology Clinics of North America*, **31**, 859–79.

Serpell, J.W., Ball, A.B., Robinson, M.H., Fryatt, I., Fisher, C., and Thomas, J.M. (1991). Factors influencing local recurrence and survival in patients with soft tissue sarcoma of the upper limb. *British Journal of Surgery*, **78**, 1368–72.

Shapeero, L.G., Couanet, D., Vanel, D., et al. (1993). Bone metastases as the presenting manifestation of rhabdomyosarcoma in childhood. *Skeletal Radiology*, **22**, 433–8.

Simon, M.A. and Enneking, W.F. (1976). The management of soft-tissue sarcomas of the extremities. *Journal of Bone and Joint Surgery, American Volume*, **58A**, 317–27.

Singer, S., Corson, J.M., Demetri, G.D., Healey, E.A., Marcus, K., and Eberlein, T.J. (1995). Prognostic factors predictive of survival for truncal and retroperitoneal soft-tissue sarcoma. *Annals of Surgery*, **221**, 185–95.

Slavotinek, J.P., Albertyn, L.E., and Oakeshott, R. (1991). A review of imaging practice in bone and soft tissue lesions. *Australasian Radiology*, **35**, 361–5.

Spanier, S.S., Shuster, J.J., and Vander, G.R. (1990). The effect of local extent of the tumor on prognosis in osteosarcoma. *Journal of Bone and Joint Surgery, American Volume*, **72A**, 643–53.

Terui, S., Terauchi, T., Abe, H., Fukuma, H., Beppu, Y., Chuman, K., and Yokoyama, R. (1994). On clinical usefulness of Tl-201 scintigraphy for the management of malignant soft tissue tumors. *Annals of Nuclear Medicine*, **8**, 55–64.

Willén, H., Åkerman, M., and Carlén, B. (1995). Fine needle aspiration (FNA) in the diagnosis of soft tissue tumours: a review of 22 years experience. *Cytopathology*, **6**, 236–47.

1.6.4   Lesions that resemble bone neoplasms
1.6.4.1 Unicameral bone cyst
Kristy Weber

Introduction

A unicameral bone cyst is a benign unilocular or partially locular fluid-filled cyst (Fig. 1). It is also referred to as a simple or solitary bone cyst (Makley and Joyce 1989). Its presentation is more consistent with a developmental or reactive lesion than a true neoplasm. It comprises less than 5 per cent of all primary bone tumors undergoing biopsy.

Most of these lytic lesions occur in the first two decades with a 2:1

Box 1

- Benign unilocular or partially locular fluid-filled cysts
- More than 90 per cent are found in the proximal humerus and femur
- Typically asymptomatic, but lead to pathologic fractures
- Often enlarge during skeletal growth and then heal spontaneously
- Current treatments of cysts that pose a risk of pathologic fracture include aspiration of cystic fluid with injection of steroids or curettage and bone grafting with or without internal fixation

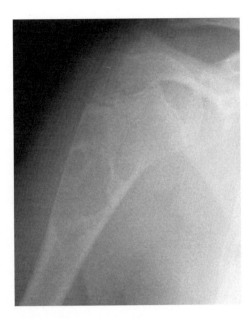

Fig. 1. Typical appearance of a proximal humeral unicameral bone cyst in a 12-year-old female. Note the central, multiloculated appearance. The cortex is minimally thinned. This lesion was followed without intervention and healed uneventfully.

male predominance (Figs 2 and 3). Most occur in the proximal ends of the humerus and femur. In older patients, half are in the ilium and calcaneous. In long bones, the cyst begins directly apposed to the growth plate in the metaphysis and gradually becomes diaphyseal as bone grows away from the lesion.

The exact pathogenesis of these cystic lesions remains unclear. Different theories include degeneration of a previous tumor such as an intraosseous lipoma or fibrous dysplasia, failure of hematoma resorption after intraosseous hemorrhage, growth plate trauma, and development from intraosseous synovial rests. Studies using electron microscopy have shown synovial-like elements in the unicameral bone cyst lining. The most widely accepted suggestion is a focal defect in metaphyseal remodeling that causes a blockage to interstitial fluid drainage. This results in elevated intraosseous pressure leading to focal bone necrosis and accumulation of fluid (Cohen 1960). Subsequent work has shown that the cyst fluid itself contributes to the bony destruction. The fluid contains prostaglandins, oxygen free radicals, interleukins, cytokines, and metalloproteinases. The prostaglandins stimulate osteoclasts to resorb bone, leading to the accumulation of more fluid.

During childhood the unicameral bone cyst will either resolve spontaneously or enlarge, causing symptoms and requiring treatment. It is a benign lesion, however, and will generally heal by the time the patient reaches adulthood.

Pathology

On gross inspection, it is usually difficult to examine more than a collection of curetted fragments. Intraoperatively the simple bone cyst is filled with clear yellow serous fluid unless a pathologic fracture has caused bleeding into the cavity. A fibrous membrane, usually less than 1 mm thick, lines the cyst wall. Bony ridges extend from the wall causing the cyst to appear multiloculated, but they do not actually cross the cavity. The cortex surrounding the cyst is often extremely thin.

On histological examination, the cyst does not have a true endothelial lining (Figs 4 and 5). The actual lining is made up of fibroblasts. Some believe that it has a synovial cell appearance. Deep to this membrane lining, the cyst wall consists of fibrovascular tissue with fragments of immature bone, osteoclast-like giant cells, mesenchymal cells, and occasional lymphocytes. No cellular atypia is seen. The lining in 10 to 15 per cent of simple cysts contains eosinophilic fibrin material amidst the loose stroma which, when calcified, resembles odontogenic cementum. Others feel that these calcified bodies, or calcospherites, form by the Liesegang phenomenon. This involves periodic supersaturation of an insoluble substance with alternating diffusion and precipitation. The calcospherites correspond to radiographic densities occasionally seen within the cyst.

The overall amount of tissue retrieved at the time of surgery is less than that from an aneurysmal bone cyst. A unicameral bone cyst with a pre-existing fracture may have a similar appearance to an aneurysmal bone cyst. There is blood-stained fluid and prominent periosteal fracture callus or granulation tissue. The cellular picture includes multinucleated giant cells, reactive bone, cholesterol clefts, and hemosiderin deposits.

Clinical presentation

Unicameral bone cysts are often asymptomatic and are only discovered when there is an associated fracture. Occasionally they are painful without an associated pathologic fracture. Other symptoms include swelling or joint stiffness. If the lesion disrupts the growth plate there may be a slight deformity, especially in the proximal humerus where the growth plate contributes the majority of the bone's length. The lesion is most active during skeletal growth and decreases with maturity, usually healing spontaneously at that time. Two-thirds of patients do present with a fracture which, in a small proportion of cases, can stimulate the cyst to heal. Unicameral bone cysts occurring in the flat bones are usually asymptomatic, found incidentally, and rarely fracture.

Imaging

Plain radiographs are often diagnostic for this benign lesion. The unicameral bone cyst appears as a purely lytic lesion with a well-defined outline. It may expand concentrically but never penetrates the cortices. It is centrally located in the canal and can grow to involve the entire bony shaft but rarely crosses the growth plate. A cyst in the ilium is often quite large before discovery. A unicameral bone cyst is usually a unilocular cystic lesion, but prominent osseous ridges on the inner cortical wall may give it a multiloculated appearance. No periosteal reaction is noted unless there has been a fracture.

Occasionally a thinned cortical fragment fractures and falls into the base of the lesion confirming its empty cystic nature. This 'fallen fragment' sign occurs only in patients with open physes and is pathognomonic for a unicameral bone cyst with a fracture. It has been proposed that minor trauma causes a nondisplaced comminuted

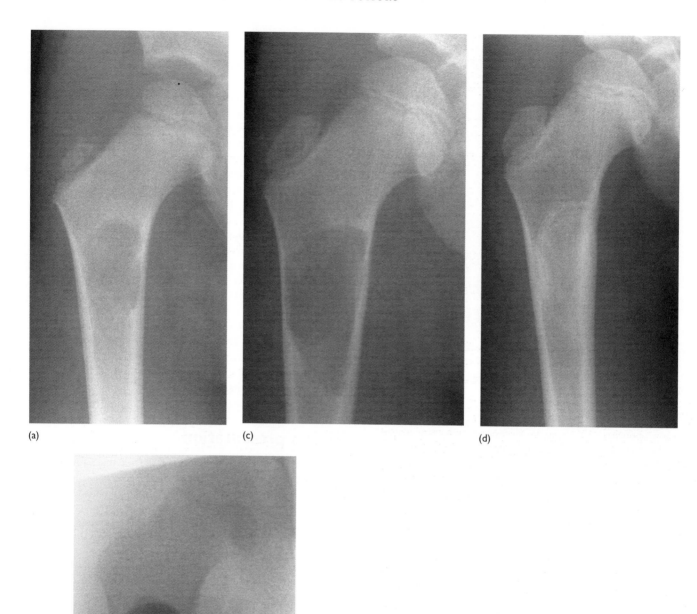

(a)

(c)

(d)

(b)

Fig. 2. (a) Anteroposterior radiograph of the proximal femur in a 4-year-old male showing a metaphyseal cystic lesion consistent with a unicameral bone cyst. (b) Fluoroscopic view showing injection of contrast material into the cyst in order to visualize the extent of the lesion before steroid injection. (c) The lesion stabilized with no change in radiographic appearance. Two years later the lesion has recurred. (d) After 1 year and two additional injections, the lesion has completely healed.

fracture in the cortex, but the intact periosteal sleeve prevents outward displacement of the fracture fragments.

The unicameral bone cyst starts as a metaphyseal lesion that abuts the epiphyseal plate in growing children. It stays in this location during its initial development as its growth is faster than the surrounding bone. It appears to move closer to the diaphysis with time when it is in either a stable or a healing phase. In addition, when the patient enters a rapid adolescent growth spurt, the bone growth is faster than that of the accompanying cyst. Unicameral bone cysts are classified as active when they are within 1 cm of the growth plate and latent when they are closer to the diaphysis. The metaphyseal bone around the cyst does not remodel normally and may always remain slightly widened though, unlike aneurysmal bone cysts, it never becomes wider than the epiphyseal plate.

A bone scan reveals a cold central spot suggesting fluid with slight peripheral uptake. CT and MRI are usually unnecessary but show nonspecific fluid levels. The CT scan can occasionally demonstrate a fallen cortical fragment. The simple bone cyst demonstrates a low signal on T_1-weighted MRI and is bright on T_2 images.

The diagnosis is often definitive by looking at the radiograph, but

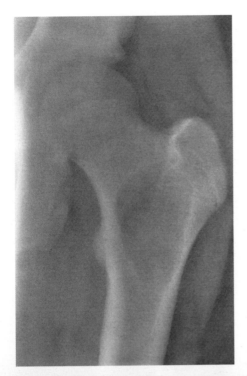

(a)

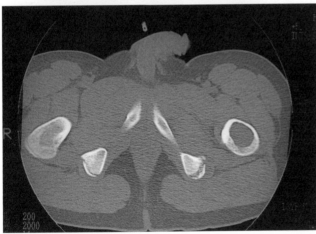

(b)

Fig. 3. (a) Anteroposterior radiograph of the proximal femur revealing a unicameral bone cyst in a 13-year-old active male. (b) CT scan through the lytic area.

occasionally a biopsy is necessary to differentiate between simple cysts, aneurysmal bone cysts, and fibrous dysplasia.

Management

Unicameral bone cysts are self-limiting benign lesions, and the only indication for treatment is to decrease the potential risk of pathologic fracture. Small lesions in nonweight-bearing bones can be watched. Treatment should be considered in large cysts or any cystic area in a site that experiences high stress and is at increased risk for fracture, such as the proximal femur. Standard options include aspiration of

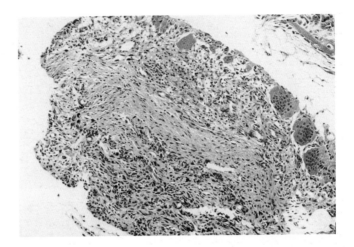

Fig. 4. Low-power view of a unicameral bone cyst. Note the large multinucleated giant cells, hemosiderin, and collagenous matrix.

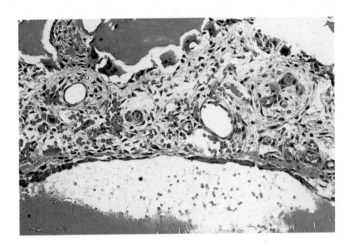

Fig. 5. High-power view of a unicameral bone cyst. Note the loose fibrovascular composition of the septae. No atypical cells are seen.

cystic fluid with injection of steroids, or curettage and bone grafting with or without internal fixation. More recently, injection of fibrosing agents, granular tricalcium phosphate, or autograft–allograft combinations have been advocated. Pathologic fractures in the upper extremity can be treated nonoperatively as the fracture may initiate cyst healing. Fractures through unicameral bone cysts in the proximal femur should be treated with curettage, bone grafting, and internal fixation (Fig. 6).

Unicameral bone cysts were initially treated with curettage and bone grafting, but the recurrence rate was 40 to 60 per cent. This led some to more radical treatment options including subtotal resection of the cyst with massive cortical grafts. This aggressive approach resulted in an unnecessarily high complication rate. When the initial results of steroid injection into unicameral bone cysts were described, a new treatment option was made available that was inexpensive and involved less morbidity (Scaglietti *et al.* 1979). The technique is thought to work either by an antiprostaglandin effect or by decreasing the pressure of the cyst after initially drilling a hole and aspirating the fluid cavity (Shindell *et al.* 1989). One cell culture study showed

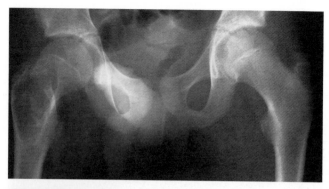

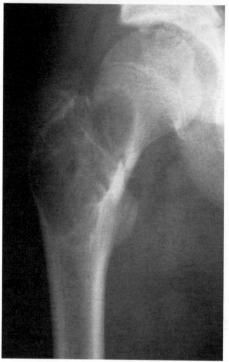

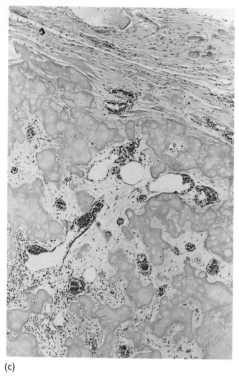

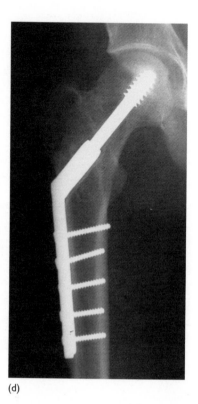

Fig. 6. (a) Anteroposterior pelvic radiograph demonstrating a right basicervical femoral neck fracture through the large multiloculated cystic lesion. (b) View of the proximal femur with clear evidence of a fracture line. (c) Histologic view of the unicameral bone cyst revealing the presence of rounded bodies of calcified fibrinous material, or calcospherites. (d) Nearly 2 years after internal fixation with curettage and bone grafting the lesion has resolved.

(a)

(b)   (c)   (d)

that steroids decreased the secretory function of the synovial-type lining cells and caused them to proliferate and fill the lesion. The length of time that the cells were exposed to the steroid was critical, with improved results after prolonged exposure. Others believe the steroid injection is not as important as decreasing the elevated pressure in the cyst by placing holes through the wall. This theory may explain why some cysts heal after a fracture causes intracystic hemorrhage and removal of the cyst fluid.

The actual treatment by steroid injection should be undertaken in the operating room with the patient under general anesthesia. Fluoroscopic guidance is essential to localize the cyst and visualize the 18-gauge spinal needle as it penetrates the cortex overlying the lesion. Any possible fluid should be removed and a second needle placed at a distance from the aspiration needle to inject radio-opaque dye into the cavity. One study demonstrated that injection of contrast can predict the response to steroid injection by identifying whether the cavity is unilocular. If the cyst is septated, it is more difficult to produce an equal amount of steroid in each compartment and the success rate decreases. Each separate cavity should be injected if pos-

sible. Most recommend using 80 to 200 mg of Depo-Medrol (Upjohn) depending on the size of the patient and lesion as well as the age of the patient. The slow, constant release of this particular steroid may be beneficial compared to the more soluble methylprednisolone. If the lesion does not show signs of radiographic healing in 2 months, repeat injections should be considered. After three injections without healing, many surgeons will treat the unicameral bone cyst with curettage and bone grafting.

Results

A review of the literature on unicameral bone cyst is confusing as 'successful' treatment has different meanings in different studies. Some refer to healing as complete radiographic obliteration of the cavity. Others state that complete radiographic healing is not necessary as long as partial healing is enough to allow unrestricted patient activity. After all, these are benign lesions that should resolve by adulthood and the cure should not be worse than the presence of the cyst. Most authors feel that a higher recurrence rate and risk of fracture is associated with radiographically active cysts and those in patients under 10 years old. The best results of surgical treatment are obtained after the unicameral bone cyst has stopped growing and becomes inactive. Studies have shown that the fluid pressure in an active cyst that has not undergone previous treatment is close to venous pressure, whereas older lesions have less fluid and low or zero pressure readings. Also, injection of dye into an active cyst causes immediate uptake and perfusion thoughout the encircling venous plexus, while inactive cysts contain the dye, and presumably the steroids, without diffusion into the surrounding tissues.

In a 3-year follow-up study (Scaglietti *et al.* 1979), 96 per cent of patients treated with steroid injection of unicameral bone cysts had partial or complete healing of the cavity although many needed repeat injections. In one of the earliest comparisons of steroid injection with curettage and bone grafting, Oppenheim and Galleno (1984) documented better results with injection of the cyst. There was a significant complication rate in the surgically treated group including coxa vara, wound infection, epiphyseal arrest, and shortening. Campanacci *et al.* (1986) compared 141 unicameral bone cysts treated by injection of steroids with 178 treated with curettage and bone grafting. Nearly half of the cysts healed after the initial steroid injection as well as after initial curettage. The poor prognostic factors identified were patients undergoing steroid injection that included multiloculated appearance, large cyst size, and radiographically active cysts. Risk factors for poor prognosis for the surgical subset included active cysts and those who had undergone previous operations. Overall, given the similar outcomes, the less invasive treatment was recommended (Campanacci *et al.* 1986). Numerous authors have confirmed that initial treatment with steroid injection is justified, although many patients will need multiple treatments prior to healing.

Results of percutaneous drilling without steroid injection for treatment of unicameral bone cysts are promising, although the reported number of patients is small and warrants further investigation.

If treating one of these lesions with curettage and bone grafting, allograft can provide excellent healing without the morbidity of autograft harvest. Various series have documented effective healing of unicameral bone cysts after using tricalcium phosphate, high-porosity hydroxyapatite, cancellous allograft mixed with autologous marrow, or injection of a fibrosing agent.

In general, patients have an excellent ultimate outcome following treatment of this benign lesion.

Further reading

Adamsbaum, C., Kalifa, G., Seringe, R., and Dubousset, J. (1993). Direct Ethibloc injection in benign bone cysts: preliminary report on four patients. *Skeletal Radiology*, 22, 317–20.

Adler, C. (1985). Tumour-like lesions in the femur with cementum-like material. *Skeletal Radiology*, 14, 26–37.

Ahn, J. and Park, J. (1994). Pathological fractures secondary to unicameral bone cysts. *International Orthopaedics*, 18, 20–2.

Altermatt, S., Schwobel, M., and Pochon, J. (1992). Operative treatment of solitary bone cysts with tricalcium phosphate ceramic. A 1 to 7 year follow-up. *European Journal of Pediatric Surgery*, 2, 180–2.

Capanna, R., Albisinni, U., Caroli, G., and Campanacci, M. (1984). Contrast

examination as a prognostic factor in the treatment of solitary bone cyst by cortisone injection. *Skeletal Radiology*, 12, 97–102.

Chigira, M., Maehara, S., Arita, S., and Udagawa, E. (1983). The aetiology and treatment of simple bone cysts. *Journal of Bone and Joint Surgery, British Volume*, 65B, 633–7.

Grabias, S. and Mankin, H. (1974). Chondrosarcoma arising in histologically proved unicameral bone cyst. *Journal of Bone and Joint Surgery, American Volume*, 56A, 1501–9.

Inoue, O., Ibaraki, K., Shimabukuro, H., and Shingaki, Y. (1993). Packing with high-porosity hydroxyapatite cubes alone for the treatment of simple bone cyst. *Clinical Orthopaedics and Related Research*, 293, 287–92.

Komiya, S., Minamitani, K., Sasaguri, Y., Hashimoto, S., Morimatsu, M., and Inoue, A. (1993). Simple bone cyst. Treatment by trepanation and studies on bone resorptive factors in cyst fluid with a theory of its pathogenesis. *Clinical Orthopaedics and Related Research*, 287, 204–11.

Komiya, S., Tsuzuki, K., Mangham, D., Sugiyama, M., and Inoue, A. (1994). Oxygen scavengers in simple bone cysts. *Clinical Orthopaedics and Related Research*, 308, 199–206.

Kragel, P., Williams, J., Garvin, D., and Goral, A. (1989). Solitary bone cyst of the radius containing Liesegang's rings. *American Journal of Clinical Pathology*, 92, 831–3.

Mirra, J. (1989). *Bone tumors*. Lea & Febiger, Philadelphia, PA.

Neer, C., Francis, K., Johnston, A., and Kiernan, H. (1973). Current concepts on the treatment of solitary unicameral bone cyst. *Clinical Orthopaedics and Related Research*, 97, 40–51.

Pentimalli, G., Tudisco, C., Scola, E., Farsetti, P., and Ippolito, E. (1987). Unicameral bone cysts—comparison between surgical and steroid injection treatment. *Archives of Orthopedic and Trauma Surgery*, 106, 251–6.

Spence, K., Sell, K., and Brown, R. (1969). Solitary bone cyst: treatment with freeze-dried cancellous bone allograft. A study of 177 cases. *Journal of Bone and Joint Surgery, American Volume*, 51A, 87–96.

Struhl, S., Edelson, C., Pritzker, H., Seimon, L., and Dorfman, H. (1989). Solitary (unicameral) bone cyst. The fallen fragment sign revisited. *Skeletal Radiology*, 18, 261–5.

Uchida, A., Araki, N., Shinto, Y., Yoshikawa, H., Kurisaki, E., and Ono, K. (1990). The use of calcium hydroxyapatite ceramic in bone tumour surgery. *Journal of Bone and Joint Surgery, British Volume*, 72B, 298–302.

Yu, C., D'Astous, J., and Finnegan, M. (1991). Simple bone cysts. The effects of methylprednisolone on synovial cells in culture. *Clinical Orthopaedics and Related Research*, 262, 34–41.

References

Campanacci, M., Capanna, R., and Picci, P. (1986). Unicameral and aneurysmal bone cysts. *Clinical Orthopaedics and Related Research*, 204, 25–36.

Cohen, J. (1960). Simple bone cysts. Studies of cyst fluid in six cases with a theory of pathogenesis. *Journal of Bone and Joint Surgery, American Volume*, 42A, 609–16.

Makley, J. and Joyce, M. (1989). Unicameral bone cyst. *Orthopedic Clinics of North America*, 20, 407–15.

Oppenheim, W. and Galleno, H. (1984). Operative treatment versus steroid injection in the management of unicameral bone cysts. *Journal of Pediatric Orthopedics*, 4, 1–7.

Scaglietti, O., Marchetti, P., and Bartolozzi, P. (1979). The effects of methylprednisolone acetate in the treatment of bone cysts. Results of 3 years follow-up. *Journal of Bone and Joint Surgery, British Volume*, 61B, 200–4.

Shindell, R., Huurman, W., Lippiello, L., and Connolly, J. (1989). Prostaglandin levels in unicameral bone cysts treated by intralesional steroid injection. *Journal of Pediatric Orthopaedics*, 9, 516–19.

1.6.4.2 **Aneurysmal bone cyst**

Kristy Weber

Introduction

An aneurysmal bone cyst is not a true neoplasm but rather a locally destructive blood-filled reactive lesion of bone (Kransdorf and Sweet 1995; Capanna *et al.* 1996). Any location may be involved but the majority of aneurysmal bone cysts are found in the metaphysis or metadiaphysis of long tubular bones, especially the proximal humerus, distal femur, proximal tibia, and ilium. Vertebral lesions, most often in the lumbar region, account for 15 to 20 per cent of these entities. The posterior elements are usually the site of the lesion, however, it frequently extends into the vertebral body or to adjacent levels. It is approximately half as common as giant cell tumors. Seventy-five per cent of aneurysmal bone cysts occur in patients under 20 years old, and there is a slight female predominance.

Aneurysmal bone cysts can arise *de novo* as a primary process or as a secondary, reactive process associated with another lesion. They are thought to occur 25 to 40 per cent of the time in association with other bone tumors including giant cell tumor, chondroblastoma, simple bone cyst, osteoblastoma, fibrous dysplasia, nonossifying fibroma, chondromyxoid fibroma, and osteosarcoma (Martinez and Sissons 1988). Some authors feel that all aneurysmal bone cysts are associated with other tumors which have often been obliterated by the hemorrhagic process, but this cannot be proved. A secondary aneurysmal bone cyst occurs in the location of the primary tumor (i.e. epiphyseal when in combination with a chondroblastoma). It should be categorized as the name of the primary lesion 'with secondary aneurysmal bone cyst changes'.

Its pathogenesis has been debated, but most agree that an aneurysmal bone cyst results from a local circulatory disturbance leading to increased venous pressure and production of local hemorrhage. The resulting reactive osteolytic process further increases the bleeding. It has been reported after a fracture or surgery which induces a subperiosteal hematoma. Some have proposed an etiology due to a localized arteriovenous malformation, but detailed flow studies have shown no communication between the lesion and the systemic circulation. The blood filling the cavity is thought to arise directly from capillaries in the cyst membrane. The usual natural history is progression to a severely destructive lesion; however, an aneurysmal bone cyst can occasionally undergo spontaneous ossification.

Examples of aneurysmal bone cysts are shown in Figs 1, 2, 3, and 4.

Box 1

- Locally destructive blood-filled reactive lesions of bone, not neoplasms
- Most commonly found in the metaphysis or metadiaphysis of long tubular bones, especially the proximal humerus, distal femur, proximal tibia, and ilium
- Can arise as a primary process or as a secondary reactive process associated with bone tumors including giant cell tumor, chondroblastoma, simple bone cyst, osteoblastoma, fibrous dysplasia, nonossifying fibroma, chondromyxoid fibroma, and osteosarcoma
- Consists of cavernous spaces filled with blood separated by a cellular stroma
- Differential diagnosis includes unicameral bone cyst, giant cell tumor, pseudotumor of hemophilia, conventional osteosarcoma, and telangiectatic osteosarcoma
- Usually presents with pain and swelling
- Most aneurysmal bone cysts are treated by curettage and bone grafting

Pathology

Grossly, an aneurysmal bone cyst is a cavitary lesion with multiple septated spaces filled with blood. It is surrounded by an extremely thin layer of bone covered by a raised periosteum. Completely excised lesions are rare, and curettings show a large amount of blood and a variable amount of solid tissue, making it difficult to reconstruct the lesional architecture.

The microscopic appearance of an aneurysmal bone cyst is of hemorrhagic tissue with cavernous spaces separated by a cellular stroma. Immunocytochemical and electron microscopic studies reveal that the spaces do not have an endothelial lining or a smooth muscle wall, but rather a lining of compressed fibroblasts and histiocytes, which negates a true vascular origin. Hemosiderin-laden macrophages, chronic inflammatory cells, and broad seams of reactive osteoid occupy the fibrohistiocytic stroma between the cavities. Multinucleated giant cells are prominent, making differentiation from a giant cell tumor difficult. The septa between cavities contain loose or dense collagen fibers and may be quite cellular. The numerous mitotic figures are not of concern in the absence of anaplastic stromal cells. The so-called 'mineralized matrix with a chondroid aura' is unique to aneurysmal bone cyst. This matrix is usually heavily calci-

Fig. 1. (a), (b) Anteroposterior and lateral radiographs of a 9-year-old female showing a cystic lesion in the proximal fibular metaphysis extending to, but not crossing, the growth plate. There is uniform expansion and thinning of the surrounding cortex. (c) T_1-weighted MRI reveals a fluid level in the lesion. No soft-tissue mass is present. (d) Low-power histologic view of the curetted lesion shows the typical appearance of an aneurysmal bone cyst. Large blood-filled spaces with extensive hemorrhage are apparent. (e) Higher power reveals abundant benign giant cells in the fibrous stroma between cavities. Reactive bone is noted on the edge of this view. (f) No atypical cells are present on high magnification. (g), (h) Postoperative radiographs after curettage and bone grafting. This lesion could also have been treated with resection of the proximal fibula.

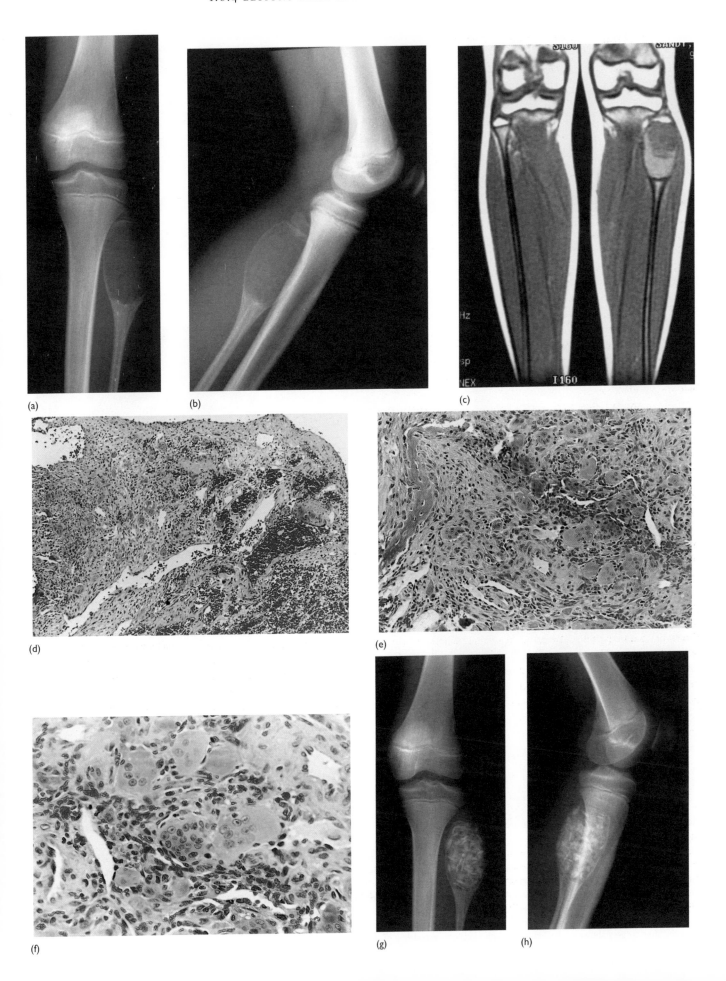

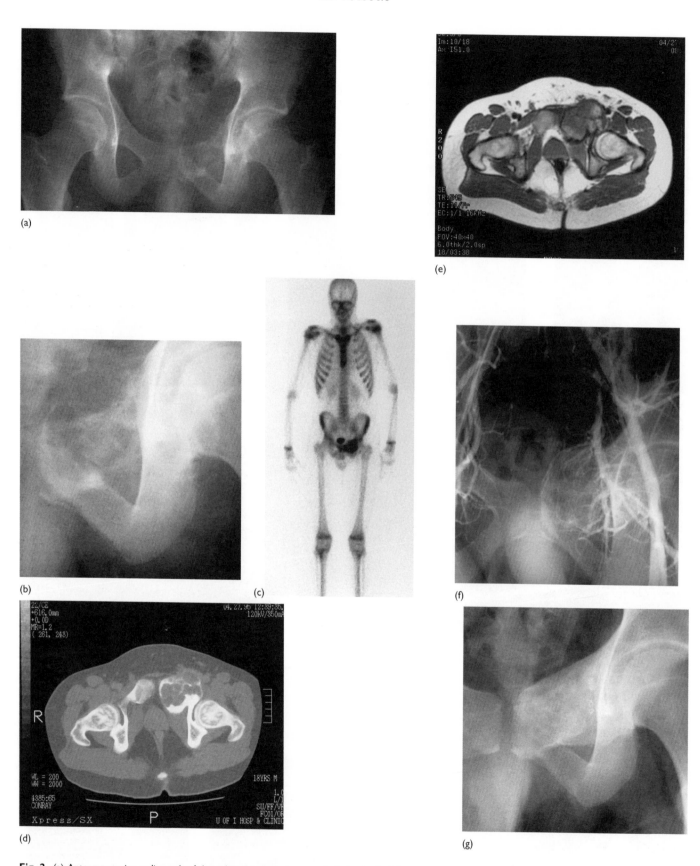

Fig. 2. (a) Anteroposterior radiograph of the pelvis showing a large cystic lesion in the left superior pubic ramus of an 18-year-old male. This aggressive appearance can be mistaken for a malignant neoplasm. (b) Coned-down view showing the location of the lesion. (c) Bone scan shows focal increased uptake in the left pubic rami. (d) Axial CT cut reveals the osteolytic destructive lesion expanding the bony cortices. (e) T_1-weighted MRI reveals a heterogeneous appearance due to the blood-filled cavities. Note the anterior expansion. (f) Angiography demonstrates the hypervascular nature of the lesion. Embolization was performed in conjunction with curettage and grafting to decrease the risk of massive intraoperative hemorrhage. (g) Anteroposterior radiograph 10 months after surgery showing a healed lesion with excellent remodeling of the pubic ramus.

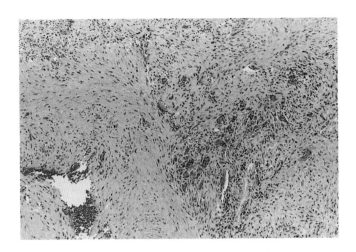

Fig. 3. Low-power view of an aneurysmal bone cyst showing the hemosiderin-laden cells.

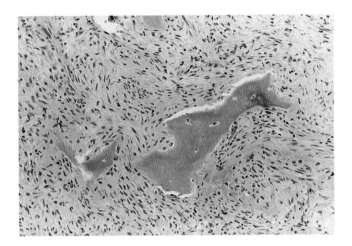

Fig. 4. High-power view of an aneurysmal bone cyst showing the benign stroma and reactive bone. No anaplasia is evident.

fied and can be used as a reliable diagnostic feature. Osteoid or mineralized bone is reactive and present along the periphery of the lesion. It may arise from the chondroid matrix or more frequently has a metaplastic quality similar to the woven bone in fibrous dysplasia. The diagnosis of aneurysmal bone cyst is one of exclusion. When associated with other bone tumors, the aneurysmal bone cyst component can be a major component and a careful search is necessary to identify areas of the underlying primary lesion.

The differential diagnosis includes unicameral bone cyst, giant cell tumor, pseudotumor of hemophilia, conventional osteosarcoma, and, most importantly, telangiectatic osteosarcoma. The unicameral bone cyst does not have large blood-filled spaces unless interrupted by a pathologic fracture. It contains a clear yellow serous fluid, and the lining consists of bland fibrous tissue. A giant cell tumor is the most likely to be associated with aneurysmal components. It is nearly impossible to differentiate histologically as it contains many of the same features as an aneurysmal bone cyst; therefore careful radiographic and clinical correlation is essential for diagnosis. Usually the osteoblastic changes seen in the trabecular areas of the cyst are not

present in giant cell tumors. The pseudotumor of hemophilia can be similar histologically but is readily differentiated by the clinical presentation. In order to prevent a potentially fatal mistake of misdiagnosing a telangiectatic osteosarcoma, it is important to study the entire specimen meticulously under high magnification. The appearance can be confusing as much of the lesion is composed of blood-filled cavities, hemorrhagic necrosis, and benign giant cells. However, there are always focal areas of markedly pleomorphic cells and atypical mitotic figures. Tumor osteoid surrounded by malignant osteoblasts is typically in a lace-like pattern instead of the broad bands found in an aneurysmal bone cyst. A completely separate consideration is a conventional osteosarcoma associated with secondary aneurysmal changes. Benign hemorrhagic cystic areas are separated from the malignant component as contrasted with the telangiectatic type which has a malignant stroma amidst the blood-filled spaces. An incisional biopsy may miss the malignant section of either type of osteosarcoma.

A solid variant of the aneurysmal bone cyst has been described with clinical and radiographic features identical to the cystic form. Except for the absence of cavernous spaces, there is no significant histological difference from the typical aneurysmal bone cyst (Vergel de Dios *et al.* 1992). The benign stromal cells are highly proliferative, giving the appearance of a giant cell reparative granuloma. Some authors feel strongly that this is not a unique lesion but actually a benign giant cell tumor with secondary aneurysmal bone cyst changes.

Clinical presentation

Patients usually present with mild pain and swelling which has been present for weeks to years depending on the activity of the lesion. Rapid growth can occur and indicates the destructive nature of an aneurysmal bone cyst. This may clinically mimic a malignancy, most commonly a telangiectatic osteosarcoma. It is important to remember that this particular malignancy is rare, comprising only 4 per cent of all osteosarcomas. Pregnancy is occasionally associated with the onset or progression of symptoms consistent with the hyperemic nature of an aneurysmal bone cyst. Spinal lesions may cause radicular compression or vertebral collapse with resultant neurologic deficits. Growth plate damage can occur from the aneurysmal bone cyst itself, surgical treatment, or radiotherapy. This can result in a leg-length discrepancy or angular deformity. An aneurysmal bone cyst presenting with a pathologic fracture in a long bone is surprisingly infrequent. Laboratory studies are normal.

Imaging studies

The radiographic picture is typically one of a radiolucent destructive cyst that expands the surrounding cortex. Along with progressive bony resorption, it elevates the periosteum but remains contained by a thin shell. An aneurysmal bone cyst can have well-defined margins, though not sclerotic, or a permeative appearance that mimics a malignancy. It is most often eccentric but can be central or subperiosteal in location. The latter type causes minimal erosion of the cortex and a soft-tissue mass. The metaphysis is the most common location of an aneurysmal bone cyst with diaphyseal and epiphyseal presentations less likely. Normally the metaphyseal lesion does not cross the growth plate in children unless it is aggressive or recurrent. An epiphyseal aneurysmal bone cyst is usually the secondary component of a chondroblastoma or giant cell tumor.

Four phases of aneurysmal bone cyst development have been described. The initial phase consists of a small lytic lesion that may have an aggressive appearance. The growth phase is typified by the typical 'blow-out' picture from rapid uncontained growth and bony destruction. The stable phase is most commonly seen; it has a multiloculated cystic appearance with expanded cortices but is contained by the periosteum. The healing phase commences with ossification of the trabeculae within the lesion.

A classification of aneurysmal bone cysts into five types based on radiographic appearance has been described (Campanacci et al. 1986). Type 1 is a central metaphyseal well-contained lesion present in long bones. The profile of the bone remains intact or only slightly expanded. Type 2 is a cyst that involves the entire segment of bone, usually in the metadiaphysis of thin long bones (i.e. fibula, radius, ulna) or flat bones. The cortex is thinned and the bone appears severely inflated with intralesional septations. Type 3 is an eccentric metaphyseal lesion that causes minimal expansion of the cortex in long bones. Type 4 is the least common and describes a cyst with subperiosteal extension and no or minimal cortical erosion. It usually occurs in the diaphysis where there is a thick cortex. Type 5 is a metadiaphyseal subperiosteal lesion of long bones that inflates the periosteum toward the soft tissues and penetrates the cancellous bone of the medullary canal.

The same authors classified aneurysmal bone cysts based on their radiographic activity. Stage 1 describes a latent or inactive lesion where the periosteal shell is intact and the inner limits of the lesion are well defined by a reactive rim. Stage 2 describes an active lesion where the periosteal shell is incomplete but the inner limit is defined. Stage 3 refers to an aggressive lesion where there is no reactive bone or periosteal shell and the inner limit is ill defined.

A bone scan shows either diffuse or peripheral tracer uptake with a central area of decreased uptake. The scintigraphy is fairly accurate in reflecting the osseous extent of an aneurysmal bone cyst. Angiography shows a persistent accumulation of contrast throughout the cyst or a marked hypervascular appearance on its peripheral aspect. No visible afferent or efferent vessels are evident which, along with findings on bone scan, supports the cyst being independent from the systemic circulation. CT demonstrates a fluid level in approximately one-third of aneurysmal bone cysts. This is a nonspecific finding, however, and often is not visualized if the patient is not immobilized for a short time before the study. CT scans are particularly helpful in delineating the cyst in areas of complex anatomy such as the spine or pelvis. MRI demonstrates the multiloculated cavities and fluid levels while also showing the occasional soft-tissue mass.

The radiographic differential diagnosis includes unicameral bone cyst, chondromyxoid fibroma, giant cell tumor, osteoblastoma when in the spine, and telangiectatic osteosarcoma.

Management

Although there are occasional instances of spontaneous healing, the accepted treatment of an aneurysmal bone cyst is surgical. The standard surgical regimen is thorough curettage and bone grafting. Incisional biopsy is usually followed by definitive treatment in the same operative session. Biopsy of the lesion may produce heavy bleeding; therefore tourniquet control is advised. Selective embolization of feeder vessels to the cyst on the day of surgery can reduce the blood loss. A large window in the cortex will facilitate complete curettage, and abundant soft tissue may be retrieved. Occasionally the mass will appear pulsatile at surgery. Local adjuvant therapy with phenol or liquid nitrogen helps to sterilize the cavity after curettage. If the aneurysmal bone cyst occurs in an expendable area such as the proximal fibula or metatarsal, it may be advisable to resect the lesion completely. If there has been aggressive growth or rapid destruction of bone after the first curettage, a second extensive curettage or resection of the lesion are the usual options. Resection may also be indicated if multiple recurrences threaten to damage an adjacent joint or physis. Arterial embolization has been utilized as definitive treatment of aneurysmal bone cysts in locations that are not amenable to surgery due to the potential for large intraoperative hemorrhage. Lesions in the spine should be treated with preoperative embolization, curettage, and stabilization as necessary. Low-dose irradiation of an aneurysmal bone cyst has been reported to be an effective method of treatment often associated with rapid ossification; however, it should be considered only in inoperable lesions because of the potential for malignant transformation. Radiation, especially in children, can cause damage to the reproductive organs, growth plate, and spinal cord. Treatment of an aneurysmal bone cyst is based on the radiographic appearance and rate of growth of the lesion. If the cyst is associated with another primary tumor, it should be classified and managed based on the primary component. The prognosis also depends on the primary tumor.

Results

The recurrence rate after curettage with or without grafting of an aneurysmal bone cyst is 18 to 34 per cent, with one report as high as 59 per cent. Different authors have used autograft or allograft to fill the curetted cavity. Recurrence is demonstrated by further bony destruction and resorption of the bone graft which usually occurs within 6 months of the first surgery. It is unusual after 2 years. Recurrences usually occur in long bones and are more likely in active or aggressive lesions. Other authors correlated recurrence with age under 15 years, centrally located aneurysmal bone cysts, and incomplete removal of the cystic cavity contents.

Most authors use adjuvant treatment such as phenol intraoperatively to minimize the risk of recurrence, as recurrent lesions can destroy the articular surface or growth plate in children. Supplementing curettage with cryotherapy has decreased the recurrence rate to 8 to 18 per cent in different studies. This use of liquid nitrogen has not been adequately studied on lesions near the open epiphyseal plate. One report documented a postoperative fracture incidence of 9.8 per cent, and the authors recommended adequate reconstruction of the cavity with polymethylmethacrylate or bone grafts as well as postoperative protective bracing in order to minimize this complication (Marcove et al. 1995). Selective arterial embolization of the nutrient vessels of an aneurysmal bone cyst with or without surgery is reported to be effective treatment. One series reported healing with complete relief of symptoms in 17 of 19 patients. Thirteen patients needed repeated embolizations to obtain satisfactory results; however, it was felt to be a much safer technique than surgery without as many potential complications (De Cristofaro *et al.* 1992). Percutaneous introduction of a paste of allograft bone and autologous bone marrow has induced healing and may be of interest for cysts in poorly accessible areas. Theoretically the cystic tissue is retained so that its intrinsic osteogenic potential can be used to promote healing. The drawback to this approach is that there is no tissue to examine for a definite diagnosis, and there is potential for further cyst progression. Injection of aneurysmal bone cysts with fibrosing agents has met with success in a small series but is concerning for the same reason. The recurrence rate with radiotherapy alone is 15 to 25 per cent in several small series. Most of the few reports concerning malignant transformation of an aneurysmal bone cyst have been related to previous radiation treatment of the lesion or were initially misdiagnosed telangiectatic osteosarcomas. The outlook is favorable for patients with this benign lesion, as the overall prognosis for acceptable function and resolution of the lesion is 90 per cent.

Further reading

Adamsbaum, C., Kalifa, G., Seringe, R., and Dubousset, J. (1993). Direct Ethibloc injection in benign bone cysts: preliminary report on four patients. *Skeletal Radiology*, **22**, 317–20.

Alles, J. and Schulz, A. (1986). Immuncytochemical markers (endothelial and histiocytic) and ultrastructure of primary aneurysmal bone cysts. *Human Pathology*, **17**, 39–45.

Bertoni, F., Bacchini, P., Capanna, R., *et al.* (1993). Solid variant of aneurysmal bone cyst. *Cancer*, **71**, 729–34.

Biesecker, J., Marcove, R., Huvos, A., and Mike, V. (1970). Aneurysmal bone cysts. A clinicopathologic study of 66 cases. *Cancer*, **26**, 615–25.

Capanna, R., Albisinni, U., Picci, P., Calderoni, P., Campanacci, M., and Springfield, D. (1985). Aneurysmal bone cyst of the spine. *Journal of Bone and Joint Surgery, American Volume*, **67A**, 527–31.

Capanna, R., Bertoni, F., Bettelli, G., *et al.* (1986). Aneurysmal bone cysts of the pelvis. *Archives of Orthopaedic and Trauma Surgery*, **105**, 279–84.

Delloye, C., De Nayer, P., Malghem, J., and Noel, H. (1996). Induced healing of aneurysmal bone cysts by demineralized bone particles. A report of two cases. *Archives of Orthopaedic and Trauma Surgery*, **115**, 141–5.

Fechner, R. and Mills, S. (1993). *Atlas of tumor pathology. Tumors of the bones and joints* (3rd series). AFIP, Washington, DC.

Freiberg, A., Loder, R., Heidelberger, K., and Hensinger, R. (1994). Aneurysmal bone cysts in young children. *Journal of Pediatric Orthopaedics*, **14**, 86–91.

Hay, M., Paterson, D., and Taylor, T. (1978). Aneurysmal bone cysts of the spine. *Journal of Bone and Joint Surgery, British Volume*, **60B**, 406–11.

Levy, W., Miller, A., Bonakdarpour, A., and Aegerter, E. (1975). Aneurysmal bone cyst secondary to other osseous lesions. Report of 57 cases. *American Journal of Clinical Pathology*, **63**, 1–8.

Nobler, M., Higinbotham, N., and Phillips, R. (1968). The cure of aneurysmal bone cyst. Irradiation superior to surgery in an analysis of 33 cases. *Radiology*, **90**, 1185–92.

Ruiter, D., van Rijssel, T., and van der Velde, E. (1977). Aneurysmal bone cysts. A clinicopathological study of 105 cases. *Cancer*, **39**, 2231–9.

Schajowicz, F. (1994). *Tumors and tumor-like lesions of bone* (2nd edn). Springer-Verlag, Berlin.

Tillman, B., Dahlin, D., Lipscomb, P., and Stewart, J. (1968). Aneurysmal bone cyst: an analysis of 95 cases. *Mayo Clinic Proceedings*, **43**, 478–95.

References

Campanacci, M., Capanna, R., and Picci, P. (1986). Unicameral and aneurysmal bone cysts. *Clinical Orthopaedics and Related Research*, **204**, 25–36.

Capanna, R., Campanacci, M., and Manfrini, M. (1996). Unicameral and aneurysmal bone cysts. *Orthopedic Clinics of North America*, **27**, 605–14.

De Cristofaro, R., Biagini, R., Boriani, S., *et al.* (1992). Selective arterial embolization in the treatment of aneurysmal bone cyst and angioma of bone. *Skeletal Radiology*, **21**, 523–7.

Kransdorf, M. and Sweet, D. (1995). Aneurysmal bone cyst: concept, controversy, clinical presentation, and imaging. *American Journal of Roentgenology*, **164**, 573–80.

Marcove, R., Sheth, D., Takemoto, S., and Healey, J. (1995). The treatment of aneurysmal bone cyst. *Clinical Orthopaedics and Related Research*, **311**, 157–63.

Martinez, V. and Sissons, H. (1988). Aneurysmal bone cyst. A review of 123 cases including primary lesions and those secondary to other bone pathology. *Cancer*, **61**, 2291–304.

Vergel De Dios, A., Bond, J., Shives, T., McLeod, R., and Unni, K. (1992). Aneurysmal bone cyst. A clinicopathologic study of 238 cases. *Cancer*, **69**, 2921–31.

1.6.4.3 Fibrous cortical defect/nonossifying fibroma

Kristy Weber

Introduction

Fibrous cortical defects are not true neoplasms, but rather developmental proliferations of fibrous tissue and histiocytes. Nonossifying fibromas are histologically identical to fibrous cortical defects but are usually larger and have a slightly different radiographic appearance. Together these lesions have been referred to as metaphyseal fibrous defects. This may correlate better with their developmental origin. Most authors feel they are fundamentally the same lesion based on their clinical course and histological similarities. Nonossifying fibromas probably originated as fibrous cortical defects. As a group, they are separate from benign fibrous histiocytomas, true neoplasms that display more aggressive behavior. Also separate are the medial supracondylar defects (cortical avulsions), normal variants that occur on the posterior medial femoral condyle.

Box 1

- Benign developmental proliferations of fibrous tissue and histiocytes
- Range from several millimeters to several centimeters in size
- Eighty per cent of lesions occur in the distal femoral, proximal tibial, and distal tibial metaphyses
- Usually discovered incidentally and remain asymptomatic
- Heal spontaneously and do not require treatment unless they substantially increase the risk of pathologic fracture

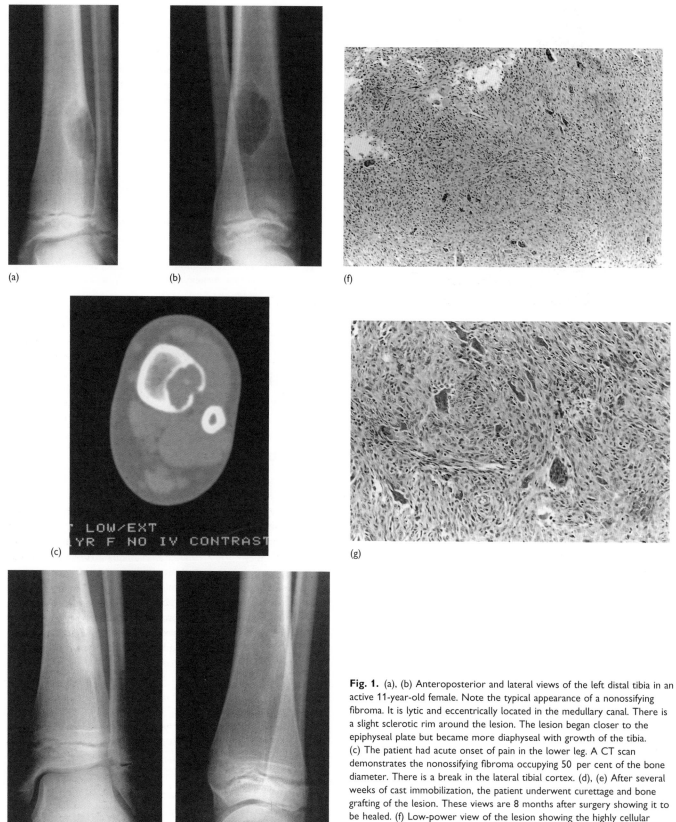

Fig. 1. (a), (b) Anteroposterior and lateral views of the left distal tibia in an active 11-year-old female. Note the typical appearance of a nonossifying fibroma. It is lytic and eccentrically located in the medullary canal. There is a slight sclerotic rim around the lesion. The lesion began closer to the epiphyseal plate but became more diaphyseal with growth of the tibia. (c) The patient had acute onset of pain in the lower leg. A CT scan demonstrates the nonossifying fibroma occupying 50 per cent of the bone diameter. There is a break in the lateral tibial cortex. (d), (e) After several weeks of cast immobilization, the patient underwent curettage and bone grafting of the lesion. These views are 8 months after surgery showing it to be healed. (f) Low-power view of the lesion showing the highly cellular fibrohistiocytic stroma in a whorled pattern. (g) Higher-power view revealing the benign stromal cells and occasional multinucleated giant cells.

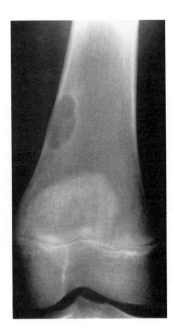

Fig. 2. Anteroposterior radiograph of the distal femur in a skeletally immature male. A well-circumscribed fibrous cortical defect is noted in the medial femoral cortex.

Fibrous cortical defects can be a few millimeters to several centimeters in diameter. Most occur in the distal femoral, proximal tibial, and distal tibial metaphyses; 10 per cent are found in the fibula. Some authors feel that these lesions only occur where there is a ligamentous or tendinous insertion (Ritschl *et al.* 1988). The flat bones, hands, feet, and spine are not affected. Fibrous cortical defects are reported to be present in over one-third of children aged 4 to 8 years and are rarely found after the age of 14. Nonossifying fibromas are found in the same sites and can occur into the fourth decade but usually present between 2 and 20 years of age. They are found much less frequently than cortical defects. Both lesions are more common in males and are usually solitary. Multifocal involvement has been reported rarely (Moser *et al.* 1987).

The etiology of these lesions is unclear, but both the clinicopathologic spectrum and natural history favor a non-neoplastic condition. Intraosseous hemorrhage undergoing resorption, vascular disturbance, and aberrant metaphyseal remodeling have been proposed as theories of pathogenesis.

The natural history of these fibrous lesions is to regress spontaneously without treatment unless, as in some large nonossifying fibromas, a pathologic fracture occurs or pain necessitates treatment. Examples of these lesions are shown in Figs 1, 2, and 3.

Pathology

These fibrous lesions are rarely seen by pathologists as they are easily diagnosed on radiographs and do not often need surgical treatment. On gross inspection, the curetted fragments are soft, well circumscribed, and either yellow or brown depending on the varying amounts of fibrous tissue, lipid-laden histiocytes, and hemosiderin

present. The surrounding cortex may be attenuated but is not disrupted except in the case of a pathologic fracture.

The histologic appearance of fibrous cortical defects and nonossifying fibromas is identical. A crowded, but unremarkable, proliferative spindle cell stroma is arranged in a whorled or storiform pattern. Collagen fibers and fibroblasts are intermixed with irregular clusters of lipid- and hemosiderin-laden histiocytes. Multinucleated giant cells are frequently seen around areas of hemorrhage. The nuclei show no atypia, although they can be plump and hyperchromatic in the spindle cells. Mitotic figures can be present in large lesions. Bone is not formed by the lesion; however, reactive new bone can form after a pathologic fracture and in older lesions undergoing regression. With time there is an increased amount of collagen and a decreased number of giant cells.

The differential diagnosis includes giant cell tumor, pigmented villinodular synovitis, brown tumor of hyperparathyroidism, and malignant fibrous histiocytoma.

Clinical presentation

Both fibrous cortical defects and nonossifying fibromas are usually noticed incidentally and remain asymptomatic. A frequent clinical scenario is a child with a sports-related injury to the knee who has an unrelated benign fibrous lesion noted on plain radiographs. Large lesions may present with pain or pathologic fracture. Mild swelling overlying a lesion close to the skin may be the only physical finding. There is no evidence for malignant transformation of these fibrous lesions.

Imaging

Fibrous cortical defects are found in the metaphysis or diaphysis of long bones as lucent defects up to 2 cm in size. They are sharply demarcated by a sclerotic rim. They can erode the cortex but cause no periosteal reaction. These fibrous lesions are usually diagnosed on plain radiographs without further need for diagnostic studies.

Nonossifying fibromas are lytic lesions eccentrically located in the medullary cavity and surrounded by a thin well-defined rim of reactive bone. In narrow bones such as the fibula, the entire width of the canal may be involved. Some can grow up to 7 cm and cause cortical expansion but no periosteal reaction. They often appear multilocular with a sharply scalloped margin.

Both lesions are elongated in the axis of long bone growth and seem to migrate from the metaphysis toward the diaphysis as endochondral ossification continues at the epiphyseal plate. Their radiographic appearance can differ with the stage of the lesion. Healing begins with sclerosis at the diaphyseal end of a lesion and progresses toward the epiphyseal side as healing progresses (Ritschl *et al.* 1988).

Bone scans show uptake of tracer only during the healing phase of these fibrous lesions or after a pathologic fracture. They should be completely inactive when healed. CT is generally not necessary but can delineate the degree of cortical expansion and thinning. The lesions have low signal enhancement on MRI and are usually seen when this study is performed for an adjacent knee abnormality. If there is high cellularity, a brighter signal may be seen.

The radiographs are distinctly diagnostic for these two lesions;

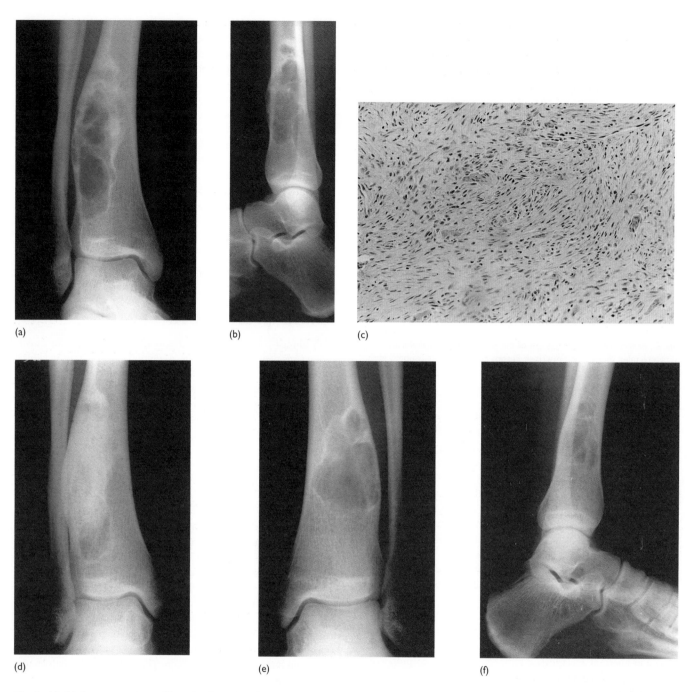

Fig. 3. (a), (b) Anteroposterior and lateral radiographs of the right distal tibia in a 14-year-old female reveal a large nonossifying fibroma. Note the eccentric location and multiloculated appearance with a prominent sclerotic border. The patient was thought to be at high risk for fracture; therefore curettage and bone grafting was performed. (c) Typical histologic appearance of the benign fibrous stroma and intermixed giant cells. (d) Anteroposterior view of the right tibia 6 months after surgery showing consolidation of the bone graft. (e), (f) The patient had multiple nonossifying fibromas throughout both lower extremities. Anteroposterior and lateral radiographs of the opposite distal tibia show a slightly smaller lesion that appears to be resolving spontaneously.

however, the differential diagnosis includes simple bone cyst, fibrous dysplasia, histiocytosis X, chondromyxoid fibroma, and low-grade central osteosarcoma. The latter lesion is differentiated by a painful clinical presentation and its microscopic appearance.

Management and results

The rule is for these lesions to heal spontaneously and disappear with time. If incidentally found when small and asymptomatic, no treatment is necessary. If on two radiographic views the lesion involves more than 50 per cent of the bony diameter or is over 33 mm in longitudinal length, an increased risk of fracture has been reported and the area should be watched carefully. Either a reduction in physical activity or prophylactic surgery may be advocated to prevent fracture (Arata *et al.* 1981). If surgery is necessary, curettage and bone grafting with autograft or allograft is the treatment of choice. Some have recently used demineralized bone matrix mixed with the patent's bone marrow to decrease autograft site morbidity. Biopsy and definitive treatment can be accomplished in the same surgical setting. Segmental resection of fibular lesions can be performed, but the distal 25 per cent of the bone should be avoided if possible to prevent ankle instability. Recurrence after surgical treatment is rare.

It is recommended that pathologic fractures be allowed to heal with closed treatment prior to surgery. If the lesion persists after fracture consolidation, curettage and grafting may be pursued if necessary. Some surgeons have treated nondisplaced pathologic fractures by immediate curettage and grafting of the lesion to decrease the period of immobilization. If a fracture is unstable and cannot be reduced in a closed fashion, curettage and grafting can be done along with internal fixation. One report described three cases of a cortical avulsion fracture though a small fibrous cortical defect. Surgery is not necessary in this situation.

Further reading

Bejarano, P. and Kyriakos, M. (1995). Nonossifying fibroma of long bones. An immunohistochemical study. *Applied Immunohistochemistry*, **3**, 257–64.

Campanacci, M., Laus, M., and Boriani, S. (1983). Multiple non-ossifying fibromata with extraskeletal anomalies: a new syndrome? *Journal of Bone and Joint Surgery, British Volume*, **65B**, 627–32.

Choong, P., Pritchard, D., Rock, M., Sim, F., McLeod, R., and Unni, K. (1996). Low grade central osteogenic sarcoma. A long-term followup of 20 patients. *Clinical Orthopaedics and Related Research*, **322**, 198–206.

Fechner, R. and Mills, S. (1993). *Atlas of tumor pathology. Tumors of the bones and joints* (3rd series). AFIP, Washington, DC.

Friedland, J., Reinus, W., Fisher, A., and Wilson, A. (1995). Quantitative analysis of the plain radiographic appearance of nonossifying fibroma. *Investigative Radiology*, **30**, 474–9.

Greyson, N. and Pang, S. (1981). The variable bone scan appearances of non-osteogenic fibroma of bone. *Clinical Nuclear Medicine*, **6**, 242–5.

Kotzot, D., Stob, H., Wagner, H., and Ulmer, R. (1994). Jaffe–Campanacci syndrome: case report and review of literature. *Clinical Dysmorphology*, **3**, 328–34.

Kumar, R., Swischuk, L., and Madewell, J. (1986). Benign cortical defect: site for an avulsion fracture. *Skeletal Radiology*, **15**, 553–5.

Schajowicz, F. (1994). *Tumors and tumor-like lesions of bone* (2nd edn). Springer-Verlag, Berlin.

Steiner, G. (1974). Fibrous cortical defect and nonossifying fibroma of bone. A study of the ultrastructure. *Archives of Pathology*, **97**, 205–10.

Young, J., Levine, A., and Dorfman, H. (1984). Case report 293. Diagnosis: nonossifying fibroma (NOF) of the upper tibial diametaphysis with a considerable increase in size over a 3-year period. *Skeletal Radiology*, **12**, 294–7.

References

Arata, M., Peterson, H., and Dahlin, D. (1981). Pathological fractures through non-ossifying fibromas. Review of the Mayo Clinic experience. *Journal of Bone and Joint Surgery, American Volume*, **63A**, 980–8.

Moser, R., Sweet, D., Haseman, D., and Madewell, J. (1987). Multiple skeletal fibroxanthomas: radiologic–pathologic correlation of 72 cases. *Skeletal Radiology*, **16**, 353–9.

Ritschl, P., Karnel, F., and Hajek, P. (1988). Fibrous metaphyseal defects—determination of their origin and natural history using a radiomorphological study. *Skeletal Radiology*, **17**, 8–15.

1.6.4.4 Bone island

Kristy Weber

Introduction

A bone island, also called a solitary enostosis, is a benign small nodule of lamellar bone located within the cancellous portion of the skeleton. It is an incidental finding and can be found within almost any bone except the cranial vault. It is primarily present, and often begins, in adulthood. Some have proposed an arrested resorption of mature bone during endochondral ossification as an etiology, whereas more recent reports agree with a proliferative process as the cause of bone islands (Hall *et al.* 1980; Brien *et al.* 1995).

Box 1

- Benign small nodules of lamellar bone located within the cancellous portion of the skeleton
- Usually 2–20 mm in diameter, but lesions over 10 cm in diameter have been reported
- Consist of mature lamellar bone with well-formed Haversian systems
- Differential diagnosis includes sclerosing osteosarcoma
- Asymptomatic stable lesions less than 2 cm do not require treatment
- Lesions that are enlarging or are symptomatic should be evaluated for possible biopsy

Pathology

These lesions are not often seen by the pathologist as they rarely need to be biopsied or excised. The gross appearance of a bone island is a round area of sharply demarcated dense bone that blends with the surrounding cancellous bone at its periphery. The edge of the lesion has a spoke-like pattern where the native and lesional bone merge. Bone islands are usually 2 to 20 mm in size but giant forms up to 10.5 cm have been reported (Brien *et al.* 1995). In order to be called a 'giant' bone island, the lesion must be at least 2 cm in size.

Microscopically the bone island consists of mature lamellar bone

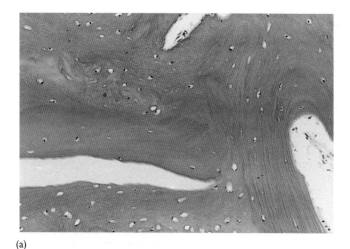

(a)

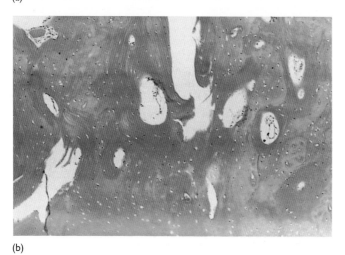

(b)

Fig. 1. (a) Typical histologic picture of a bone island with thickened lamellar bone. No sign of increased metabolic activity is seen. (b) This reveals the overall architecture of a bone island demonstrating the well-formed Haversian systems.

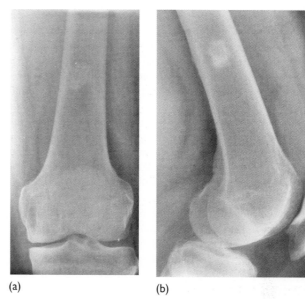

(a)   (b)

Fig. 2. (a) This anteroposterior view of the distal femur in a 50-year-old male shows a typical bone island in the medullary canal. It was completely asymptomatic and discovered incidentally. (b) Lateral view. Note the radiating spicules of lesional bone blending into the surrounding native trabeculae.

bone islands with follow-up as long as 23 years showing 32 per cent of lesions slowly enlarging over time. Growth occurred after the epiphyseal plates had closed. A lesion thought to be a bone island radiographically but causing pain should raise suspicion of a more aggressive disease.

Osteopoikilosis is a rare sclerosing bone dysplasia consisting of multiple small periarticular bone islands throughout the skeleton. They are identical in every way with solitary bone islands. Both autosomal dominant and sporadic forms of the syndrome have been identified.

with well-formed Haversian systems (Fig. 1). Where this cortical bone meets the surrounding medullary bone, there is no sclerosis. No evidence of endochondral ossification or cartilage is apparent. Occasionally woven bone is a minor part of the lesion. In some bone islands that show increased tracer uptake on bone scan, there is increased osteoblastic activity and blood flow indicating a higher degree of remodeling. The giant forms are histologically identical to the smaller examples. Bone islands are significant in terms of the differential diagnosis which includes sclerosing well-differentiated osteosarcoma. This malignant tumor should be recognized microscopically by its fibroblastic stroma and compact osteoid that permeates and replaces the normal marrow space.

Clinical presentation

Bone islands are asymptomatic and found incidentally in adults (Figs 2 and 3). There have been reports of growing lesions as well as islands that disappear with time. Onitsuka (1977) reported on 189

Imaging

A bone island can usually be diagnosed on its characteristic plain radiographic features, preventing further invasive diagnostic studies. It is typically a small round or oval area of homogeneous increased density within the cancellous bone. Radiating spicules on the periphery of the bone island merge with the native bone creating a brush-like border. No bony destruction or periosteal reaction is noted.

There have been several reviews documenting the appearance of bone islands with technetium bone scanning. A scan is usually 'cold' as this is an inert lesion, but it can have increased uptake in larger bone islands. Therefore an abnormal scan does not exclude the diagnosis. Sickles *et al.* (1976) felt that tracer uptake was proportional to the size of the lesion, though Hall *et al.* (1980) reported two histologically proven large bone islands with normal scintographic uptake. One study showed a direct relationship between increased tracer uptake and the degree of histological activity in six lesions (Greenspan *et al.* 1991). Given the inconsistent findings, bone scans may not be the best study to confirm the diagnosis of bone island.

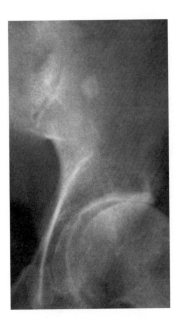

(a)

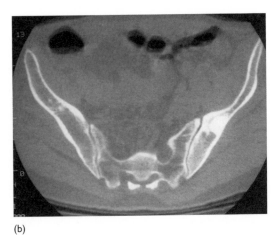

(b)

Fig. 3. (a) A bone island in the ilium of a 54-year-old male. The lesion was asymptomatic and noted incidentally on radiographs taken for mild left hip pain. Note the degenerative changes in the hip which is the most likely cause of the patient's pain. (b) This CT scan through the pelvis demonstrates the iliac lesion to be intramedullary and well circumscribed. No surrounding reaction or cortical destruction is seen.

Plain films and, if needed, CT scans can demonstrate the classic morphologic features of this benign entity.

The main importance of recognizing bone islands is to differentiate them from more aggressive lesions. The radiologic differential includes osteoid osteoma, bone infarct, sclerosing osteosarcoma, blastic metastases, and sclerotic myeloma. The lack of clinical symptoms or radiographic evidence of growth makes these options less likely; however, large islands are indistinguishable from the well-differentiated osteosarcoma and therefore prompt a biopsy.

Management and results

Mirra (1989) initially suggested repeating radiographs at 1, 3, 6, and 12 months to determine if the lesion is growing. He felt that an increase in size of 25 per cent in 6 months or 50 per cent in 1 year should lead to a surgical biopsy. A more recent report from this group added that lesions 2 to 4 cm in size with increased radionuclide uptake thought to be bone islands should be followed serially for at least 10 years. If they undergo a 50 per cent increase in size and have greater tracer uptake at any time during the decade, they should be biopsied. Lesions over 4 cm with increased bone scan activity when initially discovered should undergo biopsy unless the physician is certain of the diagnosis based on clinical and radiographic features (Brien *et al.* 1995). If the lesion is less than 2 cm, asymptomatic, and inert, no treatment is indicated.

Further reading

Blank, N. and Lieber, A. (1965). The significance of growing bone islands. *Radiology*, **85**, 508–11.

Greenspan, A. and Klein, M. (1996). Giant bone island. *Skeletal Radiology*, **25**, 67–9.

Mungovan, J., Tung, G., Lambiase, R., Noto, R., and Davis, R. (1994). Tc-99m MDP uptake in osteopoikilosis. *Clinical Nuclear Medicine*, **19**, 6–8.

Smith, J. (1973). Giant bone islands. *Radiology*, **107**, 35–6.

References

Brien, E., Mirra, J., Latanza, L., Fedenko., and Luck, J. (1995). Giant bone island of femur. *Skeletal Radiology*, **24**, 546–50.

Greenspan, A., Steiner, G., and Knutzon, R. (1991). Bone island (enostosis): clinical significance and radiologic and pathologic correlations. *Skeletal Radiology*, **20**, 85–90.

Hall, F., Goldberg, R., Davies, J., and Fansinger, M. (1980). Scintigraphic assessment of bone islands. *Radiology*, **135**, 737–42.

Mirra, J. (1989). *Bone tumors*, pp. 182–90. Lea & Febiger, Philadelphia, PA.

Onitsuka, H. (1977). Roentgenologic aspects of bone islands. *Radiology*, **123**, 607–12.

Sickles, E., Genant, H., and Hoffer, P. (1976). Increased localization of 99m-Tc-pyrophosphate in a bone island: case report. *Journal of Nuclear Medicine*, **17**, 113–15.

1.6.4.5 Fibrous dysplasia

Kristy Weber

Introduction

Fibrous dysplasia is thought by many to be a developmental abnormality rather than a true neoplasm. It is a slow-growing lesion of metaplastic bone and fibrous tissue that replaces normal bone marrow (Kransdorf *et al.* 1990; Hudson *et al.* 1993). It is known as a great imitator as its radiographic appearance can mimic many other lesions. It occurs in both monostotic (82 per cent) and polyostotic

Box 1

- Developmental abnormality that consists of a slow-growing mass of metaplastic bone and fibrous tissue that replaces normal bone marrow

- Occurs in both monostotic and polyostotic forms

- Most commonly occurs in the ribs, craniofacial bones, proximal femur, tibia, and humerus

- Consists of dense fibrous tissue with a firm gritty quality due to intermixed osteoid

- Often asymptomatic, but may cause skeletal deformity and pathologic fractures

- Active during skeletal growth but usually becomes inactive after skeletal maturity

- Surgical intervention is indicated for persistently painful lesions, lesions causing severe or progressive deformity, lesions causing or increasing the risk of pathologic fractures, and nonunion of pathologic fractures

- Treatment is internal fixation with or without bone grafting of the lesion

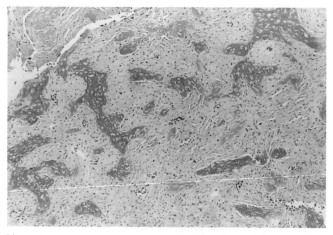

(a)

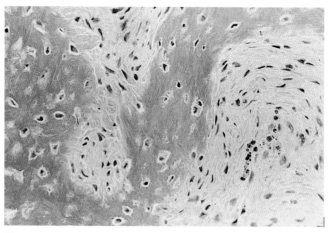

(b)

Fig. 1. (a) Low-power view of fibrous dysplasia demonstrates the irregular truncated segments of metaplastic woven bone. No cartilage is seen in this lesion though it can be present. (b) The higher-power view reveals the benign appearing stromal cells. There is an absence of osteoblasts rimming the woven bone.

(18 per cent) forms. Females are affected slightly more than males. The solitary lesions are found in adolescents, with 75 per cent occurring before the age of 30. The ribs and craniofacial bones are the most commonly affected in the axial skeleton, with the proximal femur, tibia, and humerus most likely in the appendicular skeleton. The polyostotic form usually presents by the age of 10 with clinical signs and symptoms; 75 to 90 per cent of lesions are in the femur, tibia, and pelvis. Craniofacial involvement occurs in nearly all patients with multiple lesions, with other common locations including the metatarsals, fibula, ribs, skull, metacarpals, humerus, radius, ulna, and phalanges.

Pathology

The pathologic appearance of fibrous dysplasia can be quite varied, and so a high level of suspicion must be maintained. Grossly it presents as dense fibrous tissue with a firm gritty quality due to the intermixed osteoid. Sharply defined benign cartilage nodules or large cysts filled with clear yellow fluid may be seen. The surrounding cortex may be expanded but is rarely disrupted.

The classic histologic appearance is of metaplastic trabecular bone arranged in a 'Chinese alphabet' pattern arising directly from benign fibrous stroma (Fig. 1). The amount of bone present is highly variable. The trabeculae are thin and arranged in a haphazard unconnected manner. The osteoid in fibrous dysplasia is woven rather than lamellar. There is only minimal osteoblastic rimming of the bone, which differentiates the lesion from osteofibrous dysplasia. However, reactive bone occurring after a pathologic fracture will have interspersed osteoblasts on the surface. Both osteoid and mature trabeculae can be calcified, and this is more commonly seen in the center of the lesion. The osteoid may be present as rounded bodies resembling cementum, especially in craniofacial locations. Occasional multi-

nucleated cells, which may function as osteoclasts, can be seen on the trabeculae.

The stroma is also highly varied and can be quite cellular with little collagen present, or the reverse may be true. Proliferating fibroblasts produce the collagenous matrix and are often arranged in a whorled or storiform pattern. The collagen is unevenly distributed rather than arranged in laminated collagen fibrils. Occasionally a myxomatous type stroma is seen. Regardless of the cellularity, the nuclei show no atypia or pleomorphism. Few mitotic figures may be present. Nodules of hyaline cartilage are present in 10 per cent of lesions and are thought to be the result of growth-plate disruption. Occasional binucleate chondrocytes are seen but there is no marked anaplasia. Such lesions are known as fibrocartilaginous dysplasia. They are similar to enchondromas and have a benign clinical course. In addition, cartilage is frequently visible after a pathologic fracture through the lesion. There can be areas of secondary aneurysmal bone cyst change with prominent lipophages and benign giant cells in the area. Fibrous dysplasia is only minimally vascular, but hemorrhage and hemosiderin are evident after a pathologic fracture.

It is normal to see fibrous dysplasia extend between the native bony trabeculae at the edge of the lesion, and this should not be mistaken for malignant change. The abnormal tissue can travel through the haversian systems and erode the cortex from within the medullary canal. Both monostotic and polyostotic lesions have the same microscopic appearance. Fibrous dysplasia exhibits a stable histologic pattern regardless of age.

The differential diagnosis includes osteofibrous dysplasia and well-differentiated intraosseous osteosarcoma.

Clinical presentation

A patient with a solitary lesion of fibrous dysplasia is usually asymptomatic with the abnormality noted incidentally on plain films (Fig. 2). It can also be discovered as the result of a pathologic fracture or bowing of an extremity. The patient with skull involvement may present with exophthalmos. Local swelling is often the only physical finding and laboratory studies are normal. Fibrous dysplasia is active during skeletal growth but usually becomes inactive after skeletal maturity. Twenty-five per cent of lesions do present in the adult, however, and some inactive lesions begin mild growth with the onset of pregnancy.

The polyostotic form is present in 20 per cent of patients, usually females. The lesions are usually unilateral with multiple areas of a single bone or multiple bones in one extremity affected. Pain with or without pathologic fracture, limb deformity, and a limp are some of the common presenting signs and symptoms. The most important

deformities are limb-length discrepancy, proximal femoral varus angulation, and tibial bowing. Progressive deformity is common with growth. Pathologic fractures occur in 85 per cent of patients, are rarely displaced, and heal well. Associated endocrine abnormalities include hyperthyroidism, acromegaly, hyperparathyroidism, Cushing's syndrome, and diabetes mellitus.

A rare condition known as oncogenic osteomalacia is described in patients with mesenchymal tumors. In a recent study of 17 cases, five involved fibrous dysplasia. Clinical symptoms of fatigue, joint pain, weakness, fractures, and lower extremity deformities are present from months to years prior to the discovery of the neoplasm. Laboratory findings include hypophosphatemia, normocalcemia, and increased levels of alkaline phosphatase. Radiographs show decreased bony density, coarse trabeculae and widened growth plates. In general the clinical and biochemical abnormalities resolve with removal of the tumor.

Albright described a rare syndrome of polyostotic fibrous dysplasia (Fig. 3), precocious puberty, and macular, pigmented skin lesions with irregular borders classically resembling the coast of Maine. The syndrome occurs more frequently in females and can present with vaginal bleeding in infancy. Premature closure of the epiphyseal plates causes resultant short stature. The skin lesions typically occur on the same side of the body as the bone lesions. Mazabraud's syndrome is a separate association of polyostotic fibrous dysplasia with benign intramuscular myxomas seen rarely in children and adolescents.

Malignant transformation of fibrous dysplasia occurs in 0.5 per cent of lesions with an increased incidence of 4 per cent reported in Albright's syndrome. It is likely that these percentages are falsely elev-

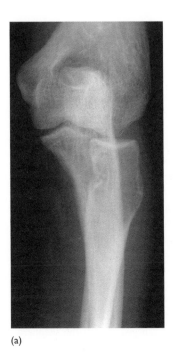
(a)

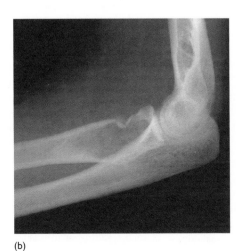
(b)

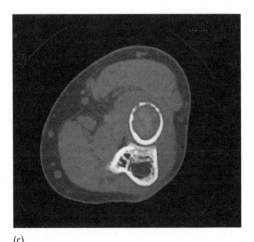
(c)

Fig. 2. (a) Anteroposterior and (b) lateral views of the elbow in a 29-year-old female. Note the lesion in the proximal radius. It has a typical ground glass density. A nondisplaced pathologic fracture with surrounding periosteal reaction is noted best on the lateral view. (c) CT scan of the lesion shows uniform medullary involvement and mild erosion of the surrounding cortex of the radius.

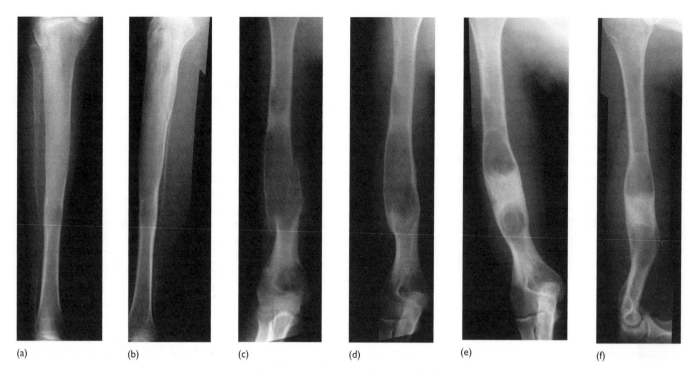

(a) (b) (c) (d) (e) (f)

Fig. 3. (a) Anteroposterior and (b) lateral radiographs of the tibia/fibula in a 20-year-old female with Albright's syndrome. Note the extensive involvement of the tibial medullary canal with mild cortical expansion. Again, the classic ground glass appearance is seen. (c) Radiograph revealing involvement of the humerus with multiple lesions. A mildly displaced pathologic fracture is evident. (d) Three months later the humeral fracture has healed with conservative management. (e), (f) Eight years later, gradual filling in of the lesions is noted. The mild angulatory deformity has no negative effect on the patient's function.

ated as many patients with fibrous dysplasia have lesions that are never discovered. It is also possible that some of the malignancies were initially misdiagnosed well-differentiated osteosarcomas. Sarcomas can develop with and without prior irradiation treatment (Ruggieri *et al.* 1994). The change is heralded by increasing pain with radiographic evidence of progressive bony erosion or development of a soft-tissue mass. High-grade malignancies, usually osteosarcomas but including chondrosarcomas, fibrosarcomas, and malignant fibrous histiocytomas, can be found 2 to 30 years after the initial diagnosis of fibrous dysplasia. They are slightly more common in patients with solitary lesions than in those with polyostotic involvement. Common locations include the jaw, femur, tibia, and pelvis. The overall survival of the patients with transformed lesions is poor.

Imaging

Fibrous dysplasia can have a multitude of radiographic appearances but the classical pattern is a diaphyseal sharply marginated lesion with a ground glass density and no sclerotic rim. The unusual homogeneous density results from dysplastic bone and fibrous stroma replacing the native cancellous bone. The appearance is actually that of the surrounding cancellous bone but without the trabecular markings. The spectrum of radiodensity is a reflection of the amount of woven bone in the tissue and the extent to which it is mineralized.

It is usually central in the intramedullary canal and symmetrically expands the surrounding cortex, seen best in rib lesions. Fibrous dysplasia is a slow-growing lesion and can involve the entire long bone from one growth plate to the other extending through the epiphysis only after growth plate closure. The periphery of the lesion blends with the thinned cortex without a reactive interface.

Variants of the classic appearance include a cystic form with a sclerotic rim surrounding a central lucent area. One type resembles pagetoid bone with a dense trabecular pattern. Another type has intralesional calcifications indicating the presence of cartilage. This type is often present in the proximal femur and diagnosed histologically as fibrocartilaginous dysplasia. Some authors believe that the classic appearance occurs in active lesions, whereas the cystic or pagetoid patterns occur in inactive lesions. The polyostotic form has the same variability in appearance as the solitary lesions. Radiographic progression has been documented in both skeletally immature and mature patients.

The structural bone strength in fibrous dysplasia is decreased, leading to common angulatory deformities. Multiple sequential fractures, each resulting in further deformity, can give rise to the shepherd's crook varus appearance of the proximal femur.

Fibrous dysplasia causes marked tracer uptake on bone scans especially in actively growing children. The intensity decreases as the lesion becomes inactive. A CT scan is used to delineate the extent of bony involvement. The appearance varies in proportion to the extent of mineralization within the lesion. Further imaging studies are rarely necessary and there is no consistent appearance noted on MRI.

The differential radiographic diagnosis includes nonossifying fibroma, enchondroma, simple and aneurysmal bone cysts, chondromyxoid fibroma, and histiocytosis X. Histologically fibrous dysplasia can be difficult to discern from a well-differentiated central osteosarcoma, therefore radiographic study may help provide the accurate diagnosis. On plain radiographs of this particular osteosarcoma there is usually a small region that is poorly marginated, exhibits periosteal reaction, or has a break in the cortex.

Management and results

Untreated lesions of fibrous dysplasia may stabilize, enlarge, or less commonly regress. The overall prognosis depends on the extent of bony involvement. Many solitary lesions do not need treatment, especially those in non-weight-bearing areas.

Surgical intervention is indicated for persistently painful lesions, lesions causing severe or progressive deformity, lesions causing pathologic femoral shaft fractures in the adult, and nonunion of pathologic fractures (Harris et al. 1962). In addition, large areas of fibrous dysplasia in high-stress weight-bearing areas prone to fracture are often treated with prophylactic internal fixation. Curettage has an extremely high local recurrence rate as the extent of disease is often not appreciated at the time of surgery. Fibrous dysplasia is best treated by biopsy followed by intramedullary fixation with or without cortical grafting to stabilize long bones. If there is a severe bony deformity, osteotomy and internal fixation may be necessary. The goal should be to strengthen and straighten the bone, not to resect the lesion. The internal fixation does not change the disease process but does provide mechanical support to the weakened bone. A patient's pain can be greatly relieved by prophylactic fixation.

Enneking and Gearen (1986) advocated an autogenous cortical fibular graft for symptomatic fibrous dysplasia with or without fracture of the femoral neck. All 15 patients in their series achieved healing with a good result regardless of age. None were treated with curettage. As none of the 12 fractures of the femoral neck were displaced and the proximal femur was relatively undeformed, no osteotomy or internal fixation was needed (Enneking and Gearen 1986). Others use allograft bone to provide a more permanent structural support as it is less likely to be resorbed. Another study recommended osteotomy and internal fixation for patients with a severe varus deformity or displaced fracture of the femoral neck.

Stephenson et al. (1987) studied various treatment methods for 65 lesions in 43 patients and found that, regardless of how they were managed, patients over the age of 18 usually had satisfactory results. Patients under the age of 18 had improved outcomes with internal fixation when compared with curettage or closed treatment (Stephenson et al. 1987). Children with large lesions or patients with severe polyostotic disease often have progressive deformity and may require multiple surgical interventions. Care must be taken when recommending an intramedullary nail for a femoral lesion in a skeletally immature patient as there have been occasional reports of avascular necrosis of the femoral head after using this technique.

Pathologic fractures or symptomatic lesions in the upper extremity and spine can often be treated in a closed fashion, whereas lower extremity fractures usually require internal fixation. Radiation ther-

apy should never be used in these lesions as it may increase the risk of malignant transformation.

Further reading

Choong, P., Pritchard, D., Rock, M., Sim, F., McLeod, R., and Unni, K. (1996). Low grade central osteogenic sarcoma: a long term follow-up of 20 patients. *Clinical Orthopaedics and Related Research*, **322**, 198–206.

Fechner, R. and Mills, S. (1993). *Atlas of tumor pathology. Tumors of the bones and joints* (3rd series). AFIP, Washington, DC.

Ishida, T. and Dorfman, H. (1993). Massive chondroid differentiation in fibrous dysplasia of bone (fibrocartilaginous dysplasia). *American Journal of Surgical Pathology*, **17**, 924–30.

McCarthy, E. (1996). *Differential diagnosis in pathology: bone and joint disorders*. Igaku-Shoin, New York.

Machida, K., Makita, K., Nishikawa, J., Ohtake, T., and Masahiro, I. (1986). Scintigraphic manifestation of fibrous dysplasia. *Clinics in Nuclear Medicine*, **6**, 426–9.

Norris, M., Kaplan, P., Pathria, M., and Greenway, G. (1990). Fibrous dysplasia: magnetic resonance imaging appearance at 1.5 tesla. *Clinical Imaging*, **14**, 211–15.

Park, Y., Unni, K., Beabout, J., and Hodgson, S. (1994). Oncogenic osteomalacia: a clinicopathologic study of 17 bone lesions. *Journal of Korean Medical Science*, **9**, 289–98.

Prayson, M. and Leeson, M. (1993). Soft-tissue myxomas and fibrous dysplasia of bone: a case report and review of the literature. *Clinical Orthopaedics and Related Research*, **291**, 222–8.

Schajowicz, F. (1994). *Tumors and tumor-like lesions of bone* (2nd edn). Springer-Verlag, Berlin.

Taconis, W. (1988). Osteosarcoma in fibrous dysplasia. *Skeletal Radiology*, **17**, 163–70.

Tsuchiya, H., Tomita, K., Matsumoto, T., and Watanabe, S. (1995). Shepherd's crook deformity with an intracapsular femoral neck fracture in fibrous dysplasia. *Clinical Orthopaedics and Related Research*, **310**, 160–4.

Uchida, A., Araki, N., Shinto, Y., Yoshikawa, H., Kurisaki, E., and Ono, K. (1990). The use of calcium hydroxyapatite ceramic in bone tumor surgery. *Journal of Bone and Joint Surgery, British Volume*, **72B**, 298–302.

Yabut, S., Kenan, S., Sissons, H., and Lewis, M. (1988). Malignant transformation of fibrous dysplasia: a case report and review of the literature. *Clinical Orthopaedics and Related Research*, **228**, 281–9.

References

Enneking, W. and Gearen, P. (1986). Fibrous dysplasia of the femoral neck: treatment by cortical bone-grafting. *Journal of Bone and Joint Surgery, American Volume*, **68A**, 1415–22.

Harris, W., Dudley, R., and Barry, R. (1962). The natural history of fibrous dysplasia. *Journal of Bone and Joint Surgery, American Volume*, **44A**, 207–33.

Hudson, T., Stiles, R., and Monson, D. (1993). Fibrous lesions of bone. *Radiologic Clinics of North America*, **31**, 279–97.

Kransdorf, M., Moser, R., and Gilkey, F. (1990). From the archives of the AFIP: fibrous dysplasia. *Radiographics*, **10**, 519–37.

Ruggieri, P., Sim, F., Bond, J., and Unni, K. (1994). Malignancies in fibrous dysplasia. *Cancer*, **73**, 1411–24.

Stephenson, R., London, M., Hankin, F., and Kaufer, H. (1987). Fibrous dysplasia: an analysis of options for treatment. *Journal of Bone and Joint Surgery, American Volume*, **69A**, 400–9.

1.6.5 Lesions that resemble soft-tissue neoplasms

1.6.5.1 Ganglion cyst

Diva R. Salamao and Antonio G. Nascimento

A ganglion cyst is a benign cystic or myxoid mass (Fig. 1) with an average diameter of 1 to 2.5 cm. It occurs around the joints without communicating with the joint cavity. Less commonly, it occurs attached to tendon sheaths.

The most common locations are the dorsal carpal area of the hands and the volar surface of the wrist (Angelides and Wallace 1976). It also occurs on the volar surface of the fingers, the dorsum of the foot, around the ankle and knee, and in the various articular and ligamentous areas of the spine.

Only half of the cases are associated with tenderness, pain, or partial disability of the joint. Occasionally, a history of injury preceding the formation of a ganglion cyst is present. Persons who overuse the wrist and fingers (pianists, typists) are prone to this condition.

Ganglion cysts develop by myxoid degeneration and cystic softening of the connective tissue of the joint capsule or tendon

Box 1

- Not neoplasms—develop by myxoid degeneration of fibrous tissues
- Consist of a thick fibrous capsule without a synovial lining containing soft myxoid tissue
- May be associated with injury or overuse
- Most common locations include the wrist, volar surfaces of the fingers, and dorsum of the foot
- May be observed or treated by excision

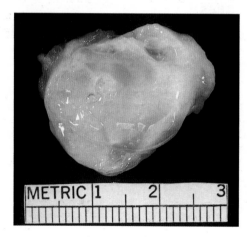

Fig. 1. Gross picture of a ganglion cyst, showing the myxoid characteristic of its cut surface.

sheath. They are characterized by an irregular thick-walled cystic space and are not lined by synovia, an important feature that differentiates them from Baker's cyst. The surrounding connective tissue can show myxoid changes.

A lesion microscopically similar to soft-tissue ganglion may occur in the subperiosteal region, the intraosseous compartment (Bauer and Dorfman 1982), the nerve sheath (intraneural), and the menisci of the knee (cystic meniscus) (Glasgow *et al.* 1993).

References

Angelides, A.C. and Wallace, P.F. (1976). The dorsal ganglion of the wrist: its pathogenesis, gross and microscopic anatomy, and surgical treatment. *Journal of Hand Surgery*, **1**, 228–35.

Bauer, T.W. and Dorfman, H.D. (1982). Intraosseous ganglion: a clinicopathologic study of 11 cases. *American Journal of Surgical Pathology*, **6**, 207–13.

Glasgow, M.M., Allen, P.W., and Blakeway, C. (1993). Arthroscopic treatment of cysts of the lateral meniscus. *Journal of Bone and Joint Surgery, British Volume*, **75B**, 299–302.

1.6.5.2 Intramuscular myxoma

Joseph A. Buckwalter, Eric A. Brandser, and Robert A. Robinson

Intramuscular myxoma, a rare benign neoplasm of the musculoskeletal soft tissues, typically occurs within the skeletal muscle of individuals more than 40 years of age. It is more common in females (Hashimoto *et al.* 1986). These lesions follow a benign course, but occasionally reach large size. In some patients they resemble soft-tissue sarcomas.

Intramuscular myxomas typically present as firm painless masses with a history of slow growth. They are freely moveable and rarely tender to firm palpation. Extremely large intramuscular myxomas may compress veins and lymphatics causing edema distal to the lesion, and large lesions can cause neurologic symptoms as a result of pressure on peripheral nerves. Myxomas develop most frequently within the buttock, thigh, leg, shoulder, and arm muscles

Box 1

- Rare benign neoplasm of the musculoskeletal soft tissues
- Typically occurs within skeletal muscle in individuals more than 40 years of age
- Consists of sparse bland appearing cells within an abundant avascular myxomatous matrix
- MRI clearly demonstrates the lesions and usually strongly suggests the diagnosis
- Generally treated by marginal excision

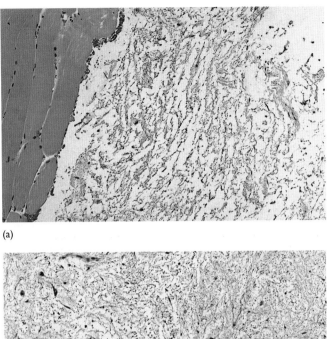

(a)

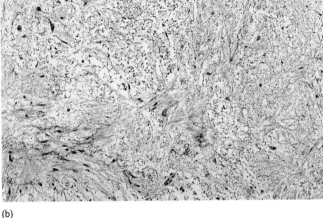

(b)

Fig. 1. Light micrographs of an intramuscular myxoma. (a) A low-magnification micrograph shows the hypocellular myxoma directly adjacent to skeletal muscle. The myxoma does not have a fibrous capsule or blood vessels. (b) A higher-magnification micrograph shows the loose reticular structure of the myxoma.

(Hashimoto *et al*. 1986). Some lesions are surrounded by skeletal muscle while others are attached to muscle fascia on one side.

Intramuscular myxomas consist of mucinous or myxomatous tissue (Meittinen *et al*. 1985; Hashimoto *et al*. 1986). Grossly the lesions are soft grayish translucent masses. They may have a thin

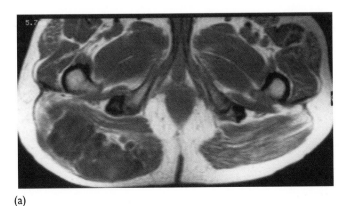

(a)

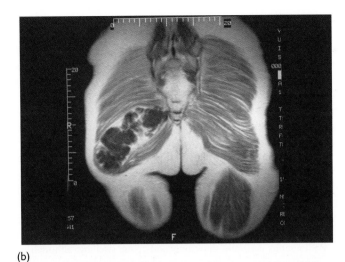

(b)

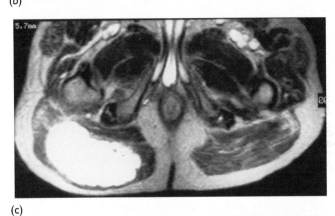

(c)

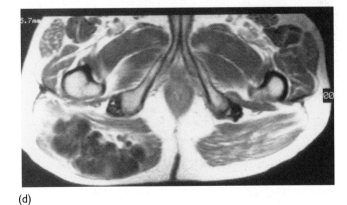

(d)

Fig. 2. MRI studies of an intramuscular myxoma of the gluteus maximus in a 61-year-old man. The patient presented with a history of a slowly enlarging painless mass in his right buttock. (a) Transverse T_1-weighted image (time of repetition, 600 ms, time of echo, 17 ms) of the pelvis shows a lobular low signal intensity mass within the gluteus maximus muscle. Notice that the mass is contained within the muscle fascia. (b) Coronal T_1-weighted image (time of repetition, 600 ms, time of echo, 17 ms) of the buttocks shows the extent of the lobular mass within the muscle. (c) Transverse T_2-weighted image (time of repetition, 2200 ms, time of echo, 80 ms) of the pelvis shows high signal intensity within the mass. This difference in signal intensity between T_1-weighted and T_2-weighted images is characteristic of myxomatous tissue. (d) Transverse T_1-weighted image (time of repetition, 600 ms, time of echo, 17 ms) following intravenous administration of gadolinium-based contrast material shows no enhancement of the central component of the mass. Minimal peripheral enhancement is seen at the interface with the surrounding skeletal muscle.

fibrous capsule or pseudocapsule, or lie directly against muscle or fascia. On cut section they often contain small fluid-filled cyst-like spaces. Light microscopy shows that they consist of sparse bland appearing cells surrounded by an abundant myxomatous matrix that has a loose fibrillar network in some areas (Fig. 1). Few, if any, blood vessels penetrate the substance of the myxomatous matrix. The cells have small nuclei and scanty neoplasm, and they do not have mitotic figures. Most of the cells resemble fibroblasts, but some of them have a striking stellate appearance (Fig. 1(b)).

Most intramuscular myxomas occur as solitary lesions, but an occasional patient has multiple lesions. Some patients with fibrous dysplasia develop multiple intramuscular myxomas, a condition referred to as Mazabraud's syndrome (Aoki *et al.* 1995; Szendroi *et al.* 1998). In most of these patients, the intramuscular myxomas appear decades after the diagnosis of fibrous dysplasia (Szendroi *et al.* 1998).

Radiographs generally show only soft-tissue swelling; although in some patients myxomas appear as areas of decreased soft-tissue density within muscle. MRI clearly demonstrates the lesions and usually strongly suggests the diagnosis (Fig. 2) (Abdelwahab *et al.* 1992; Swartz and Walker 1997). The myxomas appear as well-defined lobular masses surrounded by skeletal muscle or muscle fascia. They have low signal intensity on T_1-weighted images and high signal intensity on T_2-weighted images (Fig. 2). In many instances, the MRI study makes biopsy unnecessary, although some soft-tissue sarcomas, including myxoid malignant fibrous histiocytomas, soft-tissue chondrosarcomas, and myxoid liposarcomas, contain large volumes of sparsely cellular myxomatous tissue and can closely resemble intramuscular myxomas (Peterson *et al.* 1991).

Most surgeons treat intramuscular myxomas by marginal excision. This is relatively easily accomplished as the lesions do not have a well-developed blood supply, and they are easily separated from the surrounding muscle and fascia. Recurrences after marginal excision are rare (Meittinen *et al.* 1985; Hashimoto *et al.* 1986; Abdelwahab *et al.* 1992) and there are no reports of metastases.

References

Abdelwahab, A.F., Kenan, S., Hermann, G., Lewis, M.M., and Klein, M.J. (1992). Intramuscular myxoma: magnetic resonance features. *British Journal of Radiology*, **65**, 485–90.

Aoki, T., Kouho, H., Hisaoka, M., Hashimoto, H., Nakata, H., and Sakai, A. (1995). Intramuscular myxoma with fibrous dysplasia: a report of two cases with a review of the literature. *Pathology International*, **45**, 165–71.

Hashimoto, H., Tsuneyoshi, M., Daimaru, Y., Enjoji, M., and Shinohara, N. (1986). Intramuscular myxoma. A clinicopathologic, immunohistochemical and electron microscopic study. *Cancer*, **58**, 740–7.

Meittinen, M., Hocherstedt, K., Reitamo, J., and Totterman, S. (1985). Intramuscular myxoma—a clinicopathologic study of twenty-three cases. *American Journal of Clinical Pathology*, **84**, 265–72.

Peterson, K.K., Renfrew, D.L., Federson, R.M., and Buckwalter, J.A. (1991). Magnetic resonance imaging of myxoid containing tumors. *Skeletal Radiology*, **20**, 245–50.

Swartz, H.S. and Walker, R. (1997). Recognizable magnetic resonance imaging characteristics of intramuscular myxoma. *Orthopedics*, **20**, 431–5.

Szendroi, M., Rahoty, P., Antal, I., and Kiss, J. (1998). Fibrous dysplasia associated with myxoma (Mazabraud's syndrome): a long-term follow-up of three cases. *Journal of Cancer Research and Clinical Oncology*, **124**, 401–6.

1.6.5.3 Myositis ossificans

Michael G. Rock

Introduction

Myositis ossificans is a benign localized reactive proliferative lesion occurring within soft tissues and usually associated with trauma. The process is usually confined to muscle although involvement of tendon and even the subcutaneous fat has been reported as being involved (Campanacci 1990; Unni 1995). Most cases are found in the quadriceps, gluteal, small muscles of the hand, and brachialis muscle of the upper extremity. These muscles are commonly subject to direct and indirect injury. Myositis ossificans can also be seen as a by-product of extensive burns, immobilization due to coma, and in traumatic paraplegics, but approximately one-third of radiographic and clinically evident myositis has no apparent antecedent traumatic event.

This condition is rare in children, where it needs to be distinguished from myositis ossificans progressiva, a rare inheritable condition and generally fatal. This distinction can often be made on unique clinical features including microdactyly, clinodactyly, short broad femoral necks, exostoses, and mandibular condyle flattening and broadening. Other conditions that may mimic myositis ossificans radiographically or clinically include hemangiomas containing phleboliths, benign or malignant tumors of bone including osteogenic sarcoma and mesenchymal chondrosarcoma, synovial sarcoma, or even a calcified lipoma.

There are three variations to this condition: the pedunculated variation has a stalk that connects to the underlying adjacent bone; the periosteal variation has a broad connection to the underlying periosteum which may have been injured in the process or become reactive

---

Box 1 Common sites for myositis ossificans

- Quadriceps
- Gluteals
- Small muscles of hands
- Brachialis

Box 2 Common causes of myositis ossificans in muscles

- Contusions
- Tearing
- Burns
- Associated with coma/paraplegia—paralysis has been associated with increased circulating cytokines that stimulate bone formation, so it may not be due to immobilization
- One-third are idiopathic

Box 3 Characteristic features of myositis ossificans progressiva

- Occurs in children
- Heritable
- Microdactyly
- Clinidactyly
- Short broad/normal neck
- Exostoses
- Mandibular condyles flat and broad

due to the inflammation of the surrounding evolving myositis; the third variant is that which is unattached to either of these structures and free with a broad-base attachment to muscle alone (Jackson 1975).

Clinical features

The patient may or may not have experienced and/or volunteered a history of a significant traumatic event. Symptoms usually appear

Box 4 Differential diagnosis of myositis ossificans

- Hemangiomas in inducing phleboliths
- Osteogenic sarcoma
- Mesenchymal chondrosarcoma
- Synovial sarcoma
- Calcified lipoma

3 days to 3 weeks from the onset of the injury (if it occurred) and include pain, swelling, and decreased motion of the contiguous joints. This acute phase which has been referred to as the pseudo-inflammatory phase of the process and is not generally associated with systemic symptoms except in the child who may show malaise and fever (Clapton *et al.* 1992). Within 2 to 3 weeks this phase evolves into the subacute or pseudotumoral phase which is characterized by a painless hard mass that may or may not be mobile depending upon its association with the underlying osseous structures. This process tends to mature in growth by 3 to 6 months and thereafter enters the chronic phase of gradual resolution.

Box 5 Phases of myositis ossificans

- 0–3 weeks: acute or pseudoinflammatory phase, pain, swelling, decreased mobility
- 3–6 weeks: subacute pseudotumor phase, painless hard mass which may or may not be mobile
- 3–6 months: resolution phase

Box 6 Distinguishing clinical features of myositis ossificans

- More rapid development than malignant conditions
- History of trauma
- Site—quadriceps is common

The greatest difficulty associated with myositis ossificans is distinguishing it from more aggressive conditions that necessitate not only a biopsy but also definitive treatment. These include soft-tissue abscesses, osteogenic sarcoma, synovial sarcoma, mesenchymal chondrosarcoma, and in the very young child, myositis ossificans progressiva (Campanacci 1990; Unni 1995). Malignant conditions of soft tissue or even infective processes rarely increase in size as rapidly as is seen with myositis ossificans. The evolution of this disease in its early phases is dramatic and accelerated beyond most pathologic conditions.

With a significant history of trauma and with a clinical picture evolving as mentioned above, appropriate treatment may be initiated. An index of suspicion of the possibility for myositis should accompany certain muscle contusions or strains especially the quadriceps.

With a definite history of direct trauma, the diagnosis is generally easy to make (Figs 1 and 2). However, patients presenting with a painful rapidly evolving mass without a history of trauma challenge the clinician to make the appropriate diagnosis (Fig. 3). In children, the evolution of myositis is fast with radiographic evidence of the process apparent within several weeks of the onset of discomfort. Therefore deferring radiographic evaluation of the anatomic part for 2 to 3 weeks may be appropriate in patients in whom the index of suspicion is high for myositis ossificans (Clapton *et al.* 1992). The degree of intensity of ossification is increased in children and young adults due to the hyperplasia of this entity being inversely proportional to the age of the subject. In the early stages of this condition the classic zonal phenomenon and peripheral calcification are generally not well developed. However, within 2 to 3 weeks the typical punctate calcification may be seen in association with a thin layer of bone differentiating the inflammatory process from the surrounding normal soft-tissue architecture. Additional imaging studies may confirm the diagnosis even prior to the classic plain radiographic features.

If it is felt to be clinically appropriate, closed needle aspiration biopsy or open biopsy may be performed. In the latter, the typical zonal phenomenon will confirm the diagnosis and in the former the presence of a benign looking matrix of mature fibroblasts and osteoclast giant cells will allow the diagnosis of myositis ossificans with some element of confidence (Fig. 4). Diagnostic confirmation of this condition is confirmed by the functional orientation of the fibroblasts to osteoblasts and the inevitable maturity of the process from the central less mature aspect of the tumor to its mature periphery. This is in direct distinction to the reverse zoning phenomenon of most malignant conditions including extraskeletal osteosarcomas in which the immature highly neoplastic component of the tumor is at its periphery.

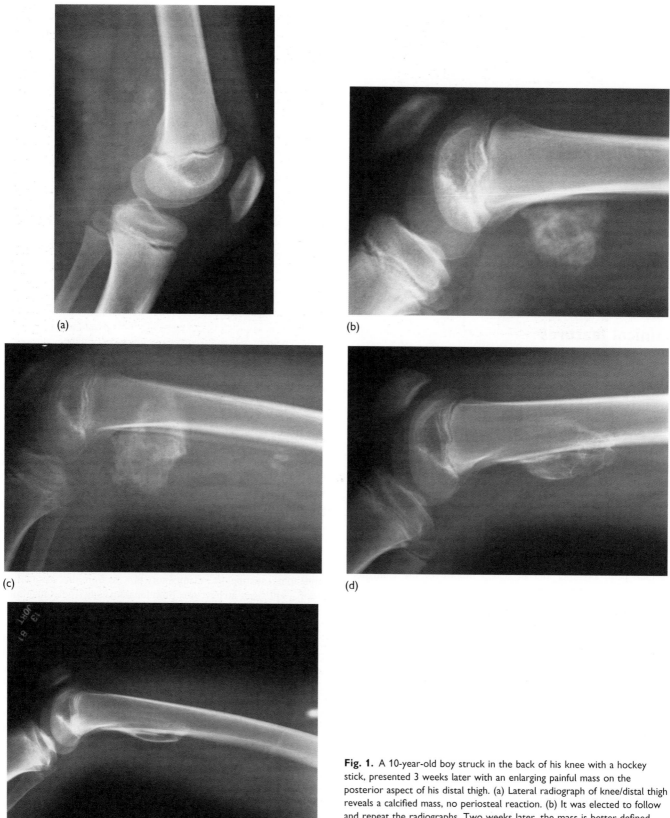

(a)

(b)

(c)

(d)

(e)

Fig. 1. A 10-year-old boy struck in the back of his knee with a hockey stick, presented 3 weeks later with an enlarging painful mass on the posterior aspect of his distal thigh. (a) Lateral radiograph of knee/distal thigh reveals a calcified mass, no periosteal reaction. (b) It was elected to follow and repeat the radiographs. Two weeks later, the mass is better defined, progressing to mineralization. Note the clear demarcation with underlying femoral cortex. (c) Ten years after the original injury further remodeling and resolution has occurred.

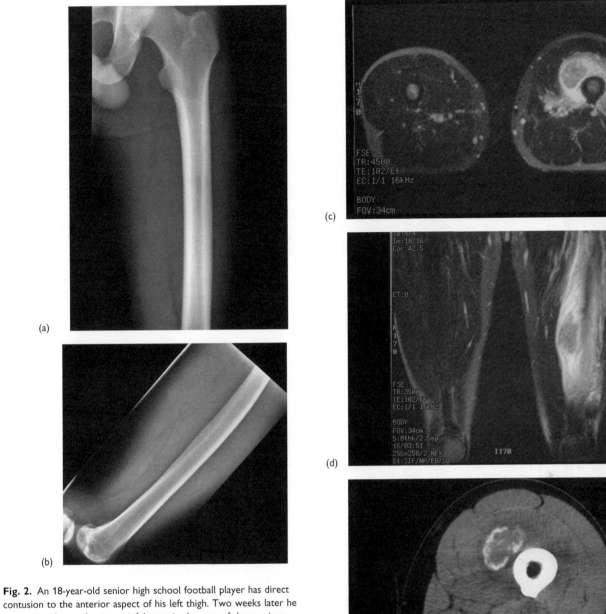

Fig. 2. An 18-year-old senior high school football player has direct contusion to the anterior aspect of his left thigh. Two weeks later he presents with an enlarging, painful mass in the area of the previous contusion. (a) Anteroposterior radiograph of the thigh reveals calcification in the distal medial thigh with loss of soft-tissue definition. (b) Lateral view of the same thigh confirms soft-tissue calcification and loss of fascial plane. (c), (d) T_2-weighted MRI axial and coronal views reveal extensive soft-tissue edema and an inhomogeneous mass in the central area of edema that appears to have a low signal periphery suggesting a zoning effect of myositis ossificans. (e) CT scan of the same extremity at the same time confirms the peripheral calcification of a myositis ossificans in evolution.

Radiographic features

In the early stages of this condition the radiographs may be entirely normal. This is despite the fact that on clinical examination there appears to be swelling, obvious discomfort, and possibly even some slight distortion to the extremity. The classic features of zonal calcification and mineralization will not become apparent for 2 to 3 weeks after the onset of symptoms and generally matures between 3 and 6 months. Thereafter gradual resolution of the process may occur, particularly if the involvement is isolated to the muscle belly and not the muscle, tendon, or even tendon regions of the muscle unit. As alluded to above, this process may be intimately associated with the underlying bone or periosteum with periosteal reaction occurring commonly with juxtacortical lesions. The periosteal reaction is that of benign lamination unlike the more aggressive appearance of surface osteosarcomas (Nuovo *et al.* 1992).

If characteristic zonal calcification is not present, other imaging modalities may need to be used to prove that it is myositis in evolu-

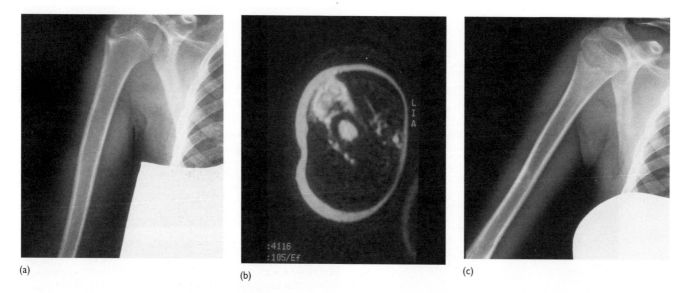

(a)   (b)   (c)

Fig. 3. A 12-year-old boy presented with a painful mass on the lateral aspect of his right dominant arm. No history of trauma was obtained. (a) Anteroposterior radiograph of the right arm suggests a mass effect lateral to the humerus with calcification. (b) MRI of the same arm at presentation confirms soft-tissue edema and a separate lesion with a low-density periphery in the center of this 'tumor'.

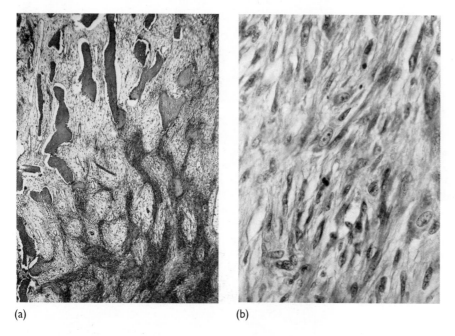

(a)   (b)

Fig. 4. Typical pathology of myositis ossificans. (a) Zonal maturation of proliferating fibroblasts into mature well-organized bone. (b) Myositis in evolution showing numerous fibroblasts, some with mitotic figures. Zonal metaplasia to osteoblasts and bone has not yet occurred. This should not be misinterpreted as a malignant soft-tissue tumor as the cells although numerous are not anaplastic. (Reproduced from Unni (1995).)

Box 7 **Distinguishing features of myositis ossificans on biopsy**

- Benign matrix of fibroblasts and osteoclast giant cells
- The most mature cells are at the periphery (contrast with malignant conditions)

tion and not something more sinister that requires immediate biopsy and treatment. The MRI has evolved as the definitive imaging modality for soft-tissue lesions (Table 1). In the acute or pseudoinflammatory phase of the condition on T_1-weighted images there appears to be a homogeneous intermediate signal, isodense with surrounding muscles. The inflammatory process often precipitates loss of fascial planes and may be associated with an increase in overall girth of the extremity relative to the opposite side. The presence of a low-signal peripheral rim consistent with bone is diagnostic for this condition. The T_2-weighted sequence will reveal a high signal enhancement

Table 1 MRI features of myositis ossificans

	T_1	T_2	Tadopentetate dineglumine enhancement
Early	Low signal rim	High signal and pronounced surrounding edema	Low signal rim is clearer
Pseudotumor	Low signal rim; central edema	High signal with patches of low signal (?mineralization); fluid levels of resolving hematoma	
Resolving phase	Central high signal from fat and bone; low signal rim		Edema resolved; no high signal

Box 8 Staged radiographic features of myositis ossificans

- Early stages: radiograph normal
- 3–6 weeks: zonal calcification and mineralization
- 3–6 months: mature benign lamination and resolution

with considerable edema in the surrounding soft tissues. The marrow of the contiguous bone should be assessed. If it shows edema and reaction the possibility of osteomyelitis as opposed to myositis would have to be seriously considered. In the acute inflammatory process of this condition the low signal peripheral rim may not be present with conventional T_1-weighted and T_2-weighted imaging on the MRI assessment but with the intravenous injection of tadopentetate dineglumine the rim is readily identified.

In the subacute or pseudotumoral stage of the condition, the T_1-weighted sequence confirms the low signal rim around the periphery with central areas of edema still present. The T_2-weighted sequence continues to show a high-signal abnormality which may have areas of low-signal intensity within the lesion suggestive of mineralization. Additionally there may be fluid levels confirming the presence of resolving hematoma. The late or chronic stage of the disease is characterized by a central area of fat with areas on T_1 that exhibit a high signal consistent with mature lamellar bone. The edema characterized in the acute phase of the process is resolved and the low signal rim is more refined, mature, and consistent with cortical bone. Additional imaging studies used to confirm this condition have included CT and ultrasonography. Bone scintigraphy is not a discriminating investigative tool but may be used to determine maturity of the process in the anticipation of its removal. CT shows the evolving mineralization and peripheral rim even more clearly, and the two imaging techniques may complement each other.

Box 9 Management of myositis ossificans

- Biopsy rarely needed
- Less than 10 per cent require removal of mature bone

Histologic features

With the history and symptoms compatible with myositis ossificans there is rarely a need to proceed with biopsy or even subsequent removal of the process. In less than 10 per cent of cases will it be necessary to remove the myositis process once chronic. When this occurs the lesion is well circumscribed within the muscle. The muscle around the peripheral rim of bone is compressed but not otherwise altered and certainly not infiltrated. It is not attached to the underlying bone and appears to have a hard shell of bone on its periphery which makes excisional biopsy of this process that much easier. When adherent to the bone, excavation of the external cortex may be evident but should not imply that the condition is more aggressive. If biopsy is performed in the acute phase, considerable edema of the surrounding normal soft-tissue architecture will be noted and as one removes a specimen for diagnosis there appears to be a grittiness to the periphery of the tumor consistent with the evolution of the cortical shell with more typical inflammatory tissue within its center. The peripheral bone maturation is clearly seen by low powered microscopic examination of the specimen. Unlike malignant conditions of soft parts in which the most malignant appearing histologic aspect of the tumor is in the periphery, in myositis the peripheral tissue is unequivocally benign. Additionally, the peripheral portion of the tumor is well marginated from the surrounding normal architecture which it is in the process of pushing out of the way and obviously not infiltrating (Unni 1995).

The zonal phenomenon becomes evident as the specimen is analyzed from the interior to the periphery. In the central portion of the lesion active proliferating fibroblasts with numerous mitotic figures, loosely arranged without organization and cytologic atypia, are commonly seen. Additionally, histiocytes, macrophages, plasma cells, and new vessels penetrating the area are evident consistent with the proliferative connective tissue repair of the process. If this were the only area biopsied, the misdiagnosis of a malignancy could be made. However, as one proceeds to the periphery of the lesion the fibroblasts become more mature and organized, with transformation into mature osteoid now becoming evident. Further to the periphery the osteoid undergoes mineralization in an organized fashion not unlike lamellar bone. There may be islands of chondroid tissue which if taken out of context could be misinterpreted as a low grade chondrosarcoma. Many of these cartilage cells will be large but they do not reveal any nuclear atypia and clearly evolves into mature osteoid.

Cystic spaces within the lesion consistent with hematomas lend an aneurysmal bone cyst-like quality to some regions of the mass (Campanacci 1990; Unni 1991).

Treatment

Without a definite history of trauma in the presence of what would appear to be an aggressive lesion of some concern in an extremity, an open or closed biopsy may be necessary to confirm the diagnosis of myositis ossificans. Once established either by biopsy in the equivocal cases as above or the classic evolving radiographic and clinical presentation, appropriate management in the acute phase includes the application of a compression dressing, ice, avoidance of additional injuries, maintenance of active range of motion, and support for the involved extremity. Recurrent injury should be avoided and therefore return to active sports should be deferred until the full range of motion of the contiguous joints has returned and the acute inflammatory process has resolved. The use of diphosphonates, indometacin, or even low-dose radiation therapy that have been applied in other conditions associated with heterotopic ossification has not found any efficacy in the classic post-traumatic myositis ossificans. The risks attended with the therapeutic options outweigh the current benefit.

If the clinical presentation, the radiographic appearance, and the evolution of this process suggests myositis ossificans apart from the treatment initiated in the acute phase of this condition, no other treatment is generally warranted or necessary. If this process is misdiagnosed clinically and/or histopathologically and the lesion is removed in the acute or subacute stage, prompt local recurrence will likely follow. As mentioned above, myositis ossificans is a self-limiting process that evolves over a period of 3 to 6 months after which gradual resolution of the process occurs. The lesion will rarely reach such a size and magnitude as to cause embarrassment and dysfunction of the contiguous muscles, joint, or neurovascular structures. Under these circumstances late removal of the ossified mass may be indicated after it has assumed maturity. This can be assessed by plain radiographs which will show mature bone deposition often with lamellar characteristics and may be confirmed by a relative decrease in the appearance on bone scintigraphy. Decreasing levels of alkaline phosphatase also imply maturity and the resolving nature of the condition and is another indicator used prior to surgical removal to minimize the possibility of local recurrence. Generally most clinicians will wait a minimum of 12, possibly 18, months from the onset of this condition before attempting removal as maturity usually occurs within this time frame.

Late sequelae of this condition include fractures through the mass. Symptoms abate quickly after the inflammation of the insult. The fractures generally go on to nonunion but are not troublesome and are not painful enough to warrant excision. Aneurysmal bone cyst degradation of this lesion more likely represents areas within the lesion that have undergone hematoma resorption and again do not mandate surgical excision. There have been few isolated reports of malignancy occurring within proximity to myositis ossificans (Pack and Braund 1942). This is an extremely rare event and should not in itself prompt the removal of the myositis anticipating this problem.

References

Campanacci, M. (1990). *Bone and soft tissue tumor*, pp. 821–30. Springer-Verlag, Vienna.

Clapton, W.K., James, C.L., Morris, L.L., Davey, R.B., Peacock, M.J., and Byard, R.W. (1992). Myositis ossificans in childhood. *Pathology*, **24**, 311–14.

Jackson, D.W. (1975). Managing myositis ossificans in the young athlete. *Physician and Sports Medicine*, **3**, 56–61.

Nuovo, M.A., Norman, A., Chumas, J., and Ackerman, L.V. (1992). Myositis ossificans with atypical clinical, radiographic, or pathological findings. A review of 23 cases. *Skeletal Radiology*, **21**, 87–101.

Pack, G.T. and Braund, R.R. (1942). The development of sarcoma in myositis ossificans: report of three cases. *Journal of the American Medical Association*, **119**, 776–9.

Unni, K.K. (1995). *Dahlin's bone tumors. General aspects and data of 11,087 cases*, pp. 395–9. Lippincott–Raven, Philadelphia, PA.

1.6.5.4 Nodular fasciitis

Diva R. Salomao and Antonio G. Nascimento

Nodular fasciitis is a benign soft-tissue lesion characterized by the proliferation of fibroblasts and myofibroblasts. Its rapid growth, high cellularity, and high mitotic activity are the factors responsible for clinical and histologic misdiagnosis. However, it follows a benign self-limiting clinical course.

The vast majority of patients complain of a rapidly growing nodule, with a duration of growth rarely exceeding 3 weeks. The lesion occurs in young adults of both sexes, commonly in the third and fourth decades of life. It is rare in patients older than 60 years and is uncommon in infants. The most frequent locations, in descending order of frequency, are the upper extremities, trunk, and head and neck region. Less frequently, it involves the lower extremities and locations such as the hands and feet.

Typically, it is a nonencapsulated but well-circumscribed nodule that rarely exceeds 3 cm in size. The nodule frequently is adherent

Box 1

- Benign proliferation of fibroblasts and myofibroblasts
- Pathogenesis remains unknown
- Typically present as rapidly growing nodules in young adults
- Frequently located in subcutaneous fat, but may occur in muscle or skin
- Follows a benign self-limiting course

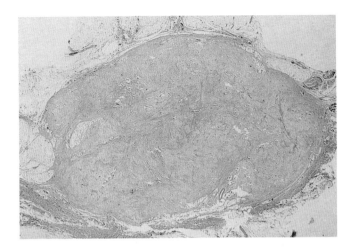

Fig. 1. Whole-mount picture of nodular fasciitis, showing the characteristic well-circumscribed nodule seated on thick fascial layer connective tissue.

to a thick layer of fibrous tissue representing the fascia (Fig. 1). The cut surface depends on the amount of myxoid or collagenous ground substance present in the lesion. The nodule frequently is located in the subcutaneous adipose tissue; however, intramuscular or exclusively dermal lesions also can occur (Lai and Lam 1993; Price *et al.* 1993).

Histologically, the lesion shows a proliferation of fibroblasts and myofibroblasts, having plump, pale-staining nuclei, somewhat prominent nucleoli, finely granular chromatin pattern, sharply delineated nuclear membrane, and elongated cytoplasm growing in short interlacing fascicles (Fig. 2). The background is typically rich in mucopolysaccharides, resulting in a loose myxoid appearance, occasionally showing microcysts. Less frequently, the stroma is more collagenous, imparting a more densely cellular appearance, a feature common in lesions from the head and neck region of children. A constant finding is the presence of a variable amount of inflammatory cells, mainly lymphocytes, dispersed among the spindled cellular elements. Multinucleated osteoclast-like giant cells are occasionally present. Typical mitotic figures are exceedingly frequent and can be numerous; how-

ever, cellular hyperchromasia and pleomorphism are not features of nodular fasciitis.

In immunohistochemical studies, the cells are positive for vimentin, smooth muscle actin, and muscle-specific actin and negative for desmin and S-100 protein.

References

Lai, F.M. and Lam, W.Y. (1993). Nodular fasciitis of the dermis. *Journal of Cutaneous Pathology*, **20**, 66–9.

Price, S.K., Kahn, L.B., and Saxe, N. (1993). Dermal and intravascular fasciitis. Unusual variants of nodular fasciitis. *American Journal of Dermatopathology*, **15**, 539–43.

1.6.6 Benign bone neoplasms
1.6.6.1 Osteoid osteoma

Kristy Weber

Introduction

Osteoid osteoma is a painful benign neoplasm of bone with an obscure etiology (Gitelis and Schajowicz 1989; Greenspan 1993; Frassica *et al.* 1996). It is a clearly demarcated lesion 1 cm or less in size with a predilection for the diaphysis of long bones. The metaphysis is less commonly involved. The femur and tibia are the most common locations, followed by the humerus, spine, talus, and hand. When the tumor presents in the spine, it is frequently found in the posterior elements of the lumbar region. Rarely, multicentric lesions have been reported occurring in the same or different bones. Osteoid osteomas make up around 10 per cent of all benign bone tumors. There is a male predominance with most lesions occurring in patients 5 to 24 years of age.

The exact origin of osteoid osteomas is unknown. The small lesions produce exquisite pain out of proportion for their size, and several explanations have been proposed. Nerve fibers associated with small blood vessels are present in the nidus of the lesion (Schulman and Dorfman 1970). An increase in prostaglandins has also been documented within the lesion, which may explain why aspirin classically relieves the pain (Wold *et al.* 1988). The vasodilation and enhanced blood flow induced by the prostaglandins may cause pres-

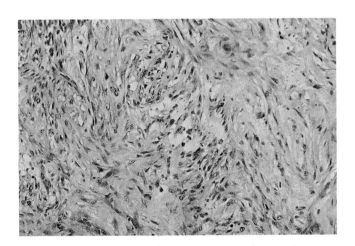

Fig. 2. Cellular spindle cell proliferation with loose myxoid background.

Box 1

- Benign bone-forming tumors usually less than 1 cm in diameter
- Most frequently develop in the femur and tibia, followed by the humerus, spine, talus, and hand bones
- Usually cause localized pain which is often relieved by aspirin or anti-inflammatory medications
- May stimulate formation of large amounts of reactive bone

sure on the local afferent nerves in the nidus and surrounding fibrous zone which causes pain. The prostaglandins have also been postulated to affect the free nerve endings in the lesion directly by lowering the threshold for nociceptive stimuli.

Pathology

The gross appearance of an osteoid osteoma is a nidus of cherry red trabecular bone surrounded by dense white bone. It has a soft or gritty consistency depending on the amount of calcification present and is usually less than 1 cm in size.

The microscopic appearance consists of uniform thin osteoid seams admixed with immature trabeculae rimmed by prominent osteoblasts. A 1- to 2-mm richly fibrovascular zone surrounds the sharply demarcated central nidus. There is an abrupt interface between the osteoid osteoma and the surrounding reactive bone. This encasing sclerotic rim can vary from thickened cancellous trabeculae to dense cortical bone with compact haversian systems. There is no permeation of the lesion into the native or reactive bone, and no atypical mitotic figures are noted. The cells are uniform in size and shape but have active appearing nuclei. Osteoclasts and occasional giant cells can be seen, but no cartilage is present unless a pathologic fracture or subarticular location is evident. No acute inflammation is noted.

Osteoid osteomas can have varied appearances microscopically as they are in a process of dynamic bone remodeling. Areas of active osteoblastic proliferation producing both osteoid and irregularly mineralized trabeculae alternate with areas of osteoclastic resorption. The center of the nidus may appear radiodense or radiolucent on imaging studies depending on whether immature mineralized bone or osteoid predominates, respectively.

A separate lesion called an osteoblastoma has an identical histo-

logic picture and is differentiated primarily on its larger size and ability to grow and destroy surrounding bone. There is no surrounding reactive bony change in an osteoblastoma.

Clinical evaluation

The most conspicuous clinical symptom is unrelenting pain related to the osteoid osteoma. It begins as a dull discomfort that is unrelated to activity, is worse at night and often progresses with time. The pain is relieved by aspirin in the majority of patients and less frequently with nonsteroidal anti-inflammatory medications. A minority present without pain, more common in children than adults, and often with a lesion in the phalanges. No erythema or warmth is noted in the area of the osteoid osteoma, but there may be tenderness or swelling especially if in a location close to the skin surface. Intra-articular tumors most frequently occur in the proximal femur, and cause a synovitis, joint effusion, or flexion contracture. In these cases the patient may be treated for presumed arthritis for a prolonged period of time before the diagnosis is recognized. Other findings may include a limp on the affected extremity, atrophy of the limb musculature, accelerated growth if the lesion is near the epiphysis in a child, or scoliosis when the lesion is located in a rib or the thoracolumbar spine.

Osteoid osteoma is a leading cause of painful scoliosis and should be considered in the young patient with back pain or radicular symptoms. In a mature patient with a spinal lesion scoliosis rarely occurs; however, neurologic compromise, paravertebral muscle spasms, and torticollis can develop. A high clinical suspicion should be present for this tumor in the young patient with back, groin, thigh, or knee pain as its location in the spine or proximal medial femur is difficult to detect with plain radiographs. Often the patient has severe pain for months before any visible radiographic changes. The clinical presentation can often be confused with spondylolysis. Osteoid osteoma is difficult to diagnose in children less than 5 years old as they may just be starting to walk and often cannot give a good history. Symptoms can be mistaken for neurologic disorders, juvenile rheumatoid arthritis, or Legg–Calvé–Perthes disease. Laboratory studies are normal.

Imaging studies

On plain radiographs, an osteoid osteoma can be classified as cortical, subperiosteal, or medullary in location. It is generally a round or oval well-circumscribed lesion with a radiolucent nidus. The center of the tumor may actually be radio-opaque but surrounded by a 2-mm radiolucent zone giving it the appearance of a ring sequestrum. There is no correlation between the duration of symptoms and presence of mineralization in the nidus. The extensive reactive sclerosis seen in the cortical type may obscure the central nidus, but this finding is

Box 5 Imaging of osteoid osteoma

- Classically oval with radiolucent nidus
- May have radiodense center with surrounding radiolucent zone

Box 7 CT scan in osteoid osteoma

- Thin cuts needed (1–2 mm)
- Good for pelvis and spine
- Helps localize for excision

not present in the medullary type. If the lesion is intra-articular, there is no surrounding periosteum to help produce a bony reaction; however, both periarticular osteoporosis and early degenerative changes can occur. In the young patient with scoliosis secondary to an osteoid osteoma, the lesion is found at the concavity of the curve.

Box 6 Bone scan in osteoid osteoma

- Increased immediate and delayed uptake
- Blood pooled images also hot

Sometimes the plain radiographs are inconclusive and the nidus is not visualized. When this occurs, technetium bone scans and CT scans are useful. There is increased tracer uptake on both immediate and delayed images of a technetium scan due to avid bone formation within the nidus. A similar pattern of uptake can be seen in symptomatic spondylolysis. In contrast, however, the blood-pooled images

will be hyperemic in the osteoid osteoma. The bone scan is especially helpful in the spine where overlapping shadows make it difficult to discern the small lesion. Although this imaging modality is extremely sensitive, it is not specific enough to be diagnostic for the osteoid osteoma and the uptake may be nonlocalized. Plain or CT scans allow exact localization of the nidus, but thin cuts (1 to 2 mm) need to be requested or the lesion may be missed. This technique is ideal for demonstrating the lesion in the pelvis or spine. Marking the CT scan in relation to an easily accessible bony landmark will help during any subsequent surgical excision. MRI is controversial at this time in the diagnosis and management of an osteoid osteoma. Enhancing soft-tissue edema surrounding the lesion makes it appear falsely aggressive. Examples of imaging are shown in Figs 1, 2, and 3.

The radiographic differential diagnosis includes stress fracture, infection, bone island, eosinophilic granuloma, osteoblastoma, and, rarely, osteosarcoma. These are usually differentiated by their clinical presentation and histology.

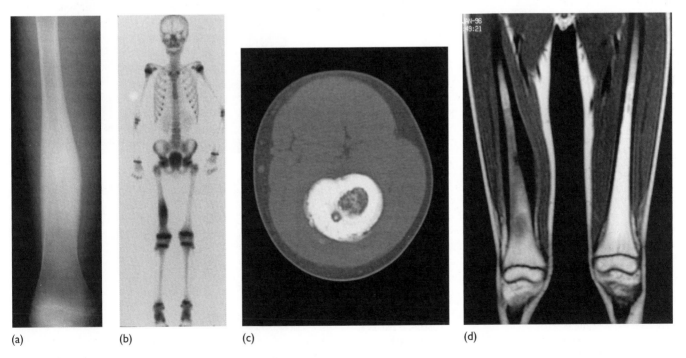

(a)　　(b)　　(c)　　(d)

Fig. 1. (a) Anteroposterior radiograph of the right distal femur in a 10-year-old male showing extensive cortical thickening that obscures the nidus of the osteoid osteoma. The patient had persistent pain worse at night. (b) Bone scan reveals diffusely increased uptake in the general area of the lesion corresponding to enhanced bone formation in the osteoid osteoma. (c) CT scan reveals the exact location of the nidus within the femoral cortex. In this case the center is mineralized and surrounded by a 1- to 2-mm radiolucent zone. (d) T_1-weighted image on MRI shows the area of the nidus with low signal intensity in the medial femoral cortex; however, note the extensive signal change throughout the medullary canal indicative of edema. This finding can be confused with a more aggressive lesion, therefore this imaging technique is rarely used for diagnosis of an osteoid osteoma.

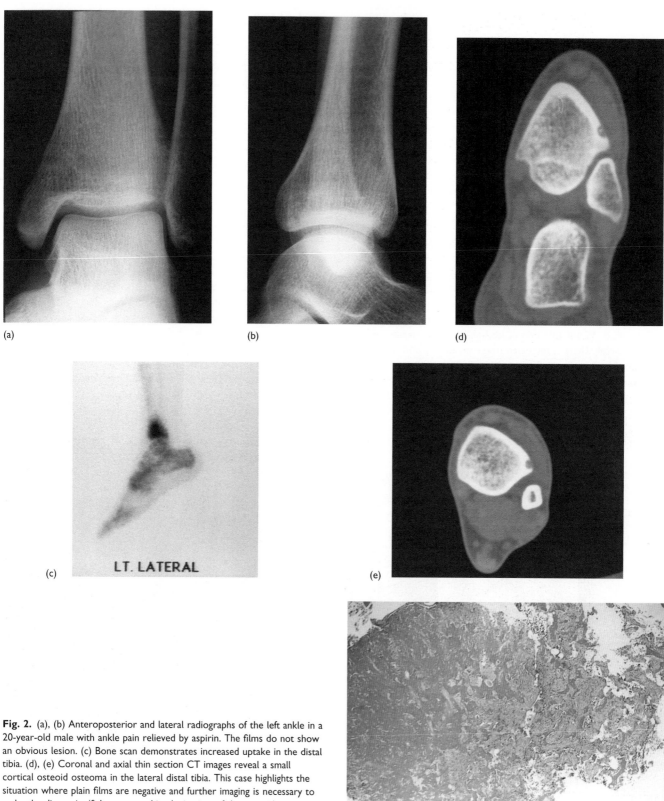

Fig. 2. (a), (b) Anteroposterior and lateral radiographs of the left ankle in a 20-year-old male with ankle pain relieved by aspirin. The films do not show an obvious lesion. (c) Bone scan demonstrates increased uptake in the distal tibia. (d), (e) Coronal and axial thin section CT images reveal a small cortical osteoid osteoma in the lateral distal tibia. This case highlights the situation where plain films are negative and further imaging is necessary to make the diagnosis. (f) Low-power histologic view of the osteoid osteoma shows immature trabeculae in the center with more compact bone surrounding the nidus.

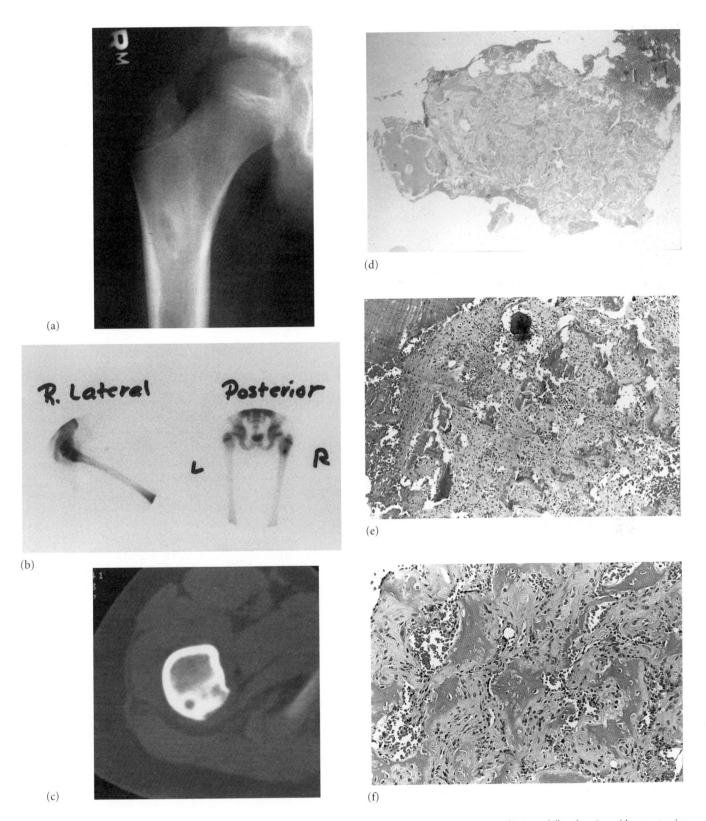

Fig. 3. (a) Anteroposterior radiograph of the proximal femur in a 10-year-old male with a radiolucent lesion noted in a medullary location without extensive reactive sclerosis. (b) Bone scan reveals intense tracer uptake around the lesion. (c) CT scan localizes the nidus just inside the cortex in the subtrochanteric region of the femur. (d) Low-power view of the nidus consisting of immature fragments of bone. This lesion was shelled out of the bone with a curette after burring through the overlying cortex. (e), (f) Higher-power views of the same lesion showing a mixture of mineralized trabeculae and seams of osteoid. Prominent osteoblasts are seen, but no cellular atypia is present.

Management

The treatment of choice is complete excision of the lesion. No attempt at resection should be undertaken, however, until the lesion is demonstrated on imaging studies. Several reports have shown that the osteoid osteoma will heal and become asymptomatic with radiographic disappearance of the nidus. This required up to 3 years of nonoperative treatment in one study (Kneisl and Simon 1992). However, the patient needs to take aspirin or nonsteroidal anti-inflammatory drugs for a prolonged period, and this is often not tolerated. For lesions that are present in surgically difficult or inaccessible locations, nonoperative treatment may be the only safe option. Children with an osteoid osteoma causing structural abnormality in the spine or extremities should be treated with excision to prevent further deformity.

Surgery is necessary for a definitive cure of the osteoid osteoma; however, the nidus is difficult to find at the time of excision. Several methods of preoperative or intraoperative localization have been advocated including radioisotope scanning, tetracycline fluorescence labeling, and CT-guided wire markers. It is claimed in several studies that tetracycline labeling is simpler and quicker than nuclear scanning; however, this is controversial. It requires the patient to take 750 to 4000 mg (4 mg/kg) of oral tetracycline 1 to 2 days prior to surgery. Ultraviolet light is used on the resected specimen to confirm removal of the nidus which takes up tetracycline in the mineralized bone. The technique has high specificity but variable sensitivity.

The standard technique of excision involves *en bloc* resection of the lesion. This gives the best assurance that the lesion has been removed; however, it involves a large amount of bone loss and the need to protect the extremity postoperatively to prevent a fracture through weakened cortex. Prophylactic internal fixation and/or bone graft may be needed depending on the size and location of lesions resected from the femur or tibia.

More recent surgical modifications include the 'burr down' technique, radiofrequency ablation, and CT-guided percutaneous resection of the lesion. The 'burr down' technique involves careful inspec-

tion of the preoperative studies to identify the lesion in relation to easily located surgical landmarks. It is best used on patients with accessible lesions. Intraoperative plain radiographs or fluoroscopy help to confirm the correct location. The cortical bone is gently burred in a circular motion until the reddish hypervascular nidus is identified. It is easily shelled out with a curette and sent to the pathology laboratory for diagnosis. Frozen sections are not needed. No more than 1 to 2 mm of the surrounding area of reactive bone, formed in response to the high local concentration of prostaglandins secreted by the nidus, needs to be removed. This minimizes the chances of later fracture, requires a shorter period of protected weight bearing, and allows an earlier return to unrestricted activity (Ward *et al.* 1993). Reports of CT-guided wire or biopsy cannula placement into the nidus and subsequent percutaneous removal of the surrounding lesion have also demonstrated a decreased need for protected weight bearing after surgery. However, up to one-quarter may recur using this technique and there is less opportunity to obtain a tissue diagnosis. Recent studies have shown excellent pain relief and minimal recurrence using radiofrequency ablation to remove the osteoid osteoma.

Results of treatment

The natural history of osteoid osteoma is not clear as a diagnosis is definitively made only after histological review of the resection specimen. These lesions do not become malignant or metastasize. Recurrence rates of less than 5 per cent are reported, these usually follow an incomplete excision. There are only a few case reports of recurrent osteoid osteomas after histologically documented *en bloc* resection of the lesion. When the lesion is completely removed, uniformly excellent results of pain relief have been noted. Removing an osteoid osteoma from the spine often causes resolution of any scoliosis caused by the lesion but depends on the age of the patient and the duration of symptoms.

The osteoid osteoma is not always found in the resected specimen. One study reported 54 patients with typical radiographic findings of this tumor who had no histological evidence of the nidus at the time of removal. Symptoms were relieved in 36 of 42 patients who still had no pathologic confirmation of the diagnosis even after some underwent several operations (Sim *et al.* 1975).

Further reading

Assoun, J., Richardi, G., Railhac, J., *et al.* (1994). Osteoid osteoma: MR imaging versus CT. *Radiology*, **191**, 217–23.

Ayala, A., Murray, J., Erling, M., and Raymond, A. (1986). Osteoid-osteoma: intraoperative tetracycline-fluorescence demonstration of the nidus. *Journal of Bone and Joint Surgery, American Volume*, **68A**, 747–51.

Fechner, R. and Mills, S. (1993). *Atlas of tumor pathology. Tumors of the bones and joints* (3rd series). AFIP, Washington D.C.

Graham, H., Laverick, M., Cosgrove, A., and Crone, M. (1993). Minimally invasive surgery for osteoid osteoma of the proximal femur. *Journal of Bone and Joint Surgery, British Volume*, **75B**, 115–18.

Greco, F., Tamburrelli, F., La Cara, A., and Di Trapani, G. (1988). Nerve fibres in osteoid osteoma. *Italian Journal of Orthopaedics and Trauma*, **14**, 89–94.

Greco, F., Tamburrelli, F., and Ciabattoni, G. (1991). Prostaglandins in osteoid osteoma. *International Orthopaedics*, **15**, 35–7.

Kirwan, E., Hutton, P., Pozo, J., and Ransford, A. (1984). Osteoid osteoma and benign osteoblastoma of the spine. *Journal of Bone and Joint Surgery, British Volume*, **66B**, 21–6.

Klein, M. and Shankman, S. (1992). Osteoid osteoma: radiologic and pathologic correlation. *Skeletal Radiology*, **21**, 23–31.

Norman, A. (1978). Persistence or recurrence of pain: a sign of surgical failure in osteoid-osteoma. *Clinical Orthopaedics and Related Research*, **130**, 263–6.

Pettine, K. and Klassen, R. (1986). Osteoid-osteoma and osteoblastoma of the spine. *Journal of Bone and Joint Surgery, American Volume*, **68A**, 354–61.

Regan, M., Galey, J., and Oakeshott, R. (1990). Recurrent osteoid osteoma. *Clinical Orthopaedics and Related Research*, **253**, 221–24.

Rosenthal, D., Wolfe, M., Jennings, L., Gebhardt, M., and Mankin, H. (1998). Percutaneous radiofrequency coagulation of osteoid osteoma compared with operative treatment. *Journal of Bone and Joint Surgery, American Volume*, **80A**, 815–21.

Schajowicz, F. (1994). *Tumors and tumorlike lesions of bone* (2nd edn). Springer-Verlag, Berlin.

Smith, F. and Gilday, D. (1980). Scintigraphic appearances of osteoid osteoma. *Radiology*, **137**, 191–5.

Vigorita, V. and Ghelman, B. (1983). Localization of osteoid osteomas—use of radionuclide scanning and autoimaging in identifying the nidus. *American Journal of Clinical Pathology*, **79**, 223–5.

Voto, S., Cook, A., Weiner, D., Ewing, J., and Arrington, L. (1990). Treatment of osteoid osteoma by computed tomography guided excision in the pediatric patient. *Journal of Pediatric Orthopaedics*, **10**, 510–13.

Worland, R., Ryder, C., and Johnston, A. (1975). Recurrent osteoid-osteoma. *Journal of Bone and Joint Surgery, American Volume*, **57A**, 277–8.

References

Frassica, F., Waltrip, R., Sponseller, P., Ma, L., and McCarthy, E. (1996). Clinicopathologic features and treatment of osteoid osteoma and osteoblastoma in children and adolescents. *Orthopedic Clinics of North America*, **27**, 559–74.

Gitelis, S. and Schajowicz, F. (1989). Osteoid osteoma and osteoblastoma. *Orthopedic Clinics of North America*, **20**, 313–24.

Greenspan, A. (1993). Benign bone-forming lesions: osteoma, osteoid osteoma, and osteoblastoma. *Skeletal Radiology*, **22**, 485–500.

Kneisl, J. and Simon, M. (1992). Medical management compared with operative treatment for osteoid-osteoma. *Journal of Bone and Joint Surgery, American Volume*, **74A**, 179–85.

Schulman, L. and Dorfman, H. (1970). Nerve fibers in osteoid osteoma. *Journal of Bone and Joint Surgery, American Volume*, **52A**, 1351–6.

Sim, F., Dahlin, D., and Beabout, J. (1975). Osteoid-osteoma: diagnostic problems. *Journal of Bone and Joint Surgery, American Volume*, **57A**, 154–9.

Ward, W., Eckardt, J., Shayestehfar, S., Mirra, J., Grogan, T., and Oppenheim, W. (1993). Osteoid osteoma diagnosis and management with low morbidity. *Clinical Orthopaedics and Related Research*, **291**, 229–35.

Wold, L., Pritchard, D., Bergert, J., and Wilson, D. (1988). Prostaglandin synthesis by osteoid osteoma and osteoblastoma. *Modern Pathology*, **1**, 129–31.

1.6.6.2 Osteoblastoma*

Panayiotis J. Papagelopoulos, Evanthia C. Galanis, Pietro Ruggieri, and Franklin H. Sim

Definition

Benign osteoblastoma is a primary bone tumor that is composed of a well-vascularized connective tissue stroma in which there is active production of osteoid and primitive woven bone (Unni 1996). Initially designated 'giant osteoid osteoma' (Dahlin and Johnson 1954) and 'osteogenic fibroma' (Golding and Sissons 1954; Kirkpatrick and Murray 1955), osteoblastoma obtained its currently accepted name in 1956 (Jaffe 1956; Lichtenstein 1956). The precise relationship between this lesion and osteoid osteoma is not clear, and in recent years an aggressive variety of osteoblastoma has been recognized (Mayer 1967; Kenan *et al.* 1985; Mitchell and Ackerman 1986).

Natural history

Osteoblastoma is a benign tumor. It grows relatively slowly, but if left without any treatment, it may attain considerable size and continue to grow for several years. After complete intralesional excision, the recurrence rate is relatively low (Lucas *et al.* 1994). Recurrences are more common in aggressive lesions, which are managed better with wide resection. Malignant change has been reported in a few cases considered to be correctly diagnosed as benign osteoblastoma (Unni 1996). It is believed that most tumors that metastasize are not osteoblastomas to begin with but instead are unrecognized low-grade osteosarcomas or osteosarcomas with atypical histologic features (Campanacci 1990; Unni 1996).

Box 1

- Rare benign bone-forming tumor that develops most frequently in long tubular bones, spine, and sacrum

- Typically causes progressively increasing pain and when located in the spine may cause muscle spasm, scoliosis, paresthesias, and weakness

- Radiographs usually show an expansile well-circumscribed partially calcified lesion that resembles a large osteoid osteoma

- Differential diagnosis includes osteoid osteoma, aneurysmal bone cyst, eosinophilic granuloma, enchondroma, fibrous dysplasia, chondromyxoid fibroma, solitary bone cyst, and in some instances osteosarcoma and Ewing's sarcoma

- Current treatment consists of surgical removal of all tumor; curettage or marginal or wide resection may be appropriate depending on the location, size, and aggressiveness of the tumor

- Local recurrence rarely occurs following complete removal of the tumor

*Part of the material in this chapter appeared in *Orthopedics*, **22**, 244–7, 1999, and is reproduced by permission of the publishers.

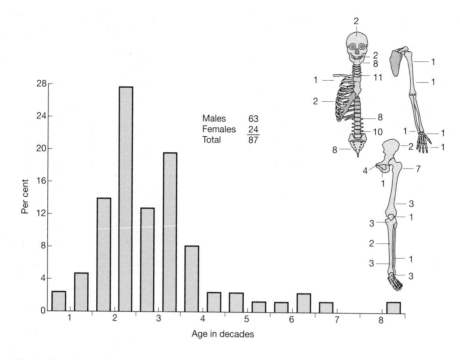

Fig. 1. Distribution of osteoblastomas according to age and sex of the patient and site of the lesion. (Reproduced from Unni (1996) by permission of the Mayo Foundation.)

Epidemiology

Osteoblastomas accounted for approximately 3.5 per cent of all benign primary tumors in the Mayo Clinic series and for less than 1 per cent of all bone neoplasms (Unni 1996). The lesion is observed most frequently in patients younger than 30 years, with an age distribution from 2 to 75 years (Fig. 1). Male patients are affected more frequently than female patients (ratio 2:1) (Lucas et al. 1994).

Osteoblastoma may affect any bone (Marsh et al. 1975; McLeod et al. 1976; Tonai et al. 1982; Lucas et al. 1994; Papagelopolous et al. 1999). The lesion has a distinct predilection for the vertebral column. The spine and the sacrum are involved in 30 per cent of cases. The long tubular bones are affected in 34 per cent of cases. Other bones affected are the skull, mandible, or maxilla (15 per cent), innominate bone (5 per cent), bones of hands and feet (10 per cent), ribs, sternum, patella, clavicle, and facial bones (Unni 1996). In the long tubular bones, the lesion is located in the diaphysis in 75 per cent of cases and in the metaphysis in the remainder; epiphyseal involvement is unusual (Lucas et al. 1994). In the spine, 55 per cent of the lesions are contained in the dorsal elements and 42 per cent in both the dorsal elements and the vertebral body (Lucas et al. 1994). Involvement of the vertebral body is less typical.

Clinical manifestations

Local pain is a common clinical manifestation of osteoblastoma (87 per cent), although generally it is mild. Pain is often progressive, and it is occasionally characterized by accentuation at night and amelioration with salicylates. Local swelling, tenderness, warmth, and gait disturbances are also mentioned (Lucas et al. 1994; Papagelopol-

ous et al. 1998). Spinal lesions may be accompanied by muscle spasm, scoliosis, and neurologic manifestations, including paresthesias and weakness. Mirra et al. (1979) described a case of osteoblastoma associated with systemic symptoms such as weight loss, chronic fever, anemia, and systemic periostosis. The symptoms abated after amputation. Yoshikawa et al. (1977) described a benign osteoblastoma as a cause of osteomalacia.

Imaging

The radiographic features of osteoblastoma are often nonspecific and may not suggest the true diagnosis. Osteolysis and osteosclerosis, alone or combined may be observed. Expansion of bone, cortical thinning, and a soft-tissue mass may accompany the lesion and in some cases may suggest a malignant process. Radiographs usually show an expansile, well-circumscribed, partially calcified lesion or a lesion similar to a large osteoid osteoma (Frassica et al. 1996; Papagelopolous et al. 1999).

In tubular bones, 65 per cent of the tumors are situated within the cortex and the remaining 35 per cent in the medullary canal (Lucas et al. 1994). The lesions have large areas of bone destruction and variable sclerosis. The margins are well defined, poorly defined, or indefinite. The size of the lesion varies from 1 to 11 cm (mean 3 cm). A calcified central nidus with a lucent halo suggestive of the diagnosis is infrequent (eight of 116 cases). Reactive sclerosis is present in more than 50 per cent of the cases. Periosteal new bone formation is frequent. According to Lucas et al. (1994), on the basis of radiographic features, 72 per cent of the lesions were thought to be benign, 10 per cent malignant, and the rest indeterminate.

In the spine, a well-defined expansile osteolytic lesion that is par-

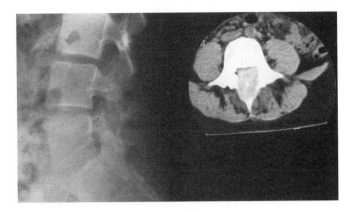

Fig. 2. Osteoblastoma of the fourth lumbar vertebra in a 10-year-old girl. In the lateral radiograph (left) the lesion is not easily seen. A CT scan in the same patient (right) shows the lesion clearly involves the dorsal vertebral elements. (Reproduced from Unni (1996) by permission of the Mayo Foundation.)

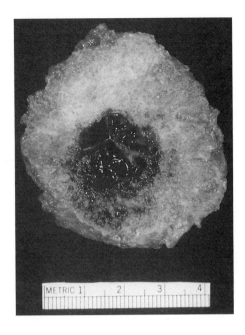

Fig. 3. Gross pathologic specimen of an osteoblastoma of the pubic bone from an 18-year-old man. The cystic quality of the lesion suggests a secondary aneurysmal bone cyst. (Reproduced from Unni (1996) by permission of the Mayo Foundation.)

tially or extensively calcified or ossified and that arises from the posterior elements, especially in the thoracic or lumbar spine (Fig. 2), should suggest the diagnosis of osteoblastoma (de Souza Dias and Frost 1973; Griffin 1978). Scoliosis may accompany osteoblastomas of the thoracic or lumbar spine or of the ribs (Lindholm *et al.* 1977; Akbarnia and Rooholamini 1981). Lucas *et al.* (1994) described 66 osteoblastomas of the spine. Their size varied from 1 to 15 cm (mean 3.5 cm).

Other imaging methods, such as bone scintigraphy, CT scanning, and MRI, may provide information about the extent of the lesion and the additional sites of involvement; however, they are unable to outline features that allow specific diagnosis (Papagelopolous *et al.* 1998). Bone scintigraphy reveals increased accumulation of the radionuclide at the site of the lesion, and CT scanning and MRI allow full delineation of the extent of the process.

Pathology

The lesions are reasonably well circumscribed and may be subperiosteal, cortical, or medullary in location (Fig. 3). Intracortical osteoblastomas are associated with extensive surrounding sclerotic bone similar to that found in an osteoid osteoma, but the nidus of an osteoblastoma is larger (Jackson *et al.* 1977; Campanacci 1990; Unni 1996). The tumor tissue is hemorrhagic, granular, purple to reddish brown, and friable because of its vascularity and its osteoid component, which shows variable calcification (McLeod *et al.* 1976; Unni 1996). Some tumors have a thin sclerotic rim, whereas others, especially those in the long bones of the extremities, have a zone of increased density as prominent as that of the ordinary osteoid osteoma. Unlike long bone osteoblastomas, which seldom extend into the soft tissue, vertebral osteoblastomas not infrequently have epidural extension and may even extend into the paraspinal tissue or involve adjacent vertebrae.

Microscopically, osteoblastoma is similar to osteoid osteoma, consisting of a well-vascularized connective tissue stroma in which there is active production of osteoid and primitive woven bone (Lichtenstein 1956; McLeod *et al.* 1976; Lucas *et al.* 1994; Unni 1996).

The bony trabeculae are variably calcified. Some osteoblastomas have abundant thick, pink osteoid trabeculae without mineralization, whereas others have much calcification with the appearance of bony trabeculae (Fig. 4). The bony trabeculae are lined with a single layer of osteoblasts, which may have small, inconspicuous nuclei with abundant cytoplasm or large, vesicular nuclei with prominent nucleoli. The intratrabecular stroma is composed of capillary proliferation and loosely arranged spindle cells without atypia. Although mitotic activity may be found within the osteoblasts, it is not prominent, and

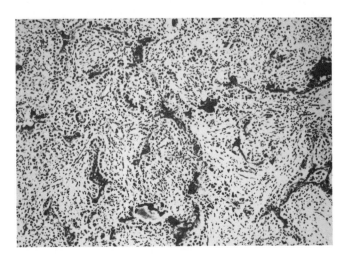

Fig. 4. Histologic specimen showing an osteoblastoma nidus composed of bony trabeculae. The mineralization is uneven. A single layer of osteoblasts is very prominent. The intertrabecular space is loose and vascular. (Hematoxylin and eosin stain.) (Reproduced from Unni (1996) by permission of the Mayo Foundation.)

atypical mitotic figures are not present (Mirra *et al.* 1989). Areas resembling secondary aneurysmal bone cysts may be seen in as many as 10 per cent of cases. Occasionally, osteoblastoma-like areas are found in an otherwise typical aneurysmal bone cyst, and this distinction sometimes is arbitrary. Although classically the bone trabeculae are thick and well formed, fine lace-like osteoid, a feature of classic osteosarcoma, may be seen focally (20 per cent of cases) (Lucas *et al.* 1994). Cartilage usually is not considered a part of the histologic spectrum of osteoblastoma, but rare examples in which the tumor contained hyaline cartilage or chondroid matrix have been reported (Bertoni *et al.* 1993).

Differential diagnosis

The radiographic features of osteoblastoma commonly do not allow the correct diagnosis. Expansile, partially calcified areas of osteolysis involving the posterior elements of the spine may be identified as osteoblastoma. In other areas, the radiographic appearance varies, and the differential diagnosis includes osteoid osteoma, aneurysmal bone cyst, eosinophilic granuloma, enchondroma, fibrous dysplasia, chondromyxoid fibroma, and solitary cyst (Campanacci 1990; Kransdorf and Sweet 1995; Unni 1996). In aggressive osteoblastomas, the osseous expansion and soft-tissue extension that are evident radiographically can simulate osteosarcoma, Ewing's sarcoma, or other malignant tumors (Papagelopolous *et al.* 1998).

The histologic features of osteoblastoma must be differentiated from those of osteoid osteoma (Marcove and Alpert 1963; Marsh *et al.* 1975; Dorfman and Weiss 1984; Frassica *et al.* 1996), aneurysmal bone cyst (Marsh *et al.* 1975; McLeod *et al.* 1976; Tonai *et al.* 1982), and osteosarcoma (Dorfman and Weiss 1984). Conventional osteosarcomas may have areas that are identical to those in osteoblastoma. The three features favoring a benign osteoblastoma are sharp circumscription with no permeation of surrounding bone, loose arrangement of the tissue with the bony trabeculae appearing embedded in loose connective tissue, and a single layer of osteoblasts surrounding bony trabeculae. Permeation of surrounding tissue with entrapment of host bone as well as sheets of osteoblasts without bone production favor osteosarcoma.

Treatment

Treatment depends on the stage and the localization of the tumor (Campanacci 1990; Lucas *et al.* 1994). In stage 1 (latent) or stage 2 (active) osteoblastoma, intralesional excision (curettage) and bone grafting of the defect may be indicated, along with local adjuvants. Curettage is especially used in vertebral localization, in a growing metaphysis, or near a functionally important epiphysis. In stage 3 (aggressive), marginal or wide resection is indicated. This is difficult in vertebral locations. In these cases, aggressive intralesional excision is used in association with fusion and internal fixation (de Souza Dias and Frost 1973; Griffin 1978; Frassica *et al.* 1996). It is doubtful whether radiation is of help. Selective arterial embolization may also be useful immediately preceding surgery (vertebral, pelvic localization) to reduce hemorrhage during the operation (Bettelli *et al.* 1989).

Prognosis

After complete removal of the tumor, recurrences are uncommon (Lucas *et al.* 1994). Instances of aggressive osteoblastoma have been described, characterized by considerable expansion and local recurrence, at times with delayed metastasis (Schajowicz and Lemos 1976; Dorfman and Weiss 1984). Many authors believe that tumors that metastasize are not osteoblastomas to begin with but rather are malignant lesions that were unrecognized because of the low grade of malignancy or because they were characterized by atypical histologic findings (Campanacci 1990). Malignant change has occurred in a few lesions considered to have been correctly diagnosed as benign osteoblastoma, for example, in one case in the Mayo Clinic series (Unni 1996). The potential hazards of radiation therapy are indicated by one case in the Mayo Clinic series in which a fatal fibrosarcoma developed 10 years after irradiation of an osteoblastoma of the fifth cervical vertebra (Unni 1996).

References

Akbarnia, B.A. and Rooholamini, S.A. (1981). Scoliosis caused by benign osteoblastoma of the thoracic or lumbar spine. *Journal of Bone and Joint Surgery, American Volume,* **63A**, 1146–55.

Bertoni, F., Unni, K.K., Lucas, D.R., and McLeod, R.A. (1993). Osteoblastoma with cartilaginous matrix. An unusual morphologic presentation in 18 cases. *American Journal of Surgical Pathology,* **17**, 69–74.

Bettelli, G., Capanna, R., van Horn, J.R., Ruggieri, P., Biagini, R., and Campanacci, M. (1989). Osteoid osteoma and osteoblastoma of the pelvis. *Clinical Orthopaedics and Related Research,* **247**, 261–71.

Campanacci, M. (1990). *Bone and soft tissue tumors.* Springer-Verlag, Vienna.

Dahlin, D.C. and Johnson, E.W., Jr (1954). Giant osteoid osteoma. *Journal of Bone and Joint Surgery, American Volume,* **36A**, 559–72.

de Souza Dias, L. and Frost, H.M. (1973). Osteoblastoma of the spine. A review and report of eight new cases. *Clinical Orthopaedics and Related Research,* **91**, 141–51.

Dorfman, H.D. and Weiss, S.W. (1984). Borderline osteoblastic tumors: problems in the differential diagnosis of aggressive osteoblastoma and low-grade osteosarcoma. *Seminars in Diagnostic Pathology,* **1**, 215–34.

Frassica, F.J., Waltrip, R.L., Sponseller, P.D., Ma, L.D., and McCarthy, E.F., Jr (1996). Clinicopathologic features and treatment of osteoid osteoma and osteoblastoma in children and adolescents. *Orthopedic Clinics of North America,* **27**, 559–74.

Golding, J.S.R. and Sissons, H.A. (1954). Osteogenic fibroma of bone: a report of two cases. *Journal of Bone and Joint Surgery, British Volume,* **36B**, 428–35.

Griffin, J.B. (1978). Benign osteoblastoma of the thoracic spine. Case report with 15-year follow-up. *Journal of Bone and Joint Surgery, American Volume,* **60A**, 833–5.

Jackson, R.P., Reckling, F.W., and Mants, F.A. (1977). Osteoid osteoma and osteoblastoma. Similar histologic lesions with different natural histories. *Clinical Orthopaedics and Related Research,* **128**, 303–13.

Jaffe, H.L. (1956). Benign osteoblastoma. *Bulletin of the Hospital for Joint Diseases,* **17**, 141–51.

Kenan, S., Floman, Y., Robin, G.C., and Laufer, A. (1985). Aggressive osteoblastoma. A case report and review of the literature. *Clinical Orthopaedics and Related Research,* **195**, 294–8.

Kirkpatrick, H.J.R. and Murray, R.C. (1955). Osteogenic fibroma of bone: report of a case. *Journal of Bone and Joint Surgery, British Volume,* **37B**, 606–11.

Kransdorf, M.J. and Sweet, D.E. (1995). Aneurysmal bone cyst: concept, controversy, clinical presentation, and imaging. *American Journal of Roentgenology*, **164**, 573–80.

Lichtenstein, L. (1956). Benign osteoblastoma: a category of osteoid- and bone-forming tumors other than classic osteoid osteoma, which may be mistaken for giant-cell tumor or osteogenic sarcoma. *Cancer*, **9**, 1044–52.

Lindholm, T.S., Snellman, O., and Österman, K. (1977). Scoliosis caused by benign osteoblastoma of the lumbar spine: a report of three patients. *Spine*, **2**, 276–81.

Lucas, D.R., Unni, K.K., McLeod, R.A., O'Connor, M.I., and Sim, F.H. (1994). Osteoblastoma: clinicopathologic study of 306 cases. *Human Pathology*, **25**, 117–34.

McLeod, R.A., Dahlin, D.C., and Beabout, J.W. (1976). The spectrum of osteoblastoma. *American Journal of Roentgenology*, **126**, 321–5.

Marcove, R.C. and Alpert, M. (1963). A pathologic study of benign osteoblastoma. *Clinical Orthopaedics and Related Research*, **30**, 175–81.

Marsh, B.W., Bonfiglio, M., Brady, L.P., and Enneking, W.F. (1975). Benign osteoblastoma: range of manifestations. *Journal of Bone and Joint Surgery, American Volume*, **57A**, 1–9.

Mayer, L. (1967). Malignant degeneration of so-called benign osteoblastoma. *Bulletin of the Hospital for Joint Diseases*, **28**, 4–13.

Mirra, J.M., Cove, K., Theros, E., Paladugu, R., and Smasson, J. (1979). A case of osteoblastoma associated with severe systemic toxicity. *American Journal of Surgical Pathology*, **3**, 463–71.

Mirra, J.M., Picci, P., and Gold, R.H. (1989). *Bone tumors: clinical, radiologic, and pathologic correlations*, Vol. 1. Lea and Febiger, Philadelphia, PA.

Mitchell, M.L. and Ackerman, L.V. (1986). Metastatic and pseudomalignant osteoblastoma: a report of two unusual cases. *Skeletal Radiology*, **15**, 213–18.

Papagelopolous, P.J., Galanis, E.C., Sim, F.H., and Unni, K.K. (1998). Osteoblastoma of the acetabulum. *Orthopedics*, **21**, 355–8.

Papagelopolous, P.J., Galanis, E.C., Sim, F.H., and Unni, K.K. (1999). Clinicopathologic features, diagnosis and treatment of osteoblastoma. *Orthopedics*, **22**, 244–7.

Schajowicz, F. and Lemos, C. (1976). Malignant osteoblastoma. *Journal of Bone and Joint Surgery, British Volume*, **58B**, 202–11.

Tonai, M., Campbell, C.J., Ahn, G.H., Schiller, A.L., and Mankin, H.J. (1982). Osteoblastoma: classification and report of 16 patients. *Clinical Orthopaedics*, **167**, 222–35.

Unni, K.K. (1996). *Dahlin's bone tumors: general aspects and data on 11,087 cases* (5th edn), pp. 131–42. Lippincott–Raven, Philadelphia, PA.

Yoshikawa, S., Nakamura, T., Takagi, M., Imamura, T., Okano, K., and Sasaki, S. (1977). Benign osteoblastoma as a cause of osteomalacia. A report of two cases. *Journal of Bone and Joint Surgery, British Volume*, **59B**, 279–86.

gave a clear definition of the tumor known today as the benign giant cell tumor of bone (Jaffe *et al.* 1940).

The giant cell tumor of bone is a mesenchymal tumor of fibrohistiocytic origin in which the primary stem cell of origin is a mononuclear fibroblastic neoplastic cell that produces type I and II collagen, has receptor sites for parathormone, and produces alkaline phosphatase (Goldring *et al.* 1986; Robinson and Einhorn 1994). A second population of cells, which are mononuclear and have an appearance similar to the neoplastic fibrohistiocytic stem cells by hemotoxylin and eosin staining, are reactive monocyte-derived macrophage cells that express monocyte–macrophage markers. The third population of cells for which the tumor is recognized are the multinucleated giant cells which possess receptors for calcitonin, a pheno-

Box 1

- Makes up about 20 per cent of benign bone tumors
- Rarely, in about 2 to 9 per cent of patients, metastasizes to the lungs and in less than 5 per cent of patients transforms into an osteosarcoma after a period of years
- Typically develops in epiphyses directly adjacent to subchondral bone
- Consists of giant cells and spindle-shaped mononuclear stromal cells
- Most commonly presents as a painful bone lesion in patients between 20 and 40 years of age
- Treatment consists of curettage, frequently with local adjuvant therapy, or *en bloc* resection

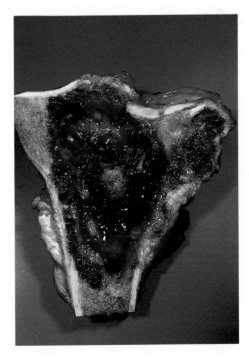

Fig. 1. Gross specimen of a typical giant cell tumor of the proximal tibial epiphyseal–metaphyseal area with extensive involvement of subchondral bone resulting in pathologic fracture.

1.6.6.3 Giant cell tumor of bone

James O. Johnston

Introduction

Soon after the use of microscopes to study the growth of neoplastic disease, it became apparent that giant cells were commonly seen in lytic destructive lesions of bone. For this reason, these tumors were classified as 'osteoclastomas', a term used by some authors even today. Considerable confusion existed until 1940 when Jaffe and Lichtenstein first developed the classification of giant cell lesions and

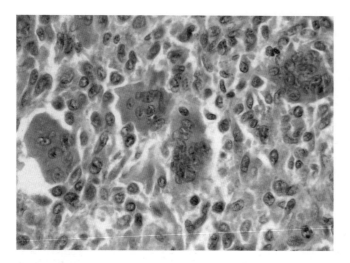

Fig. 2. Typical microscopic appearance of a giant cell tumor of bone with polyhedral stromal cells with a nuclear pattern similar to the nuclei of the benign appearing giant cells.

typic marker for osteoclasts. It is the presence of these large osteoclastic giant cells that gives the giant cell tumor of bone its clinical features of an osteolytic hemorrhagic aneurysmal lesion of the skeletal system that can lead to pathologic fracture. It is important to note that cellular characteristics of giant cell tumor of bone are also found in the so-called giant cell variants which include the aneurysmal bone cyst, osteoblastoma, chondroblastoma, and osteoid osteoma. Monocyte-derived macrophages and osteoclastic-like giant cells are seen in all these giant cell variants found typically in children, and they were found by Schajowicz (1961) to have similar histochemical staining characteristics. Giant cell lesions in general are known to produce inflammatory substances such as prostaglandin E_2 (Gebhardt *et al.* 1985) which also helps these tumors to destroy bone matrix resulting in an aneurysmal dilatation of surrounding reactive bone.

Giant cell tumor of bone is usually considered a benign neoplasm; however, it may metastasize to the lung in 2 to 9 per cent of cases (Tubbs *et al.* 1991; Kay *et al.* 1994; Rao *et al.* 1995; Cheng and Johnston 1997). This is considered to be a benign process and the prognosis for survival is quite good compared to the metastasis of malignant tumors. It is also of interest to note that less than 5 per cent of giant cell tumors of bone will spontaneously convert to a malignant osteosarcoma after lying dormant for a period of many years (Campanacci 1990).

Incidence

Giant cell tumor of bone is a relatively common bone tumor which represented 5 per cent of all bone tumors and 21 per cent of benign bone tumors in the Mayo Clinic series (Dahlin and Unni 1986).

Pathology

The giant cell tumor of bone is soft and friable with large areas of hemorrhagic response that give it the reddish-brown coloration seen in Fig. 1. The tumor is nearly always in contact with subchondral

bone of an adjacent joint and can result in intra-articular fracture (Fig. 1). The tumor is usually seen in the center of epiphyseal bone and is aggressively permeative into the surrounding cortical bone and commonly breaks through beneath the overlying periosteum. In time, this results in an aneurysmal appearance as the bone becomes dilated. It is common to see multiple hemorrhagic cysts within the giant cell tumor, and at times a large hemorrhagic cyst will give the appearance of an aneurysmal bone cyst adjacent to the main fleshy body of the tumor mass. In less aggressive lesions, one will find areas of firm fibrosis and even cholesterol deposits that might show as yellow patches in the tumor.

The cellular features of the giant cell tumor include a fairly uniform field of polyhedral to short spindle-shaped mononuclear stromal cells with a benign nuclear pattern similar to that of the nuclei seen in the numerous giant cells (Fig. 2). It is not unusual to see a few mitotic figures in the stromal cells that can cause concern when considering the differential diagnosis of a hemorrhagic osteosarcoma which typically shows many mitotic figures per high power field. There is minimal evidence of matrix production except for small amounts of collagen fiber. Occasionally areas of osteoid production can be found, especially at the periphery of the lesion. The presence of chondroid matrix should make one think more of a chondroblastoma or even an osteosarcoma. In lower-grade lesions, foam cells can be found which suggest an involutional process and a better prognosis with less chance of recurrence.

Previously pathologists attempted to classify giant cell tumor microscopically in order to prognosticate the chance for local recurrence or metastasis but without much success (Dahlin and Unni 1986).

Clinical evaluation

The giant cell tumor of bone is unique because of its presence in the epiphyseal end of long bones in young adults. Most patients are aged between 20 and 40 years. The condition is almost unheard of in patients under 13 years of age, and only 10 per cent of cases occur in patients over 65 years of age. It is more common in females and will grow faster in a pregnant female. The most common location is about the knee joint, with the distal femur being more common than the proximal tibia. After the knee, the sacrum is the next most common location, with the distal radius being the fourth most common location according to Mayo Clinic data (Dahlin and Unni 1986). It is rare to find a giant cell tumor in the spine but, if found there, it will be in the vertebral body. It is rarely seen in the hand or foot. It is interesting to note the rare occurrence of multifocal giant cell tumor usually associated with hand lesions (Peimer *et al.* 1980; Cummins *et al.* 1996). Pain is a frequent symptom of giant cell tumor in the early stages and, in most cases, swelling will be noted about the affected joint after several months. If an early diagnosis is not made, a pathologic fracture into the adjacent joint is inevitable making treatment more difficult.

Imaging studies

Routine radiographs are quite helpful in making the diagnosis of a giant cell tumor because they will localize a lytic lesion seen in the

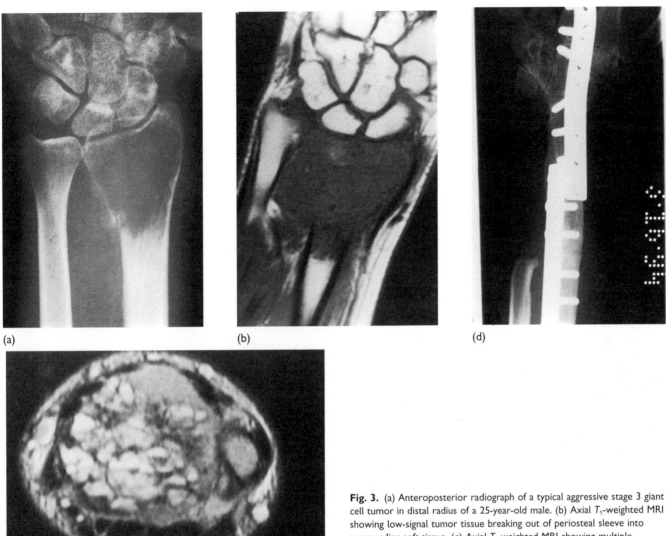

(a)　　　　　　　　　(b)　　　　　　　　　(d)

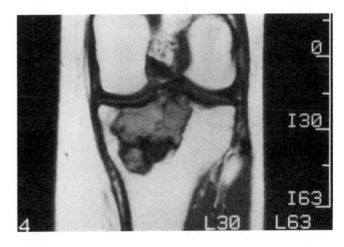

(c)

Fig. 3. (a) Anteroposterior radiograph of a typical aggressive stage 3 giant cell tumor in distal radius of a 25-year-old male. (b) Axial T_1-weighted MRI showing low-signal tumor tissue breaking out of periosteal sleeve into surrounding soft tissue. (c) Axial T_2-weighted MRI showing multiple hemorrhagic cysts in low-signal stromal tissue laden with hemosiderin. (d) Postoperative radiographic appearance with distal ulnar transposition and carpal arthrodesis with side plates for stability.

epiphyseal end of a long bone such as the one seen in the distal radius in Fig. 3(a). The lesion is purely lytic in nature and in most cases will have a fuzzy permeative interface with surrounding bone (Kricun 1993). With the additional assistance of MRI, one can also evaluate the soft-tissue involvement outside the cortex (Fig. 3(b)). Figure 3(c) is a T_2-weighted axial image which demonstrates multiple small hemorrhagic cysts with fluid–fluid levels along with the low signal characteristics of the stromal tissue laden with hemosiderin (Aoki *et al.* 1996).

Campanacci has attempted to define a staging system based on these imaging studies (Campanacci 1990). A stage 1, or quiescent stage, lesion (Fig. 4) is contained in cancellous bone with minimal, if any, cortical involvement. This is a rare stage that may be asymptomatic and tends to favor a better prognosis. The most common stage is stage 2, or the active stage (Fig. 5), which shows extensive cortical thinning and may create a slight aneurysmal appearance as the periosteal cover attempts to contain the peripheral tumor growth. Stage 3, the aggressive form of the disease, is shown in Fig. 3, where

Fig. 4. Coronal T_1-weighted MRI of small asymptomatic quiescent stage 1 giant cell tumor of proximal tibia in a 41-year-old female.

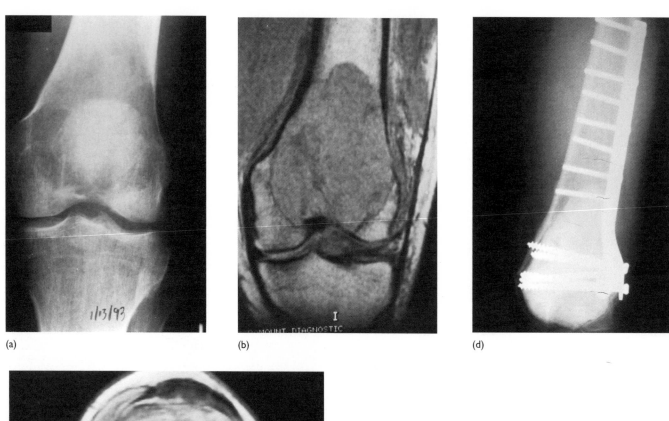

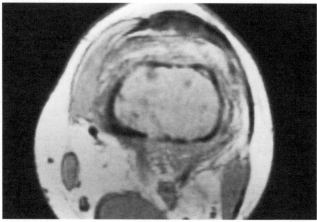

(a)   (b)   (d)

(c)

Fig. 5. (a) Anteroposterior radiograph of a typical active stage 2 giant cell tumor of distal femur in a 50-year-old male with extensive thinning of the surrounding cortices. (b) Coronal T_1-weighted MRI showing minimal cortical breakthrough under the periosteum that would still allow for a cementation procedure. (c) An axial proton density MRI demonstrating cortical breakthrough and minimal periosteal reaction. (d) Anteroposterior radiograph of the distal femur following aggressive curettage and cementation with a side plate and screws for stabilization.

the MRI demonstrates extensive extracortical involvement outside the periosteal cover. This final stage runs a greater risk of local recurrence and suggests a more aggressive surgical approach such as a wide resection instead of a simple curettage.

Management

Prior to 1989, the gold standard for the surgical management of giant cell tumor of bone was curettage and bone grafting. In 1989, a large international study was carried out involving both the American and European musculoskeletal tumor societies in which the results of 677 surgically treated giant cell tumor cases were analyzed (Miller *et al.* 1990). This study showed that curettage and bone grafting alone resulted in an unacceptable recurrence rate of 45 per cent. This same study showed that when adjuvants such as liquid nitrogen, phenol, hydrogen peroxide, or bone cement were added to the surgical curet-

tage, the recurrence rate dropped to 17 per cent. The best result from that study was a combination of curettage, phenol, and bone cement with a recurrence rate of only 3 per cent. Over the past 5 years, there have been many literature reports suggesting that bone cement instead of bone graft has now become the gold standard for the surgical management of giant cell tumor of bone (O'Donnell *et al.* 1994; Bini *et al.* 1995; Dreinhofer *et al.* 1995).

However, it is important to pay attention to surgical detail when performing this new cementation technique. Figure 6 illustrates the important details of this procedure performed on a 23-year-old woman with a stage 3 giant cell tumor of the proximal tibia (Fig. 6(a)). Firstly, the surgeon grossly debulks the tumor through a large window to gain good visualization of the entire tumor cavity (Fig. 6(b)). Then the margins are advanced with a high speed dental burr and the cavity is washed extensively with a high-pressure water lavage, followed by phenol, hydrogen peroxide (3 per cent), or liquid nitrogen. At this point, the tumor cavity should look clean

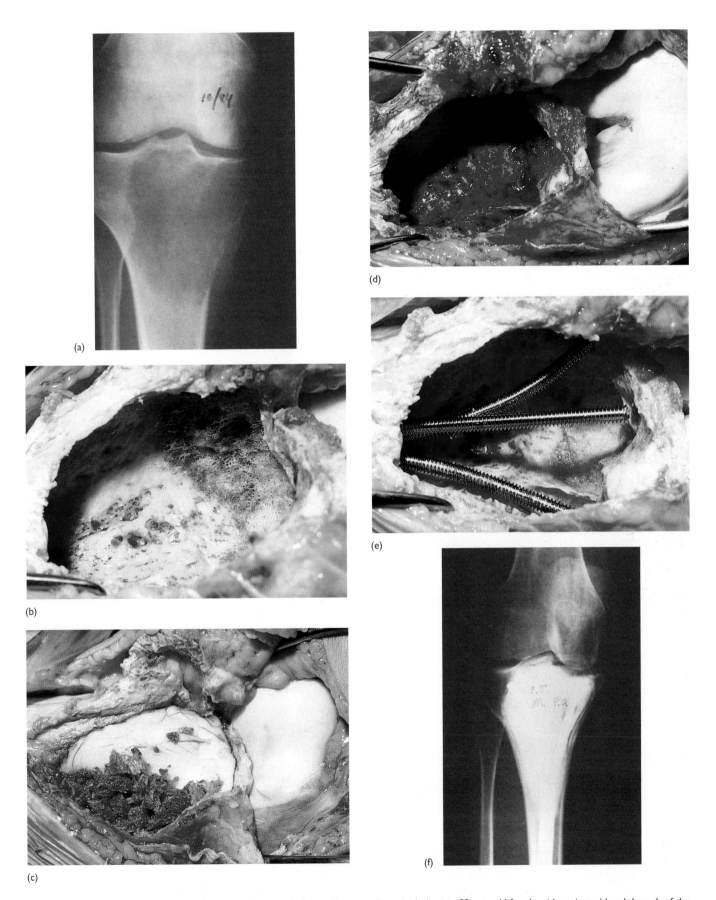

Fig. 6. (a) Anteroposterior radiograph of an aggressive stage 3 giant cell tumor of proximal tibia in a 23-year-old female with periosteal breakthrough of the medial cortex. (b) Appearance of tumor cloaca with large cortical window with a great deal of tumor left behind. (c) Appearance of tumor cavity after meticulous cleaning with water, high-speed burr, and H_2O_2. (d) Placement of Steinman pins (rebar) to reinforce bone cement. (e) Cementation completed and cancellous autograft is placed over exposed cement to form reactive involucrum. (f) Radiographic appearance 18 months later.

(Fig. 6(c)). Reconstruction may require reinforcement with Steinmann pins (rebar) for large defects (Fig. 6(d)), following which the cavity is filled with bone cement (Fig. 6(e)). With extensive exposure of articular cartilage, as in this case, it is wise to open the adjacent joint and place a small batch of cement on the subchondral area and allow it to set up first. The articular cartilage should be cooled with cold saline to prevent cartilage damage. Then, the remainder of the cavity is filled with a second batch of cement. In a case of this magnitude with a very large window, placement of a thin layer of cancellous autograft over the cement surface is advised to encourage involucrum formation (Fig. 6(f)).

In cases of large stage 3 lesions (Fig. 3), the cementation procedure is not possible and a more aggressive approach should be taken such as a wide resection followed by an osteoarticular allograft (Smith and Mankin 1977; Kattapuram *et al.* 1986; Musculo *et al.* 1993; Bell *et al.* 1994) or, as in this case, a transposition of the distal ulna as a vascularized bone segment to arthrodese the wrist with the use of sideplates (Seradge 1982; Lalla and Bhupathi 1987; Vander Griend and Funderburk 1993). Allograft reconstruction and even megaprostheses can be considered if a cementation procedure is unsuccessful.

In the case of a large giant cell tumor of the spine or sacrum, the proximity of the giant cell tumor to the spinal cord or cauda equina make the cementation technique less desirable because of thermal activity created by the use of cement. Figure 7 is an example of a giant cell tumor of the sacrum treated with aggressive curettage followed by 50 Gy (5000 rad) of radiation therapy. This patient was doing well 9 years later (Fig. 7(b)). In the older literature from the Mayo Clinic (Dahlin and Unni 1986) and the Rizzoli Institute in Bologna, Italy (Campanacci *et al.* 1987), an incidence as high as 27 per cent has been reported for irradiation sarcoma following treatment with greater than 40 Gy (4000 rad) to the tumor bed. However, more recent literature reviews indicate the percentage of irradiation sarcomas arising from the treatment of giant cell tumor with higher energy radiation sources has been negligible and the prevention of local recurrence is excellent (Bennett *et al.* 1993; Sanjay *et al.* 1993; Hug *et al.* 1995; Malone *et al.* 1995).

Summary

A great deal has been learned about the basic cellular biology of the giant cell tumor of bone over the past decade, and in the decade to follow more information will be derived from the science of molecular genetics. There is already some early information about a defect in the p53 suppressor gene on chromosome 17 in giant cell tumor which is similar to the defect seen in many osteosarcomas that would suggest a common pathogenesis between the giant cell tumor and the osteosarcoma (Matthews *et al.* 1995). Further research is needed in this area that may possibly lead to a form of gene therapy to help replace or delete the defective gene that may be the cause of this fascinating tumor.

References

Aoki, J., Tanikawa, H., Ishii, K., *et al.* (1996). MR findings indicative of hemosiderin in giant-cell tumor of bone; frequency, cause, and diagnostic significance. *American Journal of Roentgenology*, **166**, 145–8.

Bell, R.S., Davis, A., Allan, D.G., Langer, F., Czitrom, A.A., and Gross, A.E. (1994). Fresh osteochondral allografts for advanced giant cell tumors at the knee. *Journal of Arthroplasty*, **9**, 603–9.

Bennett, C.J., Jr, Marcus, R.B., Jr, Million, R.R., and Ennecking, W.F. (1993). Radiation therapy for giant cell tumor of bone. *International Journal of Radiation Oncology, Biology, Physics*, **26**, 299–304.

Bini, S.A., Gill, K., and Johnston, J.O. (1995). Giant cell tumor of bone curettage and cement reconstruction *Clinical Orthopaedics and Related Research*, **321**, 245–50.

Campanacci, M. (1990). Giant cell tumor. In *Bone and soft tissue tumors*, pp. 117–51. Springer-Verlag, Berlin.

Campanacci, M., Baldini, N., Boriani, S., *et al.* (1987). Giant-cell tumor of bone. *Journal of Bone and Joint Surgery, American Volume*, **69A**, 106–14.

Cheng, J.C. and Johnston, J.O. (1997). Giant cell tumor of bone. Prognosis and treatment of pulmonary metastases. *Clinical Orthopaedics and Related Research*, **338**, 205–14.

Cummins, C.A., Scarborough, M.T., and Enneking, W.F. (1996). Multicentric giant cell tumor of bone. *Clinical Orthopaedics and Related Research*, **322**, 245–52.

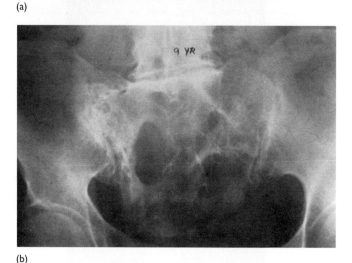

(a)

(b)

Fig. 7. (a) Anteroposterior radiograph of sacral giant cell tumor in a 56-year-old female treated with aggressive curettage followed postoperatively with 50 Gy (5000 rad) of external beam radiation therapy. (b) Anteroposterior radiograph 9 years later with no recurrence and no signs of irradiation sarcoma.

Dahlin, D. and Unni, K. (1986). Giant cell tumor (osteoclastoma). In *Bone tumors* (4th edn), pp. 119–40. C.C. Thomas, Springfield, IL.

Dreinhofer, K.E., Rydholm, A., Bauer, H.C., and Kreicbergs, A. (1995). Giant-cell tumors with fracture at diagnosis. Curettage and acrylic cementing in ten cases. *Journal of Bone and Joint Surgery, British Volume*, **77B**, 189–93.

Gebhardt, M., Lipiello, L., Bringhurst, F.R., and Mankin, H.J. (1985). Prostaglandin E₂ synthesis by human primary and metastatic bone tumors in culture. *Clinical Orthopaedics and Related Research*, **196**, 300–5.

Goldring, S.R., Schiller, A., Mankin, H.J., and Dayer, J.-M. (1986). Characterization of cells from human giant cell tumor of bone. *Clinical Orthopaedics and Related Research*, **204**, 59–75.

Hug, E.B., Fitzek, M.M., Liebsch, N.J., and Munzenrider, J.E. (1995). Locally challenging osteo- and chondrogenic tumors of the axial skeleton; results of combined proton and photon radiation therapy using three-dimensional treatment planning. *International Journal of Radiation Oncology, Biology, Physics*, **31**, 467–76.

Jaffe, H.L., Lichtenstein, L., and Porter, R.B. (1940). Giant cell tumor of bone: its pathologic appearance grading, supposed variants and treatment. *Archives of Pathology*, **30**, 993–1031.

Kattapuram, S.V., Phillips, W.C., and Mankin, H.J. (1986). Giant cell tumor of bone: radiographic changes following local excision and allograft replacement. *Radiology*, **161**, 493–8.

Kay, R.M., Eckardt, J.J., Seeger, L.L., Mirra, J.M., and Hak, D.J. (1994). Pulmonary metastasis of benign giant cell tumor of bone. Six histologically confirmed cases, including one of spontaneous regression. *Clinical Orthopaedics and Related Research*, **302**, 219–30.

Kricun, M.E. (1993). Tumors of long bones. In *Imaging of bone tumors*, pp. 84–8. W.B. Saunders, Philadelphia, PA.

Lalla, R.N. and Bhupathi, S.C. (1987). Treatment of giant cell tumors of distal radius by ulnar translocation. *Orthopedics*, **10**, 735–9.

Malone, S., O'Sullivan, B., Catton, C., Bell, R., Fornasier, V., and Davis, A. (1995). Long-term follow-up of efficacy and safety of megavoltage radiotherapy in high-risk giant cell tumors of bone. *International Journal of Radiation Oncology, Biology, Physics*, **33**, 689–94.

Mathews, C.H.E., Bini, S., and Johnston, J.O. (1995). P53 staining in giant cell tumors. *Transactions of the Orthopaedic Research Society*, **20**, 207.

Miller, G., Beteili, G., Fabbri, N., et al. (1990). Joint study of the European Musculoskeletal Oncology Society and Musculoskeletal Tumor Society on curettage of giant cell tumor of bone. In *La Chirurgica degli Organi di Movimento, Proceedings of the European Musculoskeletal Oncology Society and Musculoskeletal Tumor Society*, pp. 203–13. Cappelli Editore, Bologna.

Muscolo, D.L., Ayerza, M.A., Calabrese, M.E., and Gruenberg, M. (1993). The use of a bone allograft for reconstruction after resection of giant-cell tumor close to the knee. *Journal of Bone and Joint Surgery, American Volume*, **75A**, 1656–62.

O'Donnell, R.J., Springfield, D.S., Motwani, H.K., Ready, J.E., Gebhardt, M.C., and Mankin, H.J. (1994). Recurrence of giant-cell tumors of the long bones after curettage and packing with cement. *Journal of Bone and Joint Surgery, American Volume*, **76A**, 1827–33.

Peimer, C.A., Schiller, A.L., Mankin, H.J., and Smith, R.J. (1980). Multicentric giant cell tumor of bone. *Journal of Bone and Joint Surgery, American Volume*, **62A**, 652–6.

Rao, V.H., Bridge, J.A., Neff, J.R., et al. (1995). Expression of 72 kDa and 92 kDa type IV collagenases from human giant-cell tumor of bone. *Clinical and Experimental Metastasis*, **13**, 420–6.

Robinson, D, and Einhorn, T. (1994). Giant cell tumor of bone: a unique paradigm of stromal-hematopoietic cellular interactions. *Journal of Cellular Biochemistry*, **55**, 300–3.

Sanjay, B.K., Frassica, F.J., Frassica, D.A., Unni, K.K., McLeod, R.A., and Sim, F.H. (1993). Treatment of giant-cell tumor of the pelvis. *Journal of Bone and Joint Surgery, American Volume*, **75A**, 1466–75.

Schajowicz, F. (1961). Giant cell tumors of bone (osteoclastoma): a pathological and histochemical study. *Journal of Bone and Joint Surgery, American Volume*, **43A**, 1–29.

Seradge, H. (1982). Distal ulnar translocation in the treatment of giant cell tumors of the distal radius. *Journal of Bone and Joint Surgery, American Volume*, **64A**, 67–72.

Smith, R.J. and Mankin, H.J. (1977). Allograft replacement of distal radius for giant cell tumor. *Journal of Hand Surgery*, **2**, 299–309.

Tubbs, W.S., Brown, L.R., Beabout, J.W., Rock, M.G., and Unni, K.K. (1992). Benign giant-cell tumor of bone with pulmonary metastases: clinical findings and radiologic appearance of metastases in 13 cases. *American Journal of Roentgenology*, **158**, 331–4.

Vander Griend, R.A. and Funderburk, C.H. (1993). The treatment of giant-cell tumors of the distal part of the radius. *Journal of Bone and Joint Surgery, American Volume*, **75A**, 899–908.

1.6.6.4 Chondromyxoid fibroma

Michael G. Rock

Introduction

Chondromyxoid fibroma is a rare benign tumor representing fewer than 1 per cent of all benign and malignant tumors of bone. As its name implies, chondromyxoid fibroma is characterized by lobulated areas of spindle-shaped or stellate cells with abundant myxoid or chondroid intercellular material with a varying number of multinucleated giant cells. Largely because of the presence of islands within the tumor that look like hyaline cartilage as well as the anatomic predisposition within long bones of epiphysis and metaphysis, it has been assumed that the tumor is of chondroid derivation (Zillmer and Dorfman 1989). Owing to the variability of histologic appearance of this tumor, many legitimate chondromyxoid fibromas have probably been overdiagnosed as chondrosarcomas. Additionally, owing to its proximity to the epiphyseal plate and often contiguous involvement of the epiphysis and metaphysis of long bones, this lesion has sometimes been confused for chondroblastoma. Although there have been sporadic reports of malignant transformation, the clinical evolution of this disease before and after treatment is that of a benign neoplasm.

Given the anatomic predisposition of this tumor and the radiographic appearance, the main differential diagnosis of this condition includes aneurysmal bone cyst, fibrous dysplasia, enchondroma, giant-cell tumor of bone, chondroblastoma, and chondrosarcoma.

Box 1

- Fewer than 1 per cent of all tumors
- Most common in males in their thirties
- Most common location proximal tibia and distal femur

Clinical presentation

This condition has a definite male predilection (2:1) with the vast majority of the tumors seen in the second and third decade of life. Approximately two-thirds of the tumors present in the long bones of the extremities with predilection to the lower extremity. The most common bone involved is that of the proximal tibia followed by the distal femur, metatarsals, phalanges and tarsal bones of the foot, and lastly the fibula. Involvement of the lower extremity and phalanges of the foot are five to six times more common than involvement of the upper extremity and phalanges of the hand.

The lesion tends to be metaphyseal which with growth approximates the old epiphyseal plate and/or extend down the metaphysis of the bone. Owing to its proximity to the growth plate and many similar features of chondroblastoma, it is assumed that chondromyxoid fibroma is probably a remnant of the epiphyseal cartilaginous plate and thereby of cartilaginous origin (Unni and Dahlin 1995). Epiphyseal involvement is after skeletal maturity, and it is generally more apt to occur with involvement of the small tubular bones of the foot and hand.

The most common presenting symptom is that of pain. Not unlike chondroblastoma, pain can be mild to moderate and can be present for many months preceding the diagnosis. Unlike chondroblastoma which is anatomically closer to the contiguous joints, symptoms referable to the joint such as recurrent effusions and nondescript pain are less common. The propensity of this tumor to involve anatomic areas that are subcutaneous allow local swelling with increased superficial warmth overlying the lesion to be a common finding. Pathologic fractures are distinctly unusual events. Increased aggressiveness of this tumor in children under 10 years of age is usually observed.

Radiographic presentation

Typically the radiographic features of chondromyxoid fibroma is that of a radiolucent, generally metaphyseal eccentric lesion that is sharply

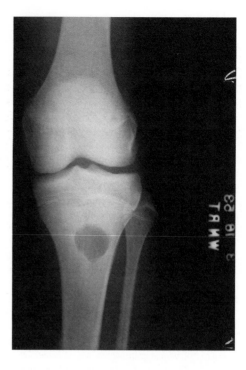

Fig. 1. Eighteen-year-old male with nondescript constant pain in the left upper calf. Anteroposterior radiograph of the left knee reveals classic well-circumscribed eccentric metaphyseal defect of chondromyxoid fibroma.

marginated from the host by a thin sclerotic rim of bone (Fig. 1). The tumor tends to be oval or round in shape, and can appear loculated due to the pseudosepti or corrugations on the surface of the defect that give it this impression. The overlying cortex appears eroded and in some cases expanded into the surrounding soft tissues (Fig. 2). Although radiographically suggestive of total cortical disruption, at the time of surgical exploration a thin film of cortex and overlying periosteum is invariably present. This expansion of the cortex can be symmetrical in the phalanges and the small bones of the foot and hand giving the bone a somewhat fusiform enlargement. In the larger bones of the lower extremity, the orientation of the tumor tends to be in line with the long axis of the bone of involvement. Calcification within these lesions is quite rare in spite of the cartilage derivation of the tumor (Fig. 3(e)).

Epiphyseal or diaphyseal involvement is rare and only seen in the skeletally mature patient. Given the slow evolution of this process, it is not surprising that periosteal new bone formation is a rare finding.

The MRI appearance of this condition, as is true of most tumors of cartilage origin, depends on the proportion of chondroid, myxoid, and fibrous tissue within the lesion. These tumors have shown enhancement after gadolinium administration suggesting increased vascularity. Although not unique, the characteristics of chondromyxoid fibroma as seen on MRI may distinguish this lesion from other bone tumors, but is likely not going to make the definitive distinction between this tumor and other tumors of chondral origin including chondrosarcoma. The MRI allows the full extent of the tumor to be appreciated as compared with plain radiographs (Adams *et al.* 1993). Therefore it has become a very effective imaging tool preoperatively to assist in surgical planning.

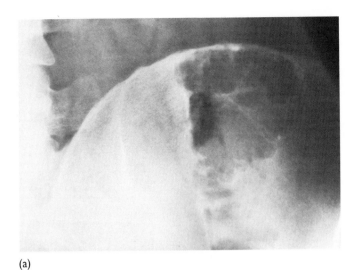

(a)

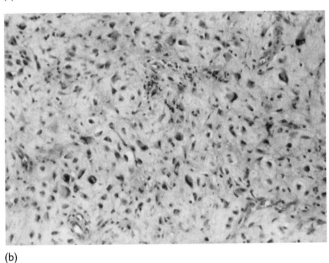

(b)

Fig. 2. Thirty-four-year-old female with left flank pain. (a) Anteroposterior radiograph of left hemipelvis shows a well-circumscribed lytic lesion with sclerotic margins and pseudoseptae consistent with chondromyxoid fibroma. (b) Open biopsy confirms the diagnosis. Despite the presence of atypical cells, the characteristic myxoid background and the presence of chondroid and fibrous bands of cells separating these areas into microlobules makes the diagnosis of chondromyxoid fibroma.

Pathologic features

At the time of tumor excision the macroscopic appearance of the mass appears to be firm, whitish-gray in color, has a very distinct lobulated appearance to it, and shells out from the medullary and cortical defect it has created quite easily (Fig. 3(b)) (Unni and Dahlin 1995). Unlike chondrosarcoma, chondromyxoid fibroma is well marginated from the host, often with a sclerotic rim of bone as well as a fibrous capsule. Although generally having an intact cortex or certainly periosteum over the lesion, approximately one-third will show small extensions of tumor into the surrounding tissues without penetration (Rahimi *et al.* 1972). Less commonly seen is entrapment by medullary bone of small foci of chondromyxoid fibroma independent of the main mass of tumor. It is these small satellites of tumor that

are more likely to be detected on MRI and missed on plain radiographs.

The microscopic appearance of this tumor, as the name implies, includes regions that appear myxomatous, fibrous, and chondroid in appearance. The lobular pattern of growth that is characteristically seen macroscopically is also evident microscopically (Fig. 3(c)). The centers of the lobules are hypocellular with a tendency towards increased cellularity at the periphery. The tumor cells which are generally spindle or stellate in shape, are embedded in the myxoid matrix with approximately half of the lobules showing scattered benign giant cells in close proximity. The sheets of cells between the lobules appearing as septi often have the cellular features of chondroblastoma. The interlobular tissue tends to be composed of oval or spindle-shaped cells with benign multinucleated giant cells becoming more apparent than is seen in the lobules themselves (Fig. 3(d)). If mitotic figures are to be found they are usually present in the cellular interlobular regions occurring in only a small proportion of tumors. Atypical mitotic figures are rarely found nor are they seen with any more frequency than three per high-power field (Unni and Dahlin 1995).

Although rarely seen radiographically, calcification is encountered histologically in approximately one-third of the tumors (Fig. 3(d)). The tendency towards calcification decreases with decreasing age of the patient. Confirming the benign nature of the radiographs, reactive new bone either between lobules or at the periphery of the lesion is not common. Soft-tissue extension was more commonly seen in lesions of the hands and feet in which symmetrical expansion of the bone occurs early along with destruction of the cortex. Secondary aneurysmal bone cyst presence in these tumors is an unusual finding. Similarly, liquefaction and necrosis of the myxoid component of the tumor commonly seen in chondrosarcomas is generally lacking in chondromyxoid fibromas.

It is not uncommon to see cellular atypia with large bizarre cells and nuclei of irregular size and shape which may be multinucleated. The histologic variability of this tumor, even in the same specimen, is a problem when distinguishing it from chondrosarcoma. However, the benign nature of chondromyxoid fibroma is reinforced by the clear and definitive margination between it and the host and the benign-appearing fibrous septa separating the tumor into numerous lobules which is not seen in chondrosarcoma.

The clinical, radiographic, and histopathologic similarities to chondroblastoma, as well as its tendency to stain positively with S-100 protein, suggest that chondromyxoid fibroma is derived from cartilage.

Treatment

Owing to the principally metaphyseal involvement of this tumor and relative sparing of the epiphysis, *en bloc* excision can be performed with either allogeneic or autograft reconstruction. This assures *en bloc* removal of the tumor and minimizes recurrences. However, the intralesional curettage continues to be the mainstay of surgical management despite a recurrence rate of around one in five. Most of these lesions are sufficiently large to warrant grafting to minimize the possibility of pathologic fracture through the defects created. Some authors have suggested that grafting itself may stimulate local recurrence. Other authors have suggested, and successfully per-

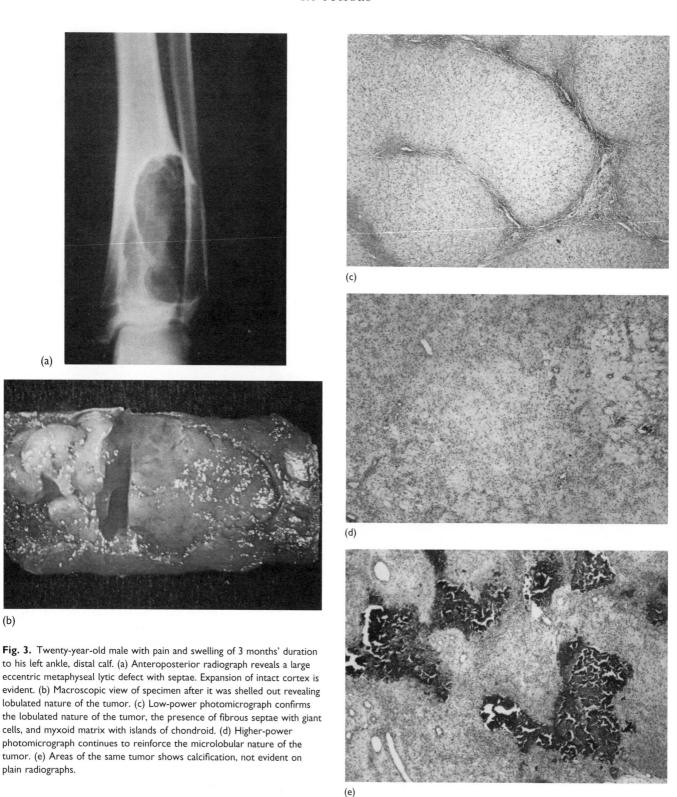

(a)

(b)

(c)

(d)

(e)

Fig. 3. Twenty-year-old male with pain and swelling of 3 months' duration to his left ankle, distal calf. (a) Anteroposterior radiograph reveals a large eccentric metaphyseal lytic defect with septae. Expansion of intact cortex is evident. (b) Macroscopic view of specimen after it was shelled out revealing lobulated nature of the tumor. (c) Low-power photomicrograph confirms the lobulated nature of the tumor, the presence of fibrous septae with giant cells, and myxoid matrix with islands of chondroid. (d) Higher-power photomicrograph continues to reinforce the microlobular nature of the tumor. (e) Areas of the same tumor shows calcification, not evident on plain radiographs.

formed without recurrence, cementation using polymethylmethacrylate into the defect, not unlike what is recommended for a giant cell tumor (Campos Filho *et al.* 1992). The interval to recurrence varies from several months to several years with an average interval of just over 3 years in one large series. Recurrences can generally be treated in similar fashion to the primary. Soft-tissue recurrences of this lesion are rare but have been reported (Troncoso *et al.* 1993). The radiographic appearance is not dissimilar from that of localized myositis ossificans. The reported soft-tissue recurrences have occurred from 4 to 19 years after the diagnosis and management of the initial lesion, and so the association to the initial underlying process may not always be made.

Unlike chondroblastoma, whose proximity to the contiguous joint and epiphyseal plate can create malformations, malalignment, leg-length discrepancies, and late osteoarthritis, these complications are distinctly rare with chondromyxoid fibroma given the metaphyseal nature of the tumor. As such functional deficits after treatment are rare.

Metastases from benign chondromyxoid fibroma have not been reported. Malignant transformation of chondromyxoid fibromas has occurred with and without adjuvant radiation therapy. It is a distinctly unusual event occurring in fewer than 1 per cent of all chondromyxoid fibromas identified to date.

References

Adams, M.J., Spencer, G.M., Totterman, S., and Hicks, D.G. (1993). Quiz: case report 776. *Skeletal Radiology*, **22**, 358–61.

Campos Filho, R., de Camargo, O.P., Croci, A.T., and de Oliveira, N.R. (1992). Chondromyxoid fibroma: a study based on 18 cases. *Revista Paulista de Medicina*, **110**, 59–62.

Rahimi, A., Beabout, J.W., Ivins, J.C., and Dahlin, D.C. (1972). Chondromyxoid fibroma: a clinicopathologic study of 76 cases. *Cancer*, **30**, 726–36.

Troncoso, A., Ro, J.Y., Edeiken, J., Carrasco, C.H., Murray, J.A., and Ayala, A.G. (1993). Case report 798. *Skeletal Radiology*, **22**, 445–8.

Unni, K.K. and Dahlin, D.C. (1995). Chondromyxoid fibroma. In *Dahlin's bone tumors: general aspects and data on 11,087 cases* (5th edn), pp. 59–69. Lippincott–Raven, Philadelphia, PA.

Zillmer, D.A. and Dorfman, H.D. (1989). Chondromyxoid fibroma of bone: 36 cases with clinicopathologic correlation. *Human Pathology*, **20**, 952–64.

1.6.6.5 Chondroblastoma

Michael G. Rock

Introduction

Benign chondroblastoma is a rare tumor of the epiphyseal portion of long bones. It can metastasize but the metastatic lesion is also typically benign. Malignant conversion of chondroblastomas has been reported, and large destructive lesions that appear radiographically malignant but histologically consistent with benign chondroblastomas have been referred to as aggressive chondroblastomas but do not have any of the clinical features of a malignant process.

Box 1 **Classical features of chondroblastoma**

- Fewer than 1 per cent of tumors
- Principally in epiphysis of long bones
- Occurs in adolescents and young adults
- Rarely metastasizes

Recognizing this entity early allows for predictable local surgical control and minimizes malformations and leg-length discrepancies as late sequelae of misdiagnosis or poor treatment.

Clinical presentation

The tumor most commonly presents in male adolescents either in the long bones of the limbs or in flat bones such as the temporal bone.

The most common presenting feature is that of pain, which is often mild, localized to the contiguous joint, and may not be activity related, and diagnosis may be delayed many months. Although less commonly seen, additional symptoms include an effusion in the adjacent joint with associated decreased range of motion, local swelling, atrophy of periarticular muscle, and distortion of the bone which may be noticed if the site of the lesion is subcutaneous. Owing to the periarticular and sometimes intra-articular location of the tumor, patients with this condition are often misdiagnosed as having an intra-articular pathology that is more commonly seen such as meniscal and/or labral tears.

One of the characteristic features of chondroblastoma is simultaneous involvement of the metaphysis and epiphysis. This is most common in the older adolescent whose epiphyseal plate is in the process of closing. Apophyseal involvement occurs less commonly.

Radiographic features

The characteristic site of involvement and the specific age group make the diagnosis of chondroblastoma easier than it otherwise

Box 3 **Radiology of chondroblastoma**

- Commonly involves secondary ossification center of epiphysis
- Commonly crosses epiphyseal plate
- Usually involves medulla of bone not cortex
- No matrix calcification

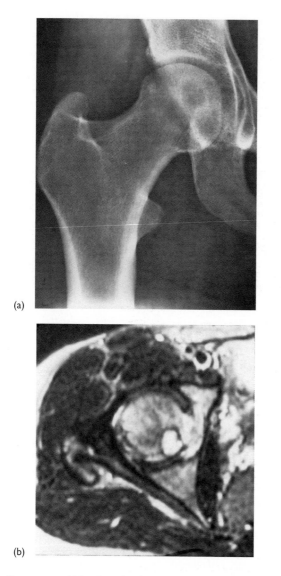

(a)

(b)

Fig. 1. Sixteen-year-old female with a 6-month history of slight groin discomfort and progressive limp. (a) Anteroposterior view of right hip reveals a poorly defined lytic lesion in the epiphysis. (b) T_2-weighted MRI confirms a subchondral lesion in the femoral head, demarcated by a thin layer of bone. Small joint effusion is also present. The hip was dislocated through an anterolateral approach allowing a transarticular access to the chondroblastoma for curettage and grafting.

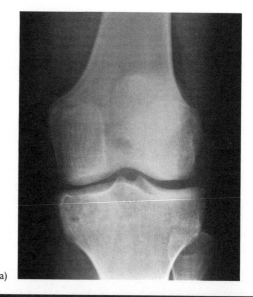

(a)

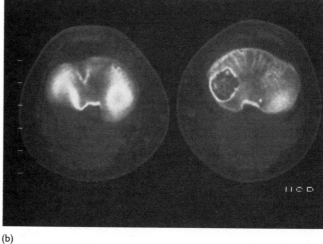

(b)

Fig. 2. Seventeen-year-old skeletally mature male presented with medial joint line pain for 2 months. (a) Anteroposterior view of left knee reveals a lytic lesion in the medial epiphysis with the suggestion of calcification within. (b) CT scan of both proximal tibias confirms a lytic lesion with a well-defined sclerotic rim and punctate calcifications suggesting a cartilage-forming tumor. The tumor was biopsied, confirming chondroblastoma, and was successfully managed with curettage and grafting.

might be. This is particularly true if the lesion involves both the epi- and metaphysis crossing what would appear to be an open epiphyseal plate. Chondroblastomas generally involve the medullary portion of bone, although cortical lesions or surface lesions have been reported. The tumors involving secondary ossification centers are eccentric, oval, well defined, and margined from the surrounding normal medullary bone with or without a sclerotic rim. The overlying cortex may be eroded from within and may even show considerable expansion without periosteal reaction. Matrix calcification is not so commonly seen in this tumor compared with other cartilage tumors. Pathologic fractures are also rare.

Examples of chondroblastoma are shown in Figs 1, 2, 3, and 4.

Imaging

The wide application of MRI has enabled more accurate diagnosis. Chondroblastoma has a low to intermediate heterogeneous signal with lobular internal architecture and fine lobular margins on T_2-weighted MRI that can be distinguished from other tumor and non-tumorous conditions of the meta-epiphysis. The variation in signal intensity likely represents the presence of chondroid matrix, fluid, and mineralization. Although not visible on plain radiographs, con-

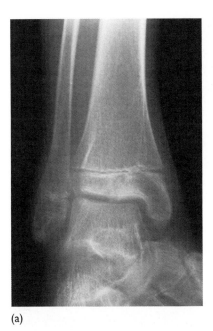 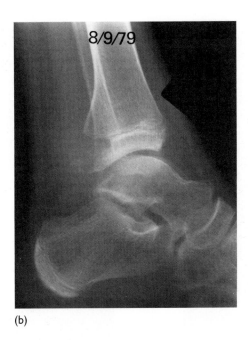 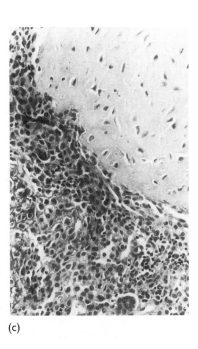

(a)　　　　　　　　　　　(b)　　　　　　　　　　　(c)

Fig. 3. Twelve-year-old male with pain and swelling in his right ankle. (a) Anteroposterior view of right ankle is non-contributory. (b) Lateral view of same ankle reveals a lytic destructive lesion of the posterior epiphysis. The radiographs suggest an aggressive, possibly malignant condition. Biopsy confirmed chondroblastoma, treated successfully with curettage and grafting. Fat was placed at the site of previous epiphyseal plate. No late sequelae. (c) Photomicrograph reveals typical pathologic features of chondroid differentiation plus mineralization between benign giant and mononuclear cells. (Reproduced from Unni and Dahlin (1995).)

tiguous medullary edema and periosteal reaction were commonly seen on MRI. There is usually evidence of periosteal reaction and significant edema in the surrounding muscles. Both of these somewhat unexpected results suggest that chondroblastomas incites an inflammatory response. This tendency decreases with age, possibly a product of epiphyseal closure and periosteal and perichondral maturation.

Histologic features

Although fine-needle aspiration is being used with greater frequency to biopsy suspect lesions, it is not often needed in chondroblastoma, a tumor that has characteristic clinical, radiographic, and MRI findings.

Surgery

The lesion itself is well demarcated from the surrounding normal medullary bone, tends to be gray–pink in color depending on the concentration of chondroid matrix to hemorrhagic areas. It is rarely possible to remove the lesion in its entirety. If present a thin sclerotic rim of bone may be noted around its periphery. There may be areas of obvious cysts suggesting an aneurysmal bone cyst quality to the lesion. Squeezing the tumor between examining fingers reveals a grittiness suggestive of underlying mineralization. Destruction of the epiphyseal plate if extension into the metaphysis has occurred may be obvious. Extension to subchondral bone may allow direct visualization of the basal layers of the articular cartilage.

The histopathologic features reveal medium-sized chondroblasts which tend to be polyhedral or round with well-defined cytoplasmic borders (Campanacci 1990; Marcove and Arlen 1992; Unni and Dahlin 1995). The nucleus is oval and may have a longitudinal groove in the middle creating a coffee-bean appearance. Mild pleomorphism may be seen as is true of frequent mitotic figures. Multinucleated giant cells are present in varying numbers dependent on the concentration of hemorrhage, calcification, or ossification. Most chondroblastomas show chondroid differentiation (Kurt *et al.* 1989). The concentration of chondroid tissue varies considerably and has a characteristic pink stain rather than the customary blue. Periodic foci of calcification may be seen in some cases and more ossification occurs. The calcified areas tend to be lace-like and are often associated with degenerated chondroblasts. This characteristic appearance has prompted the descriptive term of chicken-wire deposition of the calcium as characteristic of this condition.

The tumor cell can have an atypical appearance such as enlarged hyperchromatic nuclei which to the unwary pathologist may suggest a malignancy. To assure the diagnosis of chondroblastoma one must identify either chondroid foci or alternatively foci of calcification. Areas of necrosis are sometimes evident although aneurysmal bone cyst patterns may be the predominant picture. Vascular invasion is rare.

Through extensive histologic review, immunohistochemical staining using peripherating cell nuclear antigen and S-100 protein, electron microscopy, and tissue culturing, it has been confirmed that the derivation of chondroblastomas is that of a chondroid germ line (Marcove and Arlen 1992; Chano *et al.* 1995). The nonepiphyseal location of some tumors imply that the epiphyseal plate may not be the sole contributor to the cell or origin (Brien *et al.* 1995). This is

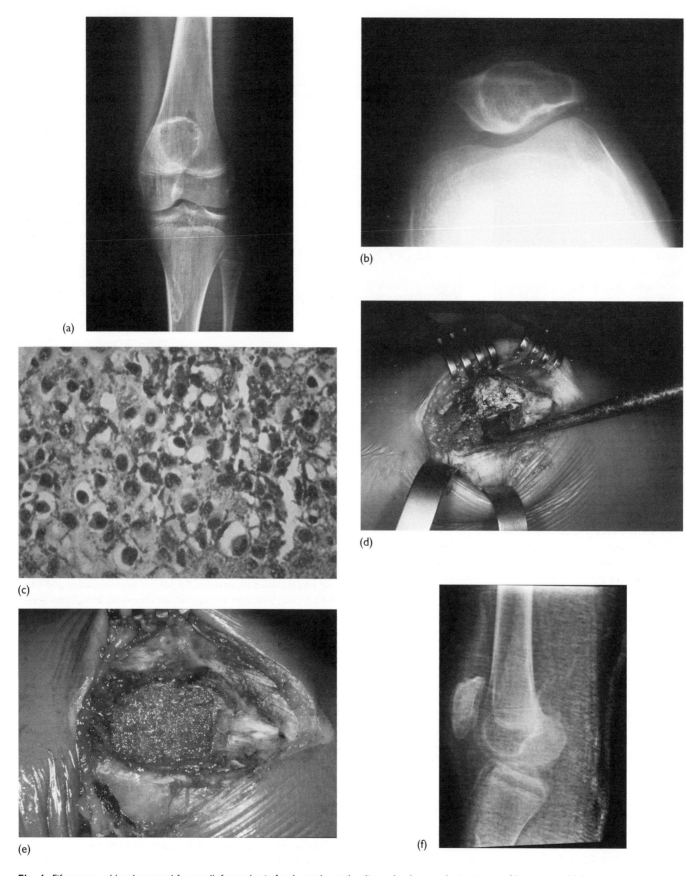

Fig. 4. Fifteen-year-old male treated for patellofemoral pain for 4 months until radiograph taken on the insistence of his parents. (a) Anteroposterior view of left knee reveals a lytic process in the body of the patella. (b) Skyline view of the left patella reveals the lytic, expansile nature of the process. (c) Open biopsy reveals the typical chicken-wire calcification within chondroid matrix and surrounding chondroblasts. (d) The lesion was exteriorized, curetted, chemically cauterized with phenol and alcohol, and grafted. (e) Autogenous graft in place prior to closure of the fascia. (f) Postoperative lateral radiograph.

further reinforced by the appearance of this tumor in the skull bone, suggesting that rarely chondroblastomas may originate from enchondrally formed bone as opposed to the physeal plate.

Treatment

As suggested by the extended time to diagnosis, a chondroblastoma is slow growing and usually does not transgress the epiphyseal plate, and the cortex. The lesions are generally small, between 2 and 4 cm, rarely more than 7 cm, and therefore local control can usually be obtained by simple excision. These include curettage and chemical cauterization in areas that are appropriate to be treated in such fashion, with or without auto- or allogeneic bone grafting. It is obviously best to avoid application of phenol or alcohol to subchondral and/ or epiphyseal plates and areas in which ligaments take origin or insert. With such techniques the local recurrence rate has varied between 10 and 20 per cent. The local recurrence rate in flat bones is higher, rising to 50 per cent in some cases. Some authors believe that the presence of aneurysmal bone cyst-like areas carries with it a higher tendency for local recurrence (Marcove and Arlen 1992). This finding is not shared by a large review of the Mayo Clinic experience (Kurt et al. 1989; Turcotte et al. 1993). Additionally increased numbers of mitotic figures have been associated with a slight increased in aggressiveness and local recurrence (Kurt et al. 1989).

Technical difficulties associated with the management of this condition include the premature closure of the growth plate and involvement of the joint. In an effort to avoid the development of osseous bars, fat, gelfoam, or other substances can be placed across the growth plate to prevent consolidation of graft material across this region. Cortical bone graft can be placed underneath the subchondral bone to add support as the remaining cavity consolidates with the autogenous cancellous bone grafting (Campanacci 1990).

Radiotherapy now has no place in the management of the condition.

The average length of time between initial management and local recurrence is usually only a few years. There appears to be a slight increase in the recurrence among patients who have open epiphyseal plates versus those that are closed or closing with extension of the tumor into the metaphysis (Springfield et al. 1985). This is not entirely unexpected given that at surgery every effort will have been made to minimize damage to the epiphyseal plate. However, there

does not seem to be any correlation with pathologic fractures, poor margination, histopathologic appearance, and vascular invasion with local recurrence (Kurt et al. 1989). Soft-tissue recurrences are rare. Recurrent disease can be treated in a similar fashion to the primary. Few patients experiencing multiple local recurrences.

There have been reports of chondroblastoma removed by arthroscope through an articular defect, when these tumors have been found by chance at surgery. There have been no local recurrences and/or evidence of intra-articular dissemination in these patients at follow-up, but the risks of incomplete excision and dissemination of cells must outweigh the advantages except in areas that are extremely difficult to address by transosseous approach.

Given the anatomic location of these tumors there is a very real concern that its presence and/or surgical management could cause eccentric growth with associated malformations, leg-length discrepancies, and possibly even the induction of degenerative arthritis as a distinct late sequela. A review of chondroblastoma at the Rizzoli Clinic revealed that 58 per cent of patients followed into skeletal maturity were asymptomatic, had a normal range of motion and normal alignment of the involved extremity. Slightly more than 35 per cent of patients had a 20 per cent restriction of motion, shortening of the extremity of less than 2 cm and/or occasional or mild pain not necessitating analgesics (Springfield et al. 1985). The remaining 7 per cent of patients had significant functional restrictions.

In those joints where the capsule inserts below the epiphysis, complications were most uncommon. These lesions are difficult to approach as they are intracapsular and surrounded by articular cartilage and the physis. Surgically the choice is of risking damaging the epiphyseal plate or the articular cartilage with a further risk to the blood supply of the area. It is usually thought better to use an extra-articular approach and risk limb growth abnormality than arthritis in the joint at some later date.

The tumor should be approached by transgressing the articular surface or through the epiphyseal plate. In an effort to avoid transgressing the articular cartilage and minimizing injury to the epiphyseal plate while also preserving blood supply to the region, the authors recommend an extra-articular approach to lesions of the hip and proximal tibia, and an attempt to do the same in the distal femur and proximal humerus. It is assumed that the possible initiation of limb-length discrepancy would be a more attractive alternative or complication than extensive chondrolysis, avascular necrosis, or significant degenerative arthritis at a future date.

One of the more unique characteristics of chondroblastoma is its capability of metastasizing in its benign form. This occurs vary rarely and most often involves the lungs although there have been reports of metastasis to viscera and to ribs (Kurt et al. 1989; Turcotte et al. 1993). Patients with metastatic chondroblastoma can be treated with local removal and anticipate long-term survival.

References

Brien, E.W., Mirra, J.M., and Ippolito, V. (1995). Chondroblastoma arising from a nonepiphyseal site. *Skeletal Radiology*, **24**, 220–2.

Campanacci, M. (1990). *Bone and soft tissue tumors*, pp. 241–52. Springer-Verlag, Vienna.

Chano, T., Ishizawa, M., Matsumoto, K., Morimoto, S., Hukuda, S., and

Okabe, H. (1995). The identity of proliferating cells in bone tumors with cartilaginous components: evaluation by double-immunohistochemical staining using proliferating cell nuclear antigen and S-100 protein. *European Journal of Histochemistry*, **39**, 21–30.

Kurt, A.M., Unni, K.K., Sim, F.H., and McLeod, R.A. (1989). Chondroblastoma of bone. *Human Pathology*, **20**, 965–76.

Marcove, R.C. and Arlen, M. (1992). *Atlas of bone pathology with clinical and radiographic correlations*, pp. 367–71. Lippincott–Raven, Philadelphia, PA.

Springfield, D.S., Capanna, R., Gherlinzoni, F., Picci, P., and Campanacci, M. (1985). Chondroblastoma. A review of 70 cases. *Journal of Bone and Joint Surgery, American Volume*, **67A**, 748–54.

Turcotte, R.E., Kurt, A.M., Sim, F.H., Unni, K.K., and McLeod, R.A. (1993). Chondroblastoma. *Human Pathology*, **24**, 944–9.

Unni, K.K. and Dahlin, D.C. (1995). Bone tumors. In *Dahlin's bone tumors: general aspects and data on 11 087 cases* (5th edn), pp. 47–57. Lippincott–Raven, Philadelphia, PA.

relatively rare skeletal disorder, representing fewer than 2 per cent of all biopsied bone lesions.

The etiology of Langerhans cell histiocytosis remains unknown. The cell of origin is the Langerhans cell, a cell of the dendritic cell system (Egeler and D'Angio 1995; Lieberman *et al.* 1996; de-Graaf and Egeler 1997), and there is some evidence that the disorder may result from a disturbance in immune regulation (Osband *et al.* 1981; Favara 1991). Langerhans cells are roughly 12 μm in diameter and typically have nuclei that are folded, indented, or lobulated (Fig. 1). They are believed to have a role in the T-cell-mediated immune system that involves transfer of antigens. The cytoplasm of the Langerhans cells in the lesions of Langerhans cell histiocytosis contain specific inclusion bodies identical to the Birbeck granules in normal Langerhans cells.

Langerhans cell histiocytosis varies in severity and prognosis from a benign localized disorder that resolves spontaneously to a dissemin-

1.6.6.6 Langerhans cell histiocytosis

Joseph A. Buckwalter, Eric A. Brandser, and Robert A. Robinson

Langerhans cell histiocytosis is a diverse group of disorders of unknown etiology that have in common the proliferation of histiocytic cells and infiltration of these cells into any tissue in the body (Salvatore *et al.* 1994; Lieberman *et al.* 1996; Willis *et al.* 1996). These disorders were formerly referred to as histiocytosis X, and have usually been divided into three syndromes based on their clinical presentation, severity, and prognosis: Letterer–Siwe disease, Hand–Schuller–Christian disease, and eosinophilic granuloma. The most commonly affected tissues are bone, skin, and lymph nodes. Langerhans cells may also invade and proliferate in the liver, lung, spleen, and bone marrow, as well as other organs. Although Langerhans cell histiocytosis involves bone more frequently than other tissues, it is a

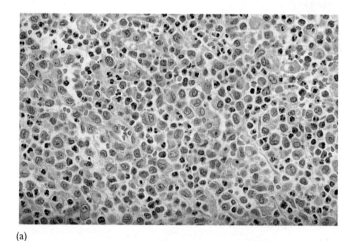

(a)

(b)

Fig. 1. Micrographs showing Langerhans cell histiocytosis. (a) A low-magnification micrograph showing a mixture of large pale cells with light-pink cytoplasm (histiocytes) and large single nuclei, and scattered eosinophils. The eosinophils have intensely bright eosinophilic granules in their cytoplasm and bilobed nuclei. A few polymorphonuclear leucocytes are also present. (b) A higher-magnification micrograph showing the mixture of histiocytes and eosinophils. The granules in the eosinophils are visible and some of the Langerhans cell histiocytes have characteristic nuclear grooves and folds.

Box 1

- A poorly defined group of disorders of unknown etiology that have in common the proliferation of Langerhans cells and infiltration of these cells into any tissue in the body

- Lesions of Langerhans cell histiocytosis consist primarily of collections of histiocytes; eosinophils are a prominent feature in some lesions, but may be difficult to find in others

- More than 75 per cent of patients have skeletal lesions

- Varies from a benign disorder that resolves spontaneously to a progressive fatal disease

- In general, the younger the individual at the time of onset of the disease, the poorer the prognosis and the more extensive the disease

- Treatment may include surgery, chemotherapy, and radiation therapy, depending on the extent and severity of the disease

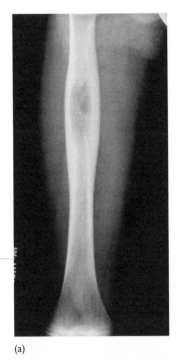

(a)

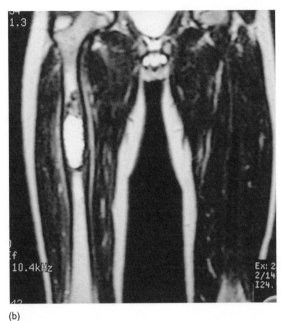

(b)

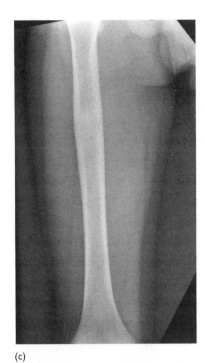

(c)

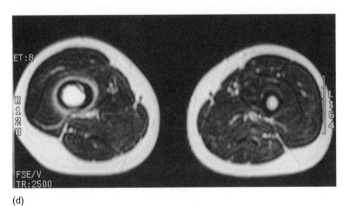

(d)

Fig. 2. Langerhans cell histiocytosis of the femoral diaphysis in a 12-year-old boy. The patient presented with a history of 6 months of increasing thigh pain. He had no systemic symptoms. A bone survey and bone scintigraphy did not show any other lesions. (a) Anteroposterior radiograph of the femur showing a central lytic lesion and expansion of the cortex. (b) Coronal MRI image of the femur showing the diaphyseal lesion. (c) Transverse MRI image of the femur showing the central lesion and a ring of periosteal reaction. (d) Anteroposterior radiograph of the femur 6 months after treatment of the lesion by curettage and grafting with demineralized bone matrix.

ated progressive fatal disease (Salvatore *et al.* 1994; Rivera-Luna *et al.* 1996; Willis *et al.* 1996). In general, the younger the patient at the time of onset of the disease, the poorer the prognosis and the more extensive the disease (Kilpatrick *et al.* 1995; Rivera-Luna *et al.* 1996). Bone lesions appear in more than 75 per cent of patients and vary from small focal collections of Langerhans cells and eosinophils in cancellous bone that can be difficult to detect to masses of cells that destroy cancellous and cortical bone (Figs 2 and 3) (Meyer *et al.* 1995; Lieberman *et al.* 1996; Hindman *et al.* 1998). In its mildest form, Langerhans cell histiocytosis is an isolated lesion in bone. In its most severe form it extends through the skeleton and mulitple viscera. Classically, the various forms of Langerhans cell histiocytosis have been grouped into three categories, although there are many patients with intermediate forms of the disease and one form may change into another form.

The most severe form of Langerhans cell histiocytosis, Letterer–Siwe disease, is most commonly seen in infants and in children less than 3 years of age. This form of the disease has an extremely poor prognosis. Although Letterer–Siwe disease may occur in older chil-

dren, most patients who develop this form of disorder do so within the first year of life. It usually involves the skeleton diffusely, and patients with this disorder commonly have fever, otitis media, papular rash, exophthalmos, hepatosplenomegaly, adenopathy, and cachexia. They are extremely vulnerable to infection. The rapid progression of the skeletal disease may cause generalized osteopenia or multiple small bone defects.

A less severe form of Langerhans cell histiocytosis, Hand–Schuller–Christian disease, occurs most commonly in children older than 1 year and less than 15 years of age. It typically causes multiple skeletal lesions including lesions of the skull as well as diabetes insipidus and exophthalmos. Any bone may be involved, but the vast majority of these patients, probably over 90 per cent, have skull lesions. The bone lesions may range in size from as little as 1 cm to involvement of an entire long bone. Otitis media is the most frequent complaint and a large portion of the patients at some point develop diabetes insipidus and may develop exophthalmos. Lymphadenopathy, hepatosplenomegaly, and anemia are also commonly seen in patients with Hand–Schuller–Christian disease.

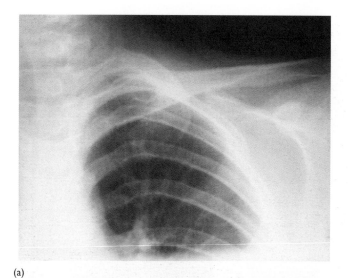

(a)

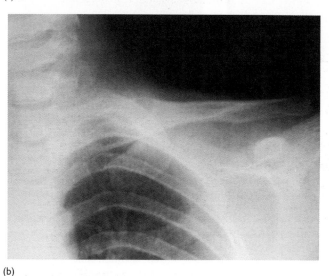

(b)

Fig. 3. Langerhans cell histiocytosis of the clavicle in a 9-year-old boy. (a) Anteroposterior radiograph shows a lucency of the superior medial left clavicle. (b) A 10° cephalic angled radiograph shows the lucent lesion more clearly.

The mildest form of Langerhans cell histiocytosis, frequently referred to as eosinophilic granuloma of bone, generally occurs in individuals between the ages of 5 and 15 years, but it has been reported in middle-aged and elderly adults. Most of the skeletal lesions involve flat bones including the skull, jaw, spine, and pelvis. However, approximately one-third of the lesions occur in long bones (Fig. 2). The common presenting complaint is bone pain. With spinal involvement, collapse of the vertebral body may develop, leading to neurologic symptoms (Fig. 4). Lesions may also cause pathologic fractures of long bones.

Microscopic examination of the lesions of Langerhans cell histiocytosis shows collections of histiocytes (Fig. 1). Eosinophils are a prominent feature in some lesions, but may be difficult to find in others. They may be seen singly, in sheets, or in focal clusters, and the proportions of eosinophils and histiocytes may vary greatly from field to field or from one lesion to another in the same individual. In some instances, eosinophils may be the predominant cell type and in others histiocytes predominate. Demonstration of Birbeck granules by electron microscopy or staining for γ CD1a and S-100 antigens by immunohistochemistry can help establish the diagnosis.

Imaging studies demonstrate the bone lesions of Langerhans cell histiocytosis, but imaging studies alone are rarely sufficient to establish the diagnosis. The radiographic appearance of Langerhans cell histiocytosis in bone varies among patients and locations, and may resemble a variety of other bone lesions. In some patients it causes diffuse osteopenia, but in others it appears as focal, sharply defined lesions or irregular destructive defects with significant reactive bone formation. Lesions of the flat bones and ribs frequently have a punched-out appearance with minimal endosteal or periosteal reaction. Many of the lesions of the long bones are circumscribed by sharply defined endosteal cortical scalloping and moderate periosteal reaction (Fig. 2), although infiltration of bone by Langerhans cells can cause a wide variety of radiographic abnormalities (Hindman et al. 1998). Lesions of the vertebral body present as collapse of the vertebral body, a condition referred to as vertebra plana (Fig. 4). Like plane radiographic studies, bone scans, CT scans and MRI scans are not diagnostic for Langerhans cell histiocytosis. However, CT and MRI (Figs 2 and 4) may be helpful in the assessment of the extent of a lesion especially in sites that are difficult to evaluate with plain radiographs. Bone scans provide a method of indentifying lesions throughout the skeleton, but in some instances they may be negative even when lesions can be demonstrated by radiography (Salvatore et al. 1994; Howarth et al. 1996).

The varied clinical presentation of Langerhans cell histiocytosis can make diagnosis difficult. The clinical and radiographic findings frequently are not specific enough to determine the diagnosis. Some patients may have an elevated erythrocyte sedimentation rate and patients with disseminated disease frequently have anemia (Salvatore et al. 1994). There are no diagnostic laboratory studies, and in many instances biopsy is necessary to establish the diagnosis. However, in patients with vertebra plana, the clinical presentation and radiographic appearance of the vertebra may be sufficient to establish a presumptive diagnosis (Salvatore et al. 1994). In these patients, biopsy is often not necessary, and it may cause a growth disturbance. Patients with diagnosis of Langerhans cell histiocytosis should be evaluated for possible systemic disease, and those with an apparently isolated skeletal lesion should be evaluated for other possible lesions. In most patients this evaluation should include a bone scan and a skeletal survey using radiographs (Howarth et al. 1996; Nieuwenhuyse et al. 1996).

The great variability in the severity and prognosis of Langerhans cell histiocytosis makes it difficult to develop uniform treatment plans. However, increasing clinical experience has helped define a general approach to the management of patients with this disorder. Individuals with isolated bone lesions can be effectively treated by biopsy and curettage of the lesion (Fig. 2). In most instances this leads to healing. In individuals with large, painful bony lesions, and lesions that may lead to pathologic fracture, internal fixation and bone grafting is appropriate. Steroid injection may also be effective treatment for selected bone lesions (Cohen et al. 1980; Capanna et al. 1985; Bernstrand et al. 1996). Individuals with widespread skeletal disease may benefit from low-dose radiotherapy. Patients with sys-

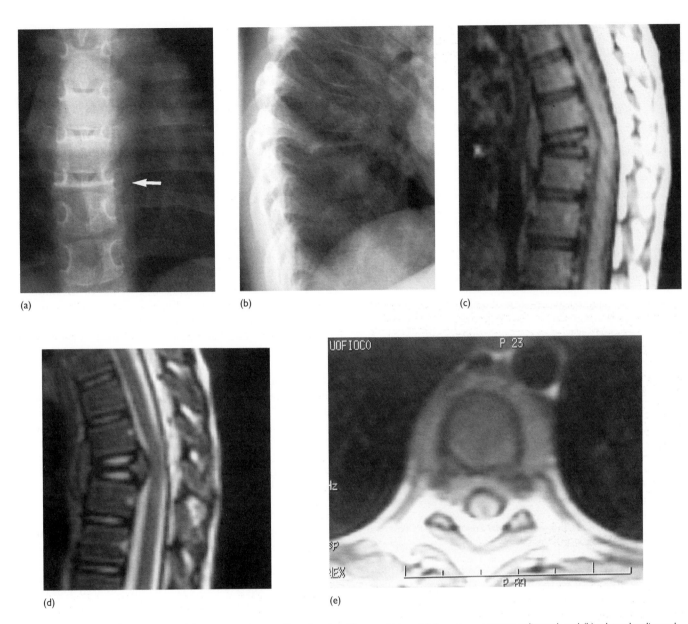

Fig. 4. Langerhans cell histiocytosis of the spine causing vertebra plana in a 12-year-old boy. (a) An anteroposterior radiograph and (b) a lateral radiograph of the thoracic spine show collapse of the T3 vertebral body. (c) T_1-weighted and (d) T_2-weighted sagittal MRI studies show collapse of the vertebral body and displacement of the spinal cord. (e) An axial T_2-weighted MRI study shows circumferential extension of the soft-tissue mass from the vertebral body.

temic symptoms and dysfunction of organs such as the liver, lungs, spleen, or bone marrow should be considered for chemotherapy. Currently accepted drug treatments include corticosteroids and etoposide, vinblastine, methotrexate, and interferon (Salvatore *et al.* 1994; Giona *et al.* 1997).

Even patients with isolated Langerhans cell skeletal histiocytosis should be followed for at least 5 years, as other lesions may appear and recurrences have been reported in approximately 10 per cent of patients (Salvatore *et al.* 1994; Willis *et al.* 1996; Giona *et al.* 1997). None the less, individuals with isolated skeletal Langerhans cell skeletal histiocytosis have an excellent prognosis.

References

Bernstrand, C., Bjork, O., Ahstrom, L., and Henter, J.I. (1996). Intralesional steroids in Langerhans cell histiocytosis of bone. *Acta Paediatrica*, **85**, 502–4.

Capanna, R., Springfield, D.S. Ruggieri, P., *et al.* (1985). Direct cortisone injection in eosinophilic granuloma of bone: a preliminary report on 11 patients. *Journal of Pediatric Orthopedics*, **5**, 339–42.

Cohen, M., Zornoza, J., Cangir, A., Murray, J.A., and Wallace, S. (1980). Direct injection of methylprednisolone sodium succinate in the treatment of solitary eosinophilic granuloma of bone: a report of 9 cases. *Radiology*, **136**, 289–93.

de-Graaf, J.H. and Egeler, R.M. (1997). New insights into the pathogenesis of Langerhans cell histiocytosis. *Current Opinion in Pediatrics*, **9**, 46–50.

Egeler, R.M. and D'Angio, G.J. (1995). Langerhans cell histiocytosis. *Journal of Pediatrics*, **127**, 1–11.

Favara, B.E. (1991). Langerhans cell histiocytosis pathobiology and pathogenesis. *Seminars in Oncoloy*, **18**, 3–7.

Giona, F., Caruso, R., Testi, A.M., *et al.* (1997). Langerhans cell histiocytosis in adults: a clinical and theraputic analysis of 11 patients from a single institution. *Cancer*, **80**, 1786–91.

Hindman, R.W., Thomas, R.D., Young, L.W., and Yu, L. (1998). Langerhans cell histiocytosis: unusual skeletal manifestations observed in thirty-four cases. *Skeletal Radiology*, **27**, 177–81.

Howarth, D.M., Mullan, B.P., Wiseman, G.A., Wenger, D.E., Forstrom, L.A., and Dunn W.L. (1996). Bone scintigraphy evaluated in diagnosing and staging Langerhans cell histiocytosis and related disorders. *Journal of Nuclear Medicine*, **37**, 1456–60.

Kilpatrick, S.E., Wenger, D.E., Gilchrist, G.S., Shives, T.C., Wollan, P.C., and Unni, K.K. (1995). Langerhans cell histiocytosis (histiocytosis X) of bone. A clinicopathologic analysis of 263 pediatric and adult cases. *Cancer*, **76**, 2471–84.

Lieberman, P.H., Jones, C.R., Steinman, R.M., *et al.* (1996). Langerhans cell (eosinophilic) granulomatosis. A clinicopathologic study encompassing 50 years. *American Journal of Surgical Pathology*, **20**, 519–52.

Meyer, J.S., Harty, M.P., Mahboubi, S., *et al.* (1995). Langerhans cell histiocytosis: presentation and evolution of radiologic findings with clinical correlation. *Radiographics*, **15**, 1135–46.

Nieuwenhuyse, J.P., Clapuyt, P., Malghem, J., *et al.* (1996). Radiographic skeletal survey and radionuclide bone scan in Langerhans cell histiocytosis of bone. *Pediatric Radiology*, **26**, 734–8.

Osband, M.E., Lipton, J.M., Lavin, P., *et al.* (1981). Histiocytosis-X: demonstration of abnormal immunity, T-cell histamine receptor deficiency and successful treatment with thymic extract. *New England Journal of Medicine*, **304**, 146–53.

Rivera-Luna, R., Alter-Molchadsky, N., and Cardenas-Cardos, R. (1996). Langerhans cell histiocytosis in children under 2 years of age. *Medical and Pediatric Oncology*, **26**, 334–43.

Salvatore, S., Sommelet, D., Lascombes, P., and Prevot, J. (1994). Treatment of Langerhans-cell histiocytosis in children. *Journal of Bone and Joint Surgery, American Volume*, **76**, 1513–25.

Willis, B., Ablin, A., Weinberg, V., Zoger, S., Wara, W.M., and Matthay, K.K. (1996). Disease course and late sequelae of Langerhans cell histiocytosis: 25-year experience at the University of California San Francisco. *Journal of Clinical Oncology*, **14**, 2073–83.

1.6.6.7 Osteochondroma

Kristy Weber

Introduction

An osteochondroma is a benign developmental defect of growth that may be better classified as a malformation rather than a true neoplasm (Greenspan 1989; Giudici *et al.* 1993; Scarborough and Moreau 1996). The lesion has a bony base and a cartilage cap extending from the surface of the bone. It occurs primarily in the metaphysis of long bones but can arise in any bone initially formed by endochondral ossification. It starts at the level of the epiphyseal plate and becomes more metadiaphyseal with growth of the patient. If more than one osteochondroma is present, a diagnosis of multiple

Box 1

- Most common primary benign bone tumors
- Benign cartilage and bone-forming tumors consisting of a bony base or stalk attached to normal bone and a hyaline cartilage cap covering the base or stalk
- Usually a solitary lesion, but some patients have multiple osteochondromas
- Malignant transformation rarely occurs in patients with solitary lesions, probably fewer than 1 per cent, but patients with multiple osteochondromas probably have a greater risk of malignant transformation
- Development of pain or enlargement following skeletal maturity suggests the possibility of malignant transformation

hereditary exostoses should be made. Solitary lesions are 10 times more common than multiple occurrences.

The most common location for a solitary lesion is the distal femur, proximal tibia, proximal humerus and pelvis. Thirty-six per cent are found about the knee. One to four per cent of solitary osteochondromas occur in the spine, but they rarely cause neurologic compromise. Symptomatic spinal lesions are most often found in the cervical area. Subungual exostoses are uniformly benign growths that arise from the distal phalanx beneath or adjacent to the nail, often in the great toe. Some authors do not consider these lesions in the same category as osteochondromas because of their frequent association with trauma or infection.

Osteochondroma is the most common primary bone tumor and was 41 per cent of benign bone tumors and 19 per cent of all tumors in one series. The true incidence cannot be calculated as so many lesions are asymptomatic and may never be identified. There is a slight male predilection and 69 per cent are found in patients less than 20 years old. Symptomatic lesions present at an even earlier age.

The etiology is felt to be from aberrant epiphyseal plate cartilage that becomes separated from the growth plate, herniates through the bony cuff and absent periosteal ring, and continues to grow via endochondral ossification at the same rate as, but perpendicular to, the adjacent bone (Milgram 1983). As the cartilage undergoes ossification, it forms cancellous bone that becomes the stalk of the lesion. The osteochondroma begins as a portion of growth-plate cartilage, and it stops growing near the time when the adjacent physis closes. Experimentally it has been shown that transplanted rabbit epiphyseal plate cartilage to a location beneath the periosteum develops into a lesion resembling an osteochondroma. However, osteochondromas have also been reported secondary to radiation of patients in the first decade of life (Libshitz and Cohen 1982). Any open growth plate is susceptible, and solitary, as well as multiple, lesions have been found to occur as late as 16 years after the radiation treatment.

Malignant transformation is rare, occurring in approximately 1 per cent of solitary lesions.

Pathology

The gross appearance of an osteochondroma is best described as resembling a cauliflower. It has an irregular surface which is capped by cartilage of varying thickness.

The primary feature on examination is the cartilage cap overlying a stalk of cancellous bone. The cap is usually 0.5 to 1.5 cm thick but thins with age, so that some older patients have only eburnated bone visible at the surface.

Microscopically the cartilage is benign and hyaline in nature with features of a typical growth plate. During skeletal growth, the base of the cartilage cap undergoes endochondral ossification. The cap may be uniform or slightly disorganized especially in the deeper zone of hypertrophic cartilage. It is covered with a well-defined perichondrium made up of fibrous tissue which blends into the periosteum of underlying bone. The bone of the stalk is continuous with the underlying medullary cavity of the native bone. The cartilage is moderately cellular with the chondrocytes evenly spaced in columns in the matrix. Typically the cells have small dark single nuclei. As with most cartilage lesions, there is a variable histologic appearance with occasional increased cellularity, binucleate cells, and mild nuclear atypia. Normal hematopoeitic or fatty marrow is interspersed between the bony trabeculae of the lesion. In particularly large lesions, small areas of cartilage trapped in the bony stalk become calcified. There may be a bursa overlying the osteochondroma which can contain fibrin deposits or calcified cartilage. Normal varients of osteochondroma include those with several cartilage caps separated by bone and others with satellite cartilage areas present deep within the stalk.

The main lesion in the differential diagnosis is a chondrosarcoma. Rarely a secondary chondrosarcoma develops in a pre-existing osteochondroma. Grossly the malignant lesion has an irregular surface with various sized cartilage lobules. It may invade the surrounding soft tissues. Most chondrosarcomas that develop in the cap of an osteochondroma are well differentiated and classified as low grade.

The histologic appearance of a chondrosarcoma is often similar to an osteochondroma, therefore differentiation may depend on clinical and radiologic factors. The previous osteochondroma may often be visible at its base, but it can also be destroyed by the chondrosarcoma. Calcification is frequently present, but at times there is no mineralization. The overall cellularity and nuclear atypia is increased along with a higher number of multinucleate forms. The cap on a grade 1 chondrosarcoma is often disorganized, has moderate cellularity, and can be up to 12 cm wide. Thick cartilage caps simply imply growth and are not a reliable indicator of neoplastic change. There is no absolute rule that correlates cap thickness with malignancy; however, careful attention should be directed toward growing lesions with large cartilage caps.

Rarely a dedifferentiated high-grade sarcoma can occur in relation to an osteochondroma and has the appearance of a malignant fibrous histiocytoma, osteosarcoma, or fibrosarcoma. There is an abrupt transition between the benign or low-grade malignant cartilage lesion and the highly malignant bordering sarcoma. The benign area may be an extremely minor part of the lesion, so the entire specimen must be carefully examined.

Examples of osteochondromas are shown in Figs 1, 2, 3, and 4.

Clinical evaluation

Most osteochondromas are asymptomatic and are noted incidentally during radiographic examination for a different problem. On clinical examination, the osteochondroma is a firm fixed nontender subcutaneous mass. If one is discovered, it is important to search for other lesions. They may be painful if in a location that irritates nearby structures or is likely to involve minor trauma. A stalk fracture can also produce symptoms. Rarely a bursa will form over the cartilage cap and become inflamed. It may be mistaken for an enlarging malignant neoplasm, therefore appropriate imaging studies should be performed to determine the correct diagnosis. If the mass is near a joint, there may be decreased motion. Some lesions are large enough that they are a cosmetic concern for the patient. After closure of the epiphyseal plates, osteochondromas should not continue to grow and may actually disappear, although some have shown slow, benign growth into the third decade. Pregnancy and lactation may stimulate mild growth of the lesion. Reported complications attributed to osteochondromas include popliteal artery pseudoaneurysm, popliteal vein thrombosis, and peroneal nerve palsy.

Malignant transformation of an osteochondroma should be suspected if there is rapid growth after skeletal maturity, increasing pain, or an enlarging mass. It is exceedingly rare to see this change in the pediatric age group and occurs more frequently in patients between 20 and 40 years of age. It is more likely to happen to lesions in axial locations, namely the scapula, pelvis, proximal humerus, and proximal femur. There has been no proven correlation between the size of an osteochondroma and its risk for secondary malignant transformation. Secondary chondrosarcomas in the pelvis may become extremely large before they are discovered. Dedifferentiated chondrosarcomas are particularly aggressive. The usual clinical scenario is long-standing mild pain which suddenly increases coincident with an enlarging mass or pathologic fracture.

Imaging studies

Plain radiographs are usually diagnostic for osteochondromas. Other studies are rarely needed for asymptomatic lesions. The cartilage lesion may be pedunculated or sessile with a broad base. The surface is round or lobulated with a radiolucent cap. The osteochondroma can be 2 to 15 cm in size and grows away from the nearest joint. The stalk consists of thin cortical bone and a medullary cavity that blends imperceptibly with the host bone in contrast to juxtacortical lesions such as periosteal chondroma or parosteal osteosarcoma. Large areas of calcified cartilage may be present throughout the lesion. Rarely, uniform ring-shaped soft-tissue calcifications can occur in a bursa on the surface of the osteochondroma having the appearance of synovial chondromatosis. This should not be mistaken for a chondrosarcoma in which the calcifications are disorganized and irregular.

Signs of malignant transformation include lucencies in the calcified cap or stalk indicating destruction of bone by unmineralized cartilage. The change is more obvious if previous films showed the areas to be mineralized. Dispersed calcifications within the cartilage cap separate from those in the stalk can be another hallmark of malignancy. The surface may have an indistinct appearance. In a more advanced form of secondary chondrosarcoma, only remnants of a bony stalk are apparent at the base of the malignant cartilage mass. In this situation the chondrosarcoma sits on the cortical surface of the affected bone. Wide-based sessile lesions are much more likely to become sarcomatous than the pedunculated forms due to their larger surface area.

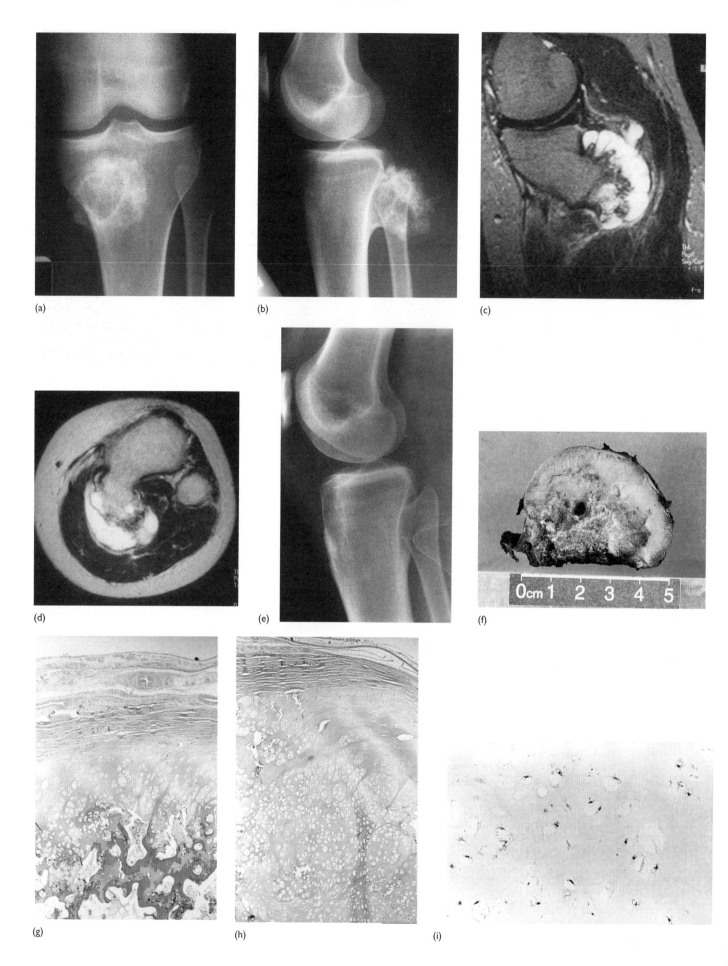

(a)

(b)

(c)

(d)

(e)

(f)

(g)

(h)

(i)

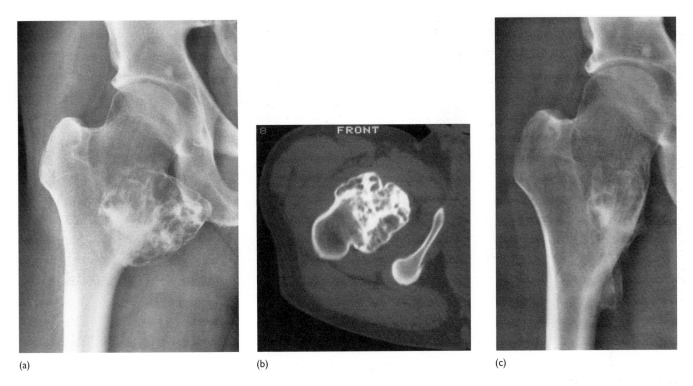

(a)   (b)   (c)

Fig. 2. (a) A proximal femoral osteochondroma in a 40-year-old male. A well-defined border is noted on the anteroposterior radiograph. (b) CT scan reveals the lobular surface and extensive calcification throughout the lesion. (c) Postoperative anteroposterior view after resection of the lesion.

Fig. 3. This histologic appearance shows how the chondrocytes in an osteochondroma are aligned in columns similar to a growth plate.

Fig. 1. (a) Radiographic appearance of an osteochondroma in a 23-year-old female. It is shown in the proximal tibia, a common location for this lesion. (b) The lateral view is necessary for better definition of the posteriorly directed osteochondroma. The medullary cavity of the lesion is continuous with that of the proximal tibia. Note the ring-like cartilage calcification at the periphery of the lesion. (c), (d) MRI T_2-weighted images demonstrate the continuity of the medullary cavity from osteochondroma to native tibia. It also nicely demonstrates the high signal intensity of the hyaline cartilage cap. (e) Postoperative lateral view after resection of the osteochondroma. (f) Gross appearance of the resected osteochondroma. The cartilage cap is approximately 1 cm thick and well circumscribed. (g) Low-power histologic view of the lesion showing chondrocytes arranged in columns with a zone of endochondral ossification at the base. The overlying perichondrium is seen at the periphery. (h) This section through the cartilage cap shows increased cellularity but no nuclear atypia. The overlying perichondrium is easily identified. (i) On higher magnification, the chondrocytes are benign with small, dark nuclei. Abundant basophilic hyaline cartilage matrix is evident.

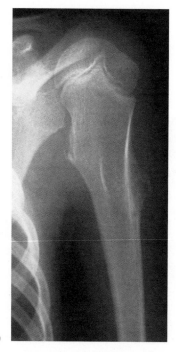

(a)

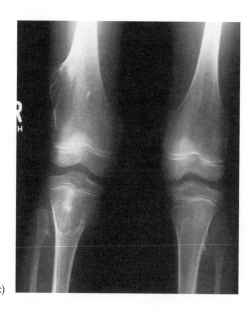

(c)

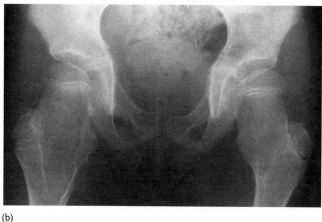

(b)

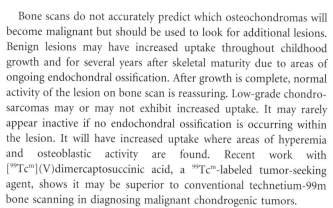

Fig. 4. (a) Radiographic appearance of osteochondromas in a 7-year-old female with the multiple hereditary form. This view shows involvement of the proximal humerus with two sessile lesions. (b) Anteroposterior radiograph of the pelvis revealing a widened proximal femoral metaphysis due to extensive disease involvement. (c) Note the sessile and pedunculated osteochondromas about both knees. Again, metaphyseal widening is characteristic in the distal femur.

Bone scans do not accurately predict which osteochondromas will become malignant but should be used to look for additional lesions. Benign lesions may have increased uptake throughout childhood growth and for several years after skeletal maturity due to areas of ongoing endochondral ossification. After growth is complete, normal activity of the lesion on bone scan is reassuring. Low-grade chondrosarcomas may or may not exhibit increased uptake. It may rarely appear inactive if no endochondral ossification is occurring within the lesion. It will have increased uptake where areas of hyperemia and osteoblastic activity are found. Recent work with $[^{99}Tc^{m}](V)$dimercaptosuccinic acid, a $^{99}Tc^{m}$-labeled tumor-seeking agent, shows it may be superior to conventional technetium-99m bone scanning in diagnosing malignant chondrogenic tumors.

Ultrasound has been used to accurately predict the size of the cartilage cap in superficial lesions. It can also differentiate a symptomatic overlying bursa from a thickened cap. CT scans are unreliable in determining the thickness of the cartilage cap. MRI is not often necessary in diagnosis but is more accurate in measuring the cartilage

cap of an osteochondroma. As mentioned earlier, however, this is not a reliable indicator of malignant degeneration. Both modalities can be used to unequivocally establish whether there is continuity of the medullary canal between the lesion and native bone. This is especially important in differentiating sessile osteochondromas from more malignant lesions as their large surface area makes this continuity difficult to assess with plain radiographs. Both CT scanning and MRI can be used to evaluate the extent of spinal lesions and their relationship to surrounding neural structures. MRI can determine the extent of soft-tissue invasion from a secondary malignancy.

Management and results

The treatment of incidentally found, asymptomatic osteochondromas is nonoperative. The patient should be educated on the rare possibility of malignant change and instructed to return for evaluation if the lesion becomes larger or painful. Resection of lesions in a child should be postponed until after skeletal maturity if possible as the cartilage cap will become smaller and further from the growth plate. The indications for resection include the following:

(1) symptomatic lesions due to an overlying bursa;

(2) lesions in a location subjected to frequent minor trauma;

(3) significant cosmetic deformity;

(4) lesions causing actual or potential damage to surrounding joints or neurovascular structures; and

(5) lesions suspicious for malignant transformation.

The cartilage cap and perichondrium are the pathologic tissues, and both should be removed to prevent recurrence which occurs in fewer than 2 per cent of solitary lesions. It is most common in the sessile forms due to their large base, therefore a wider resection is recommended in these types. Spinal lesions causing neurologic compromise should be resected either *en bloc* or in piecemeal fashion. Most patients have excellent recovery of function and rare likelihood of recurrence.

Rapid growth after maturity or increasing pain in an osteochondroma are suspicious symptoms for sarcomatous degeneration occurring in only 1 per cent of solitary lesions. Most resulting neoplasms are chondrosarcomas but osteosarcomas have also been reported. One study of 75 secondary chondrosarcomas included 40 solitary and 35 multiple lesions (Garrison *et al.* 1982). Although the lesions were usually low grade, simple excision resulted in a 78 per cent recurrence rate. Amputation or resection including a cuff of surrounding tissue generally resulted in a cure, although there was still a 15 per cent recurrence rate. The increased recurrence is likely due to the difficulty in determining the local extent of the lesion. These tumors have a predilection for the pelvic bones where the anatomy complicates the resection. Recurrences were noted up to 10 years after the original treatment. Twelve patients died of their tumor, usually from a complication of local recurrence. Only two patients were known to have developed metastases. In general, higher-grade lesions are associated with a poorer prognosis and a higher frequency of metastases.

Dedifferentiated chondrosarcomas develop extremely rarely from osteochondromas. The surgical treatment is wide resection or amputation. In one study, five of seven affected patients died of metastases, four within 1 year of surgical treatment. The remaining two are surviving without evidence of disease. In a different study of 78 dedifferentiated chondrosarcomas, eight were considered peripheral and five of those occurred in an osteochondroma. The overall 5-year survival rate for the dedifferentiated lesion in general is approximately 10 per cent.

Multiple osteochondromas

This condition is inherited as an autosomal dominant skeletal dysplasia with a prevalence of approximately one case per 50 000 population. If a person whose family is affected has not developed an osteochondroma by age 12, they will most likely remain free of lesions. Multiple osteochondroma is the most common skeletal dysplasia and is associated with short stature and long bone deformities. The affected patient is usually diagnosed after age 2 with noticeable palpable lesions numbering up to 30. The sexes are equally affected in recent studies, but males have more severe manifestations and seek medical attention more frequently. The lesions are present in the metaphysis of almost all long bones but can be diaphyseal. Flat bones, with the exception of the craniofacial skeleton, can also be affected. Spinal osteochondromas comprise 7 per cent of the lesions and are more likely to cause neurologic compromise than in patients with solitary lesions.

Histologic features of the individual lesions are similar to solitary osteochondromas. Radiographically the lesions are often larger and there is characteristic metaphyseal widening due to a lack of bony remodeling when multiple lesions are present.

Clinically there are multiple manifestations and deformities. The main orthopedic concerns stem from deformities in the forearm and lower leg where the paired bones (radius–ulna, tibia–fibula) are affected in differing degrees. This creates growth discrepancies. Removal of osteochondromas throughout the skeleton should be selective and focus on those growing or causing symptoms secondary to their anatomic location.

In the upper extremities a snapping scapula is due to osteochondromas on the vertebral margin. Proximal humeral lesions are commonly seen. Forearm deformities can be severe and are due to involvement of the distal ulna. Numerous studies have addressed treatment options. The deformities of the forearm are classified into three groups. Group 1 is the most common and includes ulnar shortening and bowing of the radius. Group 2 also has ulnar shortening in combination with radial head dislocation. Group 3 involves relative radial shortening. Peterson (1994) feels that these deformities should be aggressively treated to reduce their progression, prevent dislocation of the radial head, and minimize functional impairment of the patient. General treatment options include resection of the lesions combined with ulnar lengthening or radial hemiepiphysiodesis, radial osteotomy, and possible radial head resection. Ilizarov techniques have been used for gradual correction of the deformities although potential complications are significant. Some advocate early intervention to prevent severe deformity whereas others delay surgical treatment until skeletal maturity to decrease the risk of recurrence. In general, surgery improves cosmetic appearance more than function. In rare, recalcitrant cases a one bone forearm can be constructed as a salvage procedure.

In the lower extremities coxa magna and coxa vara deformities are seen in the proximal femur often predisposing the patient to early degenerative disease. The knee is often in valgus due to a valgus deformity within the tibia. A short fibula is common. The ankle can be in valgus and compensated by a varus deformity of the talus. Leg-length discrepancy is 4 cm. Patients frequently require multiple lower extremity surgeries at a young age. Treatment includes deformity correction by epiphysiodeses or osteotomies in severe cases.

Reports of malignant transformation in this condition have varied from 1 to 25 per cent. Many of the reports are falsely high owing to the referral nature of the reporting centers; therefore the likelihood of malignancy is probably closer to 1 per cent (Schmale *et al.* 1994). It is possible that this percentage increases with the length of follow-up or that it varies among affected families, reflecting genetic heterogeneity. Most malignant lesions are chondrosarcomas, although there have been reports of osteosarcomas and malignant fibrous histiocytomas developing in patients with multiple osteochondromas. In solitary lesions, both long and flat bones are equally affected, but in osteochondromatosis, central lesions in the shoulder girdle and pelvis are more likely to become sarcomatous.

Genetic studies have suggested that genes causing multiple osteochondromas may have a tumor-suppressor function, the loss of which may lead to the development of malignancy. Further research should provide more concrete chromosomal localization of these genes.

Further reading

Albrecht, S., Crutchfield, J., and SeGall, G. (1992). On spinal osteochondromas. *Journal of Neurosurgery*, **77**, 247–52.

Bertoni, F., Present, D., Bacchini, P., *et al.* (1989). Dedifferentiated peripheral chondrosarcomas. *Cancer*, **63**, 2054–9.

Borges, A., Huvos, A., and Smith, J. (1981). Bursa formation and synovial chondrometaplasia associated with osteochondromas. *American Journal of Clinical Pathology*, **75**, 648–53.

Burgess, R. and Cates, H. (1993). Deformities of the forearm in patients who have multiple cartilaginous exostoses. *Journal of Bone and Joint Surgery, American Volume*, **75A**, 13–18.

Dahl, M. (1993). The gradual correction of forearm deformities in multiple hereditary exostoses. *Hand Clinics*, **9**, 707–18.

D'Ambrosia, R. and Ferguson, A. (1968). The formation of osteochondroma by epiphyseal cartilage transplantation. *Clinical Orthopaedics and Related Research*, **61**, 103–15.

El-Khoury, G. and Bassett, G. (1979). Symptomatic bursa formation with osteochondromas. *American Journal of Roentgenology*, **133**, 895–98.

Frassica, F., Unni, K., Beabout, J., and Sim, F. (1986). Dedifferentiated chondrosarcoma. A report of the clinicopathological features and treatment of seventy-eight cases. *Journal of Bone and Joint Surgery, American Volume*, **68A**, 1197–205.

Griffiths, H., Thompson, R., Galloway, H., Everson, L., and Suh, J. (1991). Bursitis in association with solitary osteochondromas presenting as mass lesions. *Skeletal Radiology*, **20**, 513–16.

Hecht, J., Hogue, D., Strong, L., Hansen, M., Blanton, S., and Wagner, M. (1995). Hereditary multiple exostosis and chondrosarcoma: linkage to chromosome 11 and loss of heterozygosity for EXT-linked markers on chromosomes 11 and 8. *American Journal of Human Genetics*, **56**, 1125–31.

Johnston, C. and Sklar, F. (1988). Multiple hereditary exostoses with spinal cord compression. *Pediatric Orthopedics*, **11**, 1213–16.

Kobayashi, H., Kotoura, Y., Hosono, M., *et al.* (1995). Diagnostic value of Tc-99m (V) DMSA for chondrogenic tumors with positive Tc-99m HMDP uptake on bone scintigraphy. *Clinical Nuclear Medicine*, **20**, 361–4.

Landon, G., Johnson, K., and Dahlin, D. (1979). Subungual exostoses. *Journal of Bone and Joint Surgery, American Volume*, **61A**, 256–9.

Lange, R., Lange, T., and Rao, B. (1984). Correlative radiographic, scintigraphic, and histological evaluation of exostoses. *Journal of Bone and Joint Surgery, American Volume*, **66A**, 1454–9.

Lizama, V., Zerbini, M., Gagliardi, R., and Howell, L. (1987). Popliteal vein thrombosis and popliteal artery pseudoaneurysm complicating osteochondroma of the femur. *American Journal of Roentgenology*, **148**, 783–4.

Malghem, J., Vande Berg, B., Noel, H., and Maldague, B. (1992). Benign osteochondromas and exostotic chondrosarcomas: evaluation of cartilage cap thickness by ultrasound. *Skeletal Radiology*, **21**, 33–7.

Masada, K., Tsuyuguchi, Y., Kawai, H., Kawabata, H., and Noguchi, K. (1989). Operations for forearm deformity caused by multiple osteochondromas. *Journal of Bone and Joint Surgery, British Volume*, **71B**, 24–9.

Mercuri, M., Picci, P., Campanacci, M., and Rulli, E. (1995). Dedifferentiated chondrosarcoma. *Skeletal Radiology*, **24**, 409–16.

Peterson, H. (1989). Multiple hereditary osteochondromata. *Clinical Orthopaedics and Related Research*, **239**, 222–30.

Raskind, W., Conrad, E., Chansky, H., and Matsushita, M. (1995). Loss of heterozygosity in chondrosarcomas for markers linked to hereditary multiple exostoses loci on chromosomes 8 and 11. *American Journal of Human Genetics*, **56**, 1132–9.

Rodgers, W. and Hall, J. (1993). One-bone forearm as a salvage procedure for recalcitrant forearm deformity in hereditary multiple exostoses. *Journal of Pediatric Orthopedics*, **13**, 587–91.

Schajowicz, F. (1994). *Tumors and tumorlike lesions of bone* (2nd edn), pp. 160–71. Springer-Verlag, Berlin.

Shapiro, F., Simon, S., and Glimcher, M. (1979). Hereditary multiple exostoses. *Journal of Bone and Joint Surgery, American Volume*, **61A**, 815–24.

Voutsinas, S. and Wynne-Davies, R. (1983). The infrequency of malignant disease in diaphyseal aclasis and neurofibromatosis. *Journal of Medical Genetics*, **20**, 345–9.

Watson, L. and Torch, M. (1993). Peroneal nerve palsy secondary to compression from an osteochondroma. *Orthopedics*, **16**, 707–9.

Wicklund, C., Pauli, R., Johnston, D., and Hecht, J. (1995). Natural history study of hereditary multiple exostoses. *American Journal of Medical Genetics*, **55**, 43–6.

References

Garrison, R., Unni, K., McLeod, R., Pritchard, D., and Dahlin, D. (1982). Chondrosarcoma arising in osteochondroma. *Cancer*, **49**, 1890–7.

Giudici, M., Moser, R., and Kransdorf, M. (1993). Cartilaginous bone tumors. *Radiologic Clinics of North America*, **31**, 237–59.

Greenspan, A. (1989). Tumors of cartilage origin. *Orthopedic Clinics of North America*, **20**, 347–66.

Libshitz, H. and Cohen, M. (1982). Radiation-induced osteochondromas. *Radiology*, **142**, 643–7.

Milgram, J. (1983). The origins of osteochondromas and enchondromas. A histopathologic study. *Clinical Orthopaedics and Related Research*, **174**, 264–84.

Peterson, H. (1994). Deformities and problems of the forearm in children with multiple hereditary osteochondromata. *Journal of Pediatric Orthopedics*, **14**, 92–100.

Scarborough, M. and Moreau, G. (1996). Benign cartilage tumors. *Orthopedic Clinics of North America*, **27**, 583–9.

Schmale, G., Conrad, E., and Raskind, W. (1994). The natural history of hereditary multiple exostoses. *Journal of Bone and Joint Surgery, American Volume*, **76A**, 986–92.

1.6.6.8 Enchondroma

Kristy Weber

Introduction

An enchondroma is a benign hyaline cartilage proliferation occurring in the central portion of the metaphysis or metadiaphysis of long bones (Giudici *et al.* 1993; Scarborough and Moreau 1996). Along with periosteal chondroma, it is a member of the larger category of chondromas. Enchondromas can be classified according to Enneking (1986) as latent or inactive benign lesions of bone. Common locations are the bones of the hand and foot followed by the humerus, femur, and tibia. It is the most common primary bone tumor in the hand and usually involves the entire shaft of the phalanx. Enchondromas are found almost exclusively in the appendicular skeleton. Epiphyseal lesions comprise 10 per cent and may resemble clear-cell chondrosarcomas. Enchondromas comprise 12 to 24 per cent of benign bone tumors and can occur at any age, although most are identified in patients aged 20 to 50 years. Males and females are affected equally. Two syndromes involving multiple lesions will be discussed later in this chapter.

The etiology of enchondromas is unproven but is thought to be the result of incomplete endochondral ossification leaving embryonic rests of dysplastic cartilage in the metaphysis (Milgram 1983). This would explain why they are found exclusively in bones formed by endochondral ossification and never in bones formed by membranous ossification such as the skull. These cartilage islands do not form bone but continue to grow and stay in the central portion of long bones. Like many other tumors occurring in childhood, the enchondroma stays in one place, but the bone continues to grow causing the area of cartilage to appear more diaphyseal with time.

There is a rare incidence of malignant transformation estimated to occur in fewer than 1 per cent of solitary lesions. No one knows exactly, as the true incidence of enchondromas is unclear.

Pathology

On gross inspection, the enchondroma is a well-circumscribed lesion with discrete cartilage lobules that measure up to 1 cm in size. The hyaline cartilage is blue–white in color with yellowish calcification seen throughout the specimen. It is rare to see an entire resected enchondroma.

Evaluation of cartilage lesions based solely on the histological picture is extremely difficult. Differentiation between enchondromas and low-grade chondrosarcomas is troublesome for even the most experienced bone pathologists. It is therefore essential to correlate the clinical and radiographic presentation of the lesion with the pathology in order to plan the best course of treatment for the patient. The histologic picture does not necessarily predict the aggressiveness of the tumor and needs to be interpreted in the context of these other disciplines.

In general, viewing the lesion under low power can elucidate the growth pattern. An enchondroma is sharply marginated and consists of small hyaline cartilage lobules with abundant extracellular matrix. There is a rim of woven or lamellar bone directly apposed to the cartilage lobules which is reminiscent of previous endochondral ossification at the lesion's edge. The lobules themselves are separated by normal marrow elements, a picture not seen in higher-grade cartilage lesions. This should not be interpreted as an infiltrative process. There is never cortical destruction or a soft-tissue mass associated with an enchondroma. As patients increase in age, the lesion tends to be more calcified.

High-power magnification is used to decide the cytologic grade. This is much less important than the overall architecture, as there is considerable overlap when viewing benign and low-grade malignant lesions under high power. Normal-appearing chondrocytes are seen in their lacunar spaces. The cells are uniform with small dark nuclei. The overall appearance is hypocellular. No necrotic cells or mitotic figures are seen. There may be occasional binucleate but no multinucleate cells. However, as the cells may rarely appear malignant, clinical and radiographic correlation is essential. Lesions in the hands and feet as well as in patients with multiple enchondromas are usually more cellular with a higher number of binucleate forms. They may also have a myxoid matrix. As the hand enchondromas present with a more aggressive picture, it is particularly important to examine the curetted specimen carefully. Cartilage tumors are positive for S-100 protein which is occasionally helpful in differentiating enchondromas from noncartilagenous lesions.

The only lesion in the differential diagnosis of an enchondroma histologically is a chondrosarcoma. Mirra *et al.* (1985) developed an important histologic approach to identify each of these two lesions. Under low-power magnification, a low-grade chondrosarcoma will have poorly identified margins. An uneven distribution of confluent cartilage lobules are separated by fibrous bands instead of normal marrow. Focal calcification may be seen but is less prevalent than in an enchondroma. No bone formation is noted on the periphery of the cartilage lobules. The lesion itself permeates through the marrow spaces and can surround the native lamellar bone. There is infiltration of the cortex and may be a soft-tissue mass.

On high power, the tissue of a chondrosarcoma is more hypercellular than an enchondroma, with common binucleate and rare multinucleate cells. Mitotic figures are rare but may be present. There is increased pleomorphism and individual cell necrosis. There can be overlapping areas of enchondroma and low-grade chondrosarcoma in the same tumor, so care must be taken in interpreting small tissue samples.

A dedifferentiated chondrosarcoma is rarely associated with an enchondroma and consists histologically of the underlying cartilage lesion juxtaposed to a high-grade noncartilaginous sarcoma. The cartilage component can be benign or malignant, and the sarcoma is most frequently malignant fibrous histiocytoma, osteosarcoma, or fibrosarcoma. There is an abrupt histologic transition between the two tumors.

There has been great interest in developing a reliable test to differentiate an enchondroma from a low-grade chondrosarcoma, as treatment options differ depending on the correct diagnosis. Traditional ways of determining aggressiveness such as cellularity or mitotic figures are not always effective in solving the problem.

Flow cytometry is a method by which researchers have tried to correlate behavior of cartilage tumors with chondrocyte DNA content. Studies have shown that the hyperploid cells are closely associated with aggressive chondrosarcomas; however, it is not as reliable for differentiating enchondromas from low-grade malignancies as both have primarily diploid cells.

Recent work with the monoclonal antibody Ki-67 has yielded promising results. The premise is that low-grade chondrosarcomas are growing slowly and enchondromas are not. Certain nuclear proteins are present in cycling but not resting cells. One of these reacts with Ki-67 and can easily be identified after staining the cells of a cartilage neoplasm. Studies on other solid tumors of the brain, colon, and uterus have demonstrated that the number of Ki-67-positive cells correlates with the aggressiveness of the lesion.

Weinstein and McCarthy (1995) examined original central cartilage tumor specimens from 36 patients after Ki-67 staining. They graded and compared the amount of Ki-67 present in the chondrocytes of 20 enchondromas (four in the hands or feet), six low-grade chondrosarcomas and 10 high-grade chondrosarcomas using fetal cartilage as a control. Positive staining of chondrocytes was noted in only three enchondromas, all located in the hand. The majority of enchondromas were treated with curettage and none had recurred 1 to 20 years later. Four of the six low-grade chondrosarcomas had positively stained chondrocytes. All patients had been treated with segmental resection of the tumor without recurrence. All 10 high-grade chondrosarcomas had Ki-67-positive chondrocytes. They were treated with resection or amputation. Four patients were either dead from the disease or alive with lung metastases. Ki-67 immunostaining is therefore a useful adjunct to routine histologic studies, as positive chondrocyte nuclear staining indicates tumor growth. Positivity in lesions of the hand or foot, however, should not be regarded as a hallmark of malignancy as enchondromas in these locations are typically more cellular but rarely undergo malignant change. The same is true of cartilage lesions in childhood.

Similar work has found another antibody, PC-10, which stains a different nuclear protein, and its presence also correlates with aggressiveness of cartilage neoplasms.

Clinical evaluation

Enchondromas are usually found incidentally in the hands or long bones when patients are undergoing radiographic evaluation for a separate concern. They are generally asymptomatic unless there has been a pathologic fracture through the lesion. Enchondromas in the hands can be painful due to small stress fractures through the lytic areas. Painless swelling of the extremity can occasionally be seen, but lesions should not exhibit growth in the skeletally mature patient. Laboratory studies are normal.

A growing lesion or pain in the absence of a pathologic fracture is highly suspicious for a more malignant lesion. Other causes of pain including recent trauma or nearby degenerative changes must be ruled out first. Malignant transformation does not generally occur in childhood or from lesions in the hand at any age.

Examples of enchondromas are shown in Figs 1 and 2.

Imaging studies

Plain radiographs are diagnostic and reveal the enchondroma to be a long, oval, lytic lesion in the intramedullary canal. It is located centrally in the metaphysis or metadiaphysis. The majority of enchondromas are solitary and well delineated. In younger patients, the lesion is purely lytic but, with the exception of hand lesions, the cartilage calcifies with age. The calcification appears as punctate stippling or 'O-rings' within the enchondroma. The cortex remains intact and there is no periosteal reaction or cortical thickening. There may be bony expansion but no endosteal scalloping in long bones. Even in the hand the cortex may be thinned, but it is not violated.

The radiographic differential diagnosis includes nonossifying fibroma, unicameral bone cyst, epidermoid cyst of the distal phalanx, chondromyxoid fibroma, bone infarct, and fibrous dysplasia, especially when there are multiple lesions. A bone infarct, especially if heavily calcified, can present radiographically as an enchondroma. The cartilage lesion can be identified by its lobular margins and lack of the sclerotic outline typically seen in an infarct. The primary lesion to distinguish from an enchondroma is a low-grade chondrosarcoma. It will usually be larger than an enchondroma with poorly defined margins and cortical destruction. Endosteal erosion can be seen. Based on radiographic and histologic evidence, some speculate that most central chondrosarcomas arise from enchondromas.

Enchondromas may or may not be 'hot' on bone scans. When the lesion is actively growing the scan is most likely to be positive and remain so into early adulthood. Technetium-99m bone scanning shows a high sensitivity for bone tumors but has poor specificity in distinguishing benign from malignant forms. A recent study evaluated the use of [^{99}Tc^m](V)dimercaptosuccinic acid, a ^{99}Tc^m-labeled tumor-seeking agent, in differentiating benign versus malignant cartilage tumors. The authors found uniform positive uptake in all chondrosarcomas and uptake in only 12 out of 27 osteochondromas and enchondromas that had previously been positive with conventional technetium-99m scanning (Kobayashi et al. 1995).

A CT scan is helpful in studying the endosteal surface of the lesion for cortical destruction. Some obtain CT scans at skeletal maturity to serve as a baseline for future comparison. MRI findings in enchondromas have low sensitivity and specificity. However, recent studies have shown characteristic T_2-weighted MRI findings in low-grade chondrosarcomas. Low-signal-intensity septa combined with a ring-and-arc enhancement pattern has a sensitivity of 92.3 per cent and specificity of 76.5 per cent for these lesions. Therefore in complicated cases MRI, in addition to plain radiographs, may be helpful.

Management and results

The management of an asymptomatic solitary enchondroma should include careful follow-up but no surgical intervention. Occasional resolution of the lesion has been reported with improvement in the radiographs. Prophylactic resection of enchondromas is inappropriate. The physician should educate the patient in terms of the less than 1 per cent risk for malignant transformation so that the patient will be alerted to any signs of pain. Some patients will be uncomfort-

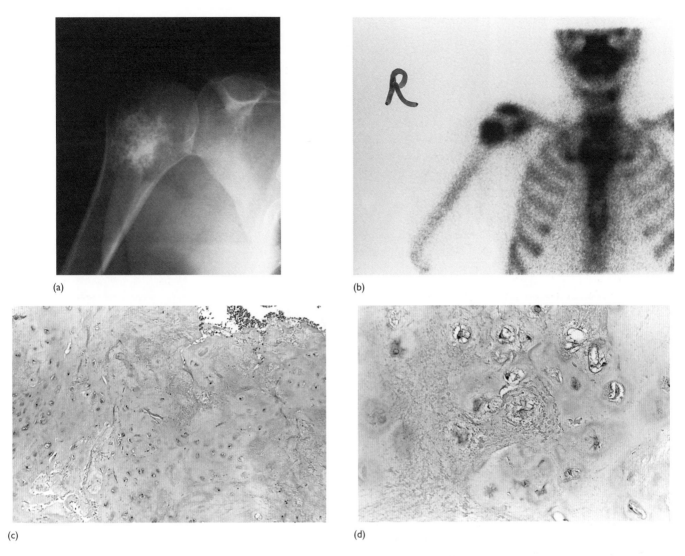

Fig. 1. (a) This is a typical presentation of an enchondroma in a 55-year-old female. The proximal humerus is a common location. Note the stippled calcifications and 'O-rings' consistent with calcified cartilage. (b) The lesion showed increased uptake on bone scan. The patient had pain in the right shoulder which could not be attributed to other causes; therefore curettage and bone grafting of the lesion was performed. (c) Histologic examination of the curetted specimen. Low-power view reveals a hyaline cartilage lesion that is relatively hypocellular. (d) High-power view shows extensive basophilic matrix and benign-appearing chondrocytes. No atypia or binucleate forms are seen.

able with the risk and request a biopsy. Incisional biopsy of an enchondroma should be interpreted with great caution. The pathologist will not have the entire lesion to study and, as discussed previously, the histologic appearance of cartilage lesions must be understood in light of the clinical and radiographic information. Lesions in the pelvis or shoulder girdle should be followed carefully and treated aggressively if symptomatic as they are associated with a higher recurrence rate and can be difficult to control. If a pathologic fracture occurs through an enchondroma, the bone should be allowed to heal prior to surgical intervention.

Enlarging lesions in mature patients or symptomatic enchondromas at any age should be treated with intralesional curettage. Bone grafting with allograft, autograft, or bone-substituting agents should be used for large defects. The recurrence rate for benign lesions after simple curettage is less than 5 per cent.

If there is a high suspicion for malignant transformation based on clinical and radiographic findings, *en bloc* resection of the lesion is recommended. As chondrosarcomas arising in enchondromas are low grade, this treatment is usually curable. Reports of malignant transformation to chondrosarcomas have generally been seen in cases involving multiple enchondromas. Only a handful of well-documented cases of this occurring in solitary enchondromas have been described.

One study reviewed 74 cases of dedifferentiated chondrosarcoma of which 64 originated from central cartilage lesions (Mercuri *et al.* 1995). Ten of these were initially enchondromas and the rest were various grades of chondrosarcomas. Sometimes, the benign cartilage component is an extremely minor portion of the entire lesion, therefore study of the entire lesion is important. In the above study, the overall 5-year survival rate was 13 per cent with a high incidence of local recurrence and metastases. Adjuvant chemotherapy or irradiation was without benefit. The surgical treatment is wide resection or

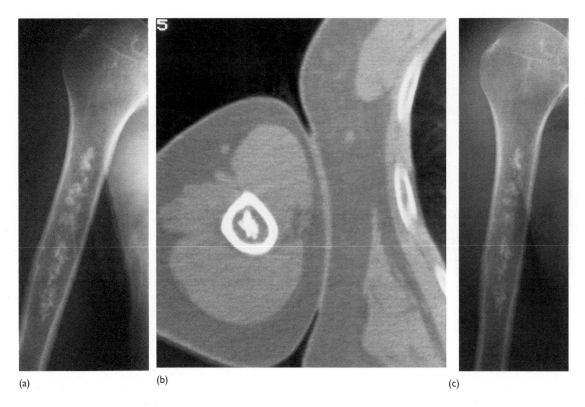

(a)   (b)   (c)

Fig. 2. (a) A humeral enchondroma in a 40-year-old male with mild right shoulder pain. Typical ring-like calcification is seen in this large diaphyseal lesion. Note that the cortex is expanded slightly but not penetrated. The mild endosteal erosion is of concern, but the patient elected continued conservative management of the lesion. (b) CT scan through the center of the lesion confirms no cortical destruction. (c) The patient was treated conservatively and 2 years later was asymptomatic with no radiographic evidence of progression.

amputation. Recurrences from skip lesions can occur despite radical surgery.

There have been numerous studies that discuss the best method of treatment for enchondromas in the hand. These lesions have been classified as central, eccentric, polycentric, associated, and giant forms. Some authors advocate nonsurgical treatment of these enchondromas, feeling they will heal regardless. A large number of lesions present after a pathologic fracture which occasionally stimulates resolution of the enchondroma. Authors agree that any surgical intervention should wait until the fracture has healed. The purpose of removing the neoplasm is to obtain a histologic diagnosis, eliminate the future risk of pathologic fracture, and avoid progressive deformity. The main controversy is whether or not to bone graft the lesion after curettage. Several studies have shown excellent results and minimal recurrence with curettage alone, but others feel that symptomatic patients, or those cases where the bone stock has been severely damaged by the enchondroma, should be grafted. Allograft has been shown to be as successful in promoting healing as autograft and eliminates the donor site morbidity. This is important in patients with multiple lesions who may undergo multiple surgeries. Studies have recently shown good results using demineralized bone powder to fill the curetted cavity. As the powder is radiolucent, any postoperative opacity in the area of the previous lesion is new bone formation. Complete healing of all lesions was seen at 9.9 weeks in one study (Whiteman *et al.* 1993).

Multiple enchondromas

Enchondromatosis, or Ollier's disease, is a rare nonhereditary developmental anomaly (Figs 3 and 4). The multiple lesions are identical to solitary enchondromas radiographically and occur in the metaphysis or diaphysis of long bones. Histologically they often have increased cellularity and more binucleate forms, therefore the distinction between a benign and malignant lesion is even more difficult. The matrix is myxoid. Clinically the enchondromas are often unilateral and may cause deformity of the limb. A shortened appearance with angular malalignment is common. The lesions occasionally grow after skeletal maturity. When initially seen by an orthopedic surgeon, a full-body skeletal survey should be ordered as a baseline study for future comparison. Severe limb deformity should be treated surgically but the enchondromas can be disregarded unless symptomatic.

The incidence of malignant transformation has differed widely in the literature, but more recent studies that have followed patients with Ollier's disease long term have reported a 25 to 30 per cent chance of sarcoma formation. Usually there is only one focus of malignancy, but there have been reports of patients having multiple foci of chondrosarcomas at various histologic stages. Regular follow-up with close attention to the onset of a painful lesion is imperative. Increasing pain or cortical destruction seen on radiographs should alert the physician to this possibility. Chondrosarcomas that develop are usually low grade, although occasionally

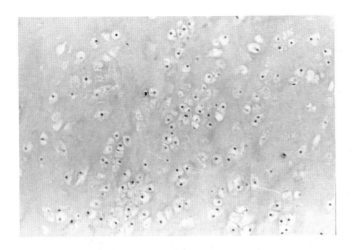

Fig. 3. (a) Enchondroma from the proximal phalanx of an 18-year-old female with Ollier's disease. Curettings demonstrate increased cellularity and binucleate chondrocytes which are often seen in enchondromas of the hand.

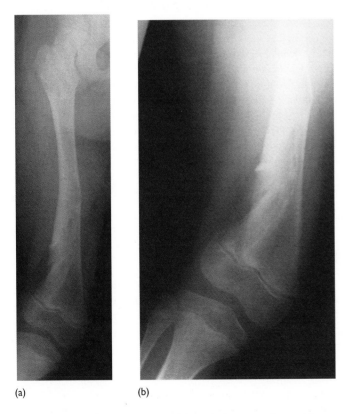

(a) (b)

Fig. 4. (a) An anteroposterior view of the right femur in a 4-year-old female with Ollier's disease. The multiple untreated lesions are asymptomatic but have caused a valgus deformity at the knee. (b) Nine months later there was progression of the valgus deformity and a corrective osteotomy was indicated.

dedifferentiation to a high-grade lesion occurs. Treatment of the malignancy requires wide surgical margins by resection or amputation. The risk of metastases and mortality is related to histologic grade of the lesion, not to size of the tumor or age of the patient. The outcome for patients with sarcomas arising in Ollier's disease is the same as if they develop in solitary enchondromas. No adjuvant therapy is necessary.

If the multiple enchondromas are associated with hemangiomas, the condition is called Maffucci's syndrome. This is a congenital, nonhereditary condition of serious concern. It is thought to represent a generalized mesodermal dysplasia. No metabolic or karyotypic abnormalities are noted. The hemangiomas are usually cavernous and occur anywhere in the skin, subcutaneous tissues or viscera. One recent study reported a group of six patients in whom the vascular counterpart of Maffucci's syndrome consisted of spindle-cell hemangioendotheliomas. Phleboliths are commonly noted on radiographs, and the vascular lesion is often the presenting sign. The enchondromas and hemangiomas do not necessarily occur in the same extremity. Histologically, the cartilage lesion is slightly more aggressive than a solitary enchondroma, and there is a myxoid matrix. The metacarpals, phalanges, and long bones are frequently affected.

As in Ollier's disease, the reported incidence of malignancy in Maffucci's syndrome varies widely based of the different methods of data collection at different centers. One study claimed a 23 per cent incidence of overall malignancy whereas a more recent report stated that sarcoma formation is inevitable if the patient with Maffucci's syndrome lives long enough (Schwartz *et al.* 1987). Chondrosarcomas that form are usually low grade. Patients are especially prone to develop both skeletal and nonskeletal malignancies, but are likely to die from the nonskeletal tumor or complications of the hemangiomatosis.

Further reading

Alho, A., Connor, J., Mankin, H., Schiller, A., and Campbell, C. (1983). Assessment of malignancy of cartilage tumors using flow cytometry. *Journal of Bone and Joint Surgery, American Volume*, **65A**, 779–85.

Bauer, H., Brosjo, O., Kreicbergs, A., and Lindholm, J. (1995). Low risk of recurrence of enchondroma and low-grade chondrosarcoma in extremities. *Acta Orthopaedica Scandinavica*, **66**, 283–8.

Bauer, R., Lewis, M., and Posner, M. (1988). Treatment of enchondromas of the hand with allograft bone. *Journal of Hand Surgery*, **13A**, 908–16.

Cannon, S. and Sweetnam, D. (1985). Multiple chondrosarcomas in dyschondroplasia (Ollier's disease). *Cancer*, **55**, 836–40.

Dahlin, D. and Salvador, A. (1974). Chondrosarcomas of bones of the hands and feet—a study of 30 cases. *Cancer*, **34**, 755–60.

De Beuckeleer, L., De Schepper, A., Ramon, F., and Somville, J. (1995). Magnetic resonance imaging of cartilaginous tumors: a retrospective study of 79 patients. *European Journal of Radiology*, **21**, 34–40.

De Beuckeleer, L., De Schepper, A., and Ramon, F. (1996). Magnetic resonance imaging of cartilaginous tumors: is it useful or necessary? *Skeletal Radiology*, **25**, 137–41.

Fanburg, J., Meis-Kindblom, J., and Rosenberg, A. (1995). Multiple enchondromas associated with spindle-cell hemangioendotheliomas. *American Journal of Surgical Pathology*, **19**, 1029–38.

Frassica, F., Unni, K., Beabout, J., and Sim, F. (1986). Dedifferentiated chondrosarcoma. A report of the clinicopathological features and treatment of seventy-eight cases. *Journal of Bone and Joint Surgery, American Volume*, **68A**, 1197–205.

Goodman, S., Bell, R., Fornasier, V., Demeter, D., and Bateman, J. (1984). Ollier's disease with multiple sarcomatous transformations. *Human Pathology*, **15**, 91–3.

Hasegawa, T., Seki, K., Yang, P., *et al.* (1995). Differentiation and proliferative activity in benign and malignant cartilage tumors of bone. *Human Pathology*, **26**, 838–45.

Hasselgren, G., Forssblad, P., and Tornvall, A. (1991). Bone grafting unnecessary in the treatment of enchondromas in the hand. *Journal of Hand Surgery*, **16A**, 139–42.

Kuur, E., Hansen, S., and Lindequist, S. (1989). Treatment of solitary enchondromas in fingers. *Journal of Hand Surgery*, **14B**, 109–12.

Lewis, R. and Ketcham, A. (1973). Maffucci's syndrome: functional and neoplastic significance. *Journal of Bone and Joint Surgery, American Volume*, **55A**, 1465–78.

Liu, J., Hudkins, P., Swee, R., and Unni, K. (1987). Bone sarcomas associated with Ollier's disease. *Cancer*, **59**, 1376–85.

Lucas, D., Tupler, R., and Enneking, W. (1990). Multicentric chondrosarcomas associated with Ollier's disease. *Journal of the Florida Medical Association*, **77**, 24–8.

McCarthy, E. (1996). *Differential diagnosis in pathology: bone and joint disorders*. Igaku-Shoin, New York.

Nelson, D., Abdul-Karim, F., Carter, J., and Makley, J. (1990). Chondrosarcomas of small bones of the hand arising from enchondroma. *Journal of Hand Surgery*, **15A**, 655–9.

Noble, J. and Lamb, D. (1974). Enchondromata of bones of the hand. A review of 40 cases. *Hand*, **6**, 275–84.

Sanerkin, N. and Woods, C. (1979). Fibrosarcomata and malignant fibrous histiocytomata arising in relation to enchondromata. *Journal of Bone and Joint Surgery, British Volume*, **61**, 366–72.

Schajowicz, F. (1994). *Tumors and tumorlike lesions of bone* (2nd edn), pp. 141–59. Springer-Verlag, Berlin.

Schiller, A. (1985). Diagnosis of borderline cartilage lesions of bone. *Seminars in Diagnostic Pathology*, **2**, 42–62.

Scotlandi, K., Serra, M., Manara, C., *et al.* (1995). Clinical relevance of Ki-67 expression in bone tumors. *Cancer*, **75**, 806–14.

Sun, T., Swee, R., Shives, T., and Unni, K. (1985). Chondrosarcoma in Maffucci's syndrome. *Journal of Bone and Joint Surgery, American Volume*, **67A**, 1214–19.

Takigawa, K. (1971). Chondroma of the bones of the hand. *Journal of Bone and Joint Surgery, American Volume*, **53A**, 1591–1600.

Tordai, P. and Lugnegard, H. (1990). Is the treatment of enchondroma in the hand by simple curettage a rewarding method? *Journal of Hand Surgery*, **15B**, 331–4.

References

Enneking, W. (1986). A system of staging musculoskeletal neoplasms. *Clinical Orthopaedics and Related Research*, **204**, 9–24.

Giudici, M., Moser, R., and Kransdorf, M. (1993). Cartilaginous bone tumors. *Radiologic Clinics of North America*, **31**, 237–59.

Kobayashi, H., Kotoura, Y., Hosono, M., *et al.* (1995). Diagnostic value of Tc-99m (V) DMSA for chondrogenic tumors with positive Tc-99m HMDP uptake on bone scintigraphy. *Clinical Nuclear Medicine*, **20**, 361–4.

Mercuri, M., Picci, P., Campanacci, L., and Rulli, E. (1995). Dedifferentiated chondrosarcoma. *Skeletal Radiology*, **24**, 409–16.

Milgram, J. (1983). The origins of osteochondromas and enchondromas. A histopathologic study. *Clinical Orthopaedics and Related Research*, **174**, 264–84.

Mirra, J., Gold, R., Downs, J., and Eckardt, J. (1985). A new histologic

approach to the differentiation of enchondroma and chondrosarcoma of the bones. *Clinical Orthopaedics and Related Research*, **201**, 214–37.

Scarborough, M. and Moreau, G. (1996). Benign cartilage tumors. *Orthopedic Clinics of North America*, **27**, 583–9.

Schwartz, H., Zimmerman, N., Simon, M., Wroble, R., Millar, E., and Bonfiglio, M. (1987). The malignant potential of enchondromatosis. *Journal of Bone and Joint Surgery, American Volume*, **69A**, 269–74.

Weinstein, L. and McCarthy, E. (1995). Ki-67 immunostaining as a tool in the diagnosis of central cartilage lesions. *Iowa Orthopedic Journal*, **16**, 39–45.

Whiteman, D., Gropper, P., Wirtz, P., and Monk, P. (1993). Demineralized bone powder. Clinical applications for bone defects of the hand. *Journal of Hand Surgery*, **18B**, 487–90.

1.6.6.9 Periosteal chondroma

Kristy Weber

Introduction

Periosteal chondroma is an extremely rare benign cartilage lesion (deSantos and Spjut 1981; Bauer *et al.* 1982; Boriani *et al.* 1983; Lewis *et al.* 1990). Also called juxtacortical chondroma, it is formed beneath the periosteum and external to the underlying cortical bone. It seems to arise from pluripotential cells deep in the periosteum that differentiate into chondroblasts instead of osteoblasts. Periosteal chondroma is not related to the epiphyseal plate. It occurs primarily in the metaphysis, but can be found in the diaphysis of any long tubular bone. The most common locations are the proximal humerus, femur, and phalanges. Periosteal chondromas comprise fewer than 1 per cent of all bone tumors but are three times more common than periosteal chondrosarcomas (Nojima *et al.* 1985). Males are affected twice as often as females and, although the lesions can be found at any age, patients in the second and third decade are generally affected. Rarely, multiple lesions can be seen.

Pathology

The gross appearance of a periosteal chondroma is a hard, sharply circumscribed lesion embedded in the underlying cortical bone. It has the typical appearance of hyaline cartilage lobules that are

Box 1

- Rare benign hyaline cartilage tumors that form between periosteum and cortical bone
- Develop most frequntly in the proximal humerus, femur, and phalanges
- May cause mild pain and swelling
- Differential diagnosis includes fibrous cortical defect, osteochondroma, periosteal chondrosarcoma, and periosteal osteosarcoma
- Marginal or wide resection is usually curative

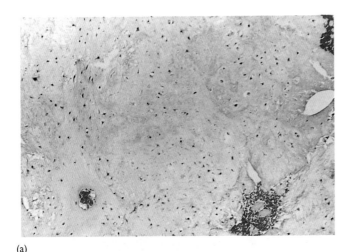

(a)

(b)

Fig. 1. (a) Low-power view of the cartilage lesion showing its lobular nature. Moderate cellularity and occasional binucleate forms are seen. (b) Higher-power view of the same lesion. The chondrocytes are abundant but no mitotic figures or necrosis is seen.

grayish-white or blue in color (Fig. 1). A thin shell of reactive periosteum may be seen covering the lesion, and no gross violation of the medullary cavity is seen.

On histologic examination, lobules of benign immature hyaline cartilage are separated by strands of fibrous connective tissue or lamellar bone (Mirra 1989). The tumor is bound by a thin fibrous capsule without obvious vascular proliferation. The surrounding soft tissues are not invaded. The microscopic appearance is more active than an enchondroma with common binucleate cells, areas of hypercellularity, and cellular atypia. As these findings may raise suspicion of a more aggressive lesion, careful attention to the clinical and radiographic findings is essential to avoid overdiagnosing malignancy. Focal calcification is identified in the majority of cases. There is no necrosis but the matrix may appear myxoid. Mitotic figures are not present. There is an active area of endochondral ossification at the base of the lesion similar to an osteochondroma. The medullary cavity of the underlying native bone is not involved, and the innermost margin of the tumor is usually encased by a rim of dense end-

osteal bone. Malignant transformation of this cartilage neoplasm does not occur; however, the histologic differential includes periosteal chondrosarcoma. In general there is a greater degree of cytological atypia in a chondrosarcoma, and the cartilage can be invasive through the capsule or into the underlying bone.

Clinical

Periosteal chondromas can be painless with their finding incidental on imaging studies taken for other concerns. Others cause mild pain, often for several years prior to diagnosis. Given their superficial location, minor trauma may cause discomfort whereas with intraosseus cartilage neoplasms pain is due to growth of the tumor. The tumor may cause swelling or an associated soft-tissue mass. It is hard, nontender, and fixed to the underlying bone on clinical examination. They can continue to grow slowly after skeletal maturity without developing into a more aggressive lesion. This differentiates it from an enchondroma or osteochondroma where growth in older patients is cause for concern.

Imaging studies

Plain radiographs are diagnostic for periosteal chondroma. It is a shallow lesion up to 4 cm in length that causes a saucerization of the cortex (Fig. 2). A well-circumscribed sclerotic rim of reactive bone is noted underlying the lesion. The cortex is eroded but remains intact, and the periosteal chondroma remains separate from the medullary cavity. It often appears as a well-circumscribed collection of ring-like densities adjacent to the cortical bone. Periosteal new bone forms buttresses that overhang the edges of the lesion. Some of the lesions are surrounded by a thin cortical shell and others have fuzzy or indistinct margins. No expansion of the native bone is seen nor have pathologic fractures been reported. One-third of cases are associated with a soft-tissue mass and approximately the same number have areas of focal ossification or calcification. MRI of periosteal chondromas is usually not necessary as it can be difficult to differentiate increased signal due to tumor invasion from marrow edema (Varma *et al.* 1991).

The radiographic differential diagnosis includes fibrous cortical defect, osteochondroma, periosteal chondrosarcoma, and periosteal osteosarcoma. Greenspan *et al.* (1993) reported two cases of periosteal chondroma that presented as osteochondromas in the popliteal region. The distinguishing feature was the intervening cortical bone which separated the periosteal chondroma from the medullary cavity. The periosteal chondrosarcoma is usually larger than 5 cm, primarily exophytic, and forms no reactive bone beneath the cortical erosion. The fibrous cortical defect and periosteal osteosarcoma are easily differentiated on the histologic findings.

Management and results

The treatment of an asymptomatic periosteal chondroma that is latent in activity is observation. For painful lesions, complete excision with a marginal or wide resection is curative in the majority of cases. Bone graft may or may not be used depending on the size of the

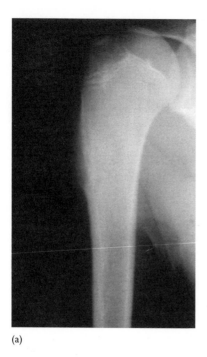
(a)

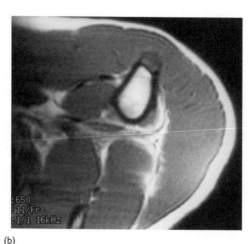
(b)

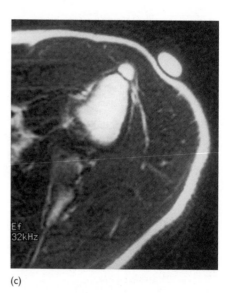
(c)

Fig. 2. (a) This is a typical radiographic appearance and presentation of a periosteal chondroma in a 15-year-old male. Note the scalloping of the underlying cortex and peripheral areas of 'buttressing' new bone arising from the mature cortex. (b) T_1 and (c) T_2 MR images demonstrate the juxtacortical nature of the lesion with a clear separation from the underlying medullary cavity.

lesion. A review of the literature shows a recurrence rate of less than 4 per cent (Nosanchuk and Kaufer 1969). Malignant transformation of periosteal chondromas has not been reported.

References

Bauer, T., Dorfman, H., and Latham, J. (1982). Periosteal chondroma. A clinicopathologic study of 23 cases. *American Journal of Surgical Pathology*, **6**, 631–7.

Boriani, M., Bacchini, P., Bertoni, F., and Campanacci, M. (1983). Periosteal chondroma. A review of 20 cases. *Journal of Bone and Joint Surgery, American Volume*, **65A**, 205–12.

deSantos, L. and Spjut, H. (1981). Periosteal chondroma: a radiographic spectrum. *Skeletal Radiology*, **6**, 15–20.

Greenspan, A., Unni, K., and Matthews, J. (1993). Periosteal chondroma masquerading as osteochondroma. *Canadian Association of Radiologists Journal*, **44**, 205–8.

Lewis, M., Kenan, S., Yabut, S., Norman, A., and Steiner, G. (1990). Periosteal chondroma. A report of ten cases and review of the literature. *Clinical Orthopaedics and Related Research*, **256**, 185–92.

Mirra, J. (1989). *Bone tumors*, pp. 1673–83. Lea and Febiger, Philadelphia, PA.

Nojima, T., Unni, K., McLeod, R., and Pritchard, D. (1985). Periosteal chondroma and periosteal chondrosarcoma. *American Journal of Surgical Pathology*, **9**, 666–77.

Nosanchuk, J. and Kaufer, H. (1969). Recurrent periosteal chondroma. *Journal of Bone and Joint Surgery, American Volume*, **51A**, 375–80.

Varma, D., Kumar, R., Carrasco, C., Guo, S., and Richli, W. (1991). MR imaging of periosteal chondroma. *Journal of Computer Assisted Tomography*, **15**, 1008–10.

1.6.6.10 Hemangioma

Diva R. Salomao and Antonio G. Nascimento

Hemangioma is one of the most common soft-tissue tumors (7 per cent of all benign tumors), and it is the most common tumor in infancy and childhood.

Most hemangiomas are superficial and have a predilection for the head and neck region, but they can also occur in the trunk or extremities or in viscera, such as the liver. They are benign neoplasms with limited growth potential, and in rare cases they regress completely.

Histologically, hemangiomas have been classified according to the caliber of the vessel involved.

Box 1

- The most common benign soft-tissue tumor in infancy and childhood
- Consists primarily of blood vessels and fibrous tissue, and may contain inflammatory cells and focal calcification
- Most commonly develops in superficial tissues, but can occur within muscle and viscera
- In selected patients, surgical excision is appropriate

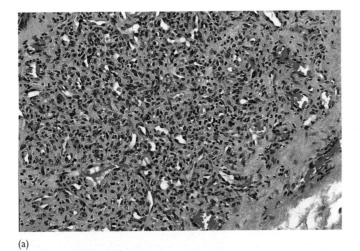

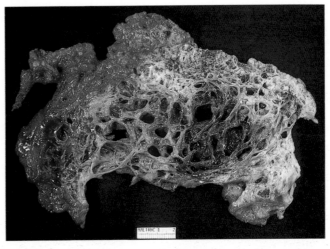

Fig. 2. Cavernous hemangioma with its typical sponge-like gross appearance.

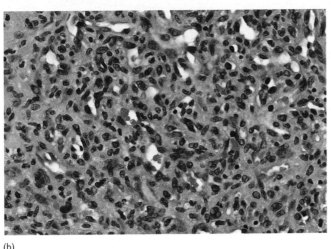

Fig. 1. (a), (b) Capillary hemangioma with endothelial proliferation forming small slit-like vascular structures with characteristic lobular arrangement.

Capillary hemangioma

Capillary hemangiomas are the largest single group of hemangiomas. They are composed of a proliferation of capillary-sized vessels lined by flattened endothelium arranged in lobules (Fig. 1). Several clinical variants of capillary hemangiomas are described.

The most distinctive and common variant is the cellular hemangioma of infancy. It is usually present at birth or appears in the first month of life, enlarges rapidly during the first few months, and stops growing only when the child is about 6 months old (Gonzalez-Crussi and Reyes-Mugica 1991). By the age of 7 years, 70 to 90 per cent of these lesions have involuted. They can be located in any part of the body, but they are most common in the head and neck region, particularly in the parotid gland.

Microscopically, capillary hemangiomas are characterized by a proliferation of plump endothelial cells lining vascular spaces, with small inconspicuous lumina (Smoller and Apfelberg 1993). Numerous mitotic figures and mast cells are a constant feature. The neoplasm can show invasive margins, and perineural involvement can

be seen (Calonje *et al.* 1995). The process of maturation and involution starts in the periphery and ultimately involves all zones, resulting in fibrosis.

Another important type to recognize is the so-called pyogenic granuloma or lobular hemangioma. It is an exophytic form of capillary hemangioma that occurs in the cutaneous and mucosal surfaces, especially in the oral cavity. The marked inflammation and myxoid background present in this tumor result in a histologic appearance of granulation tissue. Very often, the tumor is demarcated by a collarette of normal or hyperplastic epithelium. Superficial ulceration with secondary bacterial colonization is a feature that can also be observed.

Cavernous hemangioma

Cavernous hemangiomas are less frequent than capillary hemangiomas but share age and anatomical distributions. They are more common in children and in the upper portions of the body. Cavernous hemangiomas are usually larger and less circumscribed (Fig. 2), and frequently they involve deep structures. They show no tendency to regress and can be locally destructive.

Cavernous hemangiomas are characterized by dilated blood-filled vessels lined by flattened endothelium (Fig. 3). The vessel walls are occasionally thickened as a result of adventitial fibrosis and scattered inflammation. Calcification is a very common finding.

Arteriovenous hemangioma

This tumor is characterized by the presence of medium-sized or large arteries and veins in close association with each other. They are divided by location: superficially located in the dermis, in which usually no significant shunting occurs, and deeply located, most frequent in young patients and regarded as arteriovenous malformation. This diagnosis is best made in conjunction with the clinical and the radiographic findings.

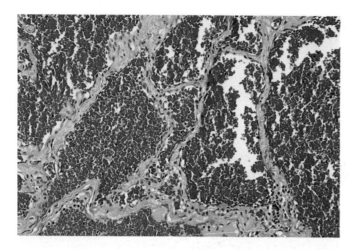

Fig. 3. Cavernous hemangioma with dilated, ectatic vascular spaces lined by flattened endothelial cells.

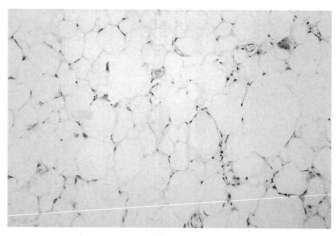

Fig. 1. Microscopic picture of typical lipoma.

References

Calonje, E., Mentzel, T., and Fletcher, C.D. (1995). Pseudomalignant perineurial invasion in cellular ('infantile') capillary haemangiomas. *Histopathology*, **26**, 159–64.

Gonzalez-Crussi, F. and Reyes-Mugica, M. (1991). Cellular hemangiomas ('hemangioendotheliomas') in infants. Light microscopic, immunohistochemical, and ultrastructural observations. *American Journal of Surgical Pathology*, **15**, 769–78.

Smoller, B.R. and Apfelberg, D.B. (1993). Infantile (juvenile) capillary hemangioma: a tumor of heterogeneous cellular elements. *Journal of Cutaneous Pathology*, **20**, 330–6.

1.6.7 Benign soft-tissue neoplasms
1.6.7.1 Lipoma

Diva R. Salomao and Antonio G. Nascimento

Lipomas are by far the most common mesenchymal tumors. Rare in children and adolescents, they are most common in the fifth and sixth decades of life. They affect a wide range of locations; however,

Box 1

- Benign slow-growing neoplasms formed primarily by fat cells
- Most common soft-tissue neoplasm
- Typically present as slowly growing masses in patients over 40 years of age
- Differential diagnosis includes well-differentiated liposarcoma
- May be treated by excision

they rarely occur on the face, hands, or feet. Their size varies according to the depth of the tumors, and because they are slow-growing lesions, they usually are asymptomatic (Enzinger and Weiss 1995). Rarely, tumors situated in the extremities can cause nerve compression leading to sensory or motor disturbances.

Grossly, lipomas are usually well-circumscribed multilobular masses that show a yellow surface. Hemorrhagic areas and zones of fat necrosis can occur in larger lesions. Histologically, they are indistinguishable from mature non-neoplastic adipose tissue (Fig. 1). However, variations occur in the form of myxoid transformation (myxolipomas), presence of variable amount of septa of connective tissue (fibrolipomas), chondroid or osseous metaplasia (chondrolipomas, osteolipomas), presence of smooth muscle proliferation (myolipomas), and nests of foamy macrophages.

It is important to recognize the existence of lipomas involving intramuscular and intermuscular compartments. The incidence rates of these lesions when compared with other tumors of adipose tissue differentiation are 1.8 and 0.3 per cent, respectively (Fletcher and Martin-Bates 1988). In those locations, they should be distinguished from well-differentiated liposarcoma.

Multiple lipomas occur in 5 to 6 per cent of patients, and in a small percentage of cases there is a hereditary trait for the development of lipomas. Hypercholesterolemia has been described in association with multiple lipomas.

Many variants of ordinary lipomas have been described, including angiolipoma, spindle cell lipoma, and pleomorphic lipoma.

Angiolipoma

Angiolipomas present as painful or tender, multiple subcutaneous nodules in the extremities and trunk of young adults (Hunt *et al.* 1990). Histologically, they are a mixture of mature fat cells and numerous branching vascular channels of uniformly small caliber containing fibrin thrombi.

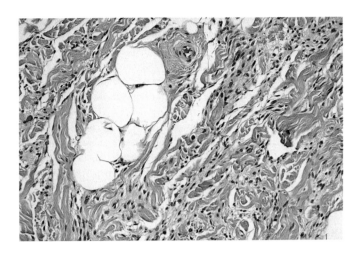

Fig. 2. Microscopic picture of spindle cell lipoma, showing a mixture of spindle cells, mature adipose tissue, and collagen bundles.

Spindle cell lipoma

This generally arises in the subcutaneous adipose tissue, representing 1.5 per cent of all lipomas. Most patients are men aged 40 to 70 years. The tumors frequently occur in the posterior neck and upper back or shoulder region. They are composed of mature adipocytes, slender spindle cells, and bundles of mature collagen, in variable proportions (Fig. 2). In most cases, the three elements are intermingled, but infrequently the tumor has an appearance of a typical lipoma presenting as a discrete nodule of spindle cells (Beham *et al.* 1989).

Pleomorphic lipoma

This is clinically identical to spindle cell lipoma. Histologically, it is composed of a mixture of mature adipocytes, spindle cells, collagen, and bizarre multinucleated giant cells showing a peculiar wreath

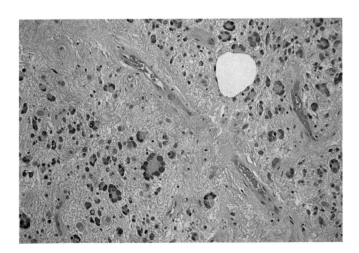

Fig. 3. Microscopic picture of pleomorphic lipoma, depicting classic 'floret-type' multinucleated giant cells.

arrangement of hyperchromatic nuclei around a deeply eosinophilic cytoplasm, the so-called floret giant cells (Fig. 3) (Digregorio *et al.* 1992).

References

Beham, A., Schmid, C., Hodl, S., and Fletcher, C.D. (1989). Spindle cell and pleomorphic lipoma: an immunohistochemical study and histogenetic analysis. *Journal of Pathology*, **158**, 219–22.

Digregorio, F., Barr, R.J., and Fretzin, D.F. (1992). Pleomorphic lipoma. Case reports and review of the literature. *Journal of Dermatologic Surgery and Oncology*, **18**, 197–202.

Enzinger, F.M. and Weiss, S.W. (1995). *Soft tissue tumors* (3rd edn). C.V. Mosby, St Louis, MO.

Fletcher, C.D. and Martin-Bates, E. (1988). Intramuscular and intermuscular lipoma: neglected diagnoses. *Histopathology*, **12**, 275–87.

Hunt, S.J., Santa Cruz, D.J., and Barr, R.J. (1990). Cellular angiolipoma. *American Journal of Surgical Pathology*, **14**, 75–81.

1.6.7.2 Cavernous lymphangioma of the extremities

William F. Blair and Joseph A. Buckwalter

Introduction

Lymphangiomas are generally classified as being of three types: simple lymphangiomas, cavernous lymphangiomas, and cystic hygromas. Simple and cavernous lymphangiomas occur in the extremities; only the cavernous type is of interest to the orthopedist. It is a neoplastic proliferation of lymph vessels and lymphoid tissues, sometimes containing some small blood vessel proliferation. The lymphangioma is a relatively uncommon tumor that presents in the pediatric age group. The location of the tumor is widely distributed, occurring in the viscera, trunk, neck, and both upper and lower extremities. Involvement in the extremities can vary considerably, from clinically inconsequential to a complex problem consisting of deformity, functional disability, and cosmetic concern (Blair *et al.* 1983; Mirra 1989). A little appreciated aspect of the clinical presentation of these tumors can be episodic extremity pain that is difficult to prevent or treat.

Box 1

- Rare, fewer than 1 per cent of benign tumors of soft tissues
- Typically present as diffuse soft-tissue masses in infancy or early childhood
- Can cause episodic pain that is difficult to treat
- Consist of lymph vessels, lymphoid tissue, and frequently blood vessels
- Local recurrence following surgical excision is common

Lymphangiomas are a subset of a larger group of tumors called angiodysplastic tumors (Schajowicz 1981). Angiodysplastic tumors include hemangiomas, hemangiolymphangiomas, as well as the lymphangiomas. These tumors are not always readily categorized on the basis of histologic criteria for a variety of reasons. The histology within a given specimen may vary from lymph channels to veins to arterioles. For this reason, the diagnosis in each clinical case should be based on the preponderance of tissue type present in the biopsy specimen. This, of course, can become a subjective determination in specific clinical circumstances. The histologic determination of a lymphangioma can also be confused in another regard. During biopsy or tissue processing bleeding can occur into lymphangiomatous channels giving a histologic picture that resembles thin-walled hemangiomas.

Primary lymphangiomas of the extremity have a very limited potential for malignancy. They do not assume malignant characteristics, either through local extension or metastasis. Lymphangiomas must be differentiated from lymphangiosarcomas, which derive from chronically lymphedematous extremities.

Epidemiology

Although lymphangiomas occur infrequently, they have typical clinical features (Stout and Little 1953). These tumors occur almost exclusively in the pediatric age group. They are equally distributed between sexes (Watson and McCarthy 1940; Nix 1954).

Clinical evaluation

Lymphangiomas are almost always diagnosed initially in infancy and early childhood, when they present as a soft-tissue mass in the extremity. The mass is soft and diffuse, with indistinct margins. It usually gradually enlarges as the infant or child matures. Rarely, cavernous lymphangiomas are associated with dermal lesions consisting of hyperpigmented skin or a vesicular dermis that can ooze transudate when gently abraded.

As the afflicted individual matures into late childhood and adolescence, pain in the involved extremity can become a problem. The pain is associated with increased levels of activity or minor trauma. Although pain can occur in both upper and lower extremity lymphangiomas, the functional demands placed upon the forearm and hand may accentuate the patient's pain experience in the upper extremities. A more problematic clinical occurrence is an episode pain syndrome consisting of palpably painful tumor, with erythema, warmth, and systemic fever (Blair *et al.* 1983).

Clinical evaluation is based on the clinical examination and imaging is usually of no value. The diagnosis is confirmed by incisional or marginal biopsy; however, a complete excisional biopsy is usually not technically possible.

Pathology

As previously mentioned, lymphangiomas are classified as simple or cavernous, or as cystic hygromas. Simple lymphangiomas are dermal in character and seldom of interest to the clinical orthopedist. By definition, cystic hygromas involve the neck and mediastinum, and not the extremities. Cavernous hemangiomas involve the extremities and are clinically significant entities to the orthopedist.

Cavernous lymphangiomas are poorly demarcated lesions that present in the skin and subcutaneous tissues, and may extend along fascial planes between muscle groups, or between muscle septae.

Superficial tumors may appear as brownish or red vesicles or warty lesions that exude a transudate when abraded (Fig. 1). Their deeper elements present as multiple diffuse compressible nodules or masses more characteristic of cavernous lymphangiomas. At surgical dissection these tumors lack a distinct capsule and their peripheral extensions are ill defined. When attempting excisional biopsy, the margins are easily violated, resulting in lymph or blood-tinged lymph that oozes from the tumor surface. When the biopsy tissue is removed, it often collapses and looses shape as fluid escapes.

Histologically a lymphangioma is composed of dilated lymphatic sinuses or channels that are filled with lymph (Jaffe 1958). After processing and sectioning, the sinuses can appear empty or even blood filled, making differentiation from hemangiomas difficult. The lymphatic sinuses have a flat endothelial lining that is described as single or multiple layers thick. The stroma is quite varied, consisting of patches of lymphoid tissue with some smooth-muscle elements (Fig. 2). Mixed forms with regional variation are present, with fatty or fibromatous elements. This tumor is noted for its tendency to have irregular extensions into adjacent muscle. When the dermis is involved, the papillary dermal projections contain lymphatic cysts (Fig. 3).

Simultaneous lymphangiomas and hemangiomas have been biopsied from separate anatomic locations within the same extremity. The presence of two tumor types is probably an unusual expression of an angiodysplasia, with neoplasias consisting of both lymphatic channels and blood vessels (Fig. 4) (Stout and Lattes 1953; Malan and Puglionisi 1965). Another observed pathologic variation has been the confirmation of cavernous lymphangioma in early childhood in a given individual. Subsequent biopsies were diagnostic of hemangioma, while the patient developed osseous dysplasia, contractures, and regional hyperhidrosis during development. This observation suggests that lymphangioma can be the first presentation of a more extensive regional dysplasia. Furthermore, lymphangiomas, with

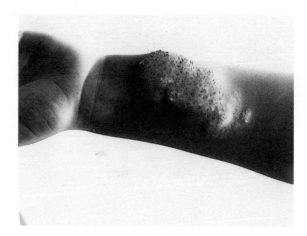

Fig. 1. Unusual dermal involvement in the forearm of a 5-year-old boy. A transudate oozed from the tumor surface.

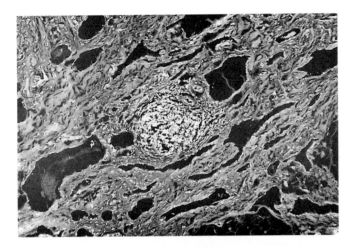

Fig. 2. Representative histology of a cavernous lymphangioma with proliferative lymph vessels, small lymphatic cysts, and lymphoid tissue.

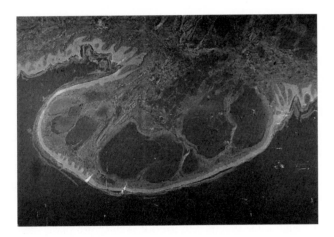

Fig. 3. In the presence of dermal involvement papillary dermal projections contain lymphatic cysts.

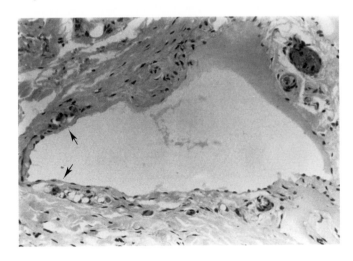

Fig. 4. An unusual histologic picture with capillaries permeating a proliferative endothelial wall in a large lymphatic cyst.

time, can histologically assume a more hemangiomatous picture. This may be in response to wound healing associated with biopsy, or it can be a consequence of a natural cellular and structural evolution of this type of angiodysplasia.

Differential diagnosis

Based upon the pathologic type of the tumor, the differential diagnosis most readily includes hemangiomas and hemangiolymphangiomas. In addition to single and cavernous lymphangiomas in the extremity, Watson and McCarthy (1940) also described a cellular or hypertrophic lymphangioma and a diffuse systemic lymphangioma.

The hypertrophic type is a slow-growing type and has a minimum of sinuses and an abundance of proliferative endothelium. The diffuse systemic type involves the entire extremity. It is slow growing over an extended period of time; the extremity appears hypertrophic, puffy, and soft.

The differential diagnosis should conceptually include lymphangiosarcoma (Taswell *et al.* 1962; Danese *et al.* 1967). This diagnosis is rare, and based on both gross and histologic features of malignancy. Lymphangiosarcomas are highly invasive, and develop in chronically lymphedematous extremities. As such, they are malignancies of adulthood, not childhood.

Although cavernous lymphangiomas present as soft-tissue masses in the extremities, bone also can be involved. In bone, lymphangioma can occur as a benign focal type, or a severe generalized lymphangiomatosis also called cystic angiomatosis of bone.

Treatment

The best treatment strategy for this tumor is not well established. In view of the range of complications and the complication rates, conservative care, to the extent possible, is always most prudent. The results of treatment vary with size and location of the lesion. For example, in a relatively small lymphangioma diagnosed by incisional biopsy, no further treatment may be indicated. Larger lesions in the proximal aspects of the extremitites are especially problematic. Once the diagnosis is confirmed by biopsy, small lymphangiomas in the extremities may need no further treatment. In larger lymphangiomas in the extremities that are bulky and unsightly, clinical management becomes a challenge. Surgical excision is the approach that is most often used. Surgical treatment utilizing wide excision is usually effective, though recurrences are a problem. Watson and McCarthy (1940) described four recurrences in 13 wide surgical excisions.

Complications after surgical excision are a concern. They include hematomas, infection, and lymphatic fistulas. Nix (1954) reported an infection rate of 19 per cent. Hypertrophic scar is certainly a subjective determination, but it can be a considerable patient concern and there may be a tendency to understate its significance. Of nine patients in Blair's series (Blair *et al.* 1983), 55 per cent complained of hypertrophic scar at final follow-up (Figs 5 and 6).

Prognosis

Cavernous lymphangioma of the upper and lower extremities presents in the pediatric age group. This tumor increases in size as the

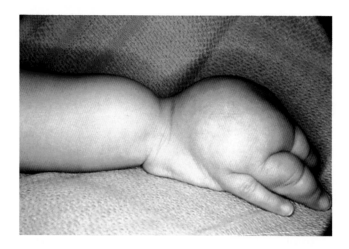

Fig. 5. Extensive lymphangioma in the distal forearm, hand, and fingers of a 2-year-old girl.

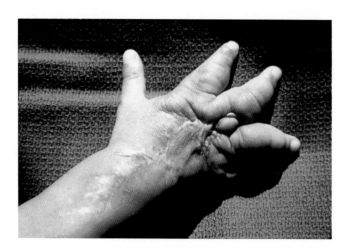

Fig. 6. Hypertrophic scarring along surgical incisions and the margins of a full-thickness skin graft.

involved individual develops. The tumor persists into adulthood. During the course of development lymphangiomas may become painful, recurrence rates after attempted surgical excision are relatively high, and pain syndromes may persist after surgical excision. The complication rate is considerable and the incidence of hypertrophic scarring following attempted surgical excision is high. Prognosis for most lymphangiomas in the extremity is fair at best. Blair stated that 'a realistic expectation for patient and surgeon and excisional biopsy is confirmation of tissue type and debulking of the tumor', but not necessarily resolution of the patient's primary clinical concerns.

References

Blair, W.F., Buckwalter, J.A., Mickelson, M.R., and Omer, G.E. (1983). Lymphangioma of the forearm and hand. *Journal of Hand Surgery*, **8**, 399–405.

Danese, C.A., Grishman, E., Oh, C., and Dreilling, D.A. (1967). Malignant vascular tumors of the lymphedematous extremity. *Annals of Surgery*, **166**, 245–53.

Jaffe, H.L. (1958). *Tumors and tumorous conditions of the bones and joints*, p. 238. Lea and Febiger, Philadelphia, PA.

Nix, J.T. (1954). Lymphangioma. *American Surgeon*, **20**, 556–62.

Malan, E. and Puglionisi, A. (1965). Congenital angiodysplasias of the extremities. *Journal of Cardiovascular Surgery*, **6**, 255–345.

Mirra, J.M. (1989). *Bone tumors. Clinical, radiologic and pathologic correlations*, pp.1422–35. Lea and Febiger, Philadelphia, PA.

Schajowicz, F. (1981). *Tumor and tumor like lesions of bone and joints*, p. 317. Springer-Verlag, New York.

Stout, A.P. and Lattes, R. (1953). *Tumors of the soft tissues. Fascicle 1: Atlas of tumor pathology*, pp. 12–13. Armed Forces Institute of Pathology, Washington, DC.

Taswell, H.P., Soule, E.H., and Coventry, M.B. (1962). Lymphangiosarcoma arising in chronic lymphedematous extremities. *Journal of Bone and Joint Surgery, American Volume*, **44A**, 277–94.

Watson, W.L. and McCarthy, W.D. (1940). Blood and lymph vessel tumors. *Surgery, Gynecology and Obstetrics*, **71**, 569–88.

1.6.7.3 Glomus tumors

David M. Oster

Introduction

Glomus tumors are benign neoplasms that closely resemble the normal glomus body. The characteristic epithelioid cell that comprises both structures is the glomus cell. Masson, in 1924, was the first to recognize the resemblance between these tumors and the glomus body (Carroll and Berman 1972).

The glomus body is a specialized form of arteriovenous anastomosis found in the stratum reticularis. It is composed of an afferent arteriole which branches into smaller vessels that transform into arteriovenous anastomoses (Sucquet–Hoyer canal) that empty into a primary collecting vein. Surrounding the arteriovenous anastomosis are smooth muscle and glomus cells. In the outer zone is loose delicate collagenous reticulum, in the meshes of which are seen numerous nonmedullated nerves. These structures are no more than 1 mm in diameter and are most numerous in the hand and foot. The function of these structures is not known, although it has been hypothesized that they regulate temperature (Popoff 1934; Couch 1941).

The glomus tumor is thought to be a hamartoma by some; however, since these lesions have been reported in locations that glomus

Box 1

- Rare benign soft-tissue neoplasms consisting of tissue that closely resembles the normal glomus body
- Usually less than 1 cm in diameter
- Typically cause pain, tenderness, and temperature sensitivity
- 30–50 per cent occur in the hand
- Surgical removal is the current optimal treatment

bodies are not found, they more likely represent a tumor. Glomus tumors are benign and rarely show local infiltration. Recurrences are secondary to incomplete excision, and metastases have not been reported (Murray and Stout 1941).

The glomus tumor is uncommon, and represented 1.6 per cent of 500 consecutive soft-tissue tumors of the extremities seen at the Mayo Clinic over a 2.5-year period (Shugart *et al.* 1963). A review at the Massachusetts General Hospital noted one occurrence per 4500 specimens of all types (Carroll and Berman 1972). The incidence in males and females is similar. The tumor has been reported in patients between the ages of 9 and 85 years with a maximum incidence in the fifth decade (Shugart *et al.* 1963).

Pathology

On gross inspection, glomus tumors are less than 1 cm in diameter and well circumscribed with a fibrous capsule. They are soft in consistency and are pink or red depending on the vascularity of the lesion.

Microscopically, glomus tumors are composed of vascular structures and glomus cells in varying proportions. The vessels are lined with endothelium and can be capillary sized or tortuous and dilated. Surrounding them are clusters of glomus cells. These cells are quite distinctive and are the distinguishing feature of this neoplasm. The cell has a rounded regular shape and a sharply defined nucleus with eosinophilic cytoplasm (Fig. 1). Initially, the glomus cell was felt to be a pericyte but recent ultrastructural analysis has revealed that they are more likely to be related to smooth muscle cells (Murray and Stout 1941; Enzinger and Weiss 1988).

The tumor is classified into three types based on the proportion of

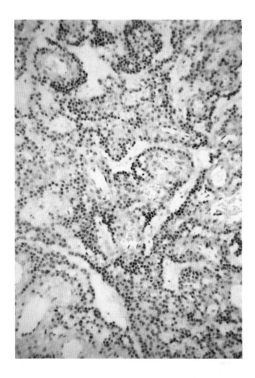

Fig. 2. Glomus tumor proper (low power).

glomus cells and vessels. The glomus tumor proper has an organoid appearance and is composed primarily of glomus cells (Fig. 2). It is the most common and accounted for 75 per cent of 507 cases reviewed by the Armed Forces Institute of Pathology. The glomangioma constitutes 20 per cent of cases. It has a greater vascular component and is composed of large veins surrounded by small clusters of glomus cells (Fig. 3). These tumors are more commonly multiple, painless, and may have a familial inheritance pattern. The glomangiomyoma is the least common type (fewer than 10 per cent) and is characterized by a gradual transition of glomus cells to smooth muscle cells (Enzinger and Weiss 1988).

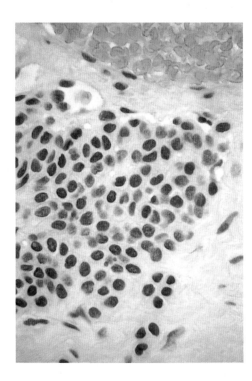

Fig. 1. Glomus cells (high power).

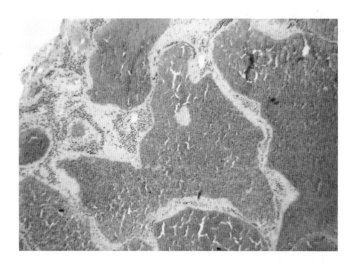

Fig. 3. Glomangioma (low power).

Clinical evaluation

The classic triad of symptoms is pain, tenderness, and temperature sensitivity. Patients complain of severe paroxysms of pain that are exacerbated by pressure and temperature exposure. These episodes of pain may be fleeting or can last as long as 3 h. The diagnosis is frequently missed; Shugart *et al.* (1963) noted that, on average, patients will have symptoms 10.9 years before the diagnosis is made.

On physical examination a mass may not be noted at the time symptoms first begin (Carroll and Berman 1972). If a mass is noted, it is well circumscribed, less than 1 cm in diameter, and located in the deep dermis. The skin over the lesion may be red–blue to red depending on its vascularity. Those in the nailbed can cause ridging and deformation of the nail. Other less frequent findings on physical examination are Hoerner's syndrome, overgrowth of an extremity, and disuse atrophy (Masson 1924; Kummel *et al.* 1972).

The distribution of glomus tumors is similar to that of glomus bodies in that they are more prevalent in the extremities, with 30 to 50 per cent located in the hand and the nailbed (Carroll and Berman 1972; Diao and Owen 1992). However, they have also been reported in areas where glomus bodies are not found, such as in the knee capsule, penis, mesentery, rectum, vagina, and bone (Grauer and Burt 1939; Hoffman and Ghormley 1941; Mackenzie 1962; Enzinger and Weiss 1988). Women have a higher incidence of subungual tumors, while men are more likely to have lesions in other locations (Shugart *et al.* 1963; Heys *et al.* 1992).

Solitary tumors occur most frequently and are usually painful. Multiple tumors have an incidence of 2.3 per cent, occur in a younger population, may not be associated with pain, and can have a familial inheritance pattern (Hueston 1946; Shugart *et al.* 1963; van der May *et al.* 1989; Tran *et al.* 1994). These multiple tumors usually have a greater vascular component and are less likely to have a discrete capsule.

Imaging studies

The diagnosis of a glomus tumor is made on history and physical examination, and imaging studies are generally not helpful. In 14 to 20 per cent of patients with subungual lesions, radiographs revealed a smooth concave erosion of the distal phalanx much like that seen with an epidermal inclusion cyst (Shugart *et al.* 1963; Carroll and Berman 1972). Disuse osteopenia may be seen in patients with extremity lesions.

Management and results of treatment

The treatment of choice is complete removal of the tumor. If a mass is not palpated or there are no overlying skin changes, the pin test may help localization. The point of a needle can be pressed very near to the lesion without causing pain, while excruciating pain will be noted with pressure within 1 cm. Biopsy is performed in the most painful area. Surgery can be performed under local anesthesia; however, epinephrine (adrenaline) should not be used as it will result in fading of the lesion and make identification difficult (Love 1944).

Complete excision of the tumor usually offers immediate pain relief with little chance of recurrence. If a recurrence does occur, it is secondary to incomplete excision and patients will note the return of pain within months of biopsy. Subungual tumors have a high recurrence rate (14 per cent) because it is difficult to distinguish the tumor from the surrounding tissue. The best way to ensure complete removal is to remove the entire nail, incise the epithelial bed, and then shell out the tumor to bleeding cancellous bone. Mild pain may persist for a few months following excision but the exquisite pain should resolve (Carroll and Berman 1972). Tumors in other areas rarely recur, as they are frequently encapsulated, and easy to distinguish from the surrounding tissue, making complete excision possible.

References

Carroll, R.E. and Berman, A.T. (1972). Glomus tumors of the hand. *Journal of Bone and Joint Surgery, American Volume*, **52A**, 691–703.

Couch, J.H. (1941). Glomus tumors: clinical picture and physiology. *Canadian Medical Association Journal*, **44**, 356–7.

Diao, E. and Owen, J.M. (1992). Common tumors. *Orthopedic Clinics of North America*, **23**, 187–96.

Enzinger, F.M. and Weiss, S.W. (1988). Glomus tumors. In *Soft tissue tumors* (2nd edn) (ed. F.M. Enzinger and S.W. Weiss), pp. 581–95. C.V. Mosby, St Louis, MO.

Grauer, R.C. and Burt, J.C. (1939). Unusual location of glomus tumor. Report of two cases. *Journal of the American Medical Association*, **112**, 1806–10.

Heys, S.D., Brittenden, J., Atkinson, P., and Eremin, O. (1992). Glomus tumor: an analysis of 43 patients and review of the literature. *British Journal of Surgery*, **79**, 345–7.

Hoffman, H.O.E. and Ghormley, R.K. (1941). *Proceedings of the Staff Meetings of the Mayo Clinic*, **16**, 13–16.

Hueston, J.T. (1946). Multiple painless glomus tumors. *British Medical Journal*, **1**, 1210–12.

Kummel, B., Stahl, D., and Fielding, J.W. (1972). Overgrowth of an extremity caused by glomus tumor. *Clinical Orthopedics and Related Research*, **82**, 80–1.

Love, J.B. (1944). Glomus tumors: diagnosis and treatment. *Proceedings of the Staff Meetings of the Mayo Clinic*, **19**, 113–22.

Mackenzie, D.H. (1962). Intraosseous glomus tumors. Report of two cases. *Journal of Bone and Joint Surgery, American Volume*, **44A**, 648–51.

Masson, P. (1924). Le glomus neuromyo-arterial des regions tactiles et ses tumeurs. *Lyon Chirurgical*, **21**, 257–80.

Murray, M.M. and Stout, A.P. (1941). The glomus tumor. Investigation of its distribution and behavior and identity of its 'epithelioid' cell. *American Journal of Pathology*, **18**, 183–203.

Popoff, N.W. (1934). The digital vascular system. With reference to the state of glomus in inflammation, arteiosclerotic gangreme, diabetic gangrene, thromboangiitis obliterans and supernumerary digits in man. *Archives of Pathology*, **18**, 295–330.

Shugart, R.R., Soule, E.H., and Johnson, E. (1963). Glomus tumor. *Surgery, Gynecology and Obstetrics*, **117**, 334–40.

Tran, L.P., Velanovich, V., and Kaufmann, C.R., (1994). Familial multiple glomus tumors: report of a pedigree and literature review. *Annals of Plastic Surgery*, **32**, 89–91.

van der May, A.G.L., Maaswinkel-Mooy, P.D., Cornelisse, C.J., Schmidt, P.H., and van de Kamp, J.J.P., (1989). Genomic imprinting in hereditary glomus tumours: evidence for new genetic theory. *Lancet*, **ii**.

1.6.7.4 **Neurofibroma**

Diva R. Salomao and Antonio G. Nascimento

Neurofibromas are benign tumors of peripheral nerves that can occur as a localized solitary tumor, sporadic form, or can be multiple associated with neurofibromatosis type 1 (von Recklinghausen's disease). Although the exact figures are unknown, it is estimated that 10 per cent of localized neurofibromas can occur in the setting of neurofibromatosis type 1.

In either form, neurofibromas can affect both sexes equally, and they usually occur in a young age group (20–30 years). Clinically, they manifest in most cases as a painless superficial mass located in the dermis and subcutaneous tissue. When occurring in deep soft tissues, they form well-circumscribed but not encapsulated tumor masses.

Grossly, neurofibromas are white–gray solid tumors that expand the structure of the nerve (Fig. 1). Secondary degenerative changes are usually not found.

Histologically, neurofibromas are composed of slender elongated cells showing wavy, darkly stained nuclei and indistinct cytoplasm. The cells are arranged in short interlacing fascicles or bundles, and

Box 1

- Benign tumors of peripheral nerves

- Expand the involved nerve

- May occur as solitary lesions or as multiple lesions in patients with neurofibromatosis type 1

- In patients with neurofibromatosis, neurofibromas may undergo malignant transformation

- Plexiform and diffuse neurofibromas occur in patients with neurofibromatosis

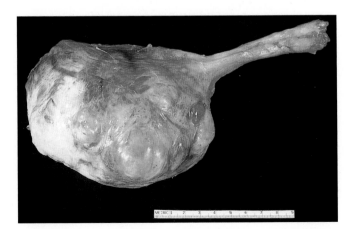

Fig. 1. A diffuse enlargement of a nerve is the characteristic picture of neurofibroma.

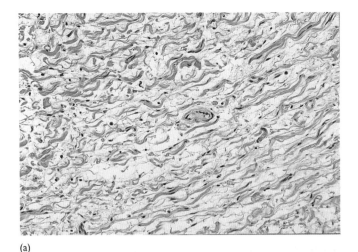

(a)

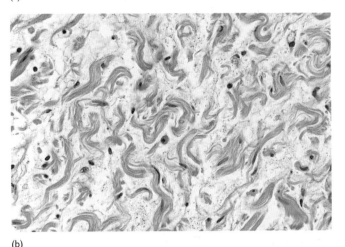

(b)

Fig. 2. (a), (b) Histologic pictures of neurofibroma showing the proliferation of slender spindle cells in a loose myxoid background.

the intercellular environment is characteristically loose and myxoid, showing thin wavy collagen fibers and inflammatory cells such as lymphocytes and mast cells (Fig. 2). The myxoid characteristic of the background varies from case to case, with lesions varying from richly myxoid background simulating myxomas to cellular lesions showing whorling or storiform arrangement. Xanthomatous changes or marked hyalinization of the stroma is observed in some tumors. Evidence of neural differentiation, such as the presence of Wagner–Meissner bodies, is sometimes present, but the finding is not associated with mitotic activity. The presence of mitosis in localized neurofibromas should raise concerns of malignant transformation. S-100 protein stain is always positive; however, the positivity is not as striking as expected in schwannomas.

Solitary neurofibromas do not have the same risk of malignant transformation as the tumors associated with neurofibromatosis; for this reason, simple excision is considered adequate therapy.

In the setting of neurofibromatosis, neurofibromas are usually multiple and may be found in deep locations. Rarely, the tumors are restricted to one area of the body (segmental neurofibromatosis).

Microscopically, the tumors associated with neurofibromatosis are usually indistinct from the solitary sporadic form. However, the plexiform variant is almost pathognomonic of neurofibromatosis type 1. It has a very peculiar gross appearance, a result of the involvement of large segments of the nerve causing thickening and distortion of the affected nerve. Histologically, it is identical to its localized counterpart, but it shows the characteristic multinodular plexiform arrangement.

Another unusual variant of neurofibroma is the diffuse form. It is most common in the head and neck region of children and young adults. It presents as a diffuse thickening of the dermis and subcutaneous tissue, due to extensive infiltration of a monomorphic population of oval cells associated with a fine, delicate fibrillary collagenous matrix.

Differing from the solitary form, tumors associated with neurofibromatosis cause significant morbidity because of their large number, the rate of recurrence, and the increased risk of developing sarcomas, estimated in different series to vary from 2 to 30 per cent of cases (Brasfield and Das Gupta 1972; Sorensen *et al.* 1986).

References

Brasfield, R.D. and Das Gupta, T.K. (1972). von Recklinghausen's disease: a clinicopathological study. *Annals of Surgery*, **175**, 86–104.

Sorensen, S.A., Mulvihill, J.J., and Nielsen, A. (1986). Long-term follow-up of von Recklinghausen neurofibromatosis: survival and malignant neoplasms. *New England Journal of Medicine*, **314**, 1010–15.

1.6.7.5 Extra-abdominal desmoid tumors

Douglas J. Pritchard

Introduction

The first report of a desmoid tumor was by MacFarlane in 1831. This report described a tumor arising in the anterior abdominal wall of a pregnant woman. It was subsequently appreciated that desmoid tumors can arise from any mesenchymal tissue (Nichols 1923). These tumors are locally aggressive and are considered by some to be low-grade sarcomas, specifically fibrosarcomas; however, they do not metastasize (Posner *et al.* 1989).

Desmoid tumor is also known as aggressive fibromatosis, extra-abdominal fibromatosis, and well-differentiated fibrosarcoma. The relatively bland histologic appearance of this tumor may result in a lack of recognition that the lesion is indeed a neoplasm (Enzinger and Weiss 1988).

Abdominal desmoid is the term applied when this tumor arises in the abdominal wall, especially in the lower portion of the rectus abdominus muscle. This tumor has the same gross and microscopic appearance as the extra-abdominal desmoid, but is considered separately because of its location and its tendency to occur in women of child-bearing age.

Intra-abdominal desmoid is the term applied to those lesions which arise in the pelvis or mesentery, or indeed, which arise from any musculoaponeurotic tissue within the abdomen.

Gardner's syndrome is the association of fibromatosis with osteomas, polyposis, and cutaneous cysts. This condition is inherited as an autosomal dominant trait.

Clinical features

Extra-abdominal desmoid is an uncommon tumor. There does not appear to be any racial or cultural prevalence.

There may be a relationship between trauma and the onset of this tumor. It is well known that desmoid tumors sometimes arise in wound scars from previous surgery. About one-third of patients recall a specific injury in the exact location of the subsequent tumor.

There may also be a hormonal relationship to this tumor; however, the exact relationship has never been completely established. Spontaneous regression has been reported following menopause (Pritchard 1990). Speculation regarding a hormonal relationship has led to anecdotal reports of hormonal treatment in an attempt to manipulate and control the tumors. Chromosomal abnormalities have been reported, supporting the concept that desmoid tumors are true neoplasms (Dal Cin *et al.* 1994).

In most series, females are more likely to have desmoid tumors than males. Any age may be afflicted, although this tumor is rare in children. The peak incidence is between ages 25 and 35.

By definition, extra-abdominal desmoid tumors do not occur in either the abdominal wall or within the abdomen. The most common area of involvement seems to be the region around the shoulder where there may be invasion of the axillary contents or the brachial plexus. The distal extremities are seldom involved (Fig. 1). These tumors may occasionally be multicentric with two or more lesions in a single extremity, or rarely may be bilateral. Most such tumors are considered to be deep rather than superficial in their location.

Most patients complain of the presence of a mass, which may grow very slowly over a long period of time, even several years. Some

Box 1

- Uncommon benign, but locally aggressive, soft-tissue tumor
- Most commonly presents as a firm slowly growing soft tissue mass in people between 25 and 35 years of age
- May be multicentric
- MRI is the best method of evaluating the extent of the lesion and its relationship with surrounding structures
- Wide surgical excision appears to offer the best chance of cure
- Local recurrence or development of metachronous disease commonly occurs following surgical excision
- Radiation therapy can provide local disease control
- Chemotherapy and hormonal therapy have been used in selected patients
- May stop growing or regress spontaneously

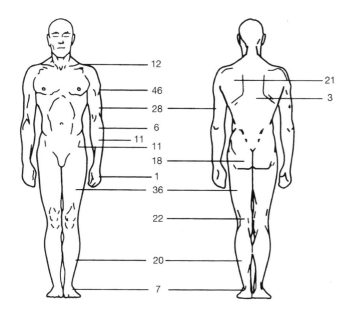

Fig. 1. The anatomic distribution of the desmoid tumor in 244 patients from two prior studies.

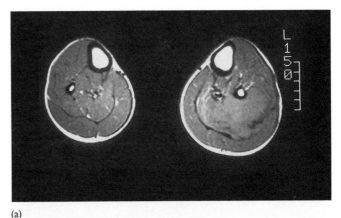

(a)

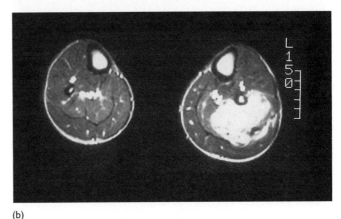

(b)

Fig. 2. (a) T_1-weighted and (b) T_2-weighted MRIs of a large desmoid tumor in the proximal part of the leg of a 37-year-old woman. The images demonstrate the relationship of adjacent important neurovascular structures. In conjunction with other views, these images allow accurate preoperative planning to achieve a wide operative margin. (Reproduced from Pritchard *et al.* (1996).)

patients complain of pain; indeed, there appears to be an unusual nature to this pain, such that patients who develop recurrent tumor following treatment can sometimes predict the recurrence before it is clinically obvious, simply by recognizing the nature of the pain. Other patients may develop neurologic complaints due to encroachment of the tumor on an adjacent nerve or they may note loss of mobility when the tumor arises in the vicinity of a major joint. Occasionally these tumors will invade adjacent bone; however, pathologic fracture from this is rare.

MRI is the modality of choice when trying to evaluate these tumors. Plain radiographs and CT scans fail to delineate these tumors from the surrounding structures. With an MRI the surgeon can get a reasonably accurate picture of the extent of the lesion and its relationship to surrounding structures (Fig. 2).

The one distinguishing finding on physical examination is the firmness of the tumor. Indeed when one palpates a soft-tissue lump and finds it to be very firm, one should include desmoid in the differential diagnosis. There are no other distinguishing features.

Pathology

Grossly these tumors are firm and white on the surface. They range in size from 1 cm to extremely large. Histologically there is a proliferation of fibroblasts. The cells have plump nuclei and mildly eosinophilic cytoplasm. The nuclei are clear. The chromatin is distributed along the nuclear membrane and the nucleoli are inconspicuous. The tumor cells are arranged in parallel rows separated by a variable amount of collagen. Some tumors are more cellular than others are

and these have less extracellular matrix. Some tumors will show an occasional mitotic figure. Necrosis is not a usual feature (Fig. 3).

Treatment and results

Management of these tumors can be difficult and frustrating for both the patient and the surgeon. Local recurrences are common and there may be considerable morbidity associated with the tumor and its treatment (Fig. 4). A previous report, which included patients managed between 1908 and 1980, noted that of 194 patients with extra-abdominal desmoid tumor, 132 developed a local recurrence following surgical resection (Rock *et al.* 1984). This occurred at an average of 1.4 years after the first treatment. In that report 120 of the 134 patients had an intralesional or a marginal resection and either developed a local recurrence or had residual disease. On the other hand, 25 of the 52 patients who had a wide excision had a local recurrence. Many of these patients with recurrent tumors had multiple procedures. It was noted that with each additional operative treatment about 20 per cent were 'cured'. In a more recent report

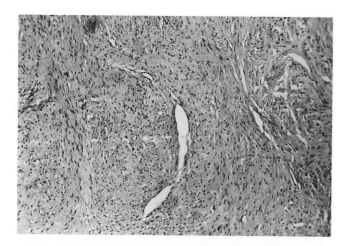

Fig. 3. Histologic appearance of a desmoid tumor. There is benign moderately cellular fibroblastic proliferation in a richly collagenized stroma (hematoxylin and eosin). (Reproduced from Pritchard *et al.* (1996).)

we noted somewhat improved local control of 44 patients with extra-abdominal desmoid tumors seen between 1981 and 1989 who underwent surgical treatment. Recurrence occurred in 14 patients at an average of 18 months. This improvement in local control may be the result of the more recent use of MRI to aid in the pretreatment planning.

Some so-called recurrences may actually be metachronous disease; that is, the patient may have the initial tumor at one site and develop a second lesion in the same extremity, but at a site remote from the original lesion. This occurs in about 10 per cent of patients. The second site may be either proximal or distal to the original site.

The histologic margin of resection appears to be the most accurate predictor of risk of subsequent local recurrence. When there is a margin of normal tissue of 2 mm or greater on all aspects of the tumor, the risk of local recurrence is lower than when tumor cells are close to the margin. It may be difficult at the time of the surgical procedure to accurately define the margin of the lesion, particularly if the patient has undergone previous surgery in that location. It may be nearly impossible to distinguish the tumor from scar tissue by gross examination and even histologically this may be a challenge for the pathologist. In our most recent experience of 13 patients who underwent wide resection alone, two developed local recurrence, whereas of 21 with marginal or intralesional resections alone, 10 developed local recurrences. Of 10 patients who underwent surgery and radiation therapy, two developed a local recurrence. One of these patients had a marginal resection and the other had an intralesional resection (Pritchard *et al.* 1996).

In an attempt to minimize the risk of local recurrence, adjuvant treatment may be considered.

There have been reports of the use of chemotherapy with agents including vincristine, dactinomycin, cyclophosphamide, methotrexate, and doxorubicin. Such chemotherapy has resulted in improvement in patients' pain and in some cases local control has been achieved. The effectiveness of chemotherapy has not, however, been completely established at this point in time. Further study of effective chemotherapy is warranted. Weiss and Lackman (1989) reported on the use of low-dose vincristine and methotrexate for eight patients with desmoid tumors who were not candidates for conservative sur-

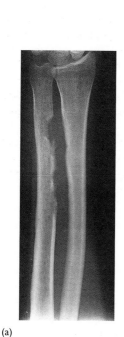

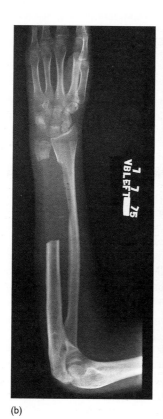

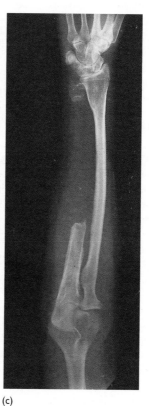

(a)　　　　　　　　(b)　　　　　　　　(c)

Fig. 4. Radiographs of the forearm of a 22-year-old woman with extra-abdominal desmoid tumor. (a) Initial image showing erosion of tumor into the ulna. (b) After the first resection. Tumor recurred 2 years later. (c) After the second procedure, at which additional bone was sacrificed. Patient has been followed for 10 additional years and has no evidence of progression. (Reproduced from Pritchard (1990).)

gery. Two patients had a complete remission, one of which persisted at 30 months, and five others had a partial or mixed response. One patient had a minimal response. Symptomatic relief was obtained in all patients. In a subsequent report, Weiss and Lackman (1996) extended their experience with unresectable desmoid tumors and concluded that 'a substantial percentage of patients with both desmoid tumor and fibromatosis have very substantial and long lasting control of their basic disease by the use of nonhormonal chemotherapy'. Some of these patients received etoposide and methotrexate rather than the vincristine–methotrexate combination. They noted that desmoid tumors involving the hands and feet were especially resistant to vincristine–methotrexate, but did respond to etoposide–methotrexate. Side-effects and toxicity were relatively mild or reversible. These investigators are conducting a trial of adjunctive chemotherapy following surgical resection for those situations where recurrence is thought to be likely, such as when surgery is known to be incomplete.

The suspected hormonal relationship of this tumor has prompted the use of hormonal therapy (Sportiello and Hoogerland 1991; Wilcken and Tattersall 1991). It has been noted that estrogen may be a growth factor for fibroblasts and fibroblastic tumors. Tamoxifen, which is an anti-estrogen, has been shown anecdotally to occasionally be effective in controlling this tumor. Various progestational agents or hormones have been tried with limited success. Side-effects may be unacceptable. Hormone treatment should also be considered investigational at this point in time.

The most promising adjuvant treatment for desmoid tumors is radiation therapy. Most would agree that radiation therapy combined with fairly conservative surgery has been effective in the local control of most soft-tissue sarcomas. One might expect that desmoid tumors would respond similarly. Several reports suggest that adjuvant radiation therapy following resection for gross residual disease has been of value. For patients with intralesional or marginal resections, the value of adjuvant radiation therapy is less clear. McCullough *et al.* (1991) reported excellent local control for patients who had radiation therapy for histologically evident residual disease after resection for primary or recurrent disease.

Radiation therapy alone may be preferable for patients with inoperable tumors or those with gross residual disease after operative debulking and even for those for whom operative management would lead to major functional disability.

The timing of radiation in relation to surgery is not well established. It is not known whether it is better to use radiation prior to surgery or following surgery. Our usual plan is to proceed with surgery with the intent to achieve a wide surgical margin. If a wide surgical margin is achieved, radiation therapy is not routinely used. However, if a less than wide margin is achieved at surgery we employ adjunctive radiation therapy. The combined results of several studies (including our own) reveal that radiation therapy with or without subtotal resection resulted in local control in 65 of 83 patients (78 per cent) who had gross disease (Keus and Bertelink 1986; Posner *et al.* 1989; Sherman *et al.* 1990; McCollough *et al.* 1991; Pritchard *et al.* 1996).

There is only one report of the transformation of an extra-abdominal desmoid to an aggressive, frankly malignant fibrosarcoma (Soule and Scanlon 1962). This occurred 11 years after the patient received radiation therapy for a desmoid of the axillary region. There have been other reports of malignant transformation following radi-

ation therapy for other benign lesions, and so caution is always advised when recommending such treatment.

It should be noted that amputation is rarely necessary for desmoid tumors and probably should only be used as a last resort. Of the 194 patients with extra-abdominal desmoid tumors seen at the Mayo Clinic between 1908 and 1980, 25 underwent amputation; however, in the more recent experience of 50 patients seen between 1981 and 1989, none underwent amputation.

Recurrent tumors are particularly difficult to manage. It is even more difficult to define the precise extent of the lesion when it occurs in an area of previous surgery. Adjuvant or neoadjuvant treatment should probably be considered for patients with recurrent disease. In our previous studies we have learned that some patients with recurrent tumors could be simply observed. Some of these patients had previously undergone multiple surgical procedures and it was the combined decision of the clinician and the patient not to undergo any additional treatment (Rock *et al.* 1984). In 60 of 68 patients who made this decision, the size of the tumor remained stable and caused few symptoms during an average follow-up of 6.3 years. In six of the patients the tumor became smaller during the period of observation and in two patients it progressed, necessitating additional treatment. Hence it may be reasonable to simply observe the patient who has undergone multiple previous procedures for recurrent desmoid tumors if the patient is not having serious symptoms or if the tumor does not threaten a vital structure (Miralbell *et al.* 1990). The patients must examine themselves frequently and return for periodic medical examinations. The main risk of this approach is that the tumor might grow to the point where it is no longer operable and might even progress to the point of threatening the life of the patient. However, this should be a rare occurrence if the patient is closely monitored.

Summary

Extra-abdominal desmoid tumors are aggressive but benign soft-tissue tumors which are difficult to manage. There is a high likelihood of local recurrence when surgical resection achieves margins that are less than wide. We advise an attempt at wide excision for previously untreated tumors. If a wide excision is confirmed by pathology, the patient is observed by periodic follow-up examinations, which include regular MRIs as well as physical examination. If a wide excision is not achieved, then adjunctive radiation therapy should be considered. If the tumor is deemed to be unresectable from the outset, then radiation therapy alone (without surgery) may be successful. For recurrent tumors, some combination of surgery and radiation is probably indicated. For patients with multiple recurrences, close observation and periodic monitoring may be advised. Finally, the role of chemotherapy in the management of this tumor appears promising, but it is as yet experimental.

References

Dal Cin, P., Sciot, R., Aly, M.S., *et al.* (1994). Some desmoid tumors are characterized by trisomy 8. *Genes, Chromosomes and Cancer*, **10**, 131–5.

Enzinger, F.M. and Weiss, S.W. (1988). Fibromatoses. In *Soft tissue tumors* (2nd edn), Chapter 6, p. 145. C.V. Mosby, St Louis, MO.

Keus, R. and Bartelink, H. (1986). The role of radiotherapy in the treatment of desmoid tumors. *Radiotherapy and Oncology*, **7**, 1–5.

McCollough, W.M., Parsons, J.T., van der Griend, R., Enneking, W.F., and Heare, T. (1991). Radiation therapy for aggressive fibromatosis. The experience at the University of Florida. *Journal of Bone and Joint Surgery, American Volume*, **73A**, 717–25.

MacFarlane, J. (1831). In *Clinical reports of the surgical practice of the Glasgow Royal Infirmary*. D. Robertson, Glasgow.

Miralbell, R., Suit, H.D., Mankin, H.J., Zuckerberg, L.R., Stracher, M.A., and Rosenberg, A.E. (1990). Fibromatoses: from postsurgical surveillance to combined surgery and radiation therapy. *International Journal of Radiation Oncology, Biology, Physics*, **18**, 535–40.

Nichols, R.W. (1923). Desmoid tumors: a report of thirty-one cases. *Archives of Surgery*, **7**, 227–36.

Posner, M.C., Shiu, M.H., Newsome, J.L., Rajdu, S.I., Gaynor, J.J., and Brennnan, M.F. (1989). The desmoid tumor. Not a benign disease. *Archives of Surgery*, **124**, 191–6.

Pritchard, D.J. (1990). Extra-abdominal desmoid tumors. In *Surgery of the musculoskeletal system* (ed. C. McCollister Evarts), pp. 4787–92. Churchill Livingstone, New York.

Pritchard, D.J., Nascimento, A.G., and Petersen, I.A. (1996). Local control of extra-abdominal desmoid tumors. *Journal of Bone and Joint Surgery, American Volume*, **78A**, 848–54.

Rock, M.G., Pritchard, D.J., Reiman, H.M., Soule, E.H., and Brewster, R.C. (1984). Extra-abdominal desmoid tumor. *Journal of Bone and Joint Surgery, American Volume*, **66A**, 1369–74.

Sherman, N.E., Romsdahl, M., Evans, H., Zagars, G., and Oswald, M.J. (1990). Desmoid tumors: a 20-year radiotherapy experience. *International Journal of Radiation Oncology, Biology, Physics*, **19**, 37–40.

Soule, E.H. and Scanlon, P.W. (1962). Fibrosarcoma arising in an extra-abdominal desmoid tumor: report of a case. *Mayo Clinic Proceedings*, **37**, 443.

Sportiello, D.J. and Hoogerland, D.L. (1991). A recurrent pelvic desmoid tumor successfully treated with tamoxifen. *Cancer*, **67**, 1443–6.

Weiss, A.J. and Lackman, R.D. (1989). Low-dose chemotherapy of desmoid tumors. *Cancer*, **64**, 1192–4.

Weiss, A.J. and Lackman, R.D. (1996). Therapy of desmoid tumors, fibromatosis and related neoplasms. *International Journal of Oncology*, **7**, 773–6.

Wilcken, N. and Tattersall, M.H. (1991). Endocrine therapy for desmoid tumors. *Cancer*, **68**, 1384–8.

1.6.7.6 Elastofibroma

Joseph A. Buckwalter and Eric A. Brandser

Elastofibroma, a neoplastic-like process, usually presents as a poorly defined soft-tissue mass fixed to the chest wall adjacent to the inferior tip of the scapula in elderly individuals (Jarvi and Saxon 1961; Giebel *et al.* 1996). It is uncertain if elastofibromas represent a benign neoplastic process or formation of reactive tissue in response to mechanical irritation of soft tissues by motion of the scapula relative to the chest wall. Although most of these lesions develop between the lower edge of the scapula and chest wall, they have been found in other locations including the region of the greater trochanter and the ischial tuberosity. They are typically painless and nontender, although some patients notice mild discomfort.

Elastofibromas rarely occur in people less than 50 years old. Many

Box 1

- A neoplastic-like process, which usually presents as a poorly defined painless soft-tissue mass fixed to the chest wall adjacent to the inferior tip of the scapula
- Rarely occurs in people less than 50 years old
- Consists of fibrous tissue with a high concentration of elastin fibers
- CT or MRI typically shows a soft-tissue mass with streaky interspersed high- and low-intensity signal
- May be treated by observation or resection

people with these lesions do not notice the presence of the mass. In these individuals the elastofibromas may be discovered during physical examinations or chest CT examinations performed for other reasons. The prevalence of elastofibromas has not been extensively investigated, but a recent autopsy study found 13 elastofibromas in 100 elderly people (Giebel *et al.* 1996), and a study of 258 chest CT scans performed on patients older than 60 years for reasons other than chest-wall abnormalities found four patients with elastofibromas (Brandser *et al.* 1998).

Most patients with elastofibromas who seek medical attention do so because they palpate a mass. Occasional individuals have mild pain or tenderness, or restriction of scapular motion. In their most common location, near the lower border of the scapula, elastofibromas are firmly attached to the chest wall. They are typically unilateral, but bilateral involvement does occur (Nagamine *et al.* 1982; Giebel *et al.* 1996; Hoffman *et al.* 1996). On physical examination the masses are firm and fixed to the chest wall. They do not involve the skin and they do not have associated erythema.

Imaging can help distinguish elastofibromas from other lesions (Fig. 1). Plain films are usually normal, but occasionally may show a soft tissue mass displacing the scapula (Fig. 1(a)) (Vande-Berg *et al.* 1966). Bone destruction or invasion has not been reported. Both CT and MRI can show the soft-tissue masses in patients with elastofibromas (Fig. 1(b)–(d)) (Kransdorf *et al.* 1992; Massengill *et al.* 1993; Yu *et al.* 1995; Naylor *et al.* 1996). With either of these imaging techniques, the tumors may have a characteristic appearance that includes streaky layers of soft tissue, similar in signal or attenuation to skeletal muscle, that are interspersed with areas of fat (Fig. 1(b)–(d)). However, some elastofibromas, especially small lesions, have a homogenous appearance (Kransdorf *et al.* 1992; Brandser *et al.* 1998) (Fig. 2). CT often shows poor differentiation of tumor edges from surrounding muscle planes and continuity with adjacent intercostal muscles (Kransdorf *et al.* 1992; Naylor *et al.* 1996).

Elastofibromas have a characteristic structure that distinguishes them from malignant soft-tissue tumors. On gross examination they are firm nodular soft-tissue masses with ill-defined margins. In most instances elastofibromas of the chest wall are adherent to the fascia and rib periosteum. They are generally grayish-white in color and may have areas of fatty tissue and cyst formation. Microscopic examination shows an extracellular matrix composed of dense fibrous tissue with prominent elastic fibers that contains occasional bland-

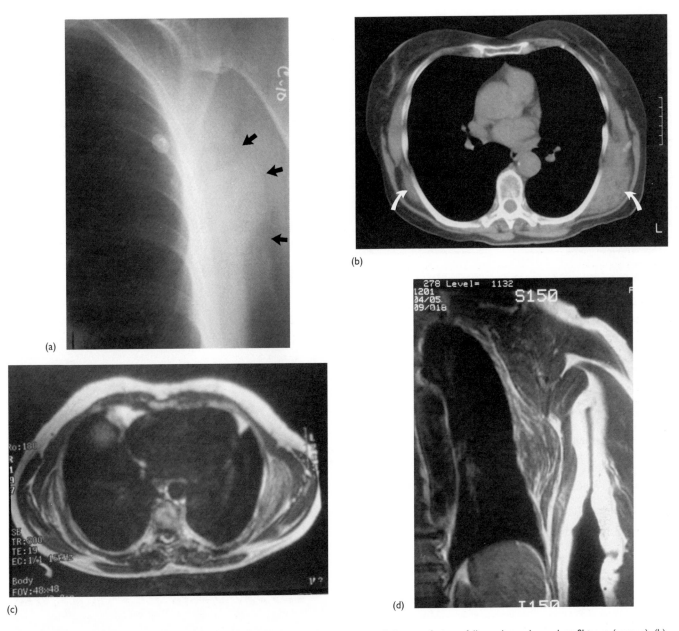

Fig. 1. Bilateral elastofibromas in a 61-year-old man. (a) Radiograph of the left chest wall shows soft-tissue fullness due to large elastofibroma (arrows). (b) Axial CT image shows larger left and smaller right masses (arrows). Note mixed attenuation due to interspersed fat and soft tissue within the larger left mass. (c) Axial T_1-weighted (TR, 800 ms; TE, 19 ms) image showing bilateral masses similar to the CT in (b). The areas of high signal intensity in the lesions represents fat. (d) Coronal T_1-weighted image (TR, 800 ms; TE, 19 ms) of left elastofibroma shows mass with interspersed layers of high and low signal intensity deep to serratus anterior and latissimus dorsi muscles. (Courtesy of Rob Danielson.)

appearing fibroblasts (Fig. 3) (Nagamine *et al.* 1982). The definitive diagnosis is based on the history, physical findings including the location of the lesion, and the microscopic demonstration of benign fibrous and fatty tissue containing a high concentration of elastic fibers (Fig. 3).

Treatment of patients with elastofibromas consists of either observation or resection of the lesion. In many patients the clinical diag-

nosis of elastofibroma can be made based on the history, physical findings, and imaging studies (Massengill *et al.* 1993; Naylor *et al.* 1996). Biopsy is indicated when the diagnosis is uncertain. Asymptomatic lesions may be observed. Local resection of the lesion generally relieves the symptoms for patients who have pain or restriction of motion, and the lesions rarely if ever recur following local resection (Nielsen *et al.* 1996).

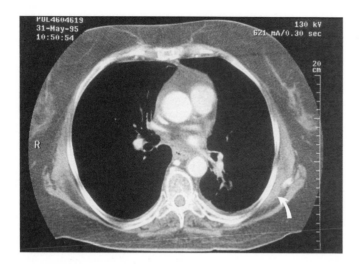

Fig. 2. Left elastofibroma dorsi in 68-year-old woman. Axial CT image at the level of left scapular tip shows soft-tissue mass involving left chest wall (arrow); right side is normal. Note that density is homogeneous in this smaller elastofibroma.

References

Brandser, E.A., Goree, J.C., and El-Khoury, G.Y. (1998). Elastofibroma dorsi: prevalence in an elderly population as revealed by CT. *American Journal of Radiology*, **171**, 977–80.

Giebel, G.D., Bierhoff, E., and Vogel, J. (1996). Elastofibroma and pre-elastofibroma—a biopsy and autopsy study. *European Journal of Surgical Oncology*, **22**, 93–6.

Hoffman, J.K., Klein, M.H., and McInerney, V.K. (1996). Bilateral elastofibroma: a case report and review of the literature. *Clinical Orthopaedics and Related Research*, **325**, 245–50.

Jarvi, O. and Saxon, A.E. (1961). Elastofibroma dorsi. *Acta Pathologica et Microbiologica Scandinavica*, **51** (Supplement 144), 83–4.

Kransdorf, M.J., Meis, J.M., and Montgomery, E. (1992). Elastofibroma: MR and CT appearance with radiologic-pathologic correlation. *American Journal of Roentgenology*, **159**, 575–9.

Massengill, A.D., Sundaram, M., Kathol, M.H., El-Khoury, G.Y., Buckwalter, J.A., and Wade, T.P. (1993). Elastofibroma dorsi: a radiological diagnosis. *Skeletal Radiology*, **22**, 121–3.

Nagamine, N., Nohara, Y., and Ito, E. (1982). Elastofibroma in Okinawa. A clinicopathologic study of 170 cases. *Cancer*, **50**, 1794–805.

Naylor, M.F., Nascimento, A.G., Sherrick, A.D., and McLeod, R.A. (1996). Elastofibroma dorsi: radiologic findings in 12 patients. *American Journal of Roentgenology*, **167**, 683–7.

Nielsen, T., Sneppen, O., Myhre-Jensen, O., Daugarrd, S., and Norback, J. (1996). Subscapular elastofibroma: a reactive pseudotumor. *Journal of Shoulder and Elbow Surgery*, **5**, 209–13.

Vande-Berg, B., Malghem, J., Leflot, J.L., Lagneaux, G., and Maldague, B. (1966). Case report: elastofibroma dorsi—pseudomalignant lesion. *Clinical Radiology*, **51**, 67–9.

Yu, J.S., Weis, L.D., Vaughan, L.M., and Resnick, D. (1995). MRI of elastofibroma dorsi. *Journal of Computer Assisted Tomography*, **19**, 601–3.

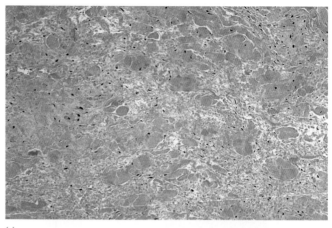

(a)

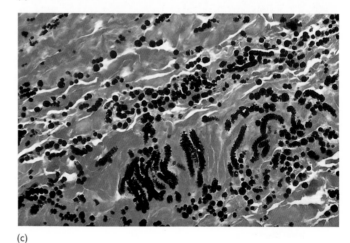

(b)

(c)

Fig. 3. Light micrographs of an elastofibroma. (a) Low-magnification light micrograph (hematoxylin and eosin stain) shows a dense collagenous extracellular matrix with scattered spindle-cell nuclei. (b) Higher-magnification light micrograph (hematoxylin and eosin stain) shows the scattered spindle cells more clearly and small round dense eosinophilic structures (elastin fibers). (c) High-magnification light micrograph (elastin stain) shows darkly stained globular and elongated elastin fibers within the collagenous matrix.

1.6.7.7 Giant cell tumor of tendon sheath

Diva R. Salomao and Antonio G. Nascimento

Giant cell tumor of the tendon sheath, or tenosynovial giant cell tumor (a term preferred by some authors) (Enzinger and Weiss 1995), can be divided into two forms, localized and diffuse, depending on the growth features.

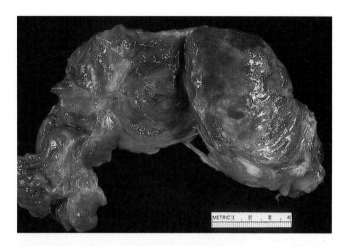

Fig. 1. Localized form of giant cell tumor of tendon sheath (nodular synovitis), showing the brown cut surface.

Localized form (nodular tenosynovitis)

This lesion can occur in any age group, although it is more common in women between 30 and 50 years old.

It is more frequent on the hand, typically located adjacent to the interphalangeal joint. Less common sites are the feet, ankles, and knees. It is a benign lesion that can recur locally if incompletely excised (Rao and Vigorita 1984).

Clinically, it presents as a painless, slow-growing mass, fixed to the deep structures. Underlying bone erosion occurs in less than 10 per cent of cases (Jones *et al.* 1969).

Grossly, giant cell tumor of the tendon sheath is usually circumscribed, with smooth lobulated contours, varying in size from 0.5 to 4 cm. The cut section is variegated, characterized by a pink–gray background flecked with yellow or brown, depending on the amount of lipid and hemosiderin (Fig. 1).

Most tumors are moderately cellular, composed of sheets of round or polygonal cells, blending with hypocellular collagenized areas containing spindle cells. Cleft-like spaces are observed. Multinucleated giant cells are scattered throughout the lesion. Foamy histiocytes and macrophages containing hemosiderin granules are also seen.

Diffuse form (pigmented villonodular synovitis)

This is a rare lesion that occurs slightly more frequently in women aged 40 years or younger.

The most common locations are the knee, ankle, and foot; frequently the finger, elbow, and temporomandibular and sacroiliac joints are involved. Rare cases involving the spine, mainly the posterior vertebral elements, have been reported (Giannini *et al.* 1996). Patients usually have a long history of a tender or painful joint, accompanied by effusion or hemarthrosis in some cases.

Grossly, the tumor presents as a diffuse expansile mass showing cleft-like or pseudoglandular spaces (Fig. 2).

Histologically, the lesion is characterized by a villous proliferation of rounded or polygonal cells, which show a clear or brown cytoplasm, a result of hemosiderin-pigmented deposition (Fig. 3). Spindle cells and xanthoma cells can also be seen intermixed with multinucleated giant cells and chronic inflammatory cells, creating a polymorphic cell population in the hypercellular areas. Hypocellular collagenized areas are often observed. Focal necrosis is a rare finding.

Although it is considered a benign lesion, the diffuse type of tenosynovial giant cell tumor has a high recurrence rate of approximately 25 per cent for the intra-articular form and 40 to 50 per cent for the extra-articular form (Schwartz *et al.* 1989). A malignant form of pigmented villonodular synovitis was reported recently (Bertoni *et al.* 1997), but it is still a debatable entity that needs to be proved by the study of a large series of cases.

Box 1

- Occurs in two forms: localized (nodular tenosynovitis) and diffuse (pigmented villonodular synovitis) that can develop within joints or in extra-articular locations

- Nodular tenosynovitis is a benign lesion consisting primarily of fibroblast-like cells, collagenous areas, giant cells, and histiocytes

- Nodular tenosynovitis develops most often in women between 30 and 50 years of age

- Nodular tenosynovitis typically presents as a circumscribed painless slow-growing mass in the hands or feet, or near the knee

- Pigmented villonodular synovitis is a benign, but potentially locally aggressive, lesion that consists of a villous proliferation of round or polygonal cells and contains spindle cells, giant cells, and inflammatory cells

- The most common locations of pigmental villonodular synovitis include the knee, ankle, and foot

- Patients with pigmental villonodular synovitis typically have a long history of a tender or painful joint, and may have had multiple hemarthroses

- Following surgical excision, the recurrance rate for pigmented villonodular synovitis is high, 25 per cent or more for intra-articular pigmented villonodular synovitis and about 40 to 50 per cent for extra-articular pigmented villonodular synovitis

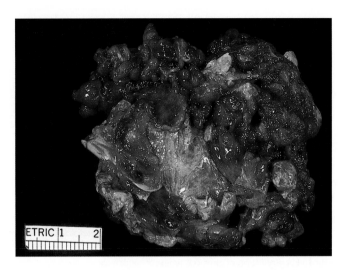

Fig. 2. Diffuse form of giant cell tumor of tendon sheath (pigmented villonodular synovitis), showing the villous poorly circumscribed nature of the process.

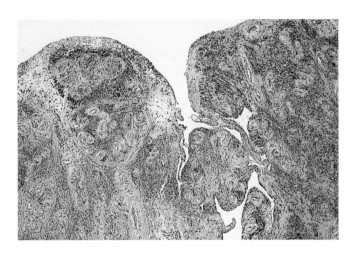

Fig. 3. Low-power view of pigmented villonodular synovitis.

References

Bertoni, F., Unni, K.K., Beabout, J.W., and Sim, F.H. (1997). Malignant giant cell tumor of the tendon sheaths and joints (malignant pigmented villonodular synovitis). *American Journal of Surgical Pathology*, **21**, 153–63.

Enzinger, F.M. and Weiss, S.W. (1995). *Soft tissue tumors* (3rd edn). C.V. Mosby, St Louis, MO.

Giannini, C., Scheithauer, B.W., Wenger, D.E., and Unni, K.K. (1996). Pigmented villonodular synovitis of the spine: a clinical, radiological, and morphological study of 12 cases. *Journal of Neurosurgery*, **84**, 592–7.

Jones, F.E., Soule, E.H., and Coventry, M.B. (1969). Fibrous xanthoma of synovium (giant-cell tumor of tendon sheath, pigmented nodular synovitis). A study of one hundred and eighteen cases. *Journal of Bone and Joint Surgery, American Volume*, **51A**, 76–86.

Rao, A.S. and Vigorita, V.J. (1984). Pigmented villonodular synovitis (giant-cell tumor of the tendon sheath and synovial membrane). A review of eighty-one cases. *Journal of Bone and Joint Surgery, American Volume*, **66A**, 76–94.

Schwartz, H.S., Unni, K.K., and Pritchard, D.J. (1989). Pigmented villonodular synovitis. A retrospective review of affected large joints. *Clinical Orthopaedics and Related Research*, **247**, 243–55.

1.6.7.8 Schwannoma

Diva R. Salomao and Antonio G. Nascimento

Schwannomas are benign encapsulated peripheral nerve sheath tumors that arise as an eccentric growth from the nerve. They can occur at any age, but they are more frequent between the ages of 20 and 50 years (Enzinger and Weiss 1995). They are more frequent in the head and neck region, involving the spinal roots and cervical nerves, and in the flexor surfaces of the extremities, involving the peroneal and ulnar nerves preferentially (Stout 1935). Deeply situated tumors are observed in the posterior mediastinum and retroperitoneum.

Schwannomas are almost always solitary lesions; however, multiple lesions can rarely be observed in patients with neurofibromatosis type 1 (von Recklinghausen's disease). In 5 per cent of cases, schwannomas have a plexiform or multinodular growth pattern

Box 1

- Benign encapsulated tumors of peripheral nerves
- Grow eccentrically from nerve
- Develop most frequently in patients between 20 and 50 years of age
- Typically present as slow-growing masses
- Surgical excision is usually curative

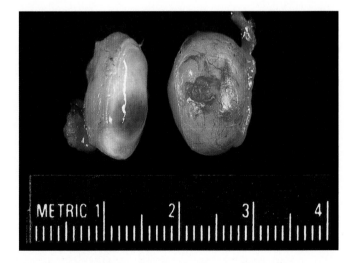

Fig. 1. A typical gross picture of schwannoma as an encapsulated eccentric growth of the associated nerve.

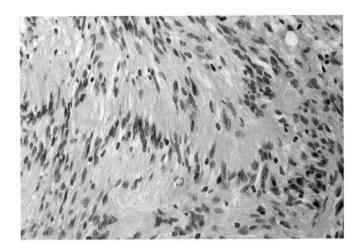

Fig. 2. Nuclear palisading with formation of typical Verocay bodies.

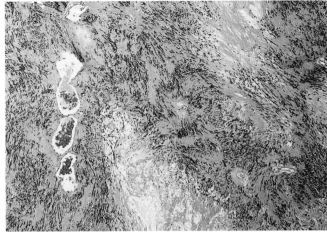

Fig. 3. Low-power picture of schwannoma depicting Antoni A and B areas and thick-walled ectatic blood vessels.

(Fletcher and Davies 1986). Schwannomas present as slow-growing tumors that are present for several years before diagnosis.

Grossly, these tumors present as an eccentric mass in the nerves, and because they arise within the nerve sheath, they are surrounded by a true capsule consisting of epineurium (Fig. 1). They are frequently smaller than 5 cm, although they can be considerably larger when located in the mediastinum and retroperitoneum.

Microscopically, they are characterized by the presence of Antoni A and B areas. The amount of each component varies from lesion to lesion. Antoni A areas are more cellular and compact, and are composed of spindle cells that have twisted nuclei with intranuclear vacuoles and indistinct cytoplasmic borders. They are arranged in short interlacing fascicles. In these areas, one can observe nuclear palisading, cell whorlings, and Verocay bodies (Fig. 2). Mitotic figures are occasionally seen in these areas. Antoni B areas are less orderly and less cellular. They are composed of spindled or oval cells arranged haphazardly within a loose matrix which can show microcystic changes, inflammatory cells, delicate collagen fibers, and large thick-walled vessels (Fig. 3).

Large tumors, usually deeply situated, can present significant degenerative changes varying from cyst formation and calcification grossly to cellular pleomorphism microscopically, with no impact in the behavior of these lesions.

An important variant is the cellular schwannoma (White *et al.* 1990). It is a schwannoma composed predominantly of Antoni A areas, resulting in increased cellularity, and has a slight increase in mitotic activity (not more than four mitotic figures per 10 high-power fields). Like classic neurilemmomas, cellular schwannomas are usually encapsulated, behave in benign fashion, and display intense and diffuse S-100 protein staining.

Schwannomas can be treated by simple excision.

References

Enzinger, F.M. and Weiss, S.W. (1995). *Soft tissue tumors* (3rd edn). C.V. Mosby, St Louis, MO.

Fletcher, C.D. and Davies, S.E. (1986). Benign plexiform (multinodular) schwannoma: a rare tumour unassociated with neurofibromatosis. *Histopathology*, **10**, 971–80.

Stout, A.P. (1935). Peripheral manifestations of specific nerve sheath tumor (neurilemoma). *American Journal of Cancer*, **24**, 751–96.

White, W., Shiu, M.H., Rosenblum, M.K., Erlandson, R.A., and Woodruff, J.M. (1990). Cellular schwannoma: a clinicopathologic study of 57 patients and 58 tumors. *Cancer*, **66**, 1266–75.

1.6.7.9 Synovial chondromatosis

J. Sybil Biermann

Introduction

Synovial chondromatosis is a benign synovial neoplasm which is usually monoarticular in adults. Metaplastic transformation of the syno-

Box 1

- Benign cartilaginous synovial neoplasm
- Cartilaginous and osteocartilaginous regions develop in synovial tissue and form synovial nodules and intra-articular loose bodies
- Most frequently occurs in the knee, hip, and shoulder
- In some instances the disease develops or extends into extra-articular tissues
- Typically presents with swelling of a single joint and limitation of motion
- Radiographs usually show multiple calcified or ossified nodules or loose bodies; air or double-contrast computed arthrotomography provides the most complete demonstration of the lesions
- Current treatment is surgical resection
- Patients may develop degenerative joint disease

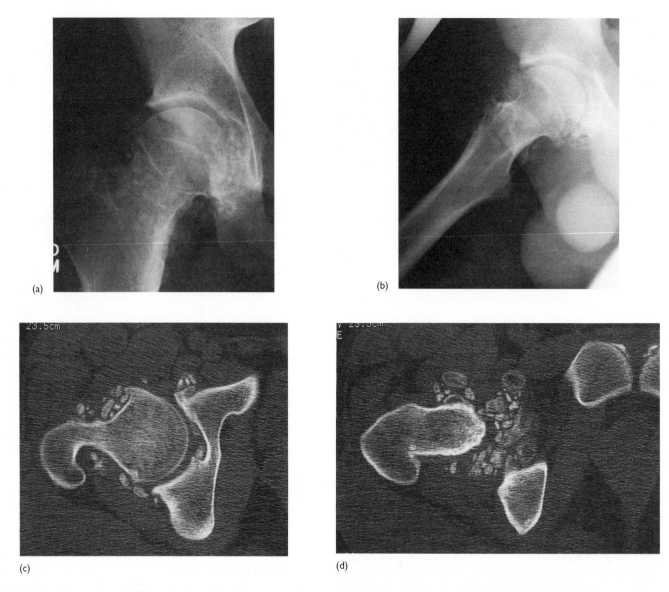

Fig. 1. (a) Anteroposterior and (b) lateral radiographs of the right hip of a 20-year-old man show multiple opacities distributed in the capsular area of the hip joint, consistent with synovial chondromatosis. Hip joint space is normal, and there are no signs of degenerative joint disease, consistent with primary synovial chondromatosis. The patient had presented with recurrent pain following arthroscopic synovectomy 3 years previously. CT scan through the level of the femoral head (c) and neck (d) show numerous round mineralized bodies in the hip joint and in the intracapsular areas surrounding the joint. Ossified bodies show a ring of ossification around their periphery. The patient remains symptom-free 2 years after open synovectomy was performed.

vium occurs, and cartilaginous or osteocartilaginous bodies are produced. Synovial chondromatosis may occur in nearly any joint; however, it is the most commonly reported about the knee, hip, and shoulder. Persons of any age may be afflicted, although the disease rarely occurs in children (Maurice *et al.* 1988). This lesion has also been referred to as 'joint chondroma', 'synovial osteochondromatosis', and 'chondromatosis of the joint capsule' (Smith 1977). Examples of synovial chondromatosis are shown in Figs 1, 2, 3, and 4.

Classification and etiology

According to Milgram (1977), in the early active stage of the disease there is intrasynovial proliferation without free loose bodies. As the disease progresses, osteochondral bodies appear and may be detached from the originating synovium. In the mature form of the disease condition, intrasynovial disease is not detectable, but the joint is filled with loose osteochondral bodies (Milgram 1977). Although the potential for disease recurrence following treatment has been postu-

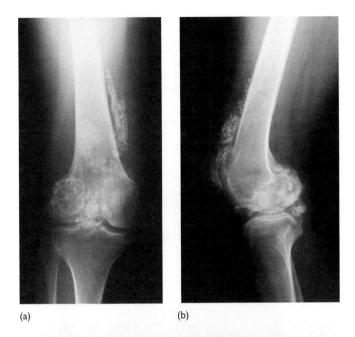

(a)   (b)

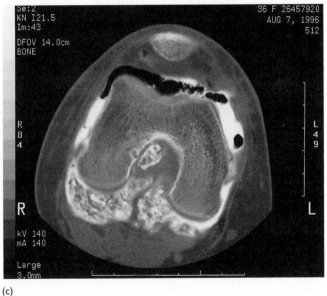

(c)

Fig. 2. A 36-year-old woman presented with a 10-year history of synovial chondromatosis of the knee. She had undergone arthroscopic synovectomy at 8 years and at 1 year prior to these radiographs. (a) Anteroposterior and (b) lateral radiographs of the knee show innumerable calcific and ossific bodies about the knee, extending proximally to the furthest reaches of the suprapatellar pouch. (c) Double-contrast air computed arthrotomography shows extensive posterior disease in the knee, behind the cruciate ligaments. Double-contrast arthrotomography can show unmineralized as well as mineralized cartilaginous bodies. Because of the extensive long-standing disease in arthroscopically inaccessible locations, the patient underwent anterior and posterior synovectomy of the knee.

lated to be related to the phase of the disease, it may be difficult to determine disease stage.

The distinction has been made between primary synovial chondromatosis and secondary synovial chondromatosis. Primary disease is diagnosed in the presence of relatively normal articular cartilage, while secondary disease is thought to arise in joints with degenerative disease (McCarthy 1982). However, this division is complicated by the fact that the disease itself may lead to degenerative changes, making the distinction difficult in advanced stages. Most authors agree that loose bodies which are created as a result of degenerative disease do not fall under the category of synovial chondromatosis.

Although synovial chondromatosis is caused by synovial metaplasia, the exact etiology of this transformation from normal synovium to synovial chondromatosis remains unclear. It has been postulated to be of neoplastic formation; however, it has also been considered to be related to degenerative joint disease, and there is evidence for both. An experimental model of cartilage injury in primates was able to elicit synovial changes similar to that seen in synovial chondromatosis (Helmy et al. 1989). Synovial chondromatosis often occurs in concert with degenerative joint disease in humans; whether this is cause and effect cannot be determined.

Synovial chondromatosis remains a relatively poorly understood process, showing some characteristics of a neoplasm and some of a reactive process when examined with immunohistochemical markers. Chondrocytes from synovial chondromatosis show a phenotype similar to chondrocytes from normal hyaline articular cartilage. Like articular cartilage, the predominant form of collagen in synovial chondromatosis is type II (Ryan et al. 1982). Cells of synovial chondromatosis do not express Ki-67, a proliferation-associated antigen present in fetal epiphyseal cartilage, and absent in adult cartilage, suggesting that there are few proliferating cells in the synovium or cartilage in these cases (Apte and Athanasou 1992). Complex chromosome changes have been reported in synovial chondromatosis, and results suggest that synovial chondromatosis is a clonal proliferation (Mertens et al. 1996).

There are some distinguishing characteristics from normal cartilage and similarities to malignant disease, however. Immunohistochemical testing for the C-erb B-2 proto-oncogene product has been found to be positive in a majority cases of synovial chondromatosis, similar to chondrosarcomas, but unlike normal hyaline cartilage or enchondromas (Davis et al. 1996).

Although the majority of cases of synovial chondromatosis occur within a joint, cases of extra-articular synovial chondromatosis have been reported. It is important to distinguish this entity, since erroneous histologic interpretation of extra-articular synovial chondromatosis may lead to a diagnosis of chondrosarcoma (Sim et al. 1977). Large, asymptomatic periarticular masses may be present without bone or joint involvement (Sviland and Malcolm 1995).

Clinical evaluation

Patients commonly present with a history of swelling about the affected joint, which may be of many years' duration. The disease usually involves only one joint or area. Involvement of deeper joints such as the shoulder or hip may present as pain with limitation of motion. Systemic complaints are absent.

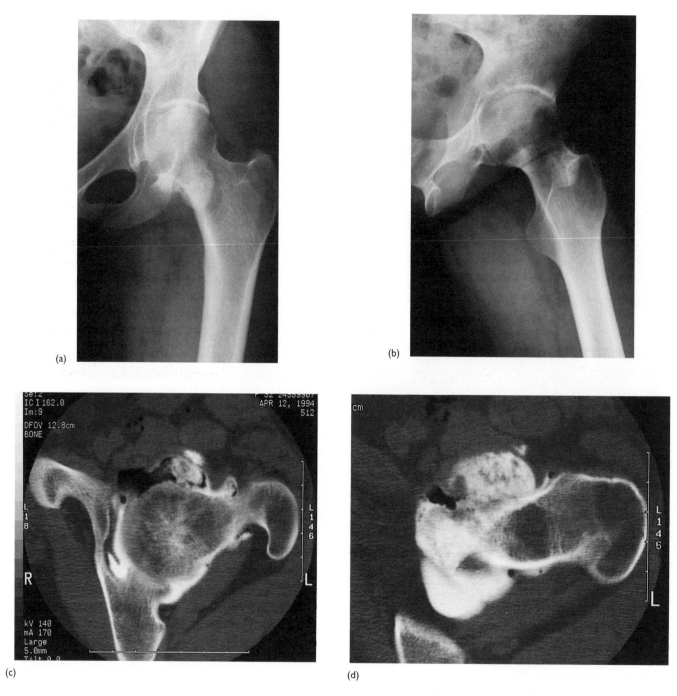

Fig. 3. (a) Anteroposterior and (b) lateral radiographs of a 32-year-old woman with a painful left hip of several months' duration show a solitary large ossific body superimposed over the femoral neck as well as some smaller opacities. (c), (d) Double-contrast computed arthrotomography shows a large ossific body anterior to the femoral neck, as well as multiple smaller loose bodies. Synovial chondromatosis occasionally presents with a solitary large intra-articular ossific body.

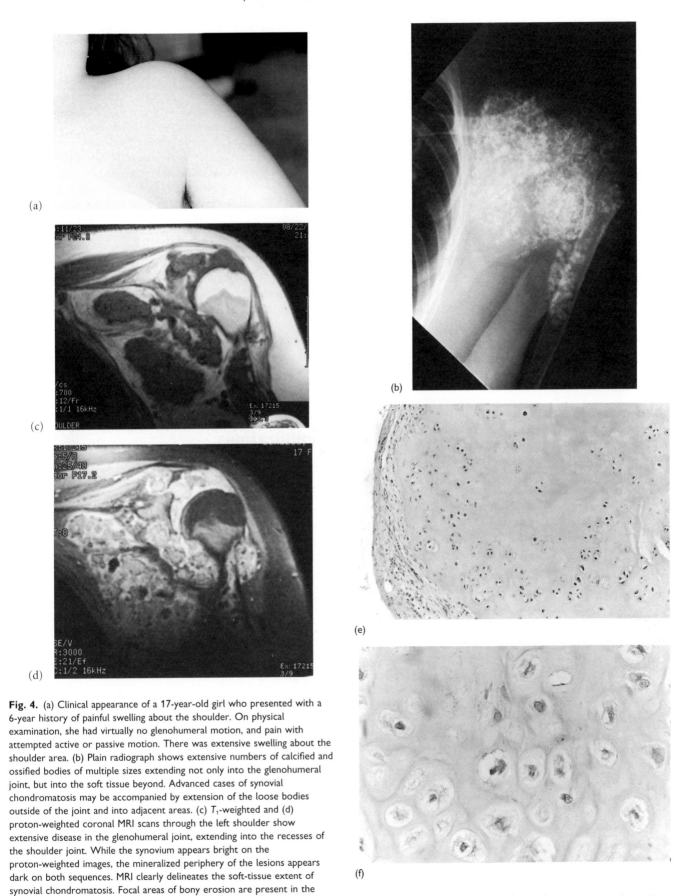

Fig. 4. (a) Clinical appearance of a 17-year-old girl who presented with a 6-year history of painful swelling about the shoulder. On physical examination, she had virtually no glenohumeral motion, and pain with attempted active or passive motion. There was extensive swelling about the shoulder area. (b) Plain radiograph shows extensive numbers of calcified and ossified bodies of multiple sizes extending not only into the glenohumeral joint, but into the soft tissue beyond. Advanced cases of synovial chondromatosis may be accompanied by extension of the loose bodies outside of the joint and into adjacent areas. (c) T_1-weighted and (d) proton-weighted coronal MRI scans through the left shoulder show extensive disease in the glenohumeral joint, extending into the recesses of the shoulder joint. While the synovium appears bright on the proton-weighted images, the mineralized periphery of the lesions appears dark on both sequences. MRI clearly delineates the soft-tissue extent of synovial chondromatosis. Focal areas of bony erosion are present in the humeral head. The patient was treated with anterior and posterior synovectomies as well as aggressive postoperative therapy; however, prognosis remains guarded in light of extensive degenerative changes already present in the joint and the attenuation of the rotator cuff. (e) Synovial chondromatosis. At the far left is seen the synovial investment of a cartilage nodule, with a histologic pattern of mature-appearing cartilage proliferation without significant atypia or mitotic activity. (Hematoxylin and eosin.) (f) High-power photomicrograph of synovial chondromatosis shows cytologic features similar to those of mature hyaline cartilage. Features are the same from one cell to the next and do not show the cellularity, atypia, or mitotic activity associated with chondrosarcomas.

Physical examination of affected joints will show limitation of range of motion, swelling, and occasionally clicking or popping. In the knee, loose bodies may be easily palpable. Superficial joints such as the knee or the small joints of the hands or feet may be notably swollen. Occasionally, synovial chondromatosis may cause nerve compression of adjacent peripheral nerves, particularly in the upper extremity (Jones *et al.* 1987).

Imaging studies

Plain radiographs show multiple juxta-articular radiodense shadows, which may have the stippled appearance of calified cartilage. Larger bodies may have peripheral linear densities, indicative of the transition to bony trabeculation in mature areas of the nodules or loose bodies. Degenerative disease may be seen, as well as pressure erosion of the bone caused by the bulky synovium or by loose bodies adherent to the bone surface (Norman and Steiner 1986). Although the disease is usually confined to the joint cavity, extensive disease may cause outpouching of the capsule and extension into adjacent soft tissues.

Occasionally, synovial chondromatosis may present with a single large solitary synovial chondroma, mimicking chondrosarcoma or parosteal osteosarcoma (Edeiken *et al.* 1994).

Air or double-contrast computed arthrotomography (air and radiographic dye) provides the most complete preoperative data for the orthopedic surgeons by outlining not only the mineralized deposits, but also the noncalified chondromatous nodules (Blacksin *et al.* 1990). Plain CT will show calcified or ossified bodies; however, unmineralized synovium will be less apparent.

Alternatively, MRI may be used to determine the extent of disease. Because of its superior soft-tissue contrast capabilities, and multiplanar imaging, MRI may show accurately the extent of unmineralized as well as mineralized disease. The MRI appearance is variable, depending on the amount of calcification or ossification (Kramer *et al.* 1993).

Management

Treatment of synovial chondromatosis is surgical. There is no role for chemotherapy or radiation. However, there is controversy regarding the optimal type of surgical treatment of synovial chondromatosis. Removal of loose bodies with synovectomy has been advocated by many investigators; others have suggested that loose body removal alone may be adequate (Shpitzer *et al.* 1990).

Synovectomy or loose body removal may be performed open (via an arthrotomy) or closed (arthroscopically). The decision to perform arthroscopic versus open synovectomy is based on the extent of disease, the anatomical areas involved in the joint, whether the patient has had previous failed surgical procedures, and surgeon preference. In one series, 14 of 18 knees with synovial chondromatosis which were treated arthroscopically were either symptom-free or had minor symptoms only at a mean follow-up of 3.5 years (Coolican and Dandy 1989). The most important prognostic factor for patients treated arthroscopically is the condition of the femoral and tibial cartilage. Reoperation may be required for recurrent cases (Dorfmann *et al.* 1989).

Arthroscopic treatment may more rapidly return the patient to function, but late in the disease course many of the bodies are adherent to the synovium and capsule and may be difficult to dislodge. Open synovectomy may be required when there is extensive disease in arthroscopically inaccessible locations, such as the far posterior locations of the knee joint, or in long-standing extensive disease. Optimal arthroscopic candidates are those with early disease limited to an arthroscopically accessible location. Two-incision synovectomy may be required to access all joint areas. In the shoulder, staged anterior and posterior synovectomy may prevent instability.

Postoperatively, an aggressive physical therapy regimen should be undertaken to restore joint mobility. Patients often have some permanent limitation of motion, related in part to the long duration of preoperative symptoms. Long-standing underuse of the extremity frequently results in atrophy of the muscles.

Recurrence following synovectomy may be due to persisting synovial activity. Patients should be followed clinically and with plain radiographs for disease recurrence, and should be aware that relapse may result in the need for additional surgeries. In advanced cases with extensive degenerative disease, arthroplasty may be considered, particularly around the hip and knee.

While synovectomy and loose body removal is indicated in the vast majority of patients, primary arthroplasty may be considered in older patients with advanced degenerative joint disease.

Complications

Although synovial chondromatosis is a benign disease, cases of transformation to synovial chondrosarcoma have been reported (Hamilton *et al.* 1987; Perry *et al.* 1988; Bertoni *et al.* 1991). However, evaluation of this type of progression is difficult due to lack of documentation of the absence of malignant disease at the time of diagnosis, and clear progression of the disease to malignancy. Malignant degeneration of the disease, if it occurs, is extremely rare. Because of extensive prior surgery and extensive spread of disease, amputation is often required.

Future directions

Improved arthoscopic techniques and equipment will likely increase the numbers of patients who may be appropriately treated arthroscopically, with earlier return to function. Advances in the understanding of cartilage development and the availability of molecular markers will improve our understanding of the etiology of this process.

Further reading

Bertoni, F., Unni, K.K., Beabout, J.W., and Sim, F. H. (1991). Chondrosarcomas of the synovium. *Cancer*, **67**, 155–62.

Ten cases of chondrosarcoma of the synovium are presented. In five of these, there is evidence of existing synovial chondromatosis, suggesting a pre-exisiting condition. Histologic features suggestive of malignancy include loss of clustering growth pattern, myxoid change in the matrix, areas of necrosis, and spindling at the periphery of chondroid lobules.

Dorfmann, H., De Bie, B., Bonvarlet, J.P., and Boyer, T. (1989). Arthroscopic treatment of synovial chondromatosis of the knee. *Arthroscopy*, **5**, 48–51. Thirty-nine patients with synovial chondromatosis of the knee underwent arthroscopy. A good result was obtained in 78 per cent with an average of 3.5 years follow-up. The essential prognostic factor for a good result was the condition of the articular cartilage at the time of arthroscopy.

Maurice, H., Crone, M., and Watt, I. (1988). Synovial chondromatosis. *Journal of Bone and Joint Surgery, British Volume*, **70B**, 807–11. Fifty-three cases of synovial chondromatosis are reviewed. Arthrography is helpful in establishing the diagnosis in early cases, and radiologic diagnosis is possible with increasing frequency as the disease progresses. Recurrence after operation was 11.5 per cent.

Milgram, J.W. (1977) Synovial osteochondromatosis. A histopathological study of thirty cases. *Journal of Bone and Joint Surgery*, **59**, 792–801. In this classic article, the author presents 30 cases of synovial chondromatosis and proposes a classification system based on three observed phases of the disease.

Smith, C.F. (1977). Synovial chondromatosis. *Orthopedic Clinics of North America*, **8**, 861–8. This review article discusses the history, pathology, radiology, and treatment of synovial chondromatosis.

Sviland, L. and Malcolm, A.J. (1995). Synovial chondromatosis presenting as a painless soft tissue mass—a report of 19 cases. *Histopathology*, **27**, 275–9. Nineteen cases of synovial chondromatosis presenting as a soft tissue mass are reviewed. The importance of making the correct diagnosis bases on clinical, radiographic, and histologic criteria, and the need to avoid confusion with chondrosarcoma, is discussed.

McCarthy, E.F. and Dorfman, H.D. (1982). Primary synovial chondromatosis. An ultrastructural study. *Clinical Orthopaedics and Related Research*, **168**, 178–86.

Maurice, H., Crone, M., and Watt, I. (1988). Synovial chondromatosis. *Journal of Bone and Joint Surgery, British Volume*, **70B**, 807–11.

Mertens, F., Jonsson, K., Willen, H., *et al.* (1996). Chromosome rearrangements in synovial chondromatous lesions. *British Journal of Cancer*, **74**, 251–4.

Milgram, J.W. (1977) Synovial osteochondromatosis. A histopathological study of thirty cases. *Journal of Bone and Joint Surgery, American Volume*, **59A**, 792–801.

Norman, A. and Steiner, G.C. (1986). Bone erosion in synovial chondromatosis. *Radiology*, **161**, 749–52.

Perry, B.E., McQueen, D.A., and Lin, J.J. (1988). Synovial chondromatosis with malignant degeneration to chondrosarcoma. Report of a case. *Journal of Bone and Joint Surgery, American Volume*, **70A**, 1259–61.

Ryan, L.M., Cheung, H.S., Schwab, J.P., and Johnson, R.P. (1982) Predominance of type II collagen in synovial chondromatosis. *Clinical Orthopaedics and Related Research*, **168**, 173–7.

Shpitzer, T., Ganel, A., and Engelberg, S. (1990). Surgery for synovial chondromatosis. 26 cases followed up for 6 years. *Acta Orthopaedica Scandanavica*, **61**, 567–9.

Sim, F.H., Dahlin, D.C., and Ivins, J.C. (1977). Extra-articular synovial chondromatosis. *Journal of Bone and Joint Surgery, American Volume*, **59A**, 492–5.

Smith, C.F. (1977). Synovial chondromatosis. *Orthopedic Clinics of North America*, **8**, 861–8.

Sviland, L. and Malcolm, A.J. (1995). Synovial chondromatosis presenting as a painless soft tissue mass—a report of 19 cases. *Histopathology*, **27**, 275–9.

References

Apte, S.S. and Athanasou, N.A. (1992). An immunohistological study of cartilage and synovium in primary synovial chondromatosis. *Journal of Pathology*, **166**, 277–81.

Bertoni, F., Unni, K.K., Beabout, J.W., and Sim, F.H. (1991). Chondrosarcomas of the synovium. *Cancer*, **67**, 155–62.

Blacksin, M.F., Ghelman, B., Freiberger, R.H., and Salvati, E. (1990). Synovial chondromatosis of the hip. Evaluation with air computed arthrotomography. *Clinical Imaging*, **14**, 315–18.

Coolican, M.R. and Dandy, D.J. (1989). Arthroscopic management of synovial chondromatosis of the knee. Findings and results in 18 cases. *Journal of Bone and Joint Surgery, British Volume*, **71B**, 498–500.

Davis, R.I., Foster, H., and Biggart, D.J. (1996). C-erb B-2 staining in primary synovial chondromatosis: a comparison with other cartilaginous tumours. *Journal of Pathology*, **179**, 392–5.

Dorfmann, H., De Bie, B., Bonvarlet, J.P., and Boyer, T. (1989). Arthroscopic treatment of synovial chondromatosis of the knee. *Arthroscopy*, **5**, 48–51.

Edeiken, J., Edeiken, B.S., Ayala, A.G., Raymond, A.K., Murray, J.A., and Guo, S. (1994). Giant solitary synovial chondromatosis. *Skeletal Radiology*, **23**, 23–9.

Hamilton, A., Davis, R.I., Hayes, D., and Mollan, R.A.B. (1987). Chondrosarcoma developing in synovial chondromatosis. A case report. *Journal of Bone and Joint Surgery, British Volume*, **69B**, 137–40.

Helmy, E.S., Bays, R.A., and Sharawy, M.M. (1989). Synovial chondromatosis associated with experimental osteoarthritis in adult monkeys. *Journal of Oral and Maxillofacial Surgery*, **47**, 823–7.

Jones, J.R., Evans, D.M., and Kaushik, A. (1987). Synovial chondromatosis presenting with peripheral nerve compression—a report of two cases. *Journal of Hand Surgery*, **12**, 25–7.

Kramer, J., Recht, M., Deely, D.M., *et al.* (1993). MR appearance of idiopathic synovial osteochondromatosis. *Journal of Computer Assisted Tomography*, **17**, 772–6.

1.6.8 Malignant bone neoplasms
1.6.8.1 Adamantinoma

Kristy Weber

Introduction

Adamantinoma is an extremely rare primary malignant bony neoplasm (Hazelbag and Hogendoorn 1996). When an adamantinoma occurs in the jaw, it is called an ameloblastoma. This discussion will focus on the extragnathic occurrence. Ninety per cent are found in

Box 1

- Rare malignant primary bone neoplasm
- About 90 per cent occur in the tibia
- Consists of epithelial cells and fibroblast-like cells
- Histologic differential diagnosis includes fibrous dysplasia, metastatic carcinoma, vascular neoplasms, synovial sarcoma, and osteofibrous dysplasia
- Typically, admantinomas grow slowly and eventually cause pain and swelling
- Plain radiographs show lobulated lytic areas surrounded by sclerotic reactive bone
- Wide surgical resection is the current optimal treatment

the diaphysis of the tibia, but they have been reported in the femur, humerus, radius, ulna, pelvis, hands, and feet. Ten per cent of patients have an ipsilateral fibular lesion. A small number of reports have noted an occasional adamantinoma in the pretibial soft tissues without an osseous component. Adamantinomas comprise less than 0.5 per cent of primary bone neoplasms and have a slight male predominance. Half of the lesions occur in the second and third decades and the remainder present throughout life. They rarely present in the first decade, however. Adamantinomas are frequently associated with osteofibrous dysplasia.

In the jaw, these tumors arise from odontogenic epithelium, although the etiology of the lesions in the remainder of the skeleton is less clear. Histologically adamantinoma has a biphasic appearance, and early reports speculated between an epithelial, mesodermal, or vascular origin. From more recent studies utilizing electron microscopy and immunohistochemical staining for specific tissue markers, there is now definite proof of an epithelial origin.

There still remains controversy over the exact pathogenesis of the lesion, however, and all hypotheses are highly speculative at this point (Hazelbag and Hogendoorn 1996). Some authors feel that trauma plays a role in implanting the overlying epidermis or dermis into the cortical bone, and this would help explain the predilection for the anterior subcutaneous border of the tibia. Antecedent trauma is reported in 60 per cent of cases involving adamantinoma. Another possibility is from embryological remnants of ectodermal epithelium displaced during early development. Others propose that the adamantinoma arises from aberrantly proliferating mesenchymal tissue. It is possible that they may have their origin from stem cells capable of differentiating into either epithelial or mesenchymal components, but then both components would be considered neoplastic. A recent study compared the two cell populations in terms of DNA aneuploidy, *p53* gene mutations, and metastatic potential, and found only the epithelial component of the adamantinoma to be malignant. It is present in association with either a reactive fibrous stroma or a separate proliferative benign fibrous component. The recent finding of chromosomal abnormalities in adamantinoma and the closely related lesion, osteofibrous dysplasia, indicate that further genetic investigations may solve some of the mystery surrounding the true pathogenesis of these lesions.

Pathology

Grossly, an adamantinoma can be firm or soft, granular or fibrotic, smooth or lobulated. It is grayish-white and may have visible necrosis, hemorrhage, or cystic spaces. It is well marginated and easily distinguishable from the surrounding normal tissue. Most are greater than 5 cm in length and can often involve the entire tibial shaft. The surrounding cortex may be eroded, and 15 per cent of lesions extend into the soft tissues.

Again, microscopically adamantinoma has a biphasic appearance with epithelial areas and a fibrous stroma. Four epithelial patterns have been described as being basaloid, spindled, tubular, or squamous (Weiss and Dorfman 1977). A mixture of several patterns is usually observed. The **basaloid** type is most common and consists of a peripheral layer of cuboidal cells with nuclear palisading surrounding inner spindle cell nests or cystic spaces. Reticulin fibers surround

entire cellular fields in this pattern giving the overall appearance a resemblance to basal cell carcinoma. The **spindled** type is difficult to recognize but usually has a storiform or 'herring-bone' pattern with the epithelial cells arranged in cords and having plump nuclei. In contrast to the basaloid type, reticulin fibers surround individual cells which is a common feature of mesenchymal tumors. The **tubular** pattern has epithelial cells branching and often having the appearance of glandular tissue. In cross-section the tubules look like lumens or vascular spaces and may be confused with a vascular neoplasm if the epithelial differentiation is not obvious. Rarely, a **squamoid** appearance is seen and ranges from immature plump cells with minimal cytoplasm in a whorl pattern to a mature squamous epithelium arranged in nests or cords that produce keratin. This type mimics squamous cell carcinoma.

Between the hyperchromatic epithelial islands, there is bland fibrous connective tissue made up of spindle-shaped collagen-producing cells. Disorganized woven bone fragments prominently lined with osteoblasts may be seen within the stroma which contrasts with the apparent epithelial origin of the tumor. The stroma can look similar to fibrous dysplasia but is less densely packed. It may even have areas of myxoid change. Regardless of which epithelial pattern is present, the nuclei throughout the lesion are bland with minimal atypia in only 15 per cent. Mitoses are infrequent in the epithelial component and absent in the fibrous areas.

The overall low-power architecture of the adamantinoma reveals the center to contain the epithelial component with a few bony trabeculae amidst the fibrous tissue. Closer to the periphery the epithelial proportion decreases with a concomitant increase in the osteofibrous component giving an appearance similar to osteofibrous dysplasia. The woven bone can be transformed to lamellar bone at the edge of the lesion.

Immunohistochemical staining and electron microscopy will confirm the lesion as an adamantinoma. Despite the multitude of appearances of the epithelial component, the cells stain strongly for keratin and other epithelial markers. Only endothelial cells stain positively for factor VIII thereby differentiating adamantinomas from vascular neoplasms. Examination by electron microscopy reveals basal membranes, microfilaments, and desmosomes in the epithelial cell cytoplasm with the desmosomes forming intercellular bridges.

The histologic differential diagnosis includes fibrous dysplasia, metastatic carcinoma, vascular neoplasms, synovial sarcoma, and osteofibrous dysplasia. A fibrous dysplasia type morphology is seen more frequently in children but careful examination of the tissue allows differentiation based on the presence of epithelial components. Metastatic carcinoma does not have the greatly diverse epithelial pattern or bland cellular appearance seen in adamantinoma. It can also be differentiated on the radiographic appearance. A vascular tumor such as an hemangioendothelioma can mimic the tubular epithelial pattern in an adamantinoma, although if enough tissue is examined, the true epithelial nature of the latter should allow the diagnosis to be made. If it is still unclear, the vascular tumor will have positive endothelial (factor VIII), but not epithelial, markers. Synovial sarcoma is difficult to discern from an adamantinoma displaying a tubular pattern with a prominent stroma as the immunohistochemical stains are not helpful. In general the stroma of a synovial sarcoma is more cellular and pleomorphic.

Osteofibrous dysplasia is characterized by a zonal pattern with a fibrous center and peripheral new bone lined by osteoblasts. It is not a healing nonossifying fibroma. An epithelioid component is not seen on routine light-microscopic examination. However, over 90 per cent contain scattered keratin-positive epithelial cells, but this finding is much less prominent than in an adamantinoma.

It is felt that adamantinoma and osteofibrous dysplasia share the same histogenetic origin, and there has been much speculation about the relationship of these two tumors. The finding of lesions clinically and radiographically identical to osteofibrous dysplasia but with larger islands of visible epithelial cells led one group to subclassify these as differentiated adamantinomas, separate from the previously described classic form (Czerniak *et al.* 1989). The differentiated form was initially diagnosed by noticing epithelial foci in tissue samples from osteofibrous dysplasia lesions that required surgical resection. It is also an attempt to keep the classical adamantinoma, with its implications for treatment and prognosis, from being overdiagnosed. The differentiated, or osteofibrous-dysplasia-like, form seems to follow a less aggressive course than its classic counterpart. Many agree that osteofibrous dysplasia and adamantinoma are related at opposite ends of a continuous spectrum. One study states that the differentiated adamantinoma develops due to a reparative process or regression of the classic form. However, most recent reports hypothesize that osteofibrous dysplasia is a precursor lesion to adamantinoma. Certainly the histologic picture becomes more aggressive with increased bony destruction and cortical penetration in the latter lesion. There have been case reports of surgically treated osteofibrous dysplasia or osteofibrous-dysplasia-like adamantinomas recurring years later as a classic adamantinoma. There is always the possibility that the initial lesions were misdiagnosed histologically but their clinical and radiographic appearances became likewise more aggressive. Some osteofibrous dysplasia lesions do arise de novo and do not progress but are self limited and may actually regress with time. Several large series confirm this finding. In general, the lesions in these studies showed no evidence of epithelial cells on light microscopy, but only after immunohistochemical staining. In summary it becomes extremely important to examine the entire tissue specimen with all available techniques to identify any epithelial areas. If found, the lesion should be treated as either a differentiated or classic adamantinoma and appropriate intervention and follow-up should ensue.

Clinical features

An adamantinoma is associated with swelling with or without pain. It is a slow-growing lesion and symptoms may be present from a few weeks to 50 years. Over one-third of patients have symptoms for more than 5 years prior to diagnosis. A mass is the only finding on physical examination. An associated local traumatic event occurs in 60 per cent of the patients but no definite causal effect has been reached. There is slow but progressive bony destruction throughout adulthood.

In the classic adamantinoma, young adults are affected, the tumor grows beyond the cortical boundary, and metastases can occur. The differentiated form affects children and young adolescents, is confined to the cortex of the bone, and has not been reported to metastasize. The clinical presentation of osteofibrous dysplasia is in the first

decade and generally asymptomatic. It is usually a self-limiting process that does not progress or metastasize.

Imaging

The plain radiographs of an adamantinoma are characteristic, demonstrating lobulated lytic areas surrounded by sclerotic reactive bone (Fig. 1). They can have intralesional opacifications and septations. The 'soap bubble' appearance is classically described with the tumor centered in the diaphysis of the tibia and asymmetrically expanding the anterior cortex. Only 15 per cent actually penetrate the cortex and develop a palpable soft-tissue mass. Ten per cent of lesions are confined completely to the cortex and are visible as shallow craters separated from the underlying medullary canal by a shell of subperiosteal bone. Though there is a dominant central lesion, the eccentric lucent areas can occur throughout the shaft separated by areas of sclerosis. This gives the adamantinoma a multiloculated appearance. The lytic areas are sharply defined and may extend into the metaphysis but never occur in the epiphysis. Plain radiographs may underestimate the extent of the neoplasm.

A bone scan is usually intensely positive because of the extensive bony reaction but no uptake is seen past the edges of the lesion. CT demonstrates if the cortical lesion has penetrated into the soft tissues or medullary canal. MRI does not add to the diagnosis but is helpful in preoperative planning.

The radiographic differential diagnosis includes fibrous cortical defect, fibrous dysplasia, and osteofibrous dysplasia. A cortical defect usually has sclerotic margins and does not cause saucerization of the cortex. Fibrous dysplasia can occur in the tibia but causes uniform expansion and occasional anterior bowing. It does not produce extensive periosteal reaction or moth-eaten destruction as can be seen in adamantinoma. A ground-glass appearance can be seen in both. In difficult cases, the diagnosis is easily made on histologic examination. Osteofibrous dysplasia is radiographically identical to the differentiated form of adamantinoma. It occurs in the tibial diaphysis as a multilocular lesion centered in the anterior cortex. It may diffusely involve the entire shaft and cause clinically apparent bowing. It differs from the classic form by not penetrating the cortex and not having satellite lesions separated by sclerotic areas throughout the length of the bone.

Management and results

Surgery is the method of choice for treating adamantinoma. In general an incisional biopsy may not be representative of the entire lesion. Either open or CT-guided biopsy techniques are acceptable, but it is important to sample the central epithelial section. Curettage is associated with a very high recurrence rate (up to 60 per cent of cases) occurring as bony or soft-tissue foci.

The goal of treatment is to achieve a wide surgical margin by resection or amputation (Moon and Mori 1986). A study specifically looking at nine children with adamantinoma found that the procedure of choice in this age group is wide resection and reconstruction with bone graft. At average 5.3 years follow-up, there were no recurrences and one patient with metastases. All of the satellite lesions must be

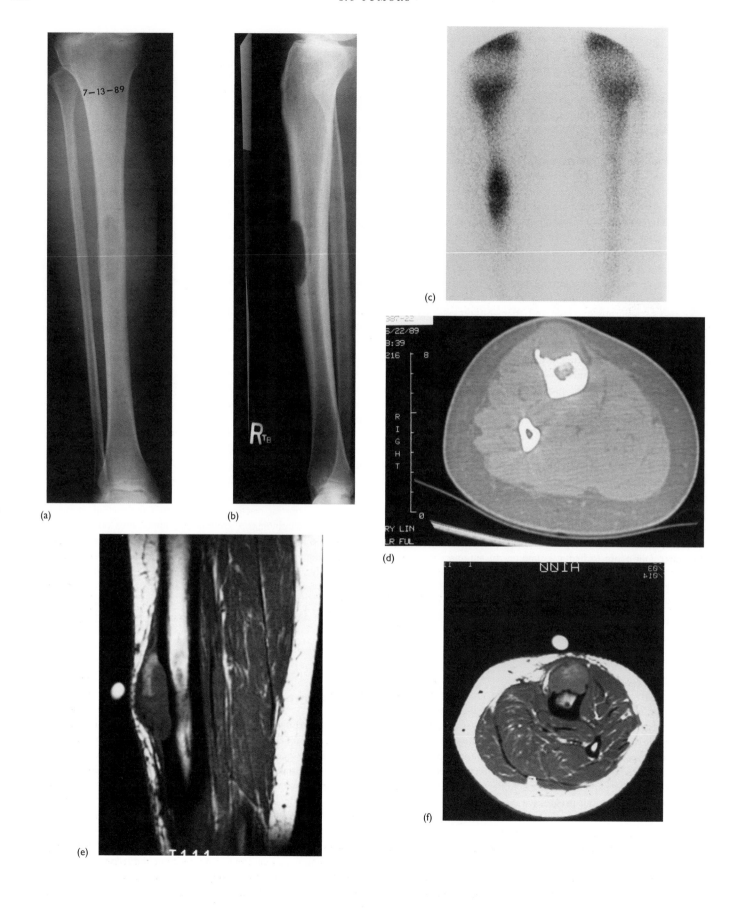

(a)

(b)

(c)

(d)

(e)

(f)

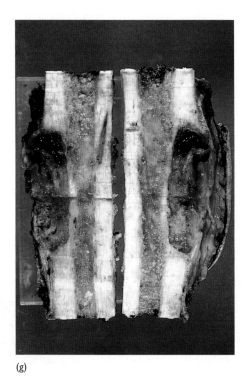

(g)

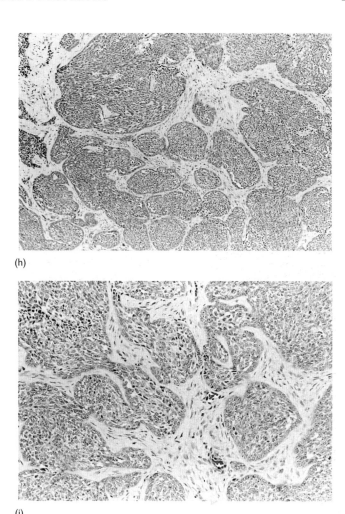

(h)

(i)

Fig. 1. (a) Anteroposterior radiograph of the tibia showing an adamantinoma as a mid-diaphyseal lytic lesion in a 39-year-old female. (b) Lateral view shows the location of the tumor within the anterior cortex. No other lesions are seen in this case. (c) Bone scan shows increased uptake only in the area of the lesion. (d) Axial CT scan through the tibia demonstrates the erosion of the anterior cortical surface. The medullary cavity is relatively uninvolved on this view. (e), (f) T_1-weighted MRI showing the soft-tissue extent of the adamantinoma. Notice how close the tumor is to the overlying skin. (g) Gross appearance of the adamantinoma. Note the distal hemorrhagic spaces. A wide surgical margin was obtained by resection. (h) Low-power view of the resected specimen showing the separate epithelial and fibrous components. The epithelioid areas show the common basaloid pattern. No woven bone is seen in this field but can often be present. (i) Higher-power view reveals the epithelial cells to be fairly uniform in size. No obvious atypia is seen. The intervening fibrous stroma is bland.

removed to decrease the chance of recurrence. If the adamantinoma is well circumscribed in the anterior cortex and has not penetrated the medullary canal, the surgeon may occasionally be able to preserve the posterior cortex to aid in the reconstruction. Reconstruction with both intercalary allografts and vascularized fibular grafts have been utilized. If the entire tibial shaft is involved, a wide resection may not be practical, therefore amputation should be considered. Other reasons to perform an amputation include extensive soft-tissue involvement of the tumor, wide local recurrence after previous surgical treatment, or pathologic fracture that increases the extent of the soft-tissue component. Adjuvant irradiation or chemotherapy have no role in the initial treatment of adamantinoma at the present time. These modalities are reserved for advanced stages of disease.

Recurrences may take from months to two decades to appear which emphasizes the need for long-term clinical and radiographic follow-up. Metastases are present in 15 to 20 per cent of all patients

and may occur up to 15 years after the initial treatment (Keeney *et al.* 1989). They are found in regional lymph nodes, distant bony sites, and lungs. There are conflicting reports of what criteria are associated with an increased risk of metastases, but they are more common in patients who have incomplete initial surgical resection or local recurrence (Hazelbag *et al.* 1994). Histologically the metastatic lesions usually show similarity to the primary tumor, although the mitotic rate may be increased and there may be a more spindled or sarcomatous appearance. Given the slow-growing nature of adamantinoma, any positive regional lymph nodes or pulmonary metastases should be excised when noticed.

If a lesion resembling osteofibrous dysplasia is noted in the young child, watchful management can be undertaken as adamantinoma is unlikely to occur in this age group. If the lesion continues to grow or begins to exhibit symptoms after skeletal maturity, surgical treatment should be employed.

Further reading

Benassi, M., Campanacci, L., Gamberi, G., et al. (1994). Cytokeratin expression and distribution in adamantinoma of the long bones and osteofibrous dysplasia of tibia and fibula. An immunohistochemical study correlated to histogenesis. *Histopathology*, **25**, 71–6.

Bloem, J., van der Heul, R., Schuttevaer, H., and Kuipers, D. (1991). Fibrous dysplasia vs adamantinoma of the tibia: differentiation based on discriminate analysis of clinical and plain film findings. *American Journal of Roentgenology*, **156**, 1017–23.

Fechner, R. and Mills, S. (1993). *Atlas of tumor pathology. Tumors of the bones and joints* (3rd series). Armed Forces Institute of Pathology, Washington, DC.

Gebhardt, M., Lord, F., Rosenberg, A., and Mankin, H. (1987). The treatment of adamantinoma of the tibia by wide resection and allograft bone transplantation. *Journal of Bone and Joint Surgery, American Volume*, **69**, 1177–88.

Hazelbag, H., Fleuren, G., Cornelisse, C., van den Broek, L., Taminiau, A., and Hogendoorn, P. (1995). DNA aberrations in the epithelial cell component of adamantinoma of long bones. *American Journal of Pathology*, **147**, 1770–9.

Knapp, R., Wick, M., Scheithauer, B., and Unni, K. (1982). Adamantinoma of bone. An electron microscopic and immunohistochemical study. *Virchows Archiv. A, Pathological Anatomy and Histopathology*, **398**, 75–86.

McCarthy, E. (1996). *Differential diagnosis in pathology. Bone and joint disorders.* Igaku-Shoin, New York.

Markel, S. (1978). Ossifying fibroma of long bone. Its distinction from fibrous dysplasia and its association with adamantinoma of long bone. *American Journal of Clinical Pathology*, **69**, 91–7.

Mills, S. and Rosai, J. (1985). Adamantinoma of the pretibial soft tissue. *American Journal of Clinical Pathology*, **83**, 108–14.

Moon, N. (1994). Adamantinoma of the appendicular skeleton in children. *International Orthopaedics*, **18**, 379–88.

Park, Y., Unni, K., McLeod, R., and Pritchard, D. (1993). Osteofibrous dysplasia: clinicopathologic study of 80 cases. *Human Pathology*, **24**, 1339–47.

Schajowicz, F. and Santini-Araujo, E. (1989). Adamantinoma of the tibia masked by fibrous dysplasia. Report of three cases. *Clinical Orthopaedics and Related Research*, **238**, 294–301.

Springfield, D., Rosenberg, A., Mankin, H., and Mindell, E. (1994). Relationship between osteofibrous dysplasia and adamantinoma. *Clinical Orthopaedics and Related Research*, **309**, 234–44.

Sweet, D., Vinh, T., and Devaney, K. (1992). Cortical osteofibrous dysplasia of long bone and its relationship to adamantinoma. A clinicopathologic study of 30 cases. *American Journal of Surgical Pathology*, **16**, 282–90.

References

Czerniak, B., Rojas-Corona, R., and Dorfman, H. (1989). Morphologic diversity of long bone adamantinoma. The concept of differentiated (regressing) adamantinoma and its relationship to osteofibrous dysplasia. *Cancer*, **64**, 2319–34.

Hazelbag, H. and Hogendoorn, P. (1996). Adamantinoma of long bones: current perspectives on clinical behaviour, histology and histogenesis. *Cancer Journal*, **9**, 26–31.

Hazelbag, H., Taminiau, A., Fleuren, G., and Hogendoorn, P. (1994). Adamantinoma of the long bones. *Journal of Bone and Joint Surgery, American Volume*, **76**, 1482–99.

Keeney, G., Unni, K., Beabout, J., and Pritchard, D. (1989). Adamantinoma of long bones. A clinicopathologic study of 85 cases. *Cancer*, **64**, 730–7.

Moon, N. and Mori, H. (1986). Adamantinoma of the appendicular skeleton—updated. *Clinical Orthopaedics and Related Research*, **204**, 215–37.

Weiss, S. and Dorfman, H. (1977). Adamantinoma of long bone. An analysis of nine new cases with emphasis on metastasizing lesions and fibrous dysplasia-like changes. *Human Pathology*, **8**, 141–53.

1.6.8.2 Osteosarcoma and variants
Mark C. Gebhardt and Francis J. Hornicek

Introduction

Sarcomas are rare malignant tumors of mesenchymal tissue. About 7000 new bone and soft-tissue sarcomas occur each year in the United States, and of these, approximately 2400 are bone sarcomas (Landis *et al.* 1998). Osteosarcoma, defined as a high-grade sarcoma which directly produces bone or osteoid matrix, accounts for nearly 900 cases annually, making it the most common primary malignant bone tumor. Its incidence is 0.3 per 100 000 population in the United States (Whelan 1997). Osteosarcoma may present at any age, but is most common in the second decade and late adulthood due primarily to osteosarcoma in Paget's disease. Osteosarcoma was once a nearly uniformly fatal disease with more than 80 to 90 per cent of children ultimately developing metastatic disease and dying of their disease within 5 years of diagnosis (McKenna *et al.* 1966). Remarkable progress has been made in our understanding and treatment of osteosarcoma. Current treatment regimens consisting of effective adjuvant chemotherapy and complete surgical excision, lead to cure in 70 to 80 per cent of patients with limb primaries who present without radiographically demonstrable metastases (Goorin *et al.* 1987). In addition, improvements in imaging modalities and surgical

Box 1

- Most common primary malignant bone tumor
- Most commonly occurs in the second decade of life
- In adults, occurs with greater frequency in patients with Paget's disease and fibrous dysplasia
- Most common sites include distal femur, proximal tibia, and proximal humerus
- Histologic diagnosis depends on identification of malignant osteoblasts that directly produce osteoid or bone
- Lungs are the most common site of metastases
- Current treatment includes systemic chemotherapy and en bloc resection of the primary tumor
- Selected patients with pulmonary metastases can benefit from resection of the metastases
- Surgical treatments of the primary tumors include amputation and en bloc resection of the tumor followed by limb reconstruction ('limb salvage')

techniques make it possible to preserve limbs in most patients with an extremity sarcoma, whereas in the past they faced amputation (Springfield *et al.* 1988; Simon and Finn 1993; Jaramillo *et al.* 1996).

The cause of osteosarcoma is unknown. Multiple members of certain families have developed osteosarcoma, suggesting that there is a genetic predisposition in some instances (Porter *et al.* 1992). Genetic predisposition to osteosarcoma is found in patients with hereditary retinoblastoma and the Li–Fraumeni syndrome. The majority of second malignancies in hereditary retinoblastoma patients are sarcomas, of which almost 50 per cent are osteosarcomas (Gebhardt 1996). Evidence for viral etiology lies in data that bone sarcomas can be induced in select animals by certain viruses. Ionizing radiation is a direct cause in 3 per cent of osteosarcomas and is being observed with greater frequency as more patients survive other cancers treated by irradiation and alkylating agents (Tucker *et al.* 1987; Frassica *et al.* 1991). The risk of subsequent bone cancer rises with increasing drug exposure, and alkylating agent chemotherapy may potentiate the radiation effect in the development of secondary osteosarcomas. Interestingly, the affected bone (as in Ewing's sarcoma) treated with irradiation seems to be more susceptible than other tissues to secondary sarcoma development. Osteosarcomas occur with higher frequency than the general population in patients with Paget's disease and certain bone diseases such as fibrous dysplasia.

The tumor location in sites and age of most rapid growth suggests that factors related to skeletal growth and development are involved in the pathogenesis of this tumor. Osteosarcoma may develop in any bone, but the most common sites are in the distal femur, proximal tibia, and humerus where the most rapid growth occurs in adolescence. Experimentally, hypophysectomy reduces the metastatic rate of tumor-bearing animals, and treatment strategies that block the growth hormone pathway are now being considered in the treatment of osteosarcoma (Polack *et al.* 1992).

Clinical evaluation

Patients with an extremity osteosarcoma usually present with pain and an enlarging soft-tissue mass. Symptoms may be present for 3 or more months and are frequently noticed following an injury. The pain persists and worsens. It is present at rest or at night and is not specifically activity related. There are usually no systemic symptoms, and no specific signs to suggest this specific tumor. A joint effusion may be present or the patient may sustain a pathologic fracture. The size of the soft-tissue mass will vary considerably, but it is frequently quite large and tender to palpation. Laboratory studies are nonspecific, but an elevated serum alkaline phosphatase or lactic dehydrogenase has been shown in some studies to be associated with a worse prognosis (Goorin and Anderson 1991; Link *et al.* 1991).

The radiographic appearance of osteosarcoma is that of an aggressive lesion usually located in the metaphysis of the bone (Fig. 1). Radiographs reveal destruction of the normal trabecular pattern with indistinct margins and no endosteal bone response. Intense, but incomplete, periosteal new bone formation and lifting of the cortex with formation of a Codman triangle or a 'starburst' appearance are characteristically seen. The soft-tissue mass is variably mineralized or ossified depending on the relative amounts of chondroblastic and osteoblastic areas. The lesions are usually a mixture of both radiodense and radiolucent areas, but may be purely radiolucent or radio-

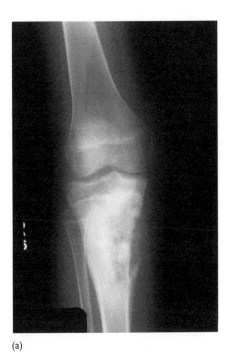 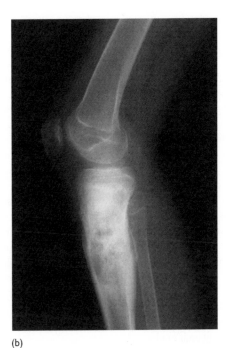 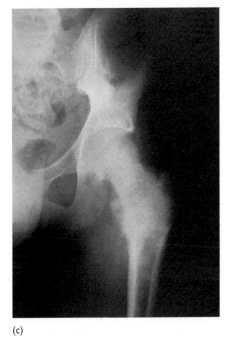

(a) (b) (c)

Fig. 1. Fourteen-year-old female with a stage IIB osteosarcoma of the proximal tibia: (a) anteroposterior and (b) lateral radiographs show a mixture of ill-defined radiodense and radiolucent regions with periosteal new bone formation. (c) Seventeen-year-old male with stage IIB osteosarcoma of the proximal femur: anteroposterior radiograph shows the destruction of the normal trabecular pattern.

dense. These characteristic radiographic features, along with clinical information and tumor location, predict the histologic diagnosis from the plain radiographs in most cases of osteosarcoma.

MRI of the involved limb will determine the local extent of the bony lesion before chemotherapy and at the time of definitive surgery (Fig. 2). The image will show the extent of the lesion within the marrow cavity and document the presence or absence of skip metastases within the bone (Jaramillo et al. 1996). Axial images will show the soft-tissue extent of the lesion beyond the cortex and the relationship of the mass to the neurovascular structures. In most instances, the MRI is the preferred modality for evaluating the primary lesion and a CT scan is unnecessary.

In 10 to 20 per cent of affected patients, radiographically detectable metastatic disease is present at diagnosis. Metastatic lesions are most frequently found in the chest and less commonly in the same or other bones. A CT scan of the chest and a bone scan are obtained to search for metastatic disease. CT scans are much more sensitive in detecting metastatic pulmonary disease than conventional chest radiographs or plane tomograms. Spiral CT offers even more sensitivity in detecting pulmonary metastases. Skeletal metastases should be considered if the patient has other bony symptoms, and occasionally asymptomatic skeletal metastases are detected by bone scan.

Pathology

Classic osteosarcoma is defined as a tumor composed of a high-grade sarcomatous stroma with malignant osteoblasts that directly produce tumor osteoid or bone (Fig. 3). The tumor cells are usually anaplastic with pleomorphic nuclei and bizarre mitoses. They can have a wide variation in cellular size and shape. Tumors may be primarily chondroblastic or fibroblastic, but the presence of a small region of tumor osteoid or bone formation is sufficient for the diagnosis of osteosarcoma.

Osteosarcomas are classified into a variety of subtypes based on their grade, number of sites, location in the bone and cause. Surface osteosarcomas may be of high or low histologic grade (Schajowicz et al. 1988). The typical parosteal osteosarcoma is a surface lesion composed of low-grade fibroblastic osteosarcoma, which produces woven or lamellar bone (Fig. 4). It occurs in an older age group than the classical osteosarcoma, usually between the ages of 20 and 40 years. The posterior aspect of the distal femur is the most common site for parosteal osteosarcomas. The tumor arises from the cortex as a broadly based lesion. With time, however, this lesion may invade the cortex and enter the endosteal cavity. Conventional high-grade osteosarcomas may also develop on the surface of the bone and may be confused with parosteal or periosteal osteosarcomas (Schajowicz et al. 1988).

The so-called periosteal osteosarcoma is a moderate-grade chondroblastic surface lesion frequently located in the proximal tibia and in the same age distribution as classic osteosarcoma (Schajowicz et al. 1988). Histologically, the tumors are relatively high grade, and are predominantly chondroblastic osteosarcomas. They may metastasize to the lungs and are treated similar to classic osteosarcoma, although the role for adjuvant chemotherapy is less clear.

Multifocal osteosarcoma is rare, but occasionally patients present with multiple synchronous sites of tumor at diagnosis (Parham et al.

1985). Each lesion resembles a primary tumor radiographically. It is not clear whether such sarcomas arise de novo in multiple sites or whether one of the lesions is the primary that has metastasized to other bony sites (Daffner et al. 1997). Multicentric osteosarcoma may also be metachronous in that other bony lesions occur years after treatment of the first.

Telangiectatic osteosarcoma is another variant of osteosarcoma that presents as a radiolucent lesion on plain radiographs with little calcification or bone formation (Fig. 5). It is a high-grade vascular lesion with little osteoid production (Huvos et al. 1982). The age distribution and treatment is identical to classic high-grade osteosarcoma. Although initially felt to be a more aggressive variant, the response to adjuvant chemotherapy appears to be similar to that of conventional osteosarcoma (Pignatti et al. 1991).

Metastases

High-grade osteosarcoma should be considered a systemic disease manifested with micrometastatic disease present at diagnosis. Approximately 10 to 20 per cent of conventional high-grade osteosarcoma patients will have radiographic evidence of metastatic disease at diagnosis (Whelan 1997). These metastatic sites will be detected by a CT scan of the chest or a bone scan. Most frequently the metastatic site will be in the lung, followed by the bone, and much less frequently by other viscera, including the pleura, pericardium, kidney, adrenal gland, lymph nodes, and brain. A small number of patients present with bone and pulmonary metastases. Patients who present with metastases only in the lung are potentially salvageable and have the chance of an event-free survival of approximately 40 per cent. One recent study has shown that cure of the metastatic patient is possible if all sites of disease can be resected in addition to the administration of aggressive chemotherapy (Meyers et al. 1993). Twenty-four patients in this study who could not be rendered surgically disease-free ultimately died, whereas seven of 22 patients who had all gross disease resected survived. Death from metastatic disease results from pulmonary failure due to widespread lung metastases, pulmonary hemorrhage, pneumothorax, and superior vena cava obstruction. Most patients who die of metastatic disease have lung involvement at the time of death. Bone metastases occur in about 25 per cent of the metastatic patients. Patients with bony metastases are probably incurable and with rare exceptions ultimately die of their disease.

Nonmetastatic patients who relapse one or more years after chemotherapy and surgical resection, usually do so in the lung and often have a better prognosis than those who present with pulmonary metastases at diagnosis. These patients are treated with pulmonary resections if surgically possible and usually receive additional chemotherapy. Results from this aggressive approach show that about 30 to 40 per cent of these patients can achieve a 5-year actuarial survival (Goorin et al.1984).

Biopsy

The technique of biopsy for osteosarcomas and all sarcomas is important to ensure that adequate tissue is obtained for diagnosis and that limb salvage surgery is not obviated. Prior to obtaining

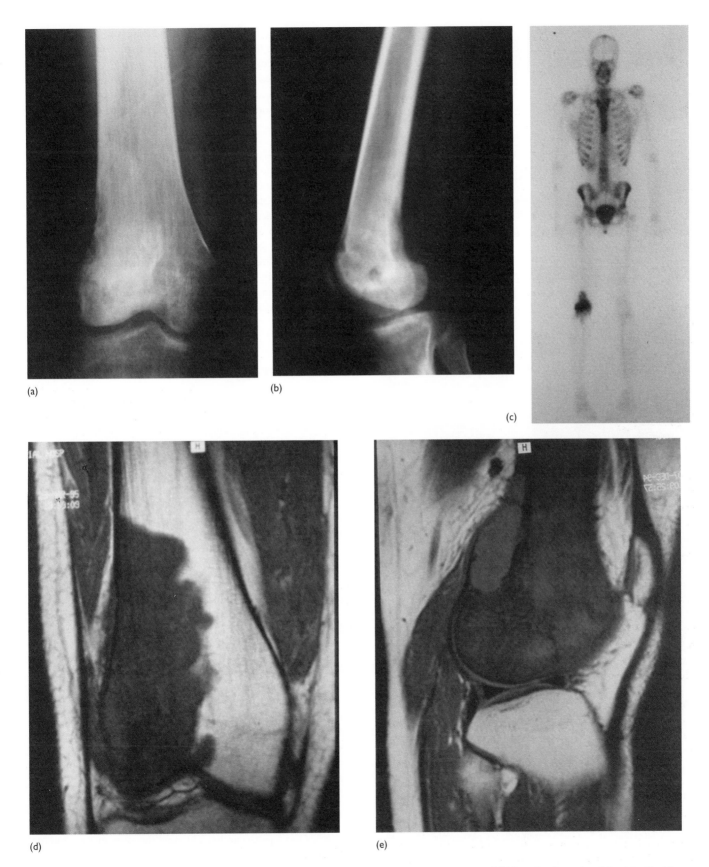

Fig. 2. Twenty-four-year-old female with stage IIB osteosarcoma of the distal femur. (a) Anteroposterior and (b) lateral radiographs of the right distal femur reveal cloudy opacities and sclerotic regions without distinct radiographic tumor margins. (c) Bone scan shows increased uptake in the distal femur and no metastatic foci. (d), (e) MRI scans show the intramedullary extent of the tumor, the distal extent of the tumor to the subchondral bone, and a small soft-tissue tumor mass. No skip lesions were identified.

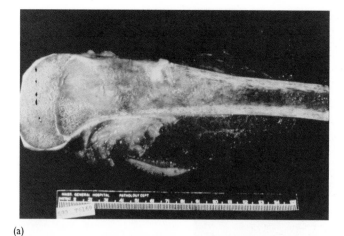

(a)

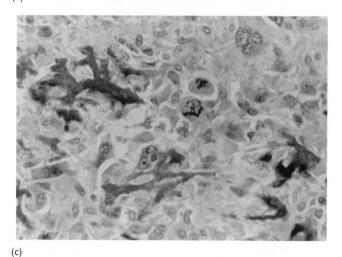

(b)

(c)

Fig. 3. (a) Gross specimen of an osteosarcoma of the distal femur. (b) Low-magnification and (c) high-magnification section of this high-grade osteosarcoma (hematoxylin and eosin stain) exhibiting the classic characteristics. These include abundance of tumor bone deposited by anaplastic cells with osteoblastic features. Some areas of immature bone will undergo mineralization. The sarcomatous cells are pleomorphic and show marked nuclear anaplasia. Note the prominent nucleoli.

tissue, the surgeon, radiologist, and pathologist should review the staging studies so that each member of the team is fully appraised of the diagnostic considerations. A core needle biopsy or open biopsy may be performed as long as adequate tissue is obtained. For CT-directed core biopsies, it is important that the surgeon and the radiologist communicate so that the biopsy tract can be placed along the line of a resection incision. Usually three or more cores are obtained. One is used for frozen section to ensure that adequate diagnostic tissue has been obtained, one is used for permanent hematoxylin and eosin sections and one preserved for special stains. Open biopsies should be performed after all the staging studies have been completed and the incision placed in accordance with the planned resection or amputation. Meticulous hemostasis and the judicious use of a drain are important to avoid the spread of hematoma containing tumor cells. If a bone defect is required to obtain tumor tissue, it should be a small, round defect and a polymethylmethacrylate plug should be employed to limit the spread of hematoma. As with core needle biopsies, a frozen section should be performed to confirm that adequate tissue has been obtained and the tissue should always be cultured.

Chemotherapy

Outcome for patients with osteosarcoma has improved significantly as a result of the administration of adjuvant systemic chemotherapy. Initial studies recognized that chemotherapy was best directed at micrometastatic disease, so it was employed postoperatively, following amputation of the primary (Goorin and Andersen 1991). High-dose methotrexate and adriamycin were the initial drugs shown to be most active in treating osteosarcoma, and subsequently cisplatin and other drugs were added. Protocols which include adriamycin, high-dose methotrexate, cisplatin, and other drugs have shown improved disease-free survival to 50 to 65 per cent of outcomes in most studies compared to a disease-free survival of 10 to 20 per cent without chemotherapy (Goorin and Andersen 1991; Link *et al.* 1991). Initially the benefit of adjuvant chemotherapy was not universally accepted by all, however, and a randomized study comparing the use of immediate postoperative adjuvant chemotherapy with delayed use (only in those patients who developed metastatic disease) was undertaken. This and other studies clearly showed an event-free and overall survival benefit in the adjuvant group(Goorin and Andersen 1991; Link *et al.* 1991).

Recent interest has focused on the use of preoperative chemotherapy (neoadjuvant chemotherapy) prior to removal of the primary tumor (Winkler *et al.* 1991; Provisor, 1997). This approach has several advantages, such as defining prognostic groups based on the observed histologic response to the chemotherapy, facilitating resection by reducing the size and increasing the amount of tumor necrosis, and possibly making limb salvage 'safer'. There are potential drawbacks, however, including the possibility that the patients who do not respond well to the treatment will develop resistant clones of cells and become refractory to the chemotherapy. A study by the Pediatric Oncology Group has addressed this issue in a randomized study and found no disease-free or survival advantage to preoperative chemotherapy. This study allayed the fear regarding the nonresponders, and neoadjuvant chemotherapy is currently the standard approach in most centers for reasons listed above. A current multi-

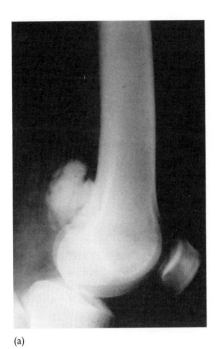

(a)

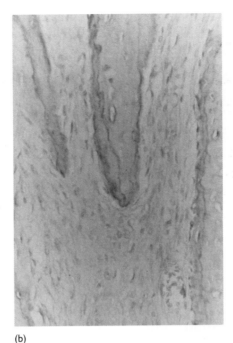

(b)

Fig. 4. (a) Lateral radiograph of the distal femur. Protruding ossified mass from the posterior cortex classic of a parosteal osteosarcoma. (b) Histology: hematoxylin and eosin stained section shows the low-grade appearance of this lesion.

institutional trial is addressing the question of whether the addition of ifosfamide and/or an immunostimulant, muramyl tripeptide-phosphatidyl ethanolamine, will improve survival beyond the 50 to 65 per cent reported in protocols using high-dose methotrexate, adriamycin, and cisplatin.

Histologic evaluation of the percentage necrosis in the excised tumor after pretreatment with chemotherapy has been demonstrated in many studies to be a prognostic indicator of drug effectiveness (Glasser *et al.* 1992). Unfavorable responders (usually defined as less than 90 to 95 per cent necrosis) were more likely to develop distant metastases despite continuation of adjuvant chemotherapy after surgery than those patients with more than 90 per cent necrosis. The prognostic value of responsiveness of the primary tumor to presurgical chemotherapy has been confirmed in several trials. Several systems for grading the effect of presurgical chemotherapy have been developed. They are based on the histologic assessment of percentage necrosis in the excised specimen. Currently, favorable responses are considered to be those tumors with extensive to complete necrosis (95 per cent or greater) of the primary tumor, whereas unfavorable histologic responses are those with the continued presence of viable tumor. Most patients with a good response do well, whereas those with an unfavorable histologic response to preoperative chemotherapy usually develop metastases. Histologic grading of response offers one means of identifying patients at high risk for the development of recurrent disease early in their treatment. Unfortunately, the initial hope that the poor responders could be 'salvaged' by adding new agents has not been realized, but it is an area of continued investigation (Whelan 1997).

Presurgical chemotherapy has been purported to increase the percentage of patients who are suitable candidates for limb-salvage surgery and to facilitate limb-sparing procedures by tumor shrinkage. To date, no randomized studies have been performed that support this contention, and osteosarcomas because of their matrix component seldom decrease in size following neoadjuvant chemotherapy.

There is the subjective impression, however, that the lesions are more safely resected following pretreatment. One study has documented an association between the risk of local recurrence and surgical margins combined with tumor necrosis (Picci *et al.* 1994). The risk of local recurrence increases in patients with less than wide margins and less than a good histologic response. In contrast, a recent unpublished study of the long-term results of a Pediatric Oncology Group study showed excellent local control in patients who had limb-sparing procedures without preoperative chemotherapy (Merkel *et al.* 1996). Most institutions are currently using presurgical chemotherapy for patients who are limb-salvage candidates. Improvements in reconstructive techniques and the increased experience and confidence of tumor surgeons have increased the number of limb-sparing procedures. Currently, about 80 per cent of patients who present with extremity osteosarcomas are limb-salvage candidates. The principles of achieving 'negative' margins of normal tissue around the tumor are important, but the necessary thickness of this cuff is unknown and many specimens contain at least a portion where the margin would be termed 'marginal'.

Despite these advances, 20 to 40 per cent of patients ultimately die of the disease. Recent investigations have identified mechanisms by which tumors become resistant to seemingly effective therapy. One of the major causes of failure is drug resistance: failure of the tumor cells to be killed by the chemotherapeutic agents administered. Multidrug resistance in osteosarcoma occurs via non-P-glycoprotein- and P-glycoprotein-mediated mechanisms (Gebhardt 1996; Whelan 1997). P-glycoprotein is a membrane-bound glycoprotein 'pump' encoded by the *MDR1* gene, and is expressed in various tumors and normal tissues. It is an adenosine-triphosphate-dependent transmembrane glycoprotein capable of pumping disparate classes of drugs, such as doxorubicin, out of the cell. It has been hypothesized that a major reason for poor chemotherapy responses is the presence of P-glycoprotein, and one recent study has shown that patients whose tumors express P-glycoprotein have a significantly lower

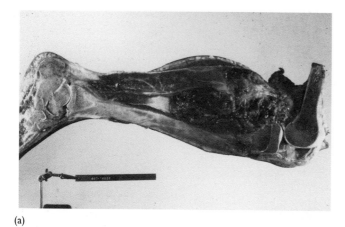

(a)

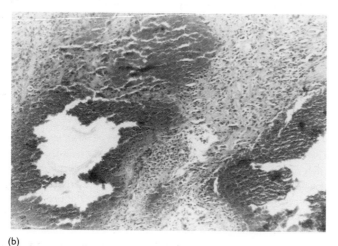

(b)

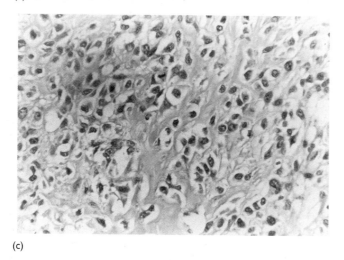

(c)

Fig. 5. A 16-year-old male underwent a transfemoral amputation for this high-grade telangiectatic osteosarcoma: (a) gross specimen; (b) hematoxylin and eosin stained sections (low magnification), abundant blood seen; (c) hematoxylin and eosin sections (higher magnification). Bizarre pleomorphic cells have clear regions in the cytoplasm which are located perinuclear. Immature tumor bone is present but to a lesser extent than that seen in convential osteosarcomas.

chance of event-free and overall survival than those whose tumors do not express detectable P-glycoprotein (Baldini *et al.* 1995). In this study, P-glycoprotein expression did not correlate with histologic necrosis, and was a more powerful prognostic indicator than necrosis. Multidrug resistance reversal agents, which are drugs that block P-glycoprotein function, have been shown to allow the accumulation of drug in the cell, further confirming the function of P-glycoprotein, and offering the possibility of overcoming its adverse effect. Unfortunately, the toxicity of the currently available drugs is significant and studies of their benefit in other types of cancers are lacking, but it is an area of intense investigation at present. It is hoped that identification of chemotherapy 'nonresponders' prospectively, in order to individualize therapy and avoid unnecessary drug toxicity, will improve outcome.

Intra-arterial routes for presurgical chemotherapy using adriamycin or cisplatin have become more popular to maximize drug delivery to the tumor (Jaffe *et al.* 1991). High local drug concentrations are achievable, and good responses in primary tumors have been reported. Appropriate angiographic support is necessary to administer repeated courses of intra-arterial therapy preoperatively. To date, no studies have documented that this approach has an advantage compared with the same agents delivered systemically.

Extent of the disease at diagnosis is very important in prognosis, and patients with overt metastatic disease have an unfavorable outcome. Patients who present with metastases have a much worse prognosis, and if they cannot be rendered surgically free of disease they seldom survive (Meyers *et al.* 1993). An aggressive approach to patients presenting with metastatic disease is warranted initially and has improved their prognosis. Patients who can be rendered surgically free of disease have a 30 to 40 per cent chance of survival when combined with aggressive chemotherapy regimens (Meyers *et al.* 1993). Newer agents are being explored to improve the outcome of the metastatic patient. Management of relapsed patients includes aggressive resection of pulmonary metastases if possible and alternative chemotherapy protocols. At times irradiation of metastatic sites may be appropriate.

Osteosarcomas may arise in pre-existent lesions or from radiation exposure (Tucker *et al.* 1987; Frassica *et al.* 1991). They are treated similarly to *de novo* lesions, but these patients and those who develop osteosarcomas with Paget's disease are usually associated with an adverse prognosis (Frassica *et al.* 1991). The primary site of disease is also an important variable, in that patients with axial skeleton primaries have a poor prognosis. Tumor size has also been cited as a powerful prognostic factor (Bieling *et al.* 1996). Skip metastases (distinct foci of tumor within the same bone as the primary lesion) are an indicator of poor prognosis, and patients behave similarly to those with pulmonary metastases (Wuisman and Enneking 1990). Patients with skip metastases usually develop local recurrence or developed distant metastases despite treatment with adjuvant chemotherapy.

Local control

Local control of an osteosarcoma requires complete *en bloc* resection with tumor-free margins (Simon 1988; Springfield *et al.* 1988; Springfield 1991). The desired margin is a wide margin as defined by Enneking *et al.* (1980). This may be achieved by amputation or limb salvage procedures, but in the past 20 years extremity osteosarcomas have been managed increasingly more frequently by limb-preserving techniques. No randomized studies have been performed to document the safety of limb-sparing resections, but several retrospective studies have failed to demonstrate a survival advantage for amputation (Goorin and Andersen 1991; Rougraff et al. 1994). The use of preoperative chemotherapy appears to make limb-salvage surgery easier because of a decrease in the peritumoral inflammation and increased mineralization in the mass, which makes the extent of the lesion easier to define at operation, although the size of the lesion seldom shrinks because of the matrix. The effect of chemotherapy in making limb sparing safer is less well documented, but one study showed an increased local recurrence rate if margins were less than wide and the chemotherapeutic response was less than good as measured by percentage histologic tumor necrosis (Picci et al. 1994).

Amputation was the only way to ensure complete eradication of the tumor prior to modern imaging techniques and the use of chemotherapy, and is still part of the standard armamentarium of operations employed today. One advantage is that local recurrence following amputation is uncommon, occurring in approximately 5 per cent of cross-bone amputations (Campanacci and Laus 1980; Springfield et al. 1988; Rougraff et al. 1994). Stump recurrence has been attributed to occult intramedullary spread of tumor and skip metastases. MRI radionuclide scans are sensitive and helpful in detecting most skip lesions (Jaramillo et al. 1996). A marrow margin of about 5 cm above the most proximal medullary extent of tumor should be achieved. It has not been clearly shown that removal of the entire bone results in enhanced survival when compared to less radical procedures done with adequate surgical margins (Rougraff et al. 1994). The functional results from cross bone amputations of the lower extremities are quite good with modern prosthetics, and patients who are desirous of high demand athletic activities are probably better served by an amputation. The same is not true for the upper extremity, where even with myoelectric prostheses the functional result of an amputation can never approach that of an intact hand. Patients with tumors in more proximal segments of the extremity, as opposed to lower extremities, have more difficulties with functional and cosmetic disabilities.

Limb-salvage surgery

Although amputations achieve adequate tumor-free margins and are functionally quite acceptable, most patients prefer to save the limb. Initial concern about the oncologic safety of resections has been addressed by several nonrandomized studies suggesting that, especially in patients with a good response to preoperative chemotherapy, local recurrence rates are below 5 to 10 per cent as long as a wide margin is achieved (Simon 1988; Rougraff et al. 1994; Picci et al. 1997). Functional outcomes compared to amputations are more difficult to assess. There is lower oxygen consumption with limb-salvage procedures compared to amputation (Otis et al. 1985), but there are no true comparisons of functional outcome between the two options. There may be psychologic benefits to limb salvage, but these are hard to assess (Greenberg et al. 1994), and no apparent benefit to limb salvage (compared to those who had amputations) could be demonstrated in one study of osteosarcoma survivors. There is clearly a higher complication rate in patients who undergo limb salvage.

The options of limb salvage must be carefully discussed with the patient and/or his or her parents so that an understanding of the expected functional results and potential complications is provided to them. In most instances, the patient is discouraged from returning to contact sports or running and jumping activities following these procedures. It is helpful in advising the patient to point out that a rotationplasty or amputation remains as an option if the primary reconstruction fails. In patients with metastatic disease at presentation, it is reasonable to consider limb salvage, even if the longevity of the reconstruction is in question, because in the fortunate situation that the patient survives, ablative procedures can be performed later if necessary.

Retrospective comparisons of patients treated by amputation to those treated by limb salvage do not suggest a reduced disease-free survival (Goorin and Andersen 1991; Rouggraff et al. 1994). A wide margin and a good histologic response (> 95 per cent) are optimal to avoid local recurrence, but a recent update of a study from Bologna suggests that surgical margin is the most important factor (Picci et al. 194). It is important to assess carefully the plane films, bone scan, and MRI following the preoperative chemotherapy to assess the resectability of the lesion. Obviously, if the nerves and vessels are encased by tumor, or if there is a large hematoma from a biopsy or fracture, resection may not be advisable. It is also very important to assess the joint to determine whether an intra-articular or extra-articular resection will be necessary, and to exclude the presence of skip metastases within the involved bone. Ideally, limb-salvage patients should have a good response to preoperative chemotherapy, although there are no proven imaging studies that reliably predict percentage tumor necrosis. MRI with gadolinium, thallium scans, and PET scans are being assessed for their worth in this regard.

The selection of appropriate patients for limb-salvage surgery is important. The type of operation should never compromise the oncologic goal. When there is doubt that adequate excision can be accomplished, amputation is the indicated procedure. A pathologic fracture may be a contraindication to limb-salvage surgery, although some investigators have reported healing of pathologic fractures during presurgical chemotherapy allowing limb-salvage surgery to be undertaken (Jaffe et al. 1987). No large studies of limb-sparing surgery following pathologic fracture have been reported, and most investigators have traditionally recommended amputation rather than limb-salvage surgery because of an unacceptably high local recurrence rate when more conservative surgical techniques are used. There is some indication, however, that nondisplaced fractures through tumors that respond well to chemotherapy may be candidates for local resection (Scully et al. 1996). Care must be exercised because local recurrence almost always leads to systemic relapse. Metastatic tumor spread invariably follows local recurrence (Rougraff et al. 1994). The incidence of subsequent systemic recurrence appears also to be higher in patients presenting with pathologic fracture.

Certain locations, such as the distal tibia, are poor locations for limb-salvage surgical resections because an adequate soft-tissue margin is difficult to achieve. Similarly, limb-salvage surgery in the lower extremity may be an inappropriate choice for young patients who have not achieved full growth potential and who would be left with a limb-length discrepancy later in life, although creative endoprosthetic devices may circumvent this relative contraindication (Finn and Simon 1991; Eckardt et al. 1993; Ward et al. 1996). Improved surgical techniques have increased the number of patients eligible for limb-salvage surgery, and a variety of novel techniques have been used to repair the defect created by resection of tumor-bearing bones. Expendable bones such as the ulna, fibula, scapula, and ribs may be resected without bony reconstruction. The functional disability from excision of these areas is minimal.

The majority of limb-salvage procedures for osteosarcoma require restoration of the structural integrity of the involved extremity, and clinical experience has centered around the use of biologic materials and metallic endoprosthetic devices. There are advantages and disadvantages to each approach, and no good comparison studies have been performed to document the superiority of one over the other. Allograft reconstructions offer the ability to restore bony defects and provide a lattice for the ingrowth of the patient's own bone tissues, as well as the ability to reconstruct articular surfaces, ligaments and tendon attachments (Gebhardt *et al.* 1991; Alman *et al.* 1995; Mankin *et al.* 1996). Endoprostheses offer immediate stability and mechanical fixation to host tissues, which allows early ambulation and usage (Eckardt *et al.* 1993; Horowitz *et al.* 1993; Malawer and Chou 1995; Ward *et al.* 1996). The decision concerning the most appropriate procedure for an individual patient reflects consideration of the age of the patient, the defect to be repaired, and the surgeon's and patient's personal preference.

The principles of the resection remain the same for all limb-sparing procedures. The lesion must be completely excised with a cuff of normal tissue completely surrounding it (Springfield *et al.* 1988). The biopsy tract should be completely excised with the tumor. The ideal thickness of the tissue is unknown and is evolving with experience. Obviously, the more muscle that can be preserved the better for soft-tissue coverage and function. Preoperative chemotherapy has led surgeons to resect less muscle than had been the case in the past. The type of marginal tissue (fascia versus muscle) is important. Fascia is a good barrier to tumor spread, whereas muscle and fat are less so. Margins are usually less thick near neurovascular structures and this seems to be acceptable given the relatively low recurrence rates following limb-sparing resections. The use of MRI has greatly enhanced the ability to determine marrow margins as well as soft-tissue extent. One should aim for 5 cm of normal marrow margin as an ideal, although 1 to 2 cm of normal marrow may be acceptable.

Autologous bone grafting is limited in tumor surgery because of the long segments of bone excised. Successful knee arthrodesis can be accomplished, even when a long segment of bone has been excised, by employing hemicylindrical grafts from the tibia or femur and using one or both fibulae (Enneking and Shirley 1977). This procedure is complicated by a high incidence of nonunion (35 per cent), fatigue fracture (45 per cent), and infection. Although the operation successfully achieves tumor-free margins, the revascularization and rehabilitation processes are prolonged and complicated. Patients must adjust their lifestyles to accommodate the arthrodesis. Once healed, however, it is a durable reconstruction that allows some athletic activity and manual labor.

Vascularized grafts are occasionally used to restore bony defects and augment other reconstruction techniques such as allograft segments (Minami *et al.* 1995). The primary indications are for irradiated wounds or repairing nonunions following primary reconstructions. The bone graft remains viable, and subsequent healing does not require the long periods of remodeling and regrowth of the tissue into the grafts. This procedure is lengthy and the vascular dissection

and reanastomosis is technically demanding. Recently this has been combined with allograft shells in some centers to quicken the healing time in metaphyseal defects where fixation techniques are limited (Capanna *et al.* 1991; Manfrini 1997). An example would be a metaphyseal resection where the epiphysis is spared. The allograft shell provides initial stability, and an intramedullary vascularized fibula augments the healing and incorporation of the graft.

One alternative for reconstruction of large bony defects is with massive allografts. Their success relates to the reduced antigenicity of nonvascularized bone that has been frozen or freeze-dried. Cryopreservation in the presence of glycerol or dimethyl sulfoxide preparations temporarily preserves at least some articular cartilage chondrocyte viability (Mankin *et al.* 1996). Tendons remain attached to the donor bone to use in the joint reconstruction. Allografts are stored in sterile conditions at low temperatures (−80 °C) in tissue banks and are thus available in a variety of sizes allowing the host and donor to be size matched. These grafts slowly become incorporated by the host, providing a structural network for creeping substitution of host bone tissue, although this probably only occurs at the osteosynthesis site and in spots along the periosteal surface of the allograft. Once the allograft–host junction heals, a stable bony reconstruction is achieved which allows the patient to pursue most non-athletic activities (Fig. 6). Satisfactory functional results are achieved in 80 to 85 per cent of patients (Gebhardt *et al.* 1991; Alman *et al.* 1995; Mankin *et al.* 1996). The complications are infection, non-union, fracture, and joint instability. The long-term fate of the articular surface is not fully established, but it is clear that some joints ultimately develop subarticular fractures or degenerative joint disease

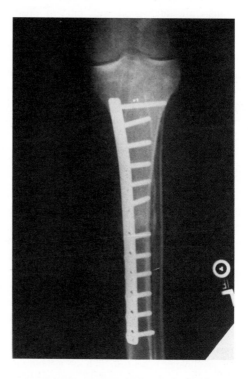

Fig. 6 A 23-year-old female underwent wide resection of an osteosarcoma of the proximal tibia with osteoarticular allograft reconstruction. After 7 years this radiograph shows a well-aligned joint without significant degenerative changes. The allograft–host junction is well healed.

and require total joint arthroplasty (Gebhardt *et al.* 1991; Mankin *et al.* 1996).

Custom-designed and modular endoprostheses are also available to reconstruct bone and joint defects created by tumor resections. They are manufactured to fit dimensions of the excised bone, and usually employ standard total joint arthroplasty components (Fig. 7) (Horowitz *et al.* 1993; Malawer and Chou 1995). One advantage of endoprostheses, especially those which are cemented in place, is that they allow for immediate weight bearing. Fatigue fracture, loosening, and infection occur with oncologic prosthesis reconstruction, and the ideal mechanism to fix these implants to host bone has not been established. The fatigue fracture potential of the metal is a design and stress problem that can be improved by manufacturing changes. Loosening at the bone–cement–prosthesis interface is a problem that is minimized by using meticulous cement technique and stress-reducing total joint mechanics such as a rotating-hinge knee design. Infection is a difficult problem with the prostheses because it acts as a large foreign body. Infection may result in a delayed amputation, although theoretically at a level no higher than if amputation had been used initially to approach the primary tumor.

Expandable endoprostheses have been employed in children to address the problem of limb-length inequality in the lower extremity in children (Fig. 8) (Gebhardt *et al.* 1991; Alman *et al.* 1995; Mankin *et al.* 1996). The concept of a telescoping unit is employed which can be expanded with a gear device or a modular design which can be lengthened by replacing a body segment with a longer one. This permits gradual expansion of the overall length of the prosthesis and makes it possible to implant the endoprosthesis in skeletally immature patients, increasing the numbers of those eligible for limb-salvage surgery. When these prostheses reach their full length, they frequently require replacement because of the loss of structural strength with full extension.

Other reconstruction options include rotationplasty and resection without reconstruction (in some sites) (Fig. 9). The Van Nes rotationplasty is a surgical technique that is essentially an intercalary amputation of the involved part of the extremity, which preserves only the nerves and sometimes the major vessels (Kotz and Salzer 1982; Merke and Gebhardt 1991). It is most commonly used for excision of distal femoral sarcomas in very young patients. The distal femur, adjacent joint, and adjacent soft tissues are resected with preservation of the lower leg (preserving the ankle and foot) by maintenance of an intact neurovascular bundle. The distal femur is replaced by 180° rotation of the distal extremity and fixation of the tibia to the proximal femur. The ankle thus functions as a knee joint. The foot is in an inverted position with the plantar surface anteriorly, and the retained foot acts as the amputation stump similar to a below-knee amputee. It has several advantages compared to above-knee amputation including a longer lever arm, an active 'knee' and durability. The functional results are excellent for athletic activities, and it solves the problem of limb-length inequality in young children. It also obviates phantom pain associated with amputation, because the nerves are preserved. The main drawback is the appearance of the limb, which is a cosmetic issue; however, with the prosthesis on, patients appear similar to standard amputees. The anticipated potential psychologic effects have not been documented in follow-up studies. Similar resections and reconstructions have been reported for the proximal femur and tibia, and the upper extremity (Winkelmann 1986; de Bari *et al.* 1990).

For extremely large tumors of the proximal humerus and shoulder girdle, the Tikhoff–Linberg resection for proximal humerus lesions is successful in eradicating the tumor with wide margins (Malawer 1991). It is an alternative to interscapulothoracic (forequarter) amputation for large tumors about the shoulder when the brachial plexus does not require resection. The proximal humerus is excised as well as the scapula, without bony replacement. The distal arm, elbow, and hand are preserved. The shoulder area is unstable, with telescoping of the intervening structures when stresses are applied to the hand or forearm. It is usually possible to stabilize the remaining humerus to the ribs or clavicle with Dacron tapes and remaining musculature,

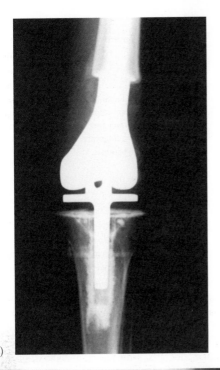

(a)

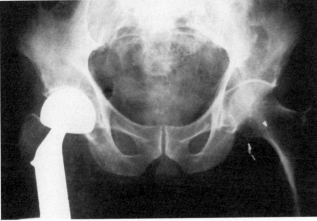

(b)

Fig. 7. Oncologic prostheses in the hip and knee. (a) A 66-year-old male following tumor resection underwent a rotating-hinge total knee arthroplasty. (b) A 54-year-old male, following resection of the proximal femur, underwent oncologic bipolar hemiarthroplasty. The greater trochanter was secured to the metal ring on the proximal femoral prosthesis.

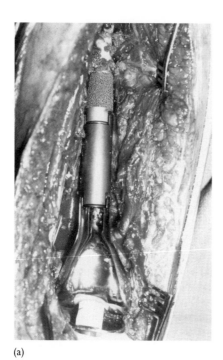

(a)

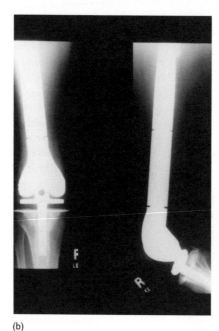

(b)

Fig. 8. Expandable prosthesis: (a) intraoperative photograph of an oncologic prosthesis replacing the distal femur and knee; (b) anteroposterior and lateral radiographs of the oncologic rotating-hinge knee prosthesis.

and the main advantage is the preservation of the hand (Malawer 1991). In most instances, a lesser resection is possible following adjuvant chemotherapy. After careful analysis of the staging studies, an intra-articular or extra-articular resection of the proximal humerus is performed and reconstructed either with a prosthesis, an osteoarticular allograft, or an allograft–prosthetic composite (Cheng and Gebhardt 1991; Malawer 1991; Alman *et al.* 1995). If the entire deltoid and rotator cuff are excised with the specimen, an arthrodesis is a more appropriate reconstruction to allow active movement of the shoulder area. (Cheng and Gebhardt 1991; Gebhardt *et al.* 1991; Alman *et al.* 1995).

Pelvic osteosarcomas present very challenging surgical dilemmas (Fig. 10). *En bloc* excision of the hemipelvis with preservation of the extremity can now be performed in some instances as an internal hemipelvectomy. The oncologic results of external and internal hemipelvectomies are similar as long as negative margins can be achieved. When the sacrum is involved as well, the functional results and the ability to achieve negative margins worsen. Metallic endoprosthesis reconstruction is available, but functional results are not very successful because fixation is extremely difficult and prosthesis loosening and migration is frequent. Allografts have also been employed to replace the resected bony segments, but the complication rate is quite high largely due to inadequate soft-tissue coverage, the proximity of the bowel, and a large dead-space. Other methods of obtaining structural integrity have included fusion of the proximal femur to the ilium or sacrum and internal hemipelvectomy with creation of a pseudoarthrosis between the proximal femur and remaining pelvis (Campanacci and Capanna 1991). When no replacement is used, the femur and pelvis are bridged by scar tissue. These procedures are not

ideal, but they do provide an alternative to external hemipelvectomy, with reasonable functional and psychologic results.

The type of reconstruction following resection depends on the patient's age and anatomic site of the tumor. In patients near or at skeletal maturity (over 12 years old in girls, and over 14 years old in boys) with lesions in the lower extremity, or for lesions in the upper extremity at any age, growth considerations are not a major concern. Osteoarticular allografts, arthrodeses, metallic implants, or, at times, vascularized bone grafts may be used to reconstruct the defects. In children with lower extremity lesions in younger ages, the consideration of growth remaining becomes a major concern. For example, a 6- to 8-year-old patient with a distal femoral osteosarcoma presents a major reconstruction challenge. The most logical option is rotationplasty or amputation, but patients and their families are often reluctant to accept such an approach. The surgeon is left with the option of reconstructing with allografts (if one of an appropriate size can be obtained) and performing standard limb-equalizing procedures at a later date, or employing metallic prostheses, which can be lengthened. Neither approach is ideal, and long-term studies of outcome in this age group are limited. Children are not as co-operative with rehabilitation protocols, nor are they as willing to limit their sports activities. Our preference has been to recommend rotationplasty for the very young patient with a lesion about the knee, and osteoarticular allografts for those at or near skeletal maturity. We believe that this biologic approach is advantageous in this young age, and prefer to restrict metallic prosthesis for adults or those who fail allograft treatment. Limb length can usually be equalized by a combination of timed epiphysiodeses, using a graft, which is 1 to 2 cm longer than the resected bone, and, on occasion, lengthening or shortening procedures.

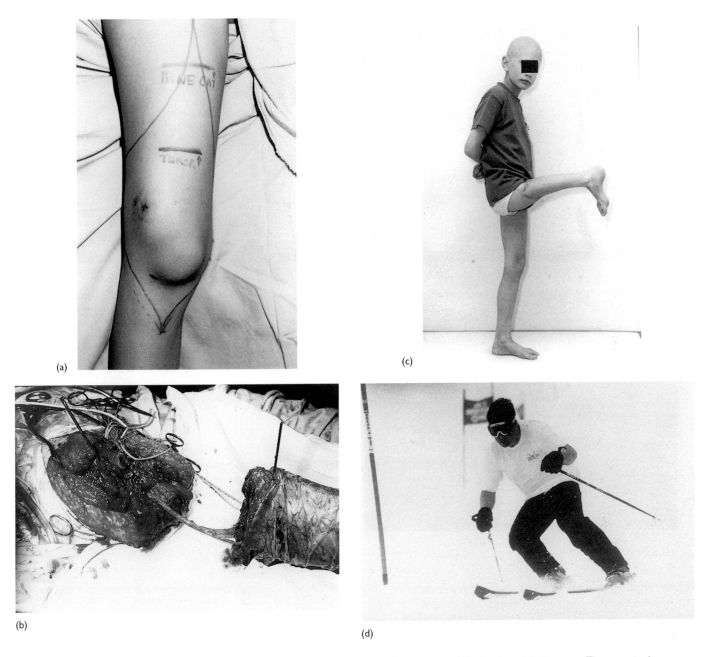

Fig. 9. Van Nes rotationplasty for distal femoral osteosarcoma in 11-year-old male. (a) Skin incision and the location of the bone cut. The tumor is shown expanding the normal contour of the distal thigh. (b) Intraoperative photograph following the wide excision of the tumor. The vessels and sciatic nerve are shown traversing the gap. The vessels can either be looped at the junction or an anastamosis of the jumped resected vessel segment is done. (c) Postoperative clinical photograph of the functional result—below-knee-like amputation with the ankle joint now functioning as the knee joint. (d) Patient skiing—excellent functional results in the appropriate patient.

Conclusion

Despite the progress in chemotherapy and limb salvage, 20 to 40 per cent of patients with high-grade osteosarcomas will ultimately relapse. Current research efforts are being directed toward better defining the high-risk patient, either by identifying biologic characteristics of the tumor or by assessing its response to neoadjuvant chemotherapy, and developing novel treatment strategies for the nonresponders. Clinical and basic research is also needed in the area

of prosthetic design and allograft biology so that better methods of limb reconstruction will be possible. We are now able to safely resect most extremity osteosarcomas, but our reconstruction techniques leave much to be desired. Tissue engineering offers an approach of the future for reconstruction using the patient's own tissues.

The prospects for understanding the biology of osteosarcoma and improving therapy are promising. New chemotherapeutic drugs promise to add further to the list of active agents. Ifosfamide is being tested in randomized trials for its worth as a front-line agent in treat-

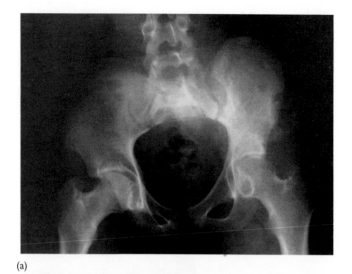

(a)

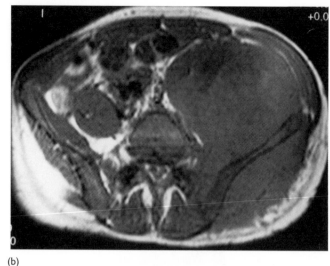

(b)

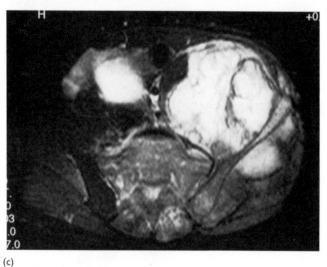

(c)

Fig. 10. An 18-year-old male with a stage III osteosarcoma of the left pelvis. (a) Anteroposterior pelvis. Tumor in the left hemipelvis. Cloudy opacities are noted in the soft tissues adjacent the left ilium. (b), (c) T_1- and T_2-weighted MRI shows the extensive soft-tissue involvement, which is not as well appreciated in the plain radiograph. Despite an aggressive chemotherapy regimen, the tumor mass continued to expand with the subsequent demise of the patient.

ment regimens, and new platinum analogs may prove to be active chemotherapeutic agents with reduced toxicity (Whelan 1997). Immunotherapy has not yet proved successful, but may in the future. Monoclonal antibodies with exquisite specificity directed against osteosarcoma antigens have been used in the detection of metastases and will be able to deliver chemotherapeutic drugs to the tumor (McGuire *et al.* 1990). Cytotoxic T cells may also provide more specific antitumor therapy. Finally, our understanding of drug resistance will likely translate into novel reversing agents to render the tumor cell sensitive or newer drugs which act through different pathways (Baldini *et al.* 1995; Whelan 1997). Dramatic improvements in the treatment of patients with osteosarcoma have been made in the past 25 years, but there is clearly a long way to go.

References

Alman, B.A., de Bari, A., and Krajbich, J.I. (1995). Massive allografts in the treatment of osteosarcoma and Ewing's sarcoma in children and adolescents. *Journal of Bone and Joint Surgery, American Volume*, **77A**, 54–64.

Baldini, N., Scotlandi, K., Barbanti-Brodano, G., *et al.* (1995). Expression of P-glycoprotein in high-grade osteosarcomas in relation to clinical outcome. *New England Journal of Medicine*, **333**, 1380–5.

Bieling, P., Rehan, N., Winkler, P., *et al.* (1996). Tumor size and prognosis in aggressively treated osteosarcoma. *Journal of Clinical Oncology*, **14**, 848–58.

Campanacci, M. and Capanna, R. (1991). Pelvic resections: the Rizzoli Institute experience. *Clinical Orthopaedics and Related Research*, **22**, 65–86.

Campanacci, M. and Laus, M. (1980). Local recurrence after amputation for osteosarcoma. *Journal of Bone and Joint Surgery, British Volume*, **62B**, 201–7.

Capanna, R., Manfrini, M., Ceruso, M., *et al.* (1991). A new reconstruction for metadiaphyseal resections. A combined graft (allograft shell plus vascularized fibula)—preliminary results. In *Complications of limb salvage. Prevention, management and outcome* (ed. K.L.B. Brown), pp. 319–21. ISOLS, Montreal.

Cheng, E.Y. and Gebhardt, M.C. (1991). Allograft reconstructions of the shoulder after bone tumor resections. *Orthopedic Clinics of North America*, **22**, 37–48.

Daffner, R.H., Kennedy, S.L., Fox, K.R., Crowley, J.J., Sauser, D.D., and Cooperstein, L.A. (1997). Synchronous multicentric osteosarcoma: the case for metastasis. *Skeletal Radiology*, **26**, 569–78.

de Bari, A., Krajbich, J.I., Langer, F., Hamilton, E.L., and Hubbard, S. (1990). Modified Van Nes rotationplasty for osteosarcoma of the proximal tibia in children. *Clinical Orthopaedics and Related Research*, **72**, 1065–9.

Eckardt, J.J., Safran, M.R., Eilber, F.R., Rosen, G., and Kabo, J.M. (1993). Expandable endoprosthetic reconstruction of the skeletally immature after malignant bone tumor resection. *Clinical Orthopaedics and Related Research*, **297**, 188–202.

Enneking, W.F. and Shirley, P.D. (1977). Resection-arthrodesis for malignant and potentially malignant lesions about the knee using an intramedullary rod and local bone grafts. *Journal of Bone and Joint Surgery, American Volume*, **59A**, 223–36.

Enneking, W.F., Spanier, S.S., and Goodman, M.A. (1980). A system for the surgical staging of musculoskeletal sarcoma. *Clinical Orthopaedics and Related Research*, **153**, 106–20.

Finn, H.A. and Simon, M.A. (1991). Limb-salvage surgery in the treatment of osteosarcoma in skeletally immature individuals. *Clinical Orthopaedics and Related Research*, **262**, 108–18.

Frassica, F.J., Sim, F.H., Frassica, D.A., and Wold, L.E. (1991). Survival and management considerations in postirradiation osteosarcoma and Paget's osteosarcoma. *Clinical Orthopaedics and Related Research*, **170**, 120–7.

Gebhardt, M.C. (1996). Molecular biology of sarcomas. *Orthopedic Clinics of North America*, **27**, 421–9.

Gebhardt, M.C., Flugstad, D.I., Springfield, D.S., and Mankin, H.J. (1991). The use of bone allografts in limb salvage in high-grade extremity osteosarcoma. *Clinical Orthopaedics and Related Research*, **270**, 181–96.

Glasser, D.B., Lane, J.M., Huvos, A.G., Marcove, R.C., and Rosen, G. (1992). Survival, prognosis, and therapeutic response in osteogenic sarcoma. The Memorial Hospital experience. *Cancer*, **69**, 698–708.

Goorin, A.M. and Andersen, J.W. (1991). Experience with multiagent chemotherapy for osteosarcoma: improved outcome. *Clinical Orthopaedics and Related Research*, **270**, 22–8.

Goorin, A.M., Delorey, M.J., Lack, E.E., et al. (1984). Prognostic significance of complete surgical resection of pulmonary metastases in patients with osteogenic sarcoma: analysis of 32 patients. *Journal of Clinical Oncology*, **2**, 425–31.

Goorin, A.M., Perez-Atayde, A., Gebhardt, M., et al. (1987). Weekly high-dose methotrexate and doxorubicin for osteosarcoma: the Dana-Farber Cancer Institute/the Children's Hospital—study III. *Journal of Clinical Oncology*, **5**, 1178–84.

Greenberg, D.B., Goorin, A.M., Gebhardt, M.C., et al. (1994). Quality of life in osteosarcoma survivors. *Oncology*, **8**, 19–25.

Horowitz, S.M., Glasser, D.B., Lane, J.M., and Healey, J.H. (1993). Prosthetic and extremity survivorship after limb salvage for sarcoma. How long do the reconstructions last? *Clinical Orthopaedics and Related Research*, **293**, 280–6.

Huvos, A.G., Rosen, G., Bretsky, S.S., and Butler, A. (1982). Telangiectatic osteogenic sarcoma: A clinicopathologic study of 124 patients. *Cancer*, **49**, 1679–89.

Jaffe, N., Spears, R., and Eftekari, F. (1987). Pathological fracture in osteosarcoma. Impact of chemotherapy on primary tumor and survival. *Cancer*, **59**, 701–9.

Jaffe, N., Smith, D.J., Jaffe, M.R., et al. (1991). Intraarterial cisplatin in the management of stage IIB osteosarcoma in the pediatric and adolescent age group. *Clinical Orthopaedics and Related Research*, **270**, 15–21.

Jaramillo, D., Laor, T., and Gebhardt, M.C. (1996). Pediatric musculoskeletal neoplasms. Evaluation with MR imaging. *MRI Clinics of North America*, **4**, 749–70.

Kotz, R. and Salzer, M. (1982). Rotation-plasty for childhood osteosarcoma of the distal part of the femur. *Journal of Bone and Joint Surgery, American Volume*, **64A**, 959–69.

Landis, S.H., Murray, T., Bolden, S., and Wingo, P.A. (1998). Cancer statistics. *CA: A Cancer Journal for Clinicians*, **48**, 6–29.

Link, M.P., Goorin, A.M., Horowitz, M., et al. (1991). Adjuvant chemotherapy of high grade osteosarcoma of the extremity. *Clinical Orthopaedics and Related Research*, **270**, 8–14.

McGuire, M.H., Ritter, R.A., Roodman, S.T., and Tsai, C.C. (1990).

TMMR-2, a monoclonal antibody to human osteosarcoma. *Chirurgia degli Organi di Movimento*, **75**, 5.

McKenna, R.J., Schwinn, C.P., Soong, K.Y., and Higinbotham, N.L. (1966). Sarcomata of the osteogenic series (osteosarcoma, fibrosarcoma, chondrosarcoma, parosteal osteogenic sarcoma, and sarcomata arising in abnormal bone). An analysis of 522 cases. *Journal of Bone and Joint Surgery, American Volume*, **48A**, 1–26.

Malawer, M.M. (1991). Tumors of the shoulder girdle. Technique of resection and description of a surgical classification. *Orthopedic Clinics of North America*, **22**, 7–35.

Malawer, M.M. and Chou, L.B. (1995). Prosthetic survival and clinical results with the use of large-segment replacements in the treatment of high-grade bone sarcomas. *Journal of Bone and Joint Surgery, American Volume*, **77A**, 1154–65.

Manfrini, M. (1997). Intraepiphyseal resection. *Mapfre Medicina*, **8**, 282–3.

Mankin, H.J., Gebhardt, M.C., Jennings, L.C., Springfield, D.S., and Tomford, W.W. (1996). Long-term results of allograft replacement in the management of bone tumors. *Clinical Orthopaedics and Related Research*, **324**, 86–97.

Merkel, K.D., Gebhardt, M.C., and Springfield, D.S. (1991). Rotationplasty as a reconstructive option after tumor resection. *Clinical Orthopaedics and Related Research*, **270**, 231–6.

Merkel, K.D., Lowen, N., Gebhardt, M.C., et al. (1996). Long-term follow-up of patients undergoing limb salvage for grade IIB osteosarcoma of the extremities. *Orthopaedic Transactions*, **20**, 173.

Meyers, P.A., Hellerm, G., Healey, J.H., et al. (1993). Osteogenic sarcoma with clinically detectable metastasis at initial presentation. *Journal of Clinical Oncology*, **11**, 449–53.

Minami, A., Kutsumi, K., Takeda, N., and Kaneda, K. (1995). Vascularized fibular graft for bone reconstruction of the extremities after tumor resection in limb-saving procedures. *Microsurgery*, **16**, 56–64.

Otis, J.C., Lane, J.M., and Kroll, M.A. (1985). Energy cost during gait in osteosarcoma patients after resection and knee replacement and after above-the-knee amputation. *Journal of Bone and Joint Surgery, American Volume*, **67A**, 606–11.

Parham, D.M., Pratt, C.B., Parvey, L.S., Webber, B.L., and Champion, J. (1985). Childhood multifocal osteosarcoma. Clinicopathologic and radiologic correlates. *Cancer*, **55**, 2653–8.

Picci, P., Sangiorgi, L., Rougraff, B.T., Neff, J.R., Casadei, R., and Campanacci, M. (1994). Relationship of chemotherapy-induced necrosis and surgical margins to local recurrence in osteosarcoma. *Journal of Clinical Oncology*, **12**, 2699–705.

Picci, P., Sangiorgi, L., Bahamonde, L., et al. (1997). Risk factors for local recurrence after limb-salvage surgery for high-grade osteosarcoma of the extremities. *Annals of Oncology*, **8**, 899–903.

Pignatti, G., Bacci, G., Picci, P., et al. (1991). Telangiectatic osteogenic sarcoma of the extremities. Results in 17 patients treated with neoadjuvant chemotherapy. *Clinical Orthopaedics and Related Research*, **270**, 99–106.

Pollack, M., Sem, A.W., Richard, M., Tetenes, E., and Bell, R. (1992). Inhibition of metastatic behavior of murine osteosarcoma by hypophysectomy. *Journal of the National Cancer Institute*, **84**, 966–71.

Porter, D.E., Holden, S.T., Steel, C.M., Cohen, B.B., Wallace, M.R., and Reid, R. (1992). A significant proportion of patients with osteosarcoma may belong to Li-Fraumeni cancer families. *Journal of Bone and Joint Surgery, British Volume*, **74B**, 883–6.

Provisor, A.J., Ettinger, L.J., Nachman, J.B., et al. (1997). Treatment of nonmetastatic osteosarcoma of the extremity with preoperative and postoperative chemotherapy: a report from the Children's Cancer Group. *Journal of Clinical Oncology*, **15**, 76–84.

Rougraff, B.T., Simon, M.A., Kniesl, J.S., Greenberg, D.B., and Mankin, H.J. (1994). Limb salvage compared with amputation for osteosarcoma of the distal end of the femur. A long-term oncological, functional, and quality-of-life study. *Clinical Orthopaedics and Related Research*, **76**, 649–56.

Schajowicz, F., McGuire, M.H., Araujo, E.S., Muscolo, D.L., and Gitelis, S.

(1988). Osteosarcomas arising on the surfaces of long bones. *Journal of Bone and Joint Surgery, American Volume*, **70A**, 555–64.

Scully, S.P., Temple, H.T., O'Keefe, R.J., Mankin, H.J., and Gebhardt, M.C. (1996). The surgical treatment of patients with osteosarcoma who sustain a pathologic fracture. *Clinical Orthopaedics and Related Research*, **324**, 227–32.

Simon, M.A. (1988). Limb salvage for osteosarcoma. *Journal of Bone and Joint Surgery, American Volume*, **70A**, 307–10.

Simon, M.A. and Finn, H.A. (1993). Diagnostic strategy for bone and soft-tissue tumors. *Journal of Bone and Joint Surgery, American Volume*, **75A**, 622–31.

Springfield, D.S. (1991). Introduction to limb-salvage surgery for sarcomas. *Orthopedic Clinics of North America*, **22**, 1–5.

Springfield, D.S., Schmidt, R., Graham-Pole, J., Marcus, R.B.J., Spanier, S.S., and Enneking, W.F. (1988). Surgical treatment for osteosarcoma. *Journal of Bone and Joint Surgery, American Volume*, **70A**, 1124–30.

Tucker, M.A., D'Angio, G.J., Boice, J.D., Jr, *et al.* (1987). Bone sarcomas linked to radiotherapy and chemotherapy in children. *New England Journal of Medicine*, **317**, 588–93.

Ward, W.G., Yang, R.-S., and Eckardt, J.J. (1996). Endoprosthetic bone reconstruction following malignant tumor resection in skeletally immature patients. *Orthopedic Clinics of North America*, **27**, 493–502.

Whelan, J.S. (1997). Osteosarcoma. *European Journal of Cancer*, **33**, 1611–19.

Winkelmann, W.W. (1986). Hip rotationplasty for malignant tumors of the proximal part of the femur. *Journal of Bone and Joint Surgery, American Volume*, **68A**, 362–9.

Winkler, K., Bieling, P., Bielack, S., *et al.* (1991). Local control and survival from the Cooperative Osteosarcoma Study Group studies of the German Society of Pediatric Oncology and the Vienna Bone Tumor Registry. *Clinical Orthopaedics and Related Research*, **270**, 79–86.

Wuisman, P. and Enneking, W.F. (1990). Prognosis for patients who have osteosarcoma with skip metastasis. *Journal of Bone and Joint Surgery, American Volume*, **72A**, 60–8.

1.6.8.3 Chondrosarcoma of bone

Steven Gitelis, Alexander Templeton, and Michael Hejna

Chondrosarcoma of bone is a malignant mesenchymal neoplasm. The World Health Organization defines chondrosarcoma as a tumor characterized by the formation of cartilage. The malignant cells of the tumor are associated with the production of varying amounts of extracellular matrix that closely resembles cartilage. This extracellular matrix is composed of collagen, principally type II and proteoglycans reminiscent of non-neoplastic cartilage such as articular cartilage, epiphyseal cartilage, and even fracture callus (Mankin *et al.* 1980*a,b*; Buckwalter 1983). There is a broad range of differentiation of this tumor from well-differentiated with easily recognizable hyaline cartilage, to poorly differentiated tumors that have scant areas of recognizable cartilage mixed with high-grade spindle cell sarcoma. The differentiation of chondrosarcoma is just one feature that predicts its biologic behavior.

Chondrosarcoma of bone has been classified in a number of ways. Currently, the most commonly used classification is the separation of chondrosarcoma into **conventional** and **variant** types (Table 1) (Campanacci 1990). Conventional chondrosarcomas are further clas-

Box 1

- Malignant tumors of cartilage-forming cells that vary considerably in aggressiveness and in histologic appearance
- Most commonly develop in the femur, pelvis, and humerus
- Patients with multiple hereditary exostoses and multiple enchondromatoses, including Ollier's and Maffucci's syndromes, have increased risk of developing a chondrosarcoma
- Typically present with increasing bone pain in middle age or older patients
- Optimal treatment is *en bloc* surgical resection with a wide margin
- In many patients a wide surgical resection can be accomplished and the limb or pelvis reconstructed ('limb salvage'); in other patients amputation is necessary
- Resection of pulmonary metastases can benefit some patients
- Chemotherapy and radiation therapy are generally ineffective
- Prognosis is related to the histologic grade of the tumor and the achievement of an *en bloc* surgical resection with a wide margin
- Because of the tendency for late local recurrence and development of metastases, patients with chondrosarcomas should be followed for more than 5 years and in many instances they should be followed for 20 years or more

Table 1 Classification of chondrosarcoma

Conventional	Variants
Central	Dedifferentiated
Peripheral	Mesenchymal
	Clear cell

sified into **central** and **peripheral** chondrosarcomas. A central chondrosarcoma generally arises *de novo* within the bone and may extend outside the bone with a large soft-tissue mass. These tumors are rarely secondary to a pre-existing benign condition and tend to have a poorer prognosis. A peripheral chondrosarcoma arises on the surface of the bone and is generally secondary to a pre-existing benign tumor such as an osteochondroma. Peripheral chondrosarcomas tend to be lower grade and have a better prognosis than central tumors. There are several well-described variants of chondrosarcoma, each with a distinctly different clinical behavior. The least aggressive of these variants is **clear cell** chondrosarcoma. It has a relatively good prognosis. The poorly differentiated chondrosarcoma variants include **mesenchymal** and **dedifferentiated** chondrosarcoma. These are extremely high-grade tumors with a poor prognosis. Owing to the broad range of clinical behavior, epidemiology, clinical presentation, radiologic appearance, pathology, imaging, treatment, and outcome, conventional chondrosarcoma and chondrosarcoma variants need to be discussed individually to understand these differences. This chapter will focus on these differences and the treatment of chondrosarcoma.

Conventional chondrosarcoma

Chondrosarcoma became a distinct pathologic entity from osteosarcoma in 1943 when Lichtenstein and Jaffe described it as a tumor that either developed from, or produced, cartilage in contradistinction to osteosarcoma which has areas of malignant cells forming osteoid. Several authors including Schajowicz then separated chondrosarcoma into central and peripheral types. These two tumors were found to differ in their position within or on the surface of the bone.

Central conventional chondrosarcoma

Central chondrosarcoma develops within the bone *de novo* and are rarely secondary tumors. In the Schajowicz (1991) series, chondrosarcoma accounted for approximately 15 per cent (339/2338) of all malignant bone tumors and 6 per cent (339/5279) of all bone tumors. In his series there were 348 primary chondrosarcomas; 306 were central tumors. Dahlin and Unni (1986) reported on 732 cases of chondrosarcoma or approximately 11 per cent (732/6514) of the Mayo Clinic malignant tumors. Eighty-seven per cent (643/732) of these chondrosarcomas were primary bone. Huvos (1991) reported on 493 chondrosarcomas; 305 were primary within bone and 168 were secondary to a pre-existing benign tumor. Males appear to be affected more commonly than females; 65 per cent (Schajowicz 1991) and 60 per cent (Dahlin and Unni 1986). Chondrosarcoma of bone, especially primary, tends to occur in older individuals. It is rarely seen in a child (Aprin *et al.* 1982; Huvos and Marcove 1987). Dahlin and Unni (1986) reported only four patients that developed a chondrosarcoma who were less than 10 years of age. We found 97 of 125 patients presenting between the age of 20 and 60 (Gitelis *et al.* 1981).

Chondrosarcoma can arise in almost any bone. The majority occur in the proximal limb or axial skeleton. The femur tends to be a common location. Ninety-six out of 360 cases reported by Schajowicz were located in the femur, 63 in the pelvis, and 27 in the humerus. Similarly, Dahlin and Unni (1986) reported a high incidence within the femur. Out of 634 tumors, 141 were located in the femur; 147 were located in the pelvis. Interestingly, 41 of these were periacetabular, a very difficult location to treat. Sixty-nine tumors occurred in the humerus and 32 in the scapula. The rib is another common site for chondrosarcoma (Fig. 1). Dahlin and Unni (1986) reported on 71 out of 634 tumors within a rib. We found 34 pelvic chondrosarcomas out of 125 patients; 36 were located in the femur and 17 in the humerus. This distribution appears to be consistent in all reported series (Gitelis *et al.* 1981).

The most common presenting symptom in chondrosarcoma is pain. The development of pain is usually insidious. This tumor is relatively slow growing, and prolonged symptoms are typical. We found the average time to presentation for chondrosarcoma to be 19 months. The lower-grade tumors tended to take longer to present (19.4 months) than the high-grade tumors (15.5 months) (Gitelis *et al.* 1981). Other presenting complaints include a soft-tissue mass that is palpable and a fracture (Fig. 2). Systemic complaints such as fever, weight loss, or loss of appetite are rare. Pain is an important symptom when evaluating a cartilaginous lesion of bone. A painful medullary cartilaginous lesion should be considered a malignancy until proven otherwise. Most benign cartilaginous tumors such as enchondroma are painless. The pain in chondrosarcoma is unremitting, pro-

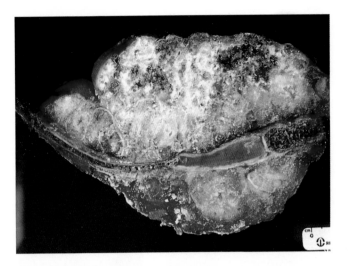

Fig. 1. Chondrosarcoma rib specimen after resection. There is a well-differentiated cartilage tumor involving the rib and soft tissues.

gressive, and characteristically present at night. Mechanical symptoms such as weight-bearing pain are not a common characteristic.

The radiologic features of chondrosarcoma include bone expansion and thickening of the cortex. The tumor typically occurs in the metaphysis or diaphysis of a long bone and may extend long distances along the medullary canal (Fig. 3) (Healey and Lane 1986). This extension is not always visible on plain radiographs and needs to be determined with other imaging techniques such as CT and MRI. A [^{99}Tc^m]diphosphonate bone scan is also useful to determine the intramedullary extent (Fig. 4). Other radiologic features of central chondrosarcoma include mineralization within the tumor. A stippled-type calcification is a common feature. Central chondrosarcoma can also extend outside the bone sometimes making it difficult to distinguish it from a peripheral or surface chondrosarcoma. CT or MRI are useful studies to fully see the soft-tissue extension.

The pathologic grading of chondrosarcoma is an important part of evaluation. The tumor is typically graded into three histologic grades (Dahlin and Unni 1986). The grade of the tumor is directly related to its prognosis and risk of metastasis. The histologic and cytologic features used for grading include the cellularity of the tumor, pleomorphism, mitotic rate, the presence of nucleoli, binucleate forms, multiple cells within lacunae, and the presence of well-defined lobules. Grade 1 chondrosarcoma has low cellularity, a single cell within a lacunae, rarely possesses mitotic figures, lacks pleomorphism, and has a distinct lobular appearance (Fig. 5). Myxomatous areas are rare in grade 1 tumors. Myxoid features include stellate cartilaginous cells with interconnecting cell processes. Grossly, myxoid tumors have a 'slimy' appearance. Grade 3 chondrosarcoma is very cellular with pleomorphism, and occasional mitotic figures, two cells within a lacuna, and binucleate forms are common (Fig. 6). Grade 3 tumors frequently have myxoid areas. Grade 2 chondrosarcoma possesses some of the features of both grade 1 and grade 3 (Fig. 7). However, the pathologic diagnosis of chondrosarcoma cannot be made with the microscope alone. It is important for the pathologist to consider the clinical presentation and the radiologic features before finalizing a diagnosis and grade. As an example, axially located tumors do not need to possess all of the above-mentioned malignant histologic

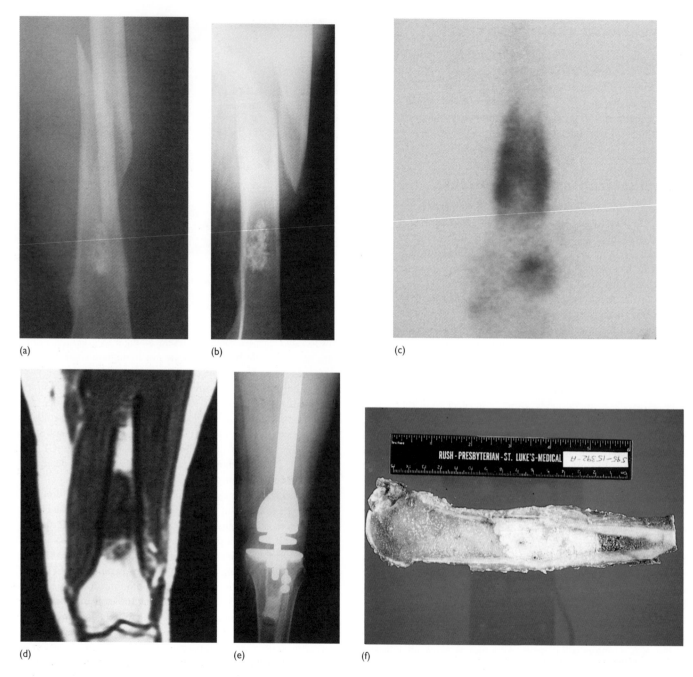

(a)   (b)   (c)

(d)   (e)   (f)

Fig. 2. Grade 1 chondrosarcoma distal femur with traumatic fracture. (a) Anteroposterior radiograph of the left distal femur in a 71-year-old female. Note the fracture through the diaphysis of the femur. Below the fracture is an area of calcification with thickening of the cortex and 'onion-skinning'-type periosteal reaction. (b) Lateral radiograph of the distal femur revealing a lytic lesion involving the metaphysis along with its calcification. There is cortical thickening and reactive periosteal changes. Above this lesion is an oblique fracture of the diaphysis of the femur. (c) [^{99}Tc^{m}]diphosphonate bone scan of the distal left femur. Note the uptake involving the lesion of the left distal femur. Also note that the area of the fracture which is acute showed no evidence of uptake. (d) Coronal T_1-weighted MRI of the left distal femur. The tumor involving the medullary bone is easily seen. Note the marrow above and below the tumor is normal. Also note that this tumor does not communicate with the traumatic fracture of the diaphysis of the left femur. (e) Postoperative anteroposterior radiograph of the left distal femur and knee joint revealing resection of the femur from the level of the fracture to the knee joint. The knee is reconstructed with a modular oncology prosthesis. (f) Specimen photograph after resection of the left distal femur. The chondrosarcoma ends well below the fracture and is apparently unrelated.

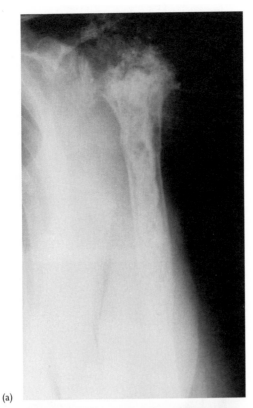

(a)

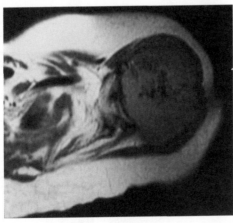

(b)

Fig. 3. Chondrosarcoma of the proximal humerus. (a) Anteroposterior radiograph of the left proximal humerus of a 62-year-old female. There is a large calcified tumor involving the left proximal humerus with an irregular margin. The tumor extends well down the medullary canal. The borders are irregular. There is also an area of osteolysis involving the left humeral head. (b) Transverse MRI of the left proximal humerus (T_1-weighted image). A chondrosarcoma with soft-tissue extension from the left proximal humerus is seen. There is marked bone expansion at the level of the glenoid and coracoid process. The tumor expands to the deltoid muscle. This tumor is a grade 2 chondrosarcoma.

features before being called chondrosarcomas. Distal tumors, on the other hand, need to show frank malignancy on histologic sections before being called chondrosarcomas. Other confusing entities for the pathologist include periosteal chondroma and enchondromas associated with Ollier's and Maffucci's syndromes. These tumors can

also share some of the features of chondrosarcoma, especially cellularity, and yet still be called benign tumors.

Staging

Prior to biopsy, chondrosarcoma of bone should be completely staged. Staging consists of a radiograph in two planes, usually anteroposterior and lateral. A [^{99}Tc^m]diphosphonate bone scan is performed to determine whether the tumor is monostotic or polyostotic. It is also useful to determine the intramedullary extent of the tumor. Three-dimensional imaging is performed with either MRI or CT scan (Fig. 8). These studies will show the intramedullary extent of the tumor along with any soft-tissue extension and its relationship to contiguous neurovascular structures. Finally, a chest radiograph and CT scan of the chest to rule out pulmonary metastases should be performed. All of these imaging studies should be performed prior to the biopsy. This is because the biopsy can distort the staging of the tumor, especially its soft-tissue staging. A biopsy can lead to a hematoma which can be confused with soft-tissue tumor extension. After staging, a biopsy is performed to determine the grade of the tumor that is necessary for ultimate staging. The Enneking staging system is the most commonly used system for chondrosarcoma (Enneking *et al.* 1980). Tumors are first determined to be low or high grade histologically. Low-grade tumors (grade 1) are stage I and high-grade tumors (grades 2 and 3) are stage II. The tumors are then determined by imaging to be either intracompartmental or extracompartmental The bone itself is defined as the compartment and any soft-tissue extension beyond the bone would make it an extracompartmental tumor. Extracompartmental tumors are stage B. A high-grade extracompartmental tumor would then be staged as a II-B tumor (Fig. 9). A low-grade intraosseous tumor would be a stage I-A. Any tumor with either bone or pulmonary metastases would be stage III.

Management

Chondrosarcoma of bone is a surgical disease (Marcove 1977; Erikkson *et al.* 1980; Gitelis *et al.* 1981). Treatments such as radiation and chemotherapy are generally ineffective. This is because the tumor is relatively avascular and, lacks the circulation necessary for radiation and chemotherapy to be effective. Most authors believe that wide surgical margins, as defined by Enneking, are required for chondrosarcoma. Wide margins are defined as *en bloc* removal of the tumor with a cuff of normal tissue (Fig. 10). Wide margins can either be achieved by amputation or limb salvage. Most limb salvage requires complex reconstruction because of the anatomic location of these tumors (Fig. 11). Frequently, the joint needs to be removed, and implants, allografts, or arthrodesis are required. If wide margins are achieved, a relatively low local recurrence rate is seen. In 1981 we found only a 6 per cent (4/63) incidence of local recurrence with wide margins; however, with contaminated operations or with less than wide margins, there was an incidence of recurrence of nearly 70 per cent (42/62) (Gitelis *et al.* 1981). Chondrosarcoma is notorious for spillage of cells. This can occur at the time of biopsy as well as definitive surgery. Tumors that are myxomatous are particularly prone to spillage. Some authors believe the biopsy is so risky that directly proceeding to definitive *en bloc* resection without biopsy should be considered in chondrosarcoma. This should be reserved for tumors where the clinical and radiologic presentation is completely

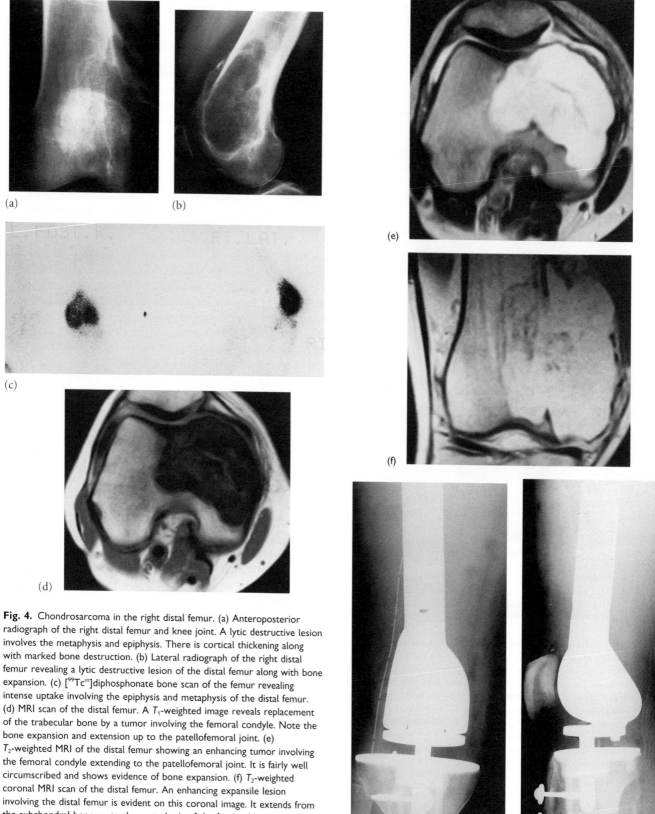

(a)

(b)

(c)

(d)

(e)

(f)

(g)

(h)

Fig. 4. Chondrosarcoma in the right distal femur. (a) Anteroposterior radiograph of the right distal femur and knee joint. A lytic destructive lesion involves the metaphysis and epiphysis. There is cortical thickening along with marked bone destruction. (b) Lateral radiograph of the right distal femur revealing a lytic destructive lesion of the distal femur along with bone expansion. (c) [$^{99}Tc^m$]diphosphonate bone scan of the femur revealing intense uptake involving the epiphysis and metaphysis of the distal femur. (d) MRI scan of the distal femur. A T_1-weighted image reveals replacement of the trabecular bone by a tumor involving the femoral condyle. Note the bone expansion and extension up to the patellofemoral joint. (e) T_2-weighted MRI of the distal femur showing an enhancing tumor involving the femoral condyle extending to the patellofemoral joint. It is fairly well circumscribed and shows evidence of bone expansion. (f) T_2-weighted coronal MRI scan of the distal femur. An enhancing expansile lesion involving the distal femur is evident on this coronal image. It extends from the subchondral bone up to the metaphysis of the femur. (g) Anteroposterior radiograph of the left knee after resection of the distal femur and reconstruction with a modular oncology prosthesis. A surgical drain is present. (h) Lateral radiograph of the left distal femur after resection and reconstruction with a modular oncology prosthesis.

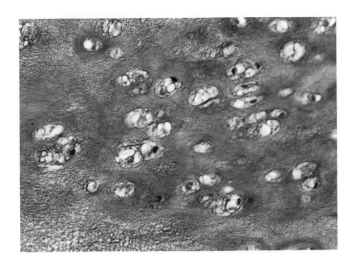

Fig. 5. Grade 1 chondrosarcoma. Hematoxylin and eosin section. Note the well-differentiated hyaline cartilage. The tumor is hypocellular with single cells within a lacunae. This section lacks pleomorphism.

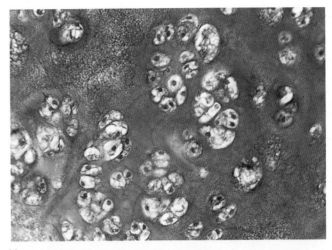

(a)

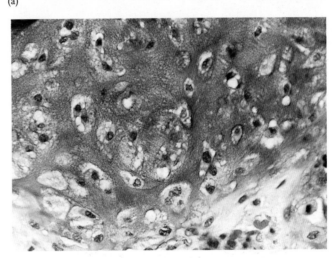

(b)

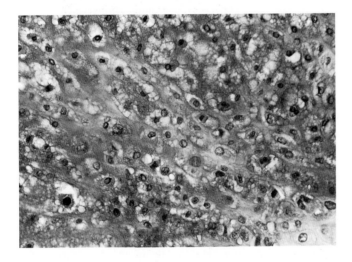

Fig. 6. Grade 3 chondrosarcoma. Hematoxylin and eosin section. Hypercellular cartilaginous tumor with pleomorphism and hyperchromatism. Some bizarre nuclei are present.

characteristic and diagnostic. One useful technique is to perform an open biopsy and a frozen section. If the frozen section is consistent with chondrosarcoma, then proceed with definitive *en bloc* resection. This technique tends to minimize the amount of spillage and hematoma associated with the biopsy and lower the risk of recurrence.

Outcome

The prognosis of chondrosarcoma is related to the grade of the tumor and the adequacy of its surgery (Marcove *et al.* 1972; Evans *et al.* 1977; Sannerkin and Gallagher 1979). Low-grade tumors have a relatively good prognosis while high-grade tumors can behave in a very aggressive manner. The rate of metastasis tends to be related directly to the grade of the tumor. In 1981 we found that 9 per cent (3/33) of grade 1 tumors metastasized while 44 per cent (7/16) of

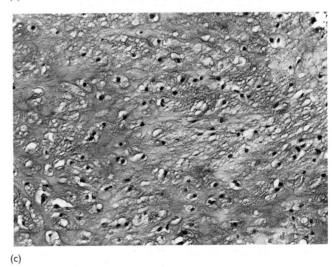

(c)

Fig. 7. Grade 2 chondrosarcoma. (a) Hematoxylin and eosin section. Binucleate cells and double cells within a lacunae are present. The cellularity is greater than grade 1. (b) Hematoxylin and eosin section. Binucleate cells are seen with hyperchromatic nucleus. (c) Hematoxylin and eosin section. Grade 2 chondrosarcoma with myxoid area. Note the cells with elongated (neuron-like) interconnecting cell processes.

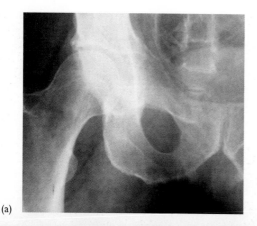

(a)

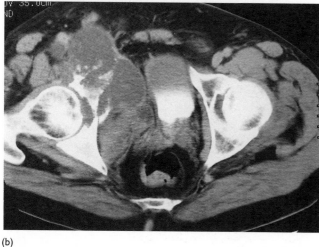

(b)

Fig. 8. Chondrosarcoma of the right pelvis. (a) Anteroposterior radiograph of the right hip and pelvis revealing a destructive lesion involving the superior pubic ramus. The lesion extends to the level of the acetabulum. The cortical margin is thin and broken in certain areas. (b) Transverse CT image of the right pelvis. Note the large destructive lesion involving the acetabulum extending anteriorly and medially to the level of the bladder. The lesion is characterized by bone destruction and bone expansion with some mineral within the tumor. This proved to be a grade 2 chondrosarcoma.

the grade 3 tumors metastasized (Gitelis *et al.* 1981). As stated earlier, local control is related to the adequacy of the surgical margin. Wide margins offer good local control whereas marginal margins or contaminated operations have a very significant risk of local recurrence. Local recurrence in general is associated with a very poor outcome. Overall, the survival for chondrosarcoma was 67 per cent (84/125) at 5 years and 50 per cent (62/125) at 10 years. Due to late relapses, it is important to follow chondrosarcoma beyond the typical 5-year time frame. Ten-year survivals for the grade 1, 2, and 3 tumors were 87 per cent (84/96), 41 per cent (39/96), and 27 per cent (26/96) respectively.

Inoperable chondrosarcomas or tumors located in inaccessible locations have been treated with neutron radiation with limited success. Since this form of radiation does not require vascularity to have an effect, it may be useful for chondrosarcoma. Chemotherapy plays little role in the treatment of chondrosarcoma. Chemotherapy has

been used for metastatic disease and for extraskeletal myxoid chondrosarcoma (Saleh *et al.* 1992; Patel *et al.* 1995) but with limited success.

Peripheral and other secondary chondrosarcoma

Most peripheral chondrosarcomas are secondary to a benign osteochondroma. Dahlin and Unni (1986) reported 89 secondary chondrosarcomas out of 732 tumors. Twenty-eight of 89 occurred in multiple hereditary exostoses (Fig. 12), 48 in an isolated exostosis, and 13 in patients with multiple enchondromas (Fig. 13). In our series, 56 of 125 patients were peripheral chondrosarcoma. These patients tended to be younger with a mean age of 33 years compared with 43.9 years for central chondrosarcoma. Fourteen of the 56 peripheral tumors had definite evidence of a pre-existing benign osteochondroma. This evidence consisted of a radiograph of a pre-existing benign lesion (osteochondroma) that ultimately underwent malignant degeneration or benign areas of cartilage seen with malignant tumor. We also found that peripheral chondrosarcoma tended to be of a lower histologic grade. Ninety-six per cent (54/56) of the tumors were grade 1 or 2 compared with 80 per cent (55/69) of the central chondrosarcomas in our series. Fewer of the peripheral chondrosarcomas were myxomatous, 7 per cent (4/56) compared with 35 per cent (24/69). The most notable difference, however, was the prognosis. The 5-year survival for the peripheral chondrosarcomas was 89 per cent (50/56). The central chondrosarcoma 5-year survival was 49 per cent (34/69) (Gitelis *et al.* 1981). Dahlin found the most common site of a secondary peripheral chondrosarcoma was the pelvic bone. Thirty-four of 76 peripheral tumors occurred in the pelvis. Fourteen occurred in the femur. Twenty-eight of 76 patients were the result of multiple exostoses, while 48 of 76 were the result of an isolated exostosis. Dahlin and Unni (1986) also found that these tumors tend to occur in younger individuals. Other than these differences, peripheral chondrosarcomas tend to be similar to central tumors. The treatment for a peripheral chondrosarcoma is the same, necessitating wide *en bloc* resection. Chemotherapy and radiation plays little role. The prognosis of a peripheral chondrosarcoma is directly related to the grade of the tumor and the adequacy of its surgical excision. Those tumors that are widely excised and are low grade have a relatively good prognosis.

Central and peripheral chondrosarcoma needs to be followed for a prolonged period of time. Late failures, after 5 years, have been reported. Follow-up consists of evaluation of the primary tumor site and the detection of metastatic disease. Chest radiographs and CTs are performed on a regular basis during the first 5 years. After 5 years, a plain chest radiograph should be performed yearly. CT, MRI, and technetium bone scan are useful techniques to evaluate the primary site for local recurrence. Physical examination is also critical to evaluate the primary tumor.

Dedifferentiated chondrosarcoma

Dedifferentiated chondrosarcoma is an extremely aggressive form of tumor with poor prognosis (Fig. 14). The World Health Organization defines it as a borderline low-grade chondrosarcoma juxtaposed to a high-grade anaplastic sarcoma. It was first described by Dahlin and Beabout (1971). They reported a series of patients who presented

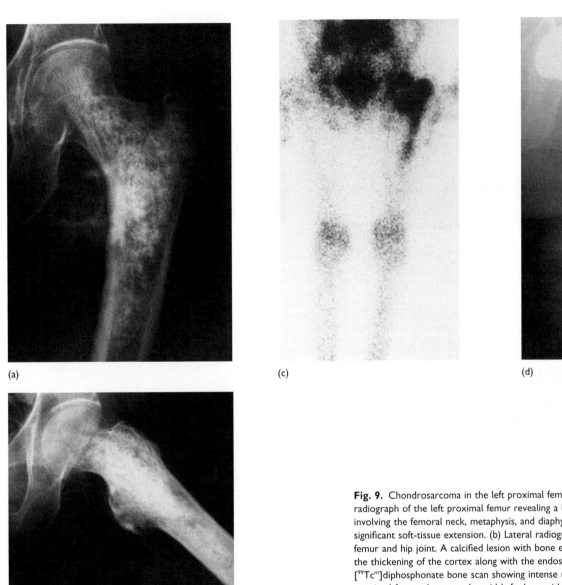

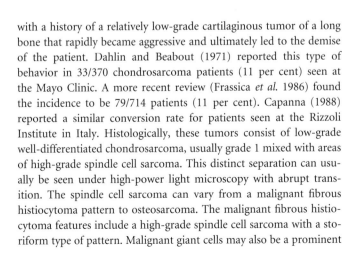

Fig. 9. Chondrosarcoma in the left proximal femur. (a) Anteroposterior radiograph of the left proximal femur revealing a large calcified lesion involving the femoral neck, metaphysis, and diaphysis of the femur. There is significant soft-tissue extension. (b) Lateral radiograph of the left proximal femur and hip joint. A calcified lesion with bone expansion is evident. Note the thickening of the cortex along with the endosteal scalloping. (c) [^{99}Tc^{m}]diphosphonate bone scan showing intense uptake involving the left proximal femur almost to the midshaft along with uptake in the soft tissues in the area of the soft-tissue extension. (d) Postoperative anteroposterior radiograph of the left proximal femur and hip joint revealing resection and reconstruction with a hip prosthesis.

with a history of a relatively low-grade cartilaginous tumor of a long bone that rapidly became aggressive and ultimately led to the demise of the patient. Dahlin and Beabout (1971) reported this type of behavior in 33/370 chondrosarcoma patients (11 per cent) seen at the Mayo Clinic. A more recent review (Frassica *et al.* 1986) found the incidence to be 79/714 patients (11 per cent). Capanna (1988) reported a similar conversion rate for patients seen at the Rizzoli Institute in Italy. Histologically, these tumors consist of low-grade well-differentiated chondrosarcoma, usually grade 1 mixed with areas of high-grade spindle cell sarcoma. This distinct separation can usually be seen under high-power light microscopy with abrupt transition. The spindle cell sarcoma can vary from a malignant fibrous histiocytoma pattern to osteosarcoma. The malignant fibrous histiocytoma features include a high-grade spindle cell sarcoma with a storiform type of pattern. Malignant giant cells may also be a prominent

feature. The spindle cells have cytologic features of malignancy. There is pleomorphism and hyperchromatism along with many mitotic figures. Johnson *et al.* (1986) reported 16/26 patients (61 per cent) with malignant fibrous histiocytoma type of dedifferentiated chondrosarcoma. Another form of dedifferentiated chondrosarcoma is a type that mixes grade 1 chondrosarcoma with osteosarcoma. In this tumor, malignant cells forming osteoid are present. Dahlin and Unni (1986) found this pattern in 43/78 patients (55 per cent). Other authors have reported the most common dedifferentiated chondrosarcoma is a fibrosarcoma type (Mirra and Marcove 1974). The risk of development of a dedifferentiated chondrosarcoma from a pre-existing low-grade cartilaginous tumor has been reported to be between 6 and 11 per cent (Daly *et al.* 1989). Most authors do not accept the concept of 'dedifferentiation'. We have reported evidence in tissue culture—the presence of multiple clonal forms in the parent

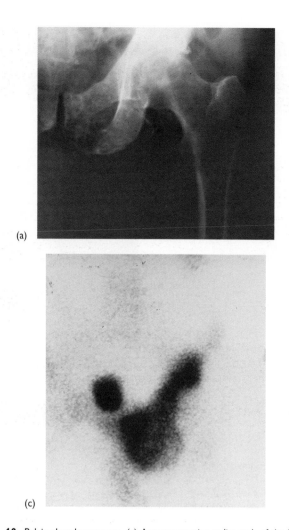

(a)

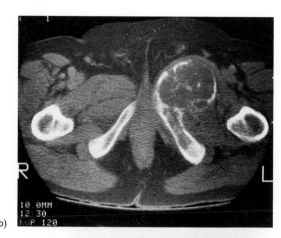

(b)

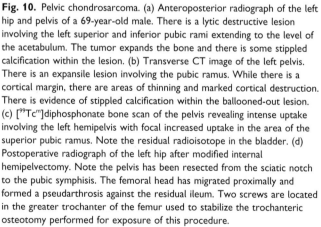

(c)

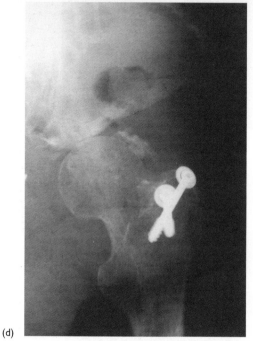

(d)

Fig. 10. Pelvic chondrosarcoma. (a) Anteroposterior radiograph of the left hip and pelvis of a 69-year-old male. There is a lytic destructive lesion involving the left superior and inferior pubic rami extending to the level of the acetabulum. The tumor expands the bone and there is some stippled calcification within the lesion. (b) Transverse CT image of the left pelvis. There is an expansile lesion involving the pubic ramus. While there is a cortical margin, there are areas of thinning and marked cortical destruction. There is evidence of stippled calcification within the ballooned-out lesion. (c) [^{99}Tc^m]diphosphonate bone scan of the pelvis revealing intense uptake involving the left hemipelvis with focal increased uptake in the area of the superior pubic ramus. Note the residual radioisotope in the bladder. (d) Postoperative radiograph of the left hip after modified internal hemipelvectomy. Note the pelvis has been resected from the sciatic notch to the pubic symphisis. The femoral head has migrated proximally and formed a pseudarthrosis against the residual ileum. Two screws are located in the greater trochanter of the femur used to stabilize the trochanteric osteotomy performed for exposure of this procedure.

chondrosarcoma. These clones vary biochemically and genetically, some with reproducible chromosome aberrations. The process of dedifferentiation we believe is the result of clonal evolution during the life of the tumor. High-grade clones predominate and take over the biology of the tumor.

Radiologically, a dedifferentiated chondrosarcoma has many of the features of a conventional central chondrosarcoma (DeLange *et al.* 1986). They occur in long bones such as the femur and humerus

which accounts for 41/79 (52 per cent) of these tumors; 23/79 (29 per cent) occur in the pelvis (Dahlin and Unni 1986). They most commonly affect patients over 40 years of age with an equal male/female incidence (Schwartz *et al.* 1987a). Radiographically, the features of a conventional chondrosarcoma consist of cortical thickening along with enlargement and expansion of the bone as well as areas of stippled calcification within the lesion. In addition to these more common radiologic features, there are areas of aggressive bone

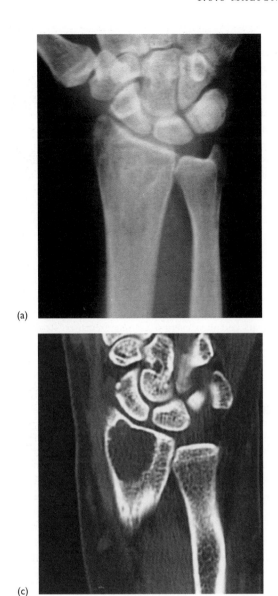

(a)

(c)

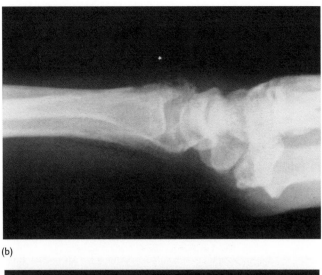

(b)

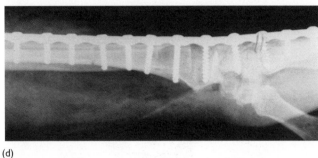

(d)

Fig. 11. Chondrosarcoma in the right distal radius. (a) Anteroposterior radiograph of the right distal radius and wrist in a 42-year-old female. There is lytic destruction of the metaphysis of the left distal radius that is well marginated, extending up to the radial styloid. (b) A lateral radiograph of the right wrist and distal forearm revealing a lytic lesion involving the distal radius. Note the cortical disruption on the dorsal surface. (c) CT image of the right distal radius. There is a lytic lesion involving the metaphysis and epiphysis of the left distal radius burrowing up to the subchondral bone plate. The lesion is fairly well circumscribed. After biopsy, this lesion proved to be a grade 1 chondrosarcoma. (d) Lateral radiograph of the right distal wrist and forearm. There has been a resection of the distal radius for a grade 1 chondrosarcoma and the wrist fused with an intercalary allograft along with internal fixation.

destruction. Large areas of osteolysis that is either moth-eaten in appearance or permeative are usually present in dedifferentiated chondrosarcoma (Frassica *et al.* 1986). In addition, it is not uncommon to see a pathologic fracture due to the amount of bone destruction. Three-dimensional imaging with either MRI or CT will frequently show the bone destruction along with a soft-tissue mass. It is not uncommon for the soft-tissue extension to be massive.

While some dedifferentiated chondrosarcomas can be diagnosed by its appearance on radiographs, most are diagnosed after complete tumor excision. It is not unusual for a surgeon to remove a central chondrosarcoma and then be informed by the pathologist that there are areas within the tumor that are high grade consisting of either malignant fibrous histiocytoma, osteosarcoma, or fibrosarcoma. The staging of dedifferentiated chondrosarcoma is the same as for all chondrosarcomas. After a careful history and physical examination, radiographs in two planes, anteroposterior and lateral, should be per-

formed. Three-dimensional imaging is important to determine soft-tissue extension and relationship to nearby neurovascular structures. These studies can include either an MRI or CT scan. [^{99}Tc^m]diphosphonate bone scan is useful to determine whether the tumor is monostotic or polyostotic. Intramedullary extension of the tumor beyond the visible bone destruction on the radiograph is not uncommon. This extension can be determined by technetium bone scanning or with a coronal image from an MRI. Skip lesions are also possible with dedifferentiated chondrosarcoma. A skip lesion is defined as a discontinuous extension within the medullary canal. Owing to the high-grade nature and aggressive biology of this tumor, systemic staging is critical. A chest radiograph along with a CT scan of the lungs is important to rule out metastatic disease. The latter is quite likely with this tumor.

The treatment of dedifferentiated chondrosarcoma is surgical. Complete removal of the tumor with wide margins as defined by

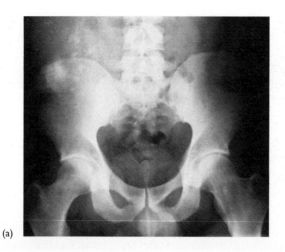

(a)

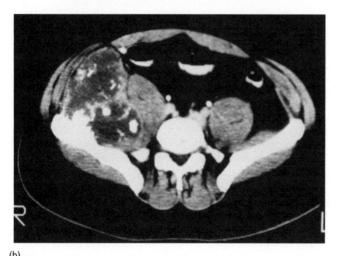

(b)

Fig. 12. Malignant degeneration in multiple hereditary exostoses. Anteroposterior radiograph of a 31-year-old male with known multiple hereditary exostoses. Note the sessile osteochondroma that involves the left femoral neck. This lesion is benign. There is a calcified lesion involving the right pelvic area that has an irregular margin. Transverse CT scan of the pelvis showing the large calcified tumor of the right ileum with a sessile-type connection to the iliac wing. There is irregular calcification within the mass and a close-pushing margin on the psoas muscle. This proved to be a grade 2 chondrosarcoma of the ileum in a patient with multiple hereditary exostoses.

Enneking *et al.* (1980) is the best form of management. This is either accomplished by amputation or limb salvage. The latter surgical approach usually requires complex reconstruction, depending upon the anatomic site. As an example, a dedifferentiated chondrosarcoma of the distal femur, without involvement of the nearby neurovascular bundle, can be treated by wide local excision of the distal femur with reconstruction using an endoprosthesis. Most of these tumors are stage II-B using the Enneking staging system (Enneking *et al.* 1980). That implies there is soft-tissue extension beyond the bone, so wide margins will require sacrifice of muscle in order to adequately remove the tumor. Patients that present with a pathologic fracture are best managed by amputation. Cartilaginous tumors including

dedifferentiated chondrosarcoma are notorious for spillage and soft-tissue extension at the time of fracture, thus making limb salvage extremely difficult, despite aggressive surgical treatment. The prognosis is extremely poor. Dahlin and Unni (1986) reported only 9/79 (11 per cent) survivors. Schajowicz (1991) reported 5-year survival less than 25 per cent. In the largest clinical review of dedifferentiated chondrosarcoma by Capanna *et al.* (1988), less than 20 per cent 5-year survivors were reported. This would suggest that other forms of therapy may be beneficial such as cytotoxic chemotherapeutic drugs. Unfortunately, effective chemotherapy has not been identified. This may be due to the age at presentation. Most patients with dedifferentiated chondrosarcoma present after the age of 40 and are less able to tolerate aggressive chemotherapy. A second reason is this tumor is extremely rare; therefore it is impossible to generate experience with any form of chemotherapeutic protocol to prove its effectiveness. The mode of tumor failure is usually osseous and pulmonary metastases. The latter should be monitored with frequent chest radiographs and CT scans. These imaging studies are performed every 3 months after surgical treatment of the primary tumor for the first 2 years and then every 6 months thereafter. Removal of pulmonary metastases by either thoracotomy or sternotomy can be performed if the patient can tolerate such a procedure.

Mesenchymal chondrosarcoma

Mesenchymal chondrosarcoma is another rare variant of chondrosarcoma that is highly malignant (Fig. 15) (Bertoni *et al.* 1983; Nakashima *et al.* 1986). The World Health Organization defines mesenchymal chondrosarcoma as a tumor composed of a well-differentiated low-grade chondrosarcoma mixed with a high-grade malignant round cell neoplasm or a vascular neoplasm resembling hemangiopericytoma. This tumor was first described by Lichtenstein and Bernstein (1959). This high-grade round cell neoplasm is reminiscent of a Ewing's sarcoma. The round cell malignant component can have a similar appearance to a hemangiopericytoma. This is because of the prominence of the round cells in a perivascular arrangement. This was first reported by Dahlin and Henderson (1962). Huvos *et al.* (1983) have divided mesenchymal chondrosarcoma into two basic types: hemangiopericytoma-like and a small dark round cell type. They found that the mean age of presentation for this tumor was 26 years. There are few large reports of mesenchymal chondrosarcoma. Christensen (1982) reviewed the published literature and found only 250 cases. Schajowicz (1991) reported on the World Health Organization experience with mesenchymal chondrosarcoma and found only 22 cases. Six of Schajowicz's cases occurred in the femur, three in the tibia, and two in the vertebra. He also reported that this tumor can occur in soft tissues, with three occurring in the thigh and one in the soft tissues of the leg. Radiologically, mesenchymal chondrosarcoma presents with a permeative type of bone destruction. Features more typical of conventional chondrosarcoma, including cortical thickening, bone expansion, and matrix mineralization, are usually absent. Some patients present with a pathologic fracture due to the bone loss present in highly stressed areas. Soft-tissue tumors are frequently heavily calcified. The prognosis for mesenchymal chondrosarcoma is extremely poor. There is little published evidence that chemotherapy should be used in this tumor. This is because the cases are so rare and clinically quite varied. However,

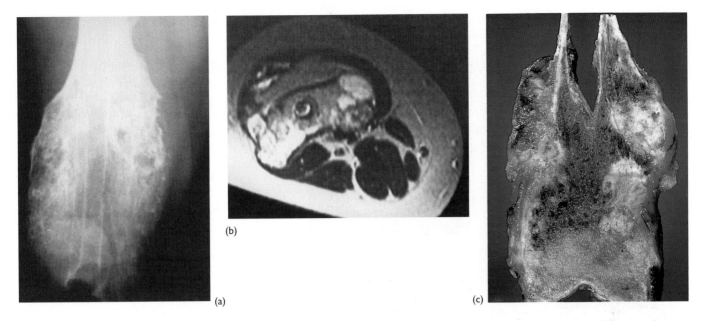

Fig. 13. (a) Malignant degeneration of enchondroma (Ollier's disease) into central chondrosarcoma. Anteroposterior radiograph of the distal femur of a 23-year-old woman with Ollier's disease (enchondromatosis). Note the marked expansion of bone due to the proliferative cartilaginous tumor. On the medial side of the distal femur, the cortical margin is irregular with evidence of destruction. The patient has a chondrosarcoma that developed in an area of a previous enchondroma. (b) MRI scan of the distal femur of a patient with enchondromatosis. This is a T_2-weighted transverse image. The cartilaginous tissue has a bright signal and extends throughout the medullary cavity with soft-tissue extension. This represents a malignant degeneration of a benign enchondroma in Ollier's disease. (c) Specimen photograph after resection of the distal femur. Note the bone expansion by the chondrosarcoma involving the femoral metaphysis.

chemotherapy does seem attractive because of the poor prognosis and the relative high incidence of metastases. Some authors suggest using a Ewing's sarcoma chemotherapeutic protocol; however, supportive data do not exist (Nakashima *et al.* 1986). Surgery for this tumor should be aggressive with wide margins by either limb salvage or amputation. Staging and follow-up is the same as dedifferentiated chondrosarcoma. Frequent chest radiographs, CT scans of the chest, and bone scans are used to follow this tumor.

Clear cell chondrosarcoma

Clear cell chondrosarcoma is a rare variant of chondrosarcoma that has a relatively good prognosis compared with dedifferentiated and mesenchymal chondrosarcoma (Fig. 16) (Bjornsson *et al.* 1984). The World Health Organization defines clear cell chondrosarcoma as a low-grade cartilage neoplasm with round cells possessing clear cytoplasm. Dahlin and Unni (1986) reported 48 clear cell chondrosarcomas; 12 occurred at the Mayo Clinic and the other 36 were in their consultation files. In their series, males predominated (34 of 48 patients). Most of their patients were in the third and fourth decades of life. The majority of clear cell chondrosarcomas occur in the femur and most notably in a juxta-articular location. In the Dahlin and Unni series, 26 out of 48 tumors were located in the femur. Twenty-four of these were in the femoral head. Another common site is the upper end of the tibia. Because of its juxta-articular location, it is frequently mistaken for a benign tumor such as a giant-cell tumor or aneurysmal bone cyst. Osteoblastoma is also considered in the differential diagnosis. Patients frequently present with symptoms for

a prolonged period of time because this tumor is slow growing. It is not uncommon for a patient to have symptoms up to 5 years before diagnosis (37 per cent (Dahlin and Unni 1986)). Radiologically, these tumors are osteolytic without evidence of matrix mineralization. They tend to burrow right up to the subchondral bone and are well circumscribed. Occasionally, they are aneurysmal with ballooning of the bone.

Pathologically, clear cell chondrosarcoma consists of areas of low-grade, well-differentiated, usually grade 1 chondrosarcoma, but there are hypercellular areas and these cells are characterized by abundant clear cytoplasm. Benign giant cells are present in clear cell chondrosarcoma which is a reason that it is often mistaken pathologically for a chondroblastoma. The latter tumor, however, is usually epiphyseal and occurs in adolescents. Some of the tumors have fine areas of calcification between the cells. Vascularity is a common feature of clear cell chondrosarcoma. Clear cell chondrosarcoma, while of relatively benign appearance pathologically, needs to be treated as a malignancy. Seven of the 48 patients in the Mayo Clinic series expired due to disease. Bjornsson *et al.* (1984) reported an overall mortality of 15 per cent in 47 patients. In the Schajowicz series of six patients with clear cell chondrosarcoma, three patients were managed by intralesional excision and one patient by *en bloc* resection of the upper end of the tibia. All patients were disease free at most recent follow-up. This tumor is generally not treated with radiation or chemotherapy. The latter is reserved only for patients with metastatic disease. The risk of metastasis in clear cell chondrosarcoma is relatively low. These patients should be followed with chest radiographs to detect pulmonary metastasis after surgery. The likelihood of local control with *en bloc* resection and reconstruction is high.

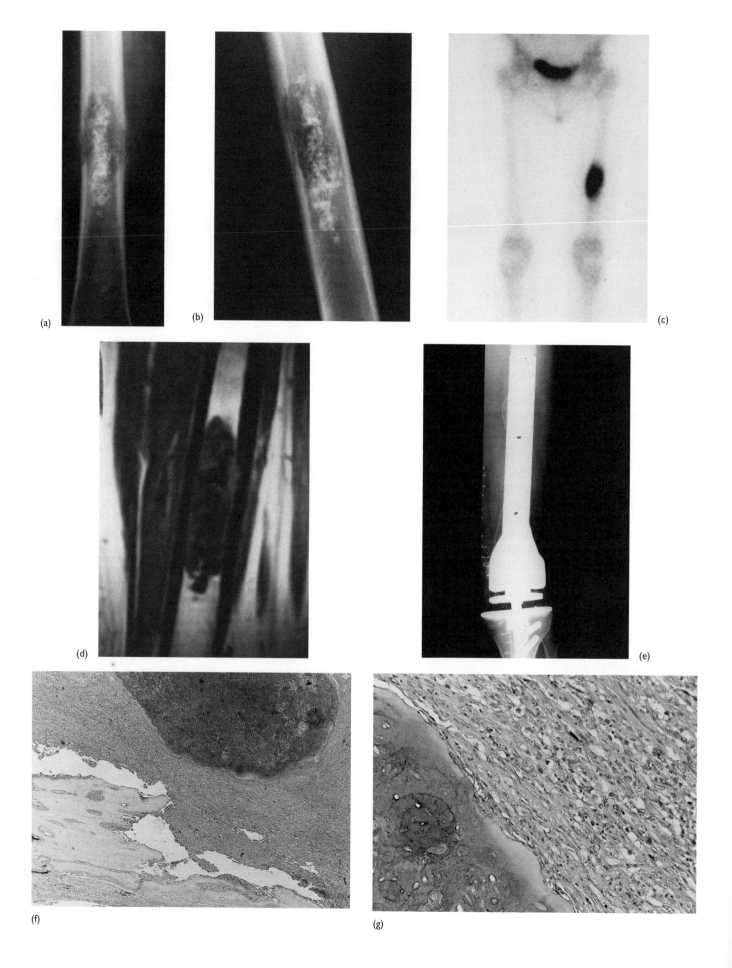

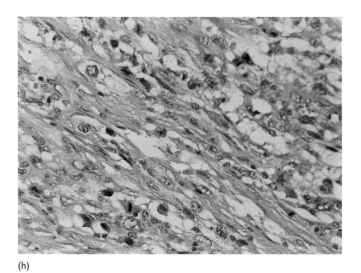

(h)

Fig. 14. Dedifferentiated chondrosarcoma in the left femur. (a) Anteroposterior radiograph of the diaphysis of the left femur in a 72-year-old female. There is a lytic destructive lesion involving the diaphysis of the left distal femur. There is mineralization within the medullary canal. There is also marked osteolysis of the surrounding cortex. There is bone expansion and cortical thickening in certain areas. There is also soft-tissue extension of the tumor. (b) Lateral radiograph of the left femur showing a lytic destructive lesion involving the midshaft of the femur with calcification. The posterior cortex is destroyed. (c) [^{99}Tc^m]diphosphonate bone scan revealing intense uptake involving the diaphysis of the left femur. (d) MRI examination of the left femur showing the marrow replacement by the chondrosarcoma. The extent up and down the medullary canal can easily be seen. (e) Anteroposterior radiograph of the left distal femur and knee joint after surgery. The distal third of the femur has been resected and reconstructed with a modular oncology prosthesis. (f) Low-power section (hematoxylin and eosin) showing low-grade chondrosarcoma (blue) surrounded by spindle cell sarcoma (pink). (g) Hematoxylin and eosin section: demarcation between chondrosarcoma and malignant fibrous histiocytoma is evident. (h) High-power section (hematoxylin and eosin) of the spindle cell sarcoma revealing malignant fibrous histiocytoma.

Because these tumors commonly effect the upper end of the femur, complex hip reconstruction is usually necessary.

Low-grade (grade $\frac{1}{2}$) central chondrosarcoma

Benign calcified lesions of the metaphysis and diaphysis of long bones is a common radiologic finding. Frequently, these lesions are picked up incidentally after a history of trauma. These lesions are calcified without evidence of bone destruction or bone reaction. They tend to be central without evidence of endosteal scalloping. They may show uptake on [^{99}Tc^m]diphosphonate bone scanning. The differential diagnosis for this lesion is either a calcifying enchondroma or a bone infarct. The latter radiographically shows a flame-shaped type of calcification without bone destruction. Once a clinical and radiographic diagnosis is made, these lesions can be followed symptomatically. They are benign and nonprogressive and rarely pose a threat to the patient. However, there is a similar lesion that represents a low-grade chondrosarcoma (Fig. 17). This tumor is characterized by location in

the metaphysis and diaphysis of long bones but is usually associated with pain. The pain is nonmechanical and quite prominent at night. The clinical features tend to be progressive. The pain starts out as mild but then becomes more significant as time passes. Radiographically, not only is the mineralization seen in the medullary canal of a long bone, endosteal scalloping is a common feature. This tumor shows areas of cortical thinning from the inside. The typical features of chondrosarcoma, including bone expansion and cortical thickening, are absent. Pathologic fracture is a rare occurrence through this tumor. [^{99}Tc^m]diphosphonate scans usually shows uptake through these lesions. Most authors now believe that these represent low-grade or grade $\frac{1}{2}$ chondrosarcoma. A biopsy reveals some of the features of grade 1 chondrosarcoma but nothing to suggest aggressiveness. The tumor tends to be somewhat more cellular than an enchondroma but pleomorphism is distinctly absent. Some binucleate forms may be present and occasionally more than one cell within a lacuna is present. A well-recognized proteoglycan matrix background is a common feature. If a biopsy includes the cortical margin, the histologic appearance of endosteal scalloping is present. The cortex is thinned by the tumor.

Some authors have suggested that these low-grade (grade $\frac{1}{2}$) chondrosarcomas can be treated in a similar manner to an aggressive benign bone tumor. They have recommended intralesional excision along with cauterization. Cauterization can be performed by freezing the bone with either liquid nitrogen or phenol (Marcove *et al.* 1977). A careful excision is performed along with burring of the tumor cavity with a high-speed dental burr. After cauterization, the cavity is either packed with methylmethacrylate or some type of bone-graft material. The results with this form of treatment have been universally good. Some authors, however, do not believe this entity exists. They believe grade $\frac{1}{2}$ chondrosarcoma is actually an enchondroma that could be managed by observation. The advantage of the above-mentioned surgical management is that histologic tissue can be obtained to confirm the diagnosis. Perhaps overtreatment is a possibility, but confirmatory tissue is obtained ruling out other more significant tumors.

Secondary chondrosarcomas

Secondary chondrosarcomas need to be considered while following some benign cartilaginous tumors of bone. The most common is a secondary peripheral chondrosarcoma. This tumor occurs in a pre-existing benign osteochondroma (Fig. 12). The risk in an isolated osteochondroma is relatively low. Most authors believe this risk is below 1 per cent. In multiple hereditary exostosis, however, the risk is between 10 and 20 per cent (Garrison *et al.* 1982; Hudson *et al.* 1984; Schmale *et al.* 1994). The usual clinical presentation is the development of pain within a previously known osteochondroma. This tumor develops during the third and fourth decades of life and are more common in an axial location. Rarely they are seen before the conclusion of skeletal growth. Growth of an osteochondroma after skeletal maturity is one of the features of a secondary chondrosarcoma; pain is the second feature. The pain, however, is rather insidious. The duration of symptoms tends to be prolonged because of the paucity of symptoms. A third clinical feature is a mass. Patients will frequently complain of the growth or development of a mass that was previously not present. Radiographically, the features of an

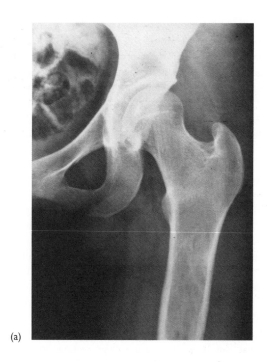

(a)

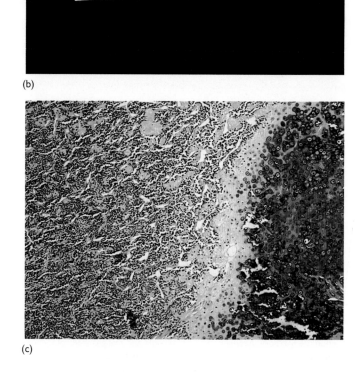

(b)

(c)

Fig. 15. Mesenchymal chondrosarcoma. (a) Anteroposterior radiograph of the left hip and proximal femur of a 17-year-old female. Note the lytic bone destruction of the proximal femur. (b) Specimen photograph after resection of the femur. The tumor involves the femoral diaphysis with cortical destruction and soft-tissue extension evident. Hematoxylin and eosin section. There is a low-grade chondrosarcoma next to a round cell malignancy. The round cell component has a hemangiopericytoma-like appearance. (Courtesy of Dr K.K. Unni, Mayo Clinic.)

osteochondroma are present. Either a sessile or pedunculated bony stalk from the surface of the bone is present. The medullary canal of the host bone communicates with the medullary canal of the tumor. The distinguishing features from a benign osteochondroma include a thick and somewhat irregular cartilaginous cap on the surface of the bony stalk (Kenney *et al.* 1981; Norman and Sissons 1984). The mineral within this calcified mass is quite irregular. Its margins are also irregular and sometimes indistinct. The cartilaginous cap can be measured with MRI scans and usually exceeds 1 cm in thickness. If the tumor involves the medullary canal, then it is quite likely to be a secondary chondrosarcoma. These exophytic chondrosarcomas tend to have pushing margins on contiguous neurovascular structures. In addition, those in the pelvis that extend into the retroperitoneum can impinge upon bowel, bladder, and other visceral organs. Secondary peripheral chondrosarcomas, however, tend to be well differentiated histologically. Most are either grade 1 or grade 2, and rarely is a high-grade tumor seen. Myxomatous tumors are rare. Their surface tends to be firm and have a cauliflower appearance. Complete surgical excision with wide margins is the treatment of choice by either amputation or limb salvage. Biopsy can lead to spillage and needs to be done very carefully. The prognosis for this tumor is good and tends to be far better than a central chondrosarcoma.

Because of the risk of malignant degeneration of an osteochondroma, patients with this tumor need to be followed both clinically and radiographically throughout their life. Since the risk is greater in multiple hereditary exostosis, these patients should be seen yearly and appropriate imaging studies ordered to rule out the development of a secondary peripheral chondrosarcoma.

Secondary central chondrosarcomas are far rarer tumors. Most central chondrosarcomas arise *de novo* and have a poorer prognosis than a peripheral chondrosarcoma. The lesions that can lead to a secondary central chondrosarcoma include an enchondroma and multiple enchondromatosis such as Ollier's or Maffucci's syndrome (Fig. 13) (Lewis and Ketcham 1973; Cannon 1985; Schwartz *et al.* 1987*b*). The risk of an isolated enchondroma undergoing secondary malignant degeneration is low. This risk is well below 1 per cent and some authors believe that it almost never occurs. However, malignant degeneration of Ollier's or Maffucci's syndromes is a significant risk. That risk ranges from 10 to 20 per cent. Interestingly, these patients also develop other epithelial cancers that pose a greater risk to the patient. The pathologic diagnosis of a secondary central chondrosarcoma requires some evidence of a pre-existing benign enchondroma along with the features of a chondrosarcoma. Some secondary chondrosarcomas are actually misdiagnosed chondrosarcomas from the

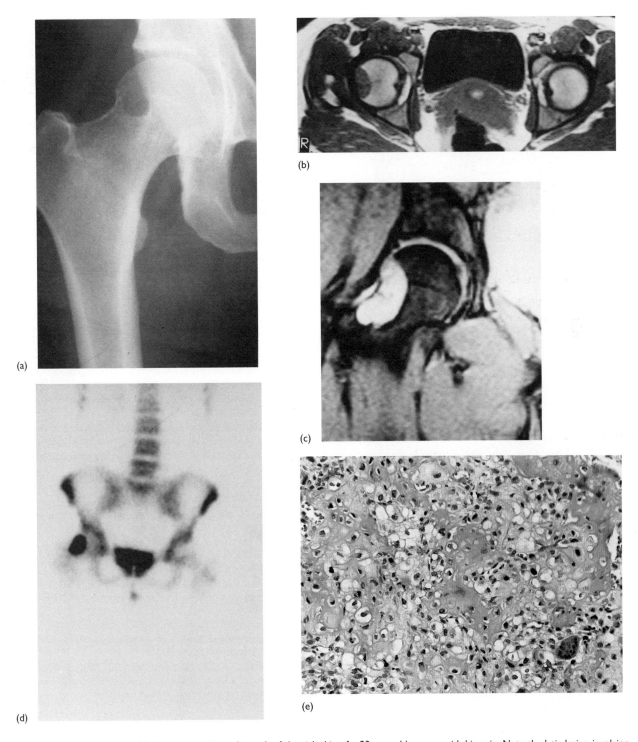

Fig. 16. Clear cell chondrosarcoma. (a) Anteroposterior radiograph of the right hip of a 23-year-old woman with hip pain. Note the lytic lesion involving the lateral aspect of the femoral head and neck. The lesion is well demarcated without evidence of mineralization. The cortical margin appears intact. There is an area of sclerosis surrounding the lytic lesion more medially. (b) Transverse T_1-weighted MRI scan of the right and left hip. There is a lesion in the femoral head, centrally located, that is well demarcated. (c) Coronal T_2-weighted MRI scan of the right hip joint. An enhancing lesion is found in the femoral head and neck corresponding with the lesion seen on the plain radiograph. The lesion is well demarcated but there is evidence of cortical disruption. (d) [^{99}Tc^m]diphosphonate bone scan of the right hip showing intense uptake in the femoral head and neck area. (e) Hematoxylin and eosin section. Chondrocytes within lacunae are scattered throughout the section. A single multinucleated giant cell is present. The most noteworthy feature is the presence of numerous cells with abundant clear cytoplasm ('clear cells').

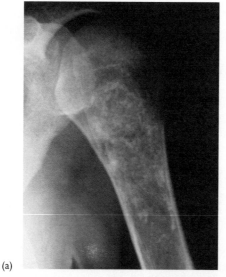

(a)

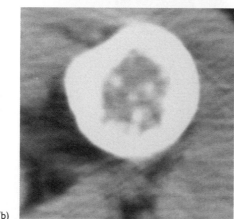

(b)

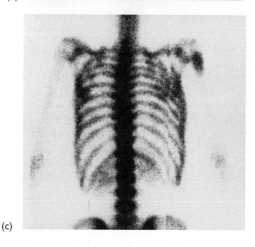

(c)

Fig. 17. Grade $\frac{1}{2}$ chondrosarcoma in the left proximal humerus. (a) Anteroposterior radiograph of the left proximal humerus in a 35-year-old female. The patient presented with pain both with activity and rest. The radiograph reveals a calcified lesion involving the upper end of the humerus with some slight endosteal bone destruction. (b) CT image of the left proximal humerus. On this transverse image there is evidence of a calcified medullary lesion with some small areas of endosteal scalloping with bony erosion. (c) [^{99}Tc^{m}]diphosphonate bone scan of the left proximal humerus showing uptake in the metaphysis. This lesion was biopsied and proved to be a grade $\frac{1}{2}$ chondrosarcoma.

beginning. The treatment of a secondary central chondrosarcoma is the same as a chondrosarcoma that arises *de novo*. Wide *en bloc* resection with reconstruction is usually necessary. Chemotherapy and radiation have a very limited role.

References

Aprin, H., Riseborough, E.J., and Hall, J.E. (1982). Chondrosarcoma in children and adolescents. *Clinical Orthopaedics and Related Research*, **166**, 226–32.

Bertoni, F., Picci, P., Bacchini, P., *et al.* (1983). Mesenchymal chondrosarcoma of bone and soft tissue. *Cancer*, **52**, 533–41.

Bjornsson, J., Unni, K.K., Dahlin, D.C., Beabout, J.W., and Sim, F.H. (1984). Clear cell chondrosarcoma of bone: observations in 47 cases. *American Journal of Surgical Pathology*, **8**, 223–30.

Buckwalter, J.A. (1983). The structure of human chondrosarcoma proteoglycans. *Journal of Bone and Joint Surgery, American Volume*, **65A**, 958–74.

Campanacci, M. (1990). *Bone and soft tissue tumors*, pp. 267–303. Springer-Verlag, New York.

Cannon, S.R. and Sweetnam, D.R. (1985). Multiple chondrosarcomas in dyschondroplasia (Ollier's disease). *Cancer*, **55**, 836–40.

Capanna, R., Bertoni, F., Betteli, G., *et al.* (1988). Dedifferentiated chondrosarcomy. *Journal of Bone and Joint Surgery, American Volume*, **70A**, 60–9.

Christensen, R.E., Jr (1982). Mesenchymal chondrosarcoma of the jaws. *Oral Surgery*, **54**, 197–206.

Dahlin, D.C. and Beabout, J.W. (1971). Dedifferentiation of low-grade chondrosarcoma. *Cancer*, **28**, 461–6.

Dahlin, D.C. and Henderson, E.D. (1962). Mesenchymal chondrosarcoma. Further observations on a new entity. *Cancer*, **15**, 410–17.

Dahlin, D.C. and Unni, K.K. (1986). *Bone tumors: general aspects and data on 8542 cases.* C.C. Thomas, Springfield, IL.

Daly, P.J., Sim, E.H., and Wold, L.E. (1989). Dedifferentiated chondrosarcoma of bone. *Orthopedics*, **12**, 763–7.

DeLange, E.E., Pope, T.L., Jr, and Fechner, R.E. (1986). Dedifferentiated chondrosarcoma: radiographic features. *Radiology*, **160**, 489–92.

Enneking, W.F., Spanier, S.S., and Goodman, M.A. (1980). A system for the surgical staging of musculoskeletal sarcoma. *Clinical Orthopaedics and Related Research*, **153**, 106–120.

Erikkson, A.I., Schiller, A., and Mankin, H.J. (1980). The management of chondrosarcoma of bone. *Clinical Orthopaedics and Related Research*, **153**, 44–60.

Evans, H.L., Ayala, A.G., and Rohmsdahl, M.D. (1977). Prognostic factors in chondrosarcoma of bone: a clinicopathologic analysis with emphasis on histologic grading. *Cancer*, **40**, 818–31.

Frassica, F.J., Unni, K.K., Beabout, J.W., *et al.* (1986). Dedifferentiated chondrosarcoma: a report of the clinicopathological features and treatment of seventy-eight cases. *Journal of Bone and Joint Surgery, American Volume*, **68A**, 1197–205.

Garrison, R.C., Unni, K.K., McLeod, R.A., Pritchard, D.J., and Dahlin, D.C. (1982). Chondrosarcoma arising in osteochondroma. *Cancer*, **49**, 1890–7.

Gitelis, S., Bertoni, F., Picci, P., and Campanacci, M. (1981). Chondrosarcoma of bone: the experience at the Istituto Ortopedico Rizzoli. *Journal of Bone and Joint Surgery, American Volume*, **63A**, 1248–57.

Healey, J.H. and Lane, J.M. (1986). Chondrosarcoma. *Clinical Orthopaedics and Related Research*, **204**, 119–29.

Hudson, T.M., Springfield, D.S., Spanier, S.S., *et al.* (1984). Benign exostoses and exostotic chondrosarcoma: evaluation of cartilage thickness by CT. *Radiology*, **12**, 595–9.

Huvos, A.G. (1991). *Bone tumors: diagnosis, treatment, prognosis.* W.B. Saunders, Philadelphia, PA.

Huvos, A.G. and Marcove, R.C. (1987). Chondrosarcoma in the young: a clinicopathologic analysis of 79 patients younger than 21 years of age. *American Journal of Surgical Pathology*, **11**, 930–42.

Huvos, A.G., Rosen, G., Dabska, M., *et al.* (1983). Mesenchymal chondrosarcoma. A clinicopathologic analysis of 35 patients with emphasis on treatment. *Cancer*, **51**, 1230–7.

Johnson, S., Tetu, B., Ayala, A.G., *et al.* (1986). Chondrosarcoma with additional mesenchymal component (dedifferentiated chondrosarcoma). 1. A clinicopathologic study of 26 cases. *Cancer*, **58**, 278–86.

Kenney P.J., Gilula, L.A., and Murphy, W.A. (1981) The use of computed tomography to distinguish osteochondroma and chondrosarcoma. *Radiology*, **139**, 129–37.

Lewis, R.J. and Ketcham, A.S. (1973). Maffucci's syndrome: functional and neoplastic significance. Case report and review of the literature. *Journal of Bone and Joint Surgery, American Volume*, **55A**, 1465–79.

Lichtenstein, L. and Jaffe, H.L. (1943). Chondrosarcoma of bone. *American Journal of Pathology*, **19**, 553–89.

Mankin, H.J., Cantley, K.P., Lippiello, L., Schiller, A.L., and Campbell, C.J. (1980*a*). The biology of human chondrosarcoma. I. Description of the cases, grading, and biochemical analyses. *Journal of Bone and Joint Surgery, American Volume*, **62A**, 160–76.

Mankin, H.J., Cantley, K.P., Schiller, A.L., and Lippiello, L. (1980*b*). The biology of human chondrosarcoma. II. Variation in chemical composition among types and subtypes of benign and malignant cartilage tumors. *Journal of Bone and Joint Surgery, American Volume*, **62A**, 176–88.

Marcove, R.C. (1977) Chondrosarcoma: diagnosis and treatment. *Orthopedic Clinics of North America*, **8**, 811–20.

Marcove, R.C., Mike, V., Hutter, R.V.P., *et al.* (1972). Chondrosarcoma of the pelvis and upper end of the femur. An analysis of factors influencing survival times in one hundred and thirteen cases. *Journal of Bone and Joint Surgery, American Volume*, **54A**, 561–72.

Marcove, R.C., Stovell, P.B., Huvos, A.G., and Bullough, P.G. (1977). The use of cryosurgery in the treatment of low and medium grade chondrosarcoma. *Clinical Orthopaedics and Related Research*, **12**, 147–55.

Mirra, J.M. and Marcove, R.C. (1974). Fibrosarcomatous dedifferentiation of primary and secondary chondrosarcoma: review of five cases. *Journal of Bone and Joint Surgery, American Volume*, **56A**, 285–96.

Nakashima, Y., Unni, K.K., Shives, T.C., *et al.* (1986). Mesenchymal chondrosarcoma of bone and soft tissue: a review of 111 cases. *Cancer*, **57**, 2444–53.

Norman, A. and Sissons, H.A. (1984). Radiographic hallmarks of peripheral chondrosarcoma. *Radiology*, **151**, 589–96.

Patel, S.R., Burgess, M.A., Papadopoulos, N.E., *et al.* (1995). Extraskeletal myxoid chondrosarcoma. Long-term experience with chemotherapy. *American Journal of Clinical Oncology*, **18**, 161–3.

Saleh, G., Evans, H.L., Ro, J.Y., *et al.* (1992). Extraskeletal myxoid chondrosarcoma: a clinicopathologic study of ten patients with long-term follow-up. *Cancer*, **70**, 2827–30.

Sannerkin, N.G. and Gallagher, P. (1979). A review of the behaviour of chondrosarcoma of bone. *Journal of Bone and Joint Surgery, British Volume*, **61B**, 395–400.

Schajowicz, F. (1991). *Tumors and tumorlike lesions of bone, pathology, radiology, and treatment* (2nd edn). Springer-Verlag, New York.

Schmale, G.A., Conrad, E.U., III, and Raskind, W.H. (1994). The natural history of hereditary multiple exostoses. *Journal of Bone and Joint Surgery, American Volume*, **76A**, 986–92.

Schwartz, H.S., Zimmerman, N.B., Simon, M.A., *et al.* (1987*a*). Dedifferentiated chondrosarcoma: a report of the clinicopathological features and treatment of seventy-eight cases. *Journal of Bone and Joint Surgery, American Volume*, **69A**, 269–74.

Schwartz, H.S., Zimmerman, N.B., Simon, M.A., *et al.* (1987*b*). The malignant potential of enchondromatosis. *Journal of Bone and Joint Surgery, American Volume*, **69A**, 269–74.

1.6.8.4 Ewing's sarcoma

Richard Vlasak and Franklin H. Sim

Introduction
Definition

Ewing's sarcoma is a malignant nonosteogenic primary tumor of bone (Fig. 1) characterized by islands of anaplastic small round cells closely associated with blood vessels (Ewing 1921; Dahlin and Unni 1986). The cell of origin of Ewing's sarcoma is unknown, but recent cytogenetic as well as immunocytochemical studies support a neural cell origin (Devaney *et al.* 1995). In a patient with the appropriate clinical presentation, the diagnosis of Ewing's sarcoma is made by excluding other round cell tumors that occur in bone in a patient with the appropriate clinical presentation.

Epidemiology

Ewing's sarcoma is the second most common primary malignant bone tumor of children and the fourth most common malignant tumor of bone overall (Pritchard *et al.* 1975). Ewing's sarcoma accounted for 6 per cent of primary malignant bone tumors at the Mayo Clinic (Dahlin and Unni 1986). It accounted for approximately 10 per cent of primary malignant bone tumors in a Swedish study

Box 1

- A malignant nonosteogenic primary tumor of bone consisting of islands of anaplastic small round cells closely associated with blood vessels

- The second most common primary malignant bone tumor of children and the fourth most common malignant tumor of bone overall

- Prior to the advent of effective chemotherapy, more than 90 per cent of patients with Ewing's sarcoma died with disseminated disease

- Tumors that must be differentiated from Ewing's sarcoma include lymphoma of bone, embryonal rhabdomyosarcoma, metastatic neuroblastoma, small cell osteogenic sarcoma, and mesenchymal chondrosarcoma

- Peak incidence of Ewing's sarcoma (65 per cent of cases) is in the second decade of life

- Most common presenting symptom is pain (90 per cent of patients), followed by swelling (70 per cent of patients)

- The current general approach to treatment includes intense chemotherapy followed by wide *en bloc* excision of the primary tumor when possible

- Radiation therapy is added postoperatively if the postoperative margin is intralesional or marginal; in anatomic sites where *en bloc* resection with wide margins is difficult, radiation therapy may be used before surgery to allow a closer margin of resection

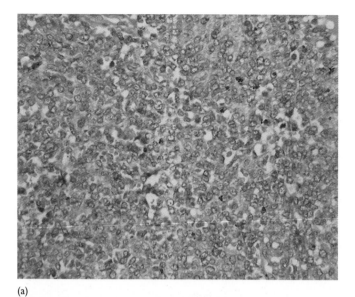

(a)

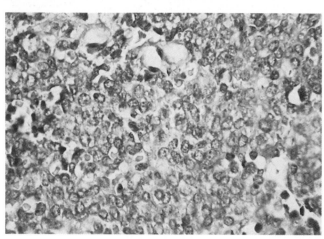

(b)

Fig. 1. (a) Low-power photomicrograph of a Ewing's sarcoma biopsy showing sheets of small round-shaped cells that are extremely undifferentiated. The cells are filed in sheets around small blood vessels with no stromal matrix. (b) High-power photomicrograph of Ewing's sarcoma cells showing the prominent nuclei with minimal cytoplasm.

(Larsson *et al.* 1973). The mean annual incidence of Ewing's sarcomas per million population is 0.6 in England and 0.8 in Sweden.

Natural history

Prior to the advent of effective chemotherapy, more than 90 per cent of patients with Ewing's sarcoma died with disseminated disease (Boyer *et al.* 1967). The development of effective multiagent chemotherapy over the past 20 years has increased the 5-year survival of Ewing's sarcoma patients from 5 to 10 per cent to the current value in excess of 70 per cent (Burgert *et al.* 1990).

Pathology

Histologically, Ewing's sarcomas are extremely undifferentiated and consist of sheets of small, round, oval, or spindle-shaped cells with prominent nuclei and poorly visualized cytoplasm (Fig. 1). The nuclei are uniform and mitotic nuclei figures are numerous. Frequently areas of necrosis are present due to a tumor outgrowing the blood supply. Often, viable cells are found in cords or masses about blood vessels with necrosis in more remote areas. A diagnosis of Ewing's sarcoma is generally made by excluding other round cell tumors that occur in bone (Dahlin and Unni 1986). The identification of glycogen in the tumor cells using the periodic acid–Schiff stain may be helpful, but this finding is neither specific nor always present in the diagnosis of Ewing's sarcoma.

The tumors that must be differentiated from Ewing's sarcoma both clinically and pathologically include primary lymphoma of bone, embryonal rhabdomyosarcoma, metastatic neuroblastoma, small cell osteogenic sarcoma, and mesenchymal chondrosarcoma (Dahlin and Unni 1986; Devaney *et al.* 1995). Osteomyelitis which can occur concurrently with Ewing's sarcoma and Langerhans' cell histiocytosis also falls into the differential diagnosis. Undifferentiated carcinoma can usually be excluded on a clinical basis as well as by special stains.

James Ewing believed that the tumor bearing his name was of vascular origin and called it diffuse endothelioma of bone. Since then, many have assumed a primitive mesenchymal cell as the cell of origin. Recent advances in cytogenetics, immunocytochemistry, and electron microscopy have allowed pathologists to incorporate Ewing's sarcoma into a unified concept of primitive neuroectodermal tumors with a neural cell origin (Devaney *et al.* 1995). Ewing's sarcoma is the least differentiated tumor of this group which includes primitive neuroectodermal tumor, atypical Ewing's tumor, Askins' tumor, and neuroepithelioma. Cytogenetic studies show that these tumors share the reciprocal translocation (11:22) (q24:q12) (Womer 1991).

The reciprocal translocation (11:22) (q24:q12) has been cloned and is identical in Ewing's sarcoma and primitive neuroectodermal tumor. In addition, these tumors produce a cell surface glycoprotein designated P30/32 MIC2 which is a product of the MIC2 gene located on the short arms of the X and Y chromosomes (Devaney *et al.* 1995). This cell surface glycoprotein can be recognized by commercially available monoclonal antibodies HBA71 and MIC2 (Signet Laboratories, Dedham, Massachusetts). Although these antibodies are not specific for Ewing's sarcoma, they can be helpful in differentiating Ewing's sarcoma from lymphomas and embryonal cell rhabdomyosarcomas using immunocytochemistry (Devaney *et al.* 1995). Approximately 90 per cent of Ewing's sarcomas react with antibodies HBA71 and MIC2.

The unified concept of primitive neuroectodermal tumors has also been supported by a clinical study from the Mayo Clinic (Siebenrock 1996). In this study, patients with the diagnosis of Ewing's sarcoma and primitive neuroectodermal tumor were compared using similar treatments and found to have statistically similar outcomes.

Primary lymphoma of bone is the most important tumor that must be differentiated from Ewing's sarcoma. Primary lymphoma of bone generally occurs in an older age group, but the age of presentation may overlap with Ewing's sarcoma. Both Ewing's sarcoma and primary lymphoma of bone can present with a large soft-tissue mass. Radiographically, Ewing's sarcoma tends to appear destructive (Figs 2(a), 3(a), 3(b), and 4(a)), while primary lymphoma of bone tends to have reactive bone formation and frequently presents with a mixed sclerotic and lytic appearance. Immunohistochemical studies can be used to help differentiate Ewing's sarcoma from primary lymphoma of bone (Devaney *et al.* 1995). Most lymphomas are

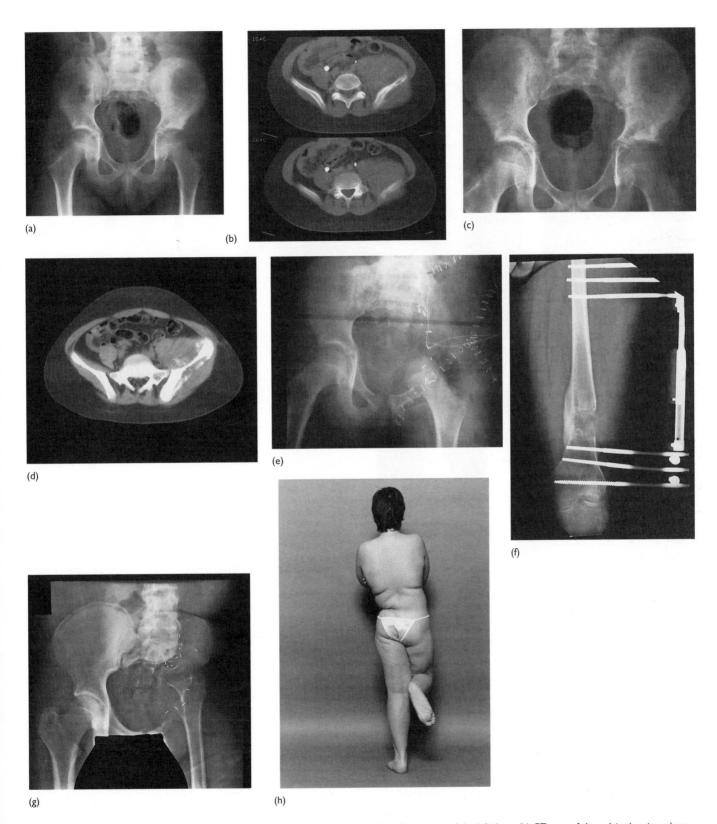

Fig. 2. (a) Anteroposterior pelvis radiograph of a 9-year-old boy presenting with Ewing's sarcoma of the left ilium. (b) CT scan of the pelvis showing a large soft-tissue extension. (c) Anteroposterior pelvis radiograph and (d) CT scan of the pelvis after two courses of preoperative chemotherapy on the Intergroup Ewing's Sarcoma Study II protocol. Note that the soft-tissue component of the tumor has considerably decreased in size. (e) Patient underwent a type I–II wide resection of Ewing's sarcoma of the left ilium. No radiation therapy was used. (f) Seven years after his left iliac resection the patient has no evidence of disease but has a 5-cm leg-length discrepancy. This was treated by limb lengthening. (g) Anteroposterior pelvis radiograph shows that the proximal femur has stabilized against the sacrum. (h) Patient's left hip function 9 years following left iliac resection. He currently has no evidence of disease. (Reproduced from Vlasak (1996).)

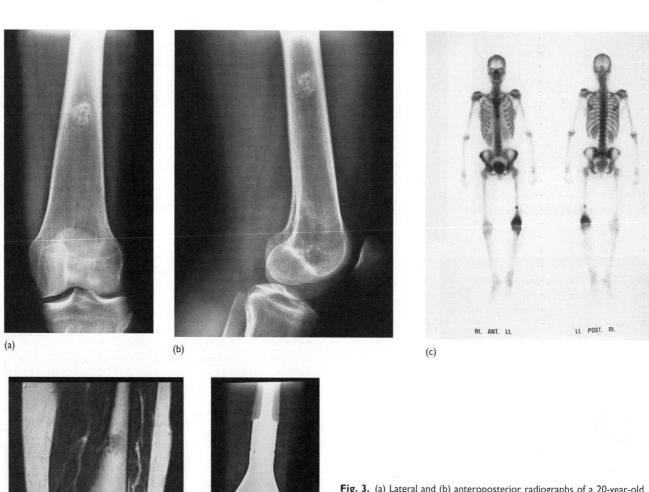

(a)   (b)   (c)

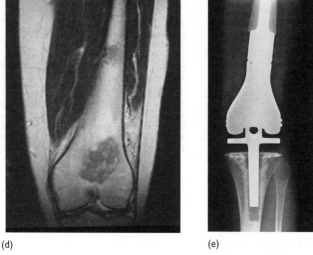

(d)   (e)

Fig. 3. (a) Lateral and (b) anteroposterior radiographs of a 20-year-old woman with Ewing's sarcoma of the left distal femur. Note the periosteal reaction along the distal lateral cortex. The enchondroma was an unrelated incidental finding. (c) Technetium bone scan showing no metastatic disease. The distal femoral uptake is from the Ewing's sarcoma and the localized more proximal uptake is from the incidental enchondroma. (d) An MRI of the distal femur showing minimal soft-tissue extension. (e) The patient underwent wide distal femoral resection after preoperative chemotherapy including doxorubicin, ifosfamide, and etoposide. She was reconstructed using a modular kinematic rotating hinge endoprosthesis and received no radiation therapy. She is now 2 years postresection and has no evidence of disease. (Reproduced from Vlasak (1996).)

common leukocyte antigen positive, distinguishing them from Ewing's sarcomas which are negative.

Metastatic embryonal rhabdomyosarcoma can be differentiated from Ewing's sarcoma by immunocytochemistry which reveals the presence of muscle markers such as actin, desmin, and myoglobin. Electron microscopy shows cytoplasmic filaments and occasionally Z-band formation in rhabdomyosarcoma, but not in Ewing's sarcoma.

Clinical evaluation

Clinical presentation

Although Ewing's sarcoma can occur at any age, the disease is uncommon before age 5 and after age 30. The peak incidence of Ewing's sarcoma (65 per cent of cases) is in the second decade of life (Pritchard *et al.* 1975; Rosen *et al.* 1981; Dahlin and Unni 1986; Toni *et al.* 1993). There is a male preponderance of approximately 1.6:1. Ewing's sarcoma rarely (fewer than 2 per cent) occurs in the black population.

Ewing's sarcoma occurs most frequently in the long bones and pelvis (Figs 2, 3, 4, and 5). In a review of all the Ewing's sarcoma cases at the Mayo Clinic, the majority of the patients had tumors of the larger bones (65 per cent). The most common site involved was the femur (22.4 per cent), followed by the pelvis (17.7 per cent), and the tibia and humerus (Dahlin and Unni 1986). Any portion of a long tubular bone may be affected and the entire shaft often is involved. In 167 cases studied at Memorial Hospital (Marcove and Rosen 1980), the most common site of involvement was the distal femoral metaphysis and diaphysis followed by the pelvis, tibia, fibula,

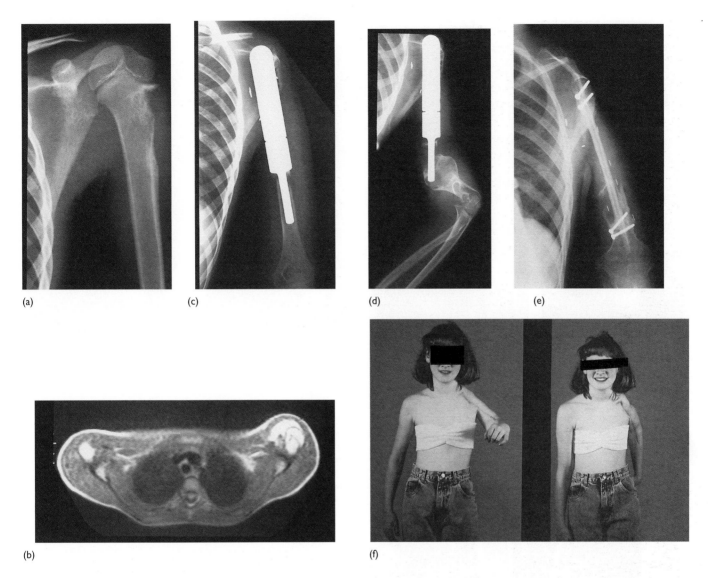

(a)   (c)   (d)   (e)

(b)   (f)

Fig. 4. (a) Anteroposterior shoulder radiograph of a 5-year-old girl presenting with Ewing's sarcoma of the left proximal humerus. (b) MRI of the shoulder shows a large anterior soft-tissue extension. (c) The patient underwent an extra-articular resection of the left shoulder and proximal half of the left humerus after receiving preoperative chemotherapy on the Intergroup Ewing's Sarcoma Study II protocol. The skeletal defect was reconstructed with a modular metallic spacer and a latissimus dorsi pedicle flap for soft-tissue coverage. No radiation therapy was used. (d) Five years after the resection, the left humeral endoprosthesis has become loose. (e) The failed humeral endoprosthesis was converted to an intercalary free vascularized fibula arthrodesis of the shoulder. (f) Ten years after her original resection and 5 years after her shoulder arthrodesis, the patient has useful function of her left upper extremity with a very acceptable cosmetic result. She has no evidence of disease 10 years after resection. (Reproduced from Vlasak (1996).)

humerus, and less often the ribs, scapula, vertebral, and small bones of the hands and feet.

The most common presenting symptom is pain, which is found in 90 per cent of patients, followed by swelling, which occurs in 70 per cent (Pritchard *et al.* 1975; Wilkins *et al.* 1986). Approximately one-fifth of the cases present with a fever, which may lead to the mistaken diagnosis of osteomyelitis.

Pathologic fractures at the site of the tumor have been reported at presentation in 5 to 10 per cent of patients. Approximately half of patients with Ewing's sarcoma of the spine present with a neurologic deficit which may initially be misdiagnosed as a lumbar disk herniation (Grubb *et al.* 1994).

Imaging studies and tests

A patient suspected of having Ewing's sarcoma is staged for both local and metastatic disease. Local disease is evaluated with plain radiographs of the bone as well as MRI imaging of the site involved (Figs 2, 3, 4, and 5). The MRI image is more sensitive than the CT scan in assessing soft-tissue involvement and bone marrow spread. The MRI or CT scan is repeated after several cycles of chemotherapy to assess the response to chemotherapy better and to help plan treatment of the primary site with surgery or radiation therapy.

Metastatic disease is evaluated at the time of presentation with chest radiographs and a chest CT, looking for pulmonary metastases. A bone scan is used to detect bone metastases (Fig. 3). A bone

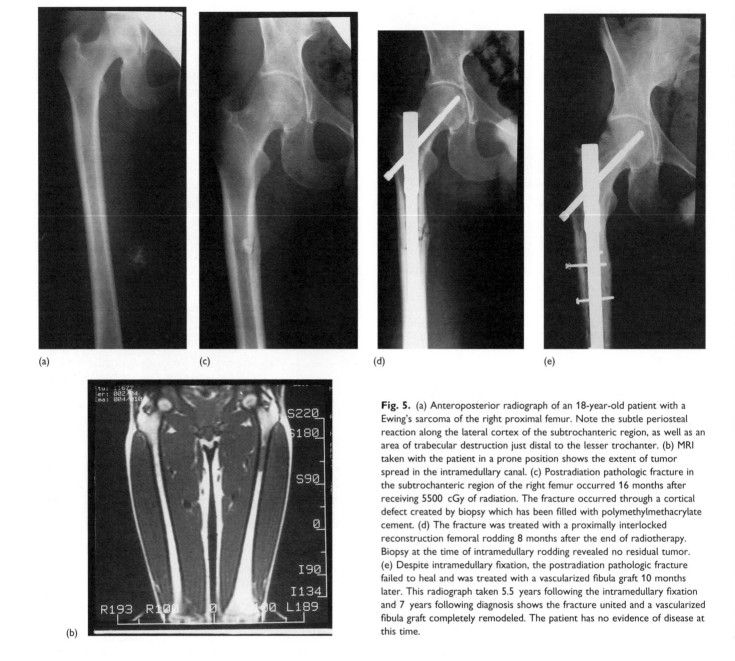

(a)   (c)   (d)   (e)

(b)

Fig. 5. (a) Anteroposterior radiograph of an 18-year-old patient with a Ewing's sarcoma of the right proximal femur. Note the subtle periosteal reaction along the lateral cortex of the subtrochanteric region, as well as an area of trabecular destruction just distal to the lesser trochanter. (b) MRI taken with the patient in a prone position shows the extent of tumor spread in the intramedullary canal. (c) Postradiation pathologic fracture in the subtrochanteric region of the right femur occurred 16 months after receiving 5500 cGy of radiation. The fracture occurred through a cortical defect created by biopsy which has been filled with polymethylmethacrylate cement. (d) The fracture was treated with a proximally interlocked reconstruction femoral rodding 8 months after the end of radiotherapy. Biopsy at the time of intramedullary rodding revealed no residual tumor. (e) Despite intramedullary fixation, the postradiation pathologic fracture failed to heal and was treated with a vascularized fibula graft 10 months later. This radiograph taken 5.5 years following the intramedullary fixation and 7 years following diagnosis shows the fracture united and a vascularized fibula graft completely remodeled. The patient has no evidence of disease at this time.

marrow aspirate and biopsy is performed at a site distant from the primary lesion to assess the spread of the disease into the bone marrow.

Prechemotherapy blood studies are performed including renal and liver function tests. Cardiac function is evaluated with an echocardiogram or a radionuclide angiogram prior to chemotherapy.

Lactate dehydrogenase levels are also measured because elevated levels have been associated with a poor prognosis and metastatic disease in some studies (Wilkins *et al.* 1986).

Plain radiographs generally show a permeative destructive lesion whose borders are not well defined (Figs 2, 3, 4, and 5). Frequently, a large soft-tissue mass may be observed with obliteration of adjacent fat planes. Usually, there is little reactive bone, but following neo-

adjuvant chemotherapy, reactive bone frequently appears at the periphery of the soft-tissue mass (Figs 2(c) and (d)).

Prognostic factors

The major prognostic factors in Ewing's sarcoma are site, volume of tumor, metastases at diagnosis, and the tumor's response to chemotherapy.

Patients with Ewing's sarcoma of distal sites, such as bones of the hands and feet, have a better prognosis than patients with central lesions, such as those of the pelvis or sacrum (Evans *et al.* 1991; Frassica *et al.* 1993; Scully *et al.* 1995). Although some of these studies show that site is an independent variable, it is very difficult to separate the effect of volume of tumor from the site of origin. Central sites are associated with larger volumes of tumor. A large initial tumor size or volume has been shown by several studies to be a poor prognostic factor (Evans *et al.* 1985; Jurgens *et al.* 1988).

Patients with tumors larger than 10 cm or having tumor volumes of 100 cm³ or greater (measured by CT) have a significantly poorer prognosis.

A third prognostic indicator of poor outcome is the presence of metastatic disease at the time of diagnosis. In a review of 140 patients at the Mayo Clinic, 25 per cent presented with metastatic disease.

The patients with metastases had a 2-year survival of 39 per cent, compared with a 69 per cent 2-year survival in patients without metastases (Wilkins *et al.* 1986).

More recently, a good pathologic response to neoadjuvant chemotherapy was shown to be a favorable prognostic sign (Picci *et al.* 1993; Wunder *et al.* 1995). These studies show the value of assessing the histopathologic response to neoadjuvant chemotherapy following surgical resection. A good clinical response to chemotherapy, as evidenced by a decrease in the size of the tumor mass, has also been shown to have a favorable prognosis (Oberlin *et al.* 1985).

Management

Modern treatment of osseous Ewing's sarcoma consists of a multidisciplinary approach in which surgeons, radiation oncologists, pediatric oncologists, medical oncologists, pathologists, and radiologists work together toward an optimal outcome. Systemic spread of the disease is controlled by aggressive multiagent chemotherapy. Local disease is controlled by surgery, radiotherapy, or both.

Local disease control

Surgery

During the past 15 years, the roll of *en bloc* excision of the primary tumor (Figs 2, 3, and 4) has expanded in an attempt to minimize the risk of local recurrence which is frequently chemotherapy resistant and leads to distant metastasis (Marcove and Rosen 1990).

With increasing long-term survival rates following the advent of modern chemotherapy, control of local disease becomes more important since patients have more time to develop local recurrences. The general philosophy is to give intense multiagent neoadjuvant chemotherapy which decreases the size of the primary tumor followed by wide *en bloc* excision (Pritchard 1980; O'Connor and Pritchard 1991). Radiation therapy is added postoperatively if it is found that the postoperative margin is intralesional or marginal. In certain anatomic sites, such as the pelvis or spine where *en bloc* resection with wide margins is very difficult, radiation therapy may be used before surgery in order to allow a closer margin of resection.

Many studies show an advantage of using surgery for primary control; however, most of these studies are noncontrolled retrospective studies and must be interpreted with caution.

A study from the Mayo Clinic showed increased 5- and 10-year survival rates in 229 patients with Ewing's sarcoma when surgery was used to control the primary tumor (Pritchard *et al.* 1975). These higher survival rates were seen regardless of the tumor's location. However, this study was performed before extensive use of multi-

agent chemotherapy. A more contemporary study from the Mayo Clinic, performed on patients receiving adjuvant chemotherapy, showed a clear survival advantage for patients who underwent complete surgical excision of the primary lesion compared with patients treated with radiation alone for local control (Wilkins *et al.* 1986).

The surgical group had a 5-year survival rate of 74 per cent versus 34 per cent for the radiation only group. A recent study of Ewing's sarcoma of the pelvis also found an increased 5-year overall survival rate for patients who had resection of their primary tumor (Frassica *et al.* 1993).

Other institutions have also shown enhanced survival of patients treated with surgical resection in addition to chemotherapy. The 5-year actuarial survival was 92 per cent in a retrospective study of 46 patients with a Ewing's sarcoma treated with surgical resection at Massachusetts General Hospital. The nonsurgical group had a 5-year actuarial survival of only 37 per cent (Sailer *et al.* 1988). A study of 18 patients with pelvic Ewing's sarcoma from Memorial Sloan-Kettering Hospital showed a twofold increase in survival rate in patients who had resection of their primary tumor in addition to radiation and chemotherapy compared with patients treated with radiation and chemotherapy alone (Li *et al.* 1983).

The reason for this higher survival rate associated with surgical excision may be the elimination of residual tumor cells that are left behind after radiation therapy or chemotherapy. The residual tumor cells, if they survive, are frequently resistant to the chemotherapy drugs that have been used. Local recurrences and late distant metastases that can develop from local recurrences have been shown to be less responsive to chemotherapy than the original tumors. It is hoped that surgical excision may remove the chemotherapy-resistant cells before they have a chance to recur clinically or to metastasize.

Tumor cells of viable appearance have been found in the irradiated primary site in 13 of 20 cases examined at autopsy (Telles *et al.* 1978). It cannot be proved that these cells were viable and capable of metastases, but they did exhibit glycogen periodic acid–Schiff staining and appeared to be active. This explanation is consistent with several studies that have shown patients treated with surgery or surgery plus radiation having a much lower recurrence rate compared with patients treated with radiation only.

Since local recurrences can occur as late as 5 years or more following treatment, the role of surgery in the treatment of primary disease will become more important as patients live longer.

Numerous retrospective studies have shown lower local recurrence rates when the primary tumor was treated with surgery and/or radiation therapy as opposed to radiation therapy alone. A study from the Rizzoli Institute, Bologna, showed a local recurrence rate of 8 per cent for patients treated with surgery or surgery plus radiation compared with 36 per cent for patients treated with radiation therapy alone (Bacci *et al.* 1989). In this study, 14 per cent of the local recurrences were diagnosed more than 4 years after the onset of treatment. At the Mayo Clinic, patients who had complete surgical excisions of their primary tumor had a 3.7 per cent recurrence rate compared with a 24 per cent recurrence rate in patients who had no surgery or incomplete excisions (Wilkins *et al.* 1986). In a series from Massachusetts General Hospital, there were eight (24 per cent) local failures in 34 cases treated with radiotherapy alone versus two (17 per cent) local recurrences in 12 patients who had primary tumor excisions along with radiotherapy (Sailer *et al.* 1988). Local recurrence is a more serious problem in Ewing's sarcoma of the pelvis where the tumors tend to be larger and wide excision can be more technically difficult (Fig. 2).

In the pelvis, most retrospective studies have shown local recurrence rates to be significantly higher in patients treated with radiation therapy alone, compared with combination therapy of surgery and radiation (Fig. 2). In both the Intergroup Ewing's Sarcoma Study I and II trials, a surgical resection resulted in an improved prognosis and decreased recurrence rate for patients with pelvic primary tumors (Evans *et al.* 1991). In this study, all patients received full-dose radiotherapy regardless of the surgical margins achieved.

In the Mayo Clinic study of Ewing's sarcoma of the pelvis, the actuarial local recurrence rate was 13 per cent in patients treated with resection versus 44 per cent in patients with nonmetastatic Ewing's sarcoma treated with radiation therapy alone. This study demonstrated a significant survival advantage to the surgical group (Frassica *et al.* 1993).

Some retrospective studies have not shown an increased survival rate and a decreased recurrence rate for patients with nonmetastatic Ewing's sarcoma of the pelvis treated with surgery and radiation.

A study from the Massachusetts General Hospital showed no statistically significant difference in the local recurrence rate and the survival of patients treated with local resection compared with patients treated without surgery (Scully *et al.* 1995).

The interpretation of these findings must be made with caution because the studies are all retrospective and the number of index patients are frequently limited. Despite these data, there appears to be a trend for prolonged survival and a decreased recurrence rate for patients treated with resection of their primary tumors. These studies also point out that the pelvis is a high-risk area for local recurrence and patients who develop a local recurrence have a very poor prognosis. In the pelvis, radiation therapy and surgery are frequently combined; however, there is still debate as to whether radiation should be given preoperatively or postoperatively.

Radiotherapy

Despite surgical resection playing a more dominant role in recent years, radiation therapy is still an important modality in treating Ewing's sarcoma locally. This is especially true for anatomic sites where surgical excision is difficult, such as the pelvis and the spine.

In these areas, radiation therapy and surgery are frequently combined and in this way the total dose of radiation given can be limited to decrease the number of complications. The risk of complications associated with radiation are becoming more apparent as patients survive longer with the use of multiagent chemotherapy.

The risks from radiation include secondary malignancy, increased risk of pathologic fracture, as well as retarded growth potential in skeletally immature patients. The risk of secondary malignancy appears especially high in patients who have received doses of radiation greater than or equal to 60 Gy, with one study reporting a 40-fold increase risk at that dose (Tucker *et al.* 1987). Another study reported that four out of 24 patients with Ewing's sarcoma of the pelvis surviving 5 years developed secondary malignancies within the radiation field (Chan *et al.* 1979). This level of risk is similar to another study which reported a cumulative risk of secondary malignancy of 35 per cent after 10 years (Strong *et al.* 1979). This study also speculated that the risk of radiation-induced sarcomas may be increased in patients who received chemotherapy.

Pathologic fractures following radiation therapy for local control are common in high-stress areas such as the proximal femur (Damron *et al.* 1996). The risk of pathologic fracture increases, especially if the cortex of the subtrochanteric level of the femur is violated during biopsy (Fig. 5). A recent review of 17 patients from the Mayo Clinic with Ewing's sarcoma of the proximal femur who were treated with radiation reported a pathologic fracture rate of 65 per cent (Damron *et al.* 1996). This study concluded that a protocol using radiation therapy for local control of Ewing's sarcoma in the proximal femur should include protected weight bearing of the involved extremity during radiotherapy and chemotherapy followed by prophylactic intramedullary fixation (Fig. 5) to minimize the potential for pathologic fracture.

In addition to these complications, others such as growth disturbances and deformities develop when radiation is used in the skeletally immature patients. This is especially true when radiotherapy is used in the lower extremities of children (Lewis *et al.* 1977). One way to minimize these complications is to shield the growth plate during radiation and to limit the radiation dose to 45 Gy (Marcus *et al.* 1991).

Indications for surgery

It is not possible to identify the indications for surgical resection of a Ewing's sarcoma precisely, but some general recommendations and principles may be given (Pritchard 1980; O'Connor and Pritchard 1991; Toni *et al.* 1993). The treatment plan, which is based on the location, stage, and size of the tumor, must be tailored for each patient. Local therapy should not take precedence over, nor interfere with, systemic chemotherapy. A patient should first receive neoadjuvant chemotherapy because it will reduce the soft-tissue component of the lesion dramatically in the majority of cases.

Following neoadjuvant chemotherapy, the patient is restaged (Fig. 2). Surgical resection should be considered in all cases in which the surgeon feels that the primary tumor can be removed completely (Figs 2, 3, and 4). If adequate margins cannot be achieved at the time of resection, then radiation therapy is used locally. The combination of surgery and radiation therapy allows a dose less than or equal to 45 Gy in most patients, which will minimize the complications of radiation. Complicated surgical reconstructions that necessitate a prolonged chemotherapy-free interlude should be avoided, since higher intensity of chemotherapy has been shown in several studies to improve survival (Fig. 2). Radiation inhibits the healing of allografts; therefore metallic intercalary and endoprosthetic replacements are generally favored when radiation is part of the treatment plan (Figs 3 and 4). Because surgical procedures for Ewing's sarcoma of the spine are frequently performed in a staged fashion and are complex, the patients should complete their full course of chemotherapy and radiation therapy before resection. In this way, the extended recuperation period and possible complications of the vertebral resection and reconstruction do not interfere with intensive multiagent chemotherapy.

Results of treatment
Chemotherapy and survival

The development of multiagent chemotherapy protocols has increased the 5-year survival rate of Ewing's sarcoma patients from

5 to 10 per cent 20 years ago to the current 5-year survival in excess of 70 per cent for patients with nonmetastatic Ewing's sarcoma. The chemotherapeutic agents most widely used for Ewing's sarcoma are vincristine, cyclophosphamide, doxorubicin, actinomycin D, ifosfamide, and etoposide.

The use of chemotherapy started in 1969 when adjuvant cyclophosphamide was used with radiation therapy to treat the primary tumor and a prolonged disease-free survival was demonstrated (Johnson and Humphreys 1969). This trial led these and other investigators to combine various chemotherapeutic agents used to treat other malignancies (Hustu *et al.* 1972; Fernandez *et al.* 1974; Pomeroy and Johnson 1975). In 1973, a trial of a four-drug sequential combination of doxorubicin, vincristine, cyclophosphamide, and actinomycin D showed superior results in 14 of 19 patients with nonmetastatic Ewing's sarcoma who remained continuously disease free at 5 to 10 years (Rosen *et al.* 1974). Sequential multidrug chemotherapy was changed to concurrent combination chemotherapy in 1975, to obtain even more activity against the primary tumor and potential metastatic disease (Pritchard *et al.* 1975; Rosen *et al.* 1981).

Co-operative multi-institutional trials began in the United States in 1973 with the first Intergroup Ewing's Sarcoma Study. The results of Intergroup Ewing's Sarcoma Study I, reported in 1981, showed that the addition of doxorubicin to the three-drug combination of vincristine, cyclophosphamide, and actinomycin D increased survival (Nesbit *et al.* 1990). Intergroup Ewing's Sarcoma Study II ran from 1978 to 1982 and tested high-dose intermittent versus moderate-dose continuous chemotherapy consisting of vincristine, actinomycin D, cyclophosphamide, and doxorubicin (Burgert *et al.* 1990). Intergroup Ewing's Sarcoma Study II demonstrated a significant disease-free survival advantage for high-dose chemotherapy compared with the less intense dosage. In this trial, the relapse-free survival was 73 per cent at a median follow-up of 5.6 years for nonmetastatic nonpelvic Ewing's sarcoma. The results of the Intergroup Ewing's Sarcoma Study III, which is evaluating the use of ifosfamide and even more intensive chemotherapeutic dosing, should be available in the near future.

Ifosfamide has emerged as a very effective chemotherapeutic agent, especially in patients who are resistant to other drugs (Miser *et al.* 1987; Meyer *et al.* 1992). The Co-operative Ewing's Sarcoma Study recently reported an increase in 3-year disease-free survival in patients in whom ifosfamide was substituted for cyclophosphamide (Jurgens *et al.* 1989). In addition to finding newer and more active chemotherapeutic agents, the intensity of dosages has been increased with the recent introduction of granulocyte colony-stimulating factor (Miser *et al.* 1988). This recombinant human cytokine glycoprotein allows more frequent and higher-dose chemotherapy delivery by stimulating bone marrow recovery.

Future directions and treatment

As long-term survival has increased, the importance of local control has become better appreciated. The role of surgery for local control has gained importance. Multi-institutional studies of perspective design are still needed to define better the indications for surgery at various anatomic sites. It will be important to find new chemotherapeutic agents to increase further the survival of Ewing's sarcoma patients, especially those in poor prognostic groups such as those presenting with metastases. In the long run, the molecular biology of the oncogenesis of Ewing's sarcoma will be defined and will allow physicians to treat this disease at the molecular level.

References

Bacci, G., Toni, A., Avella, M., *et al.* (1989). Long-term results in 144 localized Ewing's sarcoma patients treated with combined therapy. *Cancer*, **63**, 1477–86.

Boyer, C., Brickner, T., Perry, R., *et al.* (1967). Ewing's sarcoma. Case against surgery. *Cancer*, **20**, 1602–6.

Burgert, E.O., Jr, Nesbit, E.M., Garnsey, L.A., *et al.* (1990). Multimodal therapy for the management of nonpelvic localized Ewing's sarcoma of bone. Intergroup study IESS-II. *Journal of Clinical Oncology*, **8**, 1514–24.

Chan, R.C., Sutow, W.W., Lindberg, R.D., *et al.* (1979). Management and results of localized Ewing's sarcoma. *Cancer*, **43**, 1001–6.

Dahlin, D.C. and Unni, K.K. (1986). *Bone tumors. General aspects and data on 8542 cases*, No. 4, pp. 269–305. C.C. Thomas, Springfield, IL.

Damron, T.A., Sim, F.H., O'Connor, M.I., *et al.* (1996). Ewing's sarcoma of the proximal femur. *Clinical Orthopaedics and Related Research*, **322**, 232–44.

Devaney, K., Abbondanzo, S.L., Shekitka, K.M., *et al.* (1995). MIC2 detection in tumors of bone and adjacent soft tissues. *Clinical Orthopaedics and Related Research*, **310**, 176–87.

Evans, R., Nesbit, M., Askin, F., *et al.* (1985). Local recurrence, rate and sites of metastases and time to relapse as a function of treatment regimen, size of primary and surgical history in 62 patients presenting with non-metastatic Ewing's sarcoma of the pelvic bones. *International Journal of Radiation Oncology, Biology, Physics*, **11**, 129–36.

Evans, R.G., Nesbit, M.E., Gehan, E.A., *et al.* (1991). Multimodal therapy for the management of localized Ewing's sarcoma of pelvic and sacral bones. A report from the second intergroup study. *Journal of Clinical Oncology*, **9**, 1173–80.

Ewing, J. (1921). Diffuse endothelioma of bone. *Proceedings of the New York Pathology Society*, **21**, 17–24.

Fernandez, C.H., Lindberg, R.D., Sutow, W.W., *et al.* (1974). Localized Ewing's sarcoma—treatment and results. *Cancer*, **34**, 143–8.

Frassica, F.J., Frassica, D.A., Pritchard, D.J., *et al.* (1993). Ewing's sarcoma of the pelvis. *Journal of Bone and Joint Surgery, American Volume*, **75A**, 1457–65.

Grubb, M.R., Currier, B.L., Pritchard, D.J., *et al.* (1994). Primary Ewing's sarcoma of the spine. *Spine*, **19**, 309–13.

Hustu, O.H., Pinkel, D., Pratt, C.B., *et al.* (1972). Treatment of clinically localized Ewing's sarcoma with radiotherapy and combination chemotherapy. *Cancer*, **30**, 1522–7.

Johnson, R. and Humphreys, S.R. (1969). Past failure and future possibilities in Ewing's sarcoma. Experimental and preliminary clinical results. *Cancer*, **23**, 161–6.

Jurgens, H., Exner, U., Gadner, H., *et al.* (1988). Multidisciplinary treatment of primary Ewing's sarcoma of bone. A 6-year experience of a European cooperative trial. *Cancer*, **61**, 23–32.

Jurgens, H., Gadner, H., Gobel, U., *et al.* (1989). Update of the Cooperative Ewing's Sarcoma Studies (CESS) of the German Society of Pediatric Oncology (GPO). *Medicine in Pediatric Oncology*, **17**, 284.

Larsson, S., Boquist, L., and Bergdahl, L. (1973). Ewing's sarcoma—a consecutive series of 64 cases diagnosed in Sweden. *Clinical Orthopaedics and Related Research*, **95**, 263–72.

Lewis, R.J., Marcove, R.C., and Rosen, G. (1977). Ewing's sarcoma—functional effects of radiation therapy. *Journal of Bone and Joint Surgery, American Volume*, **59A**, 325–31.

Li, W.K., Lane, J.M., Rosen, G., *et al.* (1983). Pelvic Ewing's sarcoma. Advances in treatment. *Journal of Bone and Joint Surgery, American Volume*, **65A**, 738–47.

Marcove, R.C. and Rosen, G. (1980). Radical *en bloc* excision of Ewing's sarcoma. *Clinical Orthopaedics and Related Research*, **153**, 86–91.

Marcus, R.B., Cantor, A., Heare, T.C., *et al.* (1991). Local control and function after twice-a-day radiotherapy for Ewing's sarcoma of bone. *International Journal of Radiation Oncology, Biology, Physics*, **21**, 1509–15.

Meyer, J.H., Kun, L., Marina, N., *et al.* (1992). Ifosfamide plus etoposide in newly diagnosed Ewing's sarcoma of bone. *Journal of Clinical Oncology*, **10**, 1737–42.

Miser, J.S., Kinsella, T.J., Triche, T.J., *et al.* (1987). Ifosfamide with mesna uroprotection and etoposide. An effective regimen in the treatment of recurrent sarcomas and other tumors of children and young adults. *Journal of Clinical Oncology*, **5**, 1191–8.

Miser, J.S., Kinsella, T.J., Triche, T.J., *et al.* (1988). Preliminary results of treatment of Ewing's sarcoma of bone in children and young adults. Six months of intensive combined modality therapy without maintenance. *Journal of Clinical Oncology*, **6**, 484–90.

Nesbit, M.E., Gehan, E.A., Burgert, E.O., *et al.* (1990). Multimodal therapy for the management of primary, nonmetastatic Ewing's sarcoma of bone. A long-term follow-up of the first Intergroup study. *Journal of Clinical Oncology*, **8**, 1664–74.

Oberlin, O., Patte, C., Demeocq, F., *et al.* (1985). The response to initial chemotherapy as a prognostic factor in localized Ewing's sarcoma. *European Journal of Cancer and Clinical Oncology*, **21**, 463–7.

O'Connor, M.I. and Pritchard, D.J. (1991). Ewing's sarcoma. Prognostic factors, disease control and the re-emerging role of surgical treatment. *Clinical Orthopaedics and Related Research*, **262**, 78–87.

Picci, P., Rougraff, B.T., Bacci, G., *et al.* (1993). Prognostic significance of histopathologic response to chemotherapy in nonmetastatic Ewing's sarcoma of the extremities. *Journal of Clinical Oncology*, **11**, 1763–9.

Pomeroy, T.C. and Johnson, R.E. (1975). Combined modality therapy of Ewing's sarcoma. *Cancer*, **35**, 36–47.

Pritchard, D.J. (1980). Indications for surgical treatment of localized Ewing's sarcoma of bone. *Clinical Orthopaedics and Related Research*, **153**, 39–43.

Pritchard, D.J., Dahlin, D.C., Dauphine, R.T., *et al.* (1975). Ewing's sarcoma. A clinicopathological and statistical analysis of patients surviving 5 years or longer. *Journal of Bone and Joint Surgery, American Volume*, **57A**, 10–16.

Rosen, G., Wollner, N., Tan, C., *et al.* (1974). Disease-free survival in children with Ewing's sarcoma treated with radiation therapy and adjuvant four-drug sequential chemotherapy. *Cancer*, **33**, 384–93.

Rosen, G., Caparros, B., Nirenberg, A., *et al.* (1981). Ewing's sarcoma. Ten year experience with adjuvant chemotherapy. *Cancer*, **47**, 2204–13.

Sailer, S.L., Harmon, D.C., Mankin, H.J., *et al.* (1988). Ewing's sarcoma. Surgical resection as a prognostic factor. *International Journal of Radiation Oncology, Biology, Physics*, **15**, 43–52.

Scully, S.P., Temple, H.T., Keefe, R.J., *et al.* (1995). The role of surgical resection in pelvic Ewing's sarcoma. *Journal of Clinical Oncology*, **13**, 2336–41.

Siebenrock, K.A., Nascimento, A.G., Rock, M.G. (1996). Comparison of soft tissue Ewing's sarcoma peripheral neuroectodermal tumor. *Clinical Orthopaedics and Related Research*, **329**, 288–99.

Strong, L.C., Herson, J., Osborne, B., *et al.* (1979). Risk of radiation-related subsequent malignant tumors in survivors of Ewing's sarcoma. *Journal of the National Cancer Institute*, **62**, 1401–6.

Telles, N.C., Rabson, A.S., and Pomeroy, T.C. (1978). Ewing's sarcoma. An autopsy study. *Cancer*, **41**, 2321–9.

Toni, A., Neff, J.R., Sudanese, A., *et al.* (1993). The role of surgical therapy in patients with nonmetastatic Ewing's sarcoma of the limbs. *Clinical Orthopaedics and Related Research*, **286**, 225–40.

Tucker, M.A., D'Angio, G.J., Boice, J.D., *et al.* (1987). Bone sarcomas linked to radiotherapy and chemotherapy in children. *New England Journal of Medicine*, **317**, 588–93.

Vlasak, R. (1996). Ewing's sarcoma. *Orthopedic Clinics of North America*, **27**, 591–603.

Wilkins, R.M., Pritchard, D.J., Burgert, E.O., *et al.* (1986). Ewing's sarcoma of bone. Experience with 140 patients. *Cancer*, **58**, 2551–5.

Womer, R.B. (1991). The cellular biology of bone tumors. *Clinical Orthopaedics and Related Research*, **262**, 12–21.

Wunder, J.S., Paulian, G., Healey, J.H., *et al.* (1995). Chemotherapy-induced tumor necrosis as a prognostic indicator in surgically treated Ewing's sarcoma. Presented at the Joint Meeting EMSOS-AMSTS, Florence, May 1995.

1.6.8.5 Malignant vascular tumors of bone

Michael Rock

Introduction

Malignant vasoformative tumors of bone are rare, but have been given many names including angiosarcoma, hemangiosarcoma, hemangioendothelioma, hemangioendotheliosarcoma, and epithelial hemangioendothelioma. This makes the area confusing, especially since their malignant potential varies from a highly aggressive generally lethal condition to one that has a benign course with little potential to metastasize. A substantial proportion of patients have multifocal lesions in the same extremity or on the same side of the body, and a variant of Maffucci's syndrome consisting of multiple enchondromas associated with spindle cell hemangioendotheliomas has been described (Fanburg *et al.* 1995).

Owing to the infrequency of these tumors, most are misinterpreted prior to surgical biopsy and/or intervention as other primary mesenchymal sarcomas or metastatic disease. This is implied by the lytic nature of the tumor, the common diaphyseal involvement, and multifocality.

Three variants of malignant vascular tumors are discussed: hemangioendothelioma (angiosarcoma), hemangiopericytoma, and epithelioid hemangioendothelioma of bone.

Hemangioendothelioma
Clinical presentation

This is a tumor of late middle age. Multiple lesions in the same extremity or synchronous involvement at remote sites are commonly seen. Most occur in the lower half of the body. If the multifocal nature of the tumor is remote from the principle site and not synchronous, this is presumed to be metastatic disease and not simply 'multifocal primary disease'.

Patients with this condition present with pain, and occasionally

Box 1

- Very rare—less than 0.2 per cent of all bone tumors
- Very variable malignancy
- Over one-third have multifocal lesions

with pathologic fracture. If the tumor is located in the region where the osseous structures are subcutaneous, there may be increased warmth, subcutaneous venous dilatation, and pain on palpation (Unni *et al.* 1971; Campanacci *et al.* 1980).

Radiographic features

Most hemangioendotheliomas (angiosarcomas) produce a purely lytic defect regardless of the grade of the tumor (Fig. 1). The lower-grade lesion may exhibit margination with the host, and little if any cortical destruction. High-grade angiosarcomas are more likely to exhibit a moth-eaten appearance and are poorly marginated. Cortical destruction occurs early, and there may be significant soft-tissue extension. With low and high-grade lesions, little if any periosteal reaction is evident. Multifocal involvement of the same limb supports the diagnosis, but metastatic disease has to be ruled out. The tumor has a predilection toward the metadiaphysis of long bones, distinguishing it from other primary mesenchymal sarcomas that have a tendency to involve the meta-epiphysis.

Histopathologic features

The histologic diagnosis of hemangioendothelioma or angiosarcoma is based on the presence of atypical endothelial cells, the numbers of which are significantly increased over those seen lining normal vessels. Vascular channels are numerous and communicate extensively lending a ventricular framework to the appearance microscopically (Campanacci 1990; Unni and Dahlin 1995). The stroma separating these channels is loose and plentiful in low-grade lesions, and concentrated and minimal in the high-grade lesions. The designation of grade to these vascular tumors has great prognostic significance and is based on cytologic atypia, the size and number of vascular channels, the presence of pleomorphic nuclei, and variations in size and shape as well as the number of mitotic figures. At one end of the spectrum mild atypia, with nuclear pleomorphism, and rare mitosis would suggest a low-grade process. The lower-grade lesions also show osteoblastic differentiation in the periphery seen as a small sclerotic rim on radiograph. Multinucleated giant cells may appear in either high or low-grade lesions. The giant cell associated with a typical grade 3 lesion tends to show areas of epithelial character.

Several markers, including factor 8, CD31, and CD34, are positive in malignant vascular tumors and negative in metastatic carcinoma and can be used to differentiate this tumor from metastatic hypernephroma (Table 1).

Treatment

The treatment of this condition has to be tailored to the grade of the lesion and the multifocal nature of the process (Table 2). Extensive imaging studies, including bone scintigraphy, plain radiographs, and

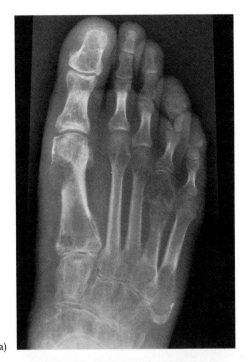

(a)

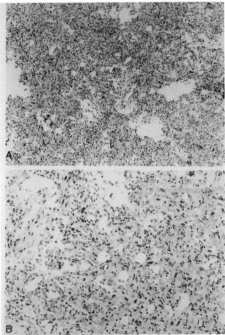

(b)

Fig. 1. An example of multifocal grade 1 hemangioendothelioma. (a) Anteroposterior radiograph of a foot showing the multiple lytic destructive lesions, some with soft-tissue extension. (b) Low- and high-power photomicrographs of a grade 1 hemangioendothelioma with hypercellularity, atypia, anastomosing vascular channels, and prominent endothelial cells. (Reproduced from Unni and Dahlin (1995).)

possibly MRI, are needed to determine how many sites are involved. Although this tumor is generally radiosensitive, the use of radiation by itself is reserved for surgically inaccessible sites as it can have late consequences including conversion to yet another malignant process.

Box 3 **Histology of hemangioendothelioma**

- Atypical endothelial cells
- Vascular in the connecting channels

Table 1 Differential diagnosis of hemangioendothelioma

	Hemangioepithelioma	Hypernephroma
Factor 8	+	−
CD31	+	−
CD34	+	−

Table 2 Treatment plans for vascular tumors

	Amputation	Limb-salvage chemotherapy	Radiotherapy
Low grade	±	+	
High grade			+
High grade disseminated	+		+

Wherever possible surgical management of this condition should be performed. Wide local excision with various reconstructive options has afforded limb sparing in most patients with grade 1 and grade 2 hemangioendotheliomas (angiosarcomas). High grade 3 hemangioendotheliomas have extensive soft-tissue extension and contamination and require radical excision or ablative surgery. Limb salvage can still be afforded in patients with multifocal disease, particularly the low grade 1 hemangioendotheliomas. In this circumstance, wide local excision plus reconstruction should be used when possible. Intralesional curettage and polymethylmethacrylate adjuvant treatment can be used in areas where a wide local excision would significantly compromise functional capabilities and/or be impossible to perform. Multifocal high-grade hemangioendotheliomas are best treated with proximal amputation assuming a margin can be obtained above the most proximal extent of the tumor. Preoperative chemotherapy may assist in decreasing tumor bulk. Postoperative radiation therapy reduces local recurrence. For high-grade lesions that are too extensive to be candidates for surgical ablation, therapeutic radiation at a dose of 50–60 Gy (5000–6000 rad) should be given along with adjuvant chemotherapy. However, there have been reports of failure of palliative high-dose radiation therapy in high-grade angiosarcomas. It is not safe to assume that all vascular tumors are radiosensitive. Patients have to be monitored carefully during and after application of radiation. Survival is very dependent on grade, varying from around 90 per cent in grade 1 to 10 per cent in grade 3 in the long term.

Hemangiopericytoma
Clinical presentation

Although commonly seen in soft tissue, hemangiopericytoma of bone is rare. This is a tumor of late middle age, and the axial skeleton including pelvis accounts for the majority of lesions. Unlike hemangioendotheliomas multifocal involvement has not been reported. The presentation of this tumor is not unlike that of other primary malignant conditions of bone with pain, swelling, and infrequently pathologic fractures. The radiographic appearance is nonspecific, predominantly osteolytic, and expansile with early cortical destruction and soft-tissue extension (Fig. 2). Periosteal reaction is generally not seen. Bony trabeculae or septae within the tumor sometimes gives this process a honeycombed appearance, particularly the lower-grade hemangiopericytomas (Backwinkel and Diddams 1970; Enzinger and Smith 1976; Wold *et al.* 1982).

Nuclear atypia and cellular pleomorphism is not marked. The malignant cells aggregate around blood vessels and in doing so distort the actual vessels to make them appear irregular and jagged, producing a stag horn appearance. The cells are round to oval and with appropriate staining techniques can be identified outside of the basal membrane of the vessels as opposed hemangioendotheliomas that occur within this structure. This condition should not be confused with other primary mesenchymal tumors that may have hemangiopericytomatous areas that are focal and discrete, and distinct from other more classic areas of fibrosarcoma, malignant fibrous histiocytoma, osteosarcoma, or mesenchymal chondrosarcoma.

The cellularity of these tumors varies considerably but the majority are considered malignant. When hemangiopericytoma of bone is diagnosed, meningeal involvement as a possible primary site always has to be ruled out. Attempts at grading this tumor have had mixed results and success. Overall the 5-year survival rate reported by Tsang and Chan (1993) after an extensive literature review was 75 per cent and the 10-year rate was 44 per cent. However, high-grade malignant hemangiopericytomas have a poor prognosis with very few surviving this condition and most experiencing metastasis. There is a definite similarity between this condition involving bone and hemangiopericytoma of soft tissues with similar survival rates.

Owing to the infrequency of the tumor and variability of clinical course and spectrum of malignancy, any definitive suggestions as to treatment becomes suspect. When feasible, wide local excision of the lesion should be performed. This becomes difficult in the axial skeleton to which this tumor has a predilection. The combination of attempt at surgical removal and radiation therapy has been recom-

Box 4 **Differential appearance of hemangiopericytoma**

- Fibrosarcoma
- Malignant fibrous histiocytoma
- Osteosarcoma
- Mesenchymal chondrosarcoma

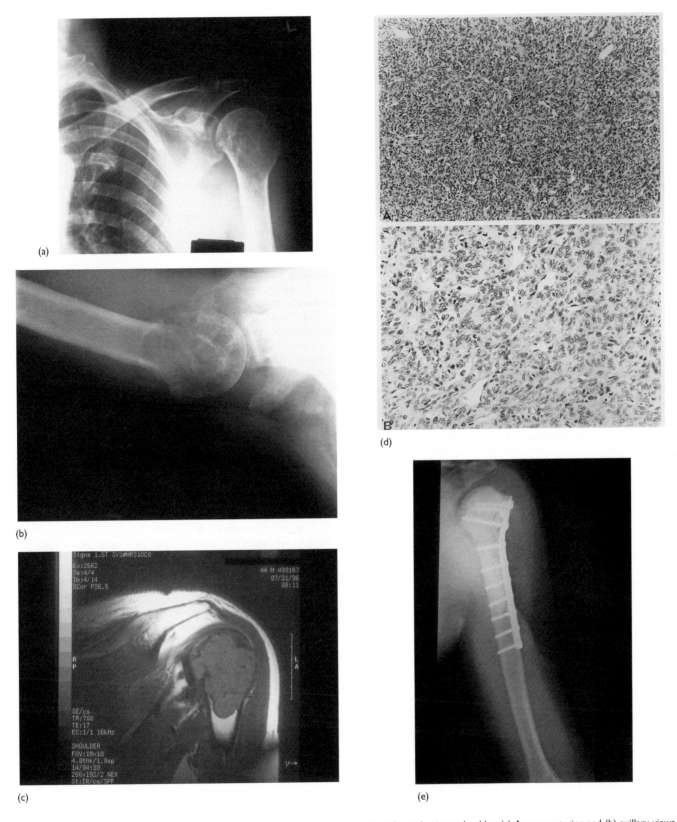

Fig. 2. A 46-year-old male presents with a 6-month history of progressive pain in his left nondominant shoulder. (a) Anteroposterior and (b) axillary views reveal a large purely lytic defect involving the proximal humeral metaphysis. (c) T_1-weighted image refines the intraosseous extent of the tumor. (d) Open biopsy confirms the presence of malignant hemangiopericytes encircling distorted blood vessels. (Reproduced from Unni and Dahlin (1995).) (e) Confirmation of low-grade hemangiopericytoma allowed for conservative curettage, cementation, and fixation with anticipated postoperative radiation.

mended but given the small numbers of patients, efficacy of such treatment cannot be assessed. It is currently not known whether chemotherapy has any benefit.

Epithelioid hemangioendothelioma of bone

This tumor is most common in the second decade, and most are multifocal occurring in the axial skeleton, pelvis, and lower limbs, as well as lung and liver. It is generally perceived to be a low-grade malignant process with a clinical course between true benign hemangioma and the conventional high-grade angiosarcomas.

Not unlike other vascular tumors, endothelial hemangioendotheliomas tend to be lytic, to involve metadiaphysis, and may or may not be well marginated from the surrounding normal bone architecture. Typically, periosteal reaction is lacking but cortical destruction and expansion are common. Soft-tissue extension is much less frequent. Multiple lesions in the same bone or certainly in the same extremity would suggest a vascular tumor, but the distinction between this and a low-grade hemangioendothelioma is impossible based on radiographs alone (Weiss and Enzinger 1982; O'Connell et al. 1993).

Microscopy

From a microscopic perspective, the consistent unique feature of this tumor is the presence of epithelioid endothelial cells. These tend to be round, sometimes cuboidal, and have abundant eosinophilic cytoplasm. Primitive attempts at forming a lumen by single cells give a signet ring appearance. Additionally vacuoles within the cytoplasm give the appearance of nuclear pseudoinclusions. Given the slow-growing nature of the tumor and the low-grade malignant potential, bone formation at its periphery as well as trabeculae of bone coursing through the substance of the tumor are commonly seen. Benign giant cells may be present.

The tumor is positive for such markers as vimentin, factor 8 related protein, CD31, and CD34.

Treatment

Before treatment starts, CT scans, bone scans, and skeletal surveys are needed to determine whether the condition is multifocal, in the skeleton, or in the viscera. Wide local excision should be performed if the tumor is accessible. In inaccessible sites such as the axial skeleton, radiation therapy and/or chemotherapy may have to be used. The efficacy of either, solely or in combination, is not known because of the small number of patients to whom such treatments have been administered.

Prognosis

There is a poor correlation between histologic appearance and the ultimate prognosis in this condition. Patients with visceral involvement tend to succumb to their disease. However, such involvement is equally distributed among histologic grade 1, 2, and 3 lesions, and therefore the histologic appearance of the tumor *per se* does not appear to have prognostic significance (Kleer *et al.* unpublished data, 1996).

References

Backwinkel, K.D. and Diddams, J.A. (1970). Hemangiopericytoma: report of a case and comprehensive review of the literature. *Cancer*, **25**, 896–901.

Campanacci, M. (1990). *Bone and soft tissue tumors*, pp. 597–615. Springer-Verlag, Vienna.

Campanacci, M., Boriani, S., and Giunti, A. (1980). Hemangioendothelioma of bone. A study of 29 cases. *Cancer*, **46**, 804–14.

Enzinger, F.M. and Smith, R.H. (1976). Hemangiopericytoma: an analysis of 106 cases. *Human Pathology*, **7**, 61–82.

Fanburg, J.C., Meis-Kindblom, J.M., and Rosenberg, A.E. (1995). Multiple enchondromas associated with spindle-cell hemangioendotheliomas: an overlooked variant of Maffucci's syndrome. *American Journal of Surgical Pathology*, **19**, 1029–38.

Kleer *et al.* (1996). *American Journal of Surgical Pathology*, **20**, 1301–11.

O'Connell, J.X., Kattapuram, S.V., Mankin, H.J., Bhan, A.K., and Rosenberg, A.E. (1993). Epithelioid hemangioma of bone: a tumor often mistaken for low-grade angiosarcoma or malignant hemangioendothelioma. *American Journal of Surgical Pathology*, **17**, 610–17.

Tsang, W.Y. and Chan, J.K. (1993). The family of epithelioid vascular tumors. *Histology and Histopathology*, **8**, 187–212.

Unni, K.K. and Dahlin, D.C. (1995). *Dahlin's bone tumors: general aspects and data on 11 087 cases* (5th edn), pp. 317–31. Lippincott–Raven, Philadelphia, PA.

Unni, K.K., Ivins, J.C., Beabout, J.W., and Dahlin, D.C. (1971). Hemangioma, hemangiopericytoma and hemangioendothelioma (angiosarcoma) of bone. *Cancer*, **27**, 1403–14.

Weiss, S.W. and Enzinger, F.M. (1982). Epithelioid hemangioendothelioma: a vascular tumor often mistaken for a carcinoma. *Cancer*, **50**, 970–81.

Wold, L.E., Sim, F.H., Unni, K.K., Dahlin, D.C., and Cooper, K.L. (1982). Hemangiopericytoma of bone. *American Journal of Surgical Pathology*, **6**, 53–8.

1.6.8.6 Myeloma of bone

*Frank J. Frassica, Deborah A. Frassica,
Steven A. Lietman, and Franklin H. Sim*

Definition

Myeloma of bone is a common cause of bone destruction in the middle-aged and geriatric patient. The disease is progressive and often causes severe destruction of the skeletal system. Myeloma is a disease that falls within the spectrum of plasma cell disorders (Table 1). Kyle (1991) has characterized the disorder as a neoplastic proliferation of a single line of plasma cells producing a specific protein as if the plasma cells were under constant antigenic stimulation. The protein which is produced is monoclonal and is also called an

Box 1

- The most common primary tumor of bone

- Caused by neoplastic proliferation of a single line of malignant plasma cells that produce a monoclonal protein

- Commonly presents with bone pain in patients over 40 years of age; many patients also have generalized weakness and tire easily

- Radiographs may show diffuse osteopenia or sharply circumscribed lytic lesions

- A rare form of myeloma causes motor disability

- Current therapy is not curative, but chemotherapy may prolong life, radiation therapy can decrease localized bone pain and slow local disease progression, and surgery can prevent or treat pathologic fractures

- Bone marrow transplantation is being investigated as a possible curative treatment

Table 1 Classification of plasma cell proliferative disorders

Monoclonal gammopathies of undetermined significance
Malignant monoclonal gammopathies
Multiple myeloma (IgG, IgA, IgD, IgE, and free light chains)
Overt multiple myeloma
Smoldering multiple myeloma
Plasma cell leukemia
Nonsecretory myeloma
IgD myeloma
Osteosclerotic myeloma (POEMS)
Plasmacytoma
Solitary plasmacytoma of bone
Extramedullary plasmacytoma
Malignant lymphoproliferative diseases
Waldenström's macroglobulinemia
Malignant lymphoma
Cryoglobulinemia
Pyroglobulinemia
Primary amyloidosis

Reproduced from Kyle (1991).

M protein or monoclonal protein. The individual protein is composed of one heavy-chain class (immunoglobulin G, A, M, D, or E) and one light-chain class (κ or λ).

There are three forms of myeloma that have clinical importance to orthopedic surgeons: multiple myeloma, solitary myeloma, and osteosclerotic myeloma (Frassica *et al.* 1994). A knowledge of the clinicopathologic features of each will allow the clinician to make an early diagnosis and plan effective treatment.

Multiple myeloma

Incidence and epidemiology

Although myeloma is the most common primary malignant tumor of bone, it accounts for only 1 per cent of the malignancies each year in the United States (approximately 15 000 new cases per year) (Boring *et al.* 1993). Myeloma is twice as common among black Americans as white Americans. The etiology of malignant plasma cell neoplasms is not known. Causes which have been implicated include genetic, occupational, and environmental factors (McPhedran *et al.* 1972; Linos *et al.* 1981).

Clinical features

Destructive lesions are common in patients in the age group 40 to 90 years. When a patient in this age group presents with a destructive malignant appearing lesion that is either solitary or multifocal, the most likely diagnosis will be either metastatic bone disease, myeloma, or lymphoma. The clinician should consider myeloma in the differential diagnosis of a patient with a destructive lesion or in the patient who has musculoskeletal pain without a diagnosis.

Patients with myeloma generally present with bone pain. The presentation may be insidious and nonspecific. Back and rib pain are common presentations and myeloma should always be considered in the older patient with back pain. Patients with myeloma will often have pain that is precipitated by movement, in contrast to pain from metastatic lesions which is usually more prominent at rest and at night. Patients often remember a single inciting episode of the pain (usually caused by a rib or vertebral fracture).

Bone pain is the initial clinical finding in about two-thirds of patients with myeloma. Weakness and fatigue are also common findings (secondary to the anemia) (Kyle 1975). Other less common findings include bacterial infections (12 per cent), gross bleeding (7 per cent), herpes zoster (2 per cent), and fever (1 per cent).

The myeloma protein may cause systemic complications such as renal insufficiency, hypercalcemia, and the deposition of amyloid. Amyloid deposition can cause congestive heart failure, nephrotic syndrome, orthostatic hypotension, peripheral neuropathy, and increased bleeding.

Myeloma may involve any bone in the skeleton (Fig. 1). The age distribution favors the fifth to eighth decades of life. Patients as young as those in the third and fourth decades may also develop myeloma. There are usually few, if any physical findings to support the diagnosis. Pallor secondary to anemia may be found by the careful examiner. Initial screening studies in patients with a solitary or multiple destructive bone lesions should include a complete blood cell count, erythrocyte sedimentation rate, chemistry group, and electrolyte panel. Patients with myeloma will often have anemia (62 per

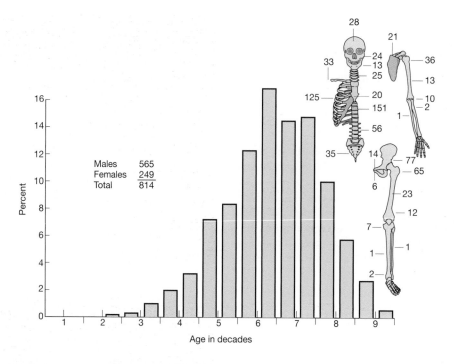

Fig. 1. Distribution of 814 lesions treated surgically in patients with myeloma. (Reproduced from Unni (1996).)

cent) and an elevated sedimentation rate (76 per cent) (Kyle 1975). Hypercalcemia and compromised renal function may also occur and should be checked prior to any surgical intervention.

Bone marrow aspirate and biopsy is the most definitive method to establish the diagnosis. Marrow plasmacytosis greater than 30 per cent is highly suggestive of multiple myeloma.

Pathology

On low-power inspection closely packed cells with little intercellular material are seen (Dahlin and Unni 1986). The cell lines are usually distinct and the nucleus is round or oval and eccentric.

Under high power the plasma cells may be well differentiated or very anaplastic. When the plasma cells are well differentiated they resemble the plasma cells seen in benign inflammatory conditions: round, eccentric nucleus with peripherally clumped chromatin (clock face or wheel spoke nucleus) (Fig. 2). A clear halo representing the Golgi apparatus is usually apparent in the cytoplasm. The undifferentiated lesions have nuclei that display large nucleoli, less prominent clumping of the chromatin, increased cytoplasmic vacuoles, and indistinct cell boundaries. In undifferentiated tumors the cell features may be difficult to differentiate from lymphomas of bone (Dahlin and Unni 1986).

Imaging studies

The classic appearance of multiple myeloma is purely lytic punched-out lesions. These lesions may vary from small to large (Fig. 3). Usu-

ally there is no reactive sclerosis. The involved cortices may be thinned and even ballooned out (Dahlin and Unni 1986). The skeleton usually appears osteopenic, and in some patients this may be the only radiographic finding.

The vertebral body findings are often very nonspecific and difficult to distinguish from osteoporosis, metastatic bone disease, lymphoma, and hyperparathyroidism. There may be loss of vertebral height and biconcave deformity with a relative increase in thickness and convexity of the disc spaces (Campanacci 1990). Multiple compression fractures may be found.

Interestingly, the bone destruction is caused by the osteoclast rather than the myeloma cells themselves. The plasma cells secrete an osteoclast-activating factor which stimulates the osteoclast to resorb the host bone. There is virtually no osteoblastic activity to match the osteoclastic resorption. This uncoupling results in the phenomenon of a negative or cold bone scan. For this reason, a skeletal survey is the best screening method when searching for myeloma lesions. A skeletal survey includes anteroposterior and lateral views of the cervical, thoracic, and lumbosacral spine, a lateral view of the skull, and anteroposterior views of the pelvis, femurs, humeri, tibiae, and radii/ulnae.

Management

The diagnosis of multiple myeloma is usually apparent. When confusion exists with regard to diagnosis the criteria outlined by Salmon and Cassady (1993) may be used (Table 2). The major criteria for diagnosis include plasmacytoma on tissue biopsy, bone marrow

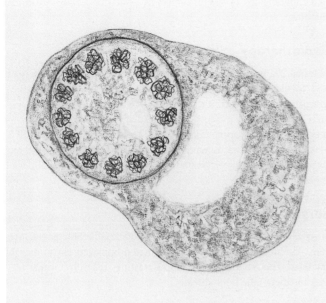

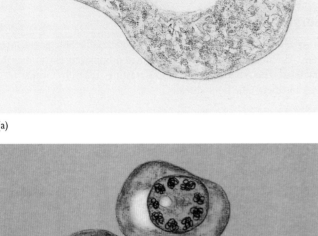

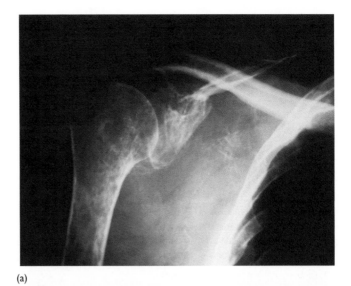

(a)

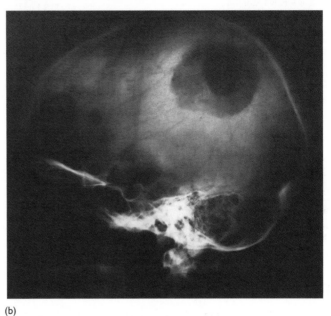

(b)

Fig. 3. (a) Anteroposterior view of the shoulder demonstrating lytic punched-out lesions in the proximal humerus with thinning of the cortices. The body of the scapula has been completely destroyed. (b) Lateral view of the skull demonstrating multiple punched-out lesions that vary in size from small (5 mm) to large (several centimeters).

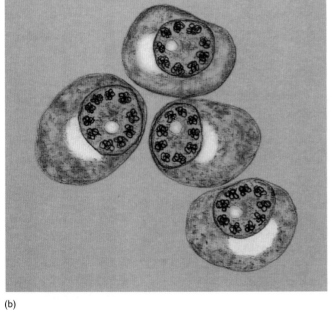

(b)

Fig. 2. Diagram of myeloma cells. (a) Plasma cells from a well-differentiated case of myeloma. The plasma cells resemble those seen in benign inflammatory cases. (b) Single plasma cell demonstrating the eccentric nucleus and peripheral chromatin pattern. The perinuclear halo represents the Golgi apparatus. (Reproduced from DeVita *et al.* (1993).)

plasmacytosis with over 30 per cent plasma cells, and a monoclonal spike on serum protein electrophoresis.

Drurie and Salmon (1975) have also developed a staging system (Table 3) that helps predict prognosis. Patients with stage I disease have a median survival greater than 60 months while patients with stage III disease have a less favorable median survival of only 23

months. Unfortunately myeloma is a slowly progressive disease with almost a 100 per cent eventual mortality.

Chemotherapy

Systemic chemotherapy is the major treatment modality for patients with multiple myeloma. Prednisone and alkylating agents such as cyclophosphamide and melphalan are the most active agents (Salmon and Cassady 1993). Vincristine, doxorubicin, and dexamethasone have been used in resistant cases. Bone marrow transplantation is

Table 2 Diagnostic criteria for multiple myeloma

Major criteria
    I Plasmacytoma on tissue biopsy
    II Bone marrow plasmacytosis with > 30% plasma cells

Minor criteria
    (a) Bone marrow plasmacytosis 10%–30% plasma cells
    (b) Monoclonal globulin spike present but less than the level defined
        above
    (c) Lytic bone lesions
    (d) Residual normal IgM < 50 mg/dl, IgA < 100 mg/dl, or
        IgG < 600 mg/dl

Diagnosis will be confirmed when any of the following features are
documented in symptomatic patients with clearly progressive disease. The
diagnosis of myeloma requires a minimum of one major and one minor
criteria or three minor criteria, which must include a + b, i.e.

    1 I + b, I + c, I + d (I + a not sufficient)
    2 II + b, II + c, II + d
    3 III + a, III + c, III + d
    4 a + b + c, a + b + d

Adapted from Salmon and Cassady (1993).

being investigated in several centers as a putative curative treatment
method.

Radiotherapy

External beam irradiation is often used for palliation on bone pain
and to halt progression of skeletal lesion that threaten structural
integrity (Mill and Griffith 1980; Bosch and Frias 1988). Approximately two-thirds of patients require radiation during the course of
their disease. The plasma cells are quite sensitive and doses of 2000 to
3000 cGy are utilized. When radiation is delivered following internal
fixation or prosthetic arthroplasty the entire bone and metal device
is generally treated.

Surgery

Surgical treatment is utilized to prevent and treat pathologic fractures
(Fig. 4). Internal fixation devices are used prophylactically to prevent
fractures. The criteria for impending fractures is similar to that utilized for metastatic bone disease:

(1) destructive lesions that exceed 50 per cent cortical bone destruc-
     tion;

(2) lesions in high stress areas;

(3) lesions which are painful despite radiotherapy.

Table 3 Myeloma staging system

Criteria	Measured myeloma cell mass (cells $\times 10^{12}$/m)
Stage I	
All of the following	
Hemoglobin value > 10 g/dl	
Serum calcium value normal (< 12 g/dl)	
On radiograph, normal bone structure or solitary plasmacytoma only	
Low M complement production rates	< 0.6 (low)
IgG value < 5 g/dl	
IgA value < 3 g/dl	
Urine light-chain M component on electrophoresis < 4 g/24 h	
Stage II	
Overall data not as minimally abnormal as shown for stage I and no single value as abnormal as defined for stage II	0.6–1.20 (intermediate)
Stage III	
One or more of the following	
Hemoglobin value < 8.5 g/dl	
Serum calcium value > 12 mg/dl	
Advanced lytic bone lesions	
High M component production rates	> 1.20 (high)
IgG value > 7 g/dl	
IgA value > 5 g/dl	
Urine light-chain M component on electrophoresis > 12 g/24 h	
Subclassification	
A = relatively normal renal function	
(serum creatinine value < 2.0 mg/dl)	
B = abnormal renal function	
(serum creatinine value 2.0 mg/dl)	

Adapted from DeVita et al. (1993).

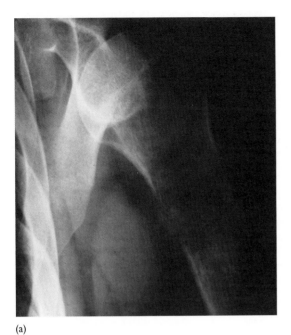

(a)

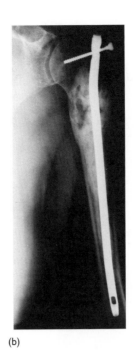

(b)

Fig. 4. (a) Anteroposterior radiograph of the shoulder demonstrating a pathologic fracture of the proximal humerus. (b) Anteroposterior radiograph of the humerus following open reduction and internal fixation with an intramedullary rod supplemented with methylmethacrylate.

Prosthetic arthroplasty is utilized in several scenarios: (a) articular surface destruction, (b) extensive lesions in which rigid internal fixation is not achievable, and (c) progressive bone destruction following adequate radiotherapy.

Solitary myeloma

Solitary myeloma is a distinct form of myeloma with a better overall prognosis (Todd 1965; Meyer and Schulz 1974; Corwin and Lindberg 1979; Woodruff *et al.* 1979; Mendenhall *et al.* 1980; Tong *et al.* 1980; Bataille and Sany 1981; Kvalow *et al.* 1983; Ray *et al.* 1983; Chak *et al.* 1987; Frassica *et al.* 1994). The authors' criteria include the following (Frassica *et al.* 1989):

(1) solitary lesion on skeletal survey;

(2) histologic confirmation of plasmacytoma;

(3) bone marrow plasmacytosis of 10 per cent or less.

Patients with serum protein abnormalities and Bence-Jones proteinuria of less than 1 g/24 h at presentation are not excluded if they meet the above criteria.

The 5- and 10-year survival rates of 74 per cent and 45 per cent respectively are much more favorable than those of multiple myeloma. However, two-thirds of patients with solitary myeloma will eventually develop multiple myeloma.

It is important to treat patients with impending and pathologic fractures aggressively as the prognosis is favorable.

Osteosclerotic myeloma

Osteosclerotic myeloma is a rare variant which is characterized by a chronic inflammatory demyelinating polyneuropathy causing prim-arily motor disability (Kelly *et al.* 1983). Patients first note sensory symptoms consisting of tingling, pins and needles, and coldness. Motor symptoms follow the sensory symptoms and both are distal, symmetric, and progressive with gradual proximal migration. Eventually severe weakness ensues and patients are unable to climb stairs, rise from a chair, or grip objects firmly.

The radiographs show a range from sclerotic to a mixed sclerotic–lytic lesions. The lesions usually involve the spine, pelvic bones, and ribs, sparing the extremities (Fig. 5). Classically numerous small sclerotic lesions are found in the pelvis and spine.

The complete syndrome is characterized by polyneuropathy, organomegaly, endocrinopathy, myeloma protein, and skin changes (the POEMS syndrome) (Bardwick *et al.* 1980).

Few clinicians are familiar with the association of the sclerotic lesions and the neurologic findings. A long delay to diagnosis is common.

Summary

Myeloma is a common disorder of the skeletal system and should be considered in the differential diagnosis of destructive lesions in the older patient. The classic radiographic appearance is that of discrete punched-out lytic lesions. Although the disease is incurable systemic chemotherapy is utilized to prolong the life of the patient and to minimize the destruction of the skeletal lesion. External beam irradiation is used to control pain and halt progression of lesions which threaten structural integrity. Surgical treatment is aimed at stabilizing lesions with internal fixation and prosthetic devices. It is important to distinguish solitary from multiple myeloma because of the more favorable prognosis. Osteosclerotic myeloma is a rare variant of myeloma in which patients have a polyneuropathy and multiple sclerotic bone lesions.

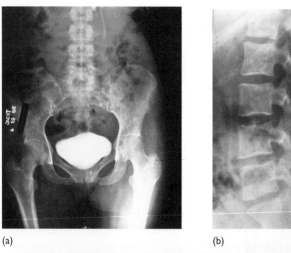

(a)   (b)

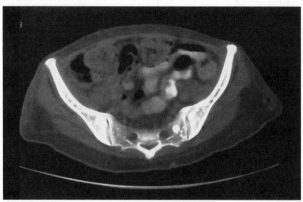

(c)

Fig. 5. (a) Anteroposterior view of the pelvis demonstrating multiple small sclerotic lesions in the pelvic and right proximal femur. (b) Lateral radiograph of the spine demonstrating multiple small sclerotic lesions. (c) CT scan of the iliac wings and sacrum demonstrating the small sclerotic lesions.

References

Bardwick, P.A., Zvaifler, N.J., Gill, G.N., *et al.* (1980). Plasma cell dyscrasia with polyneuropathy, organomegaly, endocrinopathy, M protein, and skin changes: the POEMS syndrome. Report on two cases and a review of the literature. *Medicine (Baltimore)*, **59**, 311–22.

Bataille, R. and Sany, J. (1981). Solitary myeloma: clinical and prognostic features of a review of 114 cases. *Cancer*, **48**, 845–51.

Boring, C.C., Squires, T.S., and Tong, T. (1993). Cancer statistics, 1993. *CA: A Cancer Journal for Clinicians*, **43**, 7–26.

Bosch, A. and Frias, Z. (1988). Radiotherapy in the treatment of multiple myeloma. *International Journal of Radiation, Oncology, Biology, Physics*, **15**, 1363–9.

Campanacci, M. (1990). *Bone and soft tissue tumors*. Springer-Verlag, New York.

Chak, I.Y., Cox, R.S., Bostwick, D.G., *et al.* (1987). Solitary plasmacytoma of bone: treatment, progression and survival. *Journal of Clinical Oncology*, **5**, 1811–15.

Corwin, J. and Lindberg, R.D. (1979). Solitary plasmacytoma of bone vs.

extramedullary plasmacytoma and their relationship to multiple myeloma. *Cancer*, **43**, 1007–13.

Dahlin, D.C. and Unni, K.K. (1986). *Bone tumors: general aspects and data on 8542 cases.* C.C. Thomas, Springfield, IL.

DeVita, V.T., Hellman, S., and Rosenberg, S.A. (ed.) (1993). *Cancer: principles and practice of oncology* (4th edn), p. 2025. J.B. Lippincott, Philadelphia, PA.

Drurie, B.G.M. and Salmon, S.E. (1975). A clinical staging system for multiple myeloma: correlation of measured myeloma cell mass with presenting clinical features, response to treatment and survival. *Cancer*, **36**, 842–52.

Frassica, D.A., Frassica, F.J., Schray, M.F., *et al.* (1989). Solitary plasmacytoma of bone: Mayo Clinic experience. *International Journal of Radiation, Oncology, Biology, Physics*, **16**, 43–8.

Frassica, F.J., Frassica, D.A., and Sim, F.H. (1994). Myeloma of bone. In *Advances in operative orthopaedics* (ed. R.N. Stauffer), pp. 357–77. C.V. Mosby, St Louis, MO.

Kelly, J.J., Kyle, R.A., Miles, J.M., *et al.* (1983). Osteosclerotic myeloma and peripheral neuropathy. *Neurology (New York)*, **33**, 202–10.

Kvalow, S., Abrahamsen, A.F., Landaas, T.O., *et al.* (1983). Solitary plasmacytoma of bone. *Scandinavian Journal of Haematology*, **30** (Supplement 39), 23–9.

Kyle, R.A. (1975). Multiple myeloma: review of 869 cases. *Mayo Clinic Proceedings*, **50**, 29–40.

Kyle, R.A. (1991). Plasma cell proliferative disorders. In *Hematology: basic principles and practice* (ed. R. Hoffman), pp. 1021–38. Churchill Livingstone, Edinburgh.

Linos, A., Kyle, R.A., O'Fallon, W.M., *et al.* (1981). Incidence and secular trend of multiple myeloma in Olmsted County, Minnesota: 1965–77. *National Cancer Institute*, **66**, 17–20.

McPhedran, P., Heath, C.W, and Garcia, J. (1972). Multiple myeloma incidence in metropolitan Atlanta, Georgia: racial and seasonal variations. *Blood*, **39**, 866–73.

Mendenhall, C.M., Thar, T.L., and Million, R.R. (1980). Solitary plasmacytoma of bone and soft tissue. *International Journal of Radiation, Oncology, Biology, Physics*, **6**, 1497–501.

Meyer, J.E. and Schulz, M.D. (1974). Solitary myeloma of bone. *Cancer*, **34**, 438–40.

Mill, W. and Griffith, R. (1980). The role of radiation therapy in the management of plasma cell tumors. *Cancer*, **45**, 647–52.

Ray, G., Fish, V., and Rabinowitz, L. (1983). Solitary plasma cell tumors of bone and soft tissue: natural history and response to radiotherapy. *Proceedings of the American Society of Clinical Oncology*, **2**, 243.

Salmon, S.A. and Cassady, J.R. (1993). Plasma cell neoplasms. In *Cancer: principles and practice of oncology* (ed. V.T. DeVita, S. Hellman, and S.A. Rosenberg) (4th edn), p. 1984. J.B. Lippincott, Philadelphia, PA.

Todd, I.D.H. (1965). Treatment of solitary plasmacytoma. *Clinical Radiology*, **16**, 395–9.

Tong, D., Griffin, T.W., Laramore, G.E., *et al.* (1980). Solitary plasmacytoma of bone and soft tissues. *Radiology*, **135**, 195–8.

Unni, K.K. (1996). *Dahlin's bone tumors: general aspects and data on 11,087 cases* (5th edn). Lippincott–Raven, Philadelphia, PA.

Woodruff, R.K., Malpas, J.S., and White, F.E. (1979). Solitary plasmacytoma II: solitary plasmacytoma of bone. *Cancer*, **43**, 2344–7.

1.6.8.7 Lymphoma of bone

J. Sybil Biermann

Non-Hodgkin's lymphoma

Incidence and prevalence

Worldwide incidence figures for lymphoma vary greatly from region to region, with rates as low as 2.4 per 100 000 in Poland and 0.4 per 100 000 in Mali, but as high as 30 per 100 000 in some parts of the United States (Kirsner and Federman 1996; Vineis 1996). For reasons that are unclear, the incidence of lymphoma appears to be increasing annually by a rate of 3 to 4 per cent per year (Vineis 1996). There is an increased rate of lymphoma in HIV-infected individuals and in populations exposed to certain organic solvents and pesticides.

However, primary lymphoma of bone is relatively rare, accounting for 5 per cent of malignant bone tumors in one series (Huvos 1991). The skeletal system is secondarily involved in a much larger number of cases, about 30 per cent of all malignant lymphomas (Clayton *et al.* 1987). Autopsy studies have similarly shown a high rate of skeletal involvement (Rosenberg *et al.* 1961).

Descriptions of the clinical behavior of lymphoma have been complicated by the nomenclature of the disease, as well as by the multiple forms of lymphoma. Formerly known in the literature as reticulum cell sarcoma, reticulosarcoma, or lymphangiosarcoma, lymphomas are now generally categorized as Hodgkin's lymphoma or non-Hodgkin's lymphoma. However, within the group of non-Hodgkin's lymphomas, there are numerous subtypes according to histology, cell of lineage, and grade.

While patients may present with skeletal manifestations of lymphoma, careful staging usually demonstrates additional lesions. Only a small minority of patients who present with bone lymphoma will have no evidence of additional disease sites. (Reimer *et al.* 1977; Sweet *et al.* 1981; Dinshaw *et al.* 1984). In order to distinguish patients with primary bone disease from those with other lesions, investigators have described several criteria for describing a bone lesion as primary bone lymphoma. Coley *et al.* (1950) suggested that there should be a minimum interval of 6 months between the onset of symptoms from the primary disease and the development of eventual regional or distant disease, and histologic confirmation from the bone lesion. However, over the years, based on the clinical behavior of non-Hodgkin's lymphoma, many investigators have broadened the category of primary lymphoma of bone to include cases where there is regional lymph node involvement as well as bone disease.

Classification

Much of the current literature for non-Hodgkin's lymphoma is based on the Rappaport classification system (Rappaport *et al.* 1956) in which lymphoma was classified on its light microscopic appearance (Table 1). Major separation was made between the nodular and diffuse types based on tissue architecture. Further subdivisions were made between the predominant cell type and differentiation. The classification does not take into account the subsequently identified separation of lymphomas into B-cell and T-cell lineage, or the ability to distinguish between lymphomas based on immunohistochemical markers.

The Ann Arbor Staging System (Table 2), developed initially for Hodgkin's lymphoma, has been widely applied to the non-Hodgkin's lymphomas (Carbone *et al.* 1971). This staging system is independent of histology, and relies on anatomic information regarding the location of the tumor. Solitary bone lesions are stage IE (extranodal, single site) in this classification system. Subsequent advances in the identification of molecular markers and the understanding of the heterogeneity of lymphomas have resulted in a myriad of new classification systems. Comparison of the efficacy of treatment regimens has been difficult because of the multiplicity of these systems. However, with continued improvement of the clinical and molecular understanding of this complex disease, efforts at international collaboration with the goal of a standardized classification system for the lymphomas is underway (Hiddemann *et al.* 1996).

Lymphoma of bone has been shown to present with a wide variety of tissue types, although most common histologic presentation in one large series was the diffuse type (Ostrowski *et al.* 1986). Immunotyping, however, has shown primary lymphoma of bone to be a B-cell neoplasm, usually of the diffuse large cell type (Clayton *et al.* 1987; Pettit *et al.* 1990).

Box 1

- Malignant neoplasms of bone which, like lymphomas in other locations, can consist of a variety of cell types, but most primary lymphomas of bone are B-cell neoplasms, usually the diffuse large cell type

- Typically present with bone pain; patients may also have a soft-tissue mass and constitutional symptoms including weight loss, fever, and fatigue

- Radiogaphs usually show a poorly defined lytic lesion, but some lesions have areas of bone formation

- Patients with lymphoma of bone should have staging studies to determine the extent of the disease

- Current treatment includes chemotherapy and, in many patients, radiation therapy

- Surgical treatment may be necessary to prevent or treat fractures

Table 1 Rappaport classification of malignant lymphomas

Pattern
Nodular
Diffuse

Cytology
Lymphocytic, well differentiated
Lymphocytic, poorly differentiated
Mixed cell (lymphocytic and histiocytic)
Histiocytic
Hodgkin's type

Table 2 Clinical staging system for lymphoma

Stage	Characteristics
I	Involvement of a single lymph node region
IE	Involvement of a single extralymphatic organ or site
II	Involvement of two or more lymph node regions on the same side of the diaphragm
IIE	Localized involvement of an extralymphatic organ or site and of one or more lymph node regions on the same side of the diaphragm
III	Involvement of lymph node regions on both sides of the diaphragm
IIIE	Stage III accompanied by localized involvement of an extralymphatic organ or site
IIIS	Stage III accompanied by involvement of the spleen
IIISE	Stage III accompanied by localized involvement of an extralymphatic organ or site and the spleen
IV	Diffuse or disseminated involvement of one or more extralymphatic organs or tissues with or without associated lymph node involvement

Clinical evaluation

The clinical evaluation of any patient presenting with a painful lesion of bone should include an adequate history as well as physical examination. History should include any previous malignancies, family history of malignancies, and any previous illness. The duration of symptoms should be noted; for lymphomas, the duration may be quite variable, from a few weeks to a few years. About 50 per cent of patients will have had symptoms for longer than 1 year, and about 10 per cent will have had symptoms for more than 3 years (Huvos 1991). The duration of swelling, if any, should be noted. Lymphomas may present with constitutional symptoms (the so-called B symptoms), and the patient should be questioned about weight loss, fever, and fatigue.

Physical examination usually shows a palpable soft-tissue mass or swelling about the involved bone, which may be mildly tender to palpation. Joint pain with effusion may also be a presenting symptom. Pathologic fracture may be present, particularly in the weight-bearing bones of the lower extremity. Careful examination of the regional lymph nodes should be undertaken, and may reveal lymphadenopathy.

Radiographic appearance

Bone lymphoma lesions are usually centrally located with ill-defined margins. They are often lytic, or a mixed lytic and sclerotic lesion (Braunstein and White 1980). Commonly seen associated radiographic features include periosteal new bone, soft-tissue swelling, soft-tissue mass, and areas of increased radiodensity of the bone. Sequestra may be present, which may be especially evident on CT scanning through the lesion. (Mulligan and Kransdorf 1993). Pathologic fracture may occur in as many as 27 per cent of lesions, and may be associated with a poorer prognosis (Phillips *et al.* 1982).

The soft-tissue mass may be extensive, especially relative to the radiographic changes in the bone. Soluble cytokine mediators produced by the tumor cells have been identified, and these have been postulated to regulate the extensive osteoclastic activity seen with these lesions. Intramedullary tumor cells extending through channels penetrating the cortex have been suggested as a mechanism for production of the large extraosseous soft-tissue mass commonly seen in osseous lymphoma lesions (Hicks *et al.* 1995).

MRI of primary bone lymphoma lesions shows marrow replacement by tumor, as well as any soft-tissue mass which is likely to be present. In contradistinction to most small cell tumors, lymphomas show inhomogeneous lesions of relatively low or intermediate signal intensity on T_2-weighted images. This may reflect the high content of fibrous tissue which correlates with histologic appearance (Stiglbauer *et al.* 1992).

Examples of bone lymphomas are shown in Figs 1, 2, 3, and 4.

Differential diagnosis

These lesions may be confused with small round cell tumors because of the aggressive appearance of the bone lesions on plain radiographs, particularly in children. The differential diagnosis of a small round cell infiltrate of bone in a child should include Ewing's sarcoma, rhabdomyosarcoma, lymphoma, neuroblastoma, and primitive neuroectodermal tumor. The presence of leukocyte common antigen can distinguish lymphomas from other types of malignancy. The distinction often requires expert pathologic consultation and careful handling of biopsy specimens. The use of modern methods of immunopathology can usually adequately distinguish between these lesions (Furman *et al.* 1989). Fresh tissue may be helpful for flow cytometry studies.

Treatment

Patients found to have lymphoma of bone should undergo staging studies to determine the extent of disease. Evaluation of the patient with suspected or documented lymphoma of bone should include plain radiographs, chest radiography or CT, CT of the abdomen and pelvis, bone scan, and routine hematologic and blood chemistry profiles (Ostrowski *et al.* 1986). Lactate dehydrogenase in particular is an important serum marker, and has been correlated with prognosis. Bilateral bone marrow biopsies should be performed to assess extent of disease in the bone marrow.

Treatment of malignant lymphoma of bone usually involves radiation, chemotherapy, or most commonly a combination of both. Unlike sarcomas, in which *en bloc* resection plays an important role in the management of disease, local control of lymphoma of bone is achieved with radiotherapy or chemotherapy, or both (Furman *et al.* 1989). Treatment of bone lymphoma lesions with these modalities

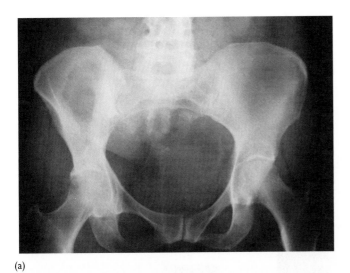

(a)

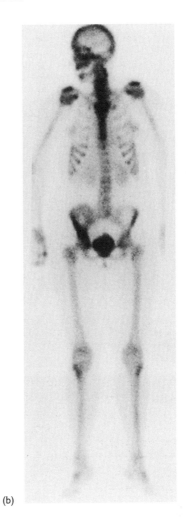

(b)

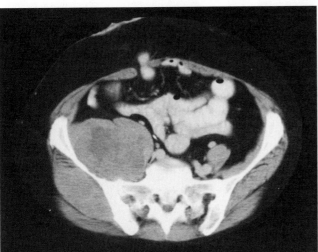

(c)

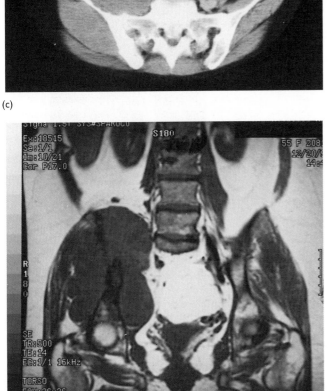

(d)

Fig. 1. (a) Plain radiograph of a 55-year-old woman who presented with a 6-month history of right pelvic pain radiating down the leg. Subtle lucency is seen in the right iliac wing with increased sclerosis of the bone in the supra-acetabular region. Radiographs of lymphoma of bone frequently show mixed lytic/sclerotic lesions. (b) Technetium bone scan shows increased uptake in the right ilium, but not elsewhere in the body. Bone scans should be performed as a staging study in patients suspected of having lymphoma of bone or metastatic carcinoma. (c) CT of the chest, abdomen, and pelvis was carried out. The chest and abdomen were free of lesions, but a large soft-tissue mass was present extending both into the pelvis and into the gluteal region. Changes in the bone are minimal relative to the extensive soft-tissue mass, a feature frequently seen in lymphoma. (d) Coronal T_1-weighted MRI of the pelvis demonstrates an extensive soft-tissue lesion arising from the ilium and extending into and out of the pelvis, and surrounding the superior portion of the acetabulum. Core needle biopsy was performed, and the diagnosis of lymphoma was confirmed. Because additional staging studies including bone marrow biopsy were negative, this is a solitary lesion or stage IE non-Hodgkin's lymphoma.

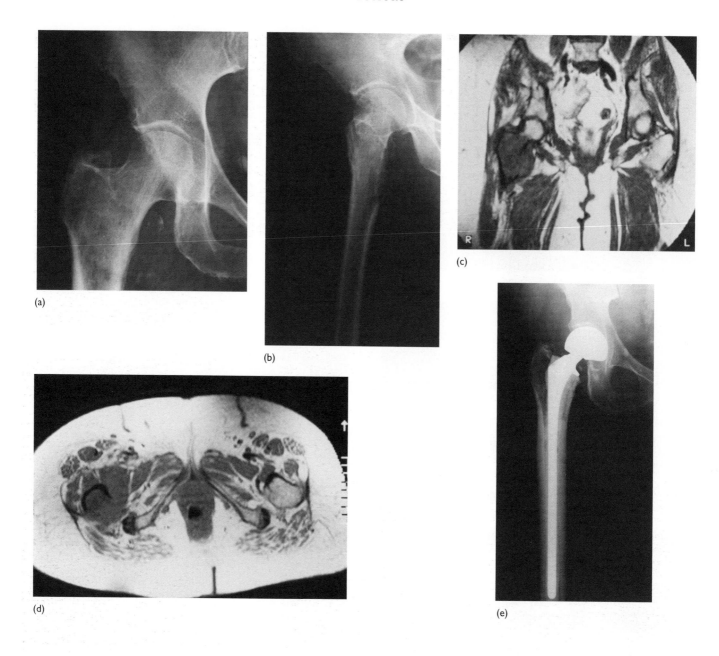

Fig. 2. (a) Anteroposterior and (b) lateral radiographs of an 83-year-old woman who presented with a 3-month history of right hip pain. Permeative destruction is seen throughout the proximal femur and femoral neck. A new lytic lesion of bone in a patient of this age is most likely to be metastatic disease. (c) Coronal and (d) axial T_1-weighted MRI shows marrow replacement of the proximal femur and an adjacent soft-tissue mass. Additional staging studies included chest, abdominal, and pelvic CT scanning which revealed retroperitoneal lymphadenopathy. (e) The patient was taken to the operating room where biopsy confirmed a diagnosis of large cell lymphoma, and hemiarthroplasty of the painful hip was carried out for palliation. The role of the orthopedic surgeon in the management of lymphoma is in obtaining tissue for diagnosis and in stabilizing pathologic fractures. Surgical intervention is for diagnosis or palliation, since the curative treatment of lymphoma is with chemotherapy and/or radiation.

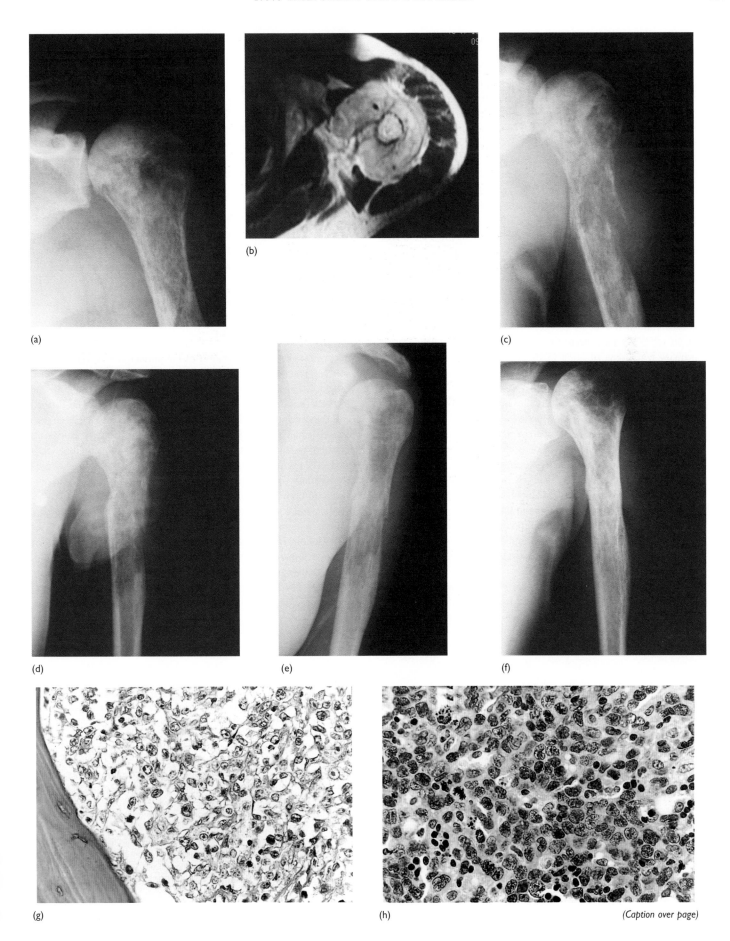

(a)

(b)

(c)

(d)

(e)

(f)

(g)

(h)

(Caption over page)

often results in radiographic improvement of the lesion with increased sclerosis (Braunstein and White 1980).

In some circumstances, stabilization of a pathologic fracture or prophylactic treatment of an impending fracture may be indicated. Surgical treatment in these cases is palliative rather than curative, and should be carefully co-ordinated with the efforts of the treating medical and radiation oncologists. Reconstitution of the involved bone often occurs with radiation or chemotherapy, bracing, immobilization, or non-weight-bearing of affected symptomatic bones may be considered as an alternative to prevent pathologic fracture.

The evaluation of the prognosis of lymphoma of bone and the relationship of stage and histologic pattern has been complicated by the rarity of the disease and the multiple treatment regimens on which reported patients have been treated. Prognosis of lymphoma of bone has been shown to be related to both stage and histologic pattern (Clayton *et al.* 1987), and to stage only (Ostrowski *et al.* 1986).

Treatment of primary of lymphoma of bone with radiation only has been reported, with a 5-year survival rate of 63 per cent and a local control rate of 84 per cent (Dosoretz *et al.*1983). Dosages of 50 to 55 Gy have been recommended for the management of primary lymphoma of bone in the absence of systemic treatment with chemotherapy (Mendenhall *et al.* 1987). Because many seemingly primary bone lymphomas may subsequently develop disease elsewhere, patients should be carefully monitored for sites of additional disease.

The use of multiagent chemotherapy in conjunction with radiation has been reported, with a 5-year survival of 83 per cent in one study (Loeffler *et al.*1986). Bacci *et al.* (1986) noted the improved prognosis and local control with combination chemotherapy and radiation therapy, and noted that these patients have a much better outcome when compared to Ewing's sarcoma of bone, another small blue cell tumor occurring in bone. Cyclophosphamide, hydroxydaunomycin, Oncovin, and prednisone (**CHOP**) and radiotherapy are the most common management methods for stage I–II histologically aggressive lesions (Tondini *et al.* 1993).

Standard chemotherapy for high-grade or advanced stage lymphoma usually consists of CHOP, which has been shown to have equivalent efficacy and less toxicity than third-generation regimens in a randomized prospective clinical trial in the United States (Fisher *et al.* 1993).

Future directions

Difficulties in the management of lymphoma revolve around the need to maintain systemic control of the disease. Although remission is relatively easy to obtain with initial therapy, durable remissions are more difficult, particularly with the low-grade lymphomas. Addition of new agents by themselves or with existing regimens will continue to be tested in patients at the time of presentation or relapse (Pohlman 1996).

Confirmation of remission remains a difficult problem, since bone deposits appear abnormal on radiographs as well as bone and gallium scans long after disease has been eradicated. Improved imaging studies may provide more reliable tools for determining the presence of viable tumor.

Hodgkin's disease

Although a skeletal presentation of lymphoma is relatively uncommon for the non-Hodgkin's lymphomas, it is even more rare for Hodgkin's disease to present with skeletal complaints (Gaudin *et al.* 1992). Because of the rarity of the lesion, diagnosis may be delayed until the development of adenopathy, even after biopsy has been performed (Chan *et al.* 1982). Only a few cases of primary Hodgkin's disease of bone in which no evidence of nodal disease could be identified have been reported (Fried *et al.* 1995). Hodgkin's disease commonly affects bone secondarily with disease progression, and frequency of bone involvement has been reported as 10 to 34 per cent (Perttala and Kijanen 1965). Osseous involvement may be identified by bone scanning, plain film radiography, bone marrow biopsy, or MRI (Gaudin *et al.* 1992).

The treatment and prognosis of Hodgkin's disease of bone is related to disease stage. Long-term survivors of Hodgkin's disease are at risk for development of secondary malignancies, including bone sarcoma and acute nonlymphocytic leukemias, at a rate of 18.7 per cent at 15 years in one study (Kushner *et al.* 1988). Patients with a

Fig. 3. (a) Plain radiograph of a 43-year-old man presenting with a 1-year history of increasing left shoulder pain with acute exacerbation of pain following minor trauma. Physical examination revealed a painful soft-tissue mass about the proximal arm. Plain radiographs show a permeative moth-eaten appearance of the proximal humerus. (b) T_2-weighted axial MRI of the proximal left arm shows an extensive soft-tissue mass of moderate signal intensity around the proximal humerus. (c) Plain radiographs taken 3 weeks later show significantly advanced disease, with pathologic fracture and periosteal reaction around the proximal humeral diaphysis. Staging studies showed that the patient had additional lesions including a bulky extradural mass which mandated immediate treatment with chemotherapy despite significant symptoms in the proximal humerus. After (d) 1 month and (e) 3 months of chemotherapy, the bone is beginning to reossify and the pathologic fracture is healing. Bone lymphomas frequently show a rapid response to appropriate chemotherapy with restitution of the bone even in the face of advanced lytic lesions. For this reason, systemic treatment of lymphomas should not be delayed for surgical management in areas which can be easily immobilized or temporarily relieved of weight bearing. Following chemotherapy, the humerus was treated with 40 Gy. (f) Two years after diagnosis, the patient is in remission from his lymphoma. He has regained full use of the extremity with minimal limitation of range of motion. Persistent changes in the bone radiographs remain. Treated bone lesions may be hot on bone scan for months or years. Distinguishing chronic changes in adequately treated bone from recurrence or inadequately treated disease remains one of the greatest challenges in the management of bone lymphoma. (g) Core needle biopsy specimen taken at the time of diagnosis shows a fragment of mature lamellar bone in the far left, associated with a population of large round cells with prominent nucleoli. (Hematoxylin and eosin stain.) (h) At higher power, a population of large anaplastic tumor cells with irregular cell contours, and readily identifiable mitotic figures, is seen. Interspersed are small mature lymphocytes (an appearance characteristic of malignant lymphoma). Immunostaining (not shown) showed a monoclonal proliferation of B-lymphocytes.

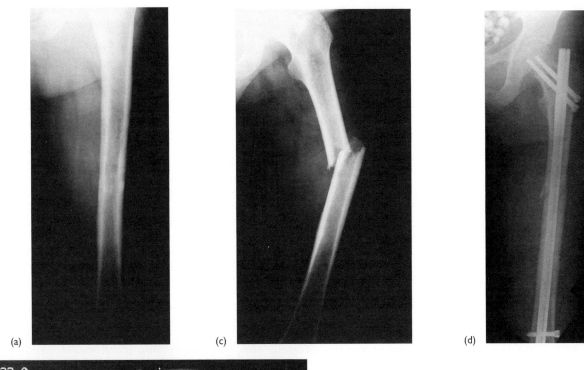

(a)   (c)   (d)

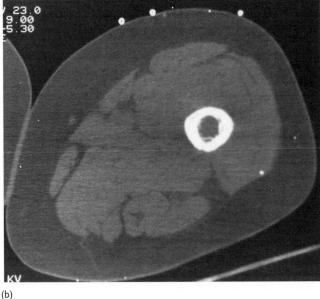

(b)

Fig. 4. (a) A 76-year-old woman presented to the orthopedic oncology clinic with complaints of left thigh pain for several months, increasing in intensity and exacerbated by weight bearing. Plain radiographs of the femur showed a mid-diaphyseal mixed lytic/sclerotic lesion. (b) CT of the mid-diaphysis revealed an intraosseous sequestrum located on the lateral portion of the endosteal cortex. Sequestra have been reported in association with lymphoma, and frequently are most evident on CT. The soft-tissue mass present underlying the vastas intermedius is difficult to appreciate. (c) Despite being placed on crutches with instructions for non-weight-bearing, she fractured her femur while undergoing her staging studies. CT of the chest, abdomen, and pelvis showed no other lesions, and there were no additional lesions identified on technetium bone scanning. (d) She was taken to the operating room where frozen-section biopsy confirmed the diagnosis of large cell lymphoma of bone. Intramedullary nailing of the femur provided immediate stability and pain relief, and she was able to begin chemotherapy within a few days. Intramedullary nailing of affected long bones with fractures or impending pathologic fractures, especially in the lower extremity, may be indicated in symptomatic lesions prior to chemotherapy, to provide pain relief and mobility.

history of Hodgkin's disease in remission who present with bone pain should be carefully evaluated with a high degree of suspicion for bone sarcoma. Pathologic fractures without secondary malignancy may occur in previously irradiated bone in areas of Hodgkin's disease.

Burkitt's lymphoma

Burkitt's lymphoma is the most common malignant disease of children in tropical Africa, and is rapidly fatal without treatment (Burkitt and O'Conor 1961). It is much less common in other parts of the

world. Unlike the endemic African type, the sporadic type occurring in other parts of the world has not been associated with the Epstein–Barr virus, high humoral antibodies, and a predilection for the jaws.

Bone lesions in the appendicular skeleton have been reported in about 4 per cent of patients with African-type Burkitt's lymphoma (Fowles *et al.* 1983). Lesions occur most commonly in the femoral and tibial diaphyses and the metaphyses around the knee. Bone lesions have radiographic appearances of aggressive lesions, with cortical destruction, periosteal reaction, and lytic areas of bone. However, the bone lesions of Burkitt's lymphoma are clinically relatively painless compared to primary bone malignancies, an important differential diagnostic feature. Lesions treated successfully with chemotherapy resulted in healed pathologic fractures and undamaged growth plates. Bone lesions have also been reported in American patients (Dunnick *et al.* 1979).

Further reading

Clayton, F., Butler, J.J., Ayala, A.G., Ro, J.Y., and Zornoza, J. (1987). Non-Hodgkin's lymphoma in bone. Pathologic and radiologic features with clinical correlates. *Cancer*, **60**, 2494–501.

Thirty-seven cases of lymphoma of bone are reviewed. Seventy-three per cent of patients with localized lymphoma were long-term survivors, in contrast to 9 per cent of those with disseminated disease. The radiographic appearance of the tumors is well described, although the findings are not specific for lymphoma.

Fisher, R.I., Gaynor, E.R., Dahlberg, S., *et al.* (1993). Comparison of a standard regimen (CHOP) with three intensive chemotherapy regimens for advanced non-Hodgkin's lymphoma. *New England Journal of Medicine*, **328**, 1002–6.

Because of the disease relapse after apparently complete remission following CHOP chemotherapy, several intensive multi-agent regimens were evaluated for the treatment of lymphoma. Although these regimens were associated with greater toxicity, they did not show improved efficacy.

Fowles, J.V., Olweny, C.L.M., Katongole-Mbidde, E., Lukanga-Ndawula, A., and Owor, R. (1983). Burkitt's lymphoma in the appendicular skeleton. *Journal of Bone and Joint Surgery, British Volume*, **65B**, 464–71.

Only 11 of 290 patients with proven Burkitt's lymphoma had lesions in the long bones or the pelvis. Although these lesions appear extremely aggressive radiologically, they are relatively painless, in contrast to other aggressive appearing lesions such as Ewing's sarcoma, osteosarcoma, or osteomyelitis.

Ostrowski, M.L., Unni, K.K., Banks, P.M., *et al.* (1986). Malignant lymphoma of bone. *Cancer*, **58**, 2646–55.

Four hundred and twenty-two patients with malignant lymphoma of bone seen over a 75-year period are reviewed. The disease stage was the most important prognostic indicator. Ten-year survival rates for primary bone lymphoma were 53 per cent, however there were significant changes in treatment over this time period.

Rosenberg, S.A., Diamond, H.D., Jaslowitz, B., and Craver, L.F. (1961). Lymphosarcoma: a review of 1269 cases. *Medicine*, **2**, 31–84.

This classic comprehensive review of 1269 cases of lymphoma was compiled from Sloan-Kettering data. Of patients with reticulum cell sarcoma 32.7 per cent had bone lesions during life or postmortem. Commonly affected sites were vertebrae, femur, ribs, and pelvis.

Vineis, P. and the Working Group on the Epidemiology of Hematolymphopoetic Malignancies in Italy (1996). Incidence and time trends for lymphomas, leukemias and myelomas: hypothesis generation. *Leukemia Research*, **20**, 285–90.

A comprehensive review of the fascinating trends in the epidemiology of the hematologic malignancies, including the variable incidence in lymphoma from country to country, and the increase in the rate of the disease everywhere. Epidemiological studies into associated factors including environmental exposures are reviewed.

References

Bacci, G., Jaffe, N., Emiliani, E., *et al.* (1986). Therapy for primary non-Hodgkin's lymphoma of bone and a comparison of results with Ewing's sarcoma. *Cancer*, **57**, 1468–72.

Braunstein, E.M. and White, S.J. (1980). Non-Hodgkin lymphoma of bone. *Radiology*, **135**, 59–63.

Burkitt, D. and O'Conor, G.T. (1961). Malignant lymphoma in African children. I: A clinical syndrome. *Cancer*, **14**, 258–69.

Carbone, P.P., Kaplan, H.S., Musshoff, K., Smithers, D.W., and Tubiana, M. (1971). Report of the Committee on Hodgkin's Disease Staging Classification. *Cancer Research*, **31**, 1860–1.

Chan, K.W., Miller, D.R., Rosen, G., and Tan, C.T.C. (1982). Hodgkin's disease in adolescents presenting as a primary bone lesion. A report of four cases and review of the literature. *American Journal of Pediatric Hematology Oncology*, **4**, 11–17.

Clayton, F., Butler, J.J., Ayala, A.G., Ro, J.Y., and Zornoza, J. (1987). Non-Hodgkin's lymphoma in bone. Pathologic and radiologic features with clinical correlates. *Cancer*, **60**, 2494–501.

Coley, B.L., Higinbotham, N.L., and Groesbeck, H.P. (1950). Primary reticulum-cell sarcoma of bone. Summary of 37 cases. *Radiology*, **55**, 641–58.

Dinshaw, K.A., Advani, S.H., Nair, C.N., Gopal, R., Talvalkar, G.V., and Desai, P.B. (1984). Primary non-Hodgkin's lymphoma of bone. *Indian Journal of Cancer*, **20**, 275–82.

Dosoretz, D.E., Murphy, G.F., Raymond, K., *et al.* (1983). Radiation therapy for primary lymphoma of bone. *Cancer*, **51**, 44–6.

Dunnick, N.R., Reaman, G.H., Head, G.L., Shawker, T.H., and Ziegler, J.L. (1979). Radiographic manifestations of Burkitt's lymphoma in American patients. *American Journal of Roentgenology*, **132**, 1–6.

Fisher, R.I., Gaynor, E.R., Dahlberg, S., *et al.* (1993). Comparison of a standard regimen (CHOP) with three intensive chemotherapy regimens for advanced non-Hodgkin's lymphoma. *New England Journal of Medicine*, **328**, 1002–6.

Fried, G., Arieh, Y.B., Haim, N., Dale, J., and Stein, M. (1995). Primary Hodgkin's disease of the bone. *Medical and Pediatric Oncology*, **24**, 204–7.

Fowles, J.V., Olweny, C.L.M., Katongole-Mbidde, E., Lukanga-Ndawula, A., and Owor, R. (1983). Burkitt's lymphoma in the appendicular skeleton. *Journal of Bone and Joint Surgery, British Volume*, **65B**, 464–71.

Furman, W.L., Fitch, S., Hustu, H.O., Callihan, T., and Murphy, S.B. (1989). Primary lymphoma of bone in children. *Journal of Clinical Oncology*, **7**, 1275–80.

Gaudin, P., Juvin, R., Rozand, Y., *et al.* (1992). Skeletal involvement as the initial disease manifestation in Hodgkin's disease: a review of 6 cases. *Journal of Rheumatology*, **19**, 146–52.

Hicks, D.G., Gokan, T., O'Keefe, R.J., *et al.* (1995). Primary lymphoma of bone. Correlation of magnetic resonance imaging features with cytokine production by tumor cells. *Cancer*, **75**, 973–80.

Hiddemann, W., Longo, D.L., Coiffier, B., *et al.* (1996). Lymphoma classification—the gap between biology and clinical management is closing. *Blood*, **88**, 4085–9.

Horan, F.T. (1969). Bone involvement in Hodgkin's disease. A survey of 201 cases. *British Journal of Surgery*, **56**, 277–81.

Huvos, A.G. (1991). Skeletal manifestations of malignant lymphomas and leukemias. In *Bone tumors: diagnosis, treatment, and prognosis* (2nd edn). W.B. Saunders, Philadelphia, PA.

Kirsner, R.S. and Federman, D.G. (1996). The epidemiology of non-Hodgkin's lymphoma. *Connecticut Medicine*, **60**, 579–82.

Kushner, B.H., Zauber, A., and Tan, C.T.C. (1988). Second malignancies after childhood Hodgkin's disease. *Cancer*, **62**, 1364–70.

Loeffler, J.S., Tarbell, N.J., Kozakewich, H., Cassady, J.R., and Weinstein, H.J. (1986) Primary lymphoma of bone in children: analysis of treatment results with Adriamycin, prednisone, Oncovin (APO), and local radiation therapy. *Journal of Clinical Oncology*, **4**, 496–501.

Mendenhall, N.P., Jones, J.J., Kramer, B.S., *et al.* (1987). The management of primary lymphoma of bone. *Radiotherapy and Oncology*, **9**, 137–45.

Mulligan, M.E. and Kransdorf, M.J. (1993). Sequestra in primary lymphoma of bone: prevalence and radiologic features. *American Journal of Roentgenology*, **160**, 1245–8.

Ostrowski, M.L., Unni, K.K., Banks, P.M., *et al.* (1986). Malignant lymphoma of bone. *Cancer*, **58**, 2646–55.

Perttala, Y. and Kijanen, I. (1965). Roentgenologic bone lesions in lymphogranulomatosis maligna. Analysis of 453 cases. *Annales Chirurgiae et Gynaecologiae Fenniae*, **54**, 414–24.

Pettit, C.K., Zukerberg, L.R., Gray, M.H., *et al.* (1990). Primary lymphoma of bone. A B-cell neoplasm with a high frequency of multilobulated cells. *American Journal of Surgical Pathology*, **14**, 329–34.

Phillips, W.C., Kattapuram, S.V., Doseretz, D.E., *et al.* (1982). Primary lymphoma of bone: relationship of radiographic appearance and prognosis. *Radiology*, **144**, 285–90.

Pohlman, B. (1996). Ifosphamide in the treatment of non-Hodgkin's lymphoma. *Seminars in Oncology*, **23**, 27–32.

Rappaport, H., Winter, W.J., and Hicks, E.B. (1956). Follicular lymphoma: a reevaluation of its position in the scheme of malignant lymphoma, based on a survey of 253 cases. *Cancer*, **9**, 792–821.

Reimer, R.R., Chabner, B.A., Young, R.C., Reddick, R., and Johnson, R.E. (1977). Lymphoma presenting in bone. Results of histopathology, staging, and therapy. *Annals of Internal Medicine*, **87**, 50–5.

Rosenberg, S.A., Diamond, H.D., Jaslowitz, B., and Craver, L.F. (1961). Lymphosarcoma: a review of 1269 cases. *Medicine*, **2**, 31–84.

Stiglbauer, R., Augustin, I., Kramer, J., Schurawitzki, H., Imhof, H., and Radaszkiewicz, T. (1992). MRI in the diagnosis of primary lymphoma of bone: correlation with histopathology. *Journal of Computer Assisted Tomography*, **16**, 248–53.

Sweet, D.L., Mass, D.P., Simon, M.A., and Shapiro, C.M. (1981). Histiocytic lymphoma (reticulum-cell sarcoma) of bone. *Journal of Bone and Joint Surgery, American Volume*, **63A**, 79–84.

Tondini, C., Zanini, M., Lombardi, F., *et al.* (1993). Combined modality treatment with primary CHOP chemotherapy followed by locoregional irradiation in stage I or II histologically aggressive non-Hodgkin's lymphomas. *Journal of Clinical Oncology*, **11**, 720–5.

Vineis, P. and the Working Group on the Epidemiology of Hematolymphopoetic Malignancies in Italy (1996). Incidence and time trends for lymphomas, leukemias and myelomas: hypothesis generation. *Leukemia Research*, **20**, 285–90.

1.6.8.8 Fibrosarcoma of bone*

Panayiotis J. Papagelopoulos, Evanthia C. Galanis, Douglas J. McDonald, and Franklin H. Sim

Introduction

Definition

Fibrosarcoma is 'a malignant tumor characterized by the formation by the spindle-shaped tumor cells of interlacing bundles of collagen fibers, and by the absence of other types of histologic differentiation, such as the formation of cartilage or bone' (World Health Organization) (Schajowicz 1994). Previous descriptions of fibrosarcoma also included examples of malignant fibrous histiocytoma, which has both histiocytic and fibroblastic features and only recently has been differentiated from fibrosarcoma of bone (Feldman and Norman 1972).

---

*Reproduced in part from Papagelopoulos, P.J., Galanis, E.C., Triantafyllidis, P., Boscainos, P.J., Sim, F.H., and Unni, K.K. Clinicopathologic features, diagnosis, and treatment of fibrosarcoma of bone: a review. *American Journal of Orthopedics* (in press). By permission of Quadrant HealthCom Inc.

Fibrosarcoma can occur *de novo* or secondary to a pre-existing lesion, such as Paget's bone disease, osteonecrosis, or chronic osteomyelitis, or be related to the dedifferentiation of other neoplasms, such as giant cell tumors, chondroma, or, especially, chondrosarcoma (Mirra and Marcove 1974; Schajowicz 1994; Unni 1996). The most common precursor condition is radiation therapy (Wilner 1982; Unni 1996). Secondary fibrosarcomas account for 15 to 25 per cent of fibrosarcomas (André *et al.* 1983; Taconis and van Rijssel 1985; Unni 1996).

Natural history

Osseous fibrosarcomas are aggressive tumors, with a tendency for one or more recurrences. The rate of such recurrence and the likelihood of patient survival correlate with the histologic grade of the neoplasm. Fibrosarcomas of bone carry a poorer prognosis than those of soft tissue (Jeffree and Price 1976; Pritchard *et al.* 1977) and behave similarly to malignant fibrous histiocytomas.

Epidemiology

Fibrosarcoma is a rare tumor. It accounts for less than 5 per cent of the total number of primary malignant bone tumors—less than one-sixth of the cases of osteosarcoma (Unni 1996). It is observed with about equal frequency in men and women, occurring most commonly between the third and sixth decades of life (Fig. 1). However, the tumor may occur in children (Lysko *et al.* 1986; Pinto *et al.* 1993) and the elderly. In the elderly, fibrosarcoma usually occurs as a late complication of a pre-existing condition.

Fibrosarcomas are considered to arise as solitary tumors in the medullary bone, but periosteal lesions (Huvos and Higinbotham 1975) and multifocal (multicentric) lesions (Steiner 1944; Nielsen and Poulsen 1962; Hernandez and Fernandez 1976) have been described.

The anatomical sites most commonly involved are the long tubular bones (70 per cent of cases): the femur in 40 per cent of cases, the tibia in 16 per cent, the humerus in 10 per cent, the fibula in 3 per cent, the radius in 1 per cent, and the ulna in 0.5 per cent (Eyre-Brook and Price 1969; Jeffree and Price 1976; Bertoni *et al.* 1984; Taconis and van Rijssel 1985; Huvos 1991). In tubular bones, a metaphyseal or metadiaphyseal location is the usual site. Epiphyseal extension of a metaphyseal tumor is not infrequent (Bertoni *et al.* 1984). The distal femur and the proximal tibia account for 33 to 80 per cent of fibrosarcomas (McLeod *et al.* 1957; Gilmer and MacEwen 1958; Cunningham and Arlen 1968; Bertoni *et al.* 1984). Rarely, the small bones of the hands and feet are affected (Dahlin and Ivins 1969). The osseous pelvis is involved in approximately 9 per cent of cases (Unni 1996). The mandible (5 per cent of cases) and the maxilla (2 per cent) are uncommon sites for fibrosarcomas (Hoggins and Brady 1962; Van Blarcom *et al.* 1971; MacFarlane 1972; Richardson *et al.* 1972; Slootweg and Muller 1984; Taconis and van Rijssel 1986). These tumors are rare in the skull without an underlying disorder such as Paget's disease or previous irradiation (Mansfield 1977; Arita *et al.* 1980).

Clinical evaluation

Clinical manifestations are similar to those associated with other bone tumors. The most common complaints include local pain,

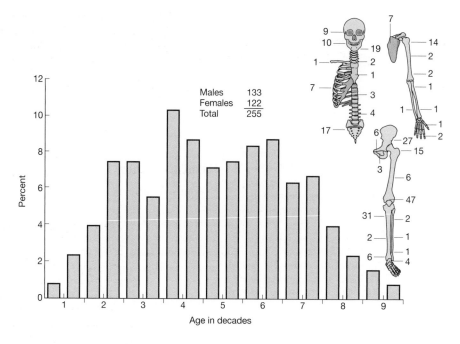

Fig. 1. Distribution of fibrosarcomas according to age and sex of the patient and site of the lesion. (Reproduced from Unni (1996) by permission of Mayo Foundation.)

swelling, and limitation of motion. Symptoms are usually of short duration (less than 6 months)with high-grade lesions, whereas in patients with slow-growing low-grade tumors the delay before diagnosis is usually long (several months to years) (Eyre-Brook and Price 1969). A mass, generally painful to palpation, is often a feature of a peripheral or high-grade malignant fibrosarcoma. Pathologic fracture is a frequent complication, because of the destructive character of the tumor, and is present in about 33 per cent of patients at the time of the initial evaluation. Patients with secondary fibrosarcomas have often had radiation therapy for a pre-exisiting condition (Unni 1996).

Imaging

Fibrosarcomas are characterized radiographically by large, eccentrically located, and purely lytic lesions with a geographic, moth-eaten, or permeative pattern of bone destruction; they are poorly marginated (Larsson *et al.* 1976). Cortical destruction and extension into adjacent soft tissues are common (Fig. 2). Rarely, there is a slight sclerotic marginal border. New bone periosteal reaction is rare (Taconis and Mulder 1984). The degree of bone destruction and the absence of significant osseous reaction are characteristic.

In tubular bones, fibrosarcomas may be central or eccentric in position and located in the metaphyseal region, extending into the epiphysis or diaphysis (Taconis and van Rijssel 1985). Eccentric epiphyseal tumors may simulate giant cell tumor.

Other imaging methods, such as scintigraphy, angiography, CT scanning, and MRI, may provide information about the extent of the lesion and the additional sites of involvement; however, they are unable to outline features that will establish histologic diagnosis.

Pathology

Fibrosarcomas are large (1.5–20 cm in size), destructive, and infiltrating tumors (McLeod *et al.* 1957; Larsson *et al.* 1976). Their macroscopic appearance depends on size and histologic differentiation. Well-differentiated neoplasms produce abundant collagen, are white or grayish-white, and have a firm and rubbery consistency. Poorly differentiated fibrosarcomas are usually soft and friable, with a fleshy consistency and myxoid foci (Huvos and Higinbotham 1975; Pritchard *et al.* 1977; Bertoni *et al.* 1984). Very large tumors may have hemorrhagic, necrotic, or cystic degeneration or myxoid areas.

Although histologic studies may reveal occasional myofibroblasts, fibrosarcoma is a tumor of malignant fibroblasts. It is characterized by poorly differentiated to well-differentiated fibrous tissue proliferation and is not associated with the production of cartilage or osteoid. Malignant fibrous histiocytoma of bone is composed of both malignant spindle-shaped fibroblast-like cells and malignant cells with histiocyte-like morphology and function. Based on an assessment of cellularity, mitotic activity, collagen production, nuclear morphology, and overall histologic pattern, fibrosarcomas are divided into 'well-differentiated', 'moderately differentiated', and 'poorly differentiated' types (Jeffree and Price 1976; Pritchard *et al.* 1977; Taconis and van Rijssel 1985; Schajowicz 1994) or into grades 1 to 4, with the higher grades representing the less differentiated tumors (McLeod *et al.* 1957; Dahlin and Ivins 1969; Taconis and van Rijssel 1985). Most fibrosarcomas are either moderately or poorly differentiated (Mirra 1980).

Well-differentiated fibrosarcomas consist of elongated and spindle-shaped tumor cells that have small uniform tapered nuclei. The cytoplasm is usually poorly defined, with indistinct borders. Intercellular collagen formation may be so abundant that the tumor may be interpreted as a desmoplastic fibroma (Dahlin and Ivins 1969; Bertoni *et*

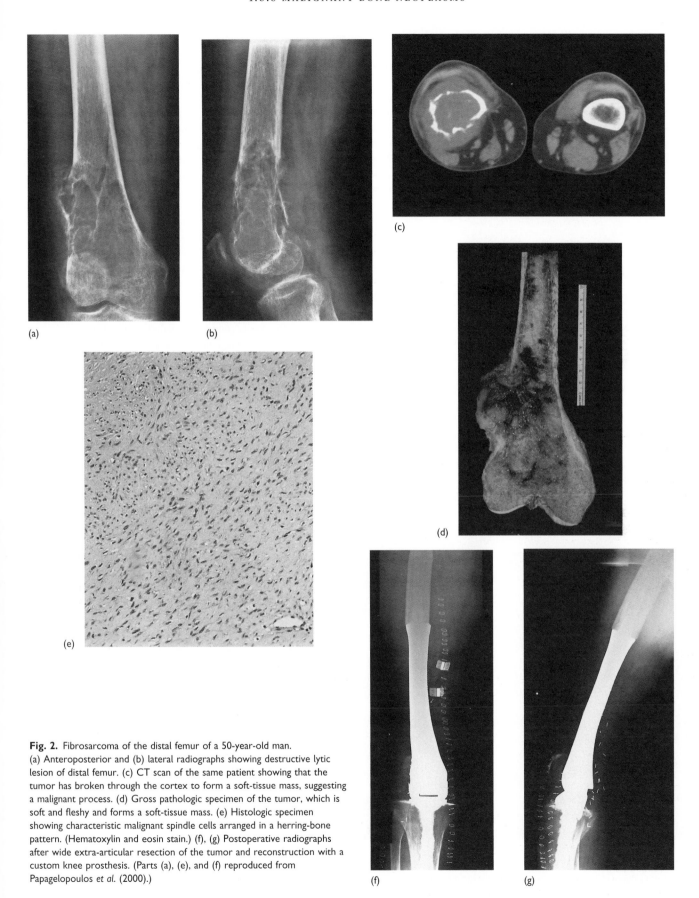

Fig. 2. Fibrosarcoma of the distal femur of a 50-year-old man.
(a) Anteroposterior and (b) lateral radiographs showing destructive lytic
lesion of distal femur. (c) CT scan of the same patient showing that the
tumor has broken through the cortex to form a soft-tissue mass, suggesting
a malignant process. (d) Gross pathologic specimen of the tumor, which is
soft and fleshy and forms a soft-tissue mass. (e) Histologic specimen
showing characteristic malignant spindle cells arranged in a herring-bone
pattern. (Hematoxylin and eosin stain.) (f), (g) Postoperative radiographs
after wide extra-articular resection of the tumor and reconstruction with a
custom knee prosthesis. (Parts (a), (e), and (f) reproduced from
Papagelopoulos *et al.* (2000).)

al. 1984). The tumor cells characteristically are arranged in intersecting fascicles, forming a 'herringbone' pattern. Rarely, a storiform configuration, as in malignant fibrous histiocytoma, is evident (Mirra 1980; Taconis and van Rijssel 1985).

In moderately or poorly differentiated fibrosarcomas, the amount of collagen is decreased and cellularity is increased. The nuclei are larger, ovoid or round, and more irregular, and the chromatin is coarse, clumped, and distributed more irregularly. Nucleoli are more common and more prominent, and mitotic activity is increased. The herringbone pattern is less evident and may be absent. Necrosis and hemorrhage are more common in the poorly differentiated tumors. Rarely, the tumor may be markedly myxoid (Unni 1996).

Differential diagnosis

The radiographic features of fibrosarcoma of bone are not specific and generally indicate an aggressive or malignant process. The absence of calcification or ossification in fibrosarcomas assumes diagnostic importance, because such findings are evident in chondrosarcomas and conventional osteosarcomas. However, the radiographic appearance of a well-differentiated fibrosarcoma may suggest the diagnosis of desmoplastic fibroma, chondromyxoid fibroma, or giant cell tumor, whereas a poorly differentiated lesion has to be distinguished from malignant fibrous histiocytoma, telangiectatic osteosarcoma, lymphoma, solitary plasmacytoma, and metastatic carcinoma (Campanacci 1990; Schajowicz 1994). The histologic features of fibrosarcoma must be distinguished from those of nonossifying fibroma, fibrous dysplasia, desmoplastic fibroma, malignant fibrous histiocytoma, fibroblastic osteosarcoma, and metastatic spindle cell carcinoma (Unni 1996).

Treatment

Surgery is accepted as the the most suitable method of treatment for both periosteal and medullary fibrosarcomas. The type of surgical procedure (*en bloc* resection, disarticulation, or amputation) depends mainly on the histologic grade of differentiation, the local conditions, and the location of the tumor. Preoperative chemotherapy and limb-sparing resection with a wide surgical margin and reconstruction are indicated, where feasible (Figs 2 and 3). Amputation may be required to achieve an adequate margin (Pritchard *et al.* 1977; Papagelopoulos *et al.* 2000).

In well-differentiated or moderately well-differentiated tumors of the extremities, without or with only limited extension into extraosseous soft tissue, wide resection is the treatment of choice, followed by allograft or prosthetic reconstruction. Currently, the treatment for high-grade tumors includes preoperative chemotherapy followed by wide resection of the tumor and postoperative chemotherapy (Huvos 1991). Amputation is indicated in the event of recurrence after *en bloc* resection.

Radiation therapy is considered ineffective and is used only as a palliative measure in surgically unresectable moderately or poorly differentiated tumors, with or without chemotherapy (Campanacci 1990). Aggressive thoracotomy is performed for pulmonary metastases whenever indicated and feasible (Ishihara 1984; Turnage *et al.* 1994).

Prognosis

Survival rates and histologic grade of differentiation are closely correlated. Patients with poorly differentiated tumors have a poorer prognosis (Jaffe 1958; Cunningham and Arlen 1968; Pritchard *et al.* 1977;

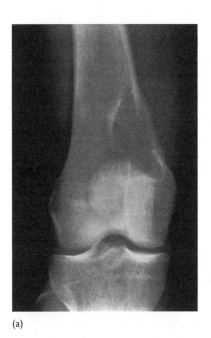
(a)

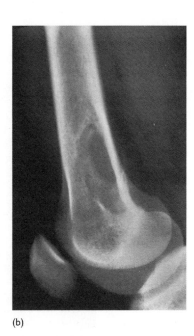
(b)

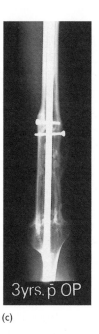
(c)

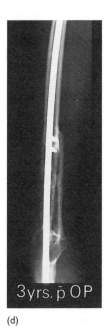
(d)

Fig. 3. Fibrosarcoma of the distal femur of a 25-year-old woman. (a) Anteroposterior and (b) lateral radiographs showing a well-demarcated lytic lesion of the distal femur. (c), (d) Three years postoperatively after wide resection of distal femur and arthrodesis using sliding bone autograft from tibia to femur and intramedullary rod fixation. (Parts (a) and (c) reproduced from Papagelopoulos *et al.* (2000).)

Bertoni *et al.* 1984; Campanacci 1990; Huvos 1991). Tumors of the long tubular bones that are located eccentrically, exhibit a geographic pattern of bone destruction, and involve only a portion of the cortex may have a more favorable prognosis than tumors without these features (Taconis and Mulder 1984).

The course of the disease is slower than that of osteosarcoma. Tumors of grade 1 or 2 grow more slowly than those of grade 3 or 4. High-grade fibrosarcomas metastasize to the lungs. Well-differentiated tumors may metastasize to the lungs and bones several years after diagnosis. Lymph metastases are uncommon (Campanacci 1990).

Overall 5-year survival rates vary from 28 per cent (Eyre-Brook and Price 1969; Pritchard *et al.* 1977) to 34 per cent (Huvos and Higinbotham 1975). In a Mayo Clinic series (Papagelopoulos *et al.* 2000), multivariate analysis showed that age 40 years or older, tumor location in the axial skeleton, and high-grade tumor were the most important risk factors that significantly affected overall survival ($p < 0.001$).

In a study from the Rizzoli Institute, the 5-year overall survival was 42 per cent, with 83 per cent survival for low-grade tumors and 34 per cent for high-grade ones (Bertoni *et al.* 1984). In the same study, local recurrence was a bad prognostic factor. In the study by The Netherlands Committee on Bone Tumors (Taconis and van Rijssel 1985), in which the treatment was similar for pure fibrosarcomas and for malignant fibrous histiocytomas, the 5-year survival was the same in both groups (34 per cent). Lung metastases developed in 63 per cent of the patients with fibrosarcomas and in 59 per cent of those with malignant fibrous histiocytomas. The histologic grade was of prognostic value in both groups: 5-year survival was 64 per cent in 14 patients with grade 1 tumors, 41 per cent in 32 patients with grade 2 tumors, and 23 per cent in 56 patients with grade 3 tumors.

References

André, S., Tomeno, B., Forest, M., and Carlioz, A. (1983). Fibrosarcoma of bone. *Revue de Chirurgie Orthopedique et de Chirurgie de l' Appareil Moteur*, **69**, 107–16.

Arita, N., Ushio, Y., Hayakawa, T., and Mogami, H. (1980). Primary fibrosarcoma of the skull. *Surgical Neurology*, **14**, 381–4.

Bertoni, F., Capanna, R., Calderoni, P., Patrizia, B., and Campanacci, M. (1984). Primary central (medullary) fibrosarcoma of bone. *Seminars in Diagnostic Pathology*, **1**, 185–98.

Campanacci, M. (1990). *Bone and soft tissue tumors*, Springer-Verlag, Vienna.

Cunningham, M.P. and Arlen, M. (1968). Medullary fibrosarcoma of bone. *Cancer*, **21**, 31–7.

Dahlin, D.C. and Ivins, J.C. (1969). Fibrosarcoma of bone. A study of 114 cases. *Cancer*, **23**, 35–41.

Eyre-Brook, A.L. and Price, C.H. (1969). Fibrosarcoma of bone. Review of fifty consecutive cases from the Bristol Bone Tumour Registry. *Journal of Bone and Joint Surgery, British Volume*, **51B**, 20–37.

Feldman, F. and Norman, D. (1972). Intra- and extraosseous malignant histiocytoma (malignant fibrous xanthoma). *Radiology*, **104**, 497–508.

Gilmer, W.S., Jr and MacEwen, G.D. (1958). Central (medullary) fibrosarcoma of bone. *Journal of Bone and Joint Surgery, American Volume*, **40**, 121–41.

Hernandez, F.J. and Fernandez, B.B. (1976). Multiple diffuse fibrosarcoma of bone. *Cancer*, **37**, 939–45.

Hoggins, G.S. and Brady, C.L. (1962). Fibrosarcoma of maxilla. *Oral Surgery*, **15**, 34–8.

Huvos, A.G. (1991). *Bone tumors: diagnosis, treatment, and prognosis* (2nd edn). W.B. Saunders, Philadelphia, PA.

Huvos, A.G. and Higinbotham, N.L. (1975). Primary fibrosarcoma of bone. A clinicopathologic study of 130 patients. *Cancer*, **35**, 837–47.

Ishihara, T. (1984). Bilateral pneumonectomy in metastatic pulmonary tumors. *Nippon Geka Gakki Zasshi*, **85**, 944–7.

Jaffe, H.L. (1958). *Tumors and tumorous conditions of the bones and joints*. Lea & Febiger, Philadelphia, PA.

Jeffree, G.M. and Price, C.H. (1976). Metastatic spread of fibrosarcoma of bone: a report on forty-nine cases, and a comparison with osteosarcoma. *Journal of Bone and Joint Surgery, British Volume*, **58B**, 418–25.

Larsson, S.E., Lorentzon, R., and Boquist, L. (1976). Fibrosarcoma of bone. A demographic, clinical and histopathological study of all cases recorded in the Swedish cancer registry from 1958 to 1968. *Journal of Bone and Joint Surgery, British Volume*, **58B**, 412–17.

Lysko, J.E., Guilford, W.B., and Siegal, G.P. (1986). Case report 362. *Skeletal Radiology*, **15**, 268–72.

MacFarlane, W.I. (1972). Fibrosarcoma of the mandible with pulmonary metastases: a case report. *British Journal of Oral Surgery*, **10**, 168–74.

McLeod, J.J., Dahlin, D.C., and Ivins, J.C. (1957). Fibrosarcoma of bone. *American Journal of Surgery*, **94**, 431–7.

Mansfield, J.B. (1977). Primary fibrosarcoma of the skull. Case report. *Journal of Neurosurgery*, **47**, 785–7.

Mirra, J.M. (1980). *Bone tumors: diagnosis and treatment*. J.B. Lippincott, Philadelphia, PA.

Mirra, J.M. and Marcove, R.C. (1974). Fibrosarcomatous dedifferentiation of primary and secondary chondrosarcoma: review of five cases. *Journal of Bone and Joint Surgery, American Volume*, **56**, 285–96.

Nielsen, A.R. and Poulsen, H. (1962). Multiple diffuse fibrosarcomata of the bones. *Acta Pathologica et Microbiologica Scandinavica*, **55**, 265–72.

Papagelopoulos, P.J., Galanis, E., Frassica, F.J., Sim, F.H., Larson, D.R., and Wold, L.E. (2000). Primary fibrosarcoma of bone: outcome after primary surgical treatment. *Clinical Orthopaedics and Related Research*, **373**, 88–103.

Pinto, A., Dold, O.R., Mueller, D., and Gilbert-Barness, E. (1993). Pathological cases of the month. Infantile fibrosarcoma. *American Journal of Diseases of Children*, **147**, 691–2.

Pritchard, D.J., Sim, F.H., Ivins, J.C., Soule, E.H., and Dahlin, D.C. (1977). Fibrosarcoma of bone and soft tissues of the trunk and extremities. *Orthopedic Clinics of North America*, **8**, 869–81.

Richardson, J.F., Fine, M.A., and Goldman, H.M. (1972). Fibrosarcoma of the mandible: a clinicopathologic controversy. Report of case. *Journal of Oral Surgery*, **30**, 664–8.

Schajowicz, F. (1994). *Tumors and tumorlike lesions of bones: pathology, radiology, and treatment* (2nd edn). Springer-Verlag, Berlin.

Slootweg, P.J. and Muller, H. (1984). Fibrosarcoma of the jaws. A study of 7 cases. *Journal of Maxillofacial Surgery*, **12**, 157–62.

Steiner, P.E. (1944). Multiple diffuse fibrosarcoma of bone. *American Journal of Pathology*, **20**, 877–93.

Taconis, W.K. and Mulder, J.D. (1984). Fibrosarcoma and malignant fibrous histiocytoma of long bones: radiographic features and grading. *Skeletal Radiology*, **11**, 237–45.

Taconis, W.K. and van Rijssel, T.G. (1985). Fibrosarcoma of long bones. A study of the significance of areas of malignant fibrous histiocytoma. *Journal of Bone and Joint Surgery, British Volume*, **67B**, 111–16.

Taconis, W.K. and van Rijssel, T.G. (1986). Fibrosarcoma of the jaws. *Skeletal Radiology*, **15**, 10–13.

Turnage, W.S., Gill-Murdoch, C., McKeown, P.P., and Conant, P. (1994). Bilateral thoracoscopy and limited thoracotomy. A combined approach for the resection of metastatic fibrosarcoma. *Chest*, **106**, 935–6.

Unni, K.K. (1996). *Dahlin's bone tumors: general aspects and data on 11,087 cases* (5th edn). Lippincott–Raven, Philadelphia, PA.

Van Blarcom, C.W., Masson, J.K., and Dahlin, D.C. (1971). Fibrosarcoma of the mandible. A clinicopathologic study. *Oral Surgery, Oral Medicine, Oral Pathology*, **32**, 428–39.

Wilner, D. (1982). *Radiology of bone tumors and allied disorders*. W.B. Saunders, Philadelphia, PA.

1.6.8.9 Malignant fibrous histiocytoma of bone*

Panayiotis J. Papagelopoulos, Evanthia C. Galanis, Douglas J. McDonald, and Franklin H. Sim

Introduction

Malignant fibrous histiocytoma is a malignant tumor with a pleomorphic spindle-celled structure but devoid of any specific pattern of histological differentiation (World Health Organization) (Schajowicz 1994).

Malignant fibrous histiocytoma of bone is a rare tumor of histiocytic origin described in 1972 (Feldman and Norman 1972). Earlier reports referred to this lesion as 'malignant fibrous histiocytoma', 'pleomorphic spindle cell sarcoma', and 'poorly differentiated fibrosarcoma of bone', among other names, until its identity was established (Spanier *et al.* 1975; Huvos 1976, 1991). Previously, many cases of malignant fibrous histiocytoma were classified as liposarcomas, pleomorphic fibrosarcomas, osteolytic osteosarcomas, anaplastic reticulosarcomas, or malignant giant cell tumors (Papagelopoulos *et al.* 2000*a*).

The segregation of fibrous histiocytomas from the broad spectrum of histiocytic lesions evolved as a result of extensive investigative work in the 1960s (Stout and Lattes 1967), and with the appreciation that malignant fibrous histiocytomas arise far more frequently in the soft tissues than in the bones and that the diagnosis is established

Box 1

- Rare malignant bone tumor that may develop in apparently normal bone or in association with bone infarcts, fibrous dysplasia, intraosseous lipoma, and Paget's disease
- Most common locations include the femur, tibia, humerus, and pelvis
- Differential diagnosis includes fibrosarcoma, malignant neural tumor, leiomyosarcoma, malignant giant cell tumor, osteosarcoma, and dedifferentiated chondrosarcoma
- Treatment is similar to the treatment of osteosarcoma

*Reproduced in part from Papagelopoulos, P.J., Galanis, E.C., Sim, F.H., and Unni, K.K. (2000). Clinicopathologic features, diagnosis, and treatment of malignant fibrous histiocytoma of bone. *Orthopedics*, **23**, 59–65. By permission of Slack Inc.

most firmly on the basis of conventional light microscopy, tissue culture, and ultrastructural studies. Certain histological criteria that were originally applied to the diagnosis of fibrous histiocytoma of soft tissue (Stout and Lattes 1967) are required for the identification of similar tumors arising in bone: bundles of fibrous and spindle-shaped fibroblast-like cells arranged in a storiform or cartwheel pattern and showing mitotic activity and nuclear atypism, round cells exhibiting features of histiocytes with ovoid nuclei, which are often indented or grooved, and well-defined cytoplasmic borders, and typical and atypical multinucleated tumor giant cells of the osteoclastic type (Schajowicz 1983).

Approximately 70 per cent of malignant fibrous histiocytomas of bone are primary tumors and 30 per cent are secondary tumors (Huvos 1991). Malignant fibrous histiocytoma of bone can occur *de novo*, in association with other osseous abnormalities (including bone infarction, fibrous dysplasia, intraosseous lipoma, and Paget's disease) (Spanier 1977; Mirra 1980), and after radiation therapy (Huvos *et al.* 1986). Some tumors also appear to be associated with orthopedic implants and may be metal induced (Ward *et al.* 1990).

Malignant fibrous histiocytoma of bone is an aggressive tumor characterized by a high frequency of local recurrence (as much as 80 per cent of tumors) and of metastases to regional lymph nodes and distant sites (especially the lungs, but also the liver, brain, heart, kidneys, intestines, and adrenal glands). Although the reported rate of 5-year survival for patients with this neoplasm has varied considerably (from zero to approximately 70 per cent) (Spanier *et al.* 1975; Spanier 1977; Mirra 1980; Ghandur-Mnaymneh *et al.* 1982; Capanna *et al.* 1984; Yuen and Saw 1985), the malignant nature of this tumor is not questioned, especially in older patients and in those with an underlying osseous abnormality (e.g. osteonecrosis) (Huvos *et al.* 1985).

Epidemiology

The tumor occurs more frequently in men than in women (approximately 3:2) and in patients of any age, although the majority of affected persons are in the fifth, sixth, and seventh decades of life (Fig. 1) (Feldman and Norman 1972; Feldman and Lattes 1977; Spanier 1977; Capanna *et al.* 1984; Ros *et al.* 1984; Huvos *et al.* 1985; Yuen and Saw 1985; Boland and Huvos 1986). The primary variety tends to affect younger patients, whereas secondary neoplasms are seen predominately in the sixth and seventh decades of life.

The skeletal distribution of malignant fibrous histiocytoma is similar to that of osteosarcoma, with the ends of the long tubular bones mainly affected (approximately 75 per cent of cases) (Newland *et al.* 1975; Spanier *et al.* 1975; Huvos 1976; Inada *et al.* 1976; Dahlin *et al.* 1977; Kahn *et al.* 1978; Takechi and Taguchi 1978; McCarthy *et al.* 1979; Martinez-Tello *et al.* 1981; Ghandur-Mnaymneh *et al.* 1982; Bayer Kristensen and Myhre Jensen 1984; Capanna *et al.* 1984; Nakashima *et al.* 1985). Slightly more than half of these neoplasms originate in the lower extremity (Huvos *et al.* 1985). The bones in the lower extremity are involved six times more frequently than those in the upper extremity. The bones about the knee account for approximately 50 per cent of all tumors involving the tubular bones. Within the long tubular bones, metaphyseal localization is the rule, with frequent extension of the tumor into the epiphysis or diaphysis, or both. Subperiosteal lesions (Dahlin *et al.* 1977) and multifocal lesions in

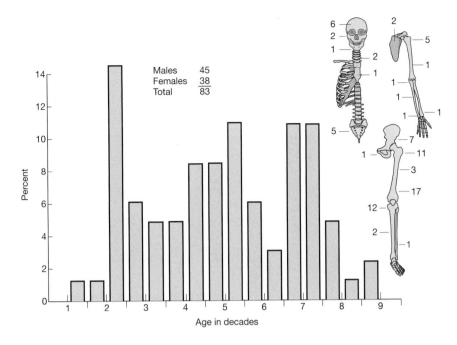

Fig. 1. Distribution of malignant fibrous histiocytomas according to age and sex of the patient and site of the lesion. (Reproduced from Unni (1996) by permission of the Mayo Foundation.)

one or more bones (Chen 1978; McCarthy *et al.* 1979; Katenkamp and Stiller 1981; Shapiro 1981; Finci *et al.* 1990) are additional rare manifestations of malignant fibrous histiocytoma.

The most common sites of tumor localization include the femur (approximately 45 per cent of cases), the tibia (20 per cent), and the humerus (9 per cent). The innominate bone is affected in approximately 10 per cent of cases; other sites of involvement are the skull and facial bones (4 per cent), ribs (3 per cent), and, less frequently, the fibula, spine, scapula, and clavicle (Barney 1972; Yumoto *et al.* 1976; Johnson *et al.* 1978; Dunham and Wilborn 1979; Nunnery *et al.* 1979; Blitzer *et al.* 1981; Chitale *et al.* 1981; Katenkamp and Stiller 1981; Kessler *et al.* 1981; Shuman *et al.* 1982). The patella and the bones of the hands and feet are rarely affected (Lopez-Barea *et al.* 1991).

Clinical evaluation

A painful fixed mass adjacent to a major joint is the most common presentation. Pain, tenderness, and localized swelling are the predominant symptoms and usually develop slowly over a period of months or even years. A more acute onset of these clinical manifestations may be indicative of a pathologic fracture (which may occur eventually in 30 to 50 per cent of patients). Discomfort and limitation of joint motion are associated with intra-articular extension of the neoplasm. A palpable and tender mass is the most common physical finding associated with malignant fibrous histiocytoma of bone.

Imaging

Osteolysis with a moth-eaten or permeative pattern of bone destruction, cortical erosion, and a soft-tissue mass represent the most char-

acteristic radiographic abnormalities of a malignant fibrous histiocytoma of bone (Taconis and Mulder 1984). Large destructive lesions, originating in weight-bearing bones, frequently lead to pathologic fracture. Periosteal new bone formation and endosteal scalloping are rarely seen.

The lesion most often arises in a metaphyseal or diaphyseal location in the affected bone (Fig. 2(a)). The lesions are variable in size, but may extend from the epiphysis to the diaphysis of a tubular bone, throughout the innominate bone, or between the body and posterior osseous elements of the vertebrae. Osseous expansion is unusual, but may be observed in the flat and irregular bones such as the ribs, scapula, and sternum (Feldman and Lattes 1977).

As in the case of most malignant neoplasms of bone, CT, MRI, and angiography (Hudson *et al.* 1979) can be used to assess the intraosseous or extraosseous extent of malignant fibrous histiocytomas. CT is useful in defining the extent of bone destruction (Paling and Hyams 1982); however, MRI with contrast enhancement of the extremity is the single study of choice to provide maximal data (Sundaram and McLeod 1990). Of these methods, MRI probably is best at defining the size of the intraosseous tumoral component; however, all three methods are beneficial to some degree in delineating soft-tissue involvement and the relationship of the tumor to adjacent vessels or nerves. In no instance are the findings specific for malignant fibrous histiocytoma.

Pathology

Macroscopically, malignant fibrous histiocytoma is usually located centrally within the bone (Fig. 2(b)), producing little or no osseous expansion (Capanna *et al.* 1984). Cortical destruction with extension of the tumor into the soft tissue is found in 80 to 100 per cent of

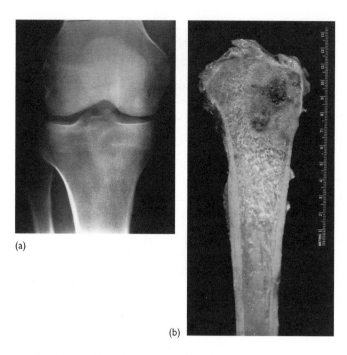

(a)

(b)

Fig. 2. Malignant fibrous histiocytoma. (a) Radiograph of right knee showing an ill-defined sclerotic area in proximal tibia. (b) Gross specimen of proximal tibia showing a large tumor destroying the cortex and occupying the proximal portion of the tibia. (Reproduced from Unni (1996) by permission of the Mayo Foundation.)

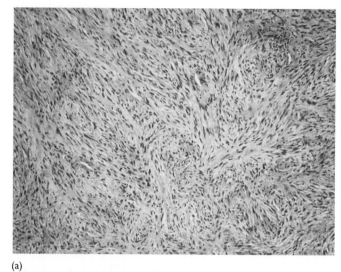

(a)

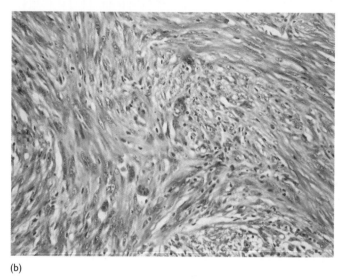

(b)

Fig. 3. Malignant fibrous histiocytoma. (a) Typical low-power appearance shows storiform arrangement of spindle cells throughout the lesion. (b) Higher-power appearance of the storiform pattern. (Hematoxylin and eosin stain.) (Reproduced from Unni (1996) by permission of the Mayo Foundation.)

cases (Huvos 1976; Spanier 1977). The soft-tissue component of the tumor may appear multinodular and pseudoencapsulated (Feldman and Lattes 1977). The neoplasm is generally 2 to 10 cm in size; lesions larger than 20 cm have been described (Saito and Caines 1977). There is variation in color and consistency of the tumor depending on the relative proportions of fibroblastic and histiocytic cells that are present and their lipid content. It may be gray, brown, yellow, or orange, and fleshy, soft, firm, or rubbery. Hemorrhagic zones are common.

The histological diagnosis of malignant fibrous histiocytoma is frequently one of exclusion, and it cannot be made with assurance when only a limited amount of biopsy tissue is available for analysis (Mirra 1980). Histologically, the tumor is composed of fibroblasts in a storiform ('whorling' or 'cartwheel') pattern with multinucleated giant cells, inflammatory cells, and histiocytes, with numerous foamy mononuclear or multinucleated giant cells (xanthomatous variant) (Fig. 3). Mitotic figures are frequent, with considerable pleomorphism. Regardless of the primary or secondary classification, most of these lesions are high-grade malignancies (grades III and IV). Only 10 per cent or fewer are low grade (grades I and II). Although malignant fibrous histiocytomas do not have a uniform histological pattern, they all share light microscopic features marked by the presence, in varying amounts, of cells with fibroblastic or histiocytic characteristics, or both. The spindle-shaped fibroblasts that are evident in the fibrous regions of a malignant fibrous histiocytoma are not arranged in the classic herringbone pattern of a fibrosarcoma; rather, the cells radiate outward in a spiral array from a central focus, producing the appearance of a nebula. In highly fibrous tumors, extensive fibrous foci create an overall mat-like or storiform appearance.

Electron microscope studies of these tumors have identified three major types of cells: fibroblast-like cells, histiocyte-like cells, and primitive undifferentiated mesenchymal cells (Inada *et al.* 1976; Saito and Caines 1977; Taxy and Battifora 1977; Chen 1978; Johnson *et al.* 1978; McCarthy *et al.* 1979; Katenkamp and Stiller 1981; Shapiro 1981; Ghandur-Mnaymneh *et al.* 1982; Nakashima *et al.* 1985). Myofibroblasts, foam cells, and multinucleated osteoclast-type giant cells also have been observed. The variability of the microscopic abnormalities of malignant fibrous histiocytomas has led to the subdivision of the soft-tissue tumors into myxoid, inflammatory, angiomatoid, and pleomorphic varieties (Kyriakos and Kempson 1976; Enzinger 1979; Poon *et al.* 1982). In most reports, however, the osseous lesions are designated simply as malignant fibrous histiocytomas.

Differential diagnosis

Histological differential diagnosis may be difficult. The presence of the storiform pattern is not specific for malignant fibrous histiocytoma because it may be found in various benign and malignant lesions. Other lesions that must be considered in the differential diagnosis of malignant fibrous histiocytoma of bone include fibrosarcoma (Taconis and van Rijssel 1985), malignant schwannoma (Jacobs and Fox 1972), leiomyosarcoma (von Hochstetter et al. 1984; Papagelopoulos et al. 2000b), malignant giant cell tumor of bone (Huvos et al. 1985), spindle cell osteosarcoma (Roessner et al. 1979), and dedifferentiated chondrosarcoma (with prominent spindle cell component) (Dahlin and Beabout 1971). Malignant fibrous histiocytoma of bone demonstrates immunoreactivity for vimentin, glycoprotein, α_1-antitrypsin, α_1-antichymotrypsin, and the bacteriolytic enzyme lysozyme (Katenkamp and Stiller 1981). These tumors are commonly negative for S-100 protein. Ultrastructurally, the lesions seem to derive from a primitive mesenchymal stem cell that may be shared with the common progenitor cell of osteosarcoma (Katenkamp and Stiller 1981). The fibroblast-like tumor cells reveal a greater degree of nuclear atypism and irregularity than is seen in a conventional fibrosarcoma. Thin bands of collagen that simulate osteoid may course between the tumor cells, making it difficult to differentiate a malignant fibrous histiocytoma from an osteosarcoma.

Radiographic features indicating an aggressive skeletal process are not specific for malignant fibrous histiocytoma. Other lesions such as metastatic carcinoma (especially of the lung or breast), plasmacytoma, lymphoma, and osteolytic osteosarcoma produce similar radiographic abnormalities. Similarities in the radiographic features of malignant fibrous histiocytoma and fibrosarcoma of bone may create a difficult diagnostic problem (Taconis and Mulder 1984). The age of the affected patient and additional clinical features will allow a malignant fibrous histiocytoma to be differentiated from other tumors.

Secondary malignant fibrous histiocytoma is by definition associated with an underlying or pre-existing condition. There appears to be a clear association with bone infarction as a pre-existing condition (Furey et al. 1960; Dorfman et al. 1966; Mirra et al. 1974, 1977; Michael and Dorfman 1976). Radiographically, the remaining punctate calcifications can be seen about the periphery of the lesion, with destruction and loss of radiographic detail evident within the lesion. Also, a contiguous soft-tissue mass is commonly present. Patients with known Paget's disease of bone, hereditary dysplasias of bone, or previous treatment with radiation therapy are at risk for the development of secondary malignant fibrous histiocytomas of bone.

Treatment

Previously, treatment was ablative surgery for all the tumors located in long limb bones, whereas in those located in bones not amenable to surgery, irradiation produced some palliation. None of the patients usually survived more than 2 years because of metastatic spread, with pulmonary involvement being the major cause of death (McCarthy et al. 1979).

Ghandur-Mnaymneh et al. (1982) reported six new patients and reviewed the literature, reporting on a total of 74 patients followed up for at least 5 years. Analysis of the data showed a 5-year survival rate of 36.5 per cent. Of these 74 patients, 13 (17.6 per cent) survived for 5 to 38 years, demonstrating certain similarities to osteosarcoma.

In the Memorial Hospital series (Huvos et al. 1985), the management of spindle cell sarcomas of bone, including malignant fibrous histiocytoma, was similar to that of osteosarcoma. The experience at the Rizzoli Institute was also similar (Campanacci 1990).

Low-grade (grades I and II) nonmetastatic malignant fibrous histiocytoma of bone is treated with wide surgical excision. Patients with a high-grade lesion (grade III or IV) are given preoperative (neoadjuvant) chemotherapy to reduce the size of the primary tumor and to make limb-sparing surgery possible. Amputations are performed less and less frequently, and are usually reserved for patients with pathologic fractures or unusually large lesions.

Nonmetastatic primary malignant fibrous histiocytoma of bone is best managed in a manner similar to that for primary osteosarcoma of adolescents and young adults. The use of neoadjuvant chemotherapy has several advantages. It permits early clinical and radiographic assessment of chemotherapy efficacy before anticipated resection, as well as pathologic assessment of the chemotherapy response of the specimen after resection, thus allowing adjustment of the chemotherapy regimen postoperatively. In addition, it permits design and development of the appropriate type of surgical reconstruction (e.g. custom prosthesis construction) and treats micrometastases early. Active chemotherapy agents include doxorubicin, cisplatin, ifosfamide, and methotrexate.

Following diagnostic biopsy, neoadjuvant chemotherapy should be considered. The primary tumor response is monitored clinically and radiographically during the administration of neoadjuvant chemotherapy (Capanna et al. 1984; Bettelli et al. 1987). Most tumors will respond clinically, with relief of pain, resolution of the associated joint contracture, diminished local edema, and reduction in the site of the soft-tissue component. Radiographic response to neoadjuvant chemotherapy is best confirmed by a decrease in the size of the soft-tissue component and diminished or absent contrast enhancement on follow-up MRI evaluation. However, lack of radiographic response does not exclude pathological response to chemotherapy (Bacci et al. 1996).

If the patient is a limb-sparing candidate, a surgical procedure with a minimum of wide margin can usually be performed following the determinants of limb-sparing surgery. The surgical determinants of limb preservation include the ability to perform a curative resection with a minimum of 'wide' margin, to maintain neural continuity, to maintain or reconstruct vascularity, to restore structural integrity, and to rotate flaps and obtain skin coverage. In these cases, most orthopedic oncologists would use a custom implant arthroplasty, a resection-arthrodesis, an allograft, an allograft–prosthetic implant composite, or rotationplasty. For lesions that prove unresectable, an ablative procedure with a minimum of a wide to compartmental margin should be performed.

The chemotherapy regimens for malignant fibrous histiocytoma of bone are evolving. Depending on the extent of tumor necrosis at the time of surgery and the type of preoperative chemotherapy, adjuvant chemotherapy can be considered. The usual approach to nonresponders (necrosis less than 70 per cent) would be the addition of drugs with known antisarcoma activity that have not previously been used.

At the Rizzoli Institute (Capanna *et al.* 1984; Campanacci 1990), a good response with preoperative chemotherapy has been obtained in nearly half of the patients. When preoperative chemotherapy was combined with wide or radical surgical resection and postoperative chemotherapy, improved survival for these patients was noted. A prospective study from the same institution showed a good response rate of 33 per cent (with more than 90 per cent tumor necrosis at the time of surgery) in patients with malignant fibrous histiocytoma of bone treated with neoadjuvant chemotherapy, including methotrexate, doxorubicin, and cisplatin with or without ifosfamide (Bacci *et al.* 1996).

A regimen of vincristine plus high-dose methotrexate with citrovorum rescue plus doxorubicin has been reported to be successful in preventing distant disease at 42 to 48 months (Weiner *et al.* 1983). Combination chemotherapy, including doxorubicin plus ifosfamide plus dacarbazine, with mesna uroprotection chemotherapy is an alternative being evaluated.

Aggressive thoracotomy should be performed for pulmonary metastases whenever feasible (Han *et al.* 1981; Ishihara 1984).

Combination chemotherapy can be considered for patients with metastatic disease not amenable to surgical treatment or palliative radiation, but it rarely results in significant survival benefit (Capanna *et al.* 1984).

Prognosis

It has been suggested that malignant fibrous histiocytomas are aggressive and rapidly growing tumors (Feldman and Lattes 1977); however, the prognosis of malignant fibrous histiocytoma is difficult to judge because in many older case reports there is a lack of follow-up data or other neoplasms with some component of malignant fibrous histiocytoma are often included.

Lung metastases are common and were noted in 31.5 per cent of the 130 patients of Huvos *et al.* (1985). Synchronous multifocal bone involvement is rare, but metachronous osseous metastases are not uncommon (10 per cent). The frequency of lymph node metastasis is low or zero in some series (Capanna *et al.* 1984; Huvos *et al.* 1985; Dahlin and Unni 1986) and relatively high in others (Spanier *et al.* 1975; Yuen and Saw 1985).

Spanier *et al.* (1975) reported on the radiographic characteristics of 11 primary bone tumors with the histopathological features of primary malignant fibrous histiocytoma of bone. The lesions involved long bones and were metaphyseal and destructive, often complicated by a pathologic fracture. Nine of the 11 patients developed pulmonary metastases and three developed regional lymph node involvement less than 2 years after diagnosis. The average survival for six of these nine patients was 12 months. Six patients who developed metastases had no further treatment. The three others received additional treatment: two patients received systemic chemotherapy, and one had additional radiation therapy. All demonstrated a partial response.

According to the Memorial Hospital series (Huvos *et al.* 1985), patients with low-grade tumors have a better prognosis than those with high-grade lesions. However, survival differs according to age, with patients aged 21 years or less having a substantially better prognosis than those who are older. This is explained by the fact that older patients are more commonly affected by secondary malignant fibrous histiocytomas, especially in association with previous irradiation or sarcoma arising in Paget's disease.

A retrospective study from the Rizzoli Institute of 90 patients with malignant fibrous histiocytoma of bone included 68 patients who received surgical therapy and 20 of 60 who received chemotherapy (Capanna *et al.* 1984). The overall survival rate was 34 per cent at 5 years and 28 per cent at 10 years. With adequate surgery (a wide margin) and chemotherapy, the 5-year survival rate improved to 57 per cent.

In a more recent prospective study from the same institution, a 71 per cent 5-year disease-free survival was reported in patients with malignant fibrous histiocytoma of bone treated with neoadjuvant chemotherapy, including methotrexate, doxorubicin, and cisplatin with or without ifosfamide (Bacci *et al.* 1996).

In a Mayo Clinic series of 81 patients with malignant fibrous histiocytoma, the 2-year, 5-year, and 10-year disease-free survivals of 69 patients with localized disease were 67.5 per cent, 58.9 per cent, and 46.0 per cent respectively (Nishida *et al.* 1997). Nine patients with metastases at presentation died at a median time of 2 years 9 months after initial treatment. Metastases developed in 36 patients; 80 per cent of metastases occurred in the lung and about 30 per cent in the bones. Survival rates were better for patients who had localized extremity lesions and radical or wide procedures, and were younger than 40 years.

In conclusion, primary modalities for the treatment of malignant fibrous histiocytoma include preoperative chemotherapy and wide surgical resection when possible. Oncological reconstruction varies with the location. Amputation may be necessary to achieve a margin in large lesions with neurovascular involvement. Neoadjuvant chemotherapy is gradually becoming the standard of care for high-grade resectable lesions. Chemotherapy for metastatic disease is palliative, with variable response rates. Thoracotomy is useful in patients with lung metastasis. Radiation therapy has been effective in some surgically inaccessible lesions.

References

Bacci, G., Gherlinzoni, F., Picci, P., *et al.* (1996). Neoadjuvant chemotherapy (NC) for malignant fibrous histiocytoma of bone of the extremities (MFHe) (abstract). *Program/Proceedings of the American Society of Clinical Oncology*, **15**, 520.

Barney, P.L. (1972). Atypical fibrous histiocytoma (fibroxanthoma) of the temporal bone. *Transactions of the American Academy of Ophthalmology and Otolaryngology*, **76**, 1392–3.

Bayer Kristensen, I. and Myhre Jensen, O. (1984). Malignant fibrous histiocytoma of bone: a clinico-pathologic study of 9 cases. *Acta Pathologica, Microbiologica, et Immunologica Scandinavica, Section A, Pathology*, **92**, 205–10.

Bettelli, G., Avella, M., Capanna, R., *et al.* (1987). Neoadjuvant chemotherapy in malignant fibrous histiocytoma of the extremities. Preliminary results in 10 cases treated preoperatively with methotrexate and cisplatin. *Chirurgia degli Organi di Movimento*, **72**, 111–17.

Blitzer, A., Lawson, W., Zak, F.G., Biller, H.F., and Som, M.L. (1981). Clinical–pathological determinants in prognosis of fibrous histiocytomas of head and neck. *Laryngoscope*, **91**, 2053–70.

Boland, P.J. and Huvos, A.G. (1986). Malignant fibrous histiocytoma of bone. *Clinical Orthopaedics and Related Research*, **204**, 130–4.

Campanacci, M. (1990). *Bone and soft tissue tumors*, pp. 885–901. Springer-Verlag, Vienna.

Capanna, R., Bertoni, F., Bacchini, P., Bacci, G., Guerra, A., and Campanacci, M. (1984). Malignant fibrous histiocytoma of bone. The experience at the Rizzoli Institute: report of 90 cases. *Cancer*, **54**, 177–87.

Chen, K.T. (1978). Multiple fibroxanthosarcoma of bone. *Cancer*, **42**, 770–3.

Chitale, V.S., Sundaresan, N., Helson, L., and Huvos, A.G. (1981). Malignant fibrous histiocytoma of the temporal bone with intracranial extension. *Acta Neurochirurgica*, **59**, 239–46.

Dahlin, D.C. and Beabout, J.W. (1971). Dedifferentiation of low-grade chondrosarcomas. *Cancer*, **28**, 461–6.

Dahlin, D.C. and Unni, K.K. (1986). *Bone tumors: general aspects and data on 8,542 cases* (4th edn). Thomas, Springfield, IL.

Dahlin, D.C., Unni, K.K., and Matsuno, T. (1977). Malignant (fibrous) histiocytoma of bone—fact or fancy? *Cancer*, **39**, 1508–16.

Dorfman, H.D., Norman, A., and Wolff, H. (1966). Fibrosarcoma complicating bone infarction in a caisson worker: a case report. *Journal of Bone and Joint Surgery, American Volume*, **48A**, 528–32.

Dunham, W.K. and Wilborn, W.H. (1979). Malignant fibrous histiocytoma of bone: report of two cases and review of the literature. *Journal of Bone and Joint Surgery, American Volume*, **61A**, 939–42.

Enzinger, F.M. (1979). Angiomatoid malignant fibrous histiocytoma: a distinct fibrohistiocytic tumor of children and young adults simulating a vascular neoplasm. *Cancer*, **44**, 2147–57.

Feldman, F. and Lattes, R. (1977). Primary malignant fibrous histiocytoma (fibrous xanthoma) of bone. *Skeletal Radiology*, **1**, 145–60.

Feldman, F. and Norman, D. (1972). Intra- and extraosseous malignant histiocytoma (malignant fibrous xanthoma). *Radiology*, **104**, 497–508.

Finci, R., Gunhan, O., Ucmakli, E., and Sarlak, O. (1990). Multiple and familial malignant fibrous histiocytoma of bone: a report of two cases. *Journal of Bone and Joint Surgery, American Volume*, **72A**, 295–8.

Furey, J.G., Ferrer-Torells, M., and Reagan, J.W. (1960). Fibrosarcoma arising at the site of bone infarcts: a report of two cases. *Journal of Bone and Joint Surgery, American Volume*, **42A**, 802–10.

Ghandur-Mnaymneh, L., Zych, G., and Mnaymneh, W. (1982). Primary malignant fibrous histiocytoma of bone: report of six cases with ultrastructural study and analysis of the literature. *Cancer*, **49**, 698–707.

Han, M.T., Telander, R.L., Pairolero, P.C., *et al.* (1981). Aggressive thoracotomy for pulmonary metastatic osteogenic sarcoma in children and young adolescents. *Journal of Pediatric Surgery*, **16**, 928–33.

Hudson, T.M., Hawkins, I.F., Jr, Spanier, S.S., and Enneking, W.F. (1979). Angiography of malignant fibrous histiocytoma of bone. *Radiology*, **131**, 9–15.

Huvos, A.G. (1976). Primary malignant fibrous histiocytoma of bone: clinicopathologic study of 18 patients. *New York State Journal of Medicine*, **76**, 552–9.

Huvos, A.G. (1991). *Bone tumors: diagnosis, treatment, and prognosis* (2nd edn), pp. 497–521. W.B. Saunders, Philadelphia, PA.

Huvos, A.G., Heilweil, M., and Bretsky, S.S. (1985). The pathology of malignant fibrous histiocytoma of bone: a study of 130 patients. *American Journal of Surgical Pathology*, **9**, 853–71.

Huvos, A.G., Woodard, H.Q., and Heilweil, M. (1986). Postradiation malignant fibrous histiocytoma of bone: a clinicopathologic study of 20 patients. *American Journal of Surgical Pathology*, **10**, 9–18.

Inada, O., Yumoto, T., Furuse, K., and Tanaka, T. (1976). Ultrastructural features of malignant fibrous histiocytoma of bone. *Acta Pathologica Japonica*, **26**, 491–501.

Ishihara, T. (1984). Bilateral pneumonectomy in metastatic pulmonary tumors. *Nippon Geka Gakkai Zasshi*, **85**, 944–7.

Jacobs, R.L. and Fox, T.A. (1972). Neurilemoma of bone: a case report with a review of the literature. *Clinical Orthopaedics and Related Research*, **87**, 248–53.

Johnson, W.W., Coburn, T.P., Pratt, C.B., Smith, J.W., Kumar, A.P., and Dahlin, D.C. (1978). Ultrastructure of malignant histiocytoma arising in the acromion. *Human Pathology*, **9**, 199–209.

Kahn, L.B., Webber, B., Mills, E., Anstey, L., and Heselson, N.G. (1978). Malignant fibrous histiocytoma (malignant fibrous xanthoma: xanthosarcoma) of bone. *Cancer*, **42**, 640–51.

Katenkamp, D. and Stiller, D. (1981). Malignant fibrous histiocytoma of bone: light microscopic and electron microscopic examination of four cases. *Virchows Archiv. A. Pathological Anatomy and Histopathology*, **391**, 323–35.

Kessler, H.P., Callihan, M.D., and van der Waal, I. (1981). Case for diagnosis: malignant fibrous histiocytoma, left maxilla. *Military Medicine*, **146**, 193, 213–14.

Kyriakos, M. and Kempson, R.L. (1976). Inflammatory fibrous histiocytoma: an aggressive and lethal lesion. *Cancer*, **37**, 1584–1606.

Lopez-Barea, F., Rodriguez-Peralto, J.L., Burgos-Lizalde, E., Gonzalez-Lopez, J., and Sanchez-Herrera, S. (1991). Case report 639: malignant fibrous histiocytoma (MFH) of the patella. *Skeletal Radiology*, **20**, 125–8.

McCarthy, E.F., Matsuno, T., and Dorfman, H.D. (1979). Malignant fibrous histiocytoma of bone: a study of 35 cases. *Human Pathology*, **10**, 57–70.

Martinez-Tello, F.J., Navas-Palacios, J.J., Calvo-Asensio, M., and Loizaga-Iriondo, J.M. (1981). Malignant fibrous histiocytoma of bone: a clinicopathological and electronmicroscopical study. *Pathology, Research and Practice*, **173**, 141–58.

Michael, R.H. and Dorfman, H.D. (1976). Malignant fibrous histiocytoma associated with bone infarcts: report of a case. *Clinical Orthopaedics and Related Research*, **118**, 180–3.

Mirra, J.M. (1980). *Bone tumors: diagnosis and treatment*. J.B. Lippincott, Philadelphia, PA.

Mirra, J.M., Bullough, P.G., Marcove, R.C., Jacobs, B., and Huvos, A.G. (1974). Malignant fibrous histiocytoma and osteosarcoma in association with bone infarcts: report of four cases, two in caisson workers. *Journal of Bone and Joint Surgery, American Volume*, **56A**, 932–40.

Mirra, J.M., Gold, R.H., and Marafiote, R. (1977). Malignant (fibrous) histiocytoma arising in association with a bone infarct in sickle-cell disease: coincidence or cause-and-effect? *Cancer*, **39**, 186–94.

Nakashima, Y., Morishita, S., Kotoura, Y., *et al.* (1985). Malignant histiocytoma of bone: a review of 13 cases and an ultrastructural study. *Cancer*, **55**, 2804–11.

Newland, R.C., Harrison, M.A., and Wright, R.G. (1975). Fibroxanthosarcoma of bone. *Pathology*, **7**, 203–8.

Nishida, J., Sim, F.H., Wenger, D.E., and Unni, K.K. (1997). Malignant fibrous histiocytoma of bone: a clinicopathologic study of 81 patients. *Cancer*, **79**, 482–93.

Nunnery, E.W., Kahn, L.B., and Guilford, W.B. (1979). Locally aggressive fibrous histiocytoma of bone: a case report. *South African Medical Journal*, **55**, 763–7.

Paling, M.R. and Hyams, D.M. (1982). Computed tomography in malignant fibrous histiocytoma. *Journal of Computer Assisted Tomography*, **6**, 785–8.

Papagelopoulos, P.J., Galanis, E., Frassica, F.J., Sim, F.H., Larson, D.R., and Wold, L.E. (2000a). Primary fibrosarcoma of bone: outcome after primary surgical treatment. *Clinical Orthopaedics and Related Research*, **373**, 88–103.

Papagelopoulos, P.J., Galanis, E., Sim, F.H., and Unni, K.K. (2000b). Clinicopathologic features, diagnosis, and treatment of malignant fibrous histiocytoma of bone. *Orthopedics*, **23**, 59–65.

Poon, M.C., Durant, J.R., Norgard, M.J., and Chang-Poon, V.Y. (1982). Inflammatory fibrous histiocytoma: an important variant of malignant fibrous histiocytoma highly responsive to chemotherapy. *Annals of Internal Medicine*, **97**, 858–63.

Roessner, A., Hobik, H.P., and Grundmann, E. (1979). Malignant fibrous histiocytoma of bone and osteosarcoma: a comparative light and electron microscopic study. *Pathology, Research and Practice*, **164**, 385–401.

Ros, P.R., Viamonte, M., Jr, and Rywlin, A.M. (1984). Malignant fibrous histiocytoma: mesenchymal tumor of ubiquitous origin. *American Journal of Roentgenology*, **142**, 753–9.

Saito, R. and Caines, M.J. (1977). Atypical fibrous histiocytoma of the humerus: a light and electron microscopic study. *American Journal of Clinical Pathology*, **68**, 409–15.

Schajowicz, F. (1983). Current trends in the diagnosis and treatment of malignant bone tumors. *Clinical Orthopaedics and Related Research*, **180**, 220–52.

Schajowicz, F. (1994). *Tumors and tumor-like lesions of bones and joints*, pp. 427–38. Springer-Verlag, New York.

Shapiro, F. (1981). Malignant fibrous histiocytoma of bone: an ultrastructural study. *Ultrastructural Pathology*, **2**, 33.

Shuman, L.S., Chuang, V.P., Wallace, S., Benjamin, R.S., and Murray, J. (1982). Intra-arterial chemotherapy of malignant fibrous histiocytoma of the pelvis. *Radiology*, **142**, 343–6.

Spanier, S.S. (1977). Malignant fibrous histiocytoma of bone. *Orthopaedic Clinics of North America*, **8**, 947–61.

Spanier, S.S., Enneking, W.F., and Enriquez, P. (1975). Primary malignant fibrous histiocytoma of bone. *Cancer*, **36**, 2084–98.

Stout, A.P. and Lattes, R. (1967). Tumors of the soft tissues. In *Atlas of tumor pathology*, Second series, Fascicle 1, p. 38. Armed Forces Institute of Pathology, Washington, DC.

Sundaram, M. and McLeod, R.A. (1990). MR imaging of tumor and tumor-like lesions of bone and soft tissue. *American Journal of Roentgenology*, **155**, 817–24.

Taconis, W.K. and Mulder, J.D. (1984). Fibrosarcoma and malignant fibrous histiocytoma of long bones: radiographic features and grading. *Skeletal Radiology*, **11**, 237–45.

Taconis, W.K. and van Rijssel, T.G. (1985). Fibrosarcoma of long bones: a study of the significance of areas of malignant fibrous histiocytoma. *Journal of Bone and Joint Surgery, British Volume*, **67B**, 111–16.

Takechi, H. and Taguchi, K. (1978). Malignant fibrous histiocytoma with skeletal involvement. *Acta Medica Okayama*, **32**, 343–54.

Taxy, J. B. and Battifora, H. (1977). Malignant fibrous histiocytoma: an electron microscopic study. *Cancer*, **40**, 254–67.

Unni, K.K. (1996). *Dahlin's bone tumors: general aspects and data on 11,087 cases* (5th edn), p. 218. Lippincott–Raven, Philadelphia, PA.

von Hochstetter, A.R., Eberle, H., and Ruttner, J.R. (1984). Primary leiomyosarcoma of extragnathic bones: case report and review of literature. *Cancer*, **53**, 2194–200.

Ward, J.J., Thornbury, D.D., Lemons, J.E., and Dunham, W.K. (1990). Metal-induced sarcoma: a case report and literature review. *Clinical Orthopaedics and Related Research*, **252**, 299–306.

Weiner, M., Sedlis, M., Johnston, A.D., Dick, H.M., and Wolff, J.A. (1983). Adjuvant chemotherapy of malignant fibrous histiocytoma of bone. *Cancer*, **51**, 25–9.

Yuen, W.W. and Saw, D. (1985). Malignant fibrous histiocytoma of bone. *Journal of Bone and Joint Surgery, American Volume*, **67A**, 482–6.

Yumoto, T., Mori, Y., Inada, O., and Tanaka, T. (1976). Malignant fibrous histiocytoma of bone. *Acta Pathologica Japonica*, **26**, 295–309.

1.6.8.10 Chordoma

Kristy Weber and Franklin H. Sim

Introduction

Chordoma is an uncommon malignant bone tumor that occurs in the midline of the axial skeleton (Mindell 1981; Healey and Lane 1989). It arises primarily at the cephalad and caudad regions of the spine, with the remainder within the cervical, thoracic, and lumbar vertebral bodies. Sacrococcygeal lesions comprise 50 per cent,

Box 1

- Uncommon malignant bone tumors that arise primarily at the cephalad and caudad regions of the spine with the remainder in the cervical, thoracic, and lumbar vertebral bodies

- Develop from notochordal remnants and tissue resembles fetal notochord

- Differential diagnosis includes liposarcoma, metastatic carcinoma, and myxoid chondrosarcoma

- Usually present with pain and often cause neurologic deficits

- *En bloc* resection of the tumor with a wide margin offers the best chance of long survival, but wide resection is often not possible

spheno-occipital lesions 35 per cent, and the rest are spread along the vertebral column. Chordomas make up only 1 to 4 per cent of primary malignant bone tumors, but have an overall somber prognosis given their poorly accessible location and frequent delay in diagnosis. The vast majority of sacral lesions present in patients between 50 and 70 years of age and are extremely unlikely in those younger than 30. The lesions arising at the base of the skull present a decade earlier than their sacral counterparts as they have less space to grow before causing symptoms. The tumors are twice as common in men than women.

Chordomas are thought to arise from primitive notochordal remnants and are epithelial in origin. During skeletal development the notochord degenerates and remains as the nucleus pulposis component of the vertebral disk. It has been proposed that there is incomplete degeneration of the residual notochord and this tissue can become neoplastic. Interestingly, the tumor seems to arise from within the vertebral body and not directly from the nucleus pulposis.

Examples of chordomas are shown in Figs 1 and 2.

Pathology

On gross inspection a chordoma may be lobulated and deceptively well circumscribed, but the tumorous tissue often extends beyond visible boundaries. It is soft and gray, and has a gelatinous consistency. Translucent areas may give it the appearance of a chondrosarcoma or mucinous carcinoma. The tumor can be focally cystic or hemorrhagic. The periosteum of the affected bone may be elevated and a large soft-tissue mass is common (Fig. 3).

Microscopically the tissue resembles fetal notochord. Lobules are separated by fibrous septa (Fig. 4(a)). The abundant basophilic extracellular matrix contains mucin and stains positively for glycogen. The cells are arranged in cords rather than isolated in individual lacunae. Occasional islands of bone or cartilage are visible. On higher magnification, the cells can be seen to be of various sizes and shapes with indistinct boundaries. The different cell types present include a square nonvacuolated cell with a central round nucleus and eosinophilic cytoplasm. Another type has a single large vacuole giving it a signet ring appearance. The most classic type, called a physaliferous cell, has a round nucleus with multivacuolated cytoplasm giving it a bubbly appearance (Fig. 4(b)). The vacuoles may displace the nucleus to the periphery of the cell. In some chordomas there is extensive nuclear pleomorphism and occasional mitotic figures. However, no

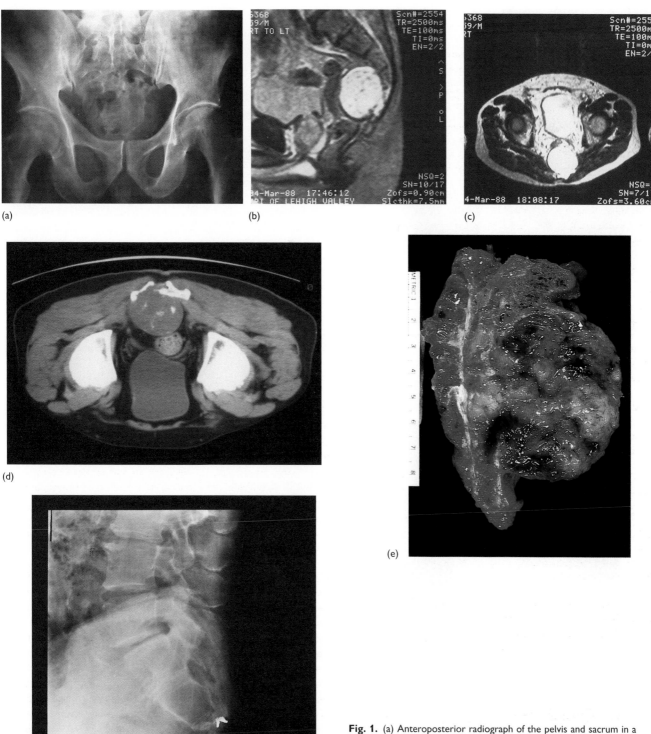

Fig. 1. (a) Anteroposterior radiograph of the pelvis and sacrum in a 59-year-old male. Overlying shadows make it difficult to see the destructive midline sacral lesion. (b), (c) Sagittal and axial T_2-weighted MRI reveals a large anterior soft-tissue mass extending from the sacrum and abutting the rectum. (d) A CT scan reveals the residual calcification present throughout the chordoma which is not appreciated on other imaging modalities. (e) Gross resected specimen shows the extensive anterior soft-tissue mass. (f) Postoperative lateral radiograph demonstrates the partial sacrectomy at the S2–3 level.

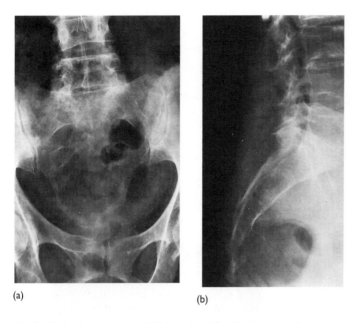

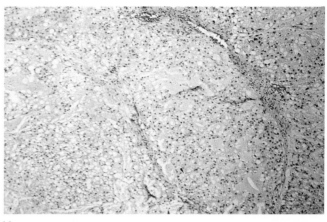

(a)

(a)   (b)

Fig. 2. (a) Anteroposterior and (b) lateral sacral radiographs reveal a more obvious sacral lytic lesion. Note how the sacral foramina caudal to S2 are obliterated.

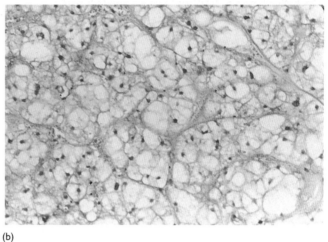

(b)

Fig. 4. (a) Low-power histologic appearance of a chordoma demonstrates lobules separated by fibrovascular connective tissue. (b) Higher-power magnification of classic bubbly physaliferous cells of various shapes and sizes.

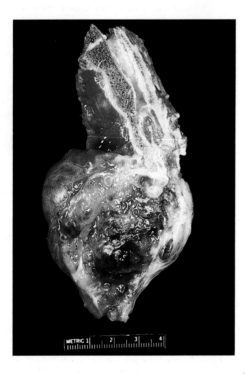

Fig. 3. Gross appearance of a resected chordoma in the coccyx and sacrum. Note the large anterior soft-tissue mass and smaller posterior mass. The chordoma extends proximally into the spinal canal, but the resected margins were negative for tumor.

compelling evidence has been found to correlate histologic features of a conventional chordoma with clinical prognosis or the ability to metastasize. Immunohistochemical stains show the chordoma to be positive for cytokeratin and epithelial membrane antigen, supporting its epithelial origin.

Two histologic variants of chordoma have been described. The first is a chondroid chordoma, found almost exclusively in the spheno-occipital region and named for its similarity to a cartilage neoplasm. Twenty-five to thirty per cent of the intracranial type of chordoma demonstrate areas resembling hyaline cartilage. The cells reside in lacunae, and the stroma is extensive and basophilic. However, immunohistochemical and ultrastructural studies have confirmed that the epithelial nature of these areas is consistent with conventional chordomas and not chondrosarcomas. The chondroid variant stains strongly for cytokeratin and epithelial membrane antigen and has visible desmosomes and tonofilaments on electron microscopy studies. It is important to examine any tissue having a cartilaginous appearance with these tests in order to make an accurate diagnosis. Otherwise, if the chondroid component is dominant, the lesion may be misdiagnosed as a skull-base chondrosarcoma. Patients having the chondroid variant of chordoma were thought to have a prolonged survival in the initial description given in 1973. That finding has not been confirmed, and more recent work shows that the long-term outcome is consistent with that of patients having a conventional chordoma (Jeffrey *et al.* 1995). The original study may have included low-grade chondrosarcoma of the skull base which does confer a more prolonged survival. It has been proposed that these variants, with features resembling cartilage but having an epithelial phenotype, be called hyalinized chordomas.

The second variant is a dedifferentiated chordoma, although it is unlikely to have actually dedifferentiated from endstage chordoma cells. It probably stems from a failure of differentiation by primitive cell types so that the neoplastic cells are capable of differentiation to either epithelial or mesenchymal phenotypes. Whereas the chondroid variant occurs in the bones of the skull base, the dedifferentiated type is found almost exclusively in the sacrococcygeal region. It is a rare biphasic lesion where a high-grade sarcoma, usually malignant fibrous histiocytoma, occurs in direct association with a conventional chordoma. Flow cytometry studies demonstrate an increased aneuploid–multiploid DNA content in these variants. The sarcoma has predominantly mesenchymal features. It is not found at initial presentation, but rather after multiple recurrences of a chordoma. Dedifferentiated chordomas have been reported to occur with and without prior irradiation used to treat a conventional chordoma.

The notochord has a dual ectodermal and mesenchymal origin, which may explain why some chordomas have a cartilaginous appearance and why the differentiated type has a mesenchymal spindle cell component.

The differential diagnosis of chordoma includes liposarcoma, metastatic carcinoma, and myxoid chondrosarcoma. The vacuolated cytoplasm of chordoma cells may be mistaken for lipoblasts; however, the presence of physaliferous cells and overall lobular pattern should help to differentiate it from liposarcoma. Differential mucin staining may also be helpful. In addition, fat stains will be positive and epithelial markers negative in adipose tumors. The reverse is true of chordomas. Glands are not present in chordomas; therefore they should be differentiated from carcinomas. Metastatic lesions do not have physaliferous cells. A myxoid chondrosarcoma may be the most difficult lesion to separate from chordoma histologically as both are lobular with cord-like cell arrangements and myxoid stroma, but the chondrosarcoma contains no physaliferous cells and is generally less pleomorphic. Although both types stain positively for S-100 protein, only chordoma is positive for epithelial markers. In addition, myxoid chondrosarcomas are rare in the axial skeleton.

Clinical

Signs and symptoms depend on the location of the chordoma. It is slow growing but relentless in its destruction of surrounding bone. Usually symptoms have been present for more than a year before a diagnosis is made. By that time, the lesions can be quite large. Chordomas at the skull base cause primarily impairment of the sixth, seventh, and eighth cranial nerves. Visual disturbances, headaches, and endocrine dysfunction from involvement of the pituitary gland are common. An anterior soft-tissue mass in the spheno-occipital region may cause breathing difficulties or dysphagia. A posterior mass may affect neurologic function.

Vertebral chordomas cause symptoms as a result of pressure on nerve roots or the spinal cord. Patients may have numbness in an extremity followed by pain. Many develop motor weakness, but paralysis is a late complication.

Sacrococcygeal lesions have room to become even larger before discovery and may be associated with a long history of vague lower back pain. This may be referred to the hip or knee with further neoplastic progression. The mass usually displaces but does not invade the rectum, and may cause constipation. Bladder symptoms such as urinary frequency are common, with incontinence a late finding. If the chordoma originates caudal to the S1 level, there is rarely any sensorimotor disturbance to the lower extremities. Late in the course, pain may become severe and intractable. For sacral lesions, a firm fixed presacral mass is usually palpable on rectal examination.

Imaging

Whether occurring in the sacrum or clivus, the plain radiographic hallmark of a chordoma is midline bony destruction with a large associated soft-tissue mass. The anterolateral mass is usually more extensive than the bony involvement. The lesions are poorly marginated and may be difficult to discern in the sacrococcygeal region. The intracranial type may destroy the sella turcica and invade the petrous and sphenoid bones. Fourteen to fifty per cent, usually in the nonchondroid intracranial type, have been noted to have focal areas of calcification. The recurrent forms of chordoma often infiltrate adjacent anatomic structures. In the vertebral body, the chordoma is lytic, centrally located, and slowly expansile. Areas of sclerosis due to reactive bone formation are seen. Adjacent vertebral bodies and the intervening disk space can be involved.

Reports vary as to the activity of a chordoma on bone scan, and accumulation of isotope in the bladder can obscure the sacral area. CT scans and MRI have been extremely helpful in determining the extent of the lesion and its proximity to vital structures. This is essential in preoperative planning. CT scans can identify calcified areas not evident on plain films. Along with myelography it is helpful in planning resection of a vertebral lesion. MRI is useful in discovering recurrent nodules after surgical resection. Angiography is only occasionally indicated to identify the proximity of a cervical chordoma to the vertebral arteries.

The radiographic differential diagnosis includes metastatic disease, multiple myeloma, giant cell tumor, and neurogenic tumors.

Management

After discovering a midline destructive lesion thought to be a chordoma, a biopsy should be done after all staging studies are completed. A posterior needle biopsy can be performed if the surgeon is experienced and comfortable with this technique, but most biopsies are done through an open posterior approach. Under no circumstances should a transrectal biopsy be performed, owing to contamination of intervening tissue planes. Usually the definitive resection should wait until a final pathologic diagnosis is made.

The mainstay of treatment and best hope for long-term survival is *en bloc* resection of the tumor with a wide margin and a surrounding cuff of normal tissue. This is more likely in sacrococcygeal lesions as the anatomy of the skull base often precludes complete excision. The following management will refer primarily to vertebral and sacral lesions, and the reader is referred to the literature for further details on treatment of spheno-occipital chordomas. The sacral nerve roots should be sacrificed if necessary to obtain an adequate margin. Given the large size, poorly accessible location, and tendency to adhere to the bowel, a wide margin is difficult to achieve, and so a marginal resection is often the best that can be done. There is a high recurrence rate with inadequate resection, and recurrent lesions carry a poor prognosis as they often infiltrate the surrounding tissues. Adjuvant radiation therapy, although not curative in itself, is often used in recurrent lesions or in cases where complete removal is not possible.

Preoperatively, a complete bowel preparation and intravenous antibiotic prophylaxis should be performed to decrease the chance of wound infection. Intraoperatively the anus should be sutured to prevent possible fecal contamination of the surgical field. The wound is only closed primarily if this can be done without undue tension. Some advocate leaving the wound packed open until the edges are able to be closed at a later date, while others perform immediate flap closure. The operative time can be prolonged with difficult resections; therefore attention to blood loss is critical. Greater loss from the middle sacral vessels and branches of the internal iliac veins can be expected in higher sacral lesions. Postoperatively, antibiotic as well as deep venous thrombosis prophylaxis is necessary.

In general, lesions below the third sacral level are approached posteriorly. Lesions more cephalad often need a combined anterior and posterior approach in the same operative setting. For high sacral lesions, a complete lumbosacral resection including plans for a colostomy should be anticipated. Surgical resection in this location is associated with high morbidity. Full sacral resection can be performed when necessary to achieve a wide margin. Current advances in skeletal reconstruction can maintain stability after extensive resections.

Thoracic lesions should be approached via thoracotomy, although combined anterior–posterior reconstruction and stabilization is often required after vertebral body excision. A retroperitoneal approach is usually adequate for middle to lower lumbar lesions.

Results

In general the results for long-term survival depend on the adequacy of the initial surgical resection. Many studies have shown increased rates of recurrence with intralesional margins compared with wide excision. One report showed an increase in recurrence rate from 28 per cent after *en bloc* resection of a chordoma to 64 per cent if the tumor was exposed during resection (Kaiser *et al.* 1984).

Chordomas are generally radio-resistant, but adjuvant treatment has been utilized for contaminated surgical margins or surgically inaccessible lesions. Given the increased recurrence rate of large lesions, attention has focused on new pre- and postoperative irradiation approaches to improve the chance of adequate surgical margins. There have been reports of increased disease-free intervals with irradiation, as well as contradictory findings that the adjuvant therapy has no effect. The real value of radiation therapy needs to be addressed in a well-designed prospective study, which is difficult given the rarity of this tumor. The amount of irradiation is limited by the sensitivity of the spinal cord in the cranial and cervical regions, and by the pelvic organs, colon, rectum, and overlying sacral skin in more caudal lesions. To facilitate the use of high local radiation doses without structural damage, proton-beam and photon-beam radiation techniques have been successful, but their long-term effectiveness is yet to be established. Wound-healing problems contribute to high morbidity after radiation therapy. In addition, there have been reports of post-irradiation high-grade sarcomas after treatment of a chordoma. Although this is a rare occurrence, thought should be given before routinely prescribing radiation therapy to all patients with this tumor.

Cryotherapy has been utilized to treat small numbers of patients with a chordoma. Anecdotal results are good, but complications of treatment include a high chance of infection spreading to the locally frozen bone and postoperative bladder dysfunction. Chemotherapy has no current role in the management of chordoma.

Function after surgery depends on the level of resection and the remaining sacral roots. If the S1 level is preserved, loss of motor function is minimal. Stener and Gunterberg (1978) reported on extirpation of high sacral tumors and believe that no deficit of urogenital or anorectal function occurs if there is only unilateral sacrifice of all sacral nerves. If only the first sacral roots are preserved, no sphincter control will remain, and the patient will need routine bladder self-catheterization. If bilateral S2 roots are maintained, up to 50 per cent may retain partial bowel and bladder control with need for catheterization. If at least one S3 root is saved, sphincter control will most likely be retained. If the tumor goes untreated, 100 per cent of patients will eventually have complete incontinence. It is important to try and preserve the pudendal nerve, if possible, in order to maintain continence. A cadaver study showed that adequate pelvic stability can be retained as long as half the first sacral body is left intact.

Chordomas with chondroid differentiation have the same prognosis as that of conventional chordomas. The dedifferentiated variant is quickly fatal, with the metastatic lesions often comprised of the sarcomatous pattern.

A recent study looked at 21 cases of sacrococcygeal chordoma (Samson *et al.* 1993). All lesions were approached posteriorly and 14 had adjuvant radiotherapy. Four patients died and 15 of the remaining 17 were disease free at average 4.5-year follow-up. There was a 19 per cent local recurrence rate which compares well with the available literature, especially as a combined operative approach was not used. It was suggested that pre- or postoperative radiation therapy may have allowed a better result with a marginal resection. There was a 5 per cent incidence of metastases at 5 years which increased to 50 per cent at 10 years.

In a study of the Mayo Clinic experience, 47 patients who had sacrococcygeal chordomas with a 9-year average follow-up were reviewed (Choudhury *et al.* 1995). Eighty-one per cent were approached posteriorly and only 19 per cent were resected with a wide margin. Fifty-two per cent received adjuvant postoperative irradiation. The cumulative probability of local recurrence was 51 per cent at 5 years and 75 per cent at 10 years. When the lesion extended to the S1 level, there was 100 per cent recurrence in seven cases. There was a 24 per cent probability of metastases at 5 years and 58 per cent at 10 years. All but one patient with distal metastases also had local recurrence.

Chordomas are known to metastasize late, with the likelihood ranging from 5 to 40 per cent in the literature. They can be found from 1 to 16 years after initial diagnosis. This finding is limited to sacral or, less likely, vertebral chordomas, as the intracranial types rarely metastasize. Accurate prediction of which tumors will metastasize is not yet possible. The spread is to the regional lymph nodes as well as to skin, lung, liver, and bone. Almost all patients die as a result of complications from local treatment failure rather than metastases, which are commonly asymptomatic. Studies show 5- and 10-year survival of patients with chordoma to be 45 to 77 per cent and 28 to 50 per cent respectively.

Further reading

Amendola, B., Amendola, M., Oliver, E., and McClatchey, K. (1986). Chordoma: role of radiation therapy. *Radiology*, **158**, 839–43.

Arbit, E. and Patterson, R. (1981). Combined transoral and median labiomandibular glossotomy approach to the upper cervical spine. *Neurosurgery*, **8**, 672–4.

Bjornsson, J., Wold, L., Ebersold, M., and Laws, E. (1993). Chordoma of the mobile spine; a clinicopathologic analysis of 40 patients. *Cancer*, **71**, 735–40.

Chambers, P. and Schwinn, C. (1979). Chordoma: a clinicopathologic study of metastasis. *American Journal of Clinical Pathology*, **72**, 765–76.

Cody, H., Marcove, R., and Quan, S. (1981). Malignant retrorectal tumors: 28 years' experience at Memorial Sloan-Kettering Cancer Center. *Diseases of the Colon and Rectum*, **24**, 501–6.

Cummings, B., Hodson, D., and Bush, R. (1983). Chordoma: the results of megavoltage radiation therapy. *International Journal of Radiation Oncology, Biology and Physics*, **9**, 633–42.

de Vries, J., Oldhoff, J., and Hadders, H. (1986). Cryosurgical treatment of sacrococcygeal chordoma: report of four cases. *Cancer*, **58**, 2348–54.

Fechner, R. and Mills, S. (1993). *Atlas of tumor pathology. Tumors of the bones and joints* (3rd series). AFIP, Washington, DC.

Gay, E., Sekhar, L., Rubinstein, E., et al. (1995). Chordomas and chondrosarcomas of the cranial base: results and follow-up of 60 patients. *Neurosurgery*, **36**, 87–896.

Gunterberg, B., Romanus, B., and Stener, B. (1976). Pelvic strength after major amputation of the sacrum: an experimental study. *Acta Orthopaedica Scandinavica*, **47**, 635–642.

Heffelfinger, M., Dahlin, D., MacCarty, C., and Beabout, J. (1973). Chordomas and cartilaginous tumors at the skull base. *Cancer*, **32**, 410–20.

Hruban, R., Traganos, F., Reuter, V., and Huvos, A. (1990). Chordomas with malignant spindle cell components: a DNA flow cytometric and immunohistochemical study with histogenetic implications. *American Journal of Pathology*, **137**, 435–47.

Karakousis, C. (1986). Sacral resection with preservation of continence. *Surgery, Gynecology and Obstetrics*, **163**, 271–3.

Klekamp, J. and Samii, M. (1996). Spinal chordomas—results of treatment over a 17-year period. *Acta Neurochirurgica*, **138**, 514–19.

MacCarty, C., Waugh, J., Mayo, C., and Coventry, M. (1952). The surgical treatment of presacral tumors: a combined problem. *Mayo Clinic Proceedings*, **27**, 73–84.

McCarthy, E. (1996). *Differential diagnosis in pathology: bone and joint disorders*. Igaku-Shoin, New York.

Meis, J., Raymond, A., Evans, H., Charles, R., and Giraldo, A. (1987). 'Dedifferentiated' chordoma: a clinicopathologic and immunohistochemical study of three cases. *American Journal of Surgical Pathology*, **11**, 516–25.

Rich, T., Schiller, A., Suit, H., and Mankin, H. (1985). Clinical and pathologic review of 48 cases of chordoma. *Cancer*, **56**, 182–7.

Romero, J., Cardenes, H., la Torre, A., et al. (1993). Chordoma: results of radiation therapy in eighteen patients. *Radiotherapy and Oncology*, **29**, 27–32.

Schajowicz, F. (1994). *Tumors and tumorlike lesions of bone* (2nd edn). Springer-Verlag, Berlin.

Schoenthaler, R., Castro, J., Petti, P., Baken-Brown, K., and Phillips, T. (1993). Charged particle irradiation of sacral chordomas. *International Journal of Radiation Oncology, Biology and Physics*, **26**, 291–8.

Simpson, A., Porter, A., Davis, A., Griffin, A., McLeod, R., and Bell, R. (1995). Cephalad sacral resection with a combined extended ilioinguinal and posterior approach. *Journal of Bone and Joint Surgery, American Volume*, **77A**, 405–11.

Smith, J., Ludwig, R., and Marcove, R. (1987). Sacrococcygeal chordoma: a clinicoradiological study of 60 patients. *Skeletal Radiology*, **16**, 37–44.

Stener, B. (1984). Musculoskeletal tumor surgery in Goteborg. *Clinical Orthopaedics and Related Research*, **191**, 8–20.

Stener, B. (1989). Complete removal of vertebrae for extirpation of tumors. *Clinical Orthopaedics and Related Research*, **245**, 72–82.

Suit, H., Goitein, M., Munzenrider, J., et al. (1982). Definitive radiation therapy for chordoma and chondrosarcoma of base of skull and cervical spine. *Journal of Neurosurgery*, **56**, 377–85.

Sundaresan, N., Huvos, A., Krol, G., Lane, J., and Brennan, M. (1987). Surgical treatment of spinal chordomas. *Archives of Surgery*, **122**, 1479–82.

Sung, H., Shu, W., Wang, H., Yuai, S., and Tsai, Y. (1987). Surgical treatment of primary tumors of the sacrum. *Clinical Orthopaedics and Related Research*, **215**, 91–8.

Wojno, K., Hruban, R., Garin-Chesa, P., and Huvos, A. (1992). Chondroid chordomas and low-grade chondrosarcomas of the craniospinal axis: an immunohistochemical analysis of 17 cases. *American Journal of Surgical Pathology*, **16**, 1144–52.

References

Choudhury, S., Emmanuel, R., Unni, K., and Rock, M. (1995). Treatment of sacrococcygeal chordoma: a review of 47 cases. Presented at the AAOS Meeting, 16 February 1995, Orlando, FL.

Healey, J. and Lane, J. (1989). Chordoma: a critical review of diagnosis and treatment. *Orthopedic Clinics of North America*, **20**, 417–26.

Jeffrey, P., Biava, C., and Davis, R. (1995). Chondroid chordoma: a hyalinized chordoma without cartilaginous differentiation. *American Journal of Clinical Pathology*, **103**, 271–9.

Kaiser, T., Pritchard, D., and Unni, K. (1984). Clinicopathologic study of sacrococcygeal chordoma. *Cancer*, **53**, 2574–8.

Mindell, E. (1981). Chordoma. *Journal of Bone and Joint Surgery, American Volume*, **63A**, 501–5.

Samson, I., Springfield, D., Suit, H., and Mankin, H. (1993). Operative treatment of sacrococcygeal chordoma. *Journal of Bone and Joint Surgery, American Volume*, **75A**, 1476–84.

Stener, B. and Gunterberg, B. (1978). High amputation of the sacrum for extirpation of tumors: principles and technique. *Spine*, **3**, 351–66.

1.6.9 Malignant soft-tissue neoplasms

1.6.9.1 Liposarcoma

Peter Choong

Introduction

The major neoplastic cell population in liposarcoma is reminiscent of lipomatous tissue. Its biological behavior closely reflects the various histological subtypes and the natural history is one of greater local and systemic aggressiveness in higher-grade lesions.

Epidemiology

Liposarcoma is the second most common soft-tissue malignancy with an incidence of 20 per cent (Chang *et al.* 1990). The incidence has decreased in comparison with earlier reports because of the reclassification of many tumors as malignant fibrous histiocytoma. The peak incidence of liposarcoma is between the sixth and seventh decades and there is a predominance of male patients (Reszel *et al.* 1966). It is rare in infants and small children, and the majority of lipomatous tumors probably represent benign lipoblastomas or lipoblastomatosis. Retroperitoneal liposarcomas appear to arise in an older age group as compared to extremity sarcomas, but this may reflect a longer delay between onset and detection of the retroperitoneal tumors.

Despite its name, liposarcoma does not necessarily arise from or in fatty tissue. The presence of adipocytes is not mandatory for the development of this tumor. The majority of tumors are found beneath the deep fascia where the amount of adipose tissue is considerably less than in the subcutaneous tissue. The position of liposarcomas in intermuscular planes further emphasize the nonfat origin of this tumor. The lower extremity and trunk are the most common sites for this tumor. The majority occur in the thigh. Other less common sites include the spermatic cord and scrotum, head and neck, and the hands and feet. Liposarcomas are also distinctive by their size, which may reach extremely large dimensions (Enzinger

and Weiss 1995). In general, the median diameter for liposarcomas is around 10 cm.

Pathology

The hallmark of liposarcoma is the lipoblast (Fig. 1) which is a primitive mesenchymal cell that reflects a commitment along the pathway of fat differentiation. Lipoblasts may be identified by the expression of aP2 protein which is detectable immunohistochemically and is therefore useful for differentiating benign and malignant lipomatous tumors, and also for distinguishing liposarcomas from other malignant mesenchymal and epithelial neoplasms (Bennet *et al.* 1995). Like most other sarcomas, it tends to be well circumscribed, encapsulated, and exhibits a lobulated pattern. Its appearance on cut section depends on the proportions of mucin, lipid, and fibrosis that are present.

Well-differentiated liposarcomas are very-low-grade malignancies which recur but do not metastasize. The term atypical lipoma has been advocated for subcutaneous tumors of this variety, because they can be controlled without radical surgery or adjuvant radiotherapy, and this label spares the patient a diagnosis of malignancy (Evans *et al.* 1979; Kindblom *et al.* 1982). The intramuscular or deep lesions retain the name well-differentiated liposarcoma because they are more likely to recur and therefore require more aggressive local therapy than their subcutaneous counterparts.

There is also a well-differentiated variant that has been subclassified into lipoma-like, sclerosing, and inflammatory variants. The

Box 2 Features of liposarcoma

- Lipoblast primitive mesenchymal
- aP2 protein on malignant liposarcoma
- Well-circumscribed, encapsulated

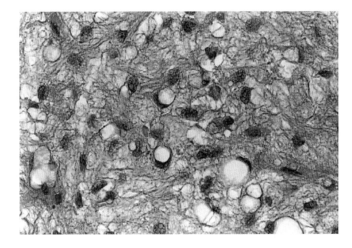

Fig. 1. The lipoblast is characterized by a plump mesenchymal cell with an eccentric nucleus that is compressed to the periphery of the cell by a large lipid globule.

Box 1

- Malignant soft-tissue tumors formed by lipoblasts
- Do not necessarily arise from or in fatty tissue
- Histologic types include well-differentiated liposarcomas, myxoid liposarcomas, round cell liposarcomas, dedifferentiated liposarcomas, and pleomorphic liposarcomas
- Prognosis associated with degree of differentiation and histologic type
- Current treatment includes wide surgical resection when possible and radiation therapy in selected patients

Box 3 Atypical liposarcoma

- Low-grade malignancy
- Subcutaneous
- May recur
- Does not metastasize

Box 5 Myxoid liposarcoma

- Most common
- Low grade
- Myxoid matrix
- Prognosis good
- Translocation of chromosome 12 and 16 is characteristic

lipoma-like liposarcoma closely mimics lipoma but the presence of lipoblasts containing atypical hyperchromatic nuclei and intracellular fat droplets differentiate this lesion from the benign lipoma. Intermingled with the lipoblasts are bands of spindle-shaped cells which form septae that separate the fat into lobules, and which can be recognized on CT scans.

The inflammatory variant of well-differentiated liposarcoma is characterized by an inflammatory infiltrate in addition to the scattered populations of lipoblasts. Lymphocytes and plasma cells are the predominant inflammatory component to the infiltrate.

Well-differentiated sclerosing liposarcomas are more often found in the groin and retroperitoneal than the extremity. As its name suggests, this tumor is characterized by prominent bands of fibrous tissue of varying density.

Characteristic chromosomal abnormalities have been detected in well-differentiated lipomas (Limon *et al.* 1986) and include rod-shaped and ring chromosomal aberrations. All may have rod- and ring-shaped chromosome abnormalities.

Myxoid liposarcoma is the most common histologic subtype and is generally regarded as low grade. The prognosis of this tumor is good although mortality from metastatic disease still occurs. The characteristic features of this tumor include different combinations of proliferating lipoblasts, plexiform capillary networks, and a distinct myxoid matrix which contains abundant nonprotein linked and non-sulfated glycosaminoglycans and hyaluronidase-sensitive muco-polysaccharides. In rare cases, less differentiated myxoid liposarcomas may have minimal distinguishing features as to be classified as malignant mesenchymomas. In contrast, the abundance of lipid within lipoblasts may be such that the lipoblasts appear signet ring-like leading to a misdiagnosis of well-differentiated liposarcoma.

Myxoid liposarcomas have few mitoses and little necrosis. With an increase in biological aggressiveness, these tumors may show an increase in spindle cells and a fascicular or storiform growth pattern signifying dedifferentiation (Fig. 2).

In the myxoid liposarcoma, a reciprocal translocation of chromosomes 12 and 16, t(12;16)(q13;p11), has been identified in 90 per cent of cases which is not present in any other subtype of liposarcoma or myxoid sarcoma (Sreekantaiah *et al.* 1992). This latter abnormality places it amongst the more important diagnostic markers in soft-

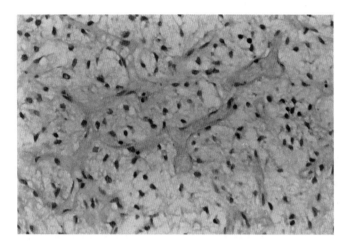

Fig. 2. Myxoid liposarcoma is dominated by a myxoid matrix with an arborizing pattern of capillaries.

tissue sarcomas and may have an etiologic role in the development of liposarcoma. In this regard, a liposarcoma tumor-specific fusion protein (*FUS-CHOP*) is produced as a result of the t(12;16) translocation (Rabbitts *et al.* 1993).

Round cell liposarcoma is a well-described but uncommon variant of liposarcoma typically associated with poor survival. It is characterized by an abundance of proliferating small round cells with vesicular nuclei (Fig. 3). The arborizing vascular pattern which is prominent

Box 4 Classification of well-differentiated liposarcoma

- Lipoma like—hyperchromatic nuclei
- Sclerosing—fibrous bands
- Inflammatory—inflammatory infiltrate

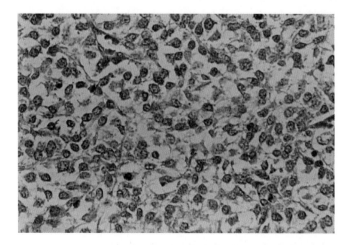

Fig. 3. Round cell liposarcoma is characterized by an abundance of small round cells with vesicular nuclei.

in myxoid liposarcoma is usually obscured by the cellular proliferation and lipoblasts are scanty. Tumor cells which are usually scattered in a haphazard array occasionally arrange themselves into cords or rows giving a trabecular pattern.

There is often a mixture of features which suggest a transition between myxoid and round cell liposarcoma. This characteristic, in association with the poorer survival of round cell liposarcoma, is the basis for the proposal that round cell liposarcoma be regarded as the poorly differentiated and thus, more aggressive form of myxoid liposarcoma (Evans 1979). Adding further support to this relationship, recent cytogenetic studies have demonstrated a recurrent nonrandom chromosomal translocation, t(12;16)(q13;p11), present in both myxoid and round cell liposarcoma (Knight *et al.* 1995). Recently, the proportion of round cells in myxoid liposarcoma was noted to correlate with clinical outcome. Tumors containing less than 25 per cent round cells were associated with better metastasis-free survival than those with a greater proportion of round cells (Kilpatrick *et al.* 1995). The phenotypic differences between myxoid liposarcoma and round cell liposarcoma may be induced by extrinsic factors or gene mutations unrelated to this typical translocation (Knight *et al.* 1995).

Pleomorphic liposarcomas are characterized by cellular pleomorphism, a disordered growth pattern, and variations in the content of tumor cell lipid (Fig. 4). The latter feature differentiates two subtypes of pleomorphic liposarcoma. The more common form accounts for 10 per cent of all liposarcomas and consists of clumps of giant lipoblasts with highly irregular nuclei, hyperchromasia, and a deeply acidophilic cytoplasm. Such histologic features can make differentiation from malignant fibrous histiocytoma difficult. The less

common variant of pleomorphic liposarcoma consists of numerous giant lipoblasts containing multiple lipid droplets which give these cells a mulberry appearance. The nuclei which are hyperchromatic are large and irregular. Both subtypes are associated with prominent mitoses and necrosis.

Dedifferentiated liposarcoma, like other dedifferentiated tumors, is characterized by the coexistence of well-differentiated and poorly differentiated components. Dedifferentiation which accounts for about 10 per cent of cases may be noted in the primary tumor or in local or distant recurrences (Weiss and Rao 1992). Malignant fibrous histiocytoma is the most common appearance of the dedifferentiated component.

A further variant, spindle cell liposarcoma, was recently described by Dei *et al.* (1994). This tumor is recognized by a prominent spindle cell component and is found around the shoulder girdle or upper limb of adults. Unlike other liposarcomas it is most commonly found in the subcutaneous tissue and is associated with multiple recurrences.

Lipsarcoma arising from pre-existing lipomas has been reported (Snover *et al.* 1982) although this is extremely rare. The common variability of subtypes within lipomas, for example spindle cell, pleomorphic, and focal myxoid variants, may be the cause for misinterpretation of benign lesions as having incipient sarcomatous foci. Trauma has also been implicated as a possible etiologic agent. The evidence for this, however, remains inconclusive. Radiation treatment has also been associated with the development of liposarcoma although this is uncommon (Arbabi and Warhol 1982).

Benign lesions that contain significant quantities of myxoid substance or lipid may be confused with well-differentiated liposarcoma. Examples of these include the different varieties of lipoma and myxomas. Malignant tumors that may mimic liposarcoma include malignant fibrous histiocytoma, myxoid chondrosarcoma, embryonal rhabdomyosarcoma, 'signet ring' lymphoma, and occasionally carcinoma.

Clinical evaluation

Liposarcomas have a rather insidious history, and present after the deep-seated mass has reached a large size. At that time, pressure symptoms and a mass effect herald its appearance. Liposarcomas are deep-seated tumors that have a propensity to arise from the

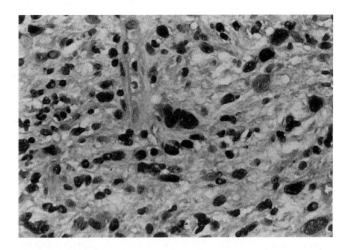

Fig. 4. Pleomorphic liposarcoma is characterized by bizarre pleomorphic cells with hyperchromatic nuclei and multiple mitoses. There is a variable amount of tumor cell lipid.

Box 8 **Dedifferentiated liposarcoma**

- 10 per cent of cases
- Occurs in primary metastases
- Looks like malignant fibrous histiocytoma

retroperitoneum and the lower extremity. Liposarcomas occurred in 11 of 50 cases reported by Gustafson (1994).

Retroperitoneal tumors often predipose to significant complications such as inferior vena cava obstruction with accompanying bilateral lower limb edema, ureteric obstruction with hydronephrosis and pyelonephritis, and subacute bowel obstruction with nausea, vomiting, constipation, or overflow diarrhea.

The lower extremity and trunk are the most common sites for this tumor. The majority occur in the thigh. Other less common sites include the spermatic cord and scrotum, head and neck, and the hands and feet. The size of liposarcomas may vary considerably, but generally they appear to be large. The majority of tumors present between 5 and 15 cm and extremely large retroperitoneal tumors have been reported.

Imaging

Plain radiographs may demonstrate a mass effect with increasing soft-tissue density and displacement of tissue planes. CT and MRI are good modalities for demonstrating the size, extent, and relationship of the lesion with surrounding vital structures. If a histologic diagnosis of liposarcoma is known, CT and MRI may be able to distinguish well-differentiated liposarcomas from other subtypes because of the predominantly fat component and thick fibrous septa of the former and the increasing heterogeneity of myxoid, round cell, and pleomorphic variants (Jelinek et al. 1993). However, these modalities are currently unable to differentiate between histologic types of sarcoma and if used alone, may not even be able to differentiate benign from malignant tumors. Staging with radio-isotope scans, plain radiographs, and CT scans of the chest are mandatory.

Management

Surgery alone or in combination with radiotherapy is the current treatment of choice. Most liposarcomas appear to be radiation sensitive; therefore this modality may be attractive preoperatively for reducing tumor size or postoperatively to prevent recurrence (Salvadori et al. 1986). Although, sporadic reports provide encouraging data to suggest that chemotherapy may have a role in the man-

agement of liposarcoma, the efficacy of chemotherapy in soft-tissue sarcomas remains unconfirmed. Bui et al. (1984) reported an increase in tumor differentiation and clinical response after induction chemotherapy in two patients. Patel et al. (1994) found a 44 per cent objective response by myxoid liposarcoma to a doxorubicin and dicarbazine-based regiment.

The treatment of well-differentiated liposarcoma or so-called 'atypical lipomas' is somewhat controversial. Simple excision of such tumors often results in poor local control (approximately 50 per cent). These tumors do not metastasize, suggesting that multiple limited excisions may be adequate for controlling this disease with only limited loss of function, in comparison to a single extensive resection. Local recurrence may be associated with an increase in tumor grade and/or dedifferentiation with the attendent risks that this carries (Hashimoto and Enjoji 1982).

Results of treatment

The overall 5-year survival of extremity liposarcoma is approximately over 50 per cent, while that for retroperitoneal lesions is significantly less than 50 per cent. The lung is the primary site for metastases and myxoid liposarcomas have the curious tendency to metastasize to the serosal surfaces of the pleura, pericardium, and diaphragm. In addition, Gustafson (1994) found that myxoid liposarcomas more commonly metastasized to soft-tissue areas other than the lung. Lymph node metastases are rare and are seen during the terminal stages of the disease.

The metastatic rate is closely linked with the differentiation of the tumor. The well-differentiated varieties are less likely to metastasize, while up to 50 per cent of the pleomorphic subtype do (Kindblom et al. 1975; Evans 1979). The histological type is an important prognostic factor with myxoid and well-differentiated liposarcomas having a more favorable outcome (70 per cent 5-year survival) than the pleomorphic or round cell variants (50 per cent 5-year survival).

Kilpatrick et al. (1996) reported that the extent of the round cell component in myxoid liposarcomas was a strongly unfavorable prognostic factor. Gustafson (1994) also showed that spontaneous tumor necrosis and vascular invasion were unfavorable for survival in liposarcoma (Gustafson 1994).

MDM2 gene amplification has been detected in a high percentage of well-differentiated liposarcomas as compared to more primitive subtypes. The identification of MDM2 amplification in deep-seated intra- or intermusuclar lipomas suggests that MDM2 amplification may play a significant role in the development of differentiated adipose tissue tumors (Nakayama et al. 1995). MDM2 amplification has also been observed in well-differentiated liposarcomas and coexistent dedifferentiated liposarcomas (Nakayama et al. 1995) and the close correlation between levels of amplification and histological grade suggests a putative role of MDM2 overexpression in tumor progression.

Local control of disease is difficult because of the tendency for the tumor to grow along tissue planes and infiltrate surrounding structures. Furthermore, satellite nodules are not uncommon features and may evade complete removal. Most recurrences have occurred by 6 years (Gustafson 1994), but delays of up to 10 years are not rare and recurrences appearing after 30 and 31 years from diagnosis have been reported. Retroperitoneal tumors are more likely to recur because of the anatomical constraints to surgery (Kinne et al. 1973).

References

Arbabi, L. and Warhol, M.J. (1982). Pleomorphic liposarcoma following radiotherapy for breast carcinoma. *Cancer*, **49**, 878–80.

Bennet, J.H., Shousha, S., Puddle, B., and Athanasou, N.A. (1995). Immunohistochemical identification of tumors of adipocytic differentiation using an antibody to aP2 protein. *Journal of Clinical Pathology*, **48**, 950–4.

Bui, N.B., Coindre, J.M., Maree, D., and Trojani, M. (1984). Liposarcoma: patterns of tumor differentiation following induction chemotherapy. *Oncology*, **41**, 170–3.

Chang, H.R., Gaynor, J., Tan, C., Hajdu, S.I., and Brennan, M.F. (1990). Multifactorial analysis of survival in primary extremity liposarcoma. *World Journal of Surgery*, **14**, 610–18.

Dei, T.A., Mentzel, T., Newman, P.L., and Fletcher, C.D. (1994). Spindle cell liposarcoma, a hitherto unrecognized variant of liposarcoma. Analysis of six cases. *American Journal of Surgical Pathology*, **18**, 913–21.

Enzinger, F.M. and Weiss, S.W. (1995). Liposarcoma. In *Soft tissue tumors* (3rd edn), pp. 431–66. C.V. Mosby, St Louis, MO.

Evans, H.L. (1979). Liposarcoma: a study of 55 cases with a reassessment of its classification. *American Journal of Surgical Pathology*, **3**, 507–23.

Evans, H.L., Soule, E.H., and Winkelmann, R.K. (1979). Atypical lipoma, atypical intramuscular lipoma, and well differentiated retroperitoneal liposarcoma: a reappraisal of 30 cases formerly classified as well differentiated liposarcoma. *Cancer*, **43**, 574–84.

Gustafson, P. (1994). Soft tissue sarcoma. Epidemiology and prognosis in 508 patients. *Acta Orthopaedica Scandinavica*, **259** (Supplement), 1–31.

Hashimoto, H. and Enjoji, M. (1982). Liposarcoma. A clinicopathologic subtyping of 52 cases. *Acta Pathologica Japonica*, **32**, 933–48.

Jelinek, J.S., Kransdorf, M.J., Shmookler, B.M., Aboulafia, A.J., and Malawer, M.M. (1993). Liposarcoma of the extremities: MR and CT findings in the histologic subtypes (see comments). *Radiology*, **186**, 455–9.

Kilpatrick, S.E., Doyon, J., Choong, P.F.M., Sim, F.H., and Nascimento, A.G. (1996). The clinicopathologic spectrum of myxoid and round cell liposarcoma. *Cancer*, **77**, 1450–8.

Kindblom, L.G., Angervall, L., and Svendsen, P. (1975). Liposarcoma a clinicopathologic, radiographic and prognostic study. *Acta Pathologica et Microbiologica Scandinavica*, **253** (Supplement), 1–71.

Kindblom, L.G., Angervall, L., and Fassina, A.S. (1982). Atypical lipoma. *Acta Pathologica Microbiologica Immunologica Scandinavica [A]*, **90**, 27–36.

Kinne, D.W., Chu, F.C., Huvos, A.G., Yagoda, A., and Fortner, J.G. (1973). Treatment of primary and recurrent retroperitoneal liposarcoma. Twenty-five-year experience at Memorial Hospital. *Cancer*, **31**, 53–64.

Knight, J.C., Renwick, P.J., Dal Cin, P., Vanden Berge, H., and Fletcher, C.D.M. (1995). Translocation t(12;16)(q13;p11) in myxoid liposarcoma and round cell liposarcoma: molecular and cytogenetic analysis. *Cancer Research*, **55**, 24–7.

Limon, J., Turc, C.C., Dal Cin, P., Rao, U., and Sandberg, A.A. (1986). Recurrent chromosome translocations in liposarcoma. *Cancer Genetics and Cytogenetics*, **22**, 93–4.

Nakayama, T., Toguchida, J., Wadayama, B., Kanoe, H., Kotoura, Y., and Sasaki, M.S. (1995). MDM2 gene amplification in bone and soft-tissue tumors: association with tumor progression in differentiated adipose-tissue tumors. *International Journal of Cancer*, **64**, 342–6.

Patel, S.R., Burgess, M.A., Plager, C., Papadopoulos, N.E., Linke, K.A., and Benjamin, R.S. (1994). Myxoid liposarcoma. Experience with chemotherapy. *Cancer*, **74**, 1265–9.

Rabbitts, T.H., Forster, A., Larson, R., and Nathan, P. (1993). Fusion of the dominant negative transcription regulator CHOP with a novel gene FUS by translocation t(12;16) in malignant liposarcoma. *Nature Genetics*, **4**, 175–80.

Reszel, P.A., Soule, E.H., and Coventry, M.B. (1966). Liposarcoma of the extremities and limb girdles: a study of 222 cases. *Journal of Bone and Joint Surgery, American Volume*, **48A**, 229–44.

Salvadori, B., Cusumano, F., Delledonne, V., De, L.R., and Conti, R. (1986). Surgical treatment of 43 retroperitoneal sarcomas. *European Journal of Surgical Oncology*, **12**, 29–33.

Snover, D.C., Sumner, H.W., and Dehner, L.P. (1982). Variability of histologic pattern in recurrent soft tissue sarcomas originally diagnosed as liposarcoma. *Cancer*, **49**, 1005–15.

Sreekantaiah, C., Karakousis, C.P., Leong, S.P., and Sandberg, A.A. (1992). Cytogenetic findings in liposarcoma correlate with histopathologic subtypes. *Cancer*, **69**, 2484–95.

Weiss, S.W. and Rao, V.K. (1992). Well differentiated liposarcoma (atypical lipoma) of deep soft tissue of the extremities, retroperitoneum and miscellaneous sites: a follow-up study of 92 cases with analysis of the incidence of 'dedifferentiation'. *American Journal of Surgical Pathology*, **16**, 1051.

1.6.9.2 Malignant fibrous histiocytoma of soft tissue

Peter Choong

Introduction

Malignant fibrous histiocytoma is the most common soft-tissue sarcoma diagnosis. There are a variety of malignant fibrous histiocytoma subtypes reflecting the heterogeneity of this tumor which include storiform–pleomorphic, myxoid, giant cell, angiomatoid, and inflammatory. The majority of malignant fibrous histiocytoma tumors are high grade. Storiform–pleomorphic tumors are regarded as high grade, while myxoid malignant fibrous histiocytoma generally behaves in a lower-grade manner.

Malignant fibrous histiocytoma may arise from the monocyte–macrophage lineage or from the fibroblastic line. They have some markers in common with both.

Some have even questioned whether malignant fibrous histiocytoma is a specific entity. A review of 159 tumors diagnosed as pleomorphic malignant fibrous histiocytoma reported that 63 per cent proved to be specific sarcomas other than malignant fibrous histiocytoma, 11 per cent were of nonmesenchymal origin, and 26 per cent were unclassifiable (Fletcher 1993).

Box 1

- Most common soft-tissue sarcoma
- Cell of origin uncertain
- Contains varying proportions and arrangements of fibroblast-like cells and large histiocyte-like cells
- May develop following radiation therapy
- Types include pleomorphic, myxoid, giant cell, angiomatoid, and inflammatory malignant fibrous histiocytomas
- Current treatment includes wide surgical resection when possible and in most patients radiation therapy

Epidemiology

The majority of tumors arise in older adults. The most common site is the lower extremity and the thigh. They are usually deep to the deep fascia and the majority are intramuscular. Malignant fibrous histiocytoma tumors are often larger than 5 cm at diagnosis. The preponderance of deep lesions and their localization in the thigh may account for the large size of this tumor as they are less easily detected at this site.

The majority of patients present with an extremity mass, pain, or both. Duration of symptoms depends upon the rate of tumor growth. Rapid increases in size from tumor growth or hemorrhage may be mistaken for abscess formation and infection. Pregnancy is one state wherein accelerated growth rates of malignant fibrous histiocytoma have been reported (Weiss and Enzinger 1978). An inflammatory syndrome characterized by fever, chills, myalgia, and leukocytosis may accompany or even precede diagnosis of the inflammatory variant of malignant fibrous histiocytoma (Kyriakos and Kempson 1976). Resolution of symptoms has been reported after removal of the tumor. Metastasis is an uncommon initial presentation.

Malignant fibrous histiocytoma may be linked with irradiation after a latent period of many years, with burns, and chronic infection.

Pathology

The characteristic histologic feature of malignant fibrous histiocytoma is its heterogeneity. The dominant cellular pattern is a mixture of storiform and pleomorphic. Many different cells shape regions which give rise to the most common variant, storiform–pleomorphic malignant fibrous histiocytoma (Fig. 1). Other subtypes include myxoid, histiocytic, inflammatory, giant cell, and angiomatoid malignant fibrous histiocytoma.

Storiform–pleomorphic malignant fibrous histiocytoma

The differential diagnosis of storiform–pleomorphic sarcoma can include pleomorphic liposarcoma, extraskeletal osteosarcoma and

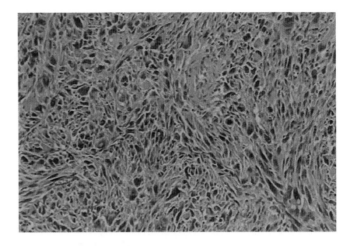

Fig. 1. A storiform and pleomorphic cellular pattern characterizes the most common form of malignant fibrous histiocytoma. Cells are large and bizarre with multiple mitoses and giant cells evident within the tumor.

chondrosarcoma, synovial sarcoma, malignant schwannoma, and leiomyosarcoma. Rarely, the large histiocytic cells of malignant fibrous histiocytoma may mimic Hodgkin's lymphoma, particularly in the presence of an inflammatory infiltrate.

Myxoid malignant fibrous histiocytoma

Myxoid malignant fibrous histiocytoma is characterized by nodular areas of myxomatous change in more than half. The differential diagnoses of myxoid malignant fibrous histiocytoma include nodular fasciitis, myxoma, and myxoid liposarcoma.

Giant cell malignant fibrous histiocytoma

The giant cell variant of malignant fibrous histiocytoma is rare. The hallmark of this tumor are the giant cells which have an abundance of eosinophilic cytoplasm and resemble osteoclasts. The differential diagnosis of this tumor is limited, but may include osteosarcoma, giant cell tumor, and malignant mesenchymoma.

Inflammatory malignant fibrous histiocytoma

Inflammatory malignant fibrous histiocytoma is an aggressive form of malignant fibrous histiocytoma which has a predisposition for the retroperitoneum. This subtype is characterized by an abundance of inflammatory and xanthomatous cells that impart a yellow discoloration to this tumor. The differential diagnosis includes non-neoplastic xanthomatous processes and lymphoma.

Angiomatoid malignant fibrous histiocytoma

Angiomatoid malignant fibrous histiocytoma has had malignant removed from its name because it is so rarely metastasizes. It arises in childhood or young adulthood and is a slowly growing mass. A characteristic feature of this tumor is the irregular hemorrhagic cystic cavities which may resemble hemangiomas or hematomas.

Imaging

Plain radiographs are always indicated, as adjacent bone changes may reflect the extrinsic nature of the tumor, while other features such as mineralization which is uncommon in malignant fibrous histiocytoma may direct the diagnosis to other calcifying lesions such as synovial sarcoma, chondrosarcoma, or a hemangiomatous lesion.

MRI provides an important method for assessing the extent and osseous involvement of the tumor. However, T_1 and T_2 signals vary widely depending upon the proportions of myxoid, fibrous, or vascular components of the tumor. In general, features suggestive of malignant soft-tissue neoplasms are poor margin definition, internal low-signal septation, and heterogeneous high-signal intensity on T_2-weighted images (Miller *et al.* 1994). Surrounding edema can be appreciated on MRI and the response to chemotherapy or radiotherapy may be important for planning resection margins.

Chest radiographs and CT scans are an essential part of staging of the tumor, as the presence of pulmonary metastases may change management to an adjuvant trial of chemotherapy and/or metastasectomy (Rosen *et al.* 1994; Choong *et al.* 1995). Radioisotope scans are helpful for identifying any osseous metastases.

Management

The primary treatment is surgery and this is commonly combined with radiotherapy (Pritchard *et al.* 1993). The local recurrence rate varies between 10 and 25 per cent The principle of achieving at least wide surgical margins may occasionally need modification if this would result in sacrifice of a major neurovascular structure or bone. If a marginal margin is employed, an additional boost of radiation can then be delivered to the questionable area. In cases where wide surgical margins, uncomplicated myectomy, or radical resection can be performed easily, consideration may be given to withhold radiotherapy (Rydholm *et al.* 1991).

Adjuvant chemotherapy for malignant fibrous histiocytoma has

not been found to be of value. Pulmonary metastasectomy is associated with prolonged survival in a major proportion of patients and now is considered part of a multidisciplinary approach to management (Choong *et al.* 1995).

Prognosis

Metastases occur in up to 40 per cent of patients despite local control of disease with the majority of metastases presenting within the first 2 years of diagnosis. The 5-year survival for patients presenting with primary localized malignant fibrous histiocytoma is approximately 60 per cent (Pritchard *et al.* 1993).

References

Choong, P.M., Pritchard, D.J., Rock, M.G., Sim, F.H., and Frassica, F.J. (1995). Survival after pulmonary metastasectomy in soft tissue sarcoma. Prognostic factors in 214 patients. *Acta Orthopaedica Scandinavica*, **66**, 561–8.

Fletcher, C.D. (1991). Angiomatoid malignant fibrous histiocytoma: an immunohistochemical study indicative of myoid differentiation. *Human Pathology*, **22**, 563–8.

Fletcher, C.D. (1993). Pleomorphic malignant fibrous histiocytoma: fact or fiction? A critical reappraisal based on 152 tumors diagnosed as pleomorphic sarcoma. *American Journal of Surgical Pathology*, **16**, 213–28.

Kyriakos, M. and Kempson, R.L. (1976). Inflammatory fibrous histiocytoma. An aggressive and lethal lesion. *Cancer*, **37**, 1584–606.

Miller, T.T., Hermann, G., Abdelwahab, I.F., Klein, M.J., Kenan, S., and Lewis, M.M. (1994). MRI of malignant fibrous histiocytoma of soft tissue: analysis of 13 cases with pathologic correlation. *Skeletal Radiology*, **23**, 271–5.

Pritchard, D.J., Reiman, H.M., Turcotte, R.E., and Ilstrup, D.M. (1993). Malignant fibrous histiocytoma of the soft tissues of the trunk and extremities. *Clinical Orthopaedics and Related Research*, **289**, 58–65.

Rosen, G., Forscher, C., Lowenbraun, S., *et al.* (1994). Synovial sarcoma. Uniform response of metastases to high dose ifosfamide. *Cancer*, **73**, 2506–11.

Rydholm, A., Gustafson, P., Rooser, B., *et al.* (1991). Limb-sparing surgery without radiotherapy based on anatomic location of soft tissue sarcoma. *Journal of Clinical Oncology*, **9**, 1757–65.

Weiss, S.W. and Enzinger, F.M. (1978). Malignant fibrous histiocytoma: an analysis of 200 cases. *Cancer*, **41**, 2250–66.

1.6.9.3 **Fibrosarcoma of soft tissue**

Peter Choong

Introduction

Fibrosarcoma is a rare soft-tissue sarcoma accounting for less than one-third of all soft-tissue sarcomas. Prior to the mid-1970s, fibrosarcoma was one of the most common diagnoses used for soft-tissue tumors (Mackenzie 1964; Cecchini 1969; Bizer 1971; Pritchard *et al.* 1974) because little distinction was made between it and other fibromatous entities, such as nodular fasciitis, desmoid tumors (Mackenzie 1964), and malignant tumors which may have a rich spindle cell population and a collagenous matrix, for example monophasic synovial sarcoma, malignant schwannoma, or malignant fibrous histiocytoma. With improvements in diagnostic modalities, such as the use of immunohistochemical staining and cytogenetics (Limon *et al.* 1991; Oshiro *et al.* 1994, 1995; Mandahl *et al.* 1995), it is now possible to differentiate between many of these entities. The evolution of this diagnosis is clearly evident in comparisons of studies from different eras. Over a period of 40 years the incidence had decreased from 65 to 12 per cent in one series (Pritchard *et al.* 1974).

Epidemiology

Heredity does not appear to be important in the pathogenesis of fibrosarcoma. In contrast, trauma has a more controversial role. Fibrosarcoma has also been observed after radiation therapy (Nageris *et al.* 1994; Bloechle *et al.* 1995; Chang *et al.* 1995), although this histotype is uncommon as a postirradiation sarcoma. The role of immunosuppressants needs consideration as tumorigenesis, including fibrosarcoma formation has been linked with allograft transplantation (Penn 1995). Like carcinomas arising in burn scars (Marjolin's ulcer), fibrosarcomas may also follow significant burns (Enzinger and Weiss 1995). The latent period for onset of fibrosarcoma (30–40 years) is similar to that of burn-associated carcinoma. The similarities between the two entities require that a desmoplastic or spindle cell

Box 1

- Malignant tumor of fibroblast-like cells that vary in degree of differentiation and mitotic activity

- May arise following radiation or severe burns

- Low-grade fibrosarcomas may resemble desmoid tumors

- Higher-grade fibrosarcomas may resemble malignant peripheral nerve sheath tumors, malignant fibrous histiocytomas, or monophasic synovial cell sarcomas

- Prognosis is related to histologic grade

- Current treatment includes wide surgical resection when possible, and radiation therapy for higher-grade tumors and in cases where a wide margin is not achieved

carcinoma be excluded before rendering a diagnosis of fibrosarcoma. Congenital fibrosarcoma will not be discussed here.

The age of onset ranges between the fourth and seventh decades, with a median age in the mid-forties. Exclusion of previously misdiagnosed malignant fibrous histiocytomas has identified a younger age group for this tumor in comparison to the more common malignant fibrous histiocytoma and liposarcomas.

Almost half of all fibrosarcomas are found in the lower extremity where they are deep-seated intra- or intermuscular tumors. Upper-extremity tumors are next most common followed by tumors of the trunk wall. Most tumors appear to arise from fibrous structures such as tendons, fascia, and aponeuroses.

Rarely have these tumors been shown to encircle the skeleton, inciting a periosteal reaction and cortical thickening, which emphasizes its slow growth rate. There may be occasional calcification within the tumor, a feature which is also characteristic of synovial sarcoma and hemangioma. Thus it is important to consider synovial sarcoma and hemangioma in the differential diagnosis of fibrosarcoma if intratumoral calcification is observed. However, this feature is uncommon.

Pathology

There are several variants of fibrosarcoma including the well-differentiated fibrosarcoma, the poorly differentiated fibrosarcoma, and a low-grade myxofibrosarcoma. An additional entity known as low-grade fibromyxoid sarcoma has been proposed as a fourth member of this group (Evans 1993).

The cut surface of fibrosarcoma exhibits a pale gray or tan colored tumor which may be lobulated. The smaller tumors tend to be well circumscribed, while larger tumors appear more invasive with tumor processes extending into the surrounding tissue. The diffuse nature of some tumors may predispose to a higher risk of recurrence after excision with minimal margins.

The histological features of fibrosarcoma are dominated by a fasciculated (herring-bone) pattern of uniform spindle cells which manifest little variation in their sizes or shape. Cellular cytoplasm is scant, and pleomorphism, storiform areas, and giant cells are rare findings in this tumor. A birefringement collagenous matrix is commonly noted and osseous metaplasia occasionally seen. Mitoses are seen and this is one feature which helps to differentiate low-grade lesions from desmoid tumors where none are usually found.

The well-differentiated fibrosarcoma is typified by clearly fibroblastic spindle cells which are arranged in an ordered herring-bone pattern. The amount of collagenous matrix may vary with small amounts in some tumors to a wiry appearance in others which may also be hyalinized. A rare variant of the well-differentiated form is the sclerosing epithelioid fibrosarcoma which is characterized by rounded cells which appear in groups or cords, and in contrast to the typical fibrosarcoma, have more cytoplasm. The sclerosing nature is reflected in the surrounding dense hyaline collagen fibers.

Another low-grade variety is the myxofibrosarcoma which is characterized by a well-differentiated tumor whose cells are richly surrounded by mature collagen and collections of myxoid material. In some tumors, alternating areas of myxoid and dense fibrous areas with a prominent capillary pattern have been described, leading to its designation as a low-grade fibromyxoid sarcoma.

The poorly differentiated fibrosarcomas are less spindle in shape and the classic herring-bone pattern is less obvious. In accordance with its higher grade, there are more numerous mitoses, and associated areas of spontaneous tumor necrosis. There is usually higher cellularity and the amount of interstitial collagen is less than would be encountered with the well-differentiated counterpart. Pleomorphism is still unusual and if present may be more suggestive of malignant fibrous histiocytoma.

The fibrotic nature of some benign lesions and many other malignant tumors can make differentiation from fibrosarcoma difficult. Nodular fasciitis is sometimes mistaken for fibrosarcoma. However, the cells are less mature, more disorganized, and arranged in short bundles as opposed to the fascicular arrangement seen with fibrosarcoma. Desmoid tumors may mimic low-grade fibrosarcoma but are often less cellular, and contain a greater abundance of collagen. Mitoses are rare and, if seen, careful inspection of other histological sections is required to exclude fibrosarcoma. Desmoid and fibrosarcoma occur in the same patient group and similar areas, thus making differentiation between the two lesions difficult.

Malignant tumors which require differentiation from fibrosarcoma include malignant peripheral nerve sheath tumor, malignant fibrous histiocytoma, and synovial sarcoma (Enzinger and Weiss 1995). Occasionally, clear cell sarcoma, dermatofibrosarcoma protuberans, liposarcoma, malignant melanoma, and some carcinomas can be confused with fibrosarcoma (Enzinger and Weiss 1995). Malignant fibrous histiocytoma is more commonly seen in elderly patients and has a median age of onset two decades later than fibrosarcoma. The storiform–pleomorphic pattern is easily distinguishable from the ordered arrangement of fibrosarcoma. Malignant peripheral nerve sheath tumors can be extremely difficult to differentiate from the poorly differentiated variety of fibrosarcoma. In such circumstances, reliance on immunohistochemistry and electronmicroscopic analysis is imperative. The former investigation will show S-100 protein positivity in approximately half of malignant peripheral nerve sheath tumors while being negative in fibrosarcomas. The monophasic spindle cell synovial sarcoma can also be difficult to differentiate from fibrosarcoma. Clinical features which may confuse the diagnosis include the relatively young age of onset of fibrosarcoma, the occasional presentation of pain, and the presence of soft-tissue calcification on radiographs in some cases. These three features are typical of synovial sarcoma. Differentiation between the two is possible employing cytogenetic or molecular genetic techniques where over 90 per cent of synovial sarcomas have a specific translocation involving chromosome X and 18 (Mandahl et al. 1995), from which a fusion gene product has been identified (Clark et al. 1994). No such chromosomal aberration has been detected in fibrosarcoma.

Clinical evaluation

Most patients give a history of 3 or more years of a lump suggesting a slow growth pattern for this tumor. However, rapid growth may also occur in some cases, and this may uncommonly cause pain, particularly in more superficial lesions. As with many other soft-tissue sarcomas, fibrosarcoma is often solitary and reaches a size between 3 and 8 cm. It is rarely found above 10 cm in diameter.

Imaging

Plain radiographs sometimes demonstrate a soft-tissue opacity if a significant mass effect is present. Intratumoral calcification may lead to a diagnosis of synovial sarcoma or hemangioma, and the periosteal thickening or reaction induced by tumors adjacent to bone may occasionally be confused with a parosteal osteosarcoma. MRI frequently demonstrate an encapsulated tumor with a low T_1-weighted signal and a high T_2-weighted signal.

Immunohistochemistry

The abundance of collagen is clearly demonstrated in reticulin preparations of tissue. Other histochemical markers include positivity for vimentin, and a lack of reactivity to antibodies for cytokeratin and S-100 protein. The expression of cell-cycle-related antigens as detected by immunohistochemistry has demonstrated that fibrosarcoma has a more proliferative nature than even desmoid tumors and dermatofibrosarcoma protuberans (Oshiro et al. 1994).

Cytogenetics

Cytogenetic findings in adults differ from congenital or infantile fibrosarcoma (Mandahl et al. 1988, 1989). The major abnormalities detected from the limited reports suggest structural changes of chromosomes X, 7, and 22 as well as clonal losses of chromosomes 9 and 11.

Electron microscopy

The main electron microscopic features of this tumor are the prominent and dilated rough endoplasmic reticulum that contain granular or amorphous material. There are also features that suggest a myofibroblastic origin, including intracytoplasmic microfilaments, dense bodies, and basal laminae (Crocker and Murad 1969; Vasudev and Harris 1978).

Treatment

The management of fibrosarcoma is the same for all soft-tissue sarcomas which includes preoperative staging with MRI of the lesion, CT of the lungs, and bone scans to exclude regional and systemic spread, prior to biopsy. Primary treatment is surgery which may be combined with radiotherapy in cases where the margin of resection was inadequate or where the tumor was seen to be high grade (Scott et al. 1989). The infiltrative nature of this tumor necessitates surgery with a wide cuff of normal tissue where possible, to ensure total removal of the tumor and its infiltrative processes. Chemotherapy has not been shown to be of specific value for this tumor and its use is confined to controlled trials.

Prognosis

The 5-year survival rates ranges between 40 and 55 per cent (Mackenzie 1964; Scott *et al.* 1989) and a close relationship is noted between the clinical outcome and the histologic grade (Scott *et al.* 1989). Low-grade tumors are clearly associated with a better survival (60 per cent) compared with high-grade lesions, where survival ranges from 34 to 21 per cent. Metastases most commonly occur to the lung and are followed by skeletal metastases in frequency (Enzinger and Weiss 1995). The majority of metastases are detected within 2 years of surgery, although late events in excess of 10 years have been reported.

References

Bizer, L.S. (1971). Fibrosarcoma. Report of sixty-four cases. *American Journal of Surgery*, **121**, 586–7.

Bloechle, C., Peiper, M., Schwarz, R., Schroeder, S., and Zornig, C. (1995). Post-irradiation soft tissue sarcoma. *European Journal of Cancer*, **31**, 31–4.

Cecchini, M. (1969). Fibrosarcomas of the soft parts of the limbs with special reference to the musculature. *Archivio Putti di Chirurgia degli Organi di Movimento*, **24**, 95–113.

Chang, S.M., Barker, F.N., Larson, D.A., Bollen, A.W., and Prados, M.D. (1995). Sarcomas subsequent to cranial irradiation. *Neurosurgery*, **36**, 685–90.

Clark, J., Rocques, P.J., Crew, A.J., *et al.* (1994). Identification of novel genes, SYT and SSX, involved in the t(X;18)(p11.2;q11.2) translocation found in human synovial sarcoma. *Nature Genetics*, **7**, 502–8.

Crocker, D.J. and Murad, T.M. (1969). Ultrastructure of fibrosarcoma in a male breast. *Cancer*, **23**, 891–9.

Enzinger, F.M. and Weiss, S.W. (1995). Fibrosarcoma. In *Soft tissue tumors* (3rd edn) (ed. F.M. Enzinger and S.W. Weiss), pp. 269–92. C.V. Mosby, St Louis, MO.

Evans, H.L. (1993). Low-grade fibromyxoid sarcoma. A report of 12 cases. *American Journal of Surgical Pathology*, **17**, 595–600.

Limon, J., Mrozek, K., Mandahl, N., *et al.* (1991). Cytogenetics of synovial sarcoma: presentation of ten new cases and review of the literature. *Genes, Chromosomes and Cancer*, **3**, 338–45.

Mackenzie, D.H. (1964). Fibroma: a dangerous diagnosis. A review of 205 cases of fibrosarcoma of soft tissues. *British Journal of Surgery*, **51**, 607–12.

Mandahl, N., Heim, S., Arheden, K., Rydholm, A., Willen, H., and Mitelman, F. (1988). Multiple karyotypic rearrangements, including t(X;18)(p11; q11), in a fibrosarcoma. *Cancer Genetics and Cytogenetics*, **30**, 323–7.

Mandahl, N., Heim, S., Arheden, K., Rydholm, A., Willen, H., and Mitelman, F. (1989). Separate karyotypic features in a local recurrence and a metastasis of a fibrosarcoma. *Cancer Genetics and Cytogenetics*, **37**, 139–40.

Mandahl, N., Limon, J., Mertens, F., *et al.* (1995). Nonrandom secondary chromosome aberrations in synovial sarcomas with t(X;18). *International Journal of Oncology*, **7**, 495–9.

Nageris, B., Elidan, J., and Sherman, Y. (1994). Fibrosarcoma of the vocal fold: a late complication of radiotherapy. *Journal of Laryngology and Otology*, **108**, 993–4.

Oshiro, Y., Fukuda, T., and Tsuneyoshi, M. (1994). Fibrosarcoma versus fibromatoses and cellular nodular fasciitis. A comparative study of their proliferative activity using proliferating cell nuclear antigen, DNA flow cytometry, and p53. *American Journal of Surgical Pathology*, **18**, 712–19.

Oshiro, Y., Fukuda, T., and Tsuneyoshi, M. (1995). Atypical fibroxanthoma versus benign and malignant fibrous histiocytoma. A comparative study of their proliferative activity using MIB-1, DNA flow cytometry, and p53 immunostaining. *Cancer*, **75**, 1128–34.

Penn, I. (1995). Sarcomas in organ allograft recipients. *Transplantation*, **60**, 1485–91.

Pritchard, D.J., Soule, E.H., Taylor, W.F., and Ivins, J.C. (1974). Fibrosarcoma—a clinicopathologic and statistical study of 199 tumors of the soft tissues of the extremities and trunk. *Cancer*, **33**, 888–97.

Scott, S.M., Reiman, H.M., Pritchard, D.J., and Ilstrup, D.M. (1989). Soft tissue fibrosarcoma. A clinicopathologic study of 132 cases. *Cancer*, **64**, 925–31.

Vasudev, K.S. and Harris, M. (1978). A sarcoma of myofibroblasts: an ultra-structural study. *Archives of Pathology and Laboratory Medicine*, **102**, 185–8.

1.6.9.4 Leiomyosarcoma of soft tissue
Peter Choong

Introduction

Leiomyosarcoma is a rare subtype of soft-tissue sarcoma, accounting for less than 10 per cent of tumors (Gustafson *et al.* 1992; Cavazzana *et al.* 1995). As the name implies, smooth muscle elements in varying degrees of differentiation are the main components of this spindle cell tumor which arises *de novo* in deep soft tissue, subcutaneous and dermal tissue, and from arterial and venous structures. Leiomyosarcoma of uterine or gastrointestinal origin differs significantly in behavior and treatment from the previous forms and will not be discussed here.

Epidemiology

The etiology of this tumor is unknown. However, an association with aberrations of the retinoblastoma gene has been implicated by reports of leiomyosarcoma arising in patients with the hereditary

Box 1

- Half are retroperitoneal
- Most common in elderly people
- Solitary and painful

Box 2

- Malignant tumor of smooth muscle cells
- May arise in deep soft tissues, subcutaneous tissues, or dermal tissues
- Superficial leiomyosarcomas are two to three times more common in males
- Current treatment includes wide surgical resection when possible and radiation therapy in selected patients

form of retinoblastoma (Font *et al.* 1983), as well as by the identification of deletions or mutations of the retinoblastoma 1 locus in sporadic forms of leiomyosarcoma (Stratton *et al.* 1989). Radiation-induced leiomyosarcomas are rarely found.

As with the majority of soft-tissue sarcomas, leiomyosarcoma is a tumor of adulthood where the highest incidence is in the sixth and seventh decade (Gustafson *et al.* 1992; Cavazzana *et al.* 1995). The gender distribution is equal in tumors arising in the extremities, but almost two-thirds to three-quarters of retroperitoneal lesions occur in females. Retroperitoneal tumors collectively account for half of all leiomyosarcomas. Other sites include an intra-abdominal location where the tumor may be attached to the mesentery or omentum and which are regarded separately from leimoyosarcoma of the gastro-intestinal tract. Superficial leiomyosarcomas are two to three times more common in males than females. The median tumor size for deep lesions is approximately 5 cm although they may range up to 25 cm. Deep-seated tumors are much larger than superficial tumors which are usually 2 cm or less in size. The inferior vena cava is the most common site for vascular leiomyosarcoma (Cavazzana *et al.* 1995). Here, leiomyosarcoma occur approximately a decade earlier than retroperitoneal sarcomas and over 80 per cent are in women.

Clinical findings

The presentation of retroperitoneal leiomyosarcomas usually follow compressive symptoms such as a mass, pain, nausea, and vomiting from involvement of intra-abdominal viscera. They often reach a large size before detection and complete removal can be difficult because of this.

Cutaneous and subcutaneous lesions are much smaller and occur with greater frequency on extensor and hair-bearing surfaces. These lesions are usually solitary and painful. Multiple regional lesions are suggestive of metastatic disease. Cutaneous tumors are slower growing than their subcutaneous counterparts, and occasionally ulcerate the overlying epidermis.

Vascular leiomyosarcomas are more commonly associated with large and medium sized vessels. While the inferior vena cava is a common site for vascular leimoyosarcomas, involvement of arteries is comparatively rare (Briggs *et al.* 1990; Delin *et al.* 1990), and the pulmonary artery is the most common arterial site. Most tumors involving the inferior vena cava originate above the liver giving rise to hepatic venous hypertension, namely the Budd–Chiari syndrome with hepatomegaly, jaundice, and ascites (Fabre *et al.* 1995). Tumors originating below the liver but above the renal vein may compromise renal function. Bilateral lower-limb edema is an accompaniment of vena caval obstruction. Leiomyosarcomas of extremity veins usually present as mass lesions without specific stigmata of venous involvement. Occasionally, symptoms of neural compression may be evident as the expanding tumor impinges on adjacent nerves which commonly accompany large veins of the extremities.

Pathology

There is little histological difference between leiomyosarcoma arising from deep, subcutaneous, or dermal sites or in association with ves-

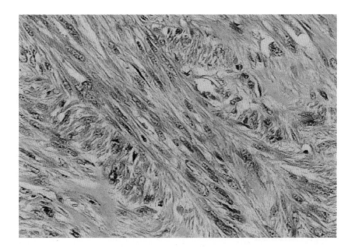

Fig. 1. Leiomyosarcoma is characterized by sweeping fascicles of spindle-shaped cells with blunt cigar-shaped nuclei.

sels. The localization of tumors to the three sites is a recognition of their varying prognostic importance.

Leiomyosarcomas are typified by spindle cells with a centrally placed blunt-ended cigar-shaped nucleus and abundant cytoplasm, arranged in intersecting bundles (Fig. 1). Nuclear palisading similar to that found in neurilemmoma is sometimes seen. More differentiated tumors exhibit numerous well-oriented myofibrils running the length of the cell. These striations are lost with poorly differentiated tumors. The majority of leiomyosarcomas are moderately well differentiated with few mitoses and the host–tumor border is usually sharply marginated. Areas of focal hyalinization can be found. Glycogen deposits and fine interstitial reticulin fibers are commonly seen.

Greater nuclear eccentricity, hyperchromatism, atypia, and size accompany more poorly differentiated cells, and prominent perinuclear vacuoles may be seen which may lead to a mistaken diagnosis of clear cell carcinoma of kidney. Pleomorphic areas resembling malignant fibrous histiocytoma can be found, and the presence of osteoclast-like giant cells together with nuclear pleomorphism can make differentiation from malignant fibrous histiocytoma difficult by light microscopy alone (Mentzel *et al.* 1995). The question as to whether these giant cells are locally induced or are part of the malignant population remains unclear (Matthews and Fisher 1994), although immunohistochemical studies have demonstrated the expression of CD68 but not markers of myogenic differentiation by the morphologically benign osteoclast-like giant cells.

Variants of leiomyosarcoma

Although leiomyosarcoma is a rare tumor, several distinct histological subtypes have been described. These include the epithelioid, myxoid, and granular cell variants.

The epithelioid subtype is characterized by cells which appear more rounded than usual and may be associated with a vacuolar or clear cell cytoplasm.

The myxoid tumors show separation of cells into cords by pools of hyaluronic acid which may be mistaken for myxoid chondrosarcoma. Myxomatous material may be so abundant in some tumors as to be grossly mistaken for chondrosarcoma. Although the number of mitoses in the myxoid variant is small (less than two per high-power field), this tumor is generally regarded as high grade because of its aggressive local and systemic behavior.

Granular cell leiomyosarcoma is the rarest form and reflects the presence of periodic acid–Schiff positive cytoplasmic granules which may represent lysosomal bodies.

Electron microscopy

Ultrastructural features of smooth muscle differentiation can be easily identified by electron microscopy (Ferenczy et al. 1971). The cells are elongated, with grooved nuclei and intracytoplasmic filaments and dense bodies. Pinocytotic vesicles are abundant and a basement membrane invests the entire cell. With less well-differentiated tumors, there is a greater proportion of rough endoplasmic reticulum and fewer myofilaments. However, myofilaments per se do not imply a smooth muscle origin as other tissues are known to contain this structure.

Immunohistochemistry

The availability of monoclonal antibodies to muscle antigens has enhanced the diagnosis of leiomyosarcomas (Parham et al. 1995; Willen et al. 1995; Schurch et al. 1996). Most leiomyosarcomas express positivity to muscle-specific actin (HHF35) and no less than half of all tumors are positive for desmin. Of note, the diffuse distribution of desmin is more diagnostic for leiomyosarcoma than focal positivity which may also be found in other malignancies as well as benign entities. Leiomyosarcoma confirmed by light microscopy and electron microscopy may lack actin or desmin positivity; therefore the diagnosis should be based on a compilation of features rather than specifically on immunohistochemistry.

Cytogenetics

Reports on the cytogenetic abnormalities of leiomyosarcoma are uncommon and no aberration has been identified which is specific for leiomyosarcoma. Generally, the chromosomal changes are complex with extensive numerical and structural changes. However, clonal patterns have been reported and hypoploidy is the most frequent abnormality noted, specifically involving chromosomes 16, 18, and 22 with recurrent structural aberrations of chromosome 1 (Sreekantaiah et al. 1993). However, non-random aberrations of chromosomes 11 and 9 have also been reported (Sait et al. 1988).

Imaging

There are no features on imaging studies which are diagnostic for leiomyosarcoma. The preoperative staging studies for this tumor are as for all other soft-tissue tumors and include chest radiographs, CT of the lungs, MRI of the lesion, and nuclear medicine. However, if biopsy suggests a leiomyosarcoma and staging studies implicate a vascular origin, preoperative arteriograms may avoid inadvertent vascular injury at surgery.

Differential diagnosis

Fibrosarcoma, monophasic synovial sarcoma, malignant schwannoma, and some malignant fibrous histiocytomas are examples of soft-tissue sarcomas that may mimic leiomyosarcoma. There are, however, features which distinguish these tumors from leiomyosarcoma. Fibrosarcoma often adopt a herring-bone pattern with cells that are more tapered than leiomyosarcoma. Monophasic synovial sarcoma have large nuclei which lack the obvious cigar shape and intersecting bundles, although it may be similar to the epithelioid subtype of leiomyosarcoma. The identification of a t(X;18) abnormality on cytogenetics or an SSX/SSY fusion gene product by molecular analysis will confirm the diagnosis of synovial sarcoma. A buckled appearance and storiform pattern differentiates malignant schwannoma from leiomyosarcoma, and the marked pleomorphism and frequent mitoses distinguishes malignant fibrous histiocytoma from leiomyosarcoma. The perinuclear vacuoles may sometimes allow leiomyosarcoma to be mistaken for clear cell carcinoma of the kidney while the myxoid variant may mimic myxoid chondrosarcoma.

Treatment

The treatment of leiomyosarcoma depends upon its position. Retroperitoneal tumors are often very large by the time diagnosis is made. Their deep and complicated position commonly make them unresectable and death by local extension may be just as important as distant metastasis. The 5-year survival ranges from less than 10 to 30 per cent (Kay and McNeill 1969; Wile et al. 1981; Shmookler and Lauer 1983).

Tumors of the extremity have a better prognosis with greater than 60 per cent survival reported at 5 years (Gustafson et al. 1992). Cutaneous and subcutaneous lesions are also associated with a good prognosis with the more superficial lesions demonstrating a lower metastatic rate (Wascher and Lee 1992). The good prognosis at this site probably reflects the easier detection of these tumors which occurs when the tumor is of a smaller size. Wide excision is the preferred treatment. Adjuvant radiotherapy is indicated if the tumor is larger than 10 cm or situated adjacent to vital neurovascular structures which if spared necessitate a marginal resection.

Vascular leiomyosarcomas which tend to occur in large and medium sized vessels cause death or morbidity by local and distant extension. Surprisingly, only half of all tumors metastasize despite their origin in a vessel (Burke and Virmani 1993). Morbidity is caused by obstruction which in the inferior vena cava may result in the Budd–Chiari syndrome or renal congestion. Tumors of the pulmonary artery may cause right-sided cardiac congestion.

Box 3

- Treatment of leiomyosarcoma of the extremities
- Wide excision
- Radiotherapy if large or in anatomically difficult site

Prognosis

In a multivariate study, Gustafson *et al.* (1992) reported that age of 60 years or greater and intratumoral vascular invasion were independent prognostic factors with relative risks of death by tumor of 8 and 4 respectively. Other prognostic factors of potential importance include DNA aneuploidy and tumor necrosis.

References

Briggs, P.J., Pooley, J., Malcolm, A.J., and Chamberlain, J. (1990). Popliteal artery leiomyosarcoma: a case report and review of the literature. *Annals of Vascular Surgery*, **4**, 365–9.

Burke, A.P. and Virmani, R. (1993). Sarcomas of the great vessels: a clinicopathologic study. *Cancer*, **71**, 1761–73.

Cavazzana, A.O., Ninfo, V., Tirabosco, R., Montaldi, A., and Frunzio, R. (1995). Leiomyosarcoma. *Current Topics in Pathology*, **89**, 313–32.

Delin, A., Johansson, G., and Silfverward, C. (1990). Vascular tumours in occlusive disease of the iliac-femoral vessels. *European Journal of Vascular Surgery*, **4**, 539–42.

Fabre, J.M., Domergue, J., Fagot, H., *et al.* (1995). Leiomyosarcoma of the inferior vena cava presenting as Budd–Chiari syndrome. Vena cava replacement under veno-venous bypass and liver hypothermic perfusion. *European Journal of Surgical Oncology*, **21**, 86–7.

Ferenczy, A., Richart, R.M., and Okagaki, T. (1971). A comparative ultrastructural study of leiomyosarcoma, cellular leiomyoma, and leiomyoma of the uterus. *Cancer*, **28**, 1004–18.

Font, R.L., Jurco, S., and Brechner, R.J. (1983). Post-radiation leiomyosarcoma of the orbit complicating bilateral retinoblastoma. *Archives of Ophthalmology*, **101**, 1557–61.

Gustafson, P., Willén, H., Baldetorp, B., Fernö, M., Åkerman, M., and Rydholm, A. (1992). Soft tissue leiomyosarcoma. A population-based epidemiologic and prognostic study of 48 patients, including cellular DNA content. *Cancer*, **70**, 114–19.

Kay, S. and McNeill, D.D. (1969). Leiomoysarcoma of the retroperitoneum. *Surgery, Gynecology and Obstetrics*, **129**, 285–8.

Matthews, T.J. and Fisher, C. (1994). Leiomyosarcoma of soft tissue and pulmonary metastasis, both with osteoclast-like giant cells. *Journal of Clinical Pathology*, **47**, 370–1.

Mentzel, T., Calonje, E., and Fletcher, C.D. (1995). Leiomyosarcoma with prominent osteoclast-like giant cells. Analysis of eight cases closely mimicking the so-called giant cell variant of malignant fibrous histiocytoma. *American Journal of Surgical Pathology*, **18**, 258–65.

Parham, D.M., Reynolds, A.B., and Webber, B.L. (1995). Use of monoclonal antibody 1H1, anticortactin, to distinguish normal and neoplastic smooth muscle cells: comparison with anti-alpha-smooth muscle actin and anti-muscle-specific actin. *Human Pathology*, **26**, 776–83.

Sait, S.N., Dal Cin, P., and Sandberg, A.A. (1988). Consistent chromosome changes in leiomyosarcoma. *Cancer Genetics and Cytogenetics*, **35**, 47–50.

Schurch, W., Begin, L.R., Seemayer, T.A., *et al.* (1996). Pleomorphic soft tissue myogenic sarcomas of adulthood. A reappraisal in the mid-1990s. *American Journal of Surgical Pathology*, **20**, 131–47.

Shmookler, B.M. and Lauer, D.H. (1983). Retroperitoneal leimoyosarcoma: a clinicopathologic analysis of 36 cases. *American Journal of Pathology*, **7**, 269–80.

Sreekantaiah, C., Davis, J.R., and Sandberg, A.A. (1993). Chromosomal abnormalities in leiomyosarcomas. *Cancer Genetics and Cytogenetics*, **142**, 293–305.

Stratton, M.R., Williams, S., and Fischer, C. (1989). Structural alterations of the RB1 gene in human soft tissue sarcomas. *British Journal of Cancer*, **60**, 202–5.

Wascher, R.A. and Lee, M.Y. (1992). Recurrent cutaneous leiomyosarcoma. *Cancer*, **70**, 490–2.

Wile, A.G., Evans, H.L., and Romsdahl, M.M. (1981). Leiomyosarcoma of the soft tissue: a clinicopathologic study. *Cancer*, **48**, 1022–32.

Willen, H., Akerman, M., and Carlen, B. (1995). Fine needle aspiration (FNA) in the diagnosis of soft tissue tumours; a review of 22 years experience. *Cytopathology*, **6**, 236–47.

1.6.9.5 Synovial sarcoma

Peter Choong

Introduction

Synovial sarcoma has previously been known as adenosarcoma, perithelial sarcoma, synovial sarcoendothelioma, sarcomesothelioma, and mesothelioma of joints. It derives its name from the histological similarity to normal or reactive synovium and may be found in the para-articular regions of the extremities but rarely within joints themselves. It is regarded as a high-grade sarcoma and metastasis is a prominent part of its natural history.

Epidemiology

Synovial sarcoma is the fourth most common (10 per cent) soft-tissue sarcoma (Enzinger and Weiss 1955). It may occur in a wide range of age groups. There is a predilection for adolescents and

Box 1

- High-grade soft-tissue sarcoma that often develops near synovial joints of the extremities but rarely within joints

- Predilection for adolescents and young adults with a peak incidence in the fourth decade

- Histological types include monophasic fibrous, monophasic epithelial, and biphasic synovial sarcomas

- Biphasic tumors contain epithelial-like cells forming cords or gland-like structures and spindle cells arranged in sheets or fascicles

- Mitoses are relatively rare despite the aggressive behavior of the tumor

- May contain areas of calcification

- In contrast with most soft-tissue sarcomas, synovial sarcomas cause pain early in the course of the disease

- Many patients have pain for years before the appearance of a detectable mass

- Current treatment includes wide surgical resection when possible and radiation therapy in selected patients

- Patients who develop pulmonary metastases may survive for years even after multiple resections

young adults with a peak in the fourth decade. Involvement below the age of 10 years is rare (Enzinger and Weiss 1995). Males are more commonly afflicted than females. The etiology of this tumor is unclear. While some reports have proposed trauma as a possible etiological agent, the evidence for this remains unconvincing and the association is most likely coincidental.

Pathology

The tumor is often well circumscribed, multinodular, and firm. The cut section may demonstrate single or multiple cysts and with particularly aggressive lesions, the tumor border may be ill defined and infiltrative. There are three histologically recognizable subtypes of synovial sarcoma (Enzinger and Weiss 1995b): a monophasic fibrous subtype which has a predominantly spindle cell population that resembles fibrosarcoma or malignant fibrous histiocytoma, a monophasic epithelial form which has a population of cuboidal epithelial-like cells in a glandular arrangement and which may be mistaken for carcinoma except for foci of spindle cells, and a biphasic variant which contains clearly distinguishable populations of either spindle or epithelial cells (Figs 1 and 2). Many monophasic tumors have previously been incorrectly diagnosed as synovial sarcoma and now have been reclassified as malignant fibrous histiocytoma. A poorly differentiated variant of synovial sarcoma has also been described.

Biphasic synovial sarcoma is the most common subtype of this tumor. The epithelial-like cells are large and ovoid with vesicular nuclei and a pale cytoplasm. These cells are arranged in solid cords or whorls and appear to line clefts which contain eosinophilic secretions giving the tumor a pseudoglandular character. Large cystic spaces within the tumor may lead to the erroneous suggestion of a synovial origin.

Occasionally, papillary structures are identified which may be mistaken for papillary carcinomas.

The spindle cell population which is the fibrous component of this biphasic tumor consists of solid compact sheets of fascicles arranged in whorls which can be mistaken for fibrosarcoma. Despite its desig-

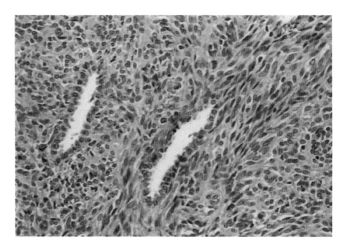

Fig. 2. Biphasic synovial sarcoma. Note cuboidal and spindle cell populations surrounding two glandular-like structures.

nation as a high-grade lesion, mitoses are not numerous except for the poorly differentiated form.

The epithelioid cells have been shown to have a higher proliferative activity as measured by the expression of Ki-67 positivity, a cell-cycle-related antigen, compared to the spindle cell component (Lopes et al. 1995). This was also verified by similar positivity to proliferating cell nuclear antigen/ cyclin PC10. The clinical significance of this difference is unknown.

Intercellular collagenous or myxoid deposits are interspersed between groups of cells and calcification is not an unusual finding. This is a characteristic feature of synovial sarcoma and is present in about one-fifth of tumors. The degree of calcification varies between tumors and may be as little as a few isolated deposits or may be extensive and involve a large proportion of the tumor. While an inflammatory response is not common in synovial sarcoma, mast cells are a typical feature in synovial sarcoma.

Monophasic fibrous synovial sarcoma is common and represents the fibrous extreme of the biphasic tumor. The lack of a herring-bone pattern, fewer mitoses, and a more nodular appearance differentiates this variant from fibrosarcoma.

The monophasic epithelioid subtype of synovial sarcoma is uncommon and may be very difficult to distinguish from carcinoma, melanoma, and other soft-tissue carcomas such as epithelioid sarcoma.

Poorly differentiated synovial sarcoma can present a diagnostic dilemma. Cells are oval or spindle shaped and small. They are tightly packed and may resemble small cell carcinomas and angiosarcomas. In some tumors, a focal rosette-like appearance may be evident which is reminiscent of peripheral neuroepithelial tumors.

Immunostaining of synovial sarcoma demonstrates high positivity for cytokeratins and, to a lesser extent, epithelial membrane antigen which is very low or nonexistent in benign synovial structures (Jorgensen et al. 1994). Electron microscopy is able to identify prominent Golgi apparatus, stacked endoplasmic reticulum, and aggregates of intermediate filaments (Mickelson et al. 1980). A continuous basal lamina is absent in normal synovium but is present in synovial sarcoma (Mickelson et al. 1980).

Cytogenetic studies have identified a characteristic translocation

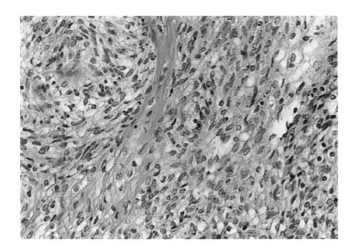

Fig. 1. Monophasic epithelial-like synovial sarcoma. Note cuboidal epithelial-like cells in a glandular arrangement.

involving chromosomes X and 18 in more than 90 per cent of synovial sarcomas (Limon *et al.* 1991), and this chromosomal aberration
is an important diagnostic tool in differentiating synovial sarcoma
from other spindle cell tumors. More recent molecular advances have
been able to identify the product of the fusion gene (*SSX/SSY*)
formed from this translocation and this provides a further avenue
for accurate diagnosis (de Leeuw *et al.* 1994). Interphase fluorescence
in situ hybridization and reverse transcription polymerase chain reaction can now be used with accuracy to identify the gene products of
synovial sarcoma (Shipley *et al.* 1996). These tools not only aid in the
diagnosis of synovial sarcoma but also may have useful application in
the identification of tumor-free margins and metastatic disease. The
presence of t(X;18) as the sole anomaly in several synovial sarcomas
suggests a central role of this aberration in tumor development.

Clinical evaluation

A painful deep-seated lump is the most common presentation. In
contrast with the majority of other soft-tissue tumors, pain is a distinguishing feature of synovial sarcomas, and occasionally these
tumors may be preceded by pain at that site for many years prior to
the appearance of a mass. The reason for this symptom is unclear.
The long duration of symptoms, which may extend from 2 to
4 years, is also noteworthy.

The majority of tumors arise in the lower extremity (70 per cent),
followed by the upper extremity (25 per cent) and the trunk (5 per
cent). Approximately 50 per cent of all tumors occur in close proximity with a joint but continuity with normal synovium is rare.
Unlike malignant fibrous histiocytoma or liposarcoma, synovial sarcoma are usually smaller (5 cm) at diagnosis and almost all are deep
to the deep fascia (Choong *et al.* 1995*b*).

Imaging

Calcification occurs in 20 per cent of tumors and may be apparent
on plain radiographs as speckled calcification or as prominent opacities. The presence of calcification is more common in synovial sarcoma than any other soft-tissue sarcoma and should alert the physician to the possibility of this tumor (Milchgrub *et al.* 1993).
Occasionally, erosion into adjacent bone is also visible on plain
radiographs but this is uncommon and if present is often associated
with poorly differentiated synovial sarcoma. Some have suggested
that synovial sarcoma should be considered when MRI demonstrate
a relatively well-defined but inhomogeneous hemorrhagic lesion near
a joint and in contact with bone (Jones *et al.* 1993). Fluid levels and
areas hyperintense, hypointense, and isointense relative to fat (triple
signal) on T_2-weighted sequences may support the diagnosis (Jones
et al. 1993).

Management

Surgery with or without radiotherapy is the preferred treatment for
synovial sarcoma (Mullen and Zagars 1994) and 5- and 10-year survival rates of 60 to 70 per cent have been reported (Mullen and
Zagars 1994; Choong *et al.* 1995*b*). Although, previous reports sug-

gested an increased incidence of lymph node metastases, lymph node
dissections should be reserved for those with clear evidence of nodal
involvement.

The role of chemotherapy has not been established, but early
results are encouraging. Kampe *et al.* (1993) reported continuous
disease-free survival after a median follow-up of 37 months in 13 of
14 patients with nonmetastatic synovial sarcoma who were treated
with a combination of surgery, local radiation, and intensive doxorubicin–cisplatin–ifosfamide-based chemotherapy. A similar finding
was reported by Ladenstein *et al.* (1993).

The role of pulmonary metastasectomy for soft-tissue sarcoma is
currently under evaluation. Initial studies suggest that this modality
may provide an alternative to or may be used in conjunction with
chemotherapy. Choong *et al.* (1995*a*) demonstrated that pulmonary
metastasectomy was associated with twice the survival rate of those
who did not undergo metastasectomy. They added that the nature of
the pulmonary lesions which included size, number, and metastasis-
free period were independently prognostic for survival. Long-term
survival after synovial sarcoma is possible after multiple thorac-
otomies, even for multiple synchronous lesions (Choong *et al.*
1995*a*).

Results of treatment

With modern multimodal therapy, an overall 5-year survival of
68 per cent and that for 10 years of 56 per cent has been reported
(Choong *et al.* 1995*b*). The vast majority of metastases are to lung
(94 per cent), and those to lymph nodes and bone occur in about
one-fifth of cases and often represent endstage disease. The continuing decline in survival rates between 5 and 10 years reflect the risk
of ongoing and late systemic spread. Older age, large size, and male
sex have been shown to be prognostically unfavorable factors
(Choong *et al.* 1995*b*). Other prognostic factors include the number
of metastatic lesions and metastasis-free interval (Choong *et al.*
1995*b*). Local recurrences occur in 30 to 40 per cent after a combination surgery and radiotherapy, and this may present up to 35 years
after the initial surgery. The indolent nature of this tumor should
not be a reason for performing less than aggressive treatment.

References

Choong, P.M., Pritchard, D.J., Rock, M.G., Sim, F.H., and Frassica, F.J.
(1995*a*). Survival after pulmonary metastasectomy in soft tissue sarcoma.
Prognostic factors in 214 patients. *Acta Orthopaedica Scandinavica*, **66**,
561–8.

Choong, P.M., Sim, F.H., Rock, M.G., Pritchard, D.J., and Nascimento, A.G.
(1995*b*). Long term survival in high grade soft tissue sarcoma: prognostic
factors in synovial sarcoma. *International Journal of Oncology*, **7**, 161–9.

de Leeuw, B., Balemans, M., Weghuis, D.O., *et al.* (1994). Molecular cloning
of the synovial sarcoma-specific translocation (X;18) (p11.2;q11.2)
breakpoint. *Human Molecular Genetics*, **3**, 745–9.

Enzinger, F.M. and Weiss, S.W. (1995). Synovial sarcoma. In *Soft tissue
tumors* (3rd edn) (ed. F.M. Enzinger and S.W. Weiss), pp. 757–86. C.V.
Mosby, St Louis, MO.

Jorgensen, L.J., Lyon, H., Myhre, J.O., Nordentoft, A., and Sneppen, O.
(1994). Synovial sarcoma. An immunohistochemical study of the epithelial
component. *APMIS*, **102**, 191–6.

Kampe, C.E., Rosen, G., Eilber, F., *et al.* (1993). Synovial sarcoma. A study of intensive chemotherapy in 14 patients with localized disease. *Cancer*, **72**, 2161–9.

Limon, J., Mrozek, K., Mandahl, N., *et al.* (1991). Cytogenetics of synovial sarcoma: presentation of ten new cases and review of the literature. *Genes, Chromosomes and Cancer*, **3**, 338–45.

Milchgrub, S., Ghandur, M.L., Dorfman, H.D., and Albores, S.J. (1993). Synovial sarcoma with extensive osteoid and bone formation. *American Journal of Surgical Pathology*, **17**, 357–63.

Mullen, J.R. and Zagars, G.K. (1994). Synovial sarcoma outcome following conservation surgery and radiotherapy. *Radiotherapy and Oncology*, **33**, 23–30.

Shipley, J., Crew, J., Birdsall, S., *et al.* (1996). Interphase fluorescence *in situ* hybridization and reverse transcription polymerase chain reaction as a diagnostic aid for synovial sarcoma. *American Journal of Pathology*, **148**, 559–67.

1.6.9.6 Malignant peripheral nerve sheath tumors

Peter Choong

Introduction

Malignant peripheral nerve sheath tumor is the term used to describe tumors arising from nerve, neurofibroma, or tumors showing nerve sheath differentiation. Previous synonyms have included malignant schwannoma, neurogenic sarcoma, neurosarcoma, and neurofibrosarcoma. There have been differences in diagnostic criteria in the literature resulting in reports of wide variation in frequency of these tumors. Some diagnoses have been based upon histology, while others have relied upon the combination of neurological symptoms and histological appearance for diagnosis. More stringent histological and immunohistochemical criteria have resulted in a decrease in the incidence of this tumor to 10 per cent or less (Ducatman *et al.* 1986).

Epidemiology

Malignant peripheral nerve sheath tumor is not common. It accounts for approximately 10 per cent of all soft-tissue sarcomas and half of these are in association with neurofibromatosis 1 (Hruban *et al.* 1990). The incidence of malignant change in neurofibromatosis 1 varies between 4 and 13 per cent and not uncommonly multiple lesions are observed (Wanebo *et al.* 1993). The latency period between diagnosis of neurofibromatosis 1 and the occurrence of malignancy is long (10–20 years).

This is a tumor of adulthood with most occurring between the third and sixth decades. However, a younger age incidence is noted for patients afflicted with neurofibromatosis 1 (Hruban *et al.* 1990). The sex distribution is similar, although there is an apparent male predominance for those with neurofibromatosis 1 because this condition is more common in males.

A genetic aberration as an etiologic factor has been suggested because of the association of this tumor with neurofibromatosis 1. Mutation or deletion of the neurofibromatosis 1 locus which is common in neurofibromatosis 1 has been implicated although this

Box 1

- Malignant tumors that arise from nerve tissue or neurofibromas or show histologic features consistent with nerve sheath tissue

- Common synonyms include malignant schwannoma, neurogenic sarcoma, neurosarcoma, and neurofibrosarcoma

- Patients with neurofibromatosis 1 have an increased risk of developing malignant peripheral nerve sheath tumours

- In patients with neurofibromatosis 1 enlargement of a neurofibroma suggests the possibility of malignancy

- Patients with neurofibromatosis 1 who develop a malignant peripheral nerve sheath tumour may have a greater risk for development of a secondary malignancy

- Current treatment includes wide surgical resection when possible and radiation therapy in selected patients

remains unproven (Jhanwar *et al.* 1994; Mertens *et al.* 1995). Another candidate gene has been the TP53 gene on chromosome 17 (Jhanwar *et al.* 1994; Mertens *et al.* 1995). Environmental causes such as chemical carcinogens and irradiation (Ducatman *et al.* 1986) have also been proposed as etiologic factors.

There are variants of this tumor including malignant triton tumor, glandular malignant schwannoma, epithelioid malignant schwannoma, and superficial epithelioid malignant peripheral nerve sheath tumor.

The triton tumor demonstrates both neural and skeletal muscle differentiation, is rare, and arises in association with neurofibromatosis 1. Therefore, patients with this tumor tend to be younger. The main areas of involvement are the head, neck, and trunk.

Glandular malignant schwannoma is now referred to as malignant peripheral nerve sheath tumor with glands because of structures demonstrating glandular differentiation within malignant peripheral nerve sheath tumor. It is the rarest variant of the group and occurs most frequently in neurofibromatosis 1. In contrast to the triton tumor, these tumors arise along major nerves such as the brachial plexus, sciatic, and median nerves.

Epithelioid malignant schwannoma is also referred to as epithelioid malignant peripheral nerve sheath tumor and as its name suggests is distinguished by cells that resemble carcinoma or melanoma. At times this tumor has been regarded as a form of melanoma, but the clinical presentation is very similar to classical malignant peripheral nerve sheath tumor.

A superficial variant of epithelioid malignant peripheral nerve sheath tumor exists which resembles its deeper counterpart but which occurs in the dermis and subcutaneous tissues. While microscopically similar to the deep variant, its gross appearance and clinical outcome varies sufficiently to regard this as a separate entity.

Clinical presentation

As with most soft-tissue sarcomas, malignant nerve sheath tumors present as an eccentric enlarging mass, often in the proximal parts of the upper and lower limbs where there is a confluence of major neural structures such as the brachial plexus, sacral plexus, and the sciatic nerve. The deep nature of the tumor often means that the tumor will have reached a large size (greater than 5 cm) prior to presentation. In patients with neurofibromatosis 1, an enlarging mass is highly suspicious of malignant transformation. Because of the close association with peripheral nerves, neurologic symptoms are common. Pain and sensory or motor symptoms are frequent accompaniments.

Pathology

The classic form of malignant peripheral nerve sheath tumor has been well described (Fig. 1). The overall appearance resembles fibrosarcoma in the long sweeping fascicles, although they lack the regularity and herring-bone appearance of fibrosarcoma. The nuclei are more irregular than fibrosarcoma, prominent and typically wavy, buckled or comma shaped. The matrix separating fascicles are commonly myxomatous, and there are frequently areas where the cells are more rounded or short fusiform. Occasionally, there is also a nodular or plexiform pattern, while in other tumors there may be a whorl-like orientation of cells and fascicles. The characteristic nuclear palisading is actually quite rare.

Less common, but distinctive, are hyalinized cords or nodules. Areas of heterologous elements within the tumor may sometimes be seen in the form of bone or cartilage. This occurrence appears to be more common with malignant peripheral nerve sheath tumors than other soft-tissue sarcomas. Tumor cells may also replace the peripheral nerve that is involved and by so doing highlight a common mode of local dissemination. Another means of spread has been the subendothelial proliferation of tumor cells which cause a bulging of the tumor into the lumen of the vessel.

In tumors arising from malignant change of neurofibromatosis 1, there are clear areas of increased aggression where cells are more pleomorphic, cellularity is greater, and mitoses are more frequent. On occasion, the level of pleomorphism may be so great as to prevent recognition of the tumor as neurogenic, or differentiation from other pleomorphic tumors such as malignant fibrous histiocytoma or pleo-

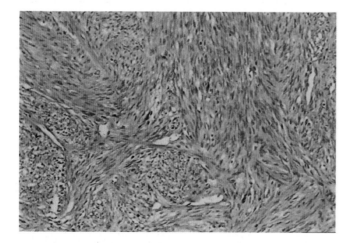

Fig. 1. Malignant peripheral nerve sheath tumor. Note long sweeping fascicles and prominent nuclei.

morphic liposarcoma. These tumors seem to occur more frequently in association with neurofibromatosis 1.

Variants of malignant peripheral nerve sheath tumor

Malignant peripheral nerve sheath tumor with rhabdomyoblastic differentiation is a rare variant (Woodruff et al. 1973). This entity is also known as a triton tumor, although any tumor with neural and skeletal muscle differentiation, such as medulloblastoma with rhabdomyosarcoma, rhabdomyosarcoma with ganglion cells, and neuromuscular hamartoma (benign triton tumor) may be referred to by the same name. Rhabdomyoblasts are found in a matrix that is typical for malignant peripheral nerve sheath tumor, and their numbers may vary between tumors and also between areas in the same tumor. Rhabdomyoblasts are large, rounded, or spindle shaped, and exhibit the characteristic cross-striations within the cytoplasm.

Malignant peripheral nerve sheath tumor with glands is characterized by glandular structures within a stroma that is typical for malignant peripheral nerve sheath tumors (Woodruff 1976). The glands are often well differentiatied with low columnar cells, sometimes also containing goblet cells. The number of glands are small but they are able to produce intra- and extracellular mucin. Difficulty is sometimes encountered, however, when the glandular structures appear more malignant and may be mistaken for biphasic synovial sarcoma. The fibrosarcoma-like spindle cells, epithelial differentiation, and t(X;18) chromosomal abnormality are features which support a diagnosis of synovial sarcoma.

The epithelioid variant of malignant peripheral nerve sheath tumor shows a vague nodular structure composed of cords of epithelioid cells (Laskin et al. 1991). The cells are large with prominent nuclei that resemble melanoma. There may be abundant myxoid component that widely separates the cell cords. The variation within this subgroup may also include tumors that have a predominance of clear cells, while in other tumors there may be a significant rhabdoid component. In other groups, marked pleomorphism may make differentiation from carcinoma difficult.

The superficial variant of epithelioid malignant nerve sheath tumor tends to be a nodular rather than a multinodular tumor (Laskin et al. 1991). Cells are gathered in small nests that are separated by a fibrous or myxoid matrix. However, the cells that comprise each nest are closely applied to each other with little intervening stroma. Individual cells retain the epithelioid appearance of the deeper tumors with their large and prominent nucleus and nucleoli.

Immunohistochemistry

Immunohistochemical techniques are helpful for identifying neural differentiation. The most commonly sought antigen is the S-100 protein which is expressed focally in groups or single cells in 50 to 90 per cent of malignant peripheral nerve sheath tumors (Fisher et al. 1992; Hirose et al. 1992). Benign tumors distinguish themselves from their malignant counterparts by a strong diffuse expression of S-100 positivity. Two other antigens which may be useful but less frequently expressed include Leu-7 and myelin basic protein (Hirose et al. 1992; Meis et al. 1993). A further marker for identifying peripheral nerve sheath neoplasms as well as their malignant transformation was proposed by Yasuda *et al.* (1991) who detected nerve growth factor expression in malignant and benign nerve sheath tumors but not in the endoneurium of normal peripheral nerves.

In glandular malignant peripheral nerve sheath tumors, differentiation from synovial sarcoma may be possible because the latter more frequently manifests keratin-positive cells with minimal S-100 positivity, while malignant peripheral nerve sheath tumors exhibit focal S-100 expression and no reaction for keratin (Rose *et al.* 1992).

The epithelioid variant of this tumor contrasts with the more typical tumor by the frequency (80 per cent) at which strong and diffuse S-100 positive expression is noted (Laskin *et al.* 1991). While this may suggest the possibility of melanoma or carcinoma, the absence of cytokeratin positivity and melanoma-associated antigen (HMB-45) supports a diagnosis of epithelioid malignant peripheral nerve sheath tumor.

Tumors with rhabdomyoblastic differentiation may show positivity for myoglobin and desmin (Rose *et al.* 1992; Maeda *et al.* 1993).

Electron microscopy

Ultrastructural examination has identified and characterized various features of neural differentiation. The most distinctive features of nerve sheath tumors are the interdigitating slender cytoplasmic processes that are covered with a continuous layer of basal lamina which reflect a Schwann cell origin (Chitale *et al.* 1991). In addition, intracytoplasmic microtubules and filaments abound, and the extensive processes form junctional complexes with other arborizing processes (Hirose *et al.* 1992). The rhabdomyoblastic variant demonstrates cross-striations, while the glandular variety has features reminiscent of intestinal epithelium with microvilli. Only a few malignant peripheral nerve sheath tumors have been karyotyped. None have demonstrated any abnormality which is unique to this tumor, although clonal chromosomal aberrations have been detected (Mertens *et al.* 1995). The most common numerical changes were a loss of a sex chromosome and loss of at least one copy of chromosomes 8, 16, and 22.

Neurofibromatosis 1 is associated with a well-described abnormality of the NF1 gene on chromosome 17. The NF1 gene may have a role in the regulation of cell proliferation and therefore is considered a putative tumor suppressor gene. Neurofibromas in neurofibromatosis 1 do not show a homozygous abnormality of chromosome 17; however, this seen in malignant nerve sheath tumors, which supports Knudson's two-hit theory of tumorigenesis (Jhanwar *et al.* 1994).

Imaging

A combination of CT and MRI provides the best preoperative evaluation of nerve sheath tumors (Verstraete *et al.* 1992). Benign nerve sheath tumors usually appear well defined, oval, spherical, or fusiform with smooth borders and distinct outlines (Cerofolini *et al.* 1991). They are often located subcutaneously and MRI is frequently able to demonstrate the nerve of origin.

CT shows these tumors to be low density on enhanced scans (Cerofolini *et al.* 1991; Verstraete *et al.* 1992). On MRI, benign tumors are isointense with muscle on T_1-weighted images and dem-

onstrate high signal intensity on T_2-weighted images (Varma *et al.* 1992; Verstraete *et al.* 1992). On both CT and MRI, contrast enhancement is often marked, but the level of homogeneity or inhomogeneity depends upon the extent of myxomatous change or necrosis that is present.

The extent of the tumor is best assessed on proton-density and T_2-weighted images where the relationships to adjacent structures and muscles are easily determined (Stull *et al.* 1991). MRI may also be able to demonstrate coexistent subtle muscle atrophy along the longitudinal axis of surrounding or distally innervated muscles (Stull *et al.* 1991), thereby suggesting the possibility of a peripheral nerve sheath neoplasm when a mass is found in the vicinity of a large nerve.

Neither CT nor MRI can establish a definite diagnosis of malignant or benign peripheral nerve sheath tumor as benign tumors may mimic malignant tumors when cystic, hemorrhagic, or necrotic. However, involvement of contiguous structures should raise suspicions of malignancy (Varma *et al.* 1992).

Treatment

Wide surgical resection and adjuvant radiotherapy remain the principal forms of treatment for this soft-tissue sarcoma. A long-term retrospective review of cases found that gross tumor resectability was the most significant prognostic factor for survival (de Cou *et al.* 1995). Sporadic tumors occurring in the extremities may be easier to treat locally than tumors arising in neurofibromatosis 1 where multiple often deep-seated and intrapelvic or intra-abdominal lesions are common. In the latter case, tumors often reach a large size prior to diagnosis and resectability may not be complete. The role of chemotherapy in this tumor is unknown. At present, off-trial chemotherapy may be considered for patients who have unresectable tumors or those who relapse following surgery (Wanebo *et al.* 1993).

Prognosis

Malignant peripheral nerve sheath tumors are commonly high grade and the overall survival of patients is poor. Wanebo *et al.* (1993) reviewed 28 cases collected over 30 years and found the 5-year survival to be less than 45 per cent. Similar rates were also reported in other series (Meis *et al.* 1993; de Cou *et al.* 1995; Vauthey *et al.* 1995). The lung is the most common site for metastasis, followed by lymph nodes, liver, bone, soft tissue, and brain with the majority occurring within 24 months from the time of diagnosis (Meis *et al.* 1993).

Large size, age over 7 years, and necrosis greater than or equal to 25 per cent have been found to be independently unfavorable prognostic features (Meis *et al.* 1993). To these Wanebo *et al.* (1993) added extent of surgery and quality of margins as important prognostic factors. A recent study from a single institution reported that the 5-year survival for patients with resectable tumors was 65 per cent, while no patient with unresectable disease survived 25 months (de Cou *et al.* 1995).

Markers of proliferation such as Ki-67 and proliferating cell nuclear antigen have been used successfully as prognostic indicators in soft-tissue sarcomas (Choong *et al.* 1994, 1995). These markers are expressed to a much greater degree in malignant peripheral nerve sheath tumors than in their benign counterparts (Kindblom *et al.*

1995). It may be possible to detect malignant transformation in some cases by the use of these proliferation markers prior ro overt histological evidence of malignancy.

There has been controversy surrounding the difference in survival between patients with and without neurofibromatosis 1. Some studies suggest that neurofibromatosis 1 may impart a more favorable outcome (Wanebo *et al.* 1993), while others suggest that neurofibromatosis 1 is more likely to be associated with poorer survival (Ducatman *et al.* 1986; Meis *et al.* 1993). Whether there is a survival difference remains unclear but it would seem more likely that patients with neurofibromatosis 1 would be reviewed on a regular basis and the availability of MRI and CT should reduce the incidence of late diagnoses of malignancy. In this regard, a review of 32 children with extremity neurofibromatosis 1 and malignancy concluded that the determining factor for survival was the resectability of the tumor (Shearer *et al.* 1994). Another study reported no difference in the survival for groups with or without neurofibromatosis 1 (Doorn *et al.* 1995). They reported, however, that patients with neurofibromatosis had a higher risk for developing a second malignant peripheral nerve sheath tumor which may in part be responsible for the apparent discrepancy in survival reported by others.

References

Cerofolini, E., Landi, A., De Santis, G., Maiorana, A., Canossi, G., and Romagnoli, R. (1991). MR of benign peripheral nerve sheath tumors. *Journal of Computer Assisted Tomography*, **15**, 593–7.

Chitale, A.R., Murthy, A.K., Desai, A.P., and Lalitha, V.S. (1991). Peripheral nerve sheath tumors: an ultrastructural study of 30 cases. *Indian Journal of Cancer*, **28**, 1–8.

Choong, P.F.M., Akerman, M., Gustafson, P., *et al.* (1994). Prognostic value of Ki-67 expression in 182 soft tissue sarcomas. Proliferation—a marker of metastasis? *Acta Pathologica Microbiologica et Immunologica Scandinavica*, **102**, 915–24.

Choong, P.F.M., Akerman, M., Rydholm, A., *et al.* (1995). Proliferating cell nuclear antigen (PCNA) and Ki-67 expression in soft tissue sarcoma. Is prognostic importance histotype specific? *Acta Pathologica et Microbiologica Immunologica Scandinavica*, **103**, 797–805.

de Cou, J.M., Rao, B.N., Parham, D.M., *et al.* (1995). Malignant peripheral nerve sheath tumors: the St Jude Children's Research Hospital experience. *Annals of Surgical Oncology*, **2**, 524–9.

Doorn, P.F., Molenaar, W.M., Buter, J., and Hoekstra, H.J. (1995). Malignant peripheral nerve sheath tumors in patients with and without neurofibromatosis. *European Journal of Surgical Oncology*, **21**, 78–82.

Ducatman, B.S., Scheithauer, B.W., and Piepgras, D.G. (1986). Malignant peripheral nerve sheath tumors: a clinicopathologic study of 120 cases. *Cancer*, **57**, 2006–21.

Fisher, C., Carter, R.L., Ramachandra, S., and Thomas, D.M. (1992). Peripheral nerve sheath differentiation in malignant soft tissue tumors: an ultrastructural and immunohistochemical study. *Histopathology*, **20**, 115–25.

Hirose, T., Hasegawa, T., Kudo, E., Seki, K., Sano, T., and Hizawa, K. (1992). Malignant peripheral nerve sheath tumors: an immunohistochemical study in relation to ultrastructural features. *Human Pathology*, **23**, 865–70.

Hruban, R.H., Shiu, M.H., Senie, R.T., and Woodruff, J.M. (1990). Malignant peripheral nerve sheath tumors of the buttock and lower extremity. A study of 43 cases. *Cancer*, **66**, 1253–65.

Jhanwar, S.C., Chen, Q., Li, F.P., Brennan, M.F., and Woodruff, J.M. (1994). Cytogenetic analysis of soft tissue sarcomas. Recurrent chromosome abnormalities in malignant peripheral nerve sheath tumors (MPNST). *Cancer Genetics and Cytogenetics*, **78**, 138–44.

Kindblom, L.G., Ahlden, M., Meis-Kindblom, J.M., and Stenman, G. (1995). Immunohistochemical and molecular analysis of p53, MDM2, proliferating cell nuclear antigen and Ki-67 in benign and malignant peripheral nerve sheath tumors. *Virchows Archiv*, **427**, 19–26.

Laskin, W.B., Weiss, S.W., and Bratthauer, G.L. (1991). Epithelioid variant of malignant peripheral nerve sheath tumor (malignant epithelioid schwannoma). *American Journal of Surgical Pathology*, **15**, 1136–45.

Maeda, M., Jozaki, T., Baba, S., Muro, H., Shirasawa, H., and Ichihashi, T. (1993). Malignant nerve sheath tumor with rhabdomyoblastic differentiation arising from the acoustic nerve. *Acta Pathologica Japonica*, **43**, 198–203.

Meis, J.M., Enzinger, F.M., Martz, K.L., and Neal, J.A. (1993). Malignant peripheral nerve sheath tumors (malignant schwannomas) in children. *American Journal of Surgical Pathology*, **17**, 531–3.

Mertens, F., Rydholm, A., Bauer, H.F., *et al.* (1995). Cytogenetic findings in malignant peripheral nerve sheath tumors. *International Journal of Cancer*, **61**, 793–8.

Rose, D.S., Wilkins, M.J., Birch, R., and Evans, D.J. (1992). Malignant peripheral nerve sheath tumor with rhabdomyoblastic and glandular differentiation: immunohistochemical features. *Histopathology*, **21**, 287–90.

Shearer, P., Parham, D., Kovnar, E., *et al.* (1994). Neurofibromatosis type 1 and malignancy: a review of 32 pediatric cases treated at a single institution. *Medical and Pediatric Oncology*, **22**, 78–83.

Stull, M.A., Moser, R.P., Kransdorf, M.J., Bogumill, G.P., and Nelson, M.C. (1991). Magnetic resonance appearance of peripheral nerve sheath tumors. *Skeletal Radiology*, **20**, 9–14.

Varma, D.G., Mouloupoulos, A., Sara, A.S., *et al.* (1992). MR imaging of extracranial nerve sheath tumors. *Journal of Computer Assisted Tomography*, **16**, 448–53.

Vauthey, J.N., Woodruff, J.M., and Brennan, M.F. (1995). Extremity malignant peripheral nerve sheath tumors (neurogenic sarcomas): a 10 year experience. *Annals of Surgical Oncology*, **2**, 126–31.

Verstraete, K.L., Achten, E., De Schepper, A., *et al.* (1992). Nerve sheath tumors: evaluation with CT and MR imaging. *Journal Belge de Radiologie*, **75**, 311–20.

Wanebo, J.E., Malik, J.M., Vanden Berg, S.R., Wanebo, H.J., Driesen, N., and Persing, J.A. (1993). Malignant peripheral nerve sheath tumors. A clinicopathologic study of 28 cases. *Cancer*, **71**, 1247–53.

Woodruff, J.M. (1976). Peripheral nerve tumors showing glandular differentiation (glandular schwannomas). *Cancer*, **37**, 2399–413.

Woodruff, J.M., Chernik, N.L., Smith, M.C., Millett, W.B., and Foote, F.J. (1973). Peripheral nerve tumors with rhabdomyosarcomatous differentiation (malignant 'triton' tumors). *Cancer*, **32**, 426–39.

Yasuda, T., Sobue, G., Ito, T., *et al.* (1991). Human peripheral nerve sheath neoplasm: expression of Schwann cell-related markers and their relation to malignant transformation. *Muscle and Nerve*, **14**, 812–19.

1.6.9.7 Malignant vascular tumors of soft tissue

Peter Choong

Introduction

Vascular neoplasms comprise a heterogeneous group of tumors that range from benign to highly malignant. Although the differences between entities may be difficult to discern, three major categories of vascular tumors have been identified: benign lesions such as hemangiomas, tumors of intermediate malignancy (hemangio-endothelioma), and highly malignant tumors (angiosarcoma). Only the latter two types will be discussed here.

Hemangioendothelioma

Hemangioendothelioma is the term used to describe vascular tumors of intermediate malignancy. Although it is a collective definition, the spectrum of intermediate tumors is wide and features between tumors may differ significantly in terms of cellularity, mitotic activity, and the closeness at which tumors may resemble the common hemangioma. Four histological subtypes are recognized: epithelioid hemangioendothelioma (Weiss et al. 1986; Kanik et al. 1995), spindle cell hemangioendothelioma (Chung et al. 1995; Pellegrini et al. 1995), kaposiform hemangioendothelioma (Tsang and Chan 1991; Zukerberg et al. 1993), and malignant endovascular papillary angioendothelioma (Ihda et al. 1995).

Epidemiology

Epithelioid hemangioendothelioma is the most common variant and arises in close association or within vessels in the extremities as well as parenchymatous organs (Weiss et al. 1986; Tsang et al. 1991). Veins are the most common vascular structure involved. This tumor may arise at any age but is rare in the young. The sex distribution in extremity lesions, is equal although tumors arising in the lung and liver are more likely to occur in women. While benign vascular tumors such as hemangiomas may be associated with the ingestion of oral contraceptives, to date, there appears to be no link between hemangioendothelioma and oral contraception. A similar lesion occurs rarely in bone (Abrahams et al. 1992; Krajca et al. 1992).

Spindle cell hemangioendothelioma was only recently described and has a predisposition for the distal extremity of young adults, particularly the hand. It commonly arises superficially in the dermis or subcutaneous tissue and may be associated with vascular abnor-

malities such as Maffucci's syndrome (Fanburg et al. 1995; Pellegrini et al. 1995) and Klippel–Trenaunay syndrome (Fletcher et al. 1991b).

Kaposiform hemangioendothelioma is another rare form of hemangioendothelioma which unlike the epithelioid form occurs most commonly in children and young adults. Although it may resemble the spindle cell variant, it occurs in deep structures as well as superficially. The retroperitoneum is a common site for deep-seated tumors and this is often associated with the Kasabach–Merritt syndrome (Tsang and Chan 1991; Zukerberg et al. 1993).

Malignant endovascular papillary angioendothelioma is a nodular or diffuse tumor that occurs superficially in young children or infants. It is the rarest of the group and no pattern of distribution has been established.

Clinical presentation

The majority of tumors are solitary lesions although the parenchymatous lesions of epithelioid hemangioendothelioma may be multifocal. They may arise in association with other cutaneous vascular abnormalities such as those found with Klippel–Trenaunay or Maffucci's syndrome. The mass is usually painless except with epithelioid hemangioendothelioma where pain may also be a feature. The deep tumors, for example retroperitoneal tumors, tend to grow to larger sizes because of late detection while those arising in the dermis or subcutis are detected early and therefore are much smaller in size. For those tumors which arise within or juxtaposed to a major vein, compressive symptoms such as thrombophlebitis or peripheral edema may be evident.

Pathology

The vessel in which endotheliomas arise usually remains intact with the tumor developing within the lumen of the vessel. The cells which resemble endothelium have a cord-like array and are embedded in a myxoid-like matrix. In some areas, nests of cells may be seen within hyalinized stroma. The cells contain vacuoles and intracytoplasmic lumina. Occasionally, vacuolization may be so extreme as to be mistaken for myxoid chondrosarcoma. Unlike hemangiomas, there is little vascular differentiation of the central core of tumor within the vessel lumen. The tumor usually shows little atypia or mitotic activity, but with increasing aggressiveness may exhibit focal necrosis and gross atypia.

Spindle cell hemangioendotheliomas have a combination of cavernous spaces juxtaposed to solid areas of spindle cells. This may resemble cavernous hemangiomas, particularly if the tumors also contain phleboliths which may be numerous. Unlike epithelioid hemangioendothelioma, there are very few epithelioid cells, and the abundance of spindle-shaped cells between vascular spaces has been one reason for their being mistaken as Kaposi's sarcoma. The cells are also vacuolated and are cord like in some areas.

The kaposiform hemangioendothelioma is characteristically infiltrating where sheets of tumor are seen to infiltrate the dermis. Within the sheets are nests of rounded or epithelioid cells merging with the spindle cells to give a nodular appearance to the tumor. Vascular-like channels are also present and appear as capillary-like or slit-like spaces. Lymphangiomatosis may also be encountered within the tumor. There is little order in the way the cells infiltrate and the picture is one of disorganization.

Malignant endovascular papillary angioendothelioma is very rare but also a quite distinct histological entity. Large vascular spaces are present lined by endothelium and filled with fluid. Within the spaces are characteristic papillary structures with marginalized cuboidal or columnar cells and a central core of hyalinization. The vascular spaces may contain lymphocytes which with the large vascular fluid-filled spaces may be mistaken for lymphangioma.

Immunohistochemistry

Immunohistochemistry has been useful for supporting a diagnosis of hemangioendothelioma (Fletcher *et al.* 1991*b*; Gonzalez and Reyes 1991; Ding *et al.* 1992; Strayer *et al.* 1992; Fukunaga *et al.* 1995; Hisaoka *et al.* 1995; Ihda *et al.* 1995). Cytokeratin is uncommon in these tumors, but factor-VIII-associated antigen can usually be demonstrated in the cytoplasm of the cells and most bind to *Ulex europeus,* a plant lectin. Kaposiform hemangioendothelioma differs from the other variants because the majority of cells express CD34 but not factor-VIII-associated antigen nor do they bind to *U. europeus.*

Angiosarcoma

Angiosarcomas are extremely rare and account for less than 1 per cent of all soft-tissue sarcomas (Haustein 1991; Flickinger and Corey 1994; Naka *et al.* 1995). Although vascular association is suggested by its name, angiosarcoma usually arises independently of major vascular structures. Angiosarcomas have been subcategorized into five groups: cutaneous angiosarcoma with and without lymphedema, angiosarcoma of breast, radiation-induced angiosarcoma, angiosarcoma of deep soft tissue, and Kaposi's sarcoma. Angiosarcomas of the breast and Kaposi's sarcoma are beyond the scope of this chapter and will not be discussed here.

Epidemiology

The majority of angiosarcomas arise in skin and other soft tissue. Despite the association between lymphedema and angiosarcoma, only one-fifth of reported skin angiosarcomas were associated with lymphedema (Kirchmann *et al.* 1994). Postmastectomy lymphedema is a common association with angiosarcoma, thereby highlighting the more common incidence of this tumor in women than men. Other infective (Aozasa *et al.* 1994), traumatic, and congenital (Offori *et al.* 1993) causes of lymphedema have also been linked with the onset of angiosarcoma.

Various theories relating the etiology of angiosarcoma to lymphedema are available. One theory suggests that chronic engorgement of the lymphatics causes deregulated proliferation of the endothelial cells. Another suggests that concentration of carcinogens within dilated lymphatics may promote and initiate neoplasia. A more recent theory suggests that the lymphatics within lymphedematous limbs are not able to function normally to remove cells that mutate spontaneously, thereby allowing clonal growth of these neoplastic or preneoplastic cells.

Radiation-induced angiosarcoma is seen in those who have undergone radiation for another malignancy such as breast, lymphoma, or cervix (Edeiken *et al.* 1992; Sessions and Smink 1992; Taat *et al.* 1992). The onset of angiosarcoma is usually long after the dose of radiation and occurs within the previously irradiated field.

Traumatic causes of angiosarcoma have been suggested by the association of cases with injury or foreign material (Jennings *et al.* 1988; Conlon *et al.* 1993). The exuberant fibrous reaction after implantation of metallic and plastic material, for example, may be important in the etiology of this tumor. As with radiation-induced tumor, there is usually a long latent period between the insult and the onset of sarcoma.

Cutaneous angiosarcoma without lymphedema is the most common variant of this tumor and occurs more frequently in those over 40 years of age. There is a greater preponderance in men with a ratio of 2:1 and the head and neck account for over 50 per cent of cases.

Cutaneous angiosarcoma with lymphedema usually follows radical breast surgery and axillary lymph node dissection. The majority are in women and occur within 10 years of surgery, and in this group of patient's angiosarcoma arises in the fourth or fifth decades.

Angiosarcoma of deep soft tissue accounts for a quarter of cases and appear to be distributed throughout the age groups equally. Once again, a 2:1 male predisposition is noted but, in contrast with cutaneous angiosarcoma, over 50 per cent of cases arise in the extremities, and head and neck lesions account for only 15 per cent of cases.

Postirradiation sarcoma is uncommon and tends to occur more frequently in women and men because of the greater incidence of malignancies requiring irradiation in women, for example breast, cervix, ovary, and uterus. Apart from the mutagenic effect of irradiation, patients also have chronic lymphedema which may in part be responsible for tumorigenesis.

Clinical presentation

Cutaneous angiosarcomas of the head and neck are usually diffuse and slightly indurated lesions. Late presentation is often with ulceration and a nodular character. The border of the tumor is rarely well defined making the true extent of the lesion difficult to define. Those tumors which arise in association with chronic lymphedema are typified by a brawny edema of the affected part which may also have a mottled purple appearance. Advanced disease is associated with nodularity and ulceration that may be quite marked. Deep soft-tissue angiosarcoma are similar in appearance to other soft-tissue sarcomas in that they are well-defined quickly growing masses which may be intra- or extramuscular structures. Aggressive or advanced disease may be associated with infiltration of surrounding structures giving the tumor a less mobile character. In rare cases of a very large tumor a consumptive coagulopathy or high-output cardiac failure may occur.

Pathology

Cutaneous angiosarcomas are usually well-differentiated or moderately well-differentiated tumors (Figs 1 and 2). They tend to form vascular-like structures that may be mistaken for hemangiomas except for the way that they infiltrate or dissect irregularly into the dermis. It is common for vascular networks to communicate with each other, trapping islands of normal tissue such as fat in between them. The vascular spaces contain papillary structures which are

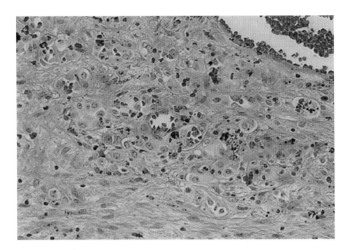

Fig. 1. Low-grade angiosarcoma (hemangio-endothelioma). Note large endothelial-like cells forming vascular-like structures.

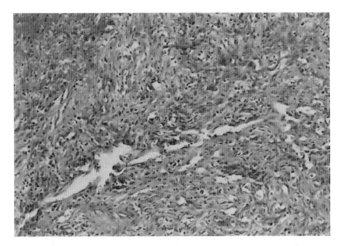

Fig. 3. High-grade angiosarcoma. Note sheets of pleomorphic epithelioid epithelial cells forming vascular-like spaces.

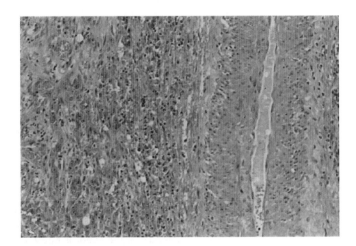

Fig. 2. Intermediate-grade angiosarcoma. Note tumor cells adjacent to large vascular-like structure. The wall of the vascular structure is invaded by tumor cells.

formed from tufting of neoplastic endothelium and which are characteristic of angiosarcoma. The cells are large and endothelial-like with nuclear hyperchromatisim. Less commonly seen are poorly differentiated lesions which have a more solid than vascular component with greater numbers of mitoses and greater cellular and nuclear pleomorphism. At times, these latter tumors may be difficult to differentiate from carcinoma.

Angiosarcomas associated with lymphedema are histologically similar to those found in the absence of lymphedema. Because of the presence of vascular spaces containing clear fluid and occasional lymphocytes this tumor has sometimes been referred to as lymphangiosarcoma. Areas of lymphangiomatosis surrounding the tumor is a feature which differentiates this variant from cutaneous angiosarcoma without lymphedema.

Deep soft-tissue angiosarcomas are often high grade and have a uniform appearance (Fig 3). Sheets of epithelioid cells with abnormal

sizes and shape are seen which contain intracytoplasmic lumina. Mitoses are frequent.

Immunohistochemistry

Tumor cells may express factor VIII antigen which is indicative of a vascular tumor, but this is not seen in all tumors (Little *et al.* 1986; Fletcher *et al.* 1991*b*; Ohsawa *et al.* 1995; Orchard *et al.* 1995). A more sensitive marker has been the binding of tumor cells to *U. europeus*. Other antibodies directed to elements of endothelium have been employed such as CD34 and thrombomodulin but these have also been expressed in various carcinomas. CD31, a platelet–endothelial adhesion molecule, may be specific for cells of the vascular lineage, as it is not expressed in nonvascular tumors.

Electron microscopy

Ultrastructural analysis is useful for identifying features of vascular differentiation which help to distinguish some tumors from carcinomas (Fletcher *et al.* 1991*a*; Ding *et al.* 1992). For example, basal lamina, tight junctions, pinocytotic vesicles, and Weibel–Palade bodies are characteristic of normal endothelium. These may be lost, however, in poorly differentiated cases, although the close topographical relationship between tumor cells and erythrocytes may persist.

Investigation

The investigation of vascular malignancies is similar to other soft-tissue sarcomas. Local and systemic staging are required to determine the extent of disease. Plain radiographs may demonstrate punctate calcification within the tumor which can be encountered in any vascular tumor. MRI may show the characteristic high-flow signals of vascular structures. Angiography is extremely useful when a malignant vascular tumor is suspected as it may help to define the feeder vessels to the tumor for preoperative embolization or intraoperative ligation. For inoperable cases, intra-arterial delivery of chemotherapy may be possible. More importantly, angiography provides preoperative (and prebiopsy) information on the vascularity of the tumor which will help to prevent unexpected and sometimes torrential hemorrhage.

Treatment

Surgery with wide margins and adjuvant radiotherapy is the preferred treatment of soft-tissue sarcomas. For the low- to intermediate-grade tumors this is associated with good local control of disease (Weiss *et al.* 1986). However, the spindle cell hemangioendothelioma may be more resistant to such measures and recurrence rates of up to 60 per cent have been reported (Weiss and Enzinger 1986).

Angiosarcomas are more difficult to control locally because of their infiltrative nature (Haustein 1991). Wide spread and/or multifocal disease is a characteristic of this tumor and achieving adequate surgical margins may be difficult (Veness and Cooper 1995). Radical surgery combined with radiotherapy appears to afford the best local control rates. Chemotherapy is of unproven benefit in the management of this tumor.

Prognosis

The prognosis for hemangioendothelioma is comparatively good. The overall survival rate exceeds 80 per cent with lung and lymph node metastases being the most common sites for dissemination (Weiss *et al.* 1986). Even for those who develop lymph node metastases, surgical removal of affected nodes appears to be compatible with longevity. Furthermore, one study suggested that with pulmonary metastasectomy, half of patients with soft-tissue sarcoma afflicted with lung metastases may experience long-term benefit (Choong *et al.* 1995). Therefore hemangioendothelioma is a tumor eminently treatable by a combination of surgery and radiotherapy. One exception is the behavior of epithelioid and kaposiform hemangioendothelioma affecting visceral structures where the frequently extensive nature of the disease and the involvement of vital structures precludes adequate resection. Death in these cases usually follows complications of local disease.

In contrast, the poor prognosis for angiosarcoma is typical of high-grade tumors, with 5-year survival rarely surpassing 20 per cent (Lydiatt *et al.* 1994; Naka *et al.* 1995). The most common sites for metastases are the lungs, liver, and spleen. Size appears to be an independent prognostic variable with small tumors (less than 5 cm) having a better prognosis than larger tumors (Maddox and Evans 1981). The relative rarity of this tumor makes adequate analysis of survival data difficult, particularly with the use of multivariate analyses.

References

Abrahams, T.G., Bula, W., and Jones, M. (1992). Epithelioid hemangioendothelioma of bone. A report of two cases and review of the literature. *Skeletal Radiology*, **21**, 509–13.

Aozasa, K., Naka, N., Tomita, Y., *et al.* (1994). Angiosarcoma developing from chronic pyothorax. *Modern Pathology*, **7**, 906–11.

Choong, P.F.M., Rock, M.G., Sim, F.H., Pritchard, D.J., and Frassica, F. (1995). Survival after pulmonary metastasectomy in soft tissue sarcoma: prognostic factors in 214 cases. *Acta Orthopaedica Scandinavica*, **66**, 561–8.

Chung, D.H., Keum, J.S., Lee, G.K., Kim, C.J., and Park, S.H. (1995). Spindle cell hemangioendothelioma—a case report. *Journal of Korean Medical Science*, **10**, 211–15.

Conlon, P.J., Daly, T., Doyle, G., and Carmody, M. (1993). Angiosarcoma at the site of a ligated arteriovenous fistula in a renal transplant recipient. *Nephrology, Dialysis, Transplantation*, **8**, 259–62.

Ding, J., Hashimoto, H., Imayama, S., Tsuneyoshi, M., and Enjoji, M. (1992). Spindle cell haemangioendothelioma: probably a benign vascular lesion not a low-grade angiosarcoma. A clinicopathological, ultrastructural and immunohistochemical study. *Virchows Archiv A. Pathology, Anatomy and Histopathology*, **420**, 77–85.

Edeiken, S., Russo, D.P., Knecht, J., Parry, L.A., and Thompson, R.M. (1992). Angiosarcoma after tylectomy and radiation therapy for carcinoma of the breast. *Cancer*, **70**, 644–7.

Fanburg, J.C., Meis, K.J., and Rosenberg, A.E. (1995). Multiple enchondromas associated with spindle-cell hemangioendotheliomas. An overlooked variant of Maffucci's syndrome. *American Journal of Surgical Pathology*, **19**, 1029–38.

Fletcher, C.D., Beham, A., Bekir, S., Clarke, A.M., and Marley, N.J. (1991*a*). Epithelioid angiosarcoma of deep soft tissue: a distinctive tumor readily mistaken for an epithelial neoplasm. *American Journal of Surgical Pathology*, **15**, 915–24.

Fletcher, C.D., Beham, A., and Schmid, C. (1991*b*). Spindle cell haemangioendothelioma: a clinicopathological and immunohistochemical study indicative of a non-neoplastic lesion. *Histopathology*, **18**, 291–301.

Flickinger, F.W. and Corey, W.J. (1994). Angiosarcoma of the extremity: pre-operative evaluation with CT, MRI, ultrasonography, and angiography. *Southern Medical Journal*, **87**, 924–7.

Fukunaga, M., Ushigome, S., Nikaido, T., Ishikawa, E., and Nakamori, K. (1995). Spindle cell hemangioendothelioma: an immunohistochemical and flow cytometric study of six cases. *Pathology International*, **45**, 589–95.

Gonzalez, C.F. and Reyes, M.M. (1991). Cellular hemangiomas ('hemangioendotheliomas') in infants. Light microscopic, immunohistochemical, and ultrastructural observations. *American Journal of Surgical Pathology*, **15**, 769–78.

Haustein, U.F. (1991). Angiosarcoma of the face and scalp. *International Journal of Dermatology*, **30**, 851–6.

Hisaoka, M., Kouho, H., Aoki, T., and Hashimoto, H. (1995). DNA flow cytometric and immunohistochemical analysis of proliferative activity in spindle cell haemangioendothelioma. *Histopathology*, **27**, 451–6.

Ihda, H., Tokura, Y., Fushimi, M., *et al.* (1995). Malignant hemangioendothelioma. *International Journal of Dermatology*, **34**, 811–16.

Jennings, T.A., Peterson, L., Axiotis, C.A., Friedlaender, G.E., Cooke, R.A., and Rosai, J. (1988). Angiosarcoma associated with foreign body material. A report of three cases. *Cancer*, **62**, 2436–44.

Kanik, A.B., Hall, J.D., and Bhawan, J. (1995). Eruptive epithelioid hemangioendothelioma with spindle cells. *American Journal of Dermatopathology*, **17**, 612–17.

Kirchmann, T.T., Smoller, B.R., and McGuire, J. (1994). Cutaneous angiosarcoma as a second malignancy in a lymphedematous leg in a Hodgkin's disease survivor. *Journal of the American Academy of Dermatology*, **31**, 861–6.

Krajca, R.J., Nicholas, R.W., and Lewis, J.M. (1992). Multifocal epithelioid hemangioendothelioma in bone. *Orthopedic Review*, **21**, 973–5.

Little, D., Said, J.W., Siegel, R.J., Fealy, M., and Fishbein, M.C. (1986). Endothelial cell markers in vascular neoplasms: an immunohistochemical study comparing factor VIII-related antigen, blood group specific antigens, 6-keto-PGF1 alpha, and *Ulex europaeus* 1 lectin. *Journal of Pathology*, **149**, 89–95.

Lydiatt, W.M., Shaha, A.R., and Shah, J.P. (1994). Angiosarcoma of the head and neck. *American Journal of Surgery*, **168**, 451–4.

Maddox, J.C. and Evans, H.L. (1981). Angiosarcoma of skin and soft tissue: a study of forty-four cases. *Cancer*, **48**, 1907–21.

Naka, N., Ohsawa, M., Tomita, Y., Kanno, H., Uchida, A., and Aozasa, K. (1995). Angiosarcoma in Japan. A review of 99 cases. *Cancer*, **75**, 989–96.

Offori, T.W., Platt, C.C., Stephens, M., and Hopkinson, G.B. (1993). Angiosarcoma in congenital hereditary lymphoedema (Milroy's disease)—

diagnostic beacons and a review of the literature. *Clinical Experience in Dermatology*, **18**, 174–7.

Ohsawa, M., Naka, N., Tomita, Y., Kawamori, D., Kanno, H., and Aozasa, K. (1995). Use of immunohistochemical procedures in diagnosing angiosarcoma. Evaluation of 98 cases. *Cancer*, **75**, 2867–74.

Orchard, G.E., Wilson, J.E., and Russell, J.R. (1995). Immunocytochemistry in the diagnosis of Kaposi's sarcoma and angiosarcoma. *British Journal of Biomedical Science*, **52**, 35–49.

Pellegrini, A.E., Drake, R.D., and Qualman, S.J. (1995). Spindle cell hemangioendothelioma: a neoplasm associated with Maffucci's syndrome. *Journal of Cutaneous Pathology*, **22**, 173–6.

Sessions, S.C. and Smink, R.J. (1992). Cutaneous angiosarcoma of the breast after segmental mastectomy and radiation therapy. *Archives of Surgery*, **127**, 1362–3.

Strayer, S.A., Yum, M.N., and Sutton, G.P. (1992). Epithelioid hemangioendothelioma of the clitoris: a case report with immunohistochemical and ultrastructural findings. *International Journal of Gynecological Pathology*, **11**, 234–9.

Taat, C.W., van Toor, B.S., Slors, J.F., Bras, J., Blank, L.E., and van Coevorden, F. (1992). Dermal angiosarcoma of the breast: a complication of primary radiotherapy? *European Journal of Surgical Oncology*, **18**, 391–5.

Tsang, W.Y. and Chan, J.K. (1991). Kaposi-like infantile hemangioendothelioma. A distinctive vascular neoplasm of the retroperitoneum. *American Journal of Surgical Pathology*, **15**, 982–9.

Tsang, W.Y., Chan, J.K., and Fletcher, C.D. (1991). Recently characterized vascular tumors of skin and soft tissues. *Histopathology*, **19**, 489–501.

Veness, M. and Cooper, S. (1995). Treatment of cutaneous angiosarcomas of the head and neck. *Australasia Radiology*, **39**, 277–81.

Weiss, S.W. and Enzinger, F.M. (1986). Spindle cell hemangioendothelioma. A low-grade angiosarcoma resembling a cavernous hemangioma and Kaposi's sarcoma. *American Journal of Surgical Pathology*, **10**, 521–30.

Weiss, S.W., Ishak, K.G., Dail, D.H., Sweet, D.E., and Enzinger, F.M. (1986). Epithelioid hemangioendothelioma and related lesions. *Seminars in Diagnostic Pathology*, **3**, 259–87.

Zukerberg, L.R., Nickoloff, B.J., and Weiss, S.W. (1993). Kaposiform hemangioendothelioma of infancy and childhood. An aggressive neoplasm associated with Kasabach–Merritt syndrome and lymphangiomatosis. *American Journal of Surgical Pathology*, **17**, 321–8.

1.6.9.8 **Rhabdomyosarcoma**

Carola A. S. Arndt

Introduction

Rhabdomyosarcoma is a complex highly malignant tumor of childhood and adolescence which arises from embryonal mesenchyma with the potential of differentiation to skeletal muscle. Despite its name, which implies an origin from tissues in which muscle is found, this tumor often arises in areas where striated muscle is not ordinarily found, such as the bladder or prostate. The most common site for rhabdomyosarcoma is the head and neck, followed by the genitourinary tract, extremities, and other sites. Primary sites of rhabdomyosarcoma in patients in Intergroup Rhabdomyosarcoma Study III are shown in Table 1 (Crist *et al.* 1995). Rhabdomyosarcoma of the bladder and vagina occur primarily in infants and nearly always have embryonal or botryoid histology, whereas sarcomas of the trunk and extremities occur in older children and have a higher incidence of

Box 1

- Most common soft-tissue sarcoma in children; accounts for about 4 per cent of all cancers in children and about 50 per cent of all soft-tissue sarcomas in children

- The most common locations are the head and neck and the genitourinary tract, but about 30 per cent occur in the extremities or trunk

- Differential diagnosis in children includes extraosseous Ewing's sarcoma and synovial cell sarcoma as well as benign lesions such as hemangioma, myositis ossificans, lipoma, and neurofibroma

- Current treatment includes chemotherapy and surgery; radiation therapy is also used in patients with microscopic or gross residual tumor

Table 1 Primary sites of rhabdomyosarcoma in Intergroup Rhabdomyosarcoma Study Group III

Site	Patients	Relative frequency (%)
Head/neck	375	35
Genitourinary	277	26
Extremity	202	19
Other	208	20
Total	1062	100

alveolar histology (Raney *et al.* 1993). Prior to the advent of multimodality chemotherapy, including multiagent chemotherapy, surgery, and radiation therapy, most patients with rhabdomyosarcoma succumbed to the disease.

Rhabdomyosarcoma is the most common soft-tissue sarcoma of childhood and accounts for 4 per cent of all cases of childhood cancer (Miller *et al.* 1994), and 50 per cent of soft-tissue sarcoma in children. Rhabdomyosarcoma occurs annually at a rate of 4 to 5 per million children under the age of 15 (Blair and Birch 1994; Gurney *et al.* 1995).

Li and Fraumeni (1969*a*) identified a familial cancer syndrome, including multiple soft-tissue sarcomas occurring in siblings and cousins with parents, grandparents, and other relatives having a higher than expected frequency of carcinoma of the breast and diverse neoplasms. However, the proportion of patients with rhabdomyosarcoma who actually have the familial cancer syndrome is quite low. An increased incidence of adrenal cortical carcinoma and brain tumors in the first-degree relatives of children with rhabdomyosarcoma was also reported (Li and Fraumeni 1969*b*). Patients with neurofibromatosis also have an increased frequency of rhabdomyosarcoma (McKeen *et al.* 1978).

Pathology, cytogenetics, and molecular genetics

Most rhabdomyosarcomas can easily be diagnosed by light microscopy on the basis of architecture and cytology. The identification of skeletal muscle differentiation with evidence of myogenesis (plump pink cytoplasm) on light microscopy, with or without cross striations, supports the diagnosis. Immunocytochemistry, electron microscopy, and cytogenetics play a significant role, especially in poorly differentiated tumors (Asmar *et al.* 1994). Desmin and muscle-specific actin are the two most commonly used markers of myogenous differentiation. Two markers, products of MyoD1 and MIC2 genes, are important in the diagnostic evaluation of rhabdomyosarcoma (Tsokos 1994). MyoD1 gene is a lineage marker for rhabdomyosarcoma (Scrable *et al.* 1989; Hosoi *et al.* 1992). MyoD1 protein can be detected with a novel monoclonal antibody even in poorly differentiated rhabdomyosarcoma (Dias *et al.* 1990, 1992). MIC2 protein has been recently identified with two antibodies in extraosseous Ewing's sarcoma and primitive neuroectodermal tumor (Kovar *et al.* 1990; Ambros *et al.* 1991; Fellinger *et al.* 1991*a*,*b*) and is useful in distinguishing those tumors from rhabdomyosarcoma which are negative for MIC2. Electron microscopy for evaluation of ultrastructural features can be helpful in the diagnosis of rhabdomyosarcoma. Diagnostic ultrastructural features include (a) well-defined sarcomas with Z bands and variable organization, (b) Z bands with or without insertion of thick and thin filaments, (c) thick and thin filaments in a hexagonal array, and (d) 'Indian file' alignment of ribosomes along thick filaments (Tsokos 1994).

The two most common variants of rhabdomyosarcoma are embryonal (80 per cent of cases) and alveolar (20 percent of cases), and have relatively distinct appearances (Fig. 1). Patients who have tumors of alveolar histology are felt to have a more unfavorable prognosis than those with tumors of embryonal histology and are generally treated more aggressively.

Cytogenetic and molecular genetic analysis also contributes to the diagnosis of rhabdomyosarcoma. Alveolar rhabdomyosarcoma has been found to have a characteristic translocation involving chromosomes 2 and 13 and, less commonly, chromosomes 1 and 13 (Seidal *et al.* 1982; Turc-Carel *et al.* 1986; Douglass *et al.* 1987, 1993; Wang-Wuu *et al.* 1988; Whang-Peng *et al.* 1992; Davis *et al.* 1994). Subsequently a novel transcript has been identified which can be detected in tumor tissue by reverse transcriptase–polymerase chain reaction (Barr *et al.* 1992, 1993; Shapiro *et al.* 1992, 1993). This can be used in conjunction with analysis for t(11;22) to differentiate Ewing's sarcoma and alveolar rhabdomyosarcoma. The value of molecular markers in diagnosis of pediatric soft-tissue sarcomas has been well summarized by Barr *et al.* (1995). Studies on loss of heterozygosity at chromosome 11p15.5 in embryonal rhabdomyosarcoma are under way (Koufos *et al.* 1985).

Clinical presentation and evaluation

The clinical manifestations are protean because rhabdomyosarcoma can present in so many different locations. The head and neck are the most common sites of rhabdomyosarcoma. A quarter of head and neck tumors arise in the orbit and may present with complaints of proptosis or ophthalmoplegia. Orbital tumors rarely metastasize, and are usually confined to the site of origin. Patients with orbital lesions have the best prognosis. Approximately one-half of head and neck rhabdomyosarcoma arise in parameningeal locations. These patients may present with symptoms of nasal, sinus, or aural obstruction. Cranial nerve palsies are not uncommon with meningeal exten-

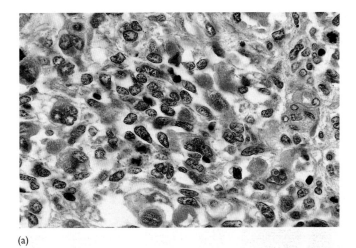

(a)

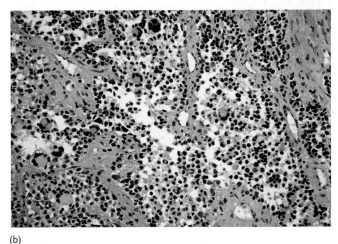

(b)

Fig. 1. Photomicrographs of subtypes of rhabdomyosarcoma: (a) alveolar; (b) embryonal.

sion. Another quarter of head and neck rhabdomyosarcoma arise in nonparameningeal sites such as scalp, face, buccal mucosa, parotid, oropharynx, larynx, and neck. Genitourinary tumors account for 20 per cent of rhabdomyosarcoma. These tumors can arise in bladder, prostate, paratesticular area, vulva, and vagina. Patients may present with hematuria, signs of bladder obstruction, asymptomatic scrotal mass, or, in the case of vaginal tumors, mucosanguinous vaginal discharge. The majority of genitourinary and head and neck rhabdomyosarcoma are of embryonal histology.

Extremity and trunk lesions, comprising 30 per cent of cases of rhabdomyosarcoma, have a much higher frequency of alveolar histology, with up to 50 per cent of tumors exhibiting this pattern. These tumors usually arise in slightly older patients than rhabdomyosarcoma in other sites. Because of the frequency of trauma to an extremity or trunk in school-age children, the diagnosis may be delayed. The differential diagnosis of a soft-tissue mass is extensive and includes both malignant tumors such as extraosseous Ewing's sarcoma or synovial cell sarcoma and non-malignant conditions such as hemangioma, myositis, ossificans, lipoma, and neurofibroma. MRI may be quite useful in suggesting malignancy with typical T_2 bright appearance (Fig. 2(a)).

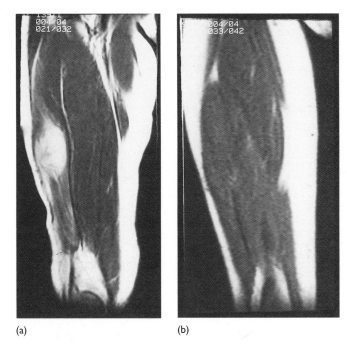

(a)   (b)

Fig. 2. MRI of alveolar rhabdomyosarcoma with (a) characteristic T_2-weighted bright appearance before chemotherapy and (b) disappearance after 9 weeks of chemotherapy.

All patients with rhabdomyosarcoma should undergo extensive evaluation for metastatic disease. This should include a chest CT scan, bone scan, bilateral bone marrow aspirate and biopsy, and imaging of local and regional lymph nodes, with biopsy of lymph nodes if possible. The existence of multiple staging systems for rhabdomyosarcoma makes comparison of different studies difficult. It is preferable to obtain the chest CT scan prior to administration of general anesthetic since even brief general anesthesia may cause atelectasis which confounds diagnosis of chest metastasis. The initial Intergroup Rhabdomyosarcoma Study staging system, as used in the first three studies, assigned patients to groups I to IV as shown in Table 2. However, this system is dependent on the initial surgical

management of the patient. The Intergroup Rhabdomyosarcoma Study is using a staging system based on a TNM staging, as well as assigning certain sites to higher or lower stages because the prognosis varies so much from one site to another. Moreover, in one study of 951 children with nonmetastatic rhabdomyosarcoma, tumor invasiveness (T stage) and site were the most important prognostic variables in a multivariate analysis (Rodary *et al.* 1991). The current Intergroup staging system is shown in Table 3.

Management

After appropriate imaging to determine the extent of disease, the management of rhabdomyosarcoma proceeds in a multidisciplinary fashion. Prior to surgical intervention, there should be consultation with the pediatric oncologist and the radiation oncologist. The initial approach to the tumor depends on the tumor site. Most parameningeal tumors are not operable at diagnosis due to their location surrounding vital structures. Thus tumors in this region are generally initially treated with chemotherapy. Radiation is the primary means of local control in this site. For genitourinary tumors, there has been an increase in the number of bladder salvages since the utilization of more aggressive chemotherapy and radiation. The traditional approach utilized by the Intergroup Rhabdomyosarcoma Study Group for other sites, particularly extremity and trunk lesions, has been to perform initial surgery in tumors considered resectable, followed by chemotherapy. For patients who present with an initial excisional biopsy, re-excision to obtain adequate margins prior to beginning chemotherapy has been recommended by the Intergroup Rhabdomyosarcoma Study Group. Radiation therapy is utilized for those patients with microscopic or gross residual disease. For patients with tumors of the extremities or in sites with easily accessible lymph nodes, the Intergroup Rhabdomyosarcoma Study has advocated lymph node sampling to evaluate for tumor.

Patients who have tumors with embryonal histology at favorable sites (e.g. nonparameningeal head and neck and nonbladder prostate genitourinary) and who have undergone complete resection or who have only microscopic residual disease, or patients with completely resected tumors at unfavorable sites, should be treated with vincris-

Table 2 Intergroup Rhabdomyosarcoma Study grouping system

Clinical group	Definition
I	A Localized, completely resected, confined to site of origin
	B Localized, completely resected, infiltrated beyond site of origin
II	A Localized
	B Regional disease, involved lymph nodes, completely resected
	C Regional disease, involved lymph nodes, grossly resected with microscopic residual
III	A Local or regional grossly visible disease after biopsy only
	B Grossly visible disease after > 50% resection of primary tumor
IV	Distant metastases present at diagnosis

Table 3 Intergroup Rhabdomyosarcoma Study staging system

Stage	Sites	T	Size	N	M
1	Orbit	T_1 or T_2	a or b	N_0 or N_1 or N_x	M_0
	Head and neck (excluding parameningeal)				
	Genitourinary—nonbladder/nonprostate				
2	Bladder/prostate	T_1 or T_2	a	N_0 or N_x	M_0
	Extremity				
	Cranial, parameningeal				
	Other (includes trunk, retroperitoneum, etc.)				
3	Bladder/prostate	T_1 or T_2	a	N_1	M_0
	Extremity		b	N_0 or N_1 or N_x	M_0
	Cranial, parameningeal				
	Other (includes trunk, retroperitoneum, etc.)				
4	All	T_1 or T_2	a or b	N_0 or N_1	M_1

Definitions

Tumor
$T(site)_1$, confined to anatomic site of origin
(a) ≤5 cm in diameter
(b) >5 cm in diameter

$T(site)_2$, extension and/or fixation to surrounding tissue
(a) ≤5 cm in diameter
(b) >5 cm in diameter

Regional nodes
N_0, regional nodes not clinically involved
N_1, regional nodes *clinically* involved by neoplasm
N_x, clinical status of regional nodes unknown (especially sites that preclude lymph node evaluation)

Metastasis
M_0, no distant metastasis
M_1, metastasis present

tine and actinomycin D for 8 to 12 months; radiation therapy is given for microscopic residual disease (Crist *et al.* 1995). Patients with similar tumors of alveolar histology require the addition of cyclophosphamide. Patients with positive lymph nodes or gross residual tumor of any site or any histology, or patients with large tumors at unfavorable sites even if completely resected, and patients with tumors at unfavorable sites with microscopic residual require therapy with at least three drugs (vincristine, actinomycin D, and cyclophosphamide) (Pappo *et al.* 1995, 1997; Arndt *et al.* 1998) as well as radiotherapy. The recently completed fourth Intergroup Rhabdomyosarcoma Study failed to show any benefit OF substitution of ifosfamide for cyclophosphamide or etoposide for actinomycin (Baker *et al.* 2000) in this group of patients.

The current fifth Intergroup Rhabdomyosarcoma Study is evaluating the addition of topotecan, a topoisomerase I inhibitor, to the standard three drug regimen for these patients. Table 4 shows the treatment algorithm for patients being treated on the current fifth Intergroup Rhabdomyosarcoma Study according to stage (depends on site, tumor size, and lymph node status (see Tables 2 and 3)), histology, and group.

Treatment for patients with rhabdomyosarcoma metastatic at diagnosis currently remains the greatest challenge. The outcome of these patients is quite dismal; therefore new approaches are being utilized. New chemotherapeutic agents are also being investigated in these patients in a 6-week up-front window prior to treatment with conventional drugs.

Results of treatment

Significant progress has been made in the past 30 years in the treatment of rhabdomyosarcoma owing to the introduction of multimodality therapy.

The four sequential Intergroup Rhabdomyosarcoma Study Group studies performed between 1972 and 1998 included more than 3000 children with rhabdomyosarcoma. The prognosis for children with rhabdomyosarcoma has improved considerably over the course of the studies (Maurer *et al.* 1988, 1993; Crist *et al.* 1995; Baker *et al.* 2000). The outcome is dependent upon many factors, including age, stage, group, and histology. The survival among 'low-risk' patients with a tumor which has been completely or nearly completely resected (with only microscopic residual) and arises in a favorable site (nonparameningeal head and neck, genitourinary tract excluding the bladder and prostate), is 90 to 95 per cent (Crist *et al.* 1995; Baker *et al.* 2000). Patients with gross residual tumors at any site other than the orbit are considered to be at intermediate risk and have a cure rate of 70 to 80 percent when treated with at least three drugs (vincristine, actinomycin D, and cyclophosphamide) and radi-

Table 4 Treatment algorithm for Intergroup Rhabdomyosarcoma Study V

Embryonal	Group I	Group II	Group III	Group IV
Stage 1	VA	N_0: VA + RT N_1: VAC + RT	Orbit only N_0: VA + RT Orbit only N_1: VAC + RT Nonorbit: VAC + RT	
Stage 2	VA	VAC + RT	VAC + RT or VAC/VTC + RT	
Stage 3	VAC + RT	VAC + RT	VAC + RT or VAC/VTC + RT	
Stage 4				> 10 years: VAC + RT or VAC/VTC + RT > 10 years: investigational window (irinotecan) + VAC

Alveolar	Group I	Group II	Group III	Group IV
Stage 1				
Stage 2		VAC + RT or VAC/VTC + RT[a]		
Stage 3				
Stage 4				Investigational window (irinotecan) + VAC

Abbreviations: V, vincristine; A, actinomycin; C, cyclophosphamide; T, topotecan; Rt, radiation therapy.
[a]Omitted if amputation.

ation therapy (Arndt *et al.* 1998; Baker *et al.* 2000). Approximately 20 per cent of patients with rhabdomyosarcoma have metastases at diagnosis. The outcome among these high risk patients is poor, with only approximately 20 per cent surviving at 5 years. However, in this high-risk group, approximately one-fifth are children under the age of 10 years who have embryonal tumors and a 5-year survival of approximately 50 per cent (Anderson *et al.* 1997).

Long-term complications as a result of surgery, radiation, and chemotherapy are being evaluated on an ongoing basis. Clearly, the extent of surgical treatment has an effect on the functional outcome. Radiation can result in fibrosis, diminished growth of underlying structures, and radiation-induced malignancies. The use of alkylating agents and etoposide can result in chemotherapy-associated leukemia. However, ongoing trials to refine the therapy for rhabdomyosarcoma and better define risk groups based on biologic prognostic indicators should enable tailoring of therapy to maximize cure and minimize late effects.

References

Ambros, I.M., Ambros, P.F., Strehl, S., *et al.* (1991). Mic2 is a specific marker for Ewing's sarcoma and peripheral primitive neuroectodermal tumors. *Cancer*, **67**, 1886–93.

Anderson, J., Ruby, E., Link, M., *et al.* (1997). Identification of a favorable subset of patients with metastatic rhabdomyosarcoma: a report from the Intergroup Rhabdomyosarcoma Study Group. *Proceedings of the Annual Meeting of the American Society of Clinical Oncology*, **16**, A510.

Arndt, C., Nascimento, A., Schroeder, G., *et al.* (1998). Treatment of intermediate risk rhabdomyosarcoma and undifferentiated sarcoma with alternating cycles of vincristine/doxorubicin/cyclophosphamide and etoposide/ifosfamide. *European Journal of Cancer*, **34**, 1224–9.

Asmar, L., Gehan, E.A., Newton, W.A., *et al.* (1994). Agreement among and within groups of pathologists in the classification of rhabdomyosarcoma and related childhood sarcomas. *Cancer*, **74**, 2579–88.

Baker, K.S., Anderson, J.R., Link, M.P., *et al.* (2000). Benefit of intensified therapy for patients with local or regional embryonal rhabdomyosarcoma. *Journal of Clinical Oncology*, **18**, 2427–34.

Barr, F.G., Holick, J., Nycum, L., *et al.* (1992). Localization of the t(2;13) breakpoint of alveolar rhabdomyosarcoma on a physical map of chromosome 2. *Genomics*, **13**, 1150–6.

Barr, F.G., Galili, N., Holick, J., *et al.* (1993). Rearrangement of the PAX3 paired box gene in the pediatric solid tumour alveolar rhabdomyosarcoma. *Nature Genetics*, **3**, 113–17.

Barr, F., Chatten, J., D'Cruz, C., *et al.* (1995). Molecular assays for chromosomal translocations in the diagnosis of pediatric soft tissue sarcomas. *Journal of the American Medical Association*, **273**, 553–7.

Blair, V. and Birch, J.M. (1994). Patterns and temporal trends in the incidence of malignant disease in children: II. Solid tumours of childhood. *European Journal of Cancer*, **30A**, 1498–511.

Crist, W., Gehan, E.A., Ragab, A.H., *et al.* (1995). The third intergroup rhabdomyosarcoma study. *Journal of Clinical Oncology*, **13**, 610–30.

Davis, R.J., D'Cruz, C.M., Lovell, M.A., *et al.* (1994). Fusion of PAX7 to FKHR by the variant t(1;13)(p36;q14) translocation in alveolar rhabdomyosarcoma. *Cancer Research*, **54**, 2869–72.

Dias, P., Parham, D.M., Shapiro, D.N., *et al.* (1990). Myogenic regulatory protein (MyoD1) expression in childhood solid tumors: diagnostic utility in rhabdomyosarcoma. *American Journal of Pathology*, **137**, 1283–91.

Dias, P., Parham, D.M., Shapiro, D.N., *et al.* (1992). Monoclonal antibodies to the myogenic regulatory protein MyoD1: epitope mapping and diagnostic utility. *Cancer Research*, **52**, 6431–9.

Douglass, E.C., Valentine, M., Etcubanas, E., *et al.* (1987). A specific chromosomal abnormality in rhabdomyosarcoma. *Cytogenetics and Cell Genetics*, **45**, 148–55.

Douglass, E.C., Shapiro, D.N., Valentine, M., *et al.* (1993). Alveolar rhabdomyosarcoma with the t(2;13): cytogenetic findings and clinicopathologic correlations. *Medical and Pediatric Oncology*, **21**, 83–7.

Fellinger, E.J., Garin-Chesa, P., Su, S.L., *et al.* (1991*a*). Biochemical and genetic characterization of the HBA71 Ewing's sarcoma cell surface antigen. *Cancer Research*, **51**, 336–40.

Fellinger, E.J., Garin-Chesa, P., Triche, T.J., *et al.* (1991*b*). Immunohistochemical analysis of Ewing's sarcoma cell surface antigen p30/32MIC2. *American Journal of Pathology*, **139**, 317–25.

Gurney, J.G., Severson, R.K., Davis, S., and Robison, L.L. (1995). Incidence of cancer in children in the United States: sex- and 1-year age-specific rates by histologic type. *Cancer*, **75**, 2186–95.

Hosoi, H., Sugimoto, T., Hayashi, Y., *et al.* (1992). Differential expression of myogenic regulatory genes, MyoD1 and myogenin, in human rhabdomyosarcoma sublines. *International Journal of Cancer*, **50**, 977–83.

Koufos, A., Hansen, M.F., Copeland, N.G., *et al.* (1985). Loss of heterozygosity in three embryonal tumors suggests a common pathogenetic mechanism. *Nature*, **316**, 330–4.

Kovar, H., Dwarzak, M., Strehl, S., *et al.* (1990). Overexpression of the pseudoautosomal gene mic2 in Ewing's sarcoma and peripheral primitive neuroectodermal tumor. *Oncogene*, **5**, 1067–70.

Li, F.P. and Fraumeni, J.F. (1969*a*). Soft tissue sarcomas, breast cancer, and other neoplasms. A familial syndrome? *Annals of Internal Medicine*, **71**, 747–53.

Li, F.P. and Fraumeni, J.F. (1969*b*). Rhabdomyosarcoma in children: epidemiologic study and identification of a familial cancer syndrome. *Journal of the National Cancer Institute*, **43**, 1365–73.

McKeen, E.A., Bordutha, J., Meadows, A.T., *et al.* (1978). Rhabdomyosarcoma complicating multiple neurofibromatosis. *Journal of Pediatrics*, **93**, 992–3.

Maurer, H.M., Beltangady, M., Gehan, E., *et al.* (1988). The Intergroup Rhabdomyosarcoma Study I. A final report. *Cancer*, **61**, 209–20.

Maurer, H.M., Gehan, E.A., Beltangady, M., *et al.* (1993). The Intergroup Rhabdomyosarcoma Study-II. *Cancer*, **71**, 1904–22.

Miller, R.W., Young, J.L., and Novakovic, B. (1994). Childhood cancer. *Cancer*, **75**, 395–405.

Pappo, A.S., Shapiro, D.N., Crist, W.M., *et al.* (1995). Biology and therapy of pediatric rhabdomyosarcoma. *Journal of Clinical Oncology*, **13**, 2123–39.

Pappo, A.S., Shapiro, D.N., and Crist, W.M. (1997). Rhabdomyosarcoma: biology and treatment. *Pediatric Clinics of North America*, **44**, 953–72.

Raney, R., Hays, D., Tefft, M., and Triche, T. (1993). Rhabdomyosarcoma and the undifferentiated sarcomas. In *Principals and practice of pediatric oncology* (ed. P. Pizzo and D. Poplack), pp. 635–58. J.B. Lippincott, Philadelphia, PA.

Rodary, C., Gehan, E., Flamant, F., *et al.* (1991). Prognostic factors in 951 non-metastatic rhabdomyosarcoma in children: a report from the international rhabdomyosarcoma workshop. *Medical and Pediatric Oncology*, **19**, 89–95.

Scrable, H., Witte, D., Shimada, H., *et al.* (1989). Molecular differential pathology of rhabdomyosarcoma. *Genes, Chromosomes and Cancer*, **1**, 23–35.

Seidal, T., Mark, J., Hagmar, B., *et al.* (1982). Alveolar rhabdomyosarcoma: a cytogenetic and correlated cytological and histological study. *Acta Pathologica, Microbiologica, et Immunologica Scandinavica, Section A, Pathology*, **90**, 345–54.

Shapiro, D.N., Valentine, M.B., Sublett, J.E., *et al.* (1992). Chromosomal sublocalization of the 2;13 translocation breakpoint in alveolar rhabdomyosarcoma. *Genes, Chromosomes and Cancer*, **4**, 241–9.

Shapiro, D.N., Sublet, J.E., Li, B., *et al.* (1993). Fusion of PAX3 to a member of the forkhead family of transcription factors in human alveolar rhabdomyosarcoma. *Cancer Research*, **53**, 5108–12.

Tsokos, M. (1994). The diagnosis and classification of childhood rhabdomyosarcoma. *Seminars in Diagnostic Pathology*, **11**, 26–38.

Turc-Carel, C., Lizard-Nacol, S., Justrabo, E., *et al.* (1986). Consistent chromosomal translocation in alveolar rhabdomyosarcoma. *Cancer, Genetics and Cytogenetics*, **19**, 361–2.

Wang-Wuu, S., Soukup, S., Ballard, E., *et al.* (1988). Chromosomal analysis of sixteen human rhabdomyosarcomas. *Cancer Research*, **48**, 983–7.

Whang-Peng, J., Knutsen, T., Theil, K., *et al.* (1992). Cytogenetic studies in subgroups of rhabdomyosarcoma. *Genes, Chromosomes and Cancer*, **5**, 299–310.

1.6.9.9 Epithelioid sarcoma

Douglas J. Pritchard

Introduction

Epithelioid sarcoma was first described by Enzinger (1970). This malignant soft-tissue tumor is frequently confused with various benign and malignant conditions including granulomas and synovial sarcoma. It occurs most commonly in the upper extremity of young adults (Chase and Enzinger 1985; Wevers *et al.* 1989). While epithelioid sarcoma may have an initial indolent course, it often behaves aggressively with a lethal outcome (Bos *et al.* 1988). Thus the tumor must be recognized and treated aggressively.

Clinical features

This is a rare tumor with no known predilection for race or culture. The peak incidence occurs in the third decade of life; however, any age may be affected. This tumor is very rare in children. Males are more commonly affected than females.

The majority of these tumors occur in the upper extremity, par-

Box 1

- Rare malignant soft-tissue tumor that can behave aggressively with a fatal outcome

- Typically presents as a soft-tissue mass in young adults, but can occur at any age

- Can present as a small subcutaneous nodule that has been present for years with minimal apparent change

- Most commonly occurs in the upper extremity, especially the hand and wrist

- Tends to spread along tendon sheaths and to regional lymph nodes

- Wide surgical excision offers the best chance of cure

ticularly in the hand and wrist. Indeed, epithelioid sarcoma is the most common soft-tissue sarcoma involving the hand and wrist. It may occasionally occur in other sites, including the trunk, buttocks, lower leg, and foot may be involved. Unusual sites of involvement include the scalp, vulva, and penis.

This tumor may occur as a superficial lesion or may be deeply seated. Those tumors that arise in the distal portion of the upper extremity tend to be superficial and may ulcerate, while those arising in the buttocks or thigh tend to be deep.

A lump or mass is usually the first indication noted by the patient. There may be pain or soreness. A typical presentation is a small subcutaneous nodule which may ulcerate. This may appear to be an innocuous benign lesion, and therefore may be ignored by the patient and occasionally by the clinician. The lump may be present for a long time before the patient seeks medical attention and its true nature is diagnosed. Indeed, in our recent report of 55 cases of epithelioid sarcoma seen between 1956 and 1991, the mean duration of symptoms was 35 months with a range from 2 months to 10 years! In this series, 39 of the 55 cases occurred in the distal upper extremity Halling *et al.* 1996).

Because this lesion often presents as a small lump, it may be mistaken for various other conditions such as an abscess or granuloma which fails to respond to antibiotic therapy. Biopsy is required to establish the diagnosis; however, the histologic pattern may also resemble that of a granuloma and thus be misdiagnosed, resulting in further delay in appropriate treatment.

In our series tumor size ranged from 0.5 to 20 cm. Over half of the tumors were less than 3 cm in diameter. The small size obscures the lethal nature of this sarcoma.

There are no diagnostic procedures specific for the diagnosis except for biopsy. MRI may be useful both to reveal the extent of the lesion and to determine its relationship with surrounding important structures, thus facilitating surgery. In addition, the initial MRI may be useful as a baseline study for future follow-up visits. This tumor has a tendency to spread along tendon sheaths and to regional nodes. Recurrence may be detected by MRI before it is clinically apparent.

Pathology

Many of these tumors are small when they are first brought to medical attention. This may be because they tend to be relatively superficial in the distal upper extremity. Larger lesions occur in other sites, such as the buttocks. About two-thirds of the lesions are located deep to the fascia and the remainder are superficial. In our most recent review, the tumor architecture was nodular in 39 of 55 patients.

Microscopically there is pseudogranulomatous palisading of the tumor cells around central areas of necrosis (Figs 1 and 2). There may a hyalinized matrix and calcification. The cells range from large epithelioid cells to spindle cells. The relative proportion of spindle to epithelial cells is variable (Figs 3 and 4). The nuclei tend to be bland and uniform, although they may have more anaplastic features. Mitotic activity is always present. Accompanying inflammatory infiltrates surrounding the tumor cells may be misleading; lesions are often misdiagnosed as granulomas. Immunohistolochemical studies include positive reactions to rifampin (rifampicin), keratin, and epithelial membrane antigen.

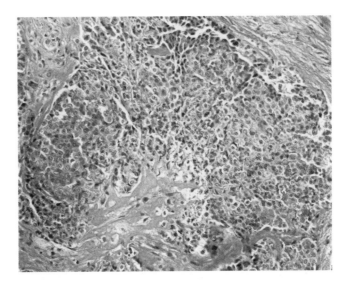

Fig. 1. Nodular arrangement in epithelioid sarcoma. The center of the nodule consists of hyalinized matrix. (Hematoxylin and eosin stain.) (Reproduced from Halling *et al.* (1996).)

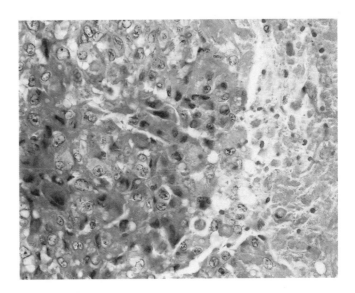

Fig. 2. Necrosis in the center of nodules in epithelioid sarcoma (a frequent finding). (Hematoxylin and eosin stain.) (Reproduced from Halling *et al.* (1996).)

Treatment and results

Surgery is the mainstay of treatment for this disease. The problem is in deciding how extensive it needs to be (Steinberg *et al.* 1992). This is particularly difficult because when this sarcoma involves the hand or wrist, there is a tendency to want to avoid mutilating surgery. In our experience, when intralesional or marginal surgery is carried out for this disease, there is a high incidence of local recurrence which may result in an increased risk of metastasis. For lesions involving an isolated digit, ray amputation is probably indicated. For lesions involving the palm or the dorsum of the hand, hemi-amputation of the hand or even below-elbow amputation may be necessary to con-

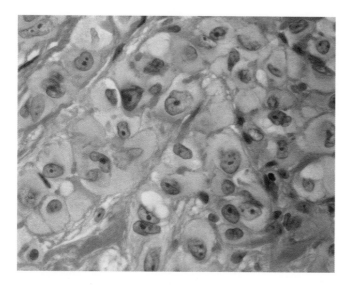

Fig. 3. Epithelioid phenotype. (Hematoxylin and eosin stain.) (Reproduced from Halling *et al.* (1996).)

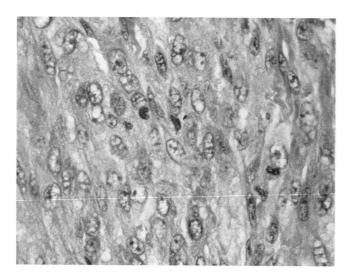

Fig. 4. Spindle cell phenotype. (Hematoxylin and eosin stain.) (Reproduced from Halling *et al.* (1996).)

trol the local disease. In other sites, it may be possible to achieve wide margins without resorting to amputation.

While there is a tendency for these tumors to involve regional nodes, there is no evidence that prophylactic lymphadenectomy plays a role in the control of this disease; however, careful physical examination on a frequent basis is indicated so that, if regional node involvement is clinically detected, lymphadenectomy can be promptly carried out. Whether or not lymphadenectomy for clinic-ally suspicious nodes will influence the final outcome is unknown.

There may be a role for adjuvant radiation therapy in the control of this disease, particularly if the margins of resection are question-able or if there is gross residual disease. In some sites such as the buttocks, where the tumor may be very large, treatment with pre-

operative radiation therapy might be considered (Shimm and Suit 1983).

The current role of chemotherapy in the initial management of the primary tumor is not established; neither neoadjuvant nor adjuvant chemotherapy is known to be effective. There may also be a role for chemotherapy in the treatment of metastatic disease; however, because this sarcoma is so rare, the precise indications for chemo-therapy have not been established.

Following treatment there may be an indolent course with delayed progression of disease. In our most recent experience 38 of 55 patients (69 per cent) had no evidence of disease after a mean follow-up interval of 118 months (range 13–300 months); however, 15 patients died of the disease and two patients are alive with disease. Twenty patients had no recurrent or metastatic lesions. Four of these had been treated by wide excision, 13 by radical excision, and three by wide excision plus adjuvant therapy. Ten patients had local recur-rences with no metastatic disease. All ten of these patients had ini-tially been treated with marginal excision; however, all of these patients were treated by subsequent wide excision plus radiation ther-apy or radical resection and all remain alive and well. Regional node involvement occurred in 15 of 55 patients and was the first mani-festation of systemic disease. Seven of these patients were alive and free of disease at last follow-up. Two additional patients died of either unknown or unrelated lesions. The remaining six patients had addi-tional metastases at various sites. The six patients who died of disease died at a mean of 20.7 months after lymphadenectomy. Ten patients had pulmonary metastatic tumors as the first manifestation of sys-temic disease. Eight of these died at a mean of 49 months after treat-ment of the metastatic disease; however, two patients had no evid-ence of disease at 75 months and 197 months respectively after surgical resection of the pulmonary tumors.

Overall, 21 patients had at least one recurrence, 11 had one recur-rence, four had two recurrences, five had three recurrences, and one had ten recurrences. The mean time to first recurrence was 24 months. The margins achieved at initial surgery affected the risk of local recurrence. Recurrence developed in 13 of 15 patients with a marginal excision, four of 11 with a wide excision, and two of 23 with a radical excision. With wide or radical excisions plus adjunctive chemotherapy or radiation therapy, none of six patients developed local recurrences. Metastatic lesions occurred in 26 patients. The mean time to metastasis was 36 months. Metastatic lesions occurred in the lungs, regional nodes, brain, and surprisingly in the scalp (four cases) (Fig. 5).

A number of clinical and pathologic findings were studied in an attempt to predict prognosis. Vascular invasion ($p = 0.001$), tumor size ($p = 0.015$), and more than 30 per cent necrosis ($p = 0.004$) were all statistically significant predictors of worse survival; however, only vascular invasion and more than 30 per cent necrosis were jointly significant ($p = 0.009$ and $p = 0.017$ respectively). Other reports have suggested that tumor depth and other factors might also predict a worse outcome; however, in our study the sex of the patient, the site of the tumor, the proportion of spindle cells, the presence of calcification, and evidence of inflammatory infiltrate were not pre-dictive of survival.

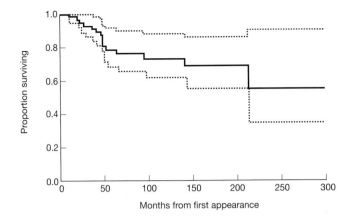

Fig. 5. Survival curve (bold line) for 55 patients with epithelioid sarcoma and 95 per cent confidence bounds (broken lines). (Reproduced from Halling *et al.* (1996).)

Discussion

This rare tumor tends to occur in the distal portion of the upper extremity in relatively young persons. The initial course appears to be slow indolent growth; however, despite this slow growth, epithelial sarcoma is a potentially lethal disease. Most recurrences take place within 2 years, but late recurrences are also noted. In addition, most metastatic tumors develop within 3 years, but again late metastatic involvement is not rare. This tumor has the potential for aggressive behavior and close follow-up for many years is necessary.

It is important to note that this tumor is often mistaken for other conditions, particularly granulomas. However, histologic features are fairly specific, and the mitotic activity and nuclear pleomorphism distinguish these cells from benign reactive histiocytes.

The treatment for this tumor should be aggressive surgical excision. There is no place for intralesional or marginal excisions unless they are followed by adjuvant radiation therapy. Anything less than wide excision is apt to result in local recurrence. However, control of local disease is not necessarily correlated with the development of metastatic disease. There may be other factors besides surgical treatment which determine subsequent metastatic disease. It may be that the clinical course is so indolent that metastasis has already occurred at the time of initial surgical treatment.

Adjuvant radiation therapy appears promising, but, because this is a rare disorder, definite evidence of its usefulness is forthcoming.

The treatment of metastatic disease is also inconclusive because of the small numbers and variability in presentation. However, it does appear that thoracotomy for excision of pulmonary nodules and chemotherapy may be helpful in salvaging some of these patients.

Summary

Epithelioid sarcoma is a rare tumor usually involving the distal upper extremity. It is deceptive in its presentation and therefore treatment is often delayed. Awareness of this tumor may lead to earlier recognition and treatment. Aggressive surgical management is indicated to achieve local control. The role of adjuvant treatment is evolving.

References

Bos, G.D., Pritchard, D.J., Reiman, H.M., Dobyns, J.H., Ilstrup, D.M., and Landon, G.C. (1988). Epithelioid sarcoma. An analysis of fifty-one cases. *Journal of Bone and Joint Surgery, American Volume*, **70A**, 862–70.

Chase, D.R. and Enzinger, F.M. (1985). Epithelioid sarcoma: diagnosis, prognostic indicators and treatment. *American Journal of Surgical Pathology*, **9**, 241–63.

Enzinger, F.M. (1970). Epithelioid sarcoma: a sarcoma simulating a granuloma or a carcinoma. *Cancer*, **26**, 1029–41.

Halling, A.C., Wollan, P.C., Pritchard, D.J., Vlasak, R., and Nascimento, A.G. (1996). Epithelioid sarcoma: a clinicopathologic review of 55 cases. *Mayo Clinic Proceedings*, **71**, 636–42.

Shimm, D.S. and Suit, H.D. (1983). Radiation therapy of epithelioid sarcoma. *Cancer*, **52**, 1022–5.

Steinberg, B.D., Gelberman, R.H., Mankin, H.J., and Rosenberg, A.E. (1992). Epithelioid sarcoma in the upper extremity. *Journal of Bone and Joint Surgery, American Volume*, **74A**, 28–35.

Wevers, A.C., Kroon, B.B.R., Albus-Lutter, C.E., and Gortzak, E. (1989). Epithelioid sarcoma. *European Journal of Surgical Oncology*, **15**, 345–9.

1.6.9.10 Clear cell sarcoma

Diva R. Salomao and Antonio G. Nascimento

Clear cell sarcoma is a malignant neuroectodermal tumor. For many years it was considered a form of malignant melanoma of soft parts, because of some overlapping histologic features. However, some evidence, including cytogenetic abnormalities (Bridge *et al.* 1990; Mrozek *et al.* 1993), has indicated that they are different entities.

It occurs mainly in young adults between the ages of 20 and 40 years (Enzinger and Weiss 1995). The most common locations are the extremities, mainly the foot and ankle, followed by the knee, hand, and wrist. The chest and the head and neck region are very uncommon sites of occurrence (Lucas *et al.* 1992). The tumor presents as a deeply situated mass, firmly attached to tendon and aponeuroses, with rare involvement of overlying skin. Patients complain

Box 1

- Rare malignant soft-tissue tumor
- Typically presents as a slow-growing mass in patients between 20 and 40 years of age
- Most frequently occurs in the foot and ankle, followed by the hand, wrist, and knee
- Consists of clusters or fascicles of round to fusiform cells, with clear or basophilic cytoplasm and prominent nucleoli, separated by fibrous septa
- May contain melanin pigment and resemble malignant melanoma
- Wide surgical excision offers the best chance of cure

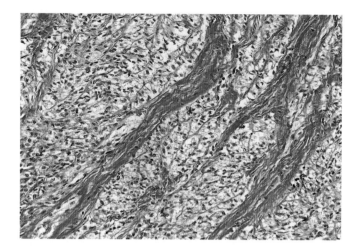

Fig. 1. Low-power view of clear cell sarcoma with clear neoplastic cells arranged in a characteristic organoid pattern.

of a slow-growing mass, which in a third of the cases is associated with pain or tenderness.

Grossly, the tumor consists of a circumscribed, although not encapsulated, lobulated or multinodular mass in the soft tissues adjacent to tendons and aponeuroses.

Histologically, clear cell sarcomas are characterized by the presence of small clusters or fascicles of round to fusiform cells with clear or basophilic cytoplasm, separated by delicate fibrous septa and arranged in an organoid neuroendocrine-like pattern (Fig. 1). The cells show prominent nucleoli and clear or pale cytoplasm (Fig. 2). Multinucleated giant cells are frequently seen. Mitotic figures and foci of necrosis are uncommon. In some cases, a focal diffuse pattern with spindle cells arranged in fascicles is observed, reminiscent of a fibrosarcoma. The amount of fibrous stroma is variable in each case. Pigment of melanin may be seen in a few cases.

Immunohistochemically, the neoplastic cells express positivity for S-100 protein and HMB-45 in approximately 70 to 80 per cent of cases (Lucas *et al.* 1992). Keratin stain is nearly always negative.

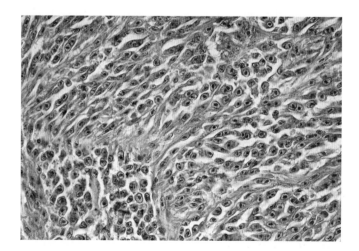

Fig. 2. High-power view of clear cell sarcoma, showing prominent eosinophilic nucleoli.

The prognosis is poor, and in most patients the disease pursues a relentlessly progressive course with frequent local recurrences ending in death due to widespread nodal and visceral metastases. The 5-year survival rate is 50 to 60 per cent in most studies (Chung and Enzinger 1983; Lucas *et al.* 1992). A large tumor and the presence of necrosis are statistically significant predictors of a poor prognosis (Lucas *et al.* 1992; Montgomery *et al.* 1993).

References

Bridge, J.A., Borek, D.A., Neff, J.R., and Huntrakoon, M. (1990). Chromosomal abnormalities in clear cell sarcoma: implications for histogenesis. *American Journal of Clinical Pathology*, **93**, 26–31.

Chung, E.B. and Enzinger, F.M. (1983). Malignant melanoma of soft parts: a reassessment of clear cell sarcoma. *American Journal of Surgical Pathology*, **7**, 405–13.

Enzinger, F.M. and Weiss, S.W. (1995). *Soft tissue tumors* (3rd edn). C.V. Mosby, St Louis, MO.

Lucas, D.R., Nascimento, A.G., and Sim, F.H. (1992). Clear cell sarcoma of soft tissues. Mayo Clinic experience with 35 cases. *American Journal of Surgical Pathology*, **16**, 1197–204.

Montgomery, E.A., Meis, J.M., Ramos, A.G., Frisman, D.M., and Martz, K.L. (1993). Clear cell sarcoma of tendons and aponeuroses: a clinicopathologic study of 58 cases with analysis of prognostic factors. *International Journal of Surgical Pathology*, **1**, 89–99.

Mrozek, K., Karakousis, C.P., Perez-Mesa, C., and Bloomfield, C.D. (1993). Translocation t(12;22) (q13;q12.2–12.3) in a clear cell sarcoma of tendons and aponeuroses. *Genes, Chromosome and Cancer*, **6**, 249–52.

1.6.9.11 Skin cancer: melanoma, basal cell carcinoma, and squamous cell carcinoma

Robert W. Demetrius, Clark C. Otley, and Randall K. Roenigk

Melanoma

Malignant melanoma is the most lethal form of skin cancer. Among Caucasians, the incidence rate for malignant melanoma has increased more than for any other cancer. Currently, melanoma is the seventh most common cancer in the United States (Parker and Zitelli 1996).

Box 1 Melanoma

- Consists of atypical melanocytes
- The most lethal form of skin cancer
- Incidence has increased steadily over the past 25 years
- Treatment of the skin lesions includes resection with a margin of normal tissue

Early detection and surgical treatment of this skin cancer affords excellent cure rates. In general, the prognosis for metastatic melanoma is very poor, although new advances in the use of immunomodulation are promising.

Definition

Malignant melanoma occurs when melanocytes undergo malignant transformation. Although the vast majority of melanomas originate in the skin, melanoma may also arise from mucosal epithelium, retina, or leptomeninges. Congenital or dysplastic nevi are associated with an increased risk of melanoma and may represent precursors of melanoma (Boyle *et al.* 1995). Although complicating variables exist, there is evidence that either intense early sun exposure or chronic intermittent sun exposure may be the initiating event in tumorogenesis (Elwood and Koh 1994; Boyle *et al.* 1995).

The biologic behavior of melanoma depends on the stage of lifecycle in which it exists. It is believed that melanoma progresses through five lifecycle stages (Brodland 1992; Barnhill *et al.* 1993):

(1) benign melanocyte or melanocytic nevus;

(2) melanocytic nevus or melanocyte with cytologic atypia (i.e. atypical nevus or atypical melanocyte);

(3) *in situ* malignant melanoma with a radial proliferation of tumor cells;

(4) invasive malignant melanoma with a vertical proliferation of tumor cells;

(5) metastasis of tumor cells to lymph nodes or distant organs.

The rapidity with which a melanoma will progress through these lifecycle phases to become invasive and ultimately metastatic depends partly on the particular subtype of melanoma (Parker and Zitelli 1996).

Epidemiology, incidence, and prevalence

There has been a steady increase in the incidence of malignant melanoma over the past 25 years (Ries *et al.* 1991; Friedman *et al.* 1996). About 38 300 new cases of malignant melanoma occur annually in the United States (Friedman *et al.* 1996), which correlates with 1 in 100 Americans developing malignant melanoma over their lifetime (Friedman *et al.* 1996), and this risk is increasing. Currently, the highest incidence for malignant melanoma occurs in Caucasians in Australia (Elwood and Koh 1994).

Except for those arising in large congenital nevi, malignant melanomas rarely occur prior to puberty. All adult age groups are affected, with a median age of 50 to 60 years at the time of diagnosis (Mackie 1992).

Epidemiologic factors associated with an increased risk of melanoma include atypical nevi, phototype I–II skin, red hair or blue eyes, personal or family history of melanoma, immunosuppression, and excessive sun exposure (Boyle *et al.* 1995). Intense periodic sun exposure may be more closely associated with superficial spreading malignant melanoma, while low-grade chronic sun exposure is more often seen with lentigo maligna melanoma (Barnhill *et al.* 1993).

Pathology

Histologically, malignant melanoma is characterized by substantial cytologic and architectural atypia of melanocytes. Differentiation of melanoma from an atypical nevus can be difficult, although several key features are useful in rendering a diagnosis of melanoma.

Histological features of malignant melanoma

These include the following (Barnhill *et al.* 1993):

(1) nesting and spread of melanocytes within the upper portion of the epidermis, known as pagetoid spread;

(2) asymmetric distribution of atypical melanocytes within the epidermis;

(3) failure of maturation by melanocytes deep in the dermis;

(4) cytologic atypia with mitotic figures.

Melanoma has been divided into multiple histological subtypes. The four classic histologic subtypes of invasive malignant melanoma with their clinical correlates are lentigo maligna melanoma, superficial spreading melanoma, nodular melanoma, and acral lentiginous melanoma. Other uncommon subtypes include amelanotic melanoma and desmoplastic melanoma (Parker and Zitelli 1996).

Histologic examination to determine tumor thickness or extent of invasion is a critical component in determining prognosis for patients with malignant melanoma (Friedman *et al.* 1996). Naturally, the deeper the melanoma, the higher is the risk of metastatic spread.

Clark (1969) developed the following system of standardizing level of tumor invasion:

- level 1: malignant melanoma cells are restricted to the epidermis and its appendages

- level 2: melanoma cells extend into the papillary dermis

- level 3: tumor cells extend throughout the papillary dermis and impinge upon the reticular dermis

- level 4: tumor cells invade through to the reticular dermis

- level 5: tumor cells invade into the subcutaneous fat.

Five-year survival for level 2 lesions is 99 per cent, compared with 75 per cent and 30 per cent respectively for level 4 and level 5 lesions (Lever and Schumberg-Lever 1990; Friedman *et al.* 1996).

However, a more accurate method of prognostication involves measuring the depth of invasion from the stratum granulosum to the deepest portion of the melanoma, known as the Breslow thickness (Lever and Schumberg-Lever 1990; Mackie 1992; Buttner *et al.* 1995). The Breslow thickness is currently the most accurate prognostic indicator for melanoma by multivariate analysis. Five-year survival for tumors of size less than or equal to 0.85 mm is 97 per cent, whereas tumors of size greater than or equal to 3.60 mm which have a 5-year survival of 48 per cent (Buttner *et al.* 1995; Friedman *et al.* 1996). In addition to depth of invasion, other factors which may be associated with a worse prognosis include ulceration, neurotropism, and lymphatic invasion (Johnson *et al.* 1995; Kohl *et al.* 1996).

Clinical evaluation

The early detection and prompt treatment of malignant melanoma significantly increases the cure rate (Johnson *et al.* 1995). Because melanoma is almost always visible on the skin surface, early recognition via cancer screening and physician and patient education may significantly decrease morbidity.

During the initial examination of a patient with possible melanoma, important historical information would include history of sun exposure, previous nonmelanoma or melanoma skin cancer, family history of melanoma skin cancer, history of atypical nevi, in addition to a general medical history (Johnson *et al.* 1995; Friedman *et al.* 1996). On physical examination, the patient should be completely undressed and cosmetics should be removed to allow for complete examination of the cutaneous and mucocutaneous surfaces (Kopf *et al.* 1995). The scalp, oral mucosa, genitalia, perirectal area, and web spaces between the toes should not be overlooked (Kopf *et al.* 1995). Regional lymph nodes should be palpated to assess possible lymph node involvement (Koh *et al.* 1996).

Distinguishing benign from malignant melanocytic neoplasms can be clinically challenging. The ABCD guidelines provide rudimentary guidance: A, asymmetry; B, border irregularity; C, color variation; D, diameter greater than 0.6 cm (about the size of a pencil eraser) (Johnson *et al.* 1995; Friedman *et al.* 1996; Koh *et al.* 1996; Mackie 1996). Asymmetry is due to the asymmetric proliferation of melanocytes within the epidermis. The irregular border is due to the irregular growth pattern of these melanocytes. Color variability is due to irregular deposits of melanin pigment within the epidermis.

A diameter greater than 0.6 cm is a common feature of early malignant melanoma (Friedman *et al.* 1996). Melanomas often have multiple ABCD features; however, melanoma can also virtually defy clinical recognition.

Clinical subtypes of melanoma

Lentigo maligna melanoma

Lentigo maligna melanoma is the least common type of melanoma among Caucasians (Barnhill *et al.* 1993). It is normally found on sun-exposed areas, frequently on the head or neck (Friedman *et al.* 1996; Parker and Zitelli 1996). Typically, there is a prolonged period of evolution with a radial growth phase lasting 3 to 15 years (Mackie 1992; Parker and Zitelli 1996). Clinically, it appears as a large irregular freckle, up to 5 to 10 cm in diameter. The color may be variable, showing areas of black, brown, and tan. Lentigo maligna (also called Hutchinson's melanotic freckle) is the *in situ* radial growth phase of lentigo maligna melanoma (Mackie 1992). With progression, a nodular component may develop which represents the vertical growth phase of the lesion (Fig. 1). Lentigo maligna melanoma often has subtle peripheral extension which can be difficult to discern clinically. Subclinical extension of tumor pigment may be better defined using a Wood's lamp (365 nm ultraviolet radiation)(Johnson *et al.* 1995; Koh *et al.* 1996).

Superficial spreading malignant melanoma

Superficial spreading malignant melanoma is the most frequent type of melanoma found in Caucasians (Barnhill *et al.* 1993). This variant of melanoma may occur anywhere on the cutaneous surface (Barnhill *et al.* 1993; Parker and Zitelli 1996). It is frequently seen on the trunk in men, while in women the lower extremities are more often involved. Diagnosis peaks in the fourth and fifth decades (Barnhill *et al.* 1993). The lesion is typically smaller than the lentigo maligna melanoma variant (Koh *et al.* 1996). There may be notching, irregu-

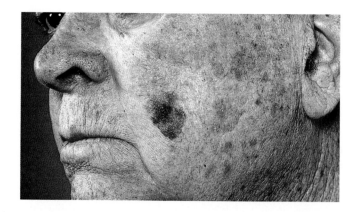

Fig. 1. Lentigo maligna melanoma: an irregular border with variable coloration is present.

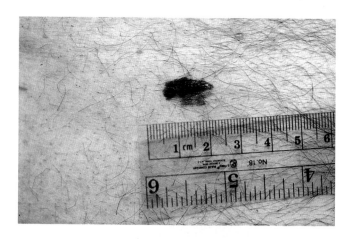

Fig. 2. Superficial spreading malignant melanoma. The lesion has an irregular 'notched' border and shows mottled coloration.

lar elevation, or mottling of color. Bleeding or serous oozing from a lesion is associated with a vertical growth phase (Fig. 2).

Nodular melanoma

Nodular melanoma is characterized by minimal radial growth prior to a rapid vertical growth phase (Koh *et al.* 1996; Parker and Zitelli 1996). Nodular melanoma is the second most prevalent type of malignant melanoma (Parker and Zitelli 1996). Because of its early invasive growth phase, this subtype carries a poor prognosis; however Breslow's thickness is still the best correlate of survival. Typically, nodular melanomas are dome-shaped, almost blueberry-like in appearance, and may have areas of ulceration and bleeding (Fig. 3).

Acral lentiginous melanoma

Acral lentiginous melanoma is the most common variant of melanoma in darker-skinned individuals (Parker and Zitelli 1996). It occurs most commonly on the soles, but can also occur on the palms and beneath the nailbed (subungual melanoma) (Koh *et al.* 1996). Acral lentiginous melanoma is frequently biologically aggressive (Barnhill *et al.* 1993) because of the delay in diagnosis of this type of melanoma. However, survival still correlates best with Breslow's

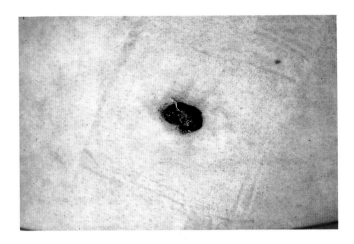

Fig. 3. Nodular melanoma: a black nodule with evidence of bleeding at the edge.

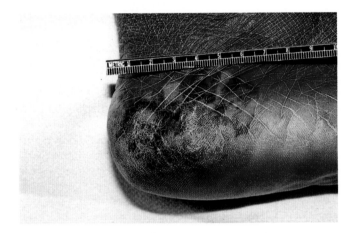

Fig. 4. Acral lentiginous melanoma: an ill-defined pigmented lesion on the heel of this darker-skinned patient.

thickness. Clinically, acral lentiginous melanoma appears as an ill-defined pigmented lesion on the plantar or palmar surface, or as a pigmented subungual streak (Fig. 4).

Epiluminescent microscopy

Epiluminescent microscopy is a noninvasive technique used as an aid in the clinical examination of pigmented lesions (Johnson *et al.* 1995). It can be helpful to differentiate benign pigmented lesions from malignant melanoma. After applying a thin layer of mineral oil on the surface of the suspicious pigmented lesion, a hand-held magnifying lens is then used to examine the lesion (Johnson *et al.* 1995). The oil renders the stratum corneum of the skin transparent, permitting better visualization of pigmented anatomic structures within the epidermis, dermoepidermal junction, and superficial papillary dermis (Kenet *et al.* 1993). Under epiluminescent microscopy, malignant melanoma tend to have irregular pigmentation, pseudopod formation, blue–gray areas, or brown globules (Johnson *et al.* 1995). Epiluminescent microscopy is an aid for judging pigmented

lesions but does not replace a careful clinical examination and history (Friedman *et al.* 1996).

Biopsy technique

Ideally, biopsy of a malignant melanoma should include total excision so that histologic examination of the whole tumor is possible (Coates *et al.* 1995; Johnson *et al.* 1995). However, an incisional biopsy may be required for very large tumors or in difficult anatomic areas (Johnson *et al.* 1995). Multiple studies have demonstrated no adverse effect on survival from incisional as opposed to excisional biopsy. Because histologic examination of the vertical thickness of melanoma is paramount for determining prognosis as well as optimal treatment, a shave biopsy, curettage, or needle biopsy should be avoided (Johnson *et al.* 1995; Friedman *et al.* 1996).

Excisional biopsies are usually easily accomplished with local anesthesia on an outpatient basis. Normally a 2-mm margin of normal skin around the lesion is sufficient for an excisional biopsy and for diagnosis (Friedman *et al.* 1996). Clinical estimation of histologic tumor thickness is often unreliable, therefore it is prudent to avoid taking large margins without histologic confirmation of depth of invasion. An elliptical incision may be oriented along the probable pathway of lymphatic drainage (Friedman *et al.* 1996). The excision should extend to the subcutaneous tissue.

Treatment

Once the diagnosis of malignant melanoma is obtained, definitive treatment depends on the histologic depth of the tumor. According to an National Institutes of Health consensus conference, melanoma *in situ* may be excised with 0.5-cm margins, while invasive melanoma less than 1 mm in thickness should have a 1-cm margin (Koh *et al.* 1996). For lesions between 1 and 4 mm in thickness, 2- to 3-cm margins should be obtained. For tumors greater than 4 mm in thickness, 3-cm margins should be obtained. Dissections should be taken down to fascia unless there is a compelling anatomic reason to compromise.

Controversy surrounds the use of elective lymph node dissection in the management of malignant melanoma. Randomized trials of elective lymph node dissection demonstrated no clear benefit compared with clinical observation (Coates *et al.* 1995; Rompel *et al.* 1995). In general, many surgeons feel that elective lymph node dissection is not indicated in patients with melanoma less than 1 mm thick or over 4 mm thick, because the odds of metastases are very low and very high respectively. Intermediate melanoma between 1 and 4 mm in thickness should be managed on a case-by-case basis.

For staging purposes, patients with thin melanomas (less than 1 mm thick) need only a history and physical examination, while patients with thicker melanomas require chest radiographs and serum lactate dehydrogenase levels. Further testing is based on findings on history and physical examination, as extensive testing is not cost-effective (Weiss *et al.* 1995).

Recent studies with adjuvant interferon-α_{2a} have shown survival benefit in a subgroup of patients with positive lymph nodes (Kirkwood *et al.* 1996). Thus these patients warrant consideration of adjuvant interferon therapy. Other adjuvant therapies have not been proven to enhance survival and are thus considered investigational.

Patients with solitary metastases have shown improved survival after metastasectomy.

Results of treatment

Prognosis is most closely predicted by the histologic tumor thickness. Eighty per cent of patients with primary melanoma will enjoy long-term disease-free survival currently, because of early detection. Surgical therapy is paramount, as adjuvant and salvage therapy is infrequently successful. Patients with metastatic nodal melanoma have approximately a 20 per cent 5-year survival after therapeutic lymphadenectomy, while the 5-year survival for distant metastatic melanoma is negligible (Ho 1995).

Basal cell carcinoma

Basal cell carcinoma is the most common form of cutaneous cancer (Mackie 1992). Approximately 500 000 to 1 million new cases of basal cell carcinoma develop in the United States each year (Miller and Weinstock 1994). Other synonyms for basal cell carcinoma include 'basal cell epithelioma', 'basalioma', and 'rodent ulcer'; however, the term basal cell carcinoma is preferable as this tumor is a locally destructive malignancy with rare metastatic potential (Carter and Lin 1993; Grande et al. 1996).

Definition

Basal cell carcinoma is a malignant neoplasm of basal epidermal keratinocytes (Mackie 1992; Carter and Lin 1993). Usually a slow-growing tumor (Grande et al. 1996), it requires months to attain a clinically appreciable size. Giant basal cell carcinoma is seen in cases of neglect or incomplete treatment (Randle 1996). Without treatment, the tumor will continue to be invasive and destructive, resulting in perineural, cartilaginous, or bone involvement. Local invasion and tumor growth of basal cell carcinoma is thought to be enhanced by enzymes which digest the surrounding matrix (Grande et al. 1996). In very rare instances basal carcinoma may metastasize (Carter and Lin 1993; Randle 1996).

Epidemiology

Risk factors for the development of basal cell carcinoma include light complexion (Randle 1996), excessive sun exposure, exposure to ionizing radiation or X-rays, the presence of chronic nonhealing ulcerations and arsenic exposure (Carter and Lin 1993; Grande et al. 1996).

Box 2 Basal cell carcinoma

- The most common form of skin cancer
- A slow-growing malignant neoplasm of basal epidermal keratinocytes
- Depending on their location and histologic type, basal cell carcinomas may be treated with a variety of modalities, such as cryotherapy, electrodesiccation and curettage, radiation therapy, excision, or Mohs micrographic surgery

Basal cell carcinomas also arise in certain genetic syndromes: basal cell nevus syndrome, xeroderma pigmentosum, Muir–Torre syndrome, Behçet's syndrome, and in patients with albinism owing to lack of photoprotective pigmentation (Carter and Lin 1993).

Basal cell carcinoma is normally found in patients over 40 years of age (Mackie 1992; Randle et al. 1993; Grande et al. 1996), but there has been an increase in the number of patients presenting in their twenties and thirties. This is felt to be in part due to increased recreational and occupational sun exposure. Most basal cell carcinomas are found in body areas subject to intense sun exposure (Randle et al. 1993), with 80 per cent on the head or neck. Approximately 50 per cent of patients with one basal cell carcinoma will develop a second one within 5 years, emphasizing the importance of close life-long follow-up.

Pathology

Twenty-six histological subtypes of basal cell carcinoma have been described (Lever and Schumburg-Lever 1990). The degree to which the histologic subtypes correlate with a clinical appearance is undefined.

Histologically, in all subtypes of basal cell carcinoma, proliferative aggregates of basaloid (bluish colored) cells of varying sizes and shapes are apparent (Lever and Schumburg-Lever 1990). In most cases, clefts separate the basaloid aggregates and the surrounding stroma. The epidermis overlying the basaloid tumor may be ulcerated or intact.

The micronodular variant of basal cell carcinoma is characterized by numerous three- to five-cell-wide finger-like extensions, while the morpheaform variant shows one- to two-cell-wide spindle-shaped extensions (Lever and Schumburg-Lever 1990; Hendrix and Parlette 1996). Metatypical basal cell carcinoma is notable for significant keratinization and may be an intermediate between basal cell and squamous cell carcinoma. These histological subtypes are particularly prone to recurrence. In the superficial variant, there are multiple budding basaloid cells with minimal dermal invasion.

Clinical evaluation

Nodular basal cell carcinoma

The nodular basal cell carcinoma is the most common clinical type of basal cell carcinoma (Leshin and White 1996). Ulceration or erosion is a frequent finding in larger lesions. Clinically one sees a waxy or pearly papule or nodule with overlying telangiectasia (Fig. 5). Eighty per cent of these tumors present on the head and neck, with the nose (40 per cent) being the most common site (Roenigk et al. 1986). Pigmented basal cell carcinomas are often nodular but may mimic melanoma.

Morpheaform basal cell carcinoma

The morpheaform variant of basal cell carcinoma clinically is seen as a scar-like dermal plaque with occasional epidermal atrophy. With long-standing growth, there may be superficial erosion or ulceration (Grande et al. 1996). Because of the atypical clinical appearance of morpheaform basal cell carcinoma, they may attain considerable size before detection.

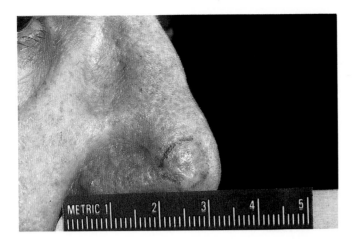

Fig. 5. Nodular basal cell carcinoma: a waxy nodule with overlying telangiectasia.

Superficial basal cell carcinoma

Superficial basal cell carcinoma is usually a pink to red scaly somewhat indurated plaque that typically presents on the trunk (Fig. 6). There may be an advancing thread-like border seen at its periphery. Clinically if there is not a high index of suspicion, it may be misdiagnosed as eczema or psoriasis (Grande *et al.* 1996).

Treatment

The optimal treatment of basal cell carcinoma is based on examination of the histologic subtype and knowledge of the associated biologic behavior. Histologic subtypes with a low propensity for recurrence, such as nodular and superficial, may be treated with a variety of modalities, such as cryotherapy, electrodesiccation and curettage, radiation therapy, excision, or Mohs micrographic surgery. Optimal treatment is also based on site, size, history of prior treatment, and desired cosmetic outcome.

Basal cell carcinoma with several well-defined characteristics has a significantly increased risk of recurrence. High-risk characteristics include history of prior treatment, location in high-risk sites (such as the eyelid, nose, nasolabial fold, lip, or ear), clinically indistinct borders, size greater than 2 cm, or aggressive histological subtype (Randle *et al.* 1993; Randle 1996). In these cases the treatment of choice is Mohs micrographic surgery because this type of procedure precisely examines 100 per cent of the excisional margin of the tumor to provide the highest cure rates. In addition, wide margins are not excised unless necessary, sparing normal tissue in some cases. This is an important consideration given the fact that many of these tumors occur in cosmetically and functionally important areas of the face (Motley and Holt 1994). Cure rates for basal cell carcinoma with Mohs micrographic surgery are 99 per cent, compared with 91 per cent for other modalitites (Randle 1996).

Squamous cell carcinoma

Squamous cell carcinoma of the skin most commonly arises on skin exposed chronically to ultraviolet light. Squamous cell carcinoma can develop *de novo* within normal skin or infrequently (approximately 20 per cent of the time) develops from premalignant lesions called actinic keratoses (Lever and Schumburg-Lever 1990). Approximately 20 per cent of all nonmelanoma cutaneous malignancies are squamous cell carcinomas (Leshin and White 1996). There has been a steady increase in incidence of squamous cell carcinoma since 1980 (Mackie 1992), with approximately 2000 deaths annually in the United States.

Definition

Squamous cell carcinoma of the skin is a malignant neoplasm derived from keratin-producing epithelial cells known as keratinocytes (Mackie 1992). Normally, if left untreated, squamous cell carcinomas cause local destruction of tissue, and in approximately 3 to 5 per cent of cases can metastasize and cause death. The biologic behavior of squamous cell carcinoma depends on the size of the tumor, its histology, and its location, as well as other concomitant disease states (Melton and Hanke 1996).

Whereas for melanoma, prognostic factors are well established by multivariate analysis, for squamous cell carcinoma, only univariate analysis has been utilized for prognostic indicators. By univariate analysis, several factors are associated with significantly increased risk of recurrence and metastasis including size greater than 2 cm, histologic thickness greater that 4 mm, poor histologic differentiation (grade III or IV), immunocompromised host, history of prior treat-

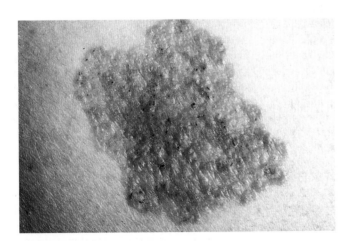

Fig. 6. Superficial basal cell carcinoma: a red scaly plaque with advancing thread-like border.

> **Box 3 Squamous cell carcinoma**
>
> - A malignant neoplasm derived from keratin-producing epithelial cells known as keratinocytes
>
> - The incidence of squamous cell carcinoma has steadily increased since 1980
>
> - Depending on the size, location, and histological grade of the tumor, as well as the age and physical condition of the patient, squamous cell carcinomas may be treated by excision, radiation therapy, electrodesiccation and curettage, or cryosurgery

ment, and origin in a chronic scarring or inflammatory process (Lever and Schumburg-Lever 1990; Brodland and Zitelli 1992; Barrett *et al.* 1993; Schwartz and Stoll 1993; Kirsner and Garland 1994; Lawrence and Cottel 1994, Bernstein *et al.* 1996; Leshin and White 1996). Squamous cell carcinoma with these high-risk features may have significant metastatic potential and should be treated aggressively. Metastasis usually occurs to regional lymph nodes, although hematogenous spread also occurs (Bernstein *et al.* 1996).

Epidemiology

Squamous cell carcinoma in the majority of cases is related to the amount of sun exposure and the degree of pigmentation of the skin (Bernstein *et al.* 1996; Leshin and White 1996; Melton and Hanke 1996). There is an increased incidence in countries closer to the equator (Mackie 1992; Leshin and White 1996). Those patients at greatest risk for developing squamous cell carcinoma include people with lighter complexions with excessive sun damage and actinic keratoses. Significant increase is also seen in patients with blue eyes, childhood freckling, and older age (Schwartz and Stoll 1993). The incidence of squamous cell carcinoma in males is higher than in females. This is probably related to men having a greater amount of sun exposure due to different clothing styles, work, and leisure activities (Schwartz and Stoll 1993). A history of arsenic exposure, as well as high doses of ultraviolet A radiation in combination with psoralens, used to treat psoriasis patients, have also been shown to increase the risk of squamous cell carcinoma (Chuang *et al.* 1992; Bernstein *et al.* 1996).

Pathology

Squamous cell carcinoma is a malignant tumor arising from the epidermal keratinocytes. Histologically, one sees irregular masses of epidermal cells invading the dermis. The tumor may be composed of well-differentiated normal squamous cells with individual cell keratinization or poorly differentiated anaplastic cells (Motley and Holt 1994). Differentiation or maturation of the tumor is characterized by its keratinization, often taking place in the form of horn pearls (Broders 1921; Lever and Schumburg-Lever 1990). Poorly differentiated squamous cell carcinoma without keratinization is a spindle cell neoplasm which mimics soft-tissue sarcomas, neural and muscle neoplasms, or desmoplastic melanoma.

The grading of squamous cell carcinoma introduced by Broders (1921) recognizes four grades of severity depending on the proportion of well-differentiated cells within the tumor (Lever and Schumburg-Lever 1990):

- grade 1: 75 per cent of keratinocytes are histologically well differentiated

- grade 2: 50 per cent

- grade 3: 25 per cent

- grade 4: less than 25 per cent.

Additional histologic information which may be helpful for prognostication and treatment decisions includes the depth of penetration and perineral invasion (Barrett *et al.* 1993; Lawrence and Cottel 1994; Bernstein *et al.* 1996)

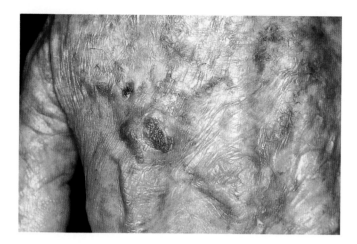

Fig. 7. Squamous cell carcinoma: a pink indurated verrucous nodule on the dorsal hand.

Clinical evaluation

Occasionally arising from a premalignant actinic keratosis, squamous cell carcinoma is a skin-colored to reddish pink papule, nodule, or plaque with a verrucous, hyperkeratotic, or ulcerated surface. The clinical margins may be indistinct. Ulceration may lead to bleeding or exudation. The most common sites for squamous cell carcinoma are those exposed to the sun. The back of the hands (Fig. 7), forearms, and upper part of the face, and, especially in males, the lower lip and pinna are areas frequently involved (Mackie 1992; Bernstein *et al.* 1996).

There are many clinical presentations of cutaneous squamous cell carcinoma. Arsenic-induced squamous cell carcinoma normally presents as discrete keratoses on the palms and soles (Maloney 1996) which may become painful, ulcerate, and bleed (Schwartz and Stoll 1993). Squamous cell carcinoma secondary to thermal or chronic heat damage may occur in the setting of brownish red patches with telangiectasias called erythema ab igne (Schwartz and Stoll 1993). When squamous cell carcinoma develops in a scar, there is usually the appearance of erosion or ulceration present for months (Schwartz and Stoll 1993). Chronic ulcers, especially on the legs, are occasionally sites of origin for squamous cell carcinoma (Schwartz and Stoll 1993; Kopf *et al.* 1995) (Fig. 8).

Solar-induced damage of the lip, more commonly seen in men, may result in squamous cell carcinoma presenting as a roughened papule or leukoplakia with hyperkeratosis involving the lower lip (Bernstein *et al.* 1996). Bowen's disease is a squamous cell carcinoma *in situ* (localized to the epidermis) which appears as a scaling erythematous patch larger than an actinic keratoses (Bernstein *et al.* 1996). Bowen's disease may develop into invasive squamous cell carcinoma in 11 per cent of the cases. Erythroplasia of Queyrat is squamous cell carcinoma *in situ* localized to the glans penis. This is more commonly seen in uncircumcised men (Melton and Hanke 1996), where clinically one sees a shiny red plaque which may be related to human papillomavirus. Verrucous carcinoma is a low-grade squamous cell carcinoma (Leshin and White 1996; Melton and Hanke 1996) which can be extensive and locally destructive. When it occurs in the oral cavity is called oral florid papillomatosis; in the anogenital region, it is called a giant condyloma of Buschke and Loewenstein. On the

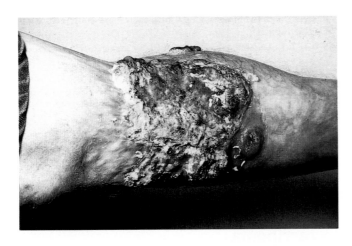

Fig. 8. Squamous cell carcinoma arising in a chronic Marjolin ulcer.

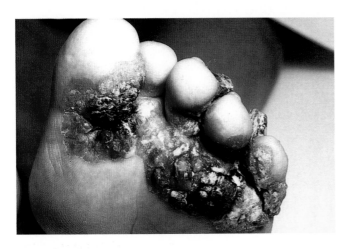

Fig. 9. Squamous cell carcinoma. Epithelioma cuniculatum—a verrucous plaque on the plantar foot.

plantar surface of the foot, it is called epithelioma cuniculatum (Fig. 9). Human papillomavirus may also play a role in these tumors.

Management

Treatment is based on several factors including size, location, the histological grade of the tumor, as well as the age and physical condition of the patient. Surgical excision, radiation therapy, electrodesiccation and curettage, and cryosurgery are all standard methods of primary treatment for squamous cell carcinoma. These modalities are associated with a 92 per cent 5-year cure rate for squamous cell carcinoma of the skin. In order for standard excisional surgery to eradicate approximately 95 per cent of squamous cell carcinomas, margins of 4 mm must be used for well-differentiated tumors, and 6 mm for poorly differentiated squamous cell carcinoma (Brodland and Zitelli 1992).

As mentioned previously, squamous cell carcinoma with high-risk features such as size greater than 2 cm, histologic thickness greater than 4 mm, poor differentiation, perineural invasion, high-risk sites (lip, ear, penis, scrotum, anus), immunocompromised host, history

of prior treatment, and origin in scarring or chronic inflammatory process have substantially increased the risk of metastasis and recurrence. For many of these tumors, the complete histologic margin control provided by Mohs micrographic surgery offers the advantage of the highest cure rates coupled with possible sparing of normal tissue. Five-year cure rates for squamous cell carcinoma of the skin excluding the lip are 97 per cent for Mohs micrographic surgery compared with 92 per cent for other modalities, including excision.

Close clinical follow-up is warranted with squamous cell carcinoma due to its metastatic potential; the vast majority of recurrences occur within the first 3 years. Regional node metastases are best managed with a therapeutic lymphadenectomy, with 5-year survival rates of approximately 25 per cent. Distant metastases of squamous cell carcinoma are managed palliatively with multimodality therapy, but the prognosis is poor.

References

Barnhill, R.L., Mihm, M.C., Jr, Fitzpatrick, T.B, *et al.* (1993). Neoplasms: malignant melanoma. In *Dermatology in general medicine* (4th edn) (ed. T.B. Fitzpatrick, A.Z. Eisen, I.M. Freedberg, *et al.*), pp. 1078–1110. McGraw-Hill, New York.

Barrett, T.L., Greenway, H.T., Jr, Massullo, V., *et al.* (1993). Treatment of basal cell carcinoma and squamous cell carcinoma with perineural invasion. *Advances in Dermatology*, **8**, 277–304.

Bernstein, S.C., Lim, K.K., Brodland, D.G., *et al.* (1996). The many phases of squamous cell carcinoma. *Dermatology Surgery*, **22**, 243–54.

Boyle, P., Maisonneuve, P., and Dore, J.-F. (1995). Epidemiology of malignant melanoma. *British Medical Bulletin*, **51**, 523–47.

Broders, A. (1921). Squamous cell epithelioma of the skin. *Annals of Surgery*, **73**, 141.

Brodland, D.G. (1992). Mechanisms of metastasis. *Journal of American Academy of Dermatology*, **27**.

Brodland, D.G. and Zitelli, J.A. (1992). Surgical margins for excision of primary cutaneous squamous cell carcinoma. *Journal of the American Academy of Dermatology*, **27**, 241–8.

Buttner, P., *et al.* (1995). Primary cutaneous melanoma. *Cancer*, **75**, 2499–505.

Carter, D.M. and Lin, A.N. (1993). Basal cell carcinoma. In *Dermatology in general medicine* (4th edn) (ed. T.B. Fitzpatrick, A.Z. Eisen, I.M. Freedberg, *et al.*), pp. 840–7. McGraw-Hill, New York.

Chuang, T.-Y., Heinrich, L.A., Schultz, M.D., *et al.* (1992). Puva and skin cancer. *Journal of the American Academy of Dermatology*, **26**, 173–7.

Clark, W., Jr (1969). The histiogenesis and biologic behavior of primary human malignant melanoma of the skin. *Cancer Research*, **29**, 705–15.

Coates, A.S., Ingvar, C.I., Petersen-Schaefer, K., *et al.* (1995). Elective lymph node dissection in patients with primary melanoma of the trunk and limbs treated at the Sydney melanoma unit from 1960 to 1991. *Journal of the American College of Surgeons*, **180**, 402–9.

Elwood, J.M. and Koh, H.K. (1994). Etiology, epidemiology, risk factors, and public health issues of melanoma. *Current Opinion in Oncology*, **6**, 179–87.

Friedman, R.J., Rigel, D.S., Silverman, S., *et al.* (1996). Malignant melanoma. In *Dermatologic surgery, principles and practice* (2nd edn) (ed. R.K. Roenigk and H.H. Roenigk Jr), pp. 551–62. Dekker, New York.

Grande, D.J., Ratner, D., and Stadecker, M.J. (1996). Basal cell carcinoma. In *Dermatology surgery, principles and practice* (2nd edn) (ed. R.K. Roenigk and H.H. Roenigk Jr), pp. 489–501. Dekker, New York.

Hendrix, J.D. and Parlette, H.L. (1996). Micronodular basal cell carcinoma. *Archives of Dermatology*, **132**, 295–8.

Ho, R.C. (1995). Medical management of stage IV malignant melanoma. Medical issues. *Cancer*, **75** (Supplement 2), 735–41.

Johnson, T.M., *et al.* (1995). Current therapy for cutaneous melanoma. *Journal of the American Academy of Dermatology*, **32**, 689–703.

Kenet, R.O., *et al.* (1993). Clinical diagnosis of pigmented lesions using digital epiluminescent microscopy. *Archives of Dermatology*, **129**, 157–74.

Kirkwood, J.M., Strawderman, M.H., Ernstoff, M.S., *et al.* (1996). Interferon alpha-2b adjuvant therapy of high-risk resected cutaneous melanoma: the Eastern Cooperative Oncology Group Trial EST 1684. *Journal of Clinical Oncology*, **14**, 7–17.

Kirsner, R.S. and Garland, L.D. (1994). Squamous cell carcinoma arising from chronic osteomyelitis treated by Mohs micrographic surgery. *Journal of Dermatologic Surgery and Oncology*, **20**, 141–3.

Koh, H.K., Barnhill, R.L., and Rogers, G.S. (1996). Melanoma. In *Cutaneous medicine and surgery*, Vol. 2 (ed. K. Arndt, P.E. Leboit, J.K. Robinson, and B.U. Wintroub), pp. 1576–600. W.B. Saunders, Philadelphia, PA.

Kopf, A.W., *et al.* (1995). Techniques of cutaneous examination for the detection of skin cancer. *Cancer*, **75**, 684–9.

Lawrence, N. and Cottel, W.I. (1994). Squamous cell carcinoma of the skin with perineural invasion. *Journal of the American Academy of Dermatology*, **31**, 30–3.

Leshin, B. and White, W.L. (1996). Malignant neoplasms of keratinocytes. In *Cutaneous medicine and surgery*, Vol. 2 (ed. K. Arndt, P.E. Leboit, J.K. Robinson, and B.U. Wintroub), pp. 1378–91. W.B. Saunders, Philadelphia, PA.

Lever, W.F. and Schumburg-Lever, G. (1990*a*). Basal cell epithelioma. In *Histopathology of the skin* (7th edn) (ed. W.F. Lever and G. Schaumburg-Lever), pp. 622–34. J.B. Lippincott, Philadelphia, PA.

Lever, W.F. and Schumburg-Lever, G. (1990*b*). Benign melanocytic tumors and malignant melanoma. In *Histopathology of the skin* (7th edn) (ed. W.F. Lever and G. Schaumburg-Lever), pp. 780–95. J.B. Lippincott, Philadelphia, PA.

Lever, W.F. and Schumburg-Lever, G. (1990*c*) Solar keratosis. In *Histopathology of the skin* (7th edn) (ed. W.F. Lever and G. Schaumburg-Lever), p. 542. J.B. Lippincott, Philadelphia, PA.

Mackie, R.M. (1992). Melanocytic naevi and malignant melanoma. In *Rook, Wilkinson, Ebling's textbook of dermatology*, Vol. 2 (5th edn) (ed. R.H. Champion, J.L. Burton, and F.J.G. Ebling), pp. 1488–1559. Blackwell Scientific, Oxford.

Maloney, M.E. (1996). Arsenic in dermatology. *Dermatologic Surgery*, **22**, 301–4.

Melton, J. and Hanke, C. (1996). Squamous cell carcinoma. In *Dermatology surgery, principles and practice*, (2nd edn) (ed. R.K. Roenigk and H.H. Roenigk Jr), pp. 503–21. Dekker, New York.

Miller, D. and Weinstock, M. (1994). Nonmelanoma skin cancer in the United States: incidence. *Journal of the American Academy of Dermatology*, **30**, 774–8.

Motley, R.J. and Holt, P.J. (1994). Micrographic surgery for basal cell carcinoma. *British Journal of Hospital Medicine*, **52**, 353–5.

Parker, T. and Zitelli, J. (1996). Malignant melanoma. *Dermatologic Surgery*, **22**, 234–40.

Randle, H.W. (1996). Basal cell carcinoma identification and treatment of the high-risk patient. *Dermatologic Surgery*, **22**, 255–61.

Randle, H.W., Roenigk, R.K., and Brodland, D.B. (1993). Giant basal cell carcinoma (T3): who is at risk? *Cancer*, **72**, 1624–9.

Ries, L., Hankey, B., Miller, B., *et al.* (1991). *Cancer statistics review 1973–1988*. NIH Publication No. 91-2789. National Cancer Institute, US Government Printing Office, Washington, DC.

Roenigk, R.K., Ratz, J.L., Bailin, P.L., *et al.* (1986). Trends in the presentation and treatment of basal cell carcinomas. *Journal of Dermatologic Surgery and Oncology*, **12**, 860–5.

Rompel, R., Garbe, C., Buttner, P., *et al.* (1995). Role of elective lymph node

dissection in stage I malignant melanoma: evaluation by matched pair analysis. *Recent Results in Cancer Research*, **139**, 323–36.

Schwartz, R.A. and Stoll, H.L. (1993). Squamous cell carcinoma. In *Dermatology in general medicine* (4th edn) (ed. T.B. Fitzpatrick, A.Z. Eisen, I.M. Freedberg, *et al.*), pp. 821–39. McGraw-Hill, New York.

Weiss, M., Loprinzi, C.L., Creagan E.T., *et al.* (1995). Utility of follow-up tests for detecting recurrent disease in patients with malignant melanomas. *Journal of the American Medical Association*, **274**, 1703–5.

1.6.10 Metastic neoplasms

1.6.10.1 Metastatic bone disease due to carcinoma

Panayiotis J. Papagelopoulos, Evanthia C. Galanis, and Franklin H. Sim

Introduction

Metastases to bone in a patient with cancer are not as common as metastases to the lungs and liver. However, bone metastases usually produce significant pain and disability early in the course of disease

Box 1

- The most common sources of bone metastases are carcinomas of the breast, prostate, kidney, lung, and thyroid, but any carcinoma can metastasize to bone

- The spine, pelvis, sternum, skull, and ribs are the most common sites of metastases

- The femur and humerus are the most frequent sites of metastases in the appendicular skeleton, and metastases distal to the elbow and knee are uncommon

- Most bone metastases present with pain, but they may present with pathologic fractures, spinal cord compression, hypercalcemia, and anemia

- Radiographs may show lytic or blastic lesions, but normal radiographs do not exclude the diagnosis of metastatic carcinoma

- Bone scans may not detect rapidly growing metastases

- MRI is the most sensitive method for evaluation of bone marrow infiltration by metastatic carcinomas

- Differential diagnosis includes primary bone tumors, osteoporosis, Paget's disease, osteomyelitis, osteoporosis, and stress or insufficiency fractures

- Systemic treatments of metastatic bone disease include cancer chemotherapy, hormonal therapy, and bisphosphonates

- Local treatments of metastatic bone lesions include radiation therapy, surgical resection, surgical stabilization to prevent or treat pathologic fractures, and surgical decompression of the spinal cord

Table 1 Incidence of skeletal metastases in autopsy studies

Primary tumor site	No. of studies	Incidence of bone metastases (%) Median	Range
Breast	5	73	47–85
Prostate	6	68	33–85
Thyroid	4	42	28–60
Kidney	3	35	33–40
Bronchus	4	36	30–55
Esophagus	3	6	5–7
Gastrointestinal tract	4	5	3–11
Rectum	3	11	9–13

as a result of pathologic fractures, anemia, and hypercalcemia. In addition, median survival after relapse in the bones is usually longer in comparison with relapse in other visceral organs. For patients with breast cancer with metastatic bone disease apparently confined to the skeleton, the median survival after the first relapse in bone is 24 months, compared with only 4 to 6 months after the first untreated relapse in the liver. Prostatic cancer metastatic bone disease can also follow a relatively long course, with patients having a median survival of about 2 years after the diagnosis of bone metastases.

Epidemiology

More than 1 million new cases of cancer are discovered in the United States each year (Silverberg *et al.* 1990). In about half of these patients, the diagnosis is carcinoma of the breast, lung, prostate, kidney, or thyroid—tumors that commonly metastasize to bone (Wirth 1979). Two-thirds of these cancer patients will have metastases at some time during their course of treatment. The incidence of bone metastases from different primary tumor sites has been recorded in postmortem studies (Table 1) (Galasko 1981).

In the last few years, the incidence of metastatic disease has increased because of the longer survival of patients with bone-seeking cancers (i.e. breast, prostate, lung, kidney, and thyroid). This may also be the reason why other cancers that traditionally have not been considered as causes of bone metastases (i.e. gastrointestinal system, uterus, adrenal gland, bladder, and testicular carcinomas) are now increasingly implicated in metastatic bone disease.

The distribution of bone metastases is predominantly to the axial skeleton, particularly the spine, pelvis, sternum, skull, and ribs, rather than the appendicular skeleton. The spine is the region most commonly affected by metastatic bone disease. Lesions in the humeri and femora are common, with the proximal long bones most commonly involved.

Pathophysiology

Mechanisms

The predominant distribution of bone metastases in the axial skeleton, where most of the active bone marrow is situated in adults, suggests that the slow blood flow at these sites could assist in the attachment of metastatic cells. The experiments of Batson (1940,

1942) in animals and human cadavers demonstrated the vertebral venous plexus and provided a good explanation for the predilection of metastatic spread from certain cancers to the skeleton.

Experimental studies on the mechanisms of vertebral metastases suggest that tumor cells lodge and grow within the sinusoids of the bone marrow and invade the spinal canal through the vertebral vein foramina. Experimentally, tumor cell lines growing as compact tumors commonly form an extradural tumor mass anteriorly and compress the cord anteriorly, whereas cell lines growing in an infiltrating fashion tend to migrate posteriorly to produce posterior compression. Of interest is the observation that tumor cells invade the extradural space through the venous foramina and not by cortical bone destruction (Arguello *et al.* 1990).

Pathogenesis

After the cancer cells lodge in bone, their biological behavior depends on both the biological activity of the cancer cells themselves and the person's immune system. Depending on the cancer cell–host interaction, cancer cells may remain controlled within the bone, may progress slowly, increasing in number and destroying the host bone, or may progress very rapidly, with relentless destruction of the bone. The damage to the skeleton is usually much more extensive than could be expected simply from the amount of malignant cells present. Accumulated evidence suggests that most of the tumor-induced destruction is mediated by osteoclasts. Tumor cells damage the skeleton in other ways, possibly by compression of the vasculature and consequent ischemia, but these processes are of less importance. In addition, tissue-specific growth factors, cytokines (i.e. tumor necrosis factor-α), and angiogenic factors (i.e. tumor growth factor-β) may contribute to metastatic growth.

Local factors

Malignant cells stimulate the production of factors with osteoclastic activity either directly or indirectly through their interaction with tumor-associated immune cells. These factors include prostaglandin E and various cytokines and growth factors.

Systemic factors

In addition to the local paracrine factors described above, osteoclastic activity can also be stimulated in malignant disease by systemic factors, particularly parathyroid-hormone-related peptide. This peptide is immunologically distinct from parathormone, but the two hormones have significant homology at the amino terminus of the molecule, which is necessary for osteoclast stimulation. Ectopic production of this hormone, particularly in lung cancer, is a cause of osteoclastic bone resorption and hypercalcemia, even in the absence of bone metastases.

Osteolytic disease is usually most evident at the sites of metastases, but osteosclerosis may predominate in some cases, particularly in prostate cancer.

Clinical evaluation

Several complications give rise to the substantial morbidity from bone metastases. They include pain, impaired mobility, pathologic fracture, spinal cord compression, cranial nerve palsies, nerve lesions, hypercalcemia, and suppression of bone marrow function.

Pain is the most common and reliable symptom of patients presenting with metastases to bone. Night pain is one of the cardinal symptoms. The pain may be intermittent in nature, but it progresses in intensity and duration. Often, the pain is in the extremities, usually activity related, but as bone destruction progresses, the pain will be present at rest. Pain is caused by several factors including periosteal stretching, compression or infiltration of nerve roots, reflex muscle spasm, and local effects of cytokines.

In patients with metastases to the spine, pain may be caused by bone destruction and by compression of both the nerve roots and the spinal cord.

The precise incidence of pathologic fracture in patients with metastatic bone disease is uncertain. Cancer of the breast is responsible for around half of pathologic fractures; the kidney, lung, thyroid, prostate, and lymphoma account for the rest.

Other manifestations of metastatic bone disease include hypercalcemia and anemia or pancytopenia. The latter can be caused by extensive infiltration of the bone marrow by metastatic disease, and it can predispose to infection or hemorrhage. Radiation therapy, often needed for treatment of bone metastases, can exacerbate this problem, which in turn may compromise effective chemotherapy. Other iatrogenic factors may also aggravate the morbidity from bone metastases; for example, ovarian ablation and corticosteroids used in the treatment of breast cancer may predispose to osteoporosis. This condition can present diagnostic problems in elderly patients in whom it may be difficult to distinguish between osteoporotic and metastatic disease as the cause of vertebral compression fracture.

Diagnostic studies

Plain radiographs

Radiographic and scintigraphic methods do not assess tumors directly; instead, they reflect skeletal reaction to metastases. A skeletal radiograph indicates the net result of bone resorption and repair. For a destructive lesion in trabecular bone to be recognized on a plain radiograph, it must be greater than 1 cm in diameter, with loss of approximately 50 per cent of the bone mineral content.

Depending on the reaction of host bone to the cancer cells, metastases may appear on radiographs as a purely lytic, purely blastic, or, most commonly, with a mixed pattern of lysis and bone formation. These differences in radiological manifestations of skeletal metastases are related to the histological types of cancer that influence the balance of dominance between osteoblastic and osteoclastic activation. Rapidly progressive bone metastases often show little or no host bone reaction, resulting in a radiographic appearance that is predominantly lytic. Lytic metastases are most common in breast, lung, thyroid, renal, melanoma, and gastrointestinal malignancies. Sclerotic metastases usually arise from the prostate but may arise from breast, lung, and carcinoid tumors. New bone formation usually appears on radiographs as nodular well-circumscribed sclerotic areas.

Normal-appearing plain radiographs do not exclude the diagnosis of metastatic spinal disease or epidural compression. Plain radiographs in patients with suspected metastatic spinal disease may show loss of definition of a pedicle or a compression deformity; however, small lesions may be difficult to detect on routine spine films.

Radionuclide bone scanning

Bone scintigraphy is considered to be the most sensitive and inexpensive skeletal radiographic survey method for bone metastases. Blood flow and reactive new bone formation usually increase around bone metastases to produce focal increase in tracer uptake, often before bone destruction can be seen in plain radiographs. If a lesion is identified on a bone scan, plain radiographs, CT, and/or MRI of the area may help clarify the diagnosis.

Lesions in the pubis, ischium, and sacrum may occasionally be obscured on a bone scan because of bladder activity. Lesion detection depends on the presence of a focal increase in osteoblast activity, so a false-negative scan can occur when pure lytic disease exists. This is typical of multiple myeloma, which is best investigated radiographically, but it also occurs in other tumors when rapid-growing lytic lesions are present. In extreme cases in which significant bone destruction has occurred, a photon-deficient area may develop ('cold spot'). Patients receiving chemotherapy may also have a false-negative scan, which is due to suppression of osteoblastic activity. Because of these false-negative scans, skeletal radiographic survey is the most effective method for radiographic follow-up in patients with these lesions.

In contrast, sclerotic metastases generally are visualized clearly on a bone scan, the only exception being very slowly growing metastases in which the alteration in metabolic activity is so subtle that it may not be distinguishable from normal background activity. When extensive skeletal metastases are present, the focal lesions may coalesce to produce diffusely increased uptake, the so-called super-scan of malignancy. This occurs most often in prostatic cancer, but it is also seen in other tumors, such as breast cancer.

Cross-sectional imaging

CT scanning may offer better definition and evaluation of bone metastases. MRI appears to be a particularly sensitive modality for directly visualizing metastases. However, both of these imaging techniques await further prospective evaluation in this regard.

CT produces images with excellent contrast and resolution of soft tissue. Bony destruction and sclerotic deposits are well shown and any soft-tissue extension of bone metastases clearly demonstrated. CT is especially helpful for evaluation of spinal lesions, but because the entire spine cannot readily be scanned, it usually is reserved for assessment of patients with positive bone scans and negative radiographs, when clinically indicated, in an attempt to clarify the lesion. In one series of such patients with breast cancer, half had obvious metastases on CT, a quarter had a benign cause, and the remainder had no abnormality that could be demonstrated and none of these patients subsequently had metastases (Muindi et al. 1983).

In spinal metastases, CT often shows evidence of bone destruction and occasionally an adjacent soft-tissue mass, whereas conventional polytomography may demonstrate only cortical destruction of a pedicle or a portion of the body of the vertebra. It also is helpful to differentiate vertebral collapse due to osteopenia from that due to neoplasm. In osteopenic collapse, there usually is intact cortical bone, relatively homogeneous bony involvement, and no soft-tissue mass, whereas a neoplasm typically results in cortical destruction and formation of a soft-tissue mass. CT also provides excellent detail of vertebrae for fixation purposes and, for this reason, may be required for preoperative planning.

MRI is excellent for demonstrating bone marrow infiltration. The solid constituents of cortical bone give no signal on MRI but the medulla gives a strong signal. So, a metastatic tumor can be visualized directly, in contrast to the indirect changes observed on radiographs or with radionuclide scanning. Like CT, MRI is useful in evaluating patients with positive bone scans and normal radiographs and for elucidating the cause of a vertebral compression fracture. It also has the advantage over CT of providing multiplanar images which permit imaging of the entire spine in the sagittal plane and may show other sites of vertebral metastases. It offers superior visualization of metastatic deposits to the vertebral bodies, epidural space, and paravertebral soft tissues. MRI has essentially replaced myelography as the method of demonstrating the level and degree of vertebral collapse and extradural compression. MRI findings were compared with those of myelography, surgical pathology, clinical course, and autopsy in patients with metastatic spinal disease (Li and Poon 1988), and MRI was 93 per cent sensitive and 97 per cent specific. MRI signal intensity of collapsed vertebrae caused by either metastases or trauma was also compared with the average signal intensity of three relatively normal adjacent vertebrae. All cases of post-traumatic vertebral collapse had a ratio of collapsed bodies to adjacent bodies greater than 0.80. Only 2 per cent of the vertebrae collapsed secondary to metastases had a ratio greater than 0.80. The sensitivity of these data was 97.6 per cent, and the accuracy was 98.2 per cent (Li and Poon 1988).

Biochemical markers

Although serial changes in biochemical markers of bone cell activity are helpful in monitoring response to treatment, no convincing reports have been published of their value in early detection of metastases nor has their superiority over bone scan been demonstrated. Markers of enhanced bone resorption include fasting excretion of calcium and hydroxyproline, which is a breakdown product of collagen, urinary excretion of hydroxypyridinium and cross-linking of amino acids of collagen, urinary levels of pyridinoline and dexopyridinoline, serum bone-specific alkaline phosphatase, and osteocalcin.

Biopsy

A needle biopsy can be useful for confirming metastatic disease. CT can be used to guide the needle. It is occasionally necessary to perform an open biopsy to sample adequate tissue, for example when the diagnosis is in question or in cases that may need immediate stabilization. Transpedicular biopsy may be performed in cases of a metastatic lesion of a vertebral body, especially when needle CT-guided biopsy results are nondiagnostic.

Several problems may arise with open biopsy procedures in long bones. When a cortical window needs to be made in the bone, it is important to make a long oval-shaped window. The window should have rounded corners. This decreases the stress-riser effect of the cortical opening. Strong consideration should be given to immediate stabilization and cementation in cases with aggressive lesions. If a fracture has already occurred, care must be taken to sample the tumorous area adequately rather than the healing area of fibrous tissue and osteoid formation.

Treatment
Nonoperative treatment
Systemic therapy

The first approach for patients with bone metastases is to use the most effective systemic anticancer therapy available. Systemic therapy for bone metastases has either direct or indirect actions. It may be directed against the tumor cell to reduce cell proliferation and, as a consequence, the production of cytokines and growth factors. Alternative systemic treatment is directed toward blocking the effect of these substances on host cells. Chemotherapy, endocrine treatment, and bone-seeking isotopes have direct antitumor effects, whereas agents such as bisphosphonates and calcitonin prevent host cells (primarily osteoclasts) from reacting to tumor products. In general, the systemic treatment for metastatic bone disease is the same as that for other metastatic manifestations of the malignancy. Thus, treatment must be discussed according to type.

Breast and prostate cancer are important because effective (palliative) systemic treatments are available and because these two tumors represent the most cases of metastatic bone disease due to solid tumors. In cases in which the tumor is refractory to anticancer therapy, bone pain due to metastases should be treated aggressively with appropriate analgesic or adjunctive therapy.

Metastatic bone disease due to breast cancer

Endocrine therapy is the initial treatment of choice for hormone receptor-positive breast cancer in patients with metastatic bone disease, except when extensive or aggressive visceral disease coexists (O'Reilly *et al.* 1990). In these situations, cytotoxic chemotherapy is the initial treatment of choice. Hormones act predominantly on cancer cells that express high affinity binding proteins (receptors) for estrogen and progesterone. These hormone–receptor complexes, in turn, act on the cell nucleus to mediate the specific cell response of the hormone. Significant (more than 50 per cent) tumor shrinkage (a complete or partial objective response) after endocrine treatment occurs in about half of the patients with steroid receptor-positive tumors. Selection of specific endocrine treatment for patients is frequently based on menopausal status. Premenopausal patients can be treated with tamoxifen, ovarian ablation, or a combination. Ovarian ablation can be achieved medically through the use of luteinizing hormone-releasing hormone agonists, surgically, or by ovarian irradiation. Tamoxifen is the preferred first-line hormonal treatment for postmenopausal patients. Although the median duration of response to endocrine therapy is 15 months, prolonged responses to first-line hormone treatments lasting several years are not uncommon in patients with metastases. Although ovarian ablation accelerates the loss of bone mass, tamoxifen, despite its classification as an anti-estrogen, can act as an antiosteoporosis agent in postmenopausal women. The choice of agents available for second- and third-line endocrine treatment is continuously increasing and includes the aromatase inhibitors anastrozole, letrozole, exemestane, and amino-glutethimide, and progestins such as megestrol acetate and medroxy-progesterone acetate. The newer aromatase inhibitors anastrozole, letrozole, and exemestane confer a survival advantage compared with megestrol acetate, and they represent the recommended second-line treatment. In patients with hormone receptor-negative breast cancer, the chance of response to hormonal treatment decreases to approximately 10 per cent.

Patients with disease that progresses after endocrine therapy and those with rapidly progressive life-threatening disease or known to have estrogen- and progesterone-negative tumors should be considered for cytotoxic chemotherapy. Responses in women with bone metastases with relief of symptoms are nearly always only partial, with a median duration of response of 9 to 12 months. Although promising in phase II studies, the use of high dose chemotherapy with autologous bone marrow or peripheral blood stem cell transplant is currently under phase III investigation and cannot yet be considered standard treatment (Vahdat and Antman 1995).

Metastatic bone disease due to prostate cancer

Most prostate tumors exhibit some degree of hormone responsiveness. The most commonly used form of endocrine therapy is orchiectomy. Many new forms of endocrine treatment have been introduced recently, including luteinizing hormone-releasing hormone agonists and antiandrogens. Patients with advanced prostate cancer tend to be elderly and to have widespread bone metastases. Their tolerance of toxic chemotherapy regimens is often poor.

As yet there is no evidence that cytotoxic drugs prolong survival in advanced prostate cancer. Therefore treatment with chemotherapy as part of clinical trials should be encouraged, with careful evaluation of pain control, mobility, and quality of life in addition to tumor response.

Bone involvement in curable malignancies is relatively uncommon. Bone involvement is seen occasionally in patients with germ cell tumors and may represent an adverse prognostic feature, but cure with chemotherapy is nevertheless usual. Patients with skeletal metastases associated with non-small-cell lung cancer or melanoma benefit most from local palliative radiation therapy. For these patients, alternative systemic treatment approaches are needed, such as the use of bisphosphonates or therapeutic radio-isotopes.

Bisphosphonates

Bisphosphonates (e.g. pamidronate) that inhibit tumor-induced osteoclastic activity are also emerging as a palliative mode of treatment for patients with generalized lytic metastases with symptoms not responding or deteriorating despite systemic treatment or local modalities. The dominant role of the osteoclast in tumor-induced osteolysis provides the rationale for the use of inhibitors of osteoclast activity for treatment of bone metastases. In recent years, the therapeutic possibilities for inhibiting osteolysis have increased considerably with the development of the bisphosphonates (e.g. etidronate, clodronate, pamidronate). These are pyrophosphate analogs containing a P–C–P backbone rather than the P–O–P bond of pyrophosphate. This biochemical substitution renders the bisphosphonates resistant to phosphatase activity. The degree of activity of individual bisphosphonates varies greatly from compound to com-pound according to the length and substitution of the aliphatic carbon backbone.

Oral bisphosphonates suffer from poor bioavailability and can cause significant gastrointestinal side-effects, such as indigestion, diarrhea, and esophagitis (Rose et al. 1992). Consequently, high dose intermittent intravenous treatment with bisphosphonates is considered superior.

Radio-isotopes

The clinical development of bone-seeking radio-isotopes is based on the rationale that medium to high energy β-particle radiation, targeted and delivered to skeletal sites involved by the tumor, can potentially result in more effective antitumor activity, while sparing normal tissues from the damaging effects of radiation. Radio-isotopes with clinical applications include iodine-131 (^{131}I), [iodine-131]monoiodobenzylguanadine ([^{131}I]MIBG), and strontium-89 (^{89}Sr). Promising radio-isotopes that are being evaluated in clinical trials include [samarium-153]ethylene-diaminetetra-methylene-phosphate ([^{153}Sm]EDTMP), and [rhenium-186]1-hydroxy-ethylidenediphosphonate ([^{186}Re]HEDP). The best results have been achieved in the treatment of blastic metastases. However, the results from the use of these radio-isotopes must be viewed cautiously because relatively few patients have been evaluated and the duration of the response is limited. Also, their use may be limited by the toxicity manifested by reversible bone marrow suppression.

Because follicular carcinoma of the thyroid commonly metastasizes to bone, the treatment of bone metastases with ^{131}I is now well established. Excellent results have been obtained with long-term palliation. Patients who do not have uptake of ^{131}I in the metastases have a poor survival rate. Treatment generally is well tolerated, although a radiation reaction of the salivary glands develops in some patients. More important, however, is the incidence of radiation-induced leukemias.

Neuroblastomas and tumors of neuroectodermal origin in general frequently metastasize to bone. Ninety per cent of these neoplasms incorporate the radiopharmaceutical [^{131}I]MIBG, and this isotope has been used to treat many children with metastatic neuroblastoma. Complete remission is possible, with nearly half achieving partial remission. Bone marrow suppression is often severe, and ideally bone marrow harvesting should be performed in patients with extensive bone metastases as a precautionary measure.

^{89}Sr is a β-emitter that imitates calcium and is taken up preferentially at sites of new bone formation. It localizes at the sites of blastic bone metastases and it has been used mainly to palliate metastatic bone disease due to prostate and breast cancer. Of great clinical significance is the low dose of radiation to the bone marrow, which is about one-tenth of that to the bone metastases. Most patients have significant pain relief for 6 months.

External beam radiation

Radiation therapy is the treatment of choice in the palliation of painful single sites. Postmortem studies have provided insight into the structural effects of irradiation on bone that contains metastases. Initially, degeneration and necrosis of tumor cells occur, followed by a proliferation of collagen. Subsequently, a rich vascular fibrous stroma is produced, within which intense osteoblast activity lays down new woven bone. This is gradually replaced by lamellar bone, and the intratrabecular stroma is repopulated by bone marrow tissue. Radiologically, recalcification of lytic areas begins to be seen 3 to 6 weeks after irradiation, with maximal recalcification occurring 2 to 3 months from the time of irradiation.

After the decision has been made to offer irradiation for bone metastases, consideration must be given to numerous other factors, such as co-ordination with surgical fixation if needed, dose and duration of treatment, volume to be treated, and potential use of more specialized types of treatment, for example hemibody irradiation or use of systemic radio-isotopes. The dose and duration (fractionation) of treatment are selected on the basis of multiple factors, including the patient's anticipated life expectancy, functional status (ability to make multiple trips to the treatment center), amount of metastatic disease (bone and visceral), and location and volume of tissue requiring treatment.

In general, simple treatment plans with single or parallel opposed fields are adequate for the palliative treatment of metastatic bone disease. However, complex planning with multiple fields and customized blocking is sometimes necessary to avoid undue late normal tissue toxic reactions, especially in patients with a longer life expectancy.

Localized metastases can be treated with external beam radiation therapy with or without operative intervention. In a patient with a solitary metastatic lesion, the ultimate prognosis is favorable and the lesion is usually treated with 40 to 50 Gy in 20 to 25 fractions. Pain relief is an excellent indicator of a good response to radiotherapy. For patients with multiple sites of metastatic disease and limited life expectancy, short courses of irradiation, such as 20 Gy in five fractions over 1 week or 30 Gy in 10 fractions over 2 weeks, are often chosen. This schedule is well suited to the treatment of patients with widespread metastatic disease, because it is generally well tolerated, less time-consuming for the patient, and equivalent in its effect to more protracted regimens. Local irradiation is definitely effective for bone pain. Overall, response rates of over 80 per cent have been reported, with complete pain relief achieved in half of patients. Pain relief usually occurs rapidly, within 1 to 2 weeks. If improvement in pain has not occurred by 6 weeks or more after treatment, it is unlikely to be achieved. Prophylactic internal fixation is often appropriate to prevent fracture during or shortly after irradiation of large lesions.

Retreatment generally is not as successful as the initial treatment but still may produce significant pain relief. Careful review of previous treatment fields, dose, and fractionation is needed to ensure that normal tissue tolerance, particularly of the spinal cord, is not exceeded. Targeted radio-isotope therapy is an alternative approach to palliation when further external beam treatment is considered hazardous.

Management of complications

Hypercalcemia

Hypercalcemia is a common metabolic complication of cancer. It is most common in patients with multiple myeloma and carcinoma of the breast, where just under half will be affected.

Hypercalcemia is related to the capacity of the tumor to secrete specific hypercalcemic factors and is not related to increased intestinal absorption of calcium. It is clear that various mechanisms are involved in malignant hypercalcemia, including increased bone resorption (osteolysis) and systemic release of humoral hypercalcemic factors such as parathyroid hormone-like peptide. Bone metastases are common but not invariably present. In tumors such as squamous cell lung cancer, humoral mechanisms are dominant, increasing both the renal tubular calcium reabsorption and phosphate excretion. In other tumors (e.g. multiple myeloma and lymphoma) osteolysis predominates, whereas in breast cancer both osteolysis and humoral mechanisms appear to be important.

The most frequent clinical symptoms associated with hypercalcemia of malignancy are anorexia, nausea, vomiting, confusion, lethargy, stupor, and coma. Because these symptoms are often nonspecific, affecting many systems in the body, they can be mistaken for symptoms of the underlying cancer or associated treatment if the oncologist is not acutely aware of the possibility of hypercalcemia. If untreated, a progressive increase in serum levels of calcium leads to a deterioration in renal function and mental status. Death ultimately occurs as a result of cardiac arrhythmias and renal failure.

Vigorous rehydration with or without diuretics is the primary treatment. For unresponsive or rapidly progressive hypercalcemia, bisphosphonates are the treatment of choice. Pamidronate is effective as a single intravenous infusion and is the current treatment of choice. Normocalcemia is usually maintained for 10 to 28 days. Repeated administration every 2 to 3 weeks will usually prevent recurrence. Other agents that can be used for the treatment of hypercalcemia include gallium nitrate, calcitonin, and steroids (mainly in hematologic malignancies).

Pathologic and impending pathologic fractures

Metastatic destruction of bone reduces its load-bearing capabilities, resulting initially in microfractures, which cause pain. Fractures of long bones and epidural extension of the tumor in the spine cause significant disability. Fractures are common through large, lytic metastases that erode the cortex. Weight-bearing bones are affected most commonly. Damage to both trabecular and cortical bone is structurally important, but cortical destruction is most relevant.

The clinical importance of aggressive management of a patient with metastases to bone is often underestimated. Pathologic fractures are not necessarily a manifestation of terminal disease, and primary internal stabilization followed by radiation therapy is usually the treatment of choice and certainly the only modality likely to restore mobility as well as to relieve pain. Failure to treat properly metastases to bone may reduce substantially the remaining quality of life of the patient. Untreated pathologic fractures rarely heal, and although radiation therapy may achieve local tumor control, bony union remains unlikely.

The operative treatment of metastases to bone remains a challenge for orthopedic surgeons. With recent advances in systemic treatment, many patients may live 1 to 3 years after the detection of their bone metastases. Therefore, the management of any pathologic and impending fractures must be sound and practical to prevent both early and late failures. The goal of surgery is to relieve pain and to maintain an independent status for the patient.

If operative treatment has been decided, special consideration needs to be given to metastatic tumor type. Lung cancer that has spread to bone is probably the most aggressive of all metastatic tumor types and should be treated more aggressively because of its destructive potential. Metastatic renal cell carcinoma and thyroid carcinoma can have extensive vascular supplies, and cases of severe bleeding have been encountered. Preoperative evaluation of these patients with arteriography and immobilization the day before definitive surgery have greatly decreased the morbidity and mortality of these procedures in these specific tumors. Preoperatively, a radionuclide bone scan and radiographs of the entire length of the affected bone should be obtained. This ensures that any other metastases that may develop subsequently into a pathologic fracture are also stabilized and included in the radiation therapy field. A pathologic fracture at the edge of a plate or an intramedullary nail, particularly when fixed with methylmethacrylate, is more difficult to treat than if no implant was placed in the bone.

Prophylactic internal fixation

Prevention of pathologic fractures is achieved through frequent follow-up examinations, including appropriate radiographs and bone scintigraphy. Early chemotherapeutic management or radiation therapy can preclude pathologic fracture; however, if the patient continues to have pain subsequent to radiation therapy or there is radiographic evidence of progression, prophylactic stabilization should be performed.

Prophylactic internal fixation must be followed by radiation therapy, to inhibit further tumor growth and to avoid further bone destruction. Depending on the primary lesion, endocrine treatment or chemotherapy may also be necessary. Provided that the lesion is irradiated, no evidence suggests that surgery increases the risk of disseminating tumor cells either locally or into the circulation. Indeed, some experimental evidence shows that pathologic fractures are associated with an increased incidence of pulmonary metastases and that prophylactic stabilization decreases this.

Indications

Increasing emphasis is being placed on attempts to predict metastatic sites at risk of fracture and the use of prophylactic surgery because the development of a fracture is so devastating to a patient with cancer. Although everyone agrees that impending fractures require prophylactic fixation, there is little agreement regarding the specific indications for these procedures. Early studies developed criteria for the treatment of these lesions. Femoral neck pure lytic lesions involving the cortex with increasing pain are at greatest risk for fracture. Patients with purely lytic metastases (e.g. lung and renal cell carcinomas) are more prone to pathologic fractures. Some authors have commented on the absence of pathologic fractures in pure blastic metastases. However, other authors have reported pathologic fractures that occurred through mixed blastic and lytic lesions.

Prophylactic internal fixation was recommended in the early 1970s for patients with breast cancer for well-defined lytic lesions of 2.5 cm or more that involved the cortex of the femur or were painful, because over half of these patients sustained fractures if they had no prophylactic internal fixation. The overall incidence of pathologic fracture has been decreased from one-third to less than one-tenth by using prophylactic internal fixation in these lesions. In another study, a fracture incidence of two-thirds was reported in patients with more than 50 per cent destruction of cortical bone, as compared with 1 in 20 in patients with less than 50 per cent cortical involvement (Fidler 1973). All of these criteria are based on attempts to correlate clinically

the biomechanical principles of a 'stress riser', in which stress concentration occurs at the edge of a defect, and the 'open section effect' resulting from a significant loss of cortical bone.

Harrington (1986a) suggested the following criteria: (a) more than 50 per cent destruction of cortical bone measured radiographically or by CT scan, (b) a lytic lesion of the proximal femur greater than 1.5 cm in diameter, and (c) avulsion of the lesser trochanter. However, in a study of patients who had painful breast cancer femoral lesions, only 5 per cent went on to have fracture after treatment with radiation despite all the lesions being larger than 2.5 cm and involving the cortex (Cheng et al. 1980).

Practical considerations for prophylactic fixation in the presence of a destructive lesion of a long bone, either known to be or presumed to be a metastatic deposit, include the need for biopsy. Frequently, biopsy of the bone lesion is the only logical method for establishing a diagnosis, and when that is necessary in a long bone deposit, concomitant internal fixation is mandatory.

The ability of the patient to modify activities is also important. Some patients are not able to protect themselves with crutches or a walker for a period sufficient to allow bone reconstitution capable of resuming unprotected weight-bearing. These patients do better with early internal fixation. However, the location of the lesion and the morbidity associated with operative fixation must be considered. Patients with lesions of the lower extremities who might respond well to radiation therapy may not be candidates for the use of crutches for protection if there is a concomitant lesion of the upper extremity.

Life expectancy is also a critical criterion for prophylactic fixation: during the last 20 years, survival after the initial pathologic fracture has improved markedly. In addition, some tumors have a poorer prognosis than others; for example, lung cancer metastatic to bone has a poor prognosis.

Operative considerations

Several advances have occurred in the treatment of metastatic lesions. These include (a) the use of methylmethacrylate to improve fixation of implants and to reconstruct bone defects, (b) improvements in the strength and design of prosthetic components, including modular devices, (c) development of interlocking nails, and (d) newer instrumentation and more aggressive management of spinal lesions.

The material properties of methylmethacrylate require that it be used to transmit compressive loads for better stress distribution. It should be used only as a complex 'filler' in conjunction with a surgical implant to promote fixation and compressive loading of the bone. It is used routinely in the upper extremity, where it is combined with intramedullary fixation to enhance the torsional stability of Rush rods and to fill large bone defects. Methylmethacrylate may be used in conjunction with a standard implant or with multiple Steinmann pins to produce a composite-like material with multiple points of fixation (e.g. for pelvic and acetabular fractures). In the lower extremity, the cement enhances the purchase of screws and intramedullary devices. It may also restore the medial cortical buttress about the hip, reducing the bending movements that fixation devices are subjected to. Methylmethacrylate greatly enhances the ability to use metal implants of either the prosthetic or the fracture-fixation type.

Extensive studies have assessed changes in the material properties of methylmethacrylate after the application of external beam radiation therapy. In general, the structural properties of methylmethacrylate appear unchanged when this material is exposed to greater than therapeutic doses of ionizing radiation (Murray *et al.* 1974; Eftekhar and Thurston 1975).

Preoperative preparation

Prior to any surgical procedure for stabilization of a pathologic fracture, great care must be taken in planning the procedure. A team approach should be used. The patient's general medical condition should be stable, life expectancy should be long enough to justify the magnitude of the procedure, and the patient and family must understand the goals of the operation. It is almost impossible to predict accurately the life expectancy of a patient with disseminated cancer. Unless death is imminent, surgical stabilization should be considered for ease of nursing care and the patient's comfort. All factors of the patient's health must be considered. Nutritional, metabolic, and hematological factors should be evaluated and treated. The patient's current condition—ambulatory potential, existence of other metastatic disease in bone, and neurologic status—should be taken into consideration. Occasionally, it is necessary to perform multiple procedures on multiple extremities in the same operation.

Surgical reconstruction

The indications for surgery must be tailored for each patient. General indications include (a) metastatic lesions that involve greater than 40 to 50 per cent of the diameter of the diaphysis of a long bone, (b) lesions greater than 2.5 cm in the femoral neck or intertrochanteric area, (c) lytic permeative lesions in high stress areas such as the subtrochanteric region, and (d) lesions that have not responded to external beam irradiation.

The type of reconstruction and internal stabilization depends on the site and extent of the metastatic lesion.

Metastatic lesions of the upper extremity

Lesions of the scapula

Most of the skeletal metastases appearing in the upper extremity develop within the proximal humerus and/or scapula.

Small lesions of the glenoid can often be treated with radiation therapy. Larger lesions of the glenoid may be managed by more permanent reconstruction techniques, using allografts or prosthetic replacement. More extensive lesions of the glenoid and scapular body that are not sensitive or manageable with radiation therapy may require forequarter amputation.

Lesions of the humerus

Those patients expected to survive longer than 3 months are best managed with internal fixation to ensure pain relief and restoration of function. Intramedullary techniques used in reconstruction of the humerus are demanding and frequently incapable of resisting torque forces.

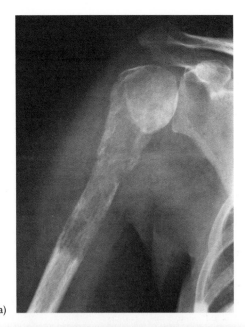

(a)

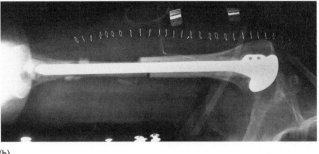

(b)

Fig. 1. Anteroposterior views of right humerus (a) showing metastatic thyroid cancer and (b) after resection and reconstruction with allograft prosthetic composite.

Proximal humerus

For lesions not amenable to radiation therapy alone, it may be reasonable to resect the area of involved bone and to reconstruct with a prosthetic device or a composite allograft prosthesis (Fig. 1). This allows the attachment of soft tissues to the allograft bone, which may be an advantage. However, the recovery time from this procedure is longer than when a prosthesis is used alone. The patient's expected survival time may help determine which device is preferable in a given situation.

Diaphyseal lesions

Diaphyseal lesions are best managed with either intramedullary fixation or plate reconstruction and supplementary methylmethacrylate (Fig. 2). Preoperative radiotherapy may help by decreasing the overall size of the mass and reducing the intraoperative blood loss.

Various techniques can be used. Perhaps the most commonly used method is fixation with a Rush rod, supplemented with methylmethacrylate. The newer interlocking rods allow fixation both proximally and distally and may be ideal for diaphyseal pathologic fractures. Some surgeons prefer to use a plate for diaphyseal lesions.

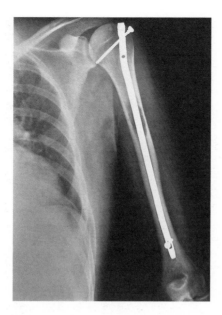

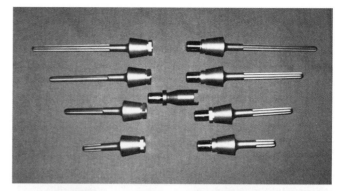

Fig. 2. Anteroposterior view of left humerus showing interlocking intramedullary rod fixation for metastatic lesion.

Either one or two plates may be used and may be supplemented with methylmethacrylate. Diaphyseal spacers may be used in selected cases of extensive diaphyseal lesions and for salvage cases after failed internal fixation with other types of devices (Fig. 3). There are modular systems that allow selection of the appropriate size spacer at the time of the surgical procedure.

Distal humerus

Lesions of the distal humerus are a difficult therapeutic challenge. One way to deal with this problem is to use two crossed Rush rods inserted in a retrograde manner. A posterior approach is used and the tumor is evacuated from the tumor cavity. Rush rods are inserted through the epicondyles in a retrograde manner, and fixation is supplemented with methylmethacrylate. This provides excellent stability and allows rapid mobilization of the elbow. If the lesion of the distal humerus is more extensive, resection of the distal end of the humerus and reconstruction using a modular prosthesis or a composite allograft total elbow prosthesis or an allograft replacement with internal fixation is preferable.

Every effort should be made to maintain either elbow or shoulder motion, short of elaborate reconstructive techniques. In most instances, external beam radiation therapy offers significant pain relief and allows sufficient healing of the fracture to retain some joint function.

Lesions of the radius and ulna

Simultaneous involvement of both the radius and ulna is uncommon, and the majority of lesions involving both of these bones lend themselves to some form of therapy short of amputation.

Lesions of the distal ulna or the proximal radius

These lesions may be excised without major reconstructive efforts or alternatively may be managed with radiation therapy alone. Efforts

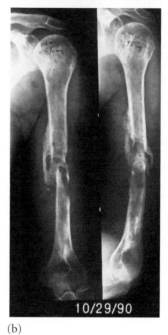
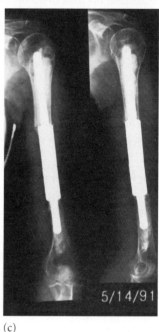

(b)   (c)

Fig. 3. (a) Modular spacer: modular segmental defect replacement prostheses for humeral prosthesis. Anteroposterior views of right humerus (b) showing extensive metastatic lesion with segmental bone loss and (c) after segmental defect replacement prosthesis.

to retain the architecture and function of the distal radius and the proximal ulna should remain a priority. Uncontrolled destructive lesions, however, may necessitate amputation.

Midshaft lesions

Midshaft lesions in either the radius or ulna most often are managed with radiation therapy alone. Some fractures may require internal fixation for stabilization and restoration of length; however, most of them also need augmentation with methylmethacrylate. When a below-elbow amputation is necessary for local control and wide margins are achieved, adjunctive external beam radiation therapy may be avoided. In patients who are expected to have prolonged survival, reconstructive efforts are justified. Satisfactory function of the upper extremity can be preserved even with stiffness in the elbow as long as the hand and limb are maintained in a functional position.

Lesions of the hand and wrist

Radiation therapy may be the treatment of choice only if limited involvement is identified in the bones of the hand or wrist. Metastases to the carpus are unusual. Extensive involvement of the carpus associated with osseous destruction is generally best managed with a wide amputation above the wrist, where methylmethacrylate and plate reconstruction are not a reasonable option. Digital metastases are best managed with amputation, and limited metacarpal involvement can also be managed with ray amputation. Adjunctive radiation therapy may also be necessary if wide margins of resection are not achieved (the plane of dissection must pass through absolutely normal tissues). In general, every effort should be made to restore as much function as possible in patients with upper extremity metastases, especially when they are located in the dominant upper extremity.

Metastatic lesions of the lower extremity

Lesions of the pelvis and periacetabular region

Pathologic fractures sustained through an area of the pelvis other than the acetabulum seldom require surgical stabilization. Most of the patients can be treated with radiation therapy. Metastatic lesions associated with pathologic fractures and deformity of the acetabulum are often best managed with preoperative radiation therapy, followed by operative reconstruction. Special attention must be given to renal cell metastatic lesions that tend to be vascular; considerable loss of blood can occur with their exposure. Preoperative embolization markedly decreases blood loss and allows for a more controlled reconstruction.

Classification

A classification of acetabular lesions has been proposed by Harrington (1981) with attendant surgical options: class I, the lateral cortices and superior and medial walls are structurally intact; class II, the medial wall is deficient; class III, the lateral cortices and dome are deficient; class IV, resection is required for cure.

Class I lesions

Given the mechanical integrity of the anterior and posterior columns as well as of the medial and superior walls, patients with this type of deficiency can be treated with routine hip replacement procedures, with cementation techniques on the acetabular and femoral side.

Surgical considerations Mesh is often incorporated to support the medial wall and to prevent migration of the polymethylmethacrylate into the pelvis. Long-stem femoral components are chosen to bypass as much of the femur as feasible with the intramedullary extent of the component, because of possible additional metastatic foci in the proximal two-thirds of the femur. These patients can be treated postoperatively in an identical fashion to those who have undergone conventional total hip replacement.

Class II lesions

These lesions usually compromise the integrity of the medial wall and present with femoral head protrusion through the medial wall,

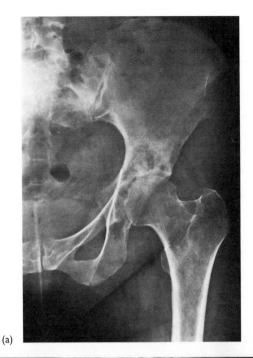

(a)

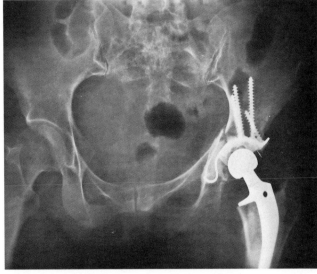

(b)

Fig. 4. Anteroposterior views of pelvis and left proximal femur (a) showing class II destruction of left acetabulum caused by metastatic breast cancer and (b) after reconstruction with Ganz ring and total hip replacement.

either initiated by the presence of tumor or possibly an osteonecrotic effect of previous radiation therapy. In reconstructing this type of acetabulum, it is important to transfer weight-bearing stresses from the central medial wall and place them onto intact anterior and posterior columns as well as the superior rim (Fig. 4). To accomplish this, there are several acetabular protrusio shell components available, such as the Oh–Harris and the Bosch–Schneider (Fig. 5).

Surgical considerations Routine approaches are used for total hip replacement for class II lesions. If the medial wall deficiency is created by the presence of a tumor, rapid removal of the tumor will

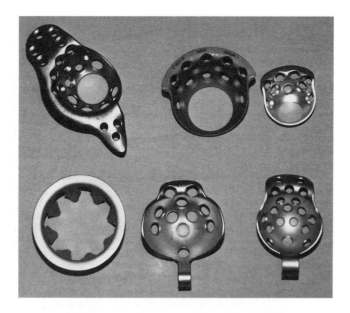

Fig. 5. Antiprotrusio devices used in the management of metastatic lesions of the acetabulum.

minimize blood loss, as will preoperative embolization. A mesh is placed over the deficient medial wall to prevent extravasation of cement into the pelvis. The acetabular protrusio shell is placed on the intact superior and anterior or inferior rims of the acetabulum before cementing the polyethylene cup into the composite. A long-neck femoral implant is used to minimize impingement of the trochanter on the protrusio ring, thereby minimizing dislocation. Trochanteric osteotomy should be avoided, given that postoperative radiation therapy is common and union under those circumstances is rare.

Class III lesions

These lesions are the more common form of presentation and by far the most challenging. Not only are the medial wall and the superior rim deficient, but the anterior and posterior columns may also be involved. Therefore there is no intact bone on which to rest the protrusio ring, making it impossible to reconstruct such deficiencies with the type of procedure recommended for class II lesions. Also, this cannot be accomplished by filling the deficiency with methylmethacrylate alone or by placing the acetabular cup high, because the diameter of the iliac bone becomes progressively smaller and affords less surface area for contact. The most effective way of transmitting the stresses up into the intact iliac wing and sacrum is to use several large threaded Steinmann pins that, in combination with methylmethacrylate, act as reinforced concrete on which the protrusio ring and acetabular component can be placed (Fig. 6).

Surgical considerations The patient is placed in the lateral decubitus position, and a conventional posterolateral incision is used. The gluteus medius and minimus are mobilized off the superior acetabular surface to allow direct access to the acetabular roof and sciatic notch. The femoral head is removed to allow access to the acetabulum. All gross tumor is removed. Often the medial wall of the acetabulum will be markedly deficient. Threaded Steinmann pins are placed appropriately into the iliac wing and sacrum. Potential dangers

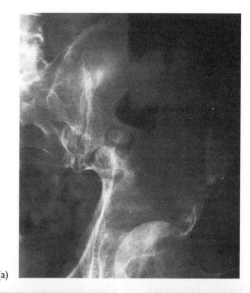
(a)

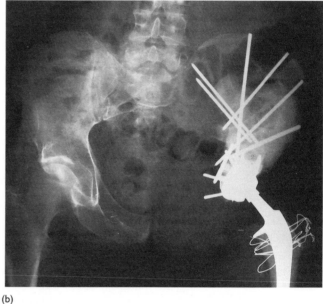
(b)

Fig. 6. (a) Anteroposterior view of left pelvis showing class III extensive destructive lesion caused by metastatic hypernephroma. (b) Anteroposterior view of pelvis and proximal femur after total hip arthroplasty with extensive acetabular reconstruction.

involve the lumbosacral plexus, femoral nerve, and gluteal vessels. The use of the index finger is necessary for guidance. The Steinmann pins are placed just above the sciatic notch in the thickened strong bone of this region, with an additional one or two Steinmann pins coursing up into the iliac wing. The addition of two or three threaded Steinmann pins placed downward into the acetabulum from the anterosuperior iliac crest has been shown to provide rotational instability of the reconstruction. A small additional stabilization at the iliac crest using Steinmann pins directed into the superior and medial aspect of the acetabulum may be necessary. These pins often can support mesh that is placed along the deficient medial wall in an effort to prevent migration of cement into the hemipelvis when the components are inserted.

After the threaded Steinmann pins are in place and positioned appropriately, the protrusio ring is applied as if there were intact anterior, posterior, and superior columns. The acetabular bed is cleansed thoroughly with a pulsating water lavage to remove any residual tumor and to expose cancellous bone surfaces to enhance the contact between the bone and the cement. Methylmethacrylate is injected from a gun into the exposed bone interstices, and pressure is maintained with finger compression. The methylmethacrylate is molded to contour around the protrusio ring and Steinmann pins. The mesh on the medial wall should prevent extravasation of methylmethacrylate into the pelvis. A polyethylene component is cemented in place. Patients are often advised to be cane-dependent, if not crutch-dependent, for the remainder of their lives in an effort to deflect stresses from the reconstruction.

Class IV lesions

There is rarely an indication to consider wide local excision of a solitary metastasis for cure. Most of these lesions are solitary metastatic hypernephromas or thyroid lesions, presenting at least 4 years after the primary tumor has been treated. Radical curative excision for unifocal hypernephroma does not carry a favorable prognosis and therefore is not recommended. The sole exception to this may be a unifocal metastasis from thyroid carcinoma or possibly unifocal lymphoma of bone previously treated with radiation and chemotherapy that continues to be symptomatic. Extensive restaging would be necessary to determine the continued unifocal nature of the disease.

Surgical considerations Internal hemipelvectomy has become a recognized reasonable alternative for patients with primary malignant tumors of the hemipelvis. The reconstruction for metastatic lesions is dependent on the anatomical area of the hemipelvis that is principally involved. Areas remote from the hip joint can be removed with no formal reconstruction and with no effective change in activity levels. Removal of the periacetabular region necessitates some form of reconstruction, stabilizing the remaining proximal femur to the hemipelvis. This is accomplished with arthrodesis to the anterior or posterior hemipelvis, saddle prosthesis supported by the iliac wing, or possibly periacetabular allograft reconstruction. These are major procedures with attendant risks, and patients should be apprised of the type and extent of the procedure and possible complications before proceeding with such an operation.

Lesions of the femur

The proximal third of the femur is the preferential site of involvement for metastatic lesions, and the subtrochanteric region of the proximal femur appears to be a common site for metastatic disease of the femur. Patients with metastatic disease of the femur are not only confronted with a poor prognosis for extended survival, but they also face the prospect of losing the ability to ambulate during their remaining months. The primary objective of the management of metastatic disease in the femur is to relieve pain and to return the patient to some sort of functional status in a safe and reliable manner. Many advances have been made in the last few years in the treatment of pathologic fractures of the hip. These include the use of methylmethacrylate for stabilization, the design of stronger and more stable fixation devices, and the development of modular proximal femoral prosthetic devices. The preoperative evaluation of these

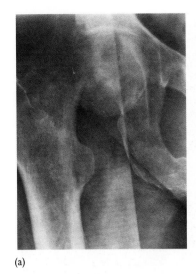
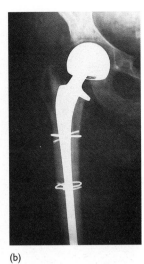

(a)   (b)

Fig. 7. Anteroposterior views of right proximal femur (a) showing pathological fracture of femoral neck and (b) after bipolar arthroplasty with long-stem component.

patients regarding the anatomical site, extent of bone loss, and anticipation of functional result assists in preoperative planning.

Fractures of the femoral head and neck

Fractures of the femoral head and neck secondary to pathologic fractures from metastatic disease may be treated by internal fixation, prosthetic replacement, or Girdlestone resection (Sim 1988). Despite advances in the design of internal fixation devices for the femoral head and neck and the use of methylmethacrylate, little progress has been made in preventing complications subsequent to pathologic fractures and internal fixation (Yazawa *et al.* 1990).

Therefore if there is extensive bony destruction that would not allow a stable construction even with bone–cement augmentation, prosthetic replacement should be considered (Fig. 7). A prosthesis with a cemented acetabular cup also should be used if there is a concomitant acetabular lesion. The dislocation rate for these prosthetic devices is higher than in the general population of hip arthroplasty patients (Yazawa *et al.* 1990). Care should be taken to protect these patients, who generally have poor muscle control and general debilitation and have undergone extensive bone and soft-tissue resection. If there is no acetabular disease, a bipolar endoprosthesis will allow greater stability.

Intertrochanteric pathologic lesions

Intertrochanteric pathologic fractures of the femur pose a specific and complex problem as a result of the tremendous forces placed on that area. In neoplastic situations, because of the tumor destruction of bone as well as the resection and removal of gross tumor for the surgical procedure, it is almost impossible to obtain bony stability. The use of methylmethacrylate has been helpful in gaining fixation and stability.

Several techniques have been used for treatment of metastatic lesions in the intertrochanteric area, including nail–plate devices, intramedullary devices, and prosthetic replacements. A nail–plate device may be used when there is enough residual bone present to

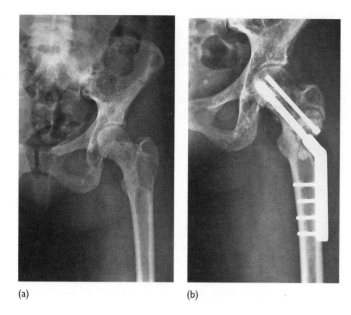

(a)   (b)

Fig. 8. Anteroposterior view of left proximal femur (a) showing metastatic destructive intertrochanteric lesion and (b) after internal fixation with sliding nail–plate apparatus and single screw.

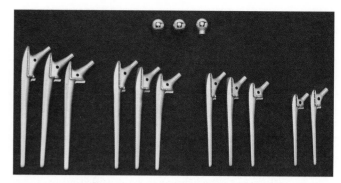

Fig. 9. Calcar replacement prostheses with various neck lengths used in intertrochanteric fractures.

allow stable bony fixation and support of body weight. With newly developed sliding nail–plate devices that have much stronger compression screws, implants may be used in these situations (Fig. 8). If these devices are used for augmentation without methylmethacrylate, the complication rate is quite high (Yazawa *et al.* 1990). The use of methylmethacrylate in the construction greatly decreases complications and improves functional results.

Surgical considerations
A standard surgical approach is used. A cortical window is made in the lateral bone cortex, and the devitalized tumor tissue is removed. Methylmethacrylate can be injected into the femoral head and neck to provide additional fixation for the sliding-screw portion of the device. The cement also can be injected down into the medullary canal to provide better fixation for the cortical screws. It is our preference to place the screws through partially hardened methylmethacrylate rather than simply injecting the cement after the screws have been placed. Care should be taken to avoid extravasation of methylmethacrylate into the soft tissues. The goal of the construction is to provide enough stability to permit immediate postoperative partial weight-bearing on the extremity.

Many intramedullary devices are now available for the fixation of intertrochanteric-type fractures. However, the standard is still the Zickel intramedullary nail (Taylor and Rush 1992). Condylocephalic intramedullary nails, such as the Ender or Harris type, generated enthusiasm early in their use, but because of subsequent complications such as loss of fixation and problems associated with rotational deformity, their use has decreased (Naiman *et al.* 1969; Chapman *et al.* 1981).

Prosthetic replacement should be considered when there is extensive bony loss in the intertrochanteric area and there is no possibility of obtaining structural stability, even with the use of methylmethacrylate. Various modular prosthetic designs are available for these applications, either in standard forms or on a custom-made basis (Fig. 9). The head and neck replacement devices have been effective for replacing most lesions that involve the calcar area (Fig. 10). This allows preservation of the lateral cortical structures if the bone is intact or reattachment of the trochanter to the prosthesis itself if bone dissolution has occurred. It is important to try to maintain the attachment of the vastus lateralis to the trochanteric area during the surgical procedure to avoid migration of the trochanter proximally and to provide better function of the abductor mechanism. Postoperatively, weight-bearing is possible immediately, and the patient can return to activities quite rapidly. Dislocation is a significant complication. Key factors to avoid dislocation include maintaining proper hip joint compression with a slightly longer prosthesis, using a bipolar cup, keeping the acetabular component more horizontal, and providing proper soft-tissue reconstruction.

Subtrochanteric lesions
Metastatic disease in the subtrochanteric area is common and much more prone to pathologic fracture because of the tremendous load applied to this area during weight-bearing. With this injury, the fracture lines often extend into the intertrochanteric area or femoral shaft. Treatment of pathologic fractures in this area is more difficult because of the usual loss of cortical support and the mechanical forces that are applied on each side of this area. The subtrochanteric area has a less copious blood supply than the intertrochanteric area, and nonunions are more common in this area.

Surgical considerations
Several different methods have been used for the treatment of fractures in this area, including nail–plate apparatus, intramedullary devices, and proximal femoral replacement arthroplasty. Previously, nail–plate devices were used extensively for subtrochanteric fractures. In cases of pathologic fracture, however, the results have been unsatisfactory because of the high incidence of implant failure (Yazawa *et al.* 1990). The addition of methylmethacrylate augmentation to this construction may improve the clinical and functional result. It is essential that medial structural support be restored. Others have shown that, even with methylmethacrylate augmentation, the failure rate remains high because of mechanical instability.

The inherent stability of an intramedullary device in the subtrochanteric area is helpful in pathologic fractures. There is usually a ring

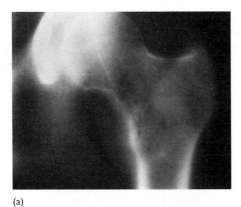

(a)

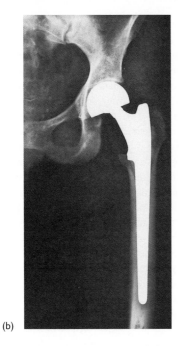

(b)

Fig. 10. (a) Anteroposterior tomogram of left proximal femur showing destructive lesion involving calcar region. (b) After replacement arthroplasty with a calcar replacement prosthesis.

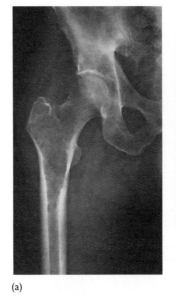

(a)

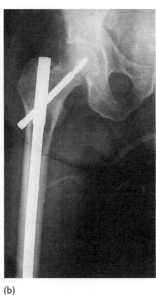

(b)

Fig. 11. Anteroposterior views of right proximal femur (a) showing extensive metastatic destruction of subtrochanteric region and (b) after internal fixation with reconstruction rod.

of good cortical bone above and below the fracture area which allows good purchase of the intramedullary device, especially when it is augmented with methylmethacrylate. The use of a standard intramedullary rod is acceptable if good cortical purchase can be accomplished above and below the fracture. However, one must remember that most patients with pathologic fractures have had preceding pain with disuse and the proximal femur is relatively osteopenic, so one cannot always rely on the proximal femoral bone to be mechanically sound. Newer intramedullary rods that have interlocking screws, such as the Gross–Kempf nail and the Russell–Taylor reconstruction rod, have been used (Fig. 11). The proximal locking screws afford fixation into the femoral neck or calcar with good intramedullary fixation through and distal to the fracture site. The most commonly used intramedullary device for this site is the Zickel nail (Zickel and Mouradian 1976). The advantage of this device over other intramedullary rods is that there is a proximal expansion of the Zickel nail that allows better fixation in the intertrochanteric area of the femur. Also, an

anatomical angulation in the proximal portion of the rod allows more stable reduction and restoration of the medial cortical structures. The apparatus allows impaction with early weight-bearing and excellent stability. The device has been used extensively with good results, especially if methylmethacrylate was used. The surgery is technically demanding and must be done with great care to avoid comminution and loss of fixation in the proximal fragment.

With the relative success of proximal femoral replacement arthroplasty for pathologic fractures of the intertrochanteric area, the indications have been extended to the subtrochanteric area. In cases in which the bone destruction is so extensive that bony stability cannot be achieved or extensive shortening would be necessary, proximal prosthetic replacement should be considered (Sim *et al.* 1974, 1976). This technique allows pain relief, early mobilization, and weight-bearing. In addition, the complete resection of the area involved with tumor prevents the risk of local progression and subsequent problems. These factors may become more important as the treatment of metastatic cancer improves with time. Proximal femoral replacement is especially applicable in patients who have extensive disease throughout the proximal femur, including the femoral head, femoral neck, and intertrochanteric and subtrochanteric areas.

In cases in which previous surgical treatment has been used for pathologic fractures and complications occurred, proximal femoral replacement is a good salvage procedure (Fig. 12) (Sim 1988). Attention needs to be given to the restoration of the abductor mechanism through soft-tissue and bony reattachment. It is essential to maintain limb length or even lengthen the limb slightly to provide enough resistance to dislocation. A bipolar acetabular component adds additional stability. Postoperatively, weight-bearing is allowed immediately, and the patient can increase this weight-bearing status as muscle strength and rehabilitation allow.

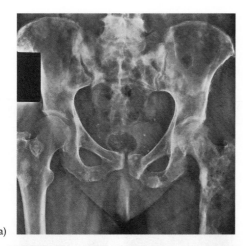

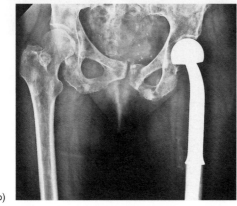

Fig. 12. Anteroposterior views of pelvis and proximal femur (a) showing extensive metastatic lesion involving left proximal femur and (b) after proximal femoral replacement prosthesis with bipolar cup.

Femoral shaft lesions

One-third of all metastatic lesions occur below the intertrochanteric region in the shaft or in the supracondylar region. Midshaft femoral metastases are often best managed with intramedullary fixation and adjunctive methylmethacrylate after preoperative radiation therapy. The design of the nail should be nearly anatomical, with an anterior bow to assist in placing the largest diameter nail possible within the femur.

Surgical considerations

Small fractures that are due to very small cortical lesions can be stabilized with a closed femoral rodding procedure. The technique does require opening the fracture site and curetting the local tumor, followed by insertion of methylmethacrylate into each side of the fractured area. Care should be taken to avoid comminution of the local area when the reaming is performed. It is important to use the largest rod possible in fixation of these fractures to obtain maximal stability.

Mechanically, two large plates placed at 90° to each other provide a more stable construct; however, problems may arise from stress shielding and fractures through other areas of metastatic disease within the femur.

When more extensive cortical destruction is involved with the pathologic fracture, more extensive procedures need to be performed. A simple intramedullary rod without cementation or additional stabilization may lead to severe complications. Two different techniques have been described for cementing pathologic fractures of the femur. The method most often used involves packing the defect with cement and subsequent introduction of the intramedullary rod through the soft cement mass. In this technique, all gross tumor is removed through curettage. Reaming and sizing of the rod are performed, and a trial reduction is done. The cement is injected either through each side of the fracture site or through the intramedullary opening proximally. Care must be taken to avoid extravasation of cement into the soft-tissue structures during rod insertion. This method allows excellent fixation of distal and proximal fragments and allows bony union in a majority of cases.

Another technique involves the removal of gross tumor, reduction of the fracture, and placement of an intramedullary rod, with subsequent packing of the cement. Additional cement can be packed proximally through the intramedullary rod opening as well as distally through a cortical window made in the supracondylar area. With this additional proximal and distal fixation, adequate stabilization can usually be obtained. This technique is somewhat less technically demanding. Methylmethacrylate may be used to fill associated osseous defects; however, if considerable length is to be restored or the fracture site appears unstable in rotation, a nail with interlocking capability should be considered to enhance fixation. These rods can be used for prophylactic placement of a rod with proximal and distal interlocking screws. They also may be used for pathologic fractures involving small cortical lesions when cementation is used. Their use in extensive femoral lesions with destruction has not been documented, because of the loss of cortical stability. Methylmethacrylate cementation should be used to augment stability and to prevent collapse and excessive stresses on the interlocking screw areas.

If stability has been achieved, patients can be mobilized soon after operation. Range of motion exercise of the hip and knee is started, and patients begin progressive weight-bearing. Their ambulatory status should be evaluated with regard to the amount of bony loss, the stability achieved at operation, and the evidence of bony healing and bridging through the fracture site.

Distal femoral lesions

Metastases to the region of the distal femur are uncommon. Lesions arising within the distal metaphysis require an interlocking intramedullary nail or either single- or double-plate reconstruction with methylmethacrylate. The most distal lesions may be dealt with using a blade–plate or a screw–plate combination with methylmethacrylate (Fig. 13). Very destructive lesions may be resected, with reconstruction using an osteoarticular allograft, an allograft–prosthesis composite, or a modular prosthesis.

Generally, fractures involving the supracondylar area of the femur can be quite difficult to manage. Bone in the area of the fracture is usually comminuted and of poor quality, and there is difficulty in obtaining reduction. In addition to these factors, the metastatic process has destroyed additional cortical bone. Small lesions may be curetted, packed with methylmethacrylate, and stabilized with rods or immobilized with a cast brace. For extensive lesions, more secure fixation is necessary. Blade–plate fixation with methylmethacrylate

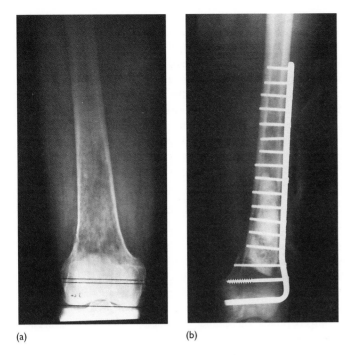

Fig. 13. Anteroposterior views of left distal femur (a) showing extensive permeative destruction caused by metastatic lung cancer and (b) after internal fixation with long condylar plate and methylmethacrylate.

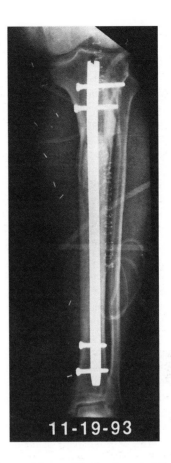

Fig. 14. Locked intramedullary rod fixation for metastatic lesion of proximal tibia; methylmethacrylate was also used.

has been an effective means of treatment for these lesions. The Zickel device has been used for the treatment of these fractures, with good functional and symptomatic results. Technically, the surgery is demanding, and attention to detail is essential.

Occasionally, because of the extensive bony loss and comminution through the fracture area, the techniques mentioned above would be ineffective. In these situations, a custom-made distal femoral replacement is recommended. With resection of the comminuted bone and cementation of the prosthesis, early range-of-motion exercise and return to functional status are possible. Large destructive lesions may require amputation with wide margins for local tumor management in an effort to rehabilitate the patient with the least overall morbidity.

Lesions of the tibia

Metastatic deposits in the tibia are not common. When identified early, most of the proximal lesions can be managed with radiation therapy alone. More destructive lesions may require joint surface reconstruction, using similar modalities as discussed for management of distal femoral involvement.

Metaphyseal lesions can be reconstructed using either single- or double-plate reconstruction with methylmethacrylate after radiation therapy. However, wound closure complications occur because of the limited soft tissues available in the leg. A medial or lateral gastrocnemius muscle flap and split-thickness skin graft may be needed for wound closure.

Midshaft lesions may require prophylactic fixation using either open or closed intramedullary nailing techniques to provide sufficient strength to prevent a pathologic fracture (Fig. 14). Most oncology surgeons prefer to consider closed intramedullary nailing only after accelerated fractionated radiation therapy to prevent tumor contamination of the entire intramedullary canal.

Distal tibial lesions may occasionally be managed with radiation therapy alone, but the majority require the addition of a plate and methylmethacrylate fixation. Some patients may need a below-knee amputation and immediate prosthetic fitting. The absence of good muscle coverage and the limited soft tissues available for wound closure prohibit major reconstructive efforts in the distal leg in most patients.

Lesions of the foot and ankle

The foot, unlike the hand, can readily be replaced with a reliable prosthesis with predictable overall excellent function. Therefore efforts to preserve the foot or the ankle involved with metastatic disease are attempted less often. Small lesions in the os calcis may be managed with radiation therapy alone, whereas lesions associated with painful pathologic fractures are often best managed with amputation and immediate prosthetic fitting. Metastatic disease to the metatarsals can be managed with ray amputation, as in the hand. Postoperative radiation therapy may be required if the margins are not free from disease. Metastases to the phalanges are best managed with amputation.

Metastatic lesions of the spine

Compression of the spinal cord or cauda equina in patients with metastatic disease of the spine is a medical emergency that requires prompt diagnosis and treatment. Its causes include pressure from an enlarging extradural mass, spinal angulation following vertebral collapse, vertebral dislocation following pathologic fracture, or, rarely, pressure from intradural metastases.

The extent and rate of progression of a neurologic deficit must be determined at the time of evaluation. Patients with severe deficits have a poorer prognosis, as do those with rapidly developing deficits. Patients with acute deterioration of neurologic status frequently have a thoracic lesion. In the thoracic spine, the ratio of canal diameter to cord size is small, resulting in early compression. Moreover, collateral circulation in the midthoracic region is limited, and metastatic involvement may produce ischemic damage to the cord, with resultant rapid worsening of the neurologic status. These data emphasize the need for urgent evaluation of patients with progressive neurologic signs or symptoms. Early recognition of cord compression permits prompt treatment and improved prognosis for restoration or preservation of neurologic function.

Spinal instability can cause excruciating pain, which is mechanical in origin. The patient is comfortable only when lying absolutely still, and any movement produces severe pain. Because the pain is due to the instability, radiation therapy or systemic treatment will not alleviate it. Stabilization is required for pain relief. An associated neurologic deficit is not a contraindication to these procedures, and in one series, 20 of 29 patients with instability of the dorsal lumbar spine and an associated neurologic deficit obtained significant recovery of function (Galasko 1991).

Classification

Harrington (1986b) categorized patients with metastatic disease of the spine into five classes, depending on the degree of neurologic involvement and bone destruction. Class I patients have asymptomatic spinal metastases. Class II patients have pain or minor neurologic deficit without bony collapse or instability (Chamberlain et al. 1990). Class III patients have major sensory or motor compromise without significant bone involvement. Patients with pain from instability or mechanical causes due to vertebral collapse and without notable neurologic deficits are categorized as class IV. Finally, patients with both a significant neurologic deficit and vertebral collapse or instability are designated class V.

Harrington used this classification system as a guide to treatment. Generally, class I and II patients respond to chemotherapy or hormonal manipulation. If improvement is not seen with these modalities, radiation therapy is considered. Class III patients usually respond to radiation therapy, and consideration may be given to supplemental systemic steroid therapy. Harrington considered surgical treatment for class IV and class V patients, emphasizing that radiation therapy is ineffective in the treatment of bony instability or epidural compression due to bony debris.

Based on tumor location, McLain and Weinstein (1990) classified primary spinal tumors according to zones of involvement and used this information to determine the optimal surgical approach. These guidelines are also applicable to metastatic lesions. Zone I includes the spinous process to the pars interarticularis and inferior facets and is best approached posteriorly. Lesions that involve the superior articular facets, transverse process, and pedicle are classified as zone II and may be resected through a posterior or posterolateral approach. Zone III tumors are located in the anterior three-quarters of the vertebral body and are best approached anteriorly. Zone IV is the most inaccessible region of the spine—the posterior quarter of the body. McClain and Weinstein recommended a combined anterior and posterior approach for zone IV lesions. This system also includes a letter designation that is useful for classification of primary neoplasms: (a) intraosseous containment; (b) extraosseous extension; (c) the presence of metastases.

Surgical indications and contraindications

Aggressive surgical treatment of metastatic disease of the spine has become popular in recent years. This popularity is due to several facts including (a) the development of new and durable spinal fixation systems and (b) further experience with the anterior approach to the spine, which allows complete removal of metastatic lesions and reconstruction of multiple vertebral bodies if necessary.

Surgery is recommended (a) when disease progression occurs despite external beam irradiation, (b) when disease involvement compromises both the anterior and posterior structures, resulting in instability and neurologic compromise, (c) when anterior disease causes significant spinal cord compression, and (d) when there is need for definitive histological diagnosis (Harrington 1986b; McLain and Weinstein 1990). Some authors also include impending pathologic vertebral fracture as an indication for surgical treatment in selected patients (Kostuik et al. 1988). After paraplegia occurs, full neurologic recovery is unlikely despite the most aggressive treatment methods. Contraindications to surgery include inadequate bone stock, more than one area of epidural compression, and life expectancy less than 3 months.

Surgical approaches

Decompression of either the cervical or thoracic spine posteriorly often results in only temporary neurologic recovery, and it may result in further instability. An anterior approach allows complete removal of the destroyed bony elements and tumor tissue. After the anterior decompression, reconstruction of the vertebral bodies using autogenous tricortical iliac grafts, bulk allografts, or methylmethacrylate metal construct will provide spinal stability. If the posterior vertebral structures are also compromised, posterior stabilization with internal fixation is necessary in addition to anterior decompression and reconstruction. Various systems are effective, including rods and plating systems.

The primary region of vertebral body destruction is often best demonstrated with CT and MRI, using both sagittal and cross-sectional reconstruction. Most patients with anterior column involvement have an anterior compression deformity and evidence of an anterior extradural tumor mass on MRI. Many of these patients require either an anterior procedure alone or a combined anteroposterior procedure and stabilization. If possible, the lesion should be treated with external beam radiation therapy before the intended operative procedure. Patients with primary involvement of the middle column often have neurologic compromise. Occasionally, radiation therapy alone suffices for treatment, especially for metastases in the lumbar spine below the level of the conus. Most often, however, the patient requires stabilization above and below the involved vertebrae with pedicle screw fixation, followed by a complete laminectomy and removal of the involved pedicle and decompression of the tumor mass. Patients with posterior column disease but without cord compression are often best managed with radiation therapy alone. Patients with evidence of posterior cord compression may require posterior decompression without internal stabilization if the facet joints remain intact. If the facet joints are either unilaterally or bilaterally involved or destroyed, pedicle screw fixation and stabilization above and below the involved segment are indicated.

Spinal cord and cauda equina compression

Spinal cord and cauda equina compression most commonly results from tumor involvement of the vertebral column and only rarely from intradural metastases. It may occur in association with spinal instability or in isolation. When there is more than 50 per cent vertebral collapse, compression of the spinal cord becomes more likely. Patients with multiple areas of epidural compression and inadequate bone stock generally are not considered for operative treatment. Patients with symptoms of acute epidural spinal cord compression may benefit from systemic steroid therapy as an adjuvant to both operative and nonoperative treatment.

The choice between surgical decompression and radiation therapy depends on several clinical features. Radiation therapy is indicated for patients either unfit for surgery or who do not fulfill the criteria for surgical decompression. Most patients with metastatic lesions of the vertebral column can be treated successfully with external beam irradiation (3000 cGy in 10 fractions). Doses beyond spinal cord tolerance (4500 cGy in 180-cGy fractions) place the patient at significant risk for transverse myelitis. Surgical decompression is indicated in patients who have recent onset of symptoms, with progressive paraplegia, and urinary retention of less than 30 h duration. The site of compression should be localized to no more than two or three segments, and the patient should have a life expectancy of at least several weeks. For those patients in whom the paraplegia has been established for several days or in whom urinary retention has been present for more than 30 h, surgical decompression rarely results in the recovery of bladder or motor function. However, some patients undoubtedly have benefited greatly from prompt surgical management. Experimentally, with gradual compression of the cord, decompression can be delayed and the patient can still retain neurologic function, whereas rapid compression necessitates immediate decompression to retain neurologic function. The use of dexamethasone to reduce vasogenic edema has been well established (Ushio et al. 1977a,b). Systemic dexamethasone may result in transient clinical improvement until operative decompression can be performed.

Postoperative external beam irradiation

Following surgical stabilization of long bone and spinal lesions, it is of paramount importance to control the metastases with external beam irradiation, otherwise metastatic disease progression within the field will result in loss of fixation and pain. Treatment can be started as soon as the patient can be moved to the radiation suite, as long as the skin incision can be blocked from the radiation fields. If the incision must be included, treatments may be delayed for 1 to 2 weeks to allow healing.

Survival

Survival after pathologic fracture varies with the type of the primary tumor. Patients with carcinoma of the lung rarely survive longer than 1 year and often do not survive 6 months, whereas those with carcinoma of the thyroid commonly live 5 years or longer.

In the experience at the authors' institution, the mean survival of patients after pathologic fracture of the long bones or pelvis was 2.5 years for those with prostate carcinoma, 2 years for those with breast metastases, 1 year for those with metastatic renal cell cancer, and only 4 months for those with metastatic lung carcinoma (Frassica and Sim 1988). Patients with metastatic involvement of the spine may have a poorer prognosis than those with extremity lesions.

As the ability to manage the primary tumor through the use of chemotherapy, radiation therapy, and surgery improves, a corresponding increase in postfracture survival time requires improved surgical methods and the development of implants to improve the management of these patients.

Some patients, usually those with a renal or a gastrointestinal primary tumor, may develop only a single isolated metastasis 18 to 24 months after surgical therapy for the primary tumor. If restaging studies, including bone scintigraphy, routine chest radiography, and CT of the abdomen and chest, indicate that the patient is otherwise free of disease, careful consideration should be given to radical surgical efforts, aiming for cure rather than palliation; in reality, only a small proportion of these patients are cured.

References

Arguello, F., Baggs, R.B., Duerst, R.E., Johnstone, L., McQueen, K., and Frantz, C.N. (1990). Pathogenesis of vertebral metastasis and epidural spinal cord compression. *Cancer*, **65**, 98–106.

Batson, O.V. (1940). The function of the vertebral veins and their role in the spread of metastases. *Annals of Surgery*, **112**, 138–49.

Batson, O.V. (1942). The role of the vertebral veins in metastatic processes. *Annals of Internal Medicine*, **16**, 38–45.

Chamberlain, M.C., Abitbol, J.J., and Garfin, S.R. (1990). Epidural spinal cord compression: treatment options. *Seminars in Spine Surgery*, **2**, 203–9.

Chapman, M.W., Bowman, W.E., Csongradi, J.J., Day, L.J., Trafton, P.G., and Bovill, E.G., Jr (1981). The use of Ender's pins in extracapsular fractures of the hip. *Journal of Bone and Joint Surgery, American Volume*, **63A**, 14–28.

Cheng, D.S., Seitz, C.B., and Eyre, H.J. (1980). Nonoperative management of femoral, humeral, and acetabular metastases in patients with breast carcinoma. *Cancer*, **45**, 1533–7.

Eftekhar, N.S. and Thurston, C.W. (1975). Effect of irradiation on acrylic cement with special reference to fixation of pathological fractures. *Journal of Biomechanics*, **8**, 53–6.

Fidler, M. (1973). Prophylactic internal fixation of secondary neoplastic deposits in long bones. *British Medical Journal*, **i**, 341–3.

Frassica, F.J. and Sim, F.H. (1988). Pathogenesis and prognosis. In *Diagnosis and management of metastatic bone disease: a multidisciplinary approach* (ed. F.H. Sim), pp. 1–6. Raven Press, New York.

Galasko, C.S.B. (1981). The anatomy and pathways of skeletal metastases. In *Bone metastasis* (ed. L. Weiss and H.A. Gilbert), pp. 49–63. G.K. Hall, Boston, MA.

Galasko, C.S.B. (1991). The role of the orthopaedic surgeon in the treatment of skeletal metastases. In *Bone metastases: diagnosis and treatment* (ed. R.D. Rubens and I. Fogelman), p. 207. Springer-Verlag, London.

Harrington, K.D. (1981). The management of acetabular insufficiency secondary to metastatic malignant disease. *Journal of Bone and Joint Surgery, American Volume*, **63A**, 653–64.

Harrington, K.D. (1986a). Impending pathologic fractures from metastatic malignancy: evaluation and management. *Instructional Course Lectures*, **35**, 357–81.

Harrington, K.D. (1986b). Metastatic disease of the spine. *Journal of Bone and Joint Surgery, American Volume*, **68A**, 1110–15.

Kostuik, J.P., Errico, T.J., Gleason, T.F., and Errico, C.C. (1988). Spinal stabilization of vertebral column tumors. *Spine*, **13**, 250–6.

Li, K.C. and Poon, P.Y. (1988). Sensitivity and specificity of MRI in detecting malignant spinal cord compression and in distinguishing malignant from benign compression fractures of vertebrae. *Magnetic Resonance Imaging*, **6**, 547–56.

McLain, R.F. and Weinstein, J.N. (1990). Tumors of the spine. *Seminars in Spine Surgery*, **2**, 157–80.

Muindi, J., Coombes, R.C., Golding, S., Powles, T.J., Khan, O., and Husband, J. (1983). The role of computed tomography in the detection of bone metastases in breast cancer patients. *British Journal of Radiology*, **56**, 233–6.

Murray, J.A., Bruels, M.C., and Lindberg, R.D. (1974). Irradiation of polymethylmethacrylate. *In vitro* gamma radiation effect. *Journal of Bone and Joint Surgery, American Volume*, **56A**, 311–12.

Naiman, P.T., Schein, A.J., and Siffert, R.S. (1969). Medial displacement fixation for severely comminuted intertrochanteric fractures. *Clinical Orthopaedics and Related Research*, **62**, 151–5.

O'Reilly, S.M., Richards, M.A., and Rubens, R.D. (1990). Liver metastases from breast cancer: the relationship between clinical, biochemical and pathological features and survival. *European Journal of Cancer*, **26**, 574–7.

Rose, C., Ford, J., Becher, R., *et al.* (1992). Pamidronate disodium (AREDIA): dose effect and tolerability evaluation in breast cancer patients with bone metastases (abstract). *Annals of Oncology*, **3** (Supplement 5), 85.

Silverberg, E., Boring, C.C., and Squires, T.S. (1990). Cancer statistics, 1990. *CA: A Cancer Journal for Clinicians*, **40**, 9–26.

Sim, F.H. (1988). *Diagnosis and management of metastatic bone disease: a multidisciplinary approach*. Raven Press, New York.

Sim, F.H., Daugherty, T.W., and Ivins, J.C. (1974). The adjunctive use of methylmethacrylate in fixation of pathological fractures. *Journal of Bone and Joint Surgery, American Volume*, **56A**, 40–8.

Sim, F.H., Hartz, C.R., and Chao, E.Y.S. (1976). Total hip arthroplasty for tumors of the hip. *Hip*, **4**, 246–59.

Taylor, A. and Rush, J. (1992). The Zickel nail in the treatment of metastatic bone disease in the upper end of the femur. *Australian and New Zealand Journal of Surgery*, **62**, 382–4.

Ushio, Y., Posner, R., Kim, J.H., Shapiro, W.R., and Posner, J.B. (1977a). Treatment of experimental spinal cord compression caused by extradural neoplasms. *Journal of Neurosurgery*, **47**, 380–90.

Ushio, Y., Posner, R., Posner, J.B., and Shapiro, W.R. (1977b). Experimental spinal cord compression by epidural neoplasm. *Neurology*, **27**, 422–9.

Vahdat, L. and Antman, K. (1995). High-dose therapy for breast cancer. *Blood Reviews*, **9**, 191–200.

Wirth, C.R. (1979). Metastatic bone cancer. *Current Problems in Cancer*, **3**, 1–36.

Yazawa, Y., Frassica, F.J., Chao, E.Y., Pritchard, D.J., Sim, F.H., and Shives, T.C. (1990). Metastatic bone disease. A study of the surgical treatment of 166 pathologic humeral and femoral fractures. *Clinical Orthopaedics and Related Research*, **251**, 213–19.

Zickel, R.E. and Mouradian, W.H. (1976). Intramedullary fixation of pathological fractures and lesions of the subtrochanteric region of the femur. *Journal of Bone and Joint Surgery, American Volume*, **58A**, 1061–6.

1.6.10.2 Metastatic neuroblastoma

Panayiotis J. Papagelopoulos, Evanthia C. Galanis, Carola A. S. Arndt, and Franklin H. Sim

Introduction

Neuroblastoma is a primitive tumor of childhood arising from the medulla of the adrenal gland or anywhere in the sympathetic nervous system. It is the third most common malignancy of childhood after acute leukemia and brain tumors. The median age at diagnosis is 2 years. The tumor has been reported slightly less frequently in boys than in girls (0.8:1) (Campanacci 1990). Familial cases occur (Roberts and Lee 1975). Neuroblastoma has also been observed in patients with neurofibromatosis, Hirschsprung's disease, Beckwith–Wiedemann syndrome, and fetal hydantoin syndrome.

Most tumors arise from the adrenal medulla and the paraspinal sympathetic ganglia but the thoracic, pelvic, and cervical ganglia are also potential sites of origin. Bone and bone marrow are common sites of metastases (Leeson *et al.* 1985). The bones mostly involved by metastatic neuroblastoma are the vertebrae, ribs, skull, femur, pelvis, humerus, tibia, and radius.

Box 1

- A primitive tumor of childhood arising from the medulla of the adrenal gland or anywhere in the sympathetic nervous system

- Most patients present with evidence of systemic disease, such as weight loss, fever, failure to thrive, pain, and anemia

- Up to 75 per cent of patients present with disseminated disease at the time of diagnosis, and the most frequent site of metastasis is the skeleton

- Pain is the most frequent presenting symptom of children with metastatic bone disease, but a few children present with pathologic fractures

- Plain radiographs of bone metastases usually show osteolytic lesions with permeative bone destruction, particularly at metaphyses

- Most metastatic bone lesions are treated by splinting and chemotherapy, although radiation therapy may be appropriate in some patients

Cytogenetics and carcinogenesis

Cytogenetic studies of neuroblastoma have demonstrated chromosomal abnormalities, commonly in chromosome 1. Amplified n-*myc* cellular oncogene (more than 10 copies/cell) occurs in around one-third of neuroblastomas and is associated with advanced disease at diagnosis and poor outcome, even in those patients who have early-stage disease or who present in infancy (Brodeur *et al.* 1984; Seeger *et al.* 1985; Tsuda *et al.* 1987). The DNA content of the tumor (ploidy) correlates with the therapeutic outcome.

Clinical evaluation

From 50 to 75 per cent of patients with neuroblastoma present with disseminated disease at the time of diagnosis, and the most frequent site of metastasis is the bones (Heisel *et al.* 1983; Daubenton *et al.* 1987). Solitary or multifocal bone metastases are common. Pain is the most frequent presenting symptom of children with metastatic bone disease. A few children may present with pathologic fractures. Fractures usually occur rather late in the course of the disease, and long-term survival after pathologic fractures is unusual. Other common sites of metastases are lymph nodes, bone marrow, liver, skin, orbit, and bone (facial bones, skull, and appendicular skeleton).

Radiographic and laboratory evaluation

When neuroblastoma is suspected, the evaluation should be conducted to establish the diagnosis, determine the extent of disease, and obtain tumor material for molecular and genetic analyses.

In neuroblastoma metastatic to bone, plain radiographs usually show symmetrical involvement and aggressive osteolytic lesions with

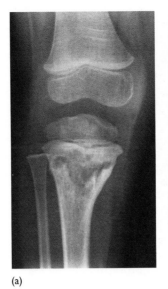
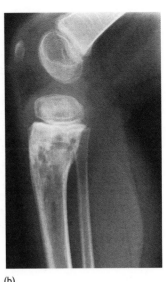

(a)   (b)

Fig. 1. (a) Anteroposterior and (b) lateral radiographs of the knee showing a lytic lesion of the proximal tibia of a 4-year-old child with metastatic neuroblastoma.

permeative bone destruction, particularly at metaphyses (Fig. 1). They may resemble Ewing's sarcoma or, rarely, leukemia or osteomyelitis (Campanacci 1990). Periosteal reaction is common with lesions in the diaphysis, and it may extend even to the entire perimeter of the diaphysis. In some cases, massive osteolysis is associated with periosteal reaction, having the radiographic appearance of Codman's triangle. In diffuse and polyostotic forms, faded osteoporosis of the metaphyses may be observed. Sutural widening in the skull and collapse of vertebral bodies with adjacent soft-tissue masses may be present (David *et al.* 1989).

Radionuclide bone scans are more sensitive than radiographic skeletal surveys. However, neuroblastoma is one of the entities in which the bone scan may be 'cold' or normal when plain radiographs show evidence of a lytic lesion. Newer radionuclide scans like iodine-131 (^{131}I) meta-iodobenzylguanidine or neural cell-specific monoclonal antibodies conjugated to ^{131}I or ^{123}I are currently investigational but may prove more accurate and sensitive for the detection of nonosseous and osseous disease, and also of any residual disease after treatment has been initiated.

Pathology

Macroscopically, the tissue is encephaloid, at times hemorrhagic, or liquescent, and yellowish due to necrosis, possibly suggesting osteomyelitic pus (Campanacci 1990). Neuroblastoma is one of the 'small blue round cell' tumors (Fig. 2). Histologically, the hallmark of neuroblastoma is rosette formation and neurofibrils. When these features are absent, light microscopy alone may be inadequate to distinguish neuroblastomas from other small round cell tumors of childhood, such as rhabdomyosarcoma, non-Hodgkin's lymphoma, Ewing's sarcoma, primitive neuroectodermal tumors, and undifferentiated soft-tissue sarcoma. In addition to the rosette formation and neurofibrils, the diagnosis is based also on the presence of more dif-

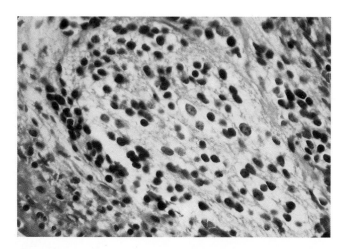

Fig. 2. Histological features of metastatic neuroblastoma of bone. These features are very similar to those of Ewing's sarcoma. (Hematoxylin and eosin stain.)

ferentiated sympathetic cells, on the absence of cellular glycogen on electron microscopy, and on the presence of neurosecretory granules (Campanacci 1990).

Neuroblastomas can be classified into three histological subgroups: neuroblastoma, ganglioneuroblastoma, and ganglioneuroma. The neuroblastoma, which is composed of sympathoblasts and is the least differentiated, consists of sheets of primitive cells with scant cytoplasm and dark-stained nuclei. The tumor cells and their fibrillar processes form so-called Homer Wright rosettes. The ganglioneuroblastoma shows signs of differentiation and maturation; it is composed of both primitive neuroblasts and mature ganglion cells. The ganglioneuroma is a mature tumor composed of fully differentiated ganglion cells embedded in Schwann cell sheaths. It is benign and lacks metastatic potential. These subgroups appear to recapitulate stages in the normal differentiation of neural crest stem cells.

Prognostic factors

In children with metastatic disease, the most significant prognostic variable is age at diagnosis; children younger than 12 months at diagnosis have a significantly greater chance for cure (Hann *et al.* 1981; Pinkel 1981). In older children with disseminated disease, the prognosis is dismal, although improvements in response and survival have been reported with modern treatment modalities.

Chemotherapy

Combination chemotherapeutic regimens including agents such as cyclophosphamide, melphalan, doxorubicin, cisplatin, epipodophyllotoxins, and vincristine are used in patients with disseminated, unresectable, or advanced disease and are more effective in producing responses than single agents.

Although improvement in the survival of infants with advanced disease and children with locally unresectable disease has resulted from the implementation of various chemotherapeutic regimens, the outlook for older children with advanced disease has not changed

Box 4 Neuroblastoma—treatment and prognosis

- Chemotherapy does not prolong survival but bone metastases may respond
- Radiotherapy may reduce pain
- Two-year survival is less than 50 per cent

significantly. Only 20 to 25 per cent of these patients survive 5 years from diagnosis. However, in the same patient population, the complete response rate and disease-free interval have increased with more intensive combination chemotherapy, encouraging the further development and refinement of such therapy.

Treatment of metastatic bone disease

Most metastatic bone lesions are treated conservatively. Splinting and protection of the involved part are the usual supportive modalities used. Chemotherapy is still the primary modality. Response to chemotherapy is frequent. In lesions not responding to chemotherapy, radiation therapy can have significant palliative benefit. Irradiation may provide pain relief, stabilize bones that have significant structural change, and help prevent neurological deterioration. In a subset of patients, radiation therapy may aid other systemic therapy in achieving long-term tumor control.

Prognosis

For patients with advanced neuroblastoma, aggressive multimodal therapy has been used. The 2-year disease-free survival of these patients is less than 50 per cent.

Autologous bone marrow transplantation is being investigated. The results of high dose chemotherapy with bone marrow transplantation in patients with a poor long-term prognosis who have achieved a complete remission or, at least, a substantial partial remission with chemotherapy are encouraging.

Because of the tendency of neuroblastoma to involve the bone marrow, purging strategies currently are being developed and undergoing clinical testing. These include use of *ex vivo* chemotherapy or monoclonal antibodies to achieve tumor cell depletion and, subsequently, increase the cure rate with autologous transplantation.

References

Brodeur, G.M., Seeger, R.C., Schwab, M., Varmus, H.E., and Bishop, J.M. (1984). Amplification of n-*myc* in untreated human neuroblastomas correlates with advanced disease stage. *Science*, **224**, 1121–4.

Campanacci, M. (1990). *Bone and soft tissue tumors*. Springer-Verlag, Vienna.

Daubenton, J.D., Fisher, R.M., Karabus, C.D., and Mann, M.D. (1987). The relationship between prognosis and scintigraphic evidence of bone metastases in neuroblastoma. *Cancer*, **59**, 1586–9.

David, R., Lamki, N., Fan, S., *et al.* (1989). The many faces of neuroblastoma. *Radiographics*, **9**, 859–82.

Hann, H.W., Evans, A.E., Cohen, I.J., and Leitmeyer, J.E. (1981). Biologic differences between neuroblastoma stages IV-S and IV. Measurement of serum ferritin and E-rosette inhibition in 30 children. *New England Journal of Medicine*, **305**, 425–9.

Heisel, M.A., Miller, J.H., Reid, B.S., and Siegel, S.E. (1983). Radionuclide bone scan in neuroblastoma. *Pediatrics*, **71**, 206–9.

Leeson, M.C., Makley, J.T., and Carter, J.R. (1985). Metastatic skeletal disease in the pediatric population. *Journal of Pediatric Orthopedics*, **5**, 261–7.

Pinkel, D. (1981). Differences between neuroblastoma stages IV-S and IV. *New England Journal of Medicine*, **305**, 1418–19.

Roberts, F.F. and Lee, K.R. (1975). Familial neuroblastoma presenting as multiple tumors. *Radiology*, **116**, 133–6.

Seeger, R.C., Brodeur, G.M., Sather, H., *et al.* (1985). Association of multiple copies of the n-*myc* oncogene with rapid progression of neuroblastomas. *New England Journal of Medicine*, **313**, 1111–16.

Tsuda, T., Obara, M., Hirano, H., *et al.* (1987). Analysis of n-*myc* amplification in relation to disease stage and histologic types in human neuroblastomas. *Cancer*, **60**, 820–6.

1.6.10.3 Wilms' tumor

Panayiotis J. Papagelopoulos, Evanthia C. Galanis, Carola A. S. Arndt, and Franklin H. Sim

Introduction

Wilms' tumor—the most common intra-abdominal tumor of childhood—is a primary renal tumor thought to arise from the metanephric blastema. Although Wilms' tumor with classic histological appearance rarely metastasizes to bone (5 per cent of cases), renal tumors with sarcomatous features, especially clear cell sarcoma ('bone-metastasizing renal tumor of childhood'), have a high incidence of metastasis to bone, with a particularly poor prognosis.

Box 1 Renal tumors of childhood metastasizing to bone

- Wilms' tumor rarely metastasizes to bone (5 per cent of cases), but childhood renal tumors with sarcomatous features, especially clear cell sarcoma ('bone-metastasizing renal tumor of childhood'), have a high incidence of metastasis to bone

- Plain radiographs of patients with renal tumor bone metastases show osteolytic areas distributed in both the axial and appendicular skeleton

- Well-differentiated Wilms' tumor resembles developing embryonic renal tissue

- Clear cell sarcoma of the kidney consists of a fibrovascular supporting network containing cells that have uniform nuclei and ill-defined 'clear' cytoplasm

- Cells of rhabdoid tumor of the kidney, unlike those of clear cell sarcoma of the kidney, have prominent acidophilic cytoplasm, often resembling that of myoblasts

- Most metastatic bone lesions from renal tumors in children are treated with splinting, radiation therapy, and chemotherapy

After neuroblastoma, Wilms' tumor is the most common retroperitoneal tumor of childhood. In 1991, Wilms' tumor represented 5 to 6 per cent of childhood cancers in the United States, where the total incidence was estimated at 460 annually (Crist and Kun 1991). Most children are 1 to 5 years old (median, 40 months) at diagnosis. Males and females are affected equally.

Children with Wilms' tumor may have associated anomalies, including aniridia, hemihypertrophy, cryptorchidism, and hypospadias (Miller *et al.* 1964). WAGR syndrome consists of Wilms' tumor, aniridia, genitourinary malformations, and mental retardation and occurs in association with an interstitial deletion of varying length on chromosome 11 (del[11p13]) (Riccardi *et al.* 1980). Children with pseudohermaphroditism and/or renal disease in whom Wilms' tumor develops may have Denys–Drash syndrome, which is associated with mutations in the same chromosomal segment as WAGR syndrome (Eddy and Mauer 1985; Coppes *et al.* 1993). Hemihypertrophy may occur as an isolated abnormality or as a component of Beckwith–Wiedemann syndrome, which includes macroglossia, omphalocele, and visceromegaly (Beckwith 1969).

Biology and cytogenetics

Wilms' tumor occurs in both heritable and sporadic forms. In children with the heritable form, the neoplasm develops at an earlier age and is more likely to be bilateral and multicentric (Kantor *et al.* 1982; Huff *et al.* 1988). Overall, approximately 15 to 20 per cent of cases of Wilms' tumor are thought to be nonsporadic (Huff *et al.* 1988). Familial cases are inherited in an autosomal dominant pattern, with variable penetrance and expressivity (Matsunaga 1981).

Clinicopathological staging

A staging system used to describe Wilms' tumor in children was employed to determine the extent of disease at diagnosis and is based on surgical pathological principles. It considers several physical features of the tumor that increase the risk of local or distant recurrence and, therefore, dictate therapeutic modifications. In the United States, the National Wilms' Tumor Study committee clinicopathologic staging system is the most widely used, relying extensively on the intraoperative determination of the extent of tumor in the abdomen (Farewell *et al.* 1981).

Clinical evaluation

Wilms' tumor most commonly occurs as an asymptomatic abdominal mass that grows insidiously. Approximately 25 per cent of the children affected experience lethargy, abdominal pain, gross hematuria (from tumor extension into the renal pelvis), and hypertension (from distortion of the renal vasculature and increased renin activity). The child may be acutely ill, having fever, anemia, and a rapidly enlarging abdomen, symptoms related to a subcapsular hemorrhage (Green 1985). A varicocele due to obstruction of the spermatic vein may be associated with the presence of a tumor thrombus in the renal vein or inferior vena cava.

Wilms' tumor, even when massive, has metastases to the lung at the time of diagnosis in fewer than 15 per cent of patients. By contrast, neuroblastoma is metastatic to bone, bone marrow, liver, skin, and retro-orbital structures at diagnosis in more than 70 per cent of patients. Thus, systemic symptoms (e.g. weight loss, cachexia, fever, and bone pain) are more characteristic of neuroblastoma than Wilms' tumor when an abdominal mass is discovered. Children with Wilms' bone metastases frequently present with pain. Uncommonly, they may present with pathologic fractures. Pathologic fractures usually occur late in the course of the disease, and long-term survival after these fractures is unusual. Most patients have involvement of multiple bones. Bones most commonly involved are the spinal column, ribs, skull, femur, pelvis, humerus, tibia, and radius. Involvement of long bone is often metaphyseal and may be bilaterally symmetrical.

Clear cell sarcoma of the kidney has a much wider distribution of bone metastases than does Wilms' tumor with favorable histology. In cases of metastatic bone disease, plain radiographs show osteolytic areas distributed in both the axial and appendicular skeleton. Osteosclerotic alterations are rarely evident (Bertoni 1984). Osteolytic defects or fusiform areas are usually found in the metaphyseal region of the long bones. Additional evidence of periosteal reaction and cortical destruction occurs, occasionally giving a radiographic appearance of an onion skin lamination or, less commonly, a sunburst phenomenon. The tumor mass may extend into the adjacent soft tissues. If metastases are generalized, the destructive lesions may resemble osteoporosis, with diffuse loss of bone mass, as seen in acute leukemia.

Pathology

Well-differentiated Wilms' tumor is the most common histological pattern and is associated with the best prognosis. All other histological patterns are associated with a poor prognosis. Microscopically well-differentiated Wilms' tumor resembles developing embryonic renal tissue. Classically, the tumor is composed of tubules surrounded by islands of compact uniform cells that comprise the blastema. The blastema, in turn, is surrounded by a proliferation of stromal elements.

When anaplastic nuclear changes are not present, the histological pattern is termed 'favorable' (**FH**) by the National Wilms' Tumor Study Group pathology center because of the generally good prognosis. They also identified an unfavorable histological subset, which includes anaplastic and sarcomatous variants. Anaplasia is recognized by the presence of gigantic polyploid nuclei with abnormal mitoses in the tumor sample. Approximately 25 per cent of treatment failures and almost 40 per cent of all tumor deaths are accounted for by children with the anaplastic variant of Wilms' tumor.

Clear cell sarcoma of the kidney

Clear cell tumors are associated with a particularly poor prognosis. Clear cell sarcoma of the kidney has a much wider distribution of metastases than FH Wilms' tumor and is unique in its tendency to metastasize to the brain and bones ('bone-metastasizing renal tumor of childhood'). MRI of the brain should be performed on all children who have clear cell sarcoma of the kidney, and radionuclide bone scanning and a skeletal survey should be performed in these children for diagnosis of metastatic bone lesions.

Metastatic bone disease

Skeletal metastasis has been regarded as uncommon in patients with Wilms' tumor, with a reported frequency of less than 5 per cent in most series. Most metastatic bone lesions are treated conservatively. Primary modalities are usually radiation therapy and chemotherapy with splinting and protection of the involved part. Painful lesions that do not respond to chemotherapy do respond to radiation. Radiation therapy can have a significant palliative benefit in a child with bone metastasis, because it can provide pain relief, stabilize bones that have marked structural change, and help prevent neurological deterioration.

The late effects of radiation are especially of concern. The effect of radiation on bone and growth depends on the patient's age, the radiation dose, the field arrangement, and the beam energy used. Children younger than 6 years and those undergoing treatment during puberty are especially vulnerable to the growth effects of radiation. For children who are long-term survivors despite the presence of metastasis, the induction of a second malignant lesion by radiation is a concern.

Late effects of trunk irradiation, including scoliosis and soft-tissue underdevelopment, have been seen since the use of megavoltage irradiation (Probert et al. 1973; Oliver et al. 1978; Wallace et al. 1990). Scoliosis was diagnosed in under one-half of patients who had entered the adolescent growth spurt, but no patient had a curve that exceeded 25 degrees. These data suggest that the frequency of spinal deformity may not decrease with the use of megavoltage radiation sources. Longer follow-up is necessary to confirm that the severity of deformities is less than that observed after orthovoltage irradiation (Heaston et al. 1979).

Second malignant neoplasms can develop in Wilms' tumor survivors. Most of these neoplasms, such as bone sarcomas, breast cancer, and thyroid cancer, have occurred in irradiated areas. The most significant risk factor for the occurrence of a second malignant neoplasm in the National Wilms' Tumor Study group cohort was treatment with irradiation. Initial treatment that included doxorubicin increased this risk. Significantly, even those patients whose therapy included only dactinomycin and vincristine, without radiation therapy, had an increased risk of cancer, compared with that of the general population.

References

Beckwith, J.B. (1969). Macroglassia, omphalocele, adrenal cytomegaly, gigantism, and hyperplastic visceromegaly. *Birth Defects*, **5**, 188–96.

Bertoni, F. (1984). Case report 287: metastatic Wilms' tumor with rhabdomyosarcomatous and osteosarcomatous elements. *Skeletal Radiology*, **12**, 218–21.

Coppes, M.J., Huff, V., and Pelletier, J. (1993). Denys–Drash syndrome: relating a clinical disorder to genetic alterations in the tumor suppressor gene WT1. *Journal of Pediatrics*, **123**, 673–8.

Crist, W.M. and Kun, L.E. (1991). Common solid tumors of childhood. *New England Journal of Medicine*, **324**, 461–71.

Eddy, A.A. and Mauer, S.M. (1985). Pseudohermaphroditism, glomerulopathy, and Wilms' tumor (Drash syndrome): frequency in end-stage renal failure. *Journal of Pediatrics*, **106**, 584–7.

Farewell, V.T., D'Angio, G.J., Breslow, N., and Norkool, P. (1981). Retrospective validation of a new staging system for Wilms' tumor. *Cancer Clinical Trials*, **4**, 167–71.

Green, D.M. (1985). *Diagnosis and management of malignant solid tumors in infants and children*, p. 129–86. Nijhoff, Boston, MA.

Heaston, D.K., Libshitz, H.I., and Chan, R.C. (1979). Skeletal effects of megavoltage irradiation in survivors of Wilms' tumor. *American Journal of Roentgenology*, **133**, 389–95.

Huff, V., Compton, D.A., Chao, L.Y., *et al.* (1988). Lack of linkage of familial Wilms' tumour to chromosomal band 11p13. *Nature*, **336**, 377–8.

Kantor, A.F., Li, F.P., Fraumeni, J.F., Jr, Curnen, M.G., and Flannery, J.T. (1982). Childhood cancer in offspring of two Wilms' tumor survivors. *Medical and Pediatric Oncology*, **10**, 85–9.

Matsunaga, E. (1981). Genetics of Wilms' tumor. *Human Genetics*, **57**, 231–46.

Miller, R.W., Fraumeni, J.F., Jr, and Manning, M.D. (1964). Association of Wilms' tumor with aniridia, hemihypertrophy and other congenital malformations. *New England Journal of Medicine*, **270**, 922–7.

Oliver, J.H., Gluck, G., Gledhill, R.B., and Chevalier, L. (1978). Musculoskeletal deformities following treatment of Wilms' tumour. *Canadian Medical Association Journal*, **119**, 459–64.

Probert, J.C., Parker, B.R., and Kaplan, H.S. (1973). Growth retardation in children after megavoltage irradiation of the spine. *Cancer*, **32**, 634–9.

Riccardi, V.M., Hittner, H.M., Francke, U., Yunis, J.J., Ledbetter, D., and Borges, W. (1980). The aniridia–Wilms' tumor association: the critical role of chromosome band 11p13. *Cancer Genetics and Cytogenetics*, **2**, 131–7.

Wallace, W.H., Shalet, S.M., Morris-Jones, P.H., Swindell, R., and Gattamaneni, H.R. (1990). Effect of abdominal irradiation on growth in boys treated for a Wilms' tumor. *Medical and Pediatric Oncology*, **18**, 441–6.

1.7   Injury and repair

1.7.1   Injury and repair

Fred F. Behrens, J. Schwappach, K. Swan, A. Levy, R. Barbieri, R. Forster, and D. Mahalick

Injuries—forces meet tissues

General concepts

The musculoskeletal system provides the supporting framework for the human body. It also protects vital internal and neurologic organs and enables us to move in space through the intricate and highly balanced arrangement of bones, ligaments, and articulations which make up our extremities. In the course of common daily and recreational activities, many diverse internal and external forces act within and upon our extremities without obvious damage to the musculoskeletal tissues.

An injury or structural tissue disruption occurs when an acting force exceeds the elastic, plastic (hard tissues), viscoelastic (soft tissues), or endurance limits (stress, overuse) of a particular tissue. According to the specific circumstances of this mismatch between tissues and forces, we distinguish between traumatic, pathologic, and stress injuries. In a **traumatic injury**, the acting internal force (e.g. a contracting hamstring muscle tearing in a sprinter) or external force (e.g. a fall from a height causing a vertebral compression fracture) exceeds the strength of a healthy or normal tissue. A **pathologic injury** occurs when a force of ordinary magnitude disrupts a tissue weakened by a pathologic process (e.g. a minor mis-step causing a fracture through a bone cyst). A **stress** or **overuse injury** occurs if ordinary forces act repeatedly on normal tissues (Tencer and Johnson 1994). In this situation, the microinjuries which are common with any impact do not have sufficient time to heal before the next submaximal event occurs. The result is either a stress injury where the tissue eventually fails because its endurance limit has been exceeded (e.g. a stress fracture of the femoral neck in a military recruit) or an overuse injury where the repeated impact causes a chronic inflammatory response (e.g. a tenosynovitis) which, by temporarily limiting the further use of an extremity, may prevent ultimate tissue failure.

Traumatic injuries

Traumatic injuries can be caused by acute exposure to mechanical, thermal, electrical, or chemical energy. They can also be due to a lack of heat or oxygen (Presswalla 1978; Committee on Trauma 1993a,b). By far the most common injuries to the musculoskeletal system are caused by mechanical trauma. These events are governed by Newton's second law of motion which states that the force acting on a body is proportional to the product of the mass of the body and its acceleration (or deceleration) (Evans 1988; Feliciano 1996). Most clinical injury events lie somewhere between the two extremes of the moving human body being suddenly decelerated (e.g. the driver in a car that hits a wall) or the human body at rest forming a barrier to a speeding projectile (e.g. a baseball) (National Research Council Committee on Trauma Research 1985). Regardless of the specific circumstances, the energetics of the traumatic event is expressed by the equation kinetic energy equals mass times velocity squared divided by two: $KE = MV^2/2$. This means that doubling the mass of a moving body will double its traumatizing kinetic energy, while doubling its velocity will quadruple the resulting traumatic impact (see also the discusion of the distinctive power of a bullet below). Depending on the circumstances, the kinetic energy imparted to an object can deform the object temporarily (elastic deformation) or permanently (plastic deformation), or cause its complete disruption (by exceeding the ultimate failure limit). A small part of the transmitted impact can be converted to thermal energy.

The hard tissues (i.e. bone) and the soft tissues (i.e. tendons, muscles, cartilage, ligaments, and neurovascular structures) of the musculoskeletal system protect each other against injury. The long bones linked by joints and the surrounding agonistic and antagonistic musculotendinous units allow for a degree of energy absorption through the extremities that far exceeds the strength of the femur

Box 1   Types of injury

- Traumatic
    - External (e.g. direct blow)
    - Internal (e.g. hamstring)
- Pathologic (e.g. tumor)
- Stress (e.g. shin splints)

and the tibia. Conversely, much of the impact of a leg hit by a car is dissipated to the osseous tibia, thus protecting the surrounding vital neurovascular structures. However, if the impacting force exceeds the failure limit of the tibia, it breaks and the sharp fracture surfaces become sharp-edged destructive instruments which may directly damage the surrounding soft tissues (Behrens 1991, 1997).

Under standard laboratory conditions, it is possible to recreate some simple musculoskeletal injury mechanisms that resemble those seen under clinical conditions (Zeitlow *et al.* 1994). However, most injury events that occur in the real world result in complex injury patterns because multiple forces commonly act in variable time sequences on different body parts (Boulanger *et al.* 1992) (Fig. 1). In addition, such variables as patient age and the rate at which the loads are applied (strain rate) affect the resulting injury patterns. Because the relative strength of musculoskeletal tissues changes with age, a lateral force applied to the knee joint in a child will most likely lead to a fracture through the epiphyseal plate or possibly a fracture of the adjacent tibial shaft, while a ligamentous injury would be extremely uncommon. The same mechanism will tear the medial–collateral ligament in a young adult and cause a tibial plateau fracture in an older person. Loading rates are another modifying factor; at higher loading rates, a bone appears stronger and thus requires more energy to fail. This also explains why a slowly applied load to a joint will probably lead to a bony avulsion, while at a faster loading rate an in-substance tear of the ligament is more common (Tencer and Johnson 1994).

A clear understanding of the principal forces that cause a particular injury pattern and the many modifying variables are key prerequisites to a complete patient evaluation, the choice of optimal treatment modes and rehabilitative strategies, and finally the prediction of expected outcomes.

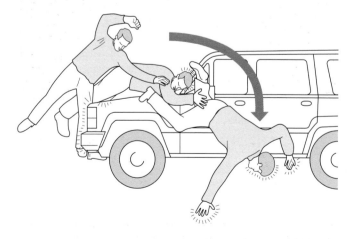

Fig. 1. Adult pedestrian injury triad.

Injuries caused by firearms

Penetrating injuries caused by firearms are an extreme example of how excessive external forces damage musculoskeletal tissues. Conceptually, bullet wounds are similar to other injuries caused by high-velocity objects, such as flying rocks, machine parts, or lawn mowers. Although firearm injuries are becoming increasingly common in civilian life, many surgeons underestimate the economic impact and the key parameters that determine firearm effects.

Economic impact

In the United States, approximately 40 000 citizens are killed by firearms every year. This approaches the total number of American servicemen killed from all causes during the 12 years of the Vietnam War (56 000) (Swan and Swan 1989). Despite a progressive clamor for gun and ammunition control, the number of civilians killed by firearms continues to increase. This is due to a general rise in civilian violence and an increase in the caliber used by both felons and law enforcement officials (Caruso *et al.* 1999). Both trends have contributed to a staggering growth in the treatment costs of firearm victims. In 1988, this cost was $429 million; by 1995 it had increased to over $4 billion (Violence Prevention Task Force 1995). Unless these trends are brought under control, firearm-related injuries will be the leading cause of trauma death in the United States by the year 2003 (Violence Prevention Task Force 1995).

Characteristics of firearms

According to specifications and effects, firearms are divided into handguns, shotguns, and rifles. Handguns (revolvers or pistols) have short barrels. Revolvers house five or six cartridges which are advanced by the movement of a trigger or hammer. Pistols have magazines containing up to 18 rounds which are fed into a receiver by the action of the previously fired round, thus making the pistol a semi-automatic weapon. Rifles have long barrels, are shoulder held when fired, and commonly discharge a single round. The barrels of most firearms have helical grooves which impart a spin to the bullet. This spin increases stability in flight and thus accuracy. Shotguns have a long and smooth barrel. The cartridges they fire contain lead or steel spheres (shot) of a specified size and number.

Velocity and kinetic energy

Velocity (distance divided by time) usually refers to the speed of a missile as it exits from the end of the barrel or muzzle. The muzzle velocity is the maximal velocity achieved by a missile. Although there is no universal agreement, bullets with muzzle velocities below 1000 ft/s (300 m/s) are considered 'low velocity'. Most rifles and shotguns

Box 4 **Ballistic injuries**

- Damage caused by a bullet is mainly related to its velocity
- 300 m/s (1000 ft/s) is the threshold between low and high velocities
- Soft-nosed bullets fragment and dissipate all their energy
- Soft-nosed bullets are banned for military use but may be used by civilians
- Secondary missiles are fragments of teeth or bone which may also cause damage
- Cavitation is an area of tissue damage around the tract related to energy transferred

Box 5 **Side-effects of cavitation**

- Injuries to tissue remote from missile track
- Foreign bodies may be sucked into the wound
- Thorough and repeated debridement is important

impart velocities in excess of 1000 ft/s, and thus are considered 'high-velocity' firearms.

Velocity on impact is important because tissue damage is proportional to a missile's kinetic energy, expressed in units of foot-pounds or joules, and its dissipation within a target. Kinetic energy is expressed by the formula

$$KE = MV^2/2$$

where M is the missile mass (in pounds or kilograms) and V is the velocity (in feet per second or meters per second). Because of its geometric progression, velocity is of greater importance than mass. For instance, the 45 caliber US Army pistol fires a 230-grain bullet with a muzzle velocity of 860 ft/s (262 m/s) and a kinetic energy of approximately 405 foot-pounds (550 J). In contrast, the M-16 rifle fires a 55-grain bullet at 3240 ft/s (988 m/s), resulting in a kinetic energy of approximately 1280 foot-pounds (1735 J). Not surprisingly, the tissue destruction caused by the two missiles is in stark contrast to their sizes.

Ballistics is the science of the movement of a projectile through a firearm, the air, and into or through a target. The tissue destruction that occurs is determined by the dissipation of the energy upon impact (ΔKE), which is given by

$$\text{mass} \times (\text{velocity})^2 \text{ on impact} - \text{mass} \times (\text{velocity})^2 \text{ at exit}$$

or

$$\Delta KE = M(V_1 - V_2)^2/2$$

where ΔKE is the change in kinetic energy, V_1 is the impact velocity, and V_2 is the terminal or exit velocity. If the bullet or its fragments have stayed within the target, the exit velocity is zero and complete energy transfer and thus maximal tissue destruction have occurred (Swan and Swan 1991).

Maximizing tissue destruction

For several centuries, man has worked persistently at increasing the damage that can be imparted by firearms. In one such effort, exit velocity has been reduced to near zero by the introduction of 'hollow-nosed' and 'soft-pointed' bullets. These missiles change their shape or fragment upon impact and thus effect an increased transfer of energy and tissue destruction. 'Soft-pointed' bullets lack a copper jacket, which contains the lead core and which minimizes deformation and fragmentation. Bullets with a copper jacket are often called 'military rounds' because the Hague Convention of 1896 mandated the 'more humane' jacketed bullets for international warfare. This mandate has been strictly adhered to in the succeeding 100 years. Because military rounds are more likely to penetrate or pass through a target, with little or no tissue deformation, injuries caused in armed conflict, paradoxically, may be less destructive than injuries caused by modified bullets used in domestic violence or urban warfare.

Secondary missiles are created when the kinetic energy of a bullet is imparted to dense tissues, such as a tooth or a foreign body (e.g. a coin in the victim's pocket), which in turn become missiles with their own ballistic properties. A tooth struck by a bullet can produce more damage within the cranial cavity than the missile itself because of the tooth's density and the fact that it is contaminated with pathological bacteria. This is important when managing missile injuries to the face. Secondary missiles, such as bone, may not be as radiographically recognizable as bullets. They also may originate from a person nearby who has been struck by a missile.

Cavitation may be the most important phenomenon concerning wound ballistics. It is caused by the rapid expansion and elastic recoil of the tissues impacted by a passing missile. Cavitation is proportional to the density of the tissue (target), the velocity of the projectile, and its kinetic energy at the time of impact. The temporal cavity may exceed the diameter of the missile by a factor of 5 to 10 and thus may lead to tissue destruction which extends many centimeters beyond the missile path. This phenomenon can be best illustrated with gelatin or clay simulants of human tissues (Figs 2, 3, and 4). Therefore cavitation can result in fractures of long bones and injury to major blood vessels and

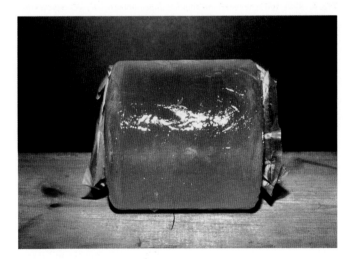

Fig. 2. Quart-sized gelatin block has plastic bags containing powdered dye at entrance (green) and exit (brown) sites. A 22 caliber rifle round will be fired from 10 m (30 ft) to the left of the block.

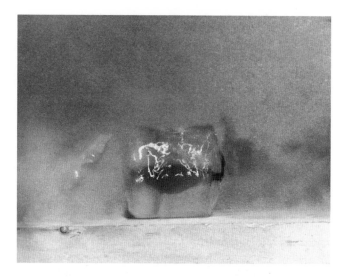

Fig. 3. Actual shot, 22 caliber rifle, 10 m (30 ft) from gelatin block.

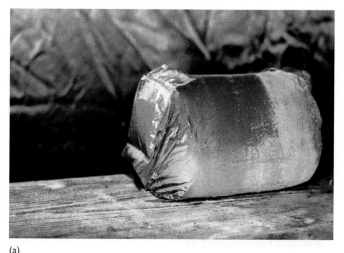

(a)

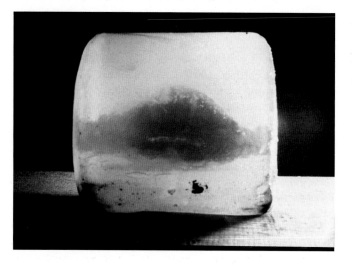

Fig. 4. Reflected light reveals an elliptical imprint of powder, well beyond the actual path of the missile through the gelatin block. This is an example of cavitation.

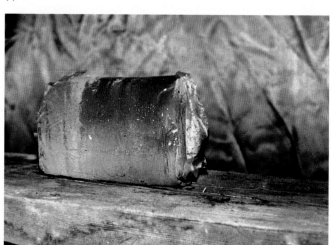

(b)

Fig. 5. Quart-sized gelatin block with (a) green dye on planned entrance and (b) red dye on planned exit wounds caused by a 222 caliber round fired from the left at 10 m (30 ft).

nerves, even if these tissues are not in direct contact with the missile or its fragments. One of the more harmful effects of cavitation is the resulting vacuum (Figs 5, 6, and 7). It brings foreign bodies and organisms into the projectile's tract, which is surrounded by a zone of damaged tissue and thus constitutes a highly susceptible medium for infection. Even if a missile has not passed through clothing or other foreign material before it penetrates an extremity, it cannot be considered sterile (Tzeng *et al.* 1981).

Clinical issues

When dealing with a firearm injury, informed diagnostic and therapeutic decisions are only possible if the relevant ballistic information is available. Such information includes the weapon (handgun, rifle, shotgun), its caliber, and the approximate range (distance between

weapon and impact). Other important parameters include the approximate path of the bullet in the victim, the presence, intensity, and location of powder burns (Fig. 8), identification of the materials through which the bullet has passed before hitting the victim, and a history of previous firearm injuries, especially the presence of retained bullets and residual disabilities. Once a careful history of the injury events and objects has been obtained, a thorough physical evaluation with special focus on the neurovascular status must follow.

Although some simple handgun injuries are now managed with local cleansing and short-term antibiotics, all firearm injuries involving vital structures and all injuries imparted by high-velocity missiles must undergo extensive evaluation in the operating room followed by thorough debridement which often must be repeated at intervals of 24 to 48 h (Behrens 1991).

Removed bullets should be marked at the base, documented in the chart, and then submitted to the surgical pathology laboratory. Only when the pathologist has logged the bullet and described its key char-

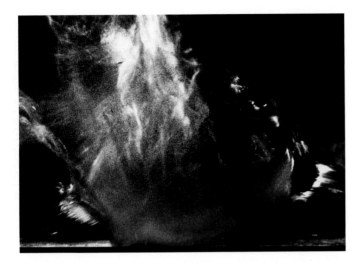

Fig. 6. Actual shot, 222 caliber rifle, 10 m (30 ft) from the gelatin block.

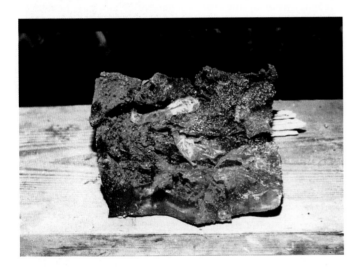

Fig. 7. Remains of the gelatin block reveal green and red dyes into its center along with remnants of the plastic bag, indicating suction from cavitation as well as the 'cloth' foreign body.

acteristics (e.g. caliber and signature) should it be turned over to law enforcement officials.

Musculoskeletal tissues—basic repair mechanisms

Tissues respond to injury

Extremity injuries limited to one tissue are rare; most disrupt several structures in close proximity to the area where the main impact occurs. If excessive traction or torsion is involved, tissue destruction at a considerable distance is common. This creates obvious diagnostic pitfalls. It also complicates treatment recommendations because different tissues may heal according to different repair mechanisms and thus require different mechanical conditions for optimal recovery

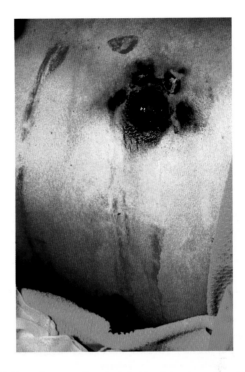

Fig. 8. M-16 gunshot wound to the left side of the chest of a soldier. The entrance wound is anterior and larger than the exit wound, which is posterior. The entrance wound is identified by powder burns which also indicate its proximity to the rifle's muzzle (point blank range).

(i.e. a periarticular fracture may require temporary immobilization to heal in a satisfactory position while the ligamentous sprain of the adjacent joint is best managed by early motion). In addition, all repair processes are influenced by patient-specific variables such as premorbid conditions, age, nutritional status, etc.

Many musculoskeletal tissues heal according to a common mechanism which involves the three phases of **inflammation**, **repair**, and **remodeling** (Cruess and Dumont 1975). However, under specific mechanical conditions (e.g. rigid fixation of a fracture) (Schenk 1992) some structures (e.g. tendons) (Lundborg and Rank 1980) can heal according to **tissue-specific healing mechanisms** which do not rely on inflammation and vascular ingrowth. Other tissues (e.g. meniscus with *in situ* tear) are incapable of repair and require removal to prevent further damage.

The surgeon must have a clear understanding of the various repair mechanisms and the preconditions for their success because they will clearly affect his or her search for an optimal treatment plan and the quality of the ultimate outcome.

Box 6 Classification of tissue repair

- Standard (most tissues)—inflammation, e.g. shin
- Tissue-specific healing mechanisms, e.g. tendons (may not involve inflammation)
- No healing, e.g. menisci

Box 7 **The standard healing model**

- Inflammation—dead tissue replaced by granulation tissue
- Repair—granulation tissue replaced by tissue-specific matrix
- Remodeling—shape and structure optimized in response to stresses

The standard healing model: inflammation–repair–remodeling

This common healing response, which is most effective in well-vascularized tissue, is usually initiated from the tissues surrounding the injury site (Buckwalter et al. 1996). It may result in a complete restitution of the defect (healing of fracture in a child), replacement of the injury site with scar tissue (muscle), or tissue restitution with severe functional limitation (ligamentous repair accompanied by local or intra-articular adhesions and joint stiffness).

Inflammation is the initial local response to an injury. The defect is quickly filled with a hematoma. Activation of the coagulation system and cytokines released by injured tissues attract polymorphonuclear leukocytes, monocytes, and T lymphocytes which remove necrotic material. They also release vasoactive mediators and activate growth factors and cytokines such as fibroblast growth factor, platelet-derived growth factor and transforming growth factor-β. These in turn promote cell migration, proliferation, and matrix differentiation. As a result of these activities, all dead tissues are removed and the hematoma is replaced by granulation tissue which consists of a dense conglomeration of capillary vessels imbedded in a fibrillar network (Freundlich et al. 1986).

Repair

In this phase, the granulation tissue is replaced by a tissue-specific matrix. The fibrillar network facilitates the rapid ingrowth of undifferentiated pluripotent mesenchymal cells from surrounding muscle, periosteum, and marrow. These stem cells, presumably under local metabolic direction, differentiate into such tissue-specific cells as osteoblasts, chondroblasts, myoblasts, fibroblasts, and other connective tissue cells which fill the injury site with repair material that closely resembles the original tissue.

Remodeling

During this phase, the often poorly shaped and organized repair tissue is optimized. This process, which goes on over many months, may be guided by the prevailing mechanical stresses and results in a tissue which approaches the preinjury status both structurally and functionally.

Fracture mechanics and new bone formation

Basic structure and failure mechanisms

Structure and mechanical properties of bone

The mechanical properties of bone and its failure mechanisms directly derive from its composition and three-dimensional structure.

As to the structure of bone, it has become customary to distinguish four levels of progressive complexity. These levels start with the chemical composition and lead to the two macroscopically distinct types of cancellous and cortical bone (Buckwalter and Cooper 1987; Buckwalter et al. 1996) (Fig. 9).

Box 8 **The structure of bone**

- Chemical—hydroxyapatite crystals linked to collagen fibers
- Electron microscope—hydroxyapatite/collagen arranged in sheets or lamellae
- Light microscope—lamellae arranged in tubular Haversian osteons
- Naked eye—cancellous or cortical bone

At the most basic level, bone is a composite of longitudinally arranged hydroxyapatite crystals connected at both ends to collagen fibrils. Together they form a composite that is not only rigid but also sufficiently ductile to allow substantial energy absorption before failure. The hydroxyapatite crystals largely determine the modulus or stiffness of the bone, while the collagen component is responsible for the ductility or capability to deform plastically (Burstein et al. 1975). With advancing age, the mineral content of bone increases. It thus becomes more brittle and less able to absorb impact loads (Currey 1969). At the second level, the hydroxyapatite–collagen elements form sheets, or lamellae, which are concentrically arranged into tubular Haversian osteons at the next level. At the fourth level, these osteons become the building blocks for either cortical or cancellous bone. Cortical bone usually consists of longitudinally arranged tight-packed osteons. The strongest lamellar or diaphyseal bone consists of a large number of relatively small osteons with essentially no porosity. In cancellous or metaphyseal bone, the osteons are shaped into small trabeculae which become part of an interconnected three-dimensional network with variable porosity. The porosities of cancellous bone range from 30 to 90 per cent of the porosity of cortical bone. The strongest metaphyseal bone is that with the lowest porosity and the trabecular architecture which is best suited to resist a particular impact (e.g. a high density of vertical trabeculae in a vertebral body will best resist compressive loads).

Beginning in the fifth decade, progressive loss of bone mass and a simultaneous change in material properties reduce bone strength and modulus and lead to a progressively greater susceptibility to fractures. This accelerated fracture tendency is less severe in men because increased endosteal resorption is partially compensated by a concomitant subperiosteal expansion. This phenomenon is particularly prominent in the femur. Under these circumstances, the loss in bone material properties typically seen with increasing age is partially counteracted by more favorable structural properties (increased polar moment of inertia) (Tencer and Johnson 1994).

Under standard conditions cortical bone as a material is weakest in shear, stronger in tension, and strongest in compression (Reilly and Burstein 1975). Trabecular bone, which has a much greater capability to deform plastically in all loading modes is, depending on its porosity, about four to 50 times weaker than cortical bone.

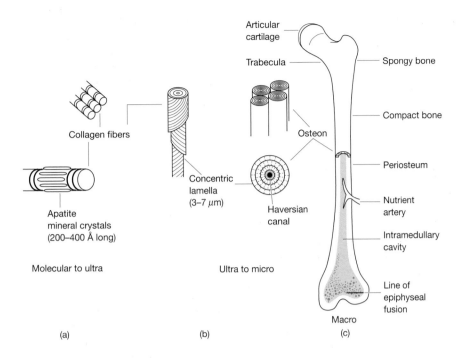

Fig. 9. The different structural levels of bone. (a) The first level is a material composed of hydroxyapatite crystals embedded between collagen fibrils. (b) The second level is an arrangement of the fibrils into sheets or lamellae with a preferred orientation. (c) In long bones, the third level consists of an arrangement of lamellae into tubular osteons (or flat sheets), which form the basic structure of cortical and trabecular bone. (Adapted from Katz (1981) and Tencer and Johnson (1994).)

Fracture mechanics

Considering the complexity of most injuries that occur in daily life and the many sophisticated mechanisms of energy absorption that characterize the musculoskeletal system, it is rarely possible to isolate specific injury mechanisms and then correlate them to particular fracture patterns.

However, by applying simple loading modes, a number of distinct fracture patterns which are clinically recognizable can be created in the laboratory (Gozna and Harrington 1982). For instance, under progressive bending, the convex side of the bone is in tension while the convex side is in compression. Failure is initiated by the formation of a small crack on the tension side (Fig. 10). As this crack progresses to the neutral axis, and then to the convex side, a transverse fracture results. The combination of bending and axial compression typically creates a comminuted fracture with a butterfly fragment (Fig. 11). Torsional forces cause spiral fractures at an angle of approximately 45° to the long axis (Fig. 12).

Box 9 **Fracture patterns in bone**

- Simple bend—transverse
- Bend with compression—butterfly
- Torsion—spiral fracture

Mechanisms of bone regeneration—overview

Three mechanisms allow for the regeneration of new bone and the healing of a fracture:

(1) secondary bone healing or bone healing through the generation of a fracture callus;

(2) primary bone healing or accelerated remodeling;

(3) distraction osteogenesis.

While these three biologic processes are quite distinct, and require specific mechanical and biologic preconditions, one or more may act in concert. Adequate blood supply and soft-tissue coverage of the bone defect appear to be shared prerequisites for all three healing modes (Brookes 1971; Perren 1979; Einhorn *et al.* 1990; Schenk 1992; Ostrum *et al.* 1994; Schenk and Hunziker 1994; Buckwalter *et al.* 1996).

Two key variables that determine the prevailing healing mechanism are the size of the fracture gap and the amount of motion between the two adjacent bony fragments. Secondary bone healing is typically seen with fractures suspended in traction or held by a cast. In this situation, initial fracture gap and fragment motion easily can exceed 1 cm. Primary bone healing is only possible with fracture gaps of less than 2 mm (Johner 1972) and motion at the fracture site of less than 1 mm or possibly only a few micrometers (Perren 1979). New bone formation generated by distraction osteogenesis requires gradual distraction of an osteotomy, a nonunion site, or an

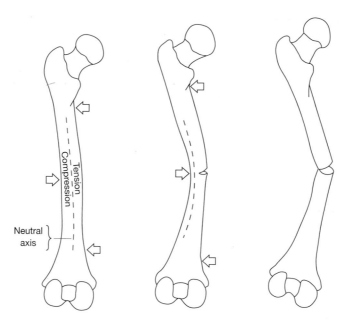

Fig. 10. Transverse fracture—bending load. Bending of long bone and resulting transverse fracture. Because cortical bone is weaker in tension than in compression, it usually fails in tension, with a crack beginning on the tensile side. As the crack progresses, the neutral axis shifts and the failure continues to advance on the tension side until the bone fails. (Reproduced from Gozna and Harrington (1982).)

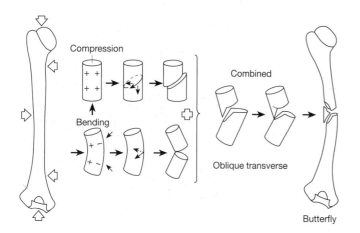

Fig. 11. Butterfly and oblique transverse fractures. The combination of axial compression and bending loads often lead to a combined transverse–butterfly fracture. (Reproduced from Gozna and Harrington (1982).)

Fracture pattern	Appearance	Mechanism of injury	Location of soft-tissue hinge	Energy
Transverse	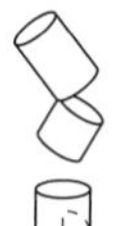	Bending	Concavity	Low
Spiral	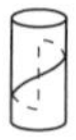	Torsion	Vertical segment	Low
Oblique transverse or butterfly	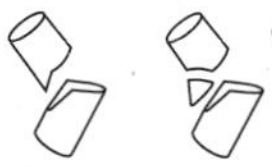	Compression + bending	Concavity or side of butterfly	Moderate
Oblique	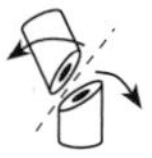	Compression + bending + torsion	Concavity (often destroyed)	Moderate
Comminuted	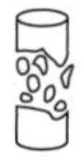	Variable	Destroyed	High
Metaphyseal compression	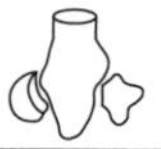	Compression	Variable	Variable

Fig. 12. Summary of long-bone fracture biomechanics. (Reproduced from Gozna and Harrington (1982).)

epiphyseal plate (epiphyseal distraction) at a rate of no more than 1 mm a day and stable conditions of both adjacent bony fragments (Ilizarov 1989a,b). These three types of bone healing are observed in cortical and, with slight modification, in cancellous bone (Uhthoff and Rahn 1981; Finnegan and Uhthoff 1987; Schatzker et al. 1989) (Table 1).

Secondary bone healing

Secondary bone healing closely follows the 'standard repair sequence' typical for many musculoskeletal tissues; an inflammatory phase is followed, within a few days, by a repair phase that lasts from several weeks to a few months, and finally a remodeling phase which often continues for several years. Rather than forming a cascade of distinct events, these three healing phases are a continuum of overlapping metabolic, cellular, vascular, electrical, and mechanical processes starting with the injury and often ending with an almost complete restoration of the fracture site years later.

Table 1 Influence of biological and mechanical variables on mechanisms of new bone formation

Biological and mechanical variables	Type of bone healing		
	Secondary	Primary	Distraction osteogenesis
Adequate blood supply/soft tissue coverage	×	×	×
Bone type			
Cortical	×	×	×
Cancellous	×	(×)	×
Fracture gap			
< 2 mm		×	NA
2 mm to > 1 cm	×		
Rigidity of fixation			
Motion at gap < 1 mm		×	
Motion at gap 1 mm to > 1 cm	×		
Distraction < 1 mm/day			×
Methods of fixation			
Casts, traction	×		
Plates		×	
Wires/metaphysis	×	(×)	
Nails	×		
External fixators	×	(×)	

NA, not applicable.

Inflammation—formation of granulation tissue

Beyond causing a fracture, most injuries lead to disruption of the surrounding periosteum, blood vessels, muscles, and other soft tissues. The plastic deformation of both fracture fragments and the terminal periosteal stripping disrupt the terminal vascular supply and render the opposing bone ends avascular. A hematoma forms in the fracture gap and quickly expands into the disrupted surrounding tissues. Inflammatory mediators generated by necrotic material and platelets attract polymorphonuclear leukocytes, macrophages, and lymphocytes. These, in turn, progressively resorb dead tissue and release cytokines which stimulate angiogenesis. The fibrillar network of the hematoma serves as a scaffold for invading fibroblasts which become part of a composite matrix that also contains fibrillar connective tissue and proliferating small vessels—granulation tissue (Anderson 1990; Gerhart *et al.* 1993) (Fig. 13).

Repair—formation of the fracture callus

During the repair phase, the fracture hematoma is replaced by the fracture callus which consists, in changing proportions, of fibroblasts, chondroblasts, and osteoblasts with their respective matrices. Accordingly, we can distinguish between a fibrinous, cartilaginous, and osseous repair phase or callus. The progressive fibrinous to osseous callus transformation closely resembles **enchondral ossification** and is typical for what happens in the center of the healing area between the two adjacent fracture fragments. In contrast with this **soft callus**, more peripherally, the cambium layer of the elevated periosteum directly generates woven bone through the mechanism of **intramembranous ossification** (Tonna and Cronkite 1963) (Fig. 14). This quickly developing circumferential bone sleeve, which is also called **hard callus**, conveys early and progressive stability to the fracture site and is a prerequisite for the normal progression of the repair process (Perren 1979) (Fig. 15).

Although many factors influence and regulate callus transforma-

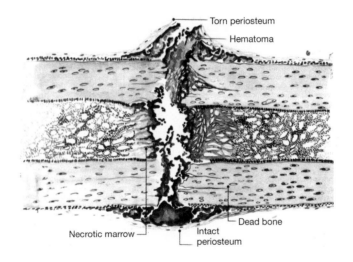

Fig. 13. Secondary bone healing: initial response after diaphyseal fracture. Periosteum remains intact over point of impact but is torn on opposite side. Hematoma forms on the periosteum and between fracture fragments. Bone ends and marrow adjacent to fracture site are necrotic. (Reproduced from Cruess and Dumont (1975).)

Box 10 Inflammation phase of bone fracture healing

- Hematoma with necrosis of bone ends from ischemia
- Necrotic material releases cytokines—attracts macrophages
- Necrotic tissue releases cytokines—attracts angiomyesis
- Granulation tissue produced

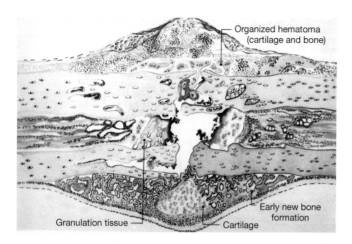

Fig. 14. Secondary bone healing: early repair phase. Organization of the hematoma. There is direct intramembranous bone formation between outer cortex and elevated periosteum; cartilage predominates in other areas. There is little callus formation between fracture fragments and in the marrow region. (Reproduced from Cruess and Dumont (1975).)

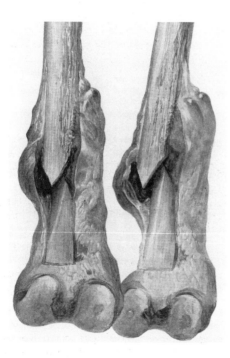

Fig. 15. Drawing of periosteal callus of a fractured femur 28 days after the injury. The central cavity contains the white ischemic bone ends which are devoid of callus. There is early formation of peripheral hard callus. (Reproduced from Charnley (1961).)

tion, the exact mechanisms that govern their interaction remain poorly understood (Brighton 1994; Brighton *et al.* 1996). At the molecular level, local mediators and growth factors and possibly changes in the metabolic, mechanical, and electrical environment appear to regulate gene expression and thus the release of specific enzymes and growth factors which are responsible for the complex sequence of tissue resorption and formation that characterizes frac-

Box 11 Repair phase of bone fracture healing

- Fibroblasts, chronoblasts, and osteoblasts invade granulation tissue
- Fibrous tissue replaced by cartilage then bone to produce callus
- Bone healing between fracture ends resembles endochondral ossification
- Peripherally bone healing from periosteum resemble membranous ossification

ture healing (Urist *et al.* 1983; Canalis *et al.* 1991). Among the growth factors, fibroblastic growth factor stimulates angiogenesis while transforming growth factor-β initiates the formation of chondroblasts and osteoblasts and thus plays an important role in the latter part of enchondral ossification (Wozney 1993; Einhorn 1994; Cook *et al.* 1995). There are recent indications that, by stimulating both angioand chondrogenesis, ultrasound may act as a 'physical growth factor' (Yang *et al.* 1996).

Histologically, in the early fibrinous stage, osteoclasts which derive from circulating monocytes and their marrow precursors resorb much of the bony debris and the avascular bone ends (Brighton and Hunt 1991). Simultaneously, pluripotent mesenchymal cells from the periosteum, the endosteum, and the surrounding injured soft tissues invade the hematoma and replace it initially with fibrinous and later with cartilaginous fracture callus (Einhorn 1992). As the fibrocartilage proliferates on all sides beyond the fracture gap, the polar moment of inertia of the callus mass increases. The resulting increase in callus strength and stiffness appears to be one of the prerequisites for the mineralization of the fibrocartilage and its subsequent transformation to woven bone. Mineralization appears to be a two-step process (Chidgey *et al.* 1986; Carter *et al.* 1988). The glycosaminoglycans which inhibit mineralization is initially removed by neutral proteoglycanases secreted by the chondrocytes. In the second stage, calcium phosphate complexes released by chondrocytes and osteoblasts initiate progressive callus mineralization and the creation of woven bone (Aro *et al.* 1989; Blenman *et al.* 1989) (Fig. 16).

Chemically, the early fracture callus consists of glycosaminoglycans and type II and type III collagen. With the transformation to hyaline and fibrocartilage, cartilage-specific proteoglycans and type II collagen become more abundant while areas of intramembranous and woven bone formation are indicated by high concentrations of alkaline phosphatase, type I collagen, and osteocalcin (Stirling 1932) (Fig. 17).

Box 12 Cytokines involved in fracture healing

- Fibroblastic growth factor stimulates angiogenesis
- Transforming growth factor-β initiates chondroblast and oesteoblast formation
- Transforming growth factor-β also stimulates enchondral ossification

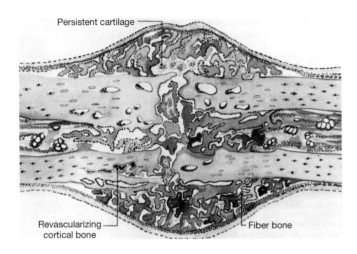

Fig. 16. Secondary bone healing: late repair phase. The fracture site is bridged by bollous callus of woven bone; residual islands of cartilage. Bone ends starting to get revascularized through the process of Haversian remodeling. (Reproduced from Cruess and Dumont (1975)).

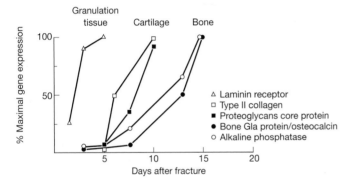

Fig. 17. Relative levels of protein gene expression during fracture repair in a rat. Expressions of laminin receptor, a protein found in blood vessels, is increased during granulation tissue formation. Expression of genes for cartilage (type II collagen and proteoglycans core protein) and bone-associated proteins (bone Gla protein, osteocalcin, alkaline phosphatase) is increased when these tissues are forming in the callus. (Reproduced from Buckwalter et al. (1996).)

Mechanically, secondary bone healing can be separated into four stages in accordance with the response of an experimental long-bone fracture to torsional loads (White et al. 1977; Goodship and Kenwright 1985; Carter et al. 1988; Blenman et al. 1989; Kenwright et al. 1991). In stage I, torsional failure occurs through the original fracture site with a low stiffness load/deformation curve typical for soft tissues. In stage II, failure is still through the fracture site but with a high stiffness pattern typical for hard tissues. In stage III, failure occurs partially through the fracture site and partially through one of the adjacent fragments, again with a hard tissue pattern. Finally, in stage IV, the bone fails through previously normal tissue adjacent to the fracture callus indicating that secondary bone healing ultimately results in an 'excessive repair' that surpasses the strength of normal bone (Matthews et al. 1974; Sarmiento et al. 1977; Markel et al. 1990).

Box 13 Stages of bone healing as measured by load–deformation curve

- Failure at fracture site—curve as for soft tissues
- Failure at fracture site—curve as for hard tissues
- Failure partially away from fracture site—curve as for hard tissue
- Failure through adjacent normal tissue—curve as for hard tissue

Remodeling: restoration of normal structure and function

Progressive mineralization of the woven callus and its protuberant shape facilitate early load and weight bearing. However, its high cellularity and water content, the amorphous arrangement of its collagen fibers, and the patchy pattern of matrix mineralization make it structurally and mechanically suboptimal. During the remodeling phase, the callus of woven bone is gradually replaced with lamellar bone through the continuous process of Haversian remodeling (Marotti and Muglia 1988; Marotti 1993). Simultaneously, osteoclastic resorption, possibly guided by electrical or mechanical strain fields, removes extraneous peripheral bone that is not necessary for optimal mechanical function. This goal-directed mechanical and functional transformation that is typical for the final phase of secondary bone healing is possibly the best example of Wolff's law in action (Wolff 1892).

Primary bone healing

After the Second World War, the development of operative fracture techniques (Allgower and Spiegel 1979; Müller et al. 1991) which require anatomic reduction of the fracture fragments and their stable fixation with metal plates and screws led to the discovery of a new 'artificial' type of bone healing—primary fracture healing (Schenk and Willenegger 1963, 1967; Schenk 1992). Clinically, the immediate stability provided by plate fixation facilitates early motion of adjacent joints and thus accelerates and often improves rehabilitation (Müller et al. 1991). Radiographically, the massive callus formation typical of secondary bone healing is absent. Often, the only radiographic sign of healing is the gradual disappearance of the small fracture lines which are still visible early after operative intervention (Schenk and Willenegger 1967).

Histologically, primary bone healing is simply a temporary acceleration of the Haversian remodeling which is responsible for the perpetual turnover of the skeleton. Haversian remodeling is a continuous process of coupled bone resorption and bone formation which is carried out by bone metabolizing units, which usually involve about 1 to 5 per cent of the resting skeleton. Bone metabolizing units

Box 14 Primary bone healing

- Temporary acceleration of Haversian remodeling
- Only occurs with rigid fixation of the fracture
- Does not involve callus formation

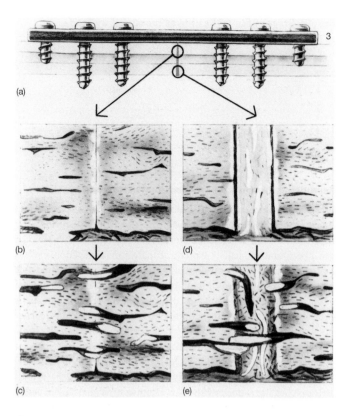

Fig. 18. Primary bone healing. (a) With the application of a plate under compression, the cortices of the two fracture fragments adjacent to the plate are in contact while there is a slight gap between the cortices opposite the plate. (b) Lag phase—contact area. Within the first week, there is little histological change between the cortices in contact. (c) Contact healing. After 4 weeks, the bone ends in contact show proliferation of bone remodeling units which go across both living and necrotic areas of the fracture end thus bridging the fracture site. (d) Lag phase—gap area. Within the first 8 days, the gap is invaded by blood vessels, followed later by osteoblasts which deposit osteoid and give rise to lamellae which are oriented at 90° to the long axis. (e) Gap healing. After the fourth week, the transversely oriented lamellae in the gap are replaced by osteons oriented along the longitudinal axis. (Modified from Müller *et al.* (1979).)

form parallel channels to the longitudinal axis of the bone. At the front end, bone metabolizing units contain cutting cones which are lined by several multicellular osteoclasts (Rahn *et al.* 1971). They have a linear rate of bone resorption of about 50 μm a day, and encompass a cross-section of about 200 μm. Behind the advancing cutting cone, the walls of the osteon are lined by osteoblasts which circumferentially appose new osteoid at the rate of about 1 μm per day. Completion of a new osteon which is about 3 mm long and has a wall thickness of about 90 μm will take 3 to 4 months. Although somewhat more complex, the same process is responsible for continuous turnover of trabecular bone. Depending on the initial fit between the reduced fracture fragments, we differentiate between contact and gap healing (Schenk and Willenegger 1967) (Fig. 18).

Contact healing

This typically occurs in areas where the fragment ends are 'perfectly' opposed. In a canine model, operative fixation is followed by a lag period of about 2 to 3 weeks (Schenk 1992). Then many new bone

metabolizing units are simultaneously activated on both sides of the fracture site so that by 4 to 5 weeks about 20 per cent and by the sixth week about 30 per cent of the fracture cross-section is taken up by crossing osteons. By the eighth week, about two-thirds of the fracture site has been connected by new osteons. It appears that after about 6 months, much of this repair activity has returned close to normal. It is assumed that, in humans, the whole process is more prolonged.

Gap healing

Owing to local comminution and imperfections in reduction, small gaps take up at least part of the interface between the two 'anatomically reduced' bony fragments. Within a few days of fracture reduction, osteoblasts enter these gaps and deposit osteoid on the viable as well as the nonviable surfaces of the fracture ends (Johner 1972). This process usually occurs without prior osteoclastic resorption. After passage of the lag period, the accelerated Haversian remodeling process bridges the fracture gap and replaces both the avascular and the gap-filling tissue with new longitudinal osteons (Schenk 1992).

Plate effects

Tightly applied plates appear to have two effects on the underlying diaphyseal bone: bone necrosis followed by osteoporosis, and stress shielding.

Initially, plate application causes a localized avascular cortex necrosis directly underneath the implant. This is most likely caused by interruption of the periosteal blood supply and plastic bone deformation that distorts or obliterates the small intraosseous vessels. However, within a few weeks or months, osteonal remodeling replaces the necrotic bone section with new lamellar bone. Plates that remain in place for a prolonged period change the load-bearing requirements of the underlying bone. The resulting stress-shielding effect is dependent on the rigidity of the plate and may lead to a permanent reduction of bone cross-section. For this reason, removal of a plate from a large bone, particularly the tibia or the femur, should be followed by a period of partial weight bearing and a delayed return to full recreational activities for up to 3 months (Uhthoff *et al.* 1993) (Fig. 19).

Mechanical aspects

Under conditions of primary bone healing, no periosteal callus is visible, although some endosteal bone may form. The fracture site regains immediate strength with the application of a plate, but fracture union usually occurs at a slower rate than would be seen under conditions of secondary bone healing. The absence of a fracture callus with its increased polar moment of inertia is an additional disadvantage. When comparing two identical fracture sites, one healing by primary and the other by secondary bone healing, and assuming identical material bone properties as well as an increased callus width of 25 per cent, the fracture that heals by secondary bone healing will initially be 66 per cent stronger and 100 per cent more rigid (Perren 1979).

Distraction osteogenesis

Distraction osteogenesis describes a process of new bone formation after the creation of an osteotomy followed by a controlled gradual distraction of the bone ends. Under optimal conditions, intramem-

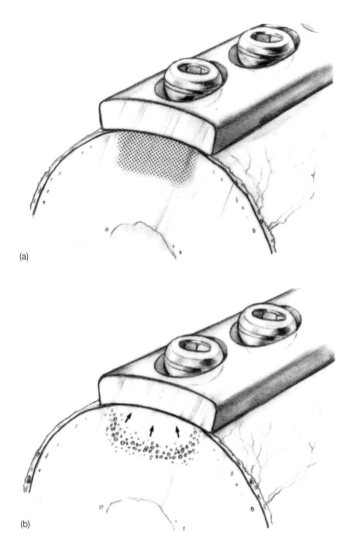

(a)

(b)

Fig. 19. Bone necrosis and remodeling after plate application. (a) Application of a plate causes regional avascular necrosis under the implant. (b) Within 3 months bone metabolizing units advancing from the intact surrounding bone will remove the necrotic bone (initial porosis) and replace it with new lamellar osteons. (Modified from Müller et al. (1991).)

branous bone develops. If the process is disturbed or the adjacent bone ends lack stability, cartilaginous tissue or fibrous tissue is seen in the distraction gap and a nonunion may develop. While distraction osteogenesis is frequently carried out with a ring fixator, the process is not device specific (Paley *et al.* 1991; Tetsworth and Paley 1995; Murray and Fitch 1996).

Prerequisites

There are several prerequisites for successful distraction osteogenesis. The fixator employed must be sturdy enough to guarantee stable fixation at both fragment ends and the distraction site throughout the distraction process. When the osteotomy is carried out, as much local blood supply as possible should be preserved. While the endosteum can be completely transected, great care must be taken to

---

Box 15 **Prerequisites for distraction osteogenesis**

- Fixator strong enough to provide stable fixation
- Blood supply to osteotomy site must be preserved
- Preserve periosteum
- Distract at 1 mm per day in steps of 0.25 mm every 8 h
- Osteogenic potential is best where cancellous bone dominates
- Allow latency of some days before starting distraction

preserve the periosteum circumferentially. In humans, the optimal distraction rate appears to be around 1 mm a day, effected in smaller steps (i.e. 0.25 mm four times a day). Osteotomy or corticotomy through the metaphysis is preferred because cancellous bone has greater osteogenic potential, forms a regenerate of better quality, and will unite more rapidly than has been observed after diaphyseal osteotomies. A latency period of 3 days in young children and 5 to 10 days in adults is recommended before the distraction process is started.

Temporal sequence

After an adequate **latency period**, the **distraction period** lasts until the desired length has been gained. During the following **consolidation period**, which may last as long as, or longer than, the distraction period, the newly formed bone matures. The fixators can be removed when the distraction gap has uniformly consolidated and at least three new cortices have formed (neocorticalization) as seen on orthogonal radiographs. While experimentally the regeneration process can be accelerated by dynamization of the fixator, dynamic loading, or the application of slight compression, these treatment modifications are only marginally effective and are rarely applied in practice.

Histologic events

After initiation of the distraction, trabeculae form on both sides of the osteotomy site (Ilizarov 1989a,b; Lascombes *et al.* 1991; Schenk and Gachter 1994). They end in a central lucent interzone which is about 5 to 10 mm wide. The conically shaped trabeculae are oriented in line with the distraction force. They end in a tip which is about 8 µm wide, but rapidly enlarges to a width of about 200 µm. The outer surfaces of the trabeculae are covered by a layer of osteoblasts. While the interzone is relatively avascular, the regions between the trabeculae contain an abundant capillary blood supply. It appears that the interzone consists of undifferentiated mesenchymal cells which, under optimal conditions, directly transform into osteoblasts (intramembranous bone formation) while under less optimal conditions, particularly in the presence of local instability, or a decreased blood supply, chondroblasts or fibroblasts emerge (Fig. 20). As in secondary bone healing, the regenerate may contain simultaneously fibrous, cartilaginous, and bony tissue. Depending on the conditions, consolidation of the regenerate may still occur, albeit at a lower rate and by a process similar to enchondral ossification. Alternatively, a fibrous nonunion may develop. After removal of the external fixator, the cortical portions of the regenerated portion are remodeled through the process of Haversian remodeling while the medullary

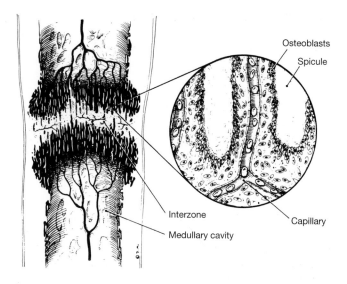

Fig. 20. Distraction osteogenesis. Region of distraction. Nutrient arteries and veins supply the richly vascular trabecular zones. These are separated by a hypovascular interzone which consists of undifferentiated mesenchymal cells. The cells surrounding the trabeculae and the cells of the interzone appear similar (insert). It is presumed that the undifferentiated mesenchymal interzone cells directly transform into the osteoblasts of the trabeculae through the process of intramembranous bone formation. (Modified from Paley *et al.* (1991).)

trabeculae are gradually resorbed until complete recanalization of the intramedullary canal has occurred.

Ligaments—injury and repair

Basic concepts

Ligaments are dense highly organized connective tissue structures that connect bone to bone. They act as primary static joint stabilizers and thus guide normal and restrict abnormal motion. As they are innervated, they are indirectly responsible for pain sensation, joint proprioception, and, through protective reflexes, the activation of musculotendinous units which act as dynamic joint stabilizers (Buckwalter *et al.* 1987; Barrack and Skinner 1990). Ligaments consist mainly of type I collagen (70 per cent dry weight). They are arranged in progressively more complex structures from fibrils to fasciculi which have a predominantly parallel (collateral ligaments) or spiral (cruciate ligaments) organization (Frank *et al.* 1988). Varying amounts of elastin are found in some ligaments such as the ligamentum flavum (Frank *et al.* 1985).

Box 16 **Characteristics of ligaments**

- Static joint stabilizers
- Innervated for pain and proprioception
- Insertion is direct by Sharpey's fibers or indirect (blending with periosteum)
- Mobilization stimulates healing

Box 17 **Behavior of ligaments**

- Viscoelastic—creep, hysteresis, and stress relaxation
- Many consist of several bands which behave independently
- Prolonged immobilization leads to decreased strength and elasticity
- Exercise increases thickness, strength, and stress

Ligament insertions into bone are classified as either direct or indirect. Direct insertions (femoral insertion of the medial collateral ligament of the knee) contain deep fibers which insert at a right angle to bone and superficial fibers which blend with the periosteum. The deep fiber insertion progresses from ligament to fibrocartilage to mineralized fibrocartilage to bone. Sharpey's fibers cross all four zones. Indirect insertions (tibial insertion of the medial collateral ligament of the knee) tend to be broader than direct insertions. The collagen fibers blend with the periosteum at an oblique angle (Cooper and Misol 1970). Clinically, indirect insertions are easily elevated off bone without actually cutting the ligament. The blood supply of ligaments originates at the insertion sites and runs longitudinally through the ligament.

The tensile properties of ligaments are similar to those of tendons, with an initial toe region produced by the nonlinear straightening of the crimped fibers and nonhomogenous recruitment of nonparallel fibers. As elongation continues, fibers become more parallel to the load. Ligaments exhibit viscoelastic properties such as creep, hysteresis, and stress relaxation. Thus the mechanical characteristics of ligaments are affected by sequential load. Clinically, this becomes relevant in anterior cruciate reconstruction where stress relaxation of graft materials may be observed in the initial hours after tensioning, and preconditioning may be appropriate prior to final tensioning (Woo *et al.* 1987 1990). Many ligaments, such as the cruciates, have multiple bands of collagen fibers attached at different points of the insertion. This allows different components of the ligament to tighten with varying joint position.

The effects of immobilization on ligamentous structures has been studied in animals. Using the medial collateral ligament, it was found that prolonged immobilization leads to decreased tensile strength and elastic modulus. Histologically, there is increased osteoclastic activity and bone resorption at the ligament insertion sites. It takes 8 months to a year for the insertion sites to normalize following resumption of motion. The mid-substance medial collateral ligament, however, recovers to normal after 2 to 3 months following remobilization. Exercise results in increased ultimate force, thickness, tensile strength, and ultimate stress (Noyes 1977; Woo *et al.* 1987; Frank *et al.* 1991*a*).

Mechanisms of injury

Ligament sprains are the most common joint injuries. Three grades of severity are usually differentiated. Grade I disruption implies pain with stress, but no increase in laxity. Grade II injuries produce a slight increase in laxity, but with a solid endpoint to stress. Grade III injuries are complete disruptions of the ligament with significant laxity and an absence of a firm endpoint to stress.

Box 18 **Classification of severity of ligament injuries**

I.	Pain on stress—no increase in laxity
II.	Slight increase in laxity, solid endpoint
III.	Complete laxity, no endpoint

Specific injury mechanisms have been best defined around the knee. Ligament injuries can be produced by contact (medial collateral disruption from a blow to the lateral aspect of the leg) or noncontact due to pivoting and decelerating activities (anterior cruciate tears from varus internal rotation or valgus external rotation). Although classic mechanisms often produce predictable isolated injuries, the continued application of a deforming force will stress and injure secondary restraints and produce combined ligamentous disruptions.

Healing of extra-articular ligaments

The medial collateral ligament has been the most extensively studied extra-articular ligament. In comparison with the anterior cruciate ligament, the medial collateral ligament has more collagen fibrils per unit area and greater mean fibril diameter. This results in increased tensile load bearing and greater resistance to elongation (Lyon *et al.* 1991). Immediately following an injury, bleeding into the region produces a fibrin clot. Within 3 days, macrophages, platelets, and neutrophils migrate into the injury site and release chemotactic, proteolytic, and angiogenic factors. In response, capillary budding and fibroblast migration occur (Buckwalter *et al.* 1996). Within the first few weeks a disorganized cellular scar is produced consisting primarily of type III collagen and proteoglycans. This proliferative scar formation continues through 6 weeks from injury with gradual shift towards production of type I collagen.

Remodeling subsequently occurs up to a year with decreased cellularity and vascularity and increased collagen alignment and bundling. However, mature ligament repair tissue only achieves 70 per cent of the tensile strength of normal ligament tissue (Frank *et al.* 1983). The increased cross-sectional area of the repair tissue appears to compensate for the diminished tensile strength (Frank *et al.* 1985). There is evidence that actin contributes to contraction and remodeling during the healing process (Rudolph 1980; Dahners *et al.* 1986; Weiss *et al.* 1991).

The healing response of extra-articular ligaments is influenced by environmental factors. Increased tensile stress and early active

Box 19 **Healing of ligaments**

- Disorganized scar (mainly type III collagen)
- Over 6 weeks shift to type I collagen
- Remodeling increases strength to 70 per cent of normal
- Extra thickness compensates for lack of strength
- Actin contributes to contraction and remodeling
- Exercise increases total collagen and organization
- Suturing of mop-end tears confers little benefit

Box 20 **Structure of articular cartilage**

- Collagen network held in tension by hydrostatic pressure from proteoglycans matrix
- Surface layer: tangential array of collagen fibers
- Middle layer: obliquely arranged fibers
- Deep layer: vertical fibers
- Base zone: calcified cartilage linked to subchondral bone

motion (Tipton *et al.* 1970; Akeson *et al.* 1977; Vailas *et al.* 1981; Hart and Dahners 1987) during the healing of a transected medial collateral ligament results in increased total collagen and improved histologic organization (Gomez *et al.* 1991). Short-term benefits have been demonstrated if sharply transected ligaments are sutured. Clinically, however, medial collateral ligament injuries result in mop-end tears with extensive overlapping of ligament ends and minimal gap formation; thus operative repair of these injuries is not always helpful (Ellsasser *et al.* 1974; Hastings 1980; Indelicato 1983; Ballmer and Jakob 1988).

Healing of intra-articular ligaments

In contrast with extra-articular ligaments, intra-articular ligaments do not heal predictably. Cells isolated from the anterior cruciate ligament show fewer mitoses and less migration than cells isolated from the medial collateral ligament. Despite an extensive vascular response, a fibrin clot is not formed after an anterior cruciate ligament injury, possibly because of synovial fluid interference. Additionally, the disruption of the synovial sleeve may contribute to extensive gap formation (Frank *et al.* 1991*b*; Lyon *et al.* 1991; Woo *et al.* 1991). Because repairs of mid-substance intra-articular ligament tears have been rarely successful, such interventions have been replaced by primary or secondary reconstructions.

Injury and repair of articular cartilage
Basic concepts

Articular cartilage is an avascular aneural tissue consisting of a limited number of chondrocytes which are surrounded by an extensive extracellular matrix. This matrix consists mainly of type II collagen and proteoglycans. The collagen network anchors the cartilage to the subchondral bone and is responsible for its shear stiffness. Charged hydrophilic groups on the proteoglycans hold water and produce the swelling pressure which gives cartilage the ability to resist compressive loads (Coletti *et al.* 1972). Shear and compression squeeze water to the articular surface and thus diminish friction during joint motion (Ateshian *et al.* 1994).

Structurally, we distinguish four layers of articular cartilage. At the surface, cells and collagen are arranged in a tangential array. In the middle zone, they are more obliquely oriented and become more vertical at the deep zone. The fourth zone is the calcified cartilage which connects the articular cartilage to the underlying subchondral bone. The tidemark, a basophilic staining line, separates the uncalcified cartilage from the calcified cartilage. Type IX cartilage appears to be important in binding type II collagen together (Mankin 1982).

Cartilage injury

Because the standard vascular–inflammatory tissue response to injury occurs only once the subchondral bone is penetrated, we distinguish between superficial cartilage injuries which do not involve the subchondral bone and deep cartilage injuries which do (Fig. 21).

Superficial injuries

Lacerations perpendicular to the tidemark may produce cell death and result in wedge-shaped matrix defects. These vertical fissures rarely progress.

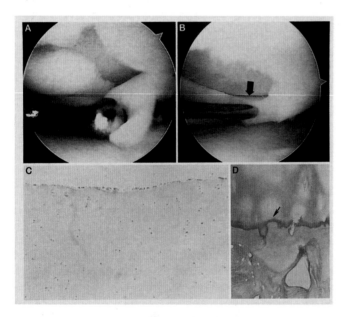

Fig. 21. (a) Arthroscopic view of the medial femoral condyle in a 22-year-old female soccer player. The chondral delamination flap is identified at the tip of the probe. (b) The same arthroscopic view after removal of the delamination flap. Further delamination (arrow) extends past the border. (c) A histologic section of the delamination flap in the same patient. The surface and superficial layers appear normal. (d) A histologic section of the delamination border from the same patient, demonstrating failure at the tidemark (arrow).

Deep cartilage injuries

Lacerations penetrating to the subchondral cartilage are rare. More often, deep injuries are due to single or repetitive blunt trauma. In the latter situation, fissuring of the calcified cartilage and then the subchondral bone can occur with secondary progression to fibrillation of the more superficial layers. A similar condition called chondral delamination, where the articular cartilage peels off the underlying calcified cartilage, has also been observed in athletes (Levy *et al.* 1996).

The initial phase of arthritic conditions is characterized by fraying of collagen bundles at the surface followed by loss of matrix proteoglycans. Later, vertical fissures extend towards the tidemark, and finally the subchondral bone is penetrated. However, in recent animal models, similar lesions were produced after repetitive impulse loading which resulted in primary changes at the subchondral plate and secondary progression to more superficial layers (Radin *et al.* 1978).

Cartilage healing

Superficial injuries

After superficial injuries which do not penetrate the subchondral plate, some chondrocyte proliferation and a regional increase in matrix synthesis is observed. Neither is sufficiently effective to repair these defects.

Deep lesions

While direct penetrating lesions down to subchondral bone occur, most of our knowledge about the spontaneous repair of lesions penetrating subchondral bone stems from such techniques as drilling and puncturing the bed of osteochondral defects and abrasion chondroplasty (Insall 1974) after delamination, osteochondritis dissecans (Mayer and Seidlein 1988), or arthritic conditions (Mink and Deutsch 1989; Buckwalter and Mow 1992). In all these techniques, the calcified cartilage is penetrated or removed down to a bleeding bed of subchondral bone which is initially covered by a fibrin clot. This is followed by formation of hyaline cartilage (type II collagen) and later fibrocartilage (type I collagen). The clinical success of this repair process is variable, unpredictable, and often not clinically satisfactory.

Tissue transplantation into osteochondral defects

Because the clinical repair process with fibrocartilage is often unsatisfactory after deep lesions, attempts have been made to transplant other tissues with functional precursor cells into the defect including rib perichondrium, tibial periosteum, and cartilage auto- and allograft. Some of these transplants have been performed with the addition of growth factors.

Transplants of rib cartilage are limited by the high propensity for calcification and poor stress profiles of the newly developed tissue. Tibial periosteal cells from the cambium layer can produce hyaline-like cartilage. This technique has been quite successful in isolated patellar and femoral lesions, particularly with the use of continuous passive motion in the postoperative period (O'Driscoll *et al.* 1988).

Preliminary reports indicate that placing cultured autogenous chondrocytes under a periosteum cover which is sutured to surrounding cartilage results in substantial reconstitution of hyaline-like cartilage (Green 1971; Grande *et al.* 1989; Brittberg *et al.* 1994). Another technique uses osteochondral plugs from the trochlear groove to fill osteochondral defects. This approach has the advantage that in addition to the chondral defect, the damaged subchondral bone is also replaced. Other efforts involve the production of collagen scaffolds to grow chondrocytes prior to implantation and the use of growth factors to foster cartilage proliferation (Freed *et al.* 1994; Vacanti *et al.* 1994).

Injury and repair of tendons

Structure and anatomy

Tendons are dense regularly arranged collagenous structures that transmit loads generated by muscle to bone. This function requires that tendons be structurally organized to resist high tensile forces. Microscopically, tendons are a complex composite material that consists of a network of parallel collagen fibers associated with proteoglycans ground substance and relatively few cells. The predominant cell type is the spindle-shaped fibroblast. These cells are arranged in parallel rows in the spaces between collagen fibrils (Fig. 22). The fibroblasts are responsible for the synthesis of connective tissue matrix precursors including collagen, elastin, and proteoglycans (Gelberman *et al.* 1988).

Collagen is the major constituent of tendon (86 per cent of dry weight) and contains a high concentration of the amino acids glycine (33 per cent), proline (15 per cent), and hydroxyproline (15 per cent). These amino acids are arranged in long sequences to form a single polypeptide chain. Currently there are 15 known different collagen types that are composed of 29 genetically distinct polypeptide chains. All types of collagen consist of three particular chains covalently cross-linked and combined with globular and nonhelical structural elements to form a rigid triple tropocollagen molecule. Normal adult tendons are composed largely of type I collagen (95 per cent) with the remaining 5 per cent consisting of type III and type IV collagen (Jimenez *et al.* 1978).

In the extracellular matrix, collagen molecules become aligned head-to-tail and side-by-side in a quarter-staggered array that aligns oppositely charged amino acids (Fig. 23). In this manner collagen molecules combine to form extremely stable highly ordered units of microfibrils and fibrils.

Proteoglycans, glycoproteins, and glycosaminoglycans, which constitute the majority of the ground substance of tendons, are then incorporated among these fibrils and bind them together to form fascicles. Their water-binding capacity influences the viscoelastic properties of tendons, and they have been found in higher concentrations in areas of tendons experiencing the greatest compressive forces (Banes *et al.* 1988).

Elastin is another structural protein found in small quantities within tendons (less than 1 per cent dry weight). Elastin, which is produced by fibroblasts, enables tendons to undergo large changes in

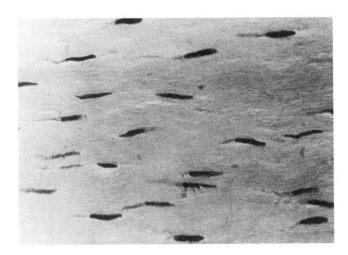

Fig. 22. Photomicrograph of a longitudinal section of a human flexor tendon showing the spindle-shaped fibroblasts (hematoxylin and eosin).

Box 22 **Structure of tendons**

- Mainly type I collagen
- Small amounts of type III and IV collagen
- Fascicles held together by endotenon
- Endotenon is continuous with periosteum—carries blood supply
- Paratenon surrounds some tendons
- Synovium surrounding tendon is called tenosynovium

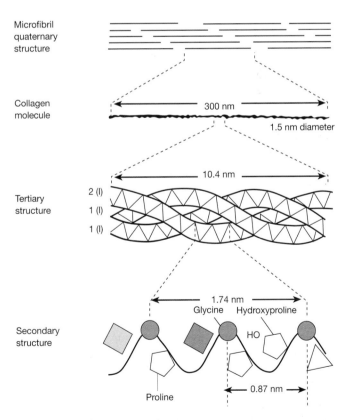

Fig. 23. Schematic drawing of the structural organization of collagen in the microfibril.

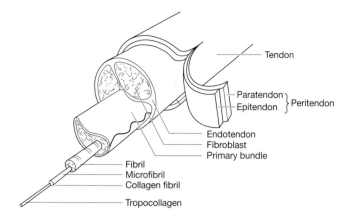

Fig. 24. Stuctural organization of tendon.

length without sustaining any permanent change in structure. The large majority of elastin is found at the fascicular surface of tendons (Rowe 1985).

The fascicles within the tendon are bound together by loose connective tissue—the endotenon, which permits longitudinal movement of collagen fascicles and carries blood vessels, lymphatics, and nerves. The endotenon is continuous with the periosteum at the tendon–bone interface where collagen fibers enter bone as Sharpey fibers. Surrounding the endotenon is a white glistening synovial-like membrane—the epitenon. In some tendons the epitenon is then circumscribed by a loose areolar tissue called the paratenon. This paratenon functions as an elastic sheath allowing free gliding of the tendon against the surrounding tissue. Together the epitenon and paratenon comprise the peritendon (Fig. 24). In some tendons the paratenon is replaced by a true synovial sheath or bursa consisting of two layers lined by synovial cells. This double-layered sheath, which is found in flexor tendons in the hand, is referred to as a tenosynovium.

Tendons surrounded by paratenon have been referred to as vascular tendons, and those surrounded by a tendon sheath as avascular tendons. In vascular tendons, vessels enter from many points on the periphery and anastomose with a longitudinal system of capillaries. The avascular tendons contained within synovial sheaths have mesotenons within these sheaths that function as vascularized conduits called vincula. This creates relatively avascular regions along the length of the tendons. The source of nutrients for these areas include diffusional pathways from the synovial fluid (Lundborg and Rank 1978). Both types of tendons receive additional blood supply from vessels in the regions of the muscle and bone attachments.

Biomechanical properties

Tendons possess one of the highest tensile strengths of all soft tissues in the body. Functionally, tendons can either generate joint motion during concentric contractions or are able to resist joint motion during eccentric contractions. By comparison, owing to their low content of ground substance, tendons have weak resistance against shear and compressive forces.

Tendons, like all other soft tissues, have viscoelastic material properties. In other words, the elongation of a tendon depends not only

on the amount of force, but also on the rate and duration of force application. These viscoelastic characteristics are due to the viscous properties of the mucopolysaccharide ground matrix found in tendons. This is important physiologically because the loading of tendons is usually cyclic. For example, when a tendon is repeatedly loaded and unloaded, its stress–strain curve shifts to the right, indicating that the tendon has become less stiff or more compliant. Clinically this is displayed by the increased laxity of tendons following exercise. In contrast, an increase in elongation speed, or a higher strain rate, will shift the curve to the left, indicating increasing stiffness. Physiologically this quality protects tendons from rupturing under extremely high eccentric forces.

As a result of its viscoelastic properties, tendons also exhibit creep. In an isometric contraction, tendon lengthening from creep allows the muscle to shorten over time. This change in length of the muscle increases muscle performance by decreasing the rate of fatigue.

Factors affecting biomechanical properties

Various factors affect the properties of tendon, including exercise, immobilization, anatomic location, and aging. Most studies have shown that exercise training results in increased collagen fibril size, ultimate tensile strength, and stiffness (Woo *et al.* 1982). On the other hand, immobilization leads to a significant decrease in water content, proteoglycans concentration, ultimate tensile strength, and stiffness (Akeson *et al.* 1977). This alteration in mechanical properties may be influenced by the location, forces, and biochemical constituents of the specific tendon involved. In a study observing the effect of exercise on swine, an increase in the tensile strength of the extensor tendons was determined to be greater than in the flexor tendons (Woo *et al.* 1981). Structural and degenerative changes as a result of aging have also been reported. The mean collagen fibril diameter and collagen content of tendons decreases with increasing age. This leads to a decline in the ultimate tensile strength (Vogel 1978). In contrast, the amount of collagen cross-linking increases, which leads to greater tendon stiffness (Eyre 1984). Other changes include decreases in total cell count, proteoglycans composition, and water content.

Tendon injury

The two major mechanisms causing tendon injury are indirect and direct trauma. Indirect injury occurs secondary to tensile overload and may manifest itself as intrasubstance tendon rupture or avulsion from bone at the tendon insertion. The mechanisms of indirect injury are multifactorial and depend on anatomic location, vascular supply, skeletal maturity, and the magnitude of the applied force. Since tendons can withstand high tensile forces, most indirect injuries occur at the bone–tendon or muscle–tendon interface. Mid-substance tendon rupture is less common and often there is a pre-existing pathologic condition. This degenerative state is often seen in chronic overuse injuries where repetitive microtrauma and incomplete healing results in a weakened tendon structure. Histologic study of these injuries reveal a lack of inflammatory cells with focal areas of collagen fragmentation and angioblastic fibroplasia. Clinically, these degenerative changes are observed most frequently in the achilles, patella, rotator cuff, and biceps tendons.

Direct injury results from a laceration or contusion and is commonly seen in the hand and upper extremity. The healing process following direct injury has been extensively studied in flexor tendons and seems to be similar for all tendons.

Tendon healing

It is currently accepted that tendons possess both an extrinsic and intrinsic capacity to heal. The extrinsic theory suggests that tendon healing depends on the generation of an inflammatory response, with subsequent scarring, by the tissues surrounding the injured tendon. Proponents of this hypothesis believed that tendon is an inert, almost avascular structure, whose cells are incapable of contributing to the healing process (Potenza 1963). In contrast, the intrinsic theory holds that the inflammatory response is nonessential, and that tendons possess an intrinsic capability to heal (Lundborg and Rank 1980). In the clinical setting both types of healing occur with the relative contribution of each depending on the type and site of the tendon injury.

As with all tissues, tendon healing proceeds in three phases: an inflammatory phase, a reparative or collagen-producing phase, and a remodeling phase. Immediately after tendon injury and repair, the defect is filled with blood clot, tissue debris, and fluid. Three days after the injury the inflammatory stage of healing predominates. Cells originating from the extrinsic peritendinous tissues (synovial sheath, deep fascia, and periosteum) and intrinsic tissue of the epitenon and endotenon migrate into the laceration site. These cells appear during the first 48 to 72 h and form granulation tissue that bridges the defect. The function of these cells is primarily phagocytic and involves the removal of cellular debris and collagen remnants. During the inflammatory phase, the strength of the tendon repair is almost entirely dependent on the suture itself with a small contribution from the fibrin clot. This inflammatory phase is evident for 8 to 10 days following injury.

Collagen synthesis begins within the first week and reaches its maximum level at approximately 4 weeks. This marks the onset of the second stage of healing—the reparative or collagen-producing phase. Fibroblasts become the predominant cell type, and they actively participate in the synthesis and resorption of collagen. Fibronectin, a glycoprotein found in plasma, serves as a chemotactic agent for fibroblasts. It promotes fibroblast adhesion to denatured collagen and fibrin. Initially the fibroblasts and collagen are oriented perpendicular to the long axis of the tendon, but by 28 days these structures are reoriented parallel to the axis of tensile loading. Strength of the reparative process increases exponentially 2 to 3 weeks following the injury. The synovial sheath, if injured, is reconstituted after 21 days, and as the wound matures a smooth gliding surface develops. If the synovial sheath is not damaged, intrinsic healing predominates and there is less chance for the extrinsic contribution of healing to lead to restrictive adhesion formation.

The remodeling phase of healing begins after 4 weeks and is char-

---

Box 24 Healing of tendons

- Inflammatory phase—fibrin clot forms
- Collagen synthesis begins in first week
- Collagen orientates over 4 weeks
- The synovial sheath repairs in 3 weeks
- Collagen production changes from type III to type I for 12 months

---

acterized by an increase in mechanical strength. Tension on the maturing granulation tissue causes remodeling of fiber architecture in a manner similar to Wolff's law for bone (Forrester *et al.* 1970). In addition, a gradual shift of collagen production from type III to type I may also contribute to the increased mechanical strength. This phase can continue for up to 6 to 12 months (Greenlee and Pike 1971).

Methods of improving tendon repair

Considerable research has been conducted in an effort to understand various factors that may influence the rate and strength of tendon healing. The most important of these involve postoperative mobilization of tendon repairs. It has been established that a healing tendon can be strengthened by the application of tension forces which may cause a more rapid realignment of collagen fibers (Takai *et al.* 1991). In a series of laboratory studies in canine flexor tendons, early passive mobilization led to a more rapid recovery of tensile strength, fewer adhesions, improved excursion, better nutrition, and minimal repair site deformation compared with immobilized repairs (Gelberman *et al.* 1986). Apparently, the rapid reinstitution of tendon gliding provides the stimulus for cellular activation of the epitenon (intrinsic response). In contrast, immobilization leads to ingrowth of cells from the surrounding tissues (extrinsic response) and adhesions predominate. Therefore the ideal postoperative protocol is one that provides the greatest tensile stress across a repair while preventing gap formation or rupture of the repair (Strickland 1995*a*).

Since the ultimate goal is to restore immediate motion and stress to a tendon repair, the limiting factor becomes the strength of the repair. This holds true whether the tendon is ruptured at its muscle–tendon junction, mid-substance, or bony insertion. The various suture and fixation techniques are too numerous to mention here, but some basic principles can be used as a guide to choosing a specific repair. The first is that each larger suture caliber increases the repair strength significantly. The next principle is that core sutures should be used that pass perpendicular to the tendon before passing

---

Box 25 Consequences of passive mobilization of tendons

- Rapid recovery of tensile strength
- Fewer adhesions
- Improved excursion
- Better nutrition

Box 26   Factors affecting suture of tendons

- Each suture increases repair strength
- Core sutures should pass perpendicular to tendon
- Increasing the number of sutures thickens the repair
- Sutures must not compromise blood supply
- Repair of tendon sheath restricts adhesion formation

Box 27   Types of nerve injury

- Neurapraxia—local conduction block
- Axonotomesis—epineurium continuity; distal degeneration
- Neurotomesis—disruption of entire nerve

it across the injury, or parallel to the tendon. Increasing the number of suture strands that cross the repair site increases the strength of the repair (Savage 1985), but this adds to the technical difficulty and increases the volume of suture material in the repair site (Strickland 1995b). The third point is that using a peripheral epitendinous suture results in a 10 to 50 per cent increase in repair strength and significantly reduces the tendency for gapping (Lin *et al.* 1988). The fifth guideline is that sutures should be placed in regions that do not compromise tendon blood supply (volar 50 per cent of flexor tendons). Finally, repair of the sheath following tendon suture has the theoretical advantage of restricting adhesion formation, restoring synovial fluid nutrition, and restoring sheath mechanics (Peterson *et al.* 1990). However, the sheath is often technically difficult to re-establish and there are few valid studies to support sheath repair (Gelberman *et al.* 1990).

Various biochemical agents have been studied in an attempt to modify adhesion formation around tendon repairs. These agents include steroids (norethandrolone), antihistamines (promethazine), anti-inflammatory drugs (ibuprofen), and hyaluronate (Douglas *et al.* 1967; St Onge *et al.* 1980; Kulick *et al.* 1986; Hagberg 1992). Although these drugs were shown to decrease adhesion formation, they all had the untoward side-effect of decreasing the rate and strength of tendon healing as well as increasing the rate of infection.

The effect of electrical current on tendon healing has also been studied (Fujita *et al.* 1992). It was shown that adhesion-causing synovial proliferation may be suppressed by the application of direct current to repaired tendons.

The most promising area of future research involves the study of cytokines that play a crucial role in the cellular sequence of tendon repair. Platelet-derived growth factor, transforming growth factor-β, and fibroblast growth factor are being studied to determine their role in both normal physiologic and pathologic processes of tendon repair.

Nerve injuries and repair
Peripheral nerve anatomy

Peripheral nerves are made up of progressively larger elements. At their most basic level, they consist of cells located in or near the spinal cord and their peripheral processes—the axons. Each axon is supported and surrounded by Schwann cells and their related connective tissue sheath—the endoneurium. Fascicles are groups of axons contained by a sleeve of connective tissue—the perineurium. Fascicles are the smallest units of a nerve which can be surgically manipulated. They form intraneural plexuses. Such networks are

more common near the spinal cord than further distal in an extremity. Groups of fascicles are bound together by the epineurium, which is the outer connective tissue layer of a peripheral nerve. It protects the nerve and provides a gliding surface (Lundborg and Dahlin 1991). Each nerve is supplied by segmental nutrient vessels which form a rich longitudinal epineural vascular plexus. This arrangement facilitates the mobilization of long segments of a peripheral nerve without compromising its function. Fascicles are vascularized segmentally by epineurial vessels and each fascicle has a longitudinally oriented perineurial and endoneurial microvascular system (Lundborg 1979).

Mechanisms of injury

Sharp lacerations cause nerve transections, while the transfer of energy through a blast, crush, or a traction injury results in variable, nonuniform nerve damage. Chronic nerve compression can cause a metabolic conduction block which may lead to paresthesias and progressive motor and sensory loss.

Classification of nerve injuries

Patterns of nerve injury may vary within a nerve from fascicle to fascicle. Seddon (1943) first described three types of nerve injury: neurapraxia, axonotomesis, and neurotomesis. Later, Sunderland (1951) defined five severity degrees with two degrees lying between axonotomesis and neurotomesis. Neurapraxia is a localized conduction block caused by the segmental demyelination of an axon that remains in continuity. Axonotomesis is an axonal injury that results in a Wallerian degeneration of the axon distal to the impact. In all forms of axonotomesis the epineurium remains in continuity. In its mildest form, a second-degree nerve injury, the endoneurial tube remains in continuity with only the axon severed. Disruption of the endoneurial tube and the axon, but with a perineurium in continuity, defines a third-degree injury. A fourth-degree injury disrupts all structures except the epineurium. Neurotomesis is a disruption of the entire nerve including the epineurium.

Healing of nerve injuries

When an axon is severed, it undergoes Wallerian degeneration distal to the injury. This process is completed when macrophages have cleared the axonal tube of degraded myelin and axoplasm. Only if the nerve cell survives can the nerve regenerate (Frykman 1993). Under these circumstances, the remaining Schwann cell tube serves as a guide for the sprouting axon. Through the production of neurotropic factors and adhesion molecules, the distal nerve stumps and target organs facilitate axonal regeneration. Under this influence, the growth-associated proteins produced by the cell body are transported distally in the regenerating axon. Within hours of injury, a regenerating axon produces sprouts from the most distal intact node of Ranvier. Each axon produces multiple sprouts. These enter Schwann cell tubes which may or may not be related to the original axonal pathway. After some pruning of the sprouts, only one axon is regenerated. There is now some evidence that, guided by a neurotropic factor from the Schwann cell, the correct type of Schwann cell tube is selected for nerve regeneration (Brushart 1993). Specificity of axon regeneration is of utmost importance. Useful regeneration only occurs when a sensory axon meets a sensory end organ and a motor axon reaches the motor end organ. The final step of successful nerve regeneration involves plasticity or re-education of the central nervous system. The cell body may be of the appropriate type but responsible for a different muscle, or a different type or area of sensation. Thus, even when a sensory axon finds a sensory end-organ, the brain must undergo some re-education to interpret the stimulus correctly (Szabo and Madison 1993).

Nerve repair

Basic principles

Mechanism of injury and physical findings help to determine when a repair is necessary or whether observation is prudent. Sharp lacerations should be explored and repaired. Blunt closed injuries are observed for recovery and repaired at 3 months if there is no evidence of recovery, there is no advancing Tinel sign, and electrical studies show no evidence of regeneration (Frykman *et al.* 1981). Open injuries with nerve deficits can be explored at the initial wound debridement and the nerve ends either repaired or tagged for later repair when local tissues will provide a better bed. Delayed repair is indicated in the face of contamination, when proper soft tissue coverage is lacking and when a blast injury or concomitant head injury prevent full initial assessment of the nerve damage (Szabo and Madison 1993). Motor recovery is unlikely if not reinnervated by 18 months, and results are worse if repair is performed 6 months after the injury. This is due to a regeneration rate of about 1 mm per day and because of ensuing muscle atrophy and fibrosis (Sunderland 1991). Partial sensory recovery may be possible for several years after injury.

The following key concepts underlie all successful nerve repair.

Box 28 Principles of nerve repair

- Sharp lacerations should be explored
- Blunt injuries should be observed
- If no recovery in 3 months, explore

Box 29 Key factors for nerve repair

- Microsurgical technique
- Adequate exposure
- Ends oppose without tension
- Primary repair if possible
- Align fascicles accurately

1. Microsurgical techniques with adequate magnification, instrumentation, and microsuture are essential.

2. Adequate exposure of both ends must be followed by debridement of the zone of injury.

3. Nerve ends must come together without tension and extreme positioning of the extremity must be avoided.

4. A primary nerve repair should be performed whenever possible.

Proper resection of the zone of injury includes the complete removal of the damaged nerve section which will otherwise heal with a scar. This is done with a sharp blade on a firm cutting surface. At the time of delayed exploration, direct palpation of the nerve reveals a firm thickened area in the zone of injury which is readily differentiated from normal nerve on either end. Scar resection is performed incrementally, removing small amounts and examining the ends for normal appearing fascicles. Examining the portion to be removed minimizes the handling of the end to be repaired.

Nerve alignment is critical for optimal outcome. Several methods are available. The simplest is alignment by anatomic landmarks such as epineural blood vessels and fascicle arrangement. For most acute injuries this is possible because functional units within the nerve follow a predictable path over a considerable distance; proper nerve repair is thus facilitated by a knowledge of the internal topography of the injured structure (Jabaley *et al.* 1980; Cook and Lubbers 1996).

Electrical stimulation in the awake patient can help delineate motor and sensory fascicles in the proximal stump and within 3 to 4 days of injury in the distal stump (Jabaley 1991). Fascicles and fascicular groups are stimulated and the patient relates sensation and location of sensation which is then carefully mapped. When stimulated, sensory fibers cause a burning pain in the corresponding dermatome while motor fibers cause a dull nonspecific feeling in the corresponding muscle belly. Stimulation by a disposable nerve stimulator may not be adequate, and equipment that allows a gradual increase in stimulus is often required. If distally no stimulation is possible, several other strategies are available. Known branches are dissected, traced back to the injury, and repaired to a corresponding area in the proximal stump or the surgeon can use topographical maps. Another option is staining of the nerve ends. Stains for acetylcholinesterase (motor) and carbonic anhydrase (sensory) are performed on sections of proximal nerve ends. This staining information allows identification of sensory and motor fascicles of the proximal stump only. Staining takes a minimum of 1 h and requires the help of a pathologist. Because of their complexity, both electrical stimulation and staining are most useful for secondary repairs.

Repair techniques

Three types of direct repair are available to the surgeon: epineural, group fascicular, and fascicular.

Epineural repair is indicated if the internal topography of the nerve is unclear. The microscope is used in conjunction with fine monofilament suture. Under high-power magnification, fascicles are aligned. Sutures are placed only through the epineurium and tied bringing its edges together without bunching. If the nerve ends stay together with one suture (8-0 nylon) in the epineurium, tension on the repair will not be excessive. Next, a second suture is placed opposite the first. The remaining sutures are then filled in, closing the gap between the ends and preventing any fascicles from

Box 30 Types of nerve repair

- Epineural—sutures in epineurium only
- Group fascicular repair—best for partial cuts

Box 32 Sources of nerve graft

- Sural nerve 30–40 cm
- Medial antebrachial cutaneous nerve
- Terminal branch of posterior interosseous nerve

puckering out between the ends. Tension is checked at the completion of the repair with the extremity taken through a gentle range of motion, and the safe limits of flexion and extension are documented.

Group fascicular repair utilizes the same techniques as epineural repair. The group to be repaired is usually identified by surface anatomy. The epineurium is split longitudinally to expose the fascicle groups. Usually two to three sutures are placed into the internal epineurium of each group. Again, there can be no tension. This repair more accurately reapproximates fascicles; however, one malaligned group can jeopardize the final result. This technique is most useful in nerves with few groups and in partial lacerations were complete fascicular groups are lacerated. To reduce error, the largest identifiable group should be repaired first. Then other groups are repaired, utilizing their anatomic relationship to the first group as an additional guide. Finally, the epineurium is repaired to take tension off the group fascicular repair.

Fascicular repair requires dissection of external and internal epineurium to expose the fascicles. This must be done under the microscope. Correct alignment of fascicles may be difficult to accomplish. The fascicles are repaired with one or two sutures of 10-0 or 11-0 nylon placed in the perineurium. This technique is useful in partial lacerations and in nerves with few fascicles. In nerves with a large number of fascicles this repair can result in malalignment and excessive scarring with results no better than simpler repairs.

Factors that influence the results of nerve repair include age, delay before repair, and level of injury. Children have the best results, possibly because of a greater plasticity of their cerebrum in adapting to a new mix of signals. The results in adults are inferior but may improve for up to 5 years. Repairs performed after 6 months have limited recovery potential. Similarly, proximal injuries have poorer results because distal muscles become fibrotic before regenerated motor axons reach their target. Mixed motor and sensory nerves have inferior recovery compared with primarily motor or sensory nerves. This is presumably due to difficulty in aligning motor and sensory fibers correctly when they are mixed throughout the nerve (Steinberg and Koman 1991).

Nerve grafts

More complex crush and blast injuries which cause segmental nerve loss and scarring are often best managed with nerve grafts. If no recovery is evident after several months, exploration and repair may

Box 31 Factors that influence success of repair

- Age—children do best
- Delay—repairs after 6 months have limited repair potential
- Level of injury—proximal injuries do less well

be indicated. For a successful grafting procedure the wound must be healed, supple, and provide a well-vascularized recipient bed. Exploration begins with dissection of normal nerve proximal and distal to the site of injury. Using the operating microscope, dissection of epineurium and fascicular groups is initiated in normal tissue and advanced into the zone of injury. A nerve stimulator can identify groups with intact motor function and awake stimulation can help to identify intact sensory fascicles. Nerve ends must be adequately trimmed and free of scar tissue. The fascicular anatomy is recorded for both ends, and appropriately matched groups of fascicles are connected by a nerve graft (Millesi *et al.* 1972). Grafts must be placed in correct anatomic alignment without any tension for successful group fascicular repair.

The most common source for a nerve graft is the sural nerve. It has tightly packed fascicles and little interfascicular tissue. It is readily identified behind the lateral malleolus and provides 30 to 40 cm of graft. Other donor nerves include the medial antebrachial cutaneous nerves and the terminal branch of the posterior interosseous nerve. These provide smaller grafts and significantly less nerve tissue than the sural nerve (Wilgis and Brushart 1993).

Postoperative care

The site of a nerve repair, or the proximal and distal ends of a nerve grafts, are carefully documented in relation to anatomic landmarks. This information is later used to monitor the progress of regeneration. The extremity is immobilized in a position that relaxes all suture lines. Immobilization is continued for 4 weeks to protect the repair site if necessary.

Regeneration is carefully monitored by physical examination and electrical studies when indicated. Since sensory axons may regenerate to sensory end-organs which are different from the preinjury end-organs, the signal the brain receives may not correspond to the actual stimulation. The patient must be re-educated to interpret the new signal. Children accomplish this much more readily than older patients. An aggressive sensory re-education program may improve the result of nerve repair by teaching the patient to adapt to their new sensory input (Dellon *et al.* 1971).

Recent developments

Alternatives to autologous nerve grafts are currently under investigation. Placing the cut nerve endings into a tube (silicone, biodegradable material, or vein) has demonstrated promising results in pure sensory nerve injuries. In one prospective randomized study of median or ulnar nerves transected at the wrist and with a 4-mm gap, similar outcomes were noted after tube or standard epineural repair in a small cohort of patients followed for 1 year (Lundborg *et al.* 1997). Allograft, various muscle preparations, and other modified synthetic tubes, as well as alternative repair techniques using fibrin glue, lasers, and the addition of neurotropic and growth factor to the local environment, are currently under investigation.

Proprioception

Proprioception provides a sense of position and movement of various body parts, in particular the extremities. Deficits in proprioception occur when afferent sensory nerve fibers are interrupted by injury or disease. These range from rare severe sensory neuropathy affecting all limbs to an isolated ligament injury affecting only one portion of proprioception feedback for one joint.

Proprioception is a complex sense that relies on information from sensory, visual, and vestibular inputs. Based on the sum of this afferent information, efferent stimuli are generated in the central nervous system. These stimuli activate appropriate agonistic and antagonistic muscle groups which reposition joints and extremity segments. This process of repositioning generates further sensory stimuli and thus maintains a feedback system which continuously monitors the motor functions of body and extremities and results in co-ordinated movements.

Sensory input comes from muscle spindles, Golgi tendon organs, Pacinian corpuscles, Meissner's corpuscles, and other receptors in muscles, tendons, ligaments, joints, and skin. The cell bodies of these nerve fibers are located outside the spinal cord in the dorsal root ganglia with their central processes entering via the dorsal root. From there, fibers connect to neurons relaying information to the cerebellum, medulla, thalamus, and the cerebral cortex (Fig. 25).

Much of our understanding of proprioception comes from evaluating patients with deficits secondary to large-fiber sensory neuropathies. In one study, upper extremity reaching tasks were evaluated in sensory-deprived subjects and controls (Gordon *et al.* 1995). Performing the task without visual input resulted in large errors. Viewing the limb just prior to but not during the task produced improved results that were quickly lost if no further visual input was allowed. Finally, visual feedback throughout the entire activity resulted in the best performance which was almost as good as controls (Ghez and Sainburg 1995). These studies indicate the important role proprioception has in controlling complex upper extremity tasks. Vision appears to be crucial in formulating an internal model at the start of a task, substituting for the absence of proprioception.

Proprioception also registers limb inertia and the effects of torque generated by one extremity segment on an adjacent joint. Deafferented patients are unable to sharply reverse the direction of multiple joint movements. Experiments where reaching motions were suddenly reversed demonstrated a decoupling of shoulder and elbow motion (Ghez *et al.* 1995). With normal proprioception, sharp changes in direction resulted in synchronized reversal of elbow and shoulder motion. Without peripheral feedback, the hand's path widened because the motions of the shoulder and elbow were desynchronized (Fig. 26). Vision before a trial and vision during a trial again improved results in patients without proprioception.

A more common loss of proprioception occurs with isolated injuries to ligaments, joints, muscles, or other end-organs, resulting in a focal loss of feedback. Injuries to the anterior cruciate ligament provide a common example of such a loss (Branch *et al.* 1989; Corrigan *et al.* 1992). The anterior cruciate ligament has sensory receptors and a neurophysiologic purpose in addition to its biomechanical func-

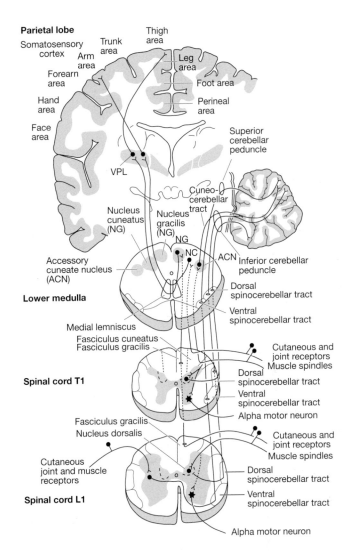

Fig. 25. The central nervous system pathways mediating proprioception and stereognosis. Note that the origin of the crossed ventral spinocerebellar tract is on the left side of the diagram and the origin of the other tracts is on the right. NG, nucleus gracilis; NC, nucleus cuneatus; ACN, accessory cuneate nucleus; VPL, thalamic nucleus ventral posterolateral.

tions (Schultz *et al.* 1984). Careful studies demonstrate that anterior cruciate ligament-deficient knees go through greater angular displacement before patients recognize that motion has occurred (Barrack *et al.* 1989). The loss of afferent signals from the anterior cruciate ligament mechanoreceptors also results in efferent changes (Beard *et al.* 1993). When, in the anterior-cruciate-ligament-deficient knee, a sudden load is applied to the tibia, the latency of the hamstring muscle reflex is increased, and thus the response that resists anterior tibial translation is delayed (Beard *et al.* 1994).

Proprioception is crucial for the recognition of the position of a joint, the motion of a joint and the forces acting on a joint. Proprioception provides the afferent data which initiate and co-ordinate the muscle functions that first stabilize a particular joint and then make it the fulcrum of a precise, co-ordinated motion. Small deficits in proprioception may lead to small changes in motor co-ordination,

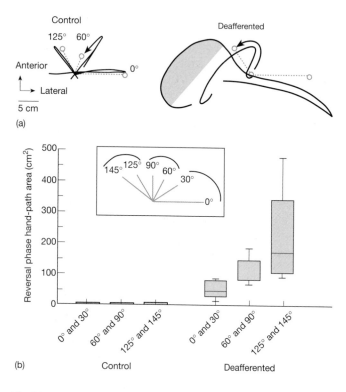

Fig. 26. Hand paths and reversal errors in controls and patient. (a) Hand paths: the target lines for all six directions are shown at the top. Hand paths for three of these directions for control (left) and deafferented patient (right). (b) Path area: median and interquartile range of the area circumscribed by the reversal phase (delimited by tangential hand velocity maxima) of the hand path (shaded above). Movements along each pair of target lines have been grouped (0° and 30°; 60° and 90°; 125° and 145°) such that each box represents 10 trials of movement. (Reproduced from Ghez and Sainburg (1995).)

while larger deficits may affect the function of entire limbs. While vision can partially substitute for proprioception, such substitution is less effective in the lower than in the upper extremity.

Head injuries—presentations and outcomes

Many patients who present with major musculoskeletal disruptions have also sustained significant head injury. While some cerebral lesions are obvious, others are missed or managed inadequately (Mahalick *et al.* 1995, 1996*a,b*).

Epidemiology

With 2 to 3 million cases every year (Beer 1992; Gaultieri 1995) in the United States alone, head injuries have been justly called a silent epidemic (Goldstein 1990). Head injuries are two to three times more common in males than in females. They also occur more frequently in the summer, at weekends, and during late afternoons or early evening hours (Kraus *et al.* 1990). As many as 60 per cent of head-injured patients have a premorbid diagnosis of attention-deficit dis-

order, learning disability, or personality/character disorder. There is also a 7 per cent recurrence rate.

Injury mechanisms and pathophysiology

Most head injuries occur as the result of motor vehicle accidents; other causes include falls, recreation- or sport-related activities (bicycles, all-terrain vehicles, in-line skating, skateboarding, football, baseball, etc.), and stab and missile wounds.

Although many head injuries present with similar symptomatology, they can be based on different pathologic lesions as follows.

Shearing/diffuse axonal injuries

Shearing is the result of acceleration, deceleration, and rotational forces which cause damage to the brain by stretching and compressing of fiber tracts, and by causing the brain to move over bony prominences. Shearing and diffuse axonal injuries are rarely visualized on initial CT scans where they may appear as small areas of 'bruising'. MRI is the best method of documenting these injuries which are associated with significant cognitive deficits.

Contusions

These are bruises or hematomas on or close to the brain's surface. They may occur in isolation or may accompany more severe lesions. They commonly afflict the frontal and temporal lobes. While some are asymptomatic, others are associated with severe neurologic and neurobehavioral deficits and seizures.

Epidural hematoma

This is a collection of blood between the dura mater and the skull. Many epidural hematomas are due to a tear of the middle meningeal artery. Epidural hematomas can cause sudden compression of the brain and may be fatal. Clinically, a short lucid interval is typically followed by loss of consciousness.

Subdural hematoma

This is an area if bleeding within the subdural space. It can be acute or, especially in the elderly, chronic. Chronic subdural hematomas are typically caused by linear and rotational forces which tear the veins between the brain and the dura mater. Most subdural hematomas result in significant focal damage of the cortex and are often accompanied by brain contusions.

Subarachnoid hemorrhage

Bleeding into the subarachnoid space is common. It is most often caused by trauma but may occur spontaneously after rupture of an aneurysm. The bleeding is usually diffuse and does not cause a space-occupying lesion.

Intracerebral hematomas and brain displacement

These are space-occupying lesions which are often accompanied by swelling of surrounding brain tissues. When they expand, they may cause life-threatening brain herniation.

Classification and assessment of head injuries

The Glasgow Coma Scale (Teasdale and Jennet 1976*a,b*) is an initial assessment of a brain injury and its probable medical outcome. Based on severity, the patient is assigned a score between 3 and 15. A score of 3 means that the patient is unresponsive while with a score of 15, the patient is alert, grossly oriented, and able to follow commands. While the Glasgow Coma Scale is an excellent predictor of gross outcome, it is less reliable in predicting neurobehavioral outcomes, particularly for initial scores in the range of 10 to 15. The most reliable predictor of neurobehavioral outcome is the duration of post-traumatic amnesia (Levin *et al.* 1982). When the patient has sustained post-traumatic amnesia of 24 h or less, the head injury is classified as mild. If the post-traumatic amnesia lasts from 24 h to 7 days, the head injury is considered moderate. Post-traumatic amnesia beyond 7 days indicates a severe head injury.

In addition to the Glasgow Coma Scale and post-traumatic amnesia, CT scans and MRI provide additional parameters to assess a head injury. For example, a patient with a Glasgow Coma Scale score of 14 to 15 and a post-traumatic amnesia of 24 to 36 h, with no cerebral involvement demonstrated on CT or MRI, will have a better prognosis than a patient with similar parameters and a left frontal lobe contusion. However, a patient with a very severe head injury who is completely unresponsive and in a protracted comatose state may have negative initial findings on both CT and MRI scans.

In summary, the key factors that determine the severity of a head injury are as follows:

- the Glasgow Coma Scale score
- duration of loss of consciousness or coma
- duration of post-traumatic amnesia
- the nature and extent of the cerebral lesion as seen on CT or MRI.

Positive prognosticators include high premorbid IQs and socio-economic status, as well as a supportive family structure (Rivara *et al.* 1993).

Clinical presentation—postconcussive syndrome

Neurobehavioral and neuropsychiatric symptoms caused by head injuries are often missed on a trauma service because of inexperience or the effects of massive pain medication which may mask the symptomatology and confuse the treating physician.

Typically, symptoms of head injury and postconcussive syndrome include inhibition, elation, euphoria, dysphoria, emotional lability, confusion, memory disturbance, disturbance of social or occupational functions, attention, concentration, and higher-order thought deficits. Often a patient whose head injury was missed initially may present 1 or 2 months later with complaints of cognitive difficulties involving memory, concentration, and higher-order thought processes. Often, the diagnosis of a head injury can be confirmed with a review of the emergency room records which may indicate that the patient was combative, was unable to follow commands, or had a 'questionable' loss of consciousness. In addition, even minimal retrograde, anterograde, or post-traumatic amnesia confirm that the patient indeed sustained a head injury.

Many head injuries have psychologic sequelae such as irritability and agitation as well as exaggerated reactions to painful stimuli such as a scheduled physical therapy session or the removal of a dressing. Protracted malaise and depression which the treating physician may consider to be residues of the musculoskeletal injuries can, in fact, be the sequelae of a concommitant head injury.

Diagnosis and management of many head injuries can be facilitated by an experienced clinical neuropsychologist who often is also skilled in cognitive–behavioral techniques such as desensitization or hypnotherapy.

Acute and chronic higher cortical deficits due to head injuries

Acute deficits

Patients with significant head injuries are initially comatose or obtunded. As the brain recovers, the level of cortical arousal becomes heightened and the mental status improves. After resolution of the coma, all patients display moderate to severe global and diffuse deficits of cognitive function which renders them incapable to execute many higher-order tasks.

Influence of age

Adult patients often languish in a comatose state for long periods of time and only gradually recover their mental capabilities. In contrast, children tend to improve quickly or perish. In addition, typical symptoms resulting from traumatic brain injury in adults are either absent or short-lived in the pediatric population.

Language functions

Most adult patients who sustain an injury to the temporal lobe, which subserves language, will experience severe aphasia, which includes decreases in fluency, difficulties in comprehension, naming, repetition, reading, and writing. If children present with aphasic symptoms at all they usually recover quickly. In the younger age group, complete mutism, which resolves in 1 or 2 weeks, may be pronounced. Similar differences have been observed with respect to visual and visuospatial dysfunction, agnostic and dyspraxic disorders, and dysfunctions of personality.

Psychiatric problems

Adults may experience a spectrum of psychiatric difficulties ranging from mild anxiety disorders to psychosis, while children under the age of 10 have a propensity for attention-deficit disorders without the hyperactive component, and adolescents tend to experience depression, anxiety, irritability, and explosive behavior. Head injuries often exacerbate pre-existing psychologic problems in both children and adolescents.

Long-term deficits

Most neurobehavioral recovery will occur within the first 12 months after injury; however, additional improvements up to 3 years is not unusual.

Residual deficits usually involve attention and concentration, short- or long-term verbal and visual memory, and higher thought processes including planning, problem solving, and strategy formation. Other long-term sequelae, in both children and adults, include anxiety, depression, acquired attention disorders (Mahalick *et al.* 1996*a*,*b*), and psychosis. Resolution of these symptoms is usually much more complete in the pediatric population.

In recent years, it has become increasingly clear that all age groups benefit significantly from outpatient cognitive rehabilitation and remediation (Ruff *et al.* 1987).

References

Akeson, W., Amiel, D., Mechanic, G., Woo, S.-Y., Harwood, F., and Hamer, M. (1977). Collagen cross-linking alterations in joint contractures: changes in the reducible cross-links in periarticular connective tissue collagen after nine weeks of immobilization. *Connective Tissue Research*, 5, 15–19.

Allgower, M. and Spiegel, P. (1979). Internal fixation of fractures: evolution of concepts. *Clinical Orthopaedics and Related Research*, 138, 26–9.

Anderson, H. (1990). The role of cells versus matrix in bone induction. *Connective Tissue Research*, 24, 3–12.

Aro, H., Wippenman, B., Hodgson, S., Whaner, H., Lewallen, D., and Chai, E. (1989). Prediction of properties of fracture callus by measurment of mineral density using micro-bone densitometry. *Journal of Bone and Joint Surgery, American Volume*, 71A, 1020–30.

Ateshian, G., Lai, W., Zhu, W., and Mow, V. (1994). An asymptotic solution for the contact of two biphasic cartilage layers. *Journal of Biomechanics*, 27, 1347–60.

Ballmer, P. and Jakob, R. (1988). The non-operative treatment of isolated complete tears of the medial collateral ligament of the knee. A prospective study. *Archives of Orthopaedic and Trauma Surgery*, 107, 273–6.

Banes, A., Link, G., Bevin, A., et al. (1988). Tendon synovial cells secrete fibronectin *in vivo* and *in vitro*. *Journal of Orthopaedic Research*, 6, 73–82.

Barrack, R. and Skinner, H. (1990). The sensory function of knee ligaments. In *Knee ligaments, structure, function, injury and repair* (ed. D. Daniel, W. Akeson, and D. O'Connor). Raven Press, New York.

Barrack, R., Skinner, H., and Buckley, S. (1989). Proprioception in the anterior cruciate deficient knee. *American Journal of Sports Medicine*, 17, 1–6.

Beard, D., Kyberd, P., Fergusson, C., and Dodd, C. (1993). Proprioception after rupture of the anterior cruciate ligament. An objective indication of the need for surgery? *Journal of Bone and Joint Surgery, British Volume*, 75B, 311–15.

Beard, D., Dodd, C., Trundle, H., and Simpson, A. (1994). Proprioception enhancement for anterior cruciate ligament deficiency. A prospective randomised trial of two physiotherapy regimes. *Journal of Bone and Joint Surgery, British Volume*, 76B, 654–9.

Beer, S. (1992). Cognitive effects of mild head injury in children and adolescents. *Neuropsychology Review*, 3, 281.

Behrens, F. (1991). Fractures with soft tissue injuries. In *Skeletal trauma* (ed. B. Browner, J. Jupiter, A. Levine, and P. Trafton), pp. 311–37. W.B. Saunders, Philadelphia, PA.

Behrens, F. (1997). Fractures with soft tissue injuries. In *Skeletal trauma in children* (2nd edn) (ed. N. Green and M. Swiontkowski), pp. 103–19. W.B. Saunders Company, Philadelphia, PA.

Blenman, P., Carter, D., and Beaupre, G. (1989). Role of mechanical loading in the progressive ossification of a fracture callus. *Journal of Orthopaedic Research*, 7, 398–407.

Boulanger, B., Milzman, D., Mitchell, K., and Rodriguez, A. (1992). Body habitus as a predictor of injury pattern after blunt trauma. *Journal of Trauma*, 33, 228.

Branch, T., Hunter, R., and Donath, M. (1989). Dynamic EMG analysis of anterior cruciate deficient legs with and without bracing during cutting. *American Journal of Sports Medicine*, 17, 35–41.

Brighton, C. (1994). Fracture callus metabolism. In *Bone formation and repair* (ed. C. Brighton, G. Friedlaender, and J. Lane), pp. 167–84. American Academy of Orthopaedic Surgeons, Rosemont, IL

Brighton, C. and Hunt, R. (1991). Early histological and ultrastructural changes in medullary fracture callus. *Journal of Bone and Joint Surgery, American Volume*, 73A, 832–47.

Brighton, C., Fisher, J., Levine, S., et al. (1996). The biochemical pathway mediating the proliferative response of bone cells to a mechanical stimulus. *Journal of Bone and Joint Surgery, American Volume*, 78A, 1337–47.

Brittberg, M., Lindahl, A., Nilsson, A., Ohlsson, C., Isaksson, O., and

Peterson, L. (1994). Treatment of deep cartilage defects in the knee with autologus chondrocyte transplantation. *New England Journal of Medicine*, 331, 889–95.

Brookes, M. (1971). *The blood supply of bone: an approach to bone biology*. Butterworths, London.

Brushart, T. (1993). Motor axons preferentially reinnervate motor pathways. *Journal of Neuroscience*, 13, 2730–8.

Buckwalter, J. and Cooper, R. (1987). Bone structure and function. In *Instructional Course Lectures*, 36, 27–48.

Buckwalter, J. and Mow, V. (1992). Cartilage repair in osteoarthritis. In *Osteoarthritis: diagnosis and medical/surgical management* (ed. R. Moskowitz, D. Howell, V. Goldberg, and H. Mankin), pp. 71–107. W.B. Saunders, Philadelphia, PA.

Buckwalter, J., Maynard, J., and Vailas, A. (1987). Skeletal fibrous tissues: tendon, joint capsule, and ligament. In *The scientific basis of orthopaedics* (ed. J. Albright and R. Brand), Appleton and Lange, Norwalk, CT.

Buckwalter, J., Einhorn, T., Bolander, M., and Cruess, R. (1996). Healing of the musculoskeletal tissues. In *Rockwood and Green's fractures in adults* (4th edn) (ed. C. Rockwood, D. Green, R. Bucholz, and J. Heckman), pp. 261–302. Lippincott–Raven, Philadelphia, PA.

Burstein, A., Zika, J., Heiple, K., and Klein, L. (1975). Contribution of collagen and mineral to the elastic–plastic properties of bone. *Journal of Bone and Joint Surgery, American Volume*, 57A, 956–61.

Canalis, E., McCarthy, T., and Centrella, M. (1991). Growth factors and cytokines in bone cell metabolism. *Annual Review of Medicine*, 42, 17–24.

Carter, D., Blenman, P., and Beaupre, G. (1988). Correlations between mechanical stress history and tissue differentiation in initial fracture healing. *Journal of Orthopaedic Research*, 6, 736–48.

Caruso, R.P., Jara, D.I., and Swan, K.G. (1999). Gunshot wounds: caliber is increasing. *Journal of Trauma*, 46, 462–5.

Charnley, J. (1961). *The closed treatment of common fractures* (3rd edn), p. 14. Churchill Livingstone, Edinburgh.

Chidgey, L., Chakkalakal, D., Blotchky, A., and Connolly, J. (1986). Vascular reorganization and return of rigidity in fracture healing. *Journal of Orthopaedic Research*, 4, 173–9.

Coletti, J., Jr, Akeson, W., and Woo, S. (1972). A comparison of the physical behavior of normal articular cartilage and the arthroplasty surface. *Journal of Bone and Joint Surgery, American Volume*, 54A, 147–60.

Committee on Trauma, American College of Surgeons (1993a). *Advanced trauma life support: course for physicians*. American College of Surgeons, Chicago, IL.

Committee on Trauma, American College of Surgeons (1993b). *Resources for optimal care of the injured patient: 1993*. American College of Surgeons, Chicago, IL.

Cook, P. and Lubbers, L. (1996). Neurorraphy at the forearm level. In *Techniques in hand surgery* (ed. W. Blair), pp. 386–97. Williams and Wilkins, Baltimore, MD

Cook, S., Wolfe, M., and Salkeid, S. (1995). Effect of recombinant human osteogenic protein-1 on healing of segmental defects in non-human primates. *Journal of Bone and Joint Surgery, American Volume*, 77A, 734–50.

Cooper, R. and Misol, S. (1970). Tendon and ligament insertions: a light and electron microscopic study. *Journal of Bone and Joint Surgery, American Volume*, 52A, 1–21.

Corrigan, J., Cashman, W., and Brady, M. (1992). Proprioception in the cruciate deficient knee. *Journal of Bone and Joint Surgery, British Volume*, 74B, 247–50.

Cruess, R. and Dumont, J. (1975). Fracture healing. *Canadian Journal of Surgery*, 18, 403–13.

Currey, J. (1969). Changes in the impact energy absorption of bone with age. *Journal of Biomechanics*, 2, 1–11.

Dahners, L., Banes, A., and Burridge, K. (1986). The relationship of actin to ligament contraction. *Clinical Orthopaedics*, 210, 246–51.

Dellon, A., Curtis, R., and Edgerton, M. (1971). Reduction of sensation in the hand following nerve injury. *Journal of Bone and Joint Surgery, American Volume*, **53A**, 813.

Douglas, L., Jackson, S., and Lindsay, W. (1967). The effects of dexamethasone, norethandrole, promethazine and a tension-relieving procedure on collagen synthesis in healing flexor tendons as estimated by tritiated proline uptake studies. *Canadian Journal of Surgery*, **40**, 36–46.

Einhorn, T. (1992). Clinical applications of recombinant gene technology: bone and cartilage repair. *Cell Materials*, **2**, 1–11.

Einhorn, T. (1994). Enhancement of fracture healing by molecular or physical means: an overview. In *Bone formation and repair* (ed. C. Brighton, G. Friedlaender, and J. Lane), pp. 223–38. American Academy of Orthopaedic Surgeons, Rosemont, IL

Einhorn, T., Levine, B., and Michel, P. (1990). Nutrition and bone. *Orthopedic Clinics of North America*, **21**, 43–50.

Ellsasser, J., Reynolds, F., and Omohundro, J. (1974). The non-operative treatment of collateral ligament injuries of the knee in professional football players: an analysis of seventy-four injuries treated non-operatively and twenty-four injuries treated surgically. *Journal of Bone and Joint Surgery, American Volume*, **56A**, 1185–90.

Evans, L. (1988). Risk of fatality from physical trauma verses sex and age. *Journal of Trauma*, **28**, 368–78.

Eyre, D. (1984). Cross-linking in collagen and elastin. *Annual Review in Biochemistry*, **53**, 717–48.

Feliciano, D. (1996). Patterns of injury. In *Trauma* (ed. D. Feliciano, E. Moore, and K. Mattox), pp. 85–103. Appleton and Lange, Stamford, CT.

Finnegan, M. and Uhthoff, H. (1987). Healing of trabecular bone. In *Fracture healing* (ed. J. Lane). Churchill Livingstone, New York.

Forrester, J., Zederfeldt, B., Hayes, T., and Hunt, T. (1970). Wolff's law in relation to the healing skin wound. *Journal of Trauma*, **10**, 770–9.

Frank, C., Woo, S., Amiel, D., Harwood, F., Gomez, M., and Akeson, W. (1983). Medial collateral ligament healing. A multidisciplinary assessment in rabbits. *American Journal of Sports Medicine*, **11**, 379–89.

Frank, C., Amiel, D., Woo, S.-Y., and Akeson, W. (1985). Normal ligament properties and ligament healing. *Clinical Orthopaedics and Related Research*, **196**, 15–25.

Frank, C., Woo, S., Andriacchi, T., *et al.* (1988). Normal ligament: structure, function and composition. In *Injury and repair of the musculoskeletal soft tissues* (ed. S. Woo and J. Buckwalter), pp. 45–103. American Academy of Orthopaedic Surgeons, Park Ridge, IL.

Frank, C., MacFarlane, B., Edwards, P., *et al.* (1991*a*). A quantitative analysis of matrix alignment in ligament scars: a comparison of movement versus immobilization in an immature rabbit model. *Journal of Orthopaedic Research*, **9**, 219–227.

Frank, C., Shrive, N., Chimich, D., *et al.* (1991*b*). The effects of surface area and gap formation on medial collateral ligament healing. *Transactions of the Orthopaedic Research Society*, **16**, 138.

Freed, L., Grande, D., Lingbin, Z., Emmanual, J., Marquis, J., and Langer, R. (1994). Joint resurfacing using allograft chondrocytes and synthetic biodegradable scaffolds. *Journal of Biomedical Materials Research*, **28**, 891–9.

Freundlich, B., Bomalski, J., Neilson, E., and Jimenez, S. (1986). Regulation of fibroblast proliferation and collagen synthesis by cytokines. *Immunology Today*, **7**, 303–6.

Frykman, G. (1993). The quest for better recovery from peripheral nerve injury: current status of nerve regeneration research. *Journal of Hand Therapy*, **6**, 83–8.

Frykman, G., Wolf, A., and Coyle, T. (1981). An algorithm for management of peripheral nerve injuries. *Orthopedic Clinics of North America*, **12**, 239–44.

Fujita, M., Hukuda, S., and Doida, Y. (1992). The effect of constant direct electrical current on intrinsic healing in the flexor tendon *in vitro*. *Journal of Hand Surgery*, **17B**, 94–8.

Gaultieri, C. (1995). The problem of mild head injury. *Neuropsychiatry, Neuropsychology, and Behavioral Neurology*, **8**, 127–36.

Gelberman, R., Botte, M., Spiegelman, J., and Akeson, W. (1986). The excursion and deformation of repaired flexor tendons treated with protected early motion. *Journal of Hand Surgery*, **11A**, 106–10.

Gelberman, R., Goldberg, V., An, K.-N., and Banes, A. (1988). Tendon. In *Injury and repair of the musculoskeletal soft tissues* (ed. S.-Y. Woo and J. Buckwalter), pp. 5–40. American Academy of Orthopaedic Surgeons, Rosemont, IL.

Gelberman, R., Woo, S.-Y., Amiel, D., Horibe, S., and Lee, D. (1990). Influences of flexor sheath continuity and early motion on tendon healing in dogs. *Journal of Hand Surgery*, **15A**, 69–77.

Gerhart, T., Kirker-Head, C., Kriz, M., *et al.* (1993). Healing segmental femoral defects in sheep using recombinant human bone morphogenetic protein. *Clinical Orthopaedics and Related Research*, **293**, 317–26.

Ghez, C. and Sainburg, R. (1995). Proprioceptive control of interjoint coordination. *Canadian Journal of Physiology and Pharmacology*, **73**, 273–84.

Ghez, C., Gordon, J., and Ghilardi, M. (1995). Impairments of reaching movements in patients without proprioception. II. Effects of visual information on accuracy. *Journal of Neurophysiology*, **73**, 361–72.

Goldstein, M. (1990). Traumatic brain injury: a silent epidemic (editorial). *Annals of Neurology*, **27**, 327.

Gomez, M., Woo, S., Amiel, D., Harwood, F., Kitabayashi, L., and Matyas, J. (1991). The effects of increased tension on healing medial collateral ligaments. *American Journal of Sports Medicine*, **19**, 347–54.

Goodship, A. and Kenwright, J. (1985). The influence of induced micromovement upon the healing experimental tibial fractures. *Journal of Bone and Joint Surgery, British Volume*, **67B**, 650–5.

Gordon, J., Ghilardi, M., and Ghez, C. (1995). Impairments of reaching movements in patients without proprioception. I. Spatial errors. *Journal of Neurophysiology*, **73**, 347–60.

Gozna, E. and Harrington, I. (1982). *Biomechanics of musculoskeletal injury*. Williams and Wilkins, Baltimore, MD.

Grande, D., Pitman, M., Peterson, L., Menche, D., and Klein, M. (1989). The repair of experimentally produced defects in rabbit articular cartilage by autologous chondrocyte transplantation. *Journal of Orthopaedic Research*, **7**, 208–18.

Green, W. (1971). Behavior of articular chondrocytes in cell culture. *Clinical Orthopaedics*, **75**, 248–60.

Greenlee, T., Jr, and Pike, D. (1971). Studies of tendon healing in the rat. *Plastic and Reconstructive Surgery*, **48**, 260–70.

Hagberg, L. (1992). Exogenous hyaluronate as an adjunct in the prevention of adhesions after flexor tendon surgery: a controlled clinical study. *Journal of Hand Surgery*, **17A**, 132–6.

Hart, D. and Dahners, L. (1987). Healing of the medial collateral in rats. The effects of repair, motion and secondary stabilizing ligaments. *Journal of Bone and Joint Surgery, American Volume*, **69A**, 1194–9.

Hastings, D. (1980). Non-operative management of collateral ligament injuries of the knee joint. *Clinical Orthopaedics*, **147**, 22–8.

Ilizarov, G. (1989*a*). The tension-stress effect on the genesis and growth of tissues: Part I. The influence of stability of fixation and soft tissue preservation. *Clinical Orthopaedics*, **283**, 249–81.

Ilizarov, G. (1989*b*). The tension-stress effect on the genesis and growth of tissues: Part II. The influence of the rate and frequency of distraction. *Clinical Orthopaedics*, **283**, 249–81.

Indelicato, P. (1983). Non-operative management of collateral ligament injuries of the knee joint. *Journal of Bone and Joint Surgery, American Volume*, **65A**, 323–9.

Insall, J. (1974). The Pridie debridement operation for osteoarthritis of the knee. *Clinical Orthopaedics*, **101**, 61–7.

Jabaley, M. (1991). Electrical nerve stimulation in the awake patient. In *Operative nerve repair and reconstruction* (ed. R. Gelberman), pp. 241–57. Lippincott, Philadelphia, PA.

Jabaley, M., Wallace, W., and Heckler, F. (1980). Internal topography of major nerves of the forearm and hand: a current view. *Journal of Hand Surgery*, **5**, 1–18.

Jimenez, S., Yankowski, R., and Bashey, R. (1978). Identification of two new collagen alpha chains in extracts of lathyritic chick embryo tendons. *Biochemical and Biophysical Research Communications*, **81**, 1298–1306.

Johner, R. (1972). Knochenheilung in Abhangigkeit von der Defektgrosse. *Helvetica Chirurgica Acta*, **39**, 409–11.

Katz, J.L. (1981). Composite material models for cortical bone. In *Mechanical properties of bone* (ed. S.C. Cowin), pp. 171–84. American Society of Mechanical Engineers, New York.

Kenwright, J., Richardson, J., Cunningham, J., White, S., Goodship, A., Adams, M., Magnussen, P., and Newman, J. (1991). Axial movement and tibial fractures: a controlled randomised trial of treatment. *Journal of Bone and Joint Surgery, British Volume*, **73B**, 654–9.

Kraus, J., Rock, A., and Hemyari, P. (1990). Brain injuries among infants, children, adolescents, and young adults. *American Journal of Diseases of Children*, **144**, 684.

Kulick, M., Smith, S., and Hadler, K. (1986). Oral ibuprofen: evaluation of its effect on peritendinous adhesions and the breaking strength of a tenorrhaphy. *Journal of Hand Surgery*, **11A**, 110–20.

Lascombes, P., Membre, H., Prevot, J., and Barrat, E. (1991). Histomorphometrie du regenerat osseux dans les allongements des membres selon la technique d'Ilizarov. (Histomorphometry of bone regenerate in limb lengthening by the Ilizarov's technique). *Revue de Chirurgie Orthopedique et Reparatrice de l'Appareil Moteur*, **77**, 141–50.

Levin, H., Benton, A., and Grossman, R. (1982). *Neurobehavioral consequences of closed head injury.* Oxford University Press, New York.

Levy, A., Lohnes, J., Lintner, S., and Garret, W. (1996). Chondral delamination of the knee in soccer players. *American Journal of Sports Medicine*, **24**, 634–9.

Lin, G.-T., An, K.-N., Amadio, P., and Cooney, W., III (1988). Biomechanical studies of running suture for flexor tendon repair in dogs. *Journal of Hand Surgery*, **13A**, 553–8.

Lundborg, G. (1979). The intrinsic vascularization of human peripheral nerves: structural and functional aspects. *Journal of Hand Surgery*, **4**, 34–41.

Lundborg, G. and Dahlin, L. (1991). Structure and function of peripheral nerve. In *Operative nerve repair and reconstruction* (ed. R. Gelberman), pp. 3–18. Lippincott, Philadelphia, PA.

Lundborg, G. and Rank, F. (1978). Experimental intrinsic healing of flexor tendons based upon synovial fluid nutrition. *Journal of Hand Surgery*, **3**, 21–31.

Lundborg, G. and Rank, F. (1980). Experimental studies on cellular mechanisms involved in healing of animal and human flexor tendon in synovial environment. *Hand*, **12**, 3–11.

Lundborg, G., Rosen, B., Dahlin, L., Damielson, M., and Holmberg, J. (1997). Tubular versus conventional repair of median and ulnar nerves in the human forearm: early results from a prospective, randomized, clinical study. *Journal of Hand Surgery*, **22A**, 99–106.

Lyon, R., Akeson, W., Amiel, D., Kitabayashi, L., and Woo, S. (1991). Ultrastructural differences between the cells of the medial collateral and the anterior cruciate ligaments. *Clinical Orthopaedics and Related Research*, **272**, 279–86.

Mahalick, D., McDonough, M., and Levitt, J. (1995). Head injuries and their outcome: an overview. *Trauma*, **27**, 27–38.

Mahalick, D., Koller, C., and Pleim, E. (1996a). Pediatric trauma and head injury. *Trauma*, **38**, 39–56.

Mahalick, D., Molofsky, W., and Bartlett, J. (1996b). Psychopharmacological treatment of children with attention disorders acquired secondary to brain injury. *Journal of the International Neuropsychology Society*, **2**, 208.

Mankin, H. (1982). The response of articular cartilage to mechanical injury. *Journal of Bone and Joint Surgery, American Volume*, **64A**, 460–6.

Markel, M., Wikenheiser, M., and Chao, E. (1990). A study of fracture callus

material properties: relationship to the torsional strength of bone. *Journal of Orthopaedic Research*, **8**, 843–50.

Marotti, G. (1993). A new theory of bone lamellation. *Calcified Tissue International*, **53** (Supplement), S47–56.

Marotti, G. and Muglia, M. (1988). A scanning electron microscope study of human bony lamellae: proposal for a new model of collagen lamellar organization. *Archivio Italiano di Anatomia di Embriologia*, **93**, 163–75.

Matthews, L., Kaufer, J., and Sonstegard, D. (1974). Manual sensing of fracture stability: a biomechanical study. *Acta Orthopaedica Scandinavica*, **45**, 373–81.

Mayer, G. and Seidlein, H. (1988). Chondral and osteochondral fractures of the knee joint-treatment and results. *Archives of Orthopaedic Trauma Surgery*, **107**, 154–7.

Millesi, H., Meissl, G., and Berger, A. (1972). The interfascicular nerve-grafting of the median and ulnar nerves. *Journal of Bone and Joint Surgery, American Volume*, **54A**, 727–50.

Mink, J. and Deutsch, A. (1989). Occult cartilage and bone injuries of the knee: detection, classification and assesssment with MR imaging. *Radiology*, **170**, 823–9.

Müller, M., Allgöwer, M., Schneider, R., and Willenegger, H. (1991). Basic aspects of internal fixation. In *Manual of internal fixation. techniques recommended by the AO-ASIF group* (3rd edn) (ed. M. Allgöwer), pp. 1–158. Springer-Verlag, Berlin.

Murray, J. and Fitch, R. (1996). Distraction histiogenesis: principles and indications. *Journal of the American Academy of Orthopaedic Surgeons*, **4**, 317–27.

National Research Council Committee on Trauma Research (1985). Injury biomechanics research and the prevention of impact injury. *Injury in America: a continuing public health problem*, pp. 48–65. National Academy Press, Washington, DC.

Noyes, F. (1977). Functional properties of knee ligaments and alterations induced by immobilization: a correlative biomechanical and histological study in primates. *Clinical Orthopaedics*, **123**, 210–42.

O'Driscoll, S., Keeley, F., and Salter, R. (1988). Durability of regenerated articular cartilage produced by free autogenous periosteal grafts in major full thickness defects in joint surfaces under the influence of continuous passive motion: a follow up at one year. *Journal of Bone and Joint Surgery, American Volume*, **70A**, 595–606.

Ostrum, R., Chao, E., Bassett, C., *et al.* (1994). Bone injury, regeneration and repair. In *Orthopaedic basic science* (ed. S. Simon), pp. 279–323. American Academy of Orthopaedic Surgeons, Rosemont, IL.

Paley, D., Rumley, T., Jr, and Kovelman, H. (1991). The Ilizarov technique: a method to regenerate bone and soft tissue. *Advances in Plastic and Reconstructive Surgery*, **7**, 1–40.

Perren, S. (1979). Physical and biological aspects of fracture healing with special reference to internal fixation. *Clinical Orthopaedics and Related Research*, **138**, 175–96.

Peterson, W., Manske, P., Dunlap, J., Horwitz, D., and Kahn, B. (1990). Effect of various methods of restoring flexor sheath integrity on the formation of adhesions after tendon injury. *Journal of Hand Surgery*, **15A**, 48–56.

Potenza, A. (1963). Critical evaluation of flexor tendon healing and adhesion formation within artificial digital sheaths. *Journal of Bone and Joint Surgery, American Volume*, **45A**, 1217–33.

Presswalla, F. (1978). The pathophysics and pathomechanics of trauma. *Medicine, Science and the Law*, **18**, 239.

Radin, E., Ehrlich, M., Chernack, R., Abernathy, P., and Rose, R. (1978). Effect of repetitive impulsive loading on the knee joints of rabbits. *Clinical Orthopaedics*, **131**, 288–93.

Rahn, B., Gallinaro, P., Baltensperger, A., and Perren, S. (1971). Primary bone healing. An experimental study in the rabbit. *Journal of Bone and Joint Surgery, American Volume*, **53A**, 783–6.

Reilly, D. and Burstein, A. (1975). The elastic and ultimate properties of compact bone tissue. *Journal of Biomechanics*, **8**, 393–405.

Rivara, J., Jaffe, K., Kay, G., *et al.* (1993). Family functioning and injury severity as predictors of child functioning one year following traumatic brain injury. *Archives of Physical Medicine and Rehabilitation*, **74**, 1047–55.

Rowe, R. (1985). The structure of rat tail tendon. *Connective Tissue Research*, **14**, 9–20.

Rudolph, R. (1980). Contraction and the control of contraction. *World Journal of Surgery*, **4**, 279–87.

Ruff, R., Baser, C.A., Johnson, J., *et al.* (1987). Neuropsychological rehabilitiation: an experimental study with head-injured patients. *Journal of Clinical and Experimental Neuropsychology*, **9**, 55.

Sarmiento, A., Schaeffer, J., Beckerman, L., Latta, L., and Enis, J. (1977). Fracture healing in rat femora as affected by functional weight-bearing. *Journal of Bone and Joint Surgery, American Volume*, **59A**, 369–75.

Savage, R. (1985). *In vitro* studies of a new method of flexor tendon repair. *Journal of Hand Surgery*, **10B**, 135–41.

Schatzker, J., Waddell, J., and Stoll, J. (1989). The effects of motion on the healing of cancellous bone. *Clinical Orthopaedics and Related Research*, **245**, 282–7.

Schenk, R. (1992). Biology of fracture repair. In *Skeletal trauma* (ed. B. Browner, J. Jupiter, A. Levine, and P. Trafton), pp. 31–75. W.B. Saunders, Philadelphia, PA.

Schenk, R. and Gachter, A. (1994). Histology of distraction osteogenesis. In *Bone formation and repair* (ed. C. Brighton, G. Friedlaender, and J. Lane), pp. 387–94. American Academy of Orthopaedic Surgeons, Rosemont, IL.

Schenk, R. and Hunziker, E. (1994). Histological and ultrastructural features of fracture healing. In *Bone formation and repair* (ed. C. Brighton, G. Friedlaender, and J. Lane), pp. 117–41. American Academy of Orthopaedic Surgeons, Rosemont, IL.

Schenk, R. and Willenegger, H. (1963). Zum histologischen Bild der sogenannten Primarheilung der Knochenkompakta nach experimentellen Osteotomien am Hund. *Experientia*, **19**, 593–5.

Schenk, R. and Willenegger, H. (1967). Morphological findings in primary fracture healing: sallus formation. *Simposia Biologica Hungarica*, **7**, 75–80.

Schultz, R., Miller, D., Kerr, C., and Micheli, L. (1984). Mechanoreceptors in human cruciate ligaments. A histological study. *Journal of Bone and Joint Surgery, American Volume*, **66A**, 1072–6.

Seddon, H. (1943). Three types of nerve injury. *Brain*, **66**, 237–88.

St Onge, R., Weiss, C., Denlinger, J., and Balazs, E. (1980). A preliminary assessment of Na-hyaluronate injection into 'no man's land' for primary flexor tendon repair. *Clinical Orthopaedics and Related Research*, **146**, 269–75.

Steinberg, D. and Koman, L. (1991). Factors affecting the results of peripheral nerve repair. In *Operative nerve repair and reconstruciton* (ed. R. Gelberman), pp. 349–64. Lippincott, New York.

Stirling, R. (1932). Healing of fractured bones: report of investigation into process of healing of fractured bones, with some clinical applications. *Transactions of the Royal Medical and Chirurgical Society of Edinburgh*, **46**, 206–28.

Strickland, J. (1995*a*). Flexor tendon injuries. I: Foundations of treatment. *Journal of the Americal Academy of Orthopaedic Surgeons*, **3**, 22–54.

Strickland, J. (1995*b*). Flexor tendon injuries: II. Operative technique. *Journal of the Americal Academy of Orthopaedic Surgeons*, **3**, 55–62.

Sunderland, S. (1951). A classification of peripheral nerve injuries producing loss of function. *Brain*, **74**, 491–516.

Sunderland, S. (1991). *Nerve injuries and their repair. a critical appraisal.* Churchill Livingstone, New York.

Swan, K. and Swan, R. (1989). *Gunshot wounds: pathophysiology and management* (2nd edn). Yearbook Medical, Chicago, IL.

Swan, K. and Swan, R. (1991). Principles of ballistics applicable to the treatment of gunshot wounds. *Surgical Clinics of North America*, **71**, 221–39.

Szabo, R. and Madison, M. (1993). Principles of nerve repair. In *Operative orthopaedics* (ed. M. Chapman and M. Madison), pp. 1411–17. Lippincott Company, Philadelphia, PA.

Takai, S., Woo, S.-Y., Horibe, S., Tung, D., and Gelberman, R. (1991). The effects of frequency and duration of controlled passive mobilization on tendon healing. *Journal of Orthopaedic Research*, **9**, 705–13.

Teasdale, G. and Jennet, B. (1976*a*). Assessment of coma and impaired consciousness: a practical scale. *Lancet*, **ii**, 81–3.

Teasdale, G. and Jennet, B. (1976*b*). Assessment prognosis of coma after head injury. *Acta Neurochirurgica (Wein)*, **34**, 45–55.

Tencer, A. and Johnson, K. (1994). *Biomechanics in orthopedic trauma.* Lippincott, Philadelphia, PA.

Tetsworth, K. and Paley, D. (1995). Basic science of distraction histogenesis. *Current Opinion in Orthopaedics*, **6**, 61–8.

Tipton, C., James, S., Mergner, W., and Tcheng, T. (1970). Influence of exercise on strength of medial collateral knee ligaments of dogs. *Americal Journal of Physiology*, **218**, 894–902.

Tonna, E. and Cronkite, E. (1963). The periosteum: autoradiographic studies on cellular proliferation and transformation utilizing tritiated thymidine. *Clinical Orthopaedics and Related Research*, **30**, 218–32.

Tzeng, S., Swan, K., and Rush, B. (1981). Bullets: a source of infection? *American Surgeon*, **48**, 239–40.

Uhthoff, H. and Rahn, B. (1981). Healing patterns of metaphyseal fractures. *Clinical Orthopaedics and Related Research*, **760**, 295–303.

Uhthoff, H., Foux, A., Yeadon, A., McAuley, J., and Black, R. (1993). Two processes of bone remodeling in plated intact femora: an experimental study in dogs. *Journal of Orthopaedic Research*, **11**, 78–91.

Urist, M., Sato, K., Brownell, A., *et al.* (1983). Human bone morphogenetic protein (hBMP). *Proceedings for the Society for Experimental Biology and Medicine*, **173**, 194–9.

Vacanti, C., Kim, W., Schloo, B., Upton, J., and Vacanti, J. (1994). Joint resurfacing with cartilage grown *in situ* from cell polymer structures. *American Journal of Sports Medicine*, **22**, 485–8.

Vailas, A., Tipton, C., Matthes, R., and Gart, M. (1981). Physical activity and its influence on the repair process of medial collateral ligaments. *Connective Tissue Research*, **9**, 25–31.

Violence Prevention Task Force (Eastern Association for the Surgery of Trauma) (1995). Violence in America: a public health crisis. *Journal of Trauma*, **38**, 163–8.

Vogel, H. (1978). Influence of maturation and age on mechanical and biochemical parameters of connective tissue of various organs in the rat. *Connective Tissue Research*, **6**, 161–6.

Weiss, J., Woo, S.-Y., Ohland, K., Horibe, S., and Newton, P. (1991). Evaluation of a new injury model to study medial collateral ligament healing: primary repair versus nonoperative treatment. *Journal of Orthopaedic Research*, **9**, 516–28.

White, A., III, Panjabi, M., and Southwick, W. (1977). The four biomechanical stages of fracture repair. *Journal of Bone and Joint Surgery, American Volume*, **59A**, 188–92.

Wilgis, E. and Brushart, T. (1993). Nerve repair and grafting. In *Operative hand surgery* (ed. D. Green and R. Hotchkiss), pp. 1315–40. Churchill Livingstone, New York.

Wolff, J. (1892). *Das Gesetz der Transformation der Knochen.* Hirschwalk, Berlin.

Woo, S.-Y., Gomez, M., Amiel, D., Ritter, M., Gelberman, R., and Akeson, W. (1981). The effects of exercise on the biomechanical and biochemical properties of swine digital flexor tendons. *Journal of Biomechanical Engineering*, **103**, 51–6.

Woo, S.-Y., Gomez, M., Woo, Y.-K., and Akeson, W. (1982). Mechanical properties of tendons and ligaments. II: The relationships of immobilization and exercise on tissue remodeling. *Biorheology*, **19**, 397–408.

Woo, S.-Y., Gomez, M., Sites, T., Newton, P., Orlando, C., and Akeson, W. (1987). The biomechanical and morphological changes in the medial collateral ligament of the rabbit after immobilization and remobilization. *Journal of Bone and Joint Surgery, American Volume*, **69A**, 1200–11.

Woo, S.-Y., Peterson, R., Ohland, K., Sites, T., and Danto, M. (1990). The effects of strain rate on the properties of the medial collateral ligament in skeletally immature and mature rabbits: a biomechanical and histological study. *Journal of Orthopaedic Research*, **8**, 712–21.

Woo, S.-Y., Hollis, J., and Adams, D. (1991). Tensile properties of the human femur–anterior cruciate ligament–tibia complex: the effects of specimen age and orientation. *American Journal Sports Medicine*, **19**, 217–25.

Wozney, J. (1993). Bone morphogenetic proteins and their gene expression. In *Cellular and molecular biology of bone* (ed. M. Noda), pp. 131–67. Academic Press, Orlando, FL.

Yang, K.-H., Parvizi, J., Wang, S.-J., *et al.* (1996). Exposure to low-intensity ultrasound increases aggrecan gene expression in a rat femur fracture model. *Journal of Orthopaedic Research*, **14**, 802–9.

Zeitlow, S., Capizzi, P., and Bannon, M. (1994). Multisystem geriatric trauma. *Journal of Trauma*, **37**, 985–8.

1.7.2   The evidence for thromboprophylaxis

Christopher Bulstrode

Most elective orthopedic operations are concerned with improving quality of life. No patient should die as a result of such an operation. This chapter looks critically at the evidence available for the cause of death after elective orthopedic operations. At the moment most of the evidence is available on total hip replacement and to a lesser extent on total knee replacement. Both serve to highlight the difficulties of this type of work, and emphasize the care which needs to be taken in drawing conclusions from small studies.

Death rate after total hip replacement

The original reports on death rates after total hip replacement included a study of 62 patients which reported a death rate of 3.4 per cent—a total of two patients (Coventry *et al.* 1974). This study is commonly reported in the introduction to studies on thromboprophylaxis as 'conventional wisdom'. The actual death rate after total hip replacement has been calculated from some very large epidemiologic studies, one based on over 10 000 consecutive cases and the other on an opportunist meta-analysis of over 100 000 cases. The total death rate comes out at a level of around 5 per thousand (0.5 per cent) cases in the first 30 days after surgery (Seagroatt *et al.* 1991; Murray *et al.* 1996). Incidentally, there is no evidence of a peak in deaths shortly after discharge from hospital (a popular misconception); the risk falls steadily from the day of surgery, and is not significantly raised after 30 days.

Cause of death after total hip replacement

Most deaths occurring after total hip replacement receive a postmortem (in the United Kingdom at least) so it is normal for the cause of death to be based on postmortem findings. Even so the cause of death is not always as clear as it appears to be when reported

Box 1   Death rate after total hip replacement in unprotected patients

- Overall deaths in 30 days approximately 5 per 1000
- Death rate from pulmonary embolus around 5 per 10 000
- The rate falls steadily from day 1 and reaches baseline by 30 days

in the literature. Over the past few years there has been a dramatic increase in interest in pulmonary embolus after total hip replacement because of the heavy advertising of new antithrombotic drugs. There has been an associated rise in the number of pulmonary emboli reported in patients dying after total hip replacement despite the fact that the proportion of patients receiving thromboprophylaxis after surgery has increased and the overall death rate has not changed. The most logical explanation for this apparent paradox was first pointed out in the early 1950s when it was noted that the finding of pulmonary embolus in patients dying in hospital from whatever cause was very high indeed (over 70 per cent). The more carefully that emboli were searched for, the more commonly they were found (Morrell and Dunnill 1968). These emboli tend to be small and are clearly not the cause of death even if they are put down on the death certificate as a subsidiary finding. They may in fact be part of the physiologic mechanism of clearing clot after trauma. Emboli that break off a resolving thrombus are naturally trapped in the lung and then removed. If the lung did not serve this function as a blood filter then emboli might end up lodged in the brain with much more serious consequences. Giving patients thromboprophylaxis for what may under normal circumstances be a normal physiologic process may at best be valueless and at worst positively damaging to a normal healing process.

Box 2

- Prevalence of small non-fatal pulmonary emboli in hospital patients is up to 70 per cent
- Death certificates may not give a clear guide to change in prevalence
- Small pulmonary emboli may be a normal physiologic process
- The most common cause of death after total hip replacement is myocardial infarct and stroke

In the study of 10 000 hips, the most common causes of death by far were myocardial infarct and stroke. Pulmonary embolus was only given as a cause of death in 10 per cent of cases. Even if this is an underestimate, the death rate from pulmonary embolus cannot be higher than the overall death rate which is itself only 5 per 1000, so the truth probably lies somewhere between 0.05 and 0.5 per cent, and is probably closer to 5 per 10 000 than 5 per 1000.

Factors affecting death rate

If there is an effect of thromboprophylaxis on the death rate from pulmonary embolus or early mobilization after total hip replacement, it is very small and is likely to be around 1 per 10 000 (25 per cent of 0.05 per cent). This low figure is very important for several reasons.

The first is that any study of the benefit of thromboprophylaxis on death rate will need to involve a randomized controlled trial with many tens of thousands of patients in each arm of the study. Any trial aimed at answering this question would be very expensive indeed and logically almost impossible to perform.

The second important issue is that pulmonary embolus may only be responsible for 10 per cent of the deaths after total hip replacement. We know that anticoagulation can have a profound effect on rates of myocardial infarction and stroke, the two major causes of death after total hip replacement. Even if this effect is only one-tenth as large as the effect on rates of pulmonary embolus, then its effect on overall death rate will be as much a result of its effect on myocardial infarction and stroke as on pulmonary embolus. It will therefore be necessary to study overall death rates as well as death from pulmonary embolus in isolation if we are to understand if thromboprophylaxis saves lives.

The third important implication is that because the overall death rate is actually much lower than previously reported, the maximum potential benefit of thromboprophylaxis will be so small that any risks involved (and risks there must be) will be of a proportionately much greater importance than previously thought. If the potential benefits are large, and they would be if the death rate in unprotected patients was 2 to 5 per cent, then the risks (if small) are unimportant. If, however, the benefits are small then small risks must also be measured, as the benefits must now be weighed against these risks. A study measuring both risks and benefits is much more complex and expensive to organize, and to date none has been attempted.

Relationship of deep vein thrombosis to pulmonary embolism

Below-knee deep vein thrombosis is very common after total hip replacement, occurring in 20 to 80 per cent of unprotected patients (depending on how this is measured). Deep vein thrombosis is therefore common and relatively easy to diagnose. It therefore makes an excellent surrogate endpoint for studies of thromboprophalaxis, and indeed small studies of thromboprophylaxis routinely show highly statistically significant reductions in the incidence of below-knee deep vein thrombosis after total hip replacement. The numbers needed for such a trial are so small that significant numbers of complications are not demonstrated but the efficacy of thromboprophylaxis in preventing deep vein thrombosis can be demonstrated (an ideal situation for a commercial organization wishing to sell a product). The problem is that the high rate of deep vein thrombosis does not appear to be associated with a high death rate. This surrogate outcome is apparently clinically irrelevant, a fact that has conveniently escaped the notice of the pharmaceutical industry and those who do research for them.

Measures that could be taken and likely efficacy

There is as yet no clear evidence that chemical anticoagulation reduces either death from pulmonary embolus or even the overall death rate after total hip replacement or total knee replacement. Equally, there is no evidence that either above- or below-knee elasticated stockings make any difference. Recently there have been strong claims for the calf and the foot pumps again based on a reduction of deep vein thrombosis rates. Once again it has not yet proved possible to perform a study large enough to measure a fall in death rate. The reduction in calf deep vein thromboses may simply mean that the pump has squeezed them all out!

It has been suggested that reducing the prevalence of deep vein thrombosis after total hip replacement will reduce the risk of postphlebitic limb. Those units with a vested interest in thromboprophylaxis research claim that they have indeed found this to be the case. Those with no vested interest have found the exact opposite. The surprise is that no properly constructed prospective trial has been performed to address this issue.

In summary, the death rate after total hip replacement is much lower than previously quoted. Any trial to test the value of thromboprophylaxis will have to be very large, look at overall death rate and measure all complications as well. Given that a trial of adequate size is unlikely to be feasible given the risk levels involved, the evidence-based surgeon will not use any thromboprophylaxis, chemical or mechanical. He or she has no idea how much good it will do (except that it cannot be much), nor how much harm.

Box 3 Benefit analysis of thromboprophylaxis

- Thromboprophylaxis is unlikely to reduce death rate by more than 1 per 10 000

- The trial size needed to demonstrate this effect is over 100 000 patients in each arm

- Death from stroke and myocardial infarction is 10 times more common than that from pulmonary embolism

- Thromboprophylaxis will affect these, so overall death rate must be studied

- The complications will need to be balanced against any benefit

- Deep vein thrombosis is a poor outcome measure for studying thromboprophylaxis

- There is no evidence for benefit of mechanical or chemical prophylaxis

References

Coventry, M.B., Beckenbaugh, R.D., Nolan, D.R., and Ilstrup, D.M. (1974). 2,012 total hip arthroplasties: a study of postoperative course and early complications. *Journal of Bone and Joint Surgery, American Volume*, **56A**, 273–84.

Morrell, M.T. and Dunnill, M.S. (1968). *British Journal of Surgery*, 55, 347–52.

Murray, D.W., Britton, A., and Bulstrode, C.J. (1996). Thrombo-prophylaxis and death after total hip replacement. *Journal of Bone and Joint Surgery, British Volume*, 78B, 863–70.

Seagroatt, V., Tan, H.S., Goldacre, M., Bulstrode, C.J.K., and Nugent, I. (1991). Elective total hip replacement: incidence, emergency readmission rate, and postoperative mortality. *British Medical Journal*, **303**, 1431–5.

1.8   Hemoglobinopathies

Paul L. F. Giangrande

Introduction

Hemoglobinopathies are inherited disorders of hemoglobin resulting from synthesis of abnormal hemoglobin molecules. In general, these conditions are encountered in people originating from tropical or subtropical areas, and it is believed that these conditions originally developed to confer protection against malaria. Although the management of these disorders is primarily the province of the hematologist, these conditions may be accompanied by orthopedic and other surgical complications. It is also important for surgeons to have an appreciation of the serious medical problems which can arise in these conditions, particularly since surgery may actually precipitate medical problems.

Sickle cell disease

This condition is due to a single mutation in the β-globin chain of the hemoglobin molecule: valine is substituted for glutamic acid at position 136. The abnormal hemoglobin is unstable and forms precipitates within the erythrocyte due to polymerization when deoxygenated. The gene is encountered predominantly in people of African-Caribbean origin, among whom the gene frequency may be as high as 5 per cent. The gene is also found with a lower frequency amongst people of the Mediterranean, Middle East, and Indian subcontinent. Carriers of this condition have no clinical problems, but homozygotes are prone to recurrent episodes of painful 'crises'. Often there is no obvious precipitating cause, but it is recognized that infections, dehydration, and exposure to cold or low levels of oxygen can provoke crises. These painful crises are due to intramedullary necrosis following occlusion of small vessels. The most frequently involved areas are the knee, lumbosacral spine, elbow, and femur. Less often the ribs, sternum, clavicles, calcaneus, and facial bones are affected. Involvement of the facial bones may be associated with impressive facial swelling. Joint effusions are commonly seen when the knees or elbows are involved. The course of sickle cell disease is variable and many patients may lead essentially normal lives punctuated by only occasional painful crises. However, in others the course can be much more serious with recurrent strokes such that bone marrow transplantation may be required in some cases of sickle cell disease (Walters *et al.* 1996). Crises in bones and joints should be treated conservatively, with bed rest, maintenance of good fluid balance, and correction of hypoxia if the lungs are affected.

Crises can be extremely painful, and opiate analgesics are often needed. Extensive sickling within the lungs can be life-threatening ('chest crisis'). This can initially present with cough, fever, and pleuritic chest pain, and a chest radiograph will show extensive infiltration of either one or both lung fields (Fig. 1).

Adults with sickle cell anemia typically have a chronic hemolytic anemia, with a hemoglobin level typically in the range of 7 to 10 g/dl. The blood film is characteristic with numerous hyperchromatic and irreversibly sickled cells (which are evident even in the absence of clinical sickling), target cells, and normoblasts (primitive nucleated red cells). The chronic hemolytic process results in consumption of folic acid, and oral supplementation is often required. Parvovirus infection in young children with sickle cell disease, and other hemolytic anemias, can trigger the onset of a profound but transient drop in the hemoglobin level ('aplastic crisis').

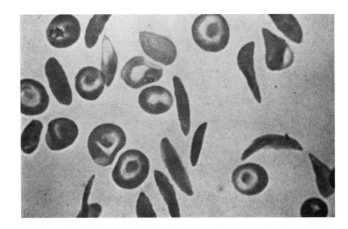

Fig. 1. Peripheral blood film from a patient with sickle cell anemia, showing the typical hyperchromatic sickled cells as well as target cells.

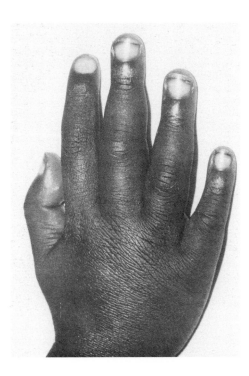

Fig. 2. Dactylitis in a young child with sickle cell disease. This is often the first manifestation of sickle cell disease, and may affect the toes as well as the fingers. In this case, the middle finger is tender, hot, and swollen.

Fetal hemoglobin (**HbF**) is composed of paired α- and γ-chains, but by approximately 6 months of age production of β-chains replaces that of fetal γ-chains and the first symptoms of the condition appear.

Dactylitis ('hand–foot syndrome') is often the first manifestation of the condition. The digits of the hand or feet become painful, swollen, hot, and tender due to sickling within the bone. There are usually no radiologic changes during the acute episode, although subperiosteal bone formation may be seen a couple of weeks afterwards. Permanent shortening of the digits may occasionally result (Fig. 2). Children born with sickle cell anemia have a normal birth weight, but often exhibit delayed growth (reflected by delayed bone age on radiologic examination) and delayed onset of sexual maturation.

Avascular necrosis of the hip is a not infrequent complication in adolescents as well as adults, and may be bilateral (Milner *et al.* 1991). The risk is particularly high in individuals with hemoglobin SC disease, and this is believed to reflect the fact that these patients tend to have higher hemoglobin concentrations and thus the whole blood viscosity is higher. Total hip replacement may certainly be carried out, but the general condition of the patient must be thoroughly evaluated in order to avoid postoperative complications (Bishop *et al.* 1988). Furthermore, the revision rate is quite high in these patients, as the poor quality of the bone may result in early loosening of the prostheses (Clarke *et al.* 1989). Core decompression of the femoral head may be of value in early cases (Camp and Colwell 1986). Osteonecrosis may also occur in other joints, such as the shoulder (Milner *et al.* 1993).

Repeated episodes of splenic infarction leads to loss of immune function with particular susceptibility to capsulated bacteria. Patients with sickle cell anemia are particularly vulnerable to pneumococcal

Box 2 Manifestations of sickle cell disease

- Dactylitis (hand–foot syndrome)
- Avascular necrosis of hip/shoulder
- Splenic infarct leads to poor immunity
- *Salmonella* osteomyelitis is common

infections, and vaccination against both *Pneumococcus pneumoniae* and *Haemophilus influenzae* as well as continuous prophylactic penicillin are important measures. Osteomyelitis due to *Salmonella* is also a recognized complication of sickle cell disease (Ortiz-Neu *et al.* 1978), involving the bones of the leg and axial skeleton in particular. Blood cultures may yield positive results, but needle aspiration of suspicious lesions is often required and presumptive antibiotic therapy should not be started until diagnostic procedures have been carried out. There is a significant risk of vaso-occlusive stroke in patients with sickle cell anemia, which may present as sudden onset of seizures, coma, visual disturbances, or hemiplegia. Gallstones formed from aggregates of bilirubin often form in sickle cell anemia, as in other chronic hemolytic anemias, and this may present as acute onset of abdominal pain. Leg ulcers are not infrequent in older patients, and tend to develop over the medial and lateral malleoli. These tend to heal very slowly, if at all, and skin grafts may be required. Early treatment of injuries to the area may prevent the development of such ulcers. Repeated infarction within the hypertonic environment of the renal medulla often results in recurrent episodes of painless hematuria.

Eventually, the ability to concentrate urine is impaired, and therefore patients are prone to dehydration. Thus it is vital that particular attention be paid to fluid balance in patients with sickle cell anemia who are admitted to hospital for any reason, particularly after surgery when oral fluid intake may be restricted.

Surgery in patients with sickle cell anemia

Elective surgery in patients with sickle cell disease is generally safe when performed by a multidisciplinary team, but it must be appreciated that despite optimal care there is a significant risk of perioperative complications, such as precipitation of a sickling crisis (including acute chest syndrome or stroke), infection, or serious transfusion reactions. Patients with sickle cell disease tend not to require regular transfusions to maintain a stable hemoglobin level, and there is no evidence that preoperative transfusion or exchange transfusion before surgery reduces the risk of perioperative complications (Vichinsky *et al.* 1995). If these patients do require a blood transfusion for any reason, it should be borne in mind that they are at particular risk of developing red cell antibodies after repeated transfusions (particularly against Kell and Duffy antigens) because of their different ethnic origin from the general donor population. Therefore screening for such antibodies is particularly important before surgery to ensure that compatible blood is made available in case it is required. Filtered blood should be used to reduce the risk of development of antibodies directed against leukocyte antigens, which may result in serious allergic reactions. Certain measures can be taken in the setting of surgery to minimize the risk of provoking a sickle crisis.

A tourniquet can be applied in procedures that require a bloodless field. The repeated postoperative use of a spirometer appears to reduce the risk of pulmonary complications, such as atelectasis or infection, presumably by promoting aeration throughout the lungs (Bellet *et al.* 1995).

Thalassemia

The thalassemias are a group of hematologic disorders in which a defect in the synthesis of one or more of the globin polypeptide chains is present, resulting in the formation of unstable aggregates of globin chains within erythrocyte precursors which are prematurely destroyed. A full classification of the thalassemias is beyond the scope of this chapter, but the principal division is between disorders involving the α- and β-chains of the hemoglobin molecule. The prevalence of the genes for thalassemia is particularly high in Mediterranean countries (particularly Greece, Italy, Cyprus, and North Africa), the Middle East, the Indian subcontinent, and Southeast Asia. Carriers of β-thalassemia, the most common form in European countries, have no clinical problems, apart from a mild and persistent microcytic anemia with a hemoglobin typically in the range from 10 to 12 g/dl. However, they are at risk of having severely affected children with β-thalassemia major if their partner is also a carrier, and so many countries with a high prevalence of the gene have developed screening programs to identify carriers.

Clinical and laboratory features

Severe anemia becomes apparent at 3 to 6 months of age in β-thalassemia major, and this is accompanied by massive enlargement of the liver and spleen due to both excessive red cell destruction and extramedullary erythropoiesis. Examination of the blood film shows severe hypochromic microcytic anemia with reticulocytosis. Normoblasts, target cells, and basophilic stippling of erythrocytes are also seen. Hemoglobin electrophoresis is required for definitive diagnosis, and the hallmark of β-thalassemia major is the absence of normal hemoglobin A, which is replaced by HbF and some HbA_2.

Skeletal changes in thalassemia

In the absence of treatment with regular blood transfusions, there is marked expansion of the bone marrow to compensate for the ineffective erythropoiesis. This is associated with both osteoporosis and

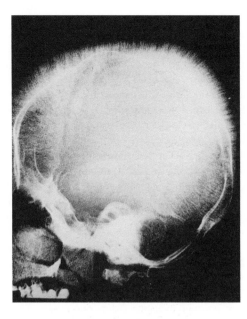

Fig. 3. Skull radiograph of a patient with severe thalassemia. The typical 'hair-on-end' appearance is due to widening of the diploë which contains hypercellular marrow.

thinning of the cortex in the bones, which can result in pathologic fractures. Striking features in untreated children include prominence of the parietal and frontal bones and protrusion of the maxillary bones, leading to malocclusion of teeth and orthodontic problems. Radiographs of the skull show a characteristic 'hair-on-end' appearance due to widening of the diploë (Fig. 3). Premature fusion of the epiphyses of the long bones, particularly the epiphyses of the proximal humerus, can result in shortening of the arms (Currarino and Erlandson 1964). Very occasionally, expansion of the hemopoietic tissue within spinal vertebrae leads to extrusion of marrow into the paravertebral area which can result in spinal cord compression. Decompressive laminectomy or even radiotherapy have been used in such cases to prevent permanent paralysis (Sorsdahl *et al.* 1964; Issaragrisil *et al.* 1981). Compression fractures of the vertebrae may also be seen.

Medical complications

Somewhat paradoxically, many of the serious medical complications seen in thalassemia actually result from treatment of the condition. In contrast with sickle cell disease, people with β-thalassemia may require regular blood transfusions. A program of regular transfusions to maintain a hemoglobin level of 10 g/dl will lead to regression of hepatosplenomegaly and skeletal changes. The skeletal changes described above are therefore unlikely to be seen by orthopedic surgeons working in developed countries, where children are adequately treated from an early age. The use of fresh blood, filtered to remove leukocytes, is associated with both better red cell survival and reduced incidence of serious allergic reactions to leukocyte antigens. As with sickle cell disease, oral supplements of folic acid should also be given. Splenectomy may occasionally be needed to reduce the requirement for blood transfusions, but this should be delayed until the patient is at least 6 years old because of the high risk of pneumococcal and other bacterial infections earlier in life. Pneumococcal vaccine should be given preoperatively in such cases, and prophylactic penicillin (250 mg twice daily) will be required for life after splenectomy. Patients should also be vaccinated against *H. influenzae.*

Regular transfusion eventually leads to iron overload, with deposition of iron in the form of hemosiderin in the tissues resulting in fibrosis. Iron overload may thus result in serious medical complications such as diabetes mellitus, cirrhosis, and cardiac complications such as arrhythmias or congestive cardiac failure. Subcutaneous infusions of the chelating agent desferrioxamine may postpone the onset of iron overload, but the side-effects of long-term therapy with this agent include retinal damage, high-tone deafness, and growth retardation. Gastroenteritis due to *Yersinia enterocolitica* infection is also a recognized complication in subjects with iron overload receiving desferrioxamine. Regular administration of vitamin C enhances excretion of iron in patients receiving desferrioxamine. Some patients with thalassemia have also been exposed to viral infections such as hepatitis C or even HIV through blood transfusions, but the prevalence of these infections is much lower than amongst hemophiliacs who received pooled coagulation factor concentrates. The combination of viral hepatitis and iron overload can hasten progression of liver disease to cirrhosis and liver failure. All patients should be vaccinated against hepatitis B. As with sickle cell anemia and other hemolytic anemias, gallstones may form at an early age in patients with thalassemia.

References

Bellet, P.S., Kalinyak, K.A., Shukla, R., Gelfand, M.J., and Rucknagel, D.L. (1995). Incentive spirometry to prevent acute pulmonary complications in sickle cell diseases. *New England Journal of Medicine*, **333**, 699–703.

Bishop, A.R., Roberson, J.R., Eckman, J.R., and Fleming, L.L. (1988). Total hip arthroplasty in patients who have sickle-cell hemoglobinopathy. *Journal of Bone and Joint Surgery, American Volume*, **70**, 853–5.

Camp, J.D. and Colwell, C.W. (1986). Core decompression of the femoral head for osteonecrosis. *Journal of Bone and Joint Surgery, American Volume*, **68**, 1313–19.

Clarke, H.J., Jinnah, R.H., Brooker, A.F., and Michaelson, J.D. (1989). Total replacement of the hip for avascular necrosis in sickle cell disease. *Journal of Bone and Joint Surgery, British Volume*, **71**, 465–70.

Currarino, G. and Erlandson, M.E. (1964). Premature fusion of epiphyses in Cooley's anemia. *Radiology*, **63**, 656.

Issaragrisil, H.C., Piankigagum, A., and Wasi, P. (1981). Spinal cord compression in thalassemia: report of 12 cases and recommendations for treatment. *Archives of Internal Medicine*, **141**, 1033–6.

Milner, P.F., Kraus, A.P., Sebes, J.I., *et al.* (1991). Sickle cell disease as a cause of osteonecrosis of the femoral head. *New England Journal of Medicine*, **325**, 1476–81.

Milner, P.F., Kraus, A.P., Sebes. J.I., *et al.* (1993). Osteonecrosis of the humeral head in sickle cell disease. *Clinical Orthopaedics and Related Research*, **289**, 136–43.

Ortiz-Neu, C., Marr, J.S., Cherubin, C.E., and Neu, H.C. (1978). Bone and joint infections due to *Salmonella. Journal of Infectious Diseases*, **138**, 820–8.

Sorsdahl, O.S., Taylor, P.E., and Noyes, W.D. (1964). Extramedullary hematopoiesis, mediastinal masses and spinal cord compression. *Journal of the American Medical Association*, **189**, 343–7.

Vichinsky, E.P., Haberkern, C.M., Neumayr, L., *et al.* (1995). A comparison of conservative and aggressive transfusion regimens in the perioperative management of sickle cell disease. *New England Journal of Medicine*, **333**, 206–13.

Walters, M.C., Patience, M., Leisenring, W., *et al.* (1996). Bone marrow transplantation for sickle cell disease. *New England Journal of Medicine*, **335**, 369–76.

1.9 Fundamentals of infection

Anthony R. Berendt and Benjamin A. Lipsky

Introduction

Infection is a 'heartsink' problem for orthopedic surgeons, especially when it is chronic or complicates a technically satisfying elective operation. Infection may destroy bone, cartilage, and soft tissue, and threatens the longevity of orthopedic implants. Thus bone and joint infection is seriously disabling and potentially limb or life threatening. In addition, it has a well-earned reputation for relapse and chronicity. Treatment may require multiple operations and prolonged courses of antibiotics, with no guarantee of a good functional outcome at the end.

Despite these obstacles, orthopedic infection can be satisfying to treat. With a rational and methodical approach, serious chronic illness can be arrested and ameliorated for long periods of time, even if most experts are unwilling to use the term 'cure' where bone infection is concerned. Basic principles of pathogenesis and host biology should be used to ensure rational use of surgery, antibiotics, and adjunctive measures in treating and preventing infection. This includes strategies to prevent cross-infection to other patients or staff. A multidisciplinary approach is essential so that diagnostic and therapeutic decisions can be co-ordinated in a coherent manner.

Fundamentals of pathogenesis
Colonization, infection, and contamination

Although infection begins with an encounter between a pathogen and its host, it is not an inevitable outcome of that encounter. **Infection** describes the physiologic state in which a pathogen multiplies within host tissues, usually causing some degree of damage and exciting an inflammatory response. Establishing infection requires the elaboration by the pathogen of a range of proteins and other molecules that together contribute to evading the host response and promoting invasion (Finlay and Falkow 1997.)

In some situations, the mechanisms responsible for invasion do not seem to operate. The result is a noninvasive association between the pathogen and the host called **colonization**. Perhaps the most dramatic example of colonization is the huge load of bacteria living in the large bowel, many of which are potential pathogens. Of more relevance to the orthopedic surgeon are the bacteria colonizing the skin, since it is these organisms (*Staphylococcus aureus*, β-hemolytic streptococci, coagulase-negative staphylococci, diphtheroids, and others) that most commonly infect orthopedic hardware.

Colonization may be transient or long lived. For example, *Staph. aureus* is carried long term in the anterior nares in up to 20 per cent of the population and transiently in some 60 per cent (Kluytmans *et al.* 1997). Staphylococcal colonization of the skin is generally a consequence of shedding from the nares. The factors that predispose to colonization are well understood, but factors such as diabetes, dialysis, eczema, and hospitalization increase the risk. Colonization is important because, while generally harmless, it locates pathogenic organisms in environments that may allow easy access to deeper host tissues, where infection can then occur. In addition to causing infection, colonizing skin flora from the patient (or from medical, nursing, or laboratory staff) may contaminate samples taken to diagnose or exclude infection. Distinguishing colonization from infection allows antibiotic therapy to be appropriately administered and targeted.

A final important concept is **contamination**. This refers to the presence of micro-organisms in a (generally sterile) host site (or in a sample) where they have not yet established an infection, but are also not in a stable colonizing relationship. Wounds may become

---

Box 1 Bone and joint infection

- Treatment involves surgical and medical inputs
- Success requires a multidisciplinary approach
- In chronic disease, 'arrest' is a preferred term to 'cure'
- Cross-infection must be avoided

Box 2 Colonization by micro-organisms

- Colonization is a universal state on epithelial and mucosal surfaces (skin, nares, bowel)
- It may be a biologically adaptive state for some organisms
- It can be transient, prolonged, or permanent
- It generally requires no treatment
- It has the potential for leading to infection, especially in orthopedics

contaminated with environmental micro-organisms through trauma, or through errant surgical or nursing practice. Contamination usually resolves into elimination of the organism or the establishment of colonization. However, it may lead to infection, with the risk rising in proportion both to the inherent virulence and to the quantitative load of bacteria present.

Microbial virulence

The severity of disease caused by a given micro-organism is determined by two factors: the characteristics of the pathogen, and the response made by the host.

Products elaborated by the pathogen that contribute to its ability to cause disease are referred to as virulence factors. They include the following:

- molecules expressed at the surface of the bacterial cell, such as adhesins (permitting attachment to host tissues)
- molecules that are secreted or otherwise released, such as toxins
- carbohydrate exoantigens that form an antiphagocytic capsule.

Genes encoding or synthesizing many such molecules have been cloned and sequenced. Complete genome sequences are already available for a number of major pathogens. These studies allow the identification of putative virulence factors on the basis of homology (i.e. relatedness) with known virulence genes from the same or other pathogens (Strauss and Falkow 1997). Furthermore, a number of powerful molecular genetic techniques now permit rapid screening (in experimental models) for virulence genes (Hensel et al. 1995) or for genes that are specifically expressed in certain environments (Slauch et al. 1994). The use of these techniques in animal models has already identified novel virulence genes without obvious homology to other known genes (Shea et al. 1996). Application of these techniques to models of orthopedic infection will elucidate which genes pathogens need to express in order to cause musculoskeletal infection.

Virulence does not appear to be an 'all or nothing' phenomenon, but one that is subject to regulation. There are at least two broad means by which this occurs. In the first, for example with the respiratory pathogen Haemophilus influenzae, genes involved in generating invasive disease each appear capable of being turned on or off independently (Moxon et al. 1994). A population of bacteria expresses many different combinations of these genes (located at so-called 'contingency loci'). This pre-existing diversity allows the pathogen to establish infection rapidly at many possible new sites within the host as they become available.

An alternative mechanism involves virulence genes that are under global regulatory control such that, in response to appropriate stimuli, the phenotype of the organism can change from colonizing to invasive. This is recognized in a number of bacteria, including Staph. aureus, and involves a phenomenon known as quorum sensing (Bassler 1999; Holden et al. 2000). The bacteria synthesize, and release into the environment, substances that act as density-dependent regulators of gene expression. Staph. aureus produces a cyclic octapeptide (Ji et al. 1995), and when a sufficient concentration of this is detected by each individual bacterium, the production of a regulatory RNA molecule is triggered (Novick et al. 1993). This changes the expression of many genes, upregulating a number of secreted exotoxins and reducing adhesin production. These co-ordinated changes in the behavior of many members of the bacterial

Box 3 Virulence regulation by contingency loci (e.g. *H. influenzae*)

- Multiple genes determine virulence
- Each can be independently regulated
- Specific permutations of active genes may be needed to invade a given tissue

population may lead to them escaping from one environment, where nutrients may be limiting, and invading another.

Box 4 Virulence regulation by quorum sensing (e.g. *Staph. aureus*)

- Multiple genes determine virulence
- Global regulators switch many genes on or off together
- Bacteria synthesize and release peptides that act as concentration-sensitive triggers of the switch from colonization to invasion

These genetic considerations are likely to be of great importance in musculoskeletal infection. Changes in the expression of global regulators or individual genes, and so in the 'invasiveness' of a population of a bacterium such as Staph. aureus, are factors that may explain the variable natural history of infection. One of the enduring mysteries in musculoskeletal infection is how patients can remain relatively well for long periods of time with deep infection and draining sinuses, only becoming ill if drainage is impaired. It may be that continuous drainage keeps the density of bacteria and of quorum-sensing molecules below critical thresholds so that a less invasive phenotype is expressed, but this hypothesis remains to be tested.

Nonspecific host response

A number of host defense mechanisms act to prevent infection, limit its extent, or resolve it. These include specific and nonspecific humoral and cellular mechanisms (Keusch 1999)

Key nonspecific responses include the generation of fever, local vasodilatation, the acute phase response, the complement system, and the recruiting and action of phagocytes.

Fever is caused by a change in the hypothalamic set-point that defines core temperature. Prostaglandin E_2 is released in the hypo-

Box 5 Host response to infection

- Nonspecific humoral (complement, mannose-binding protein, acute phase proteins)
- Nonspecific cellular (phagocytes, platelets)
- Specific humoral (antibodies)
- Specific cellular (T cells, neutrophils, macrophages in presence of specific antibody)

Box 6 Nonspecific responses to infection

- Fever
- Local vasodilatation
- Acute phase response
- Complement
- Platelet microbicidal proteins
- Phagocyte recruitment and action

thalamus in response to a number of inflammatory cytokines, including interleukin 1 and tumor necrosis factor (Dinarello *et al.* 1999). Tumor necrosis factor is synthesized by macrophages and monocytes in response, among other things, to bacterial lipopolysaccharide, also known as endotoxin. When produced in excess it may initiate a cytokine cascade resulting in septic shock (Tracey *et al.* 1987; Cerami 1993). Although this is an example of a deleterious effect of the host response, a less severe response is an important part of the fight against infection. Fever may damage or directly kill bacteria, it promotes phagocytosis by increasing the rate of metabolic processes and cellular motility, and it increases the activity of some antimicrobial agents. Tumor necrosis factor has many other effects on the immune system that also enhance function (Tracey and Cerami 1994).

The **acute phase response** involves the increased synthesis of a range of proteins, some of which have antibacterial actions.

When activated to completion, the **complement system** leads to the formation of an unregulated pore in the membrane of the target cell. The resulting loss of homeostasis leads to cell death. Complement also plays an important role in defense because the degradation products of some of the components are potent stimulators of neutrophil recruitment (C3a, C5a) and phagocytosis (C3b).

Other host proteins also function either as opsonins (enhancing phagocytosis) or in killing bacteria. Recently, much attention has been focused on **mannose-binding protein**, a primitive opsonin that binds to bacterial cell walls. Certain natural polymorphisms are associated with susceptibility to specific infections (Hibberd *et al.* 1999). The **defensins** are a group of antimicrobial polypeptides that directly kill many bacteria (Ganz and Lehrer 1998). They are released by phagocytes and cells present in epithelia. Platelets also release **platelet microbicidal proteins** and bacteria may vary in resistance to these (Bayer *et al.* 1998).

The **neutrophil** and the **monocyte** are cells of particular importance in nonspecific defenses. These cells are dedicated phagocytes and carry a range of surface proteins involved in cell–cell recognition and cellular ingestion. They are potent agents in destroying and clearing bacteria, but their internal enzyme complement is as able to destroy host cells and tissues as it is bacteria; indeed, one of their functions is to clear away dead tissue and promote healing. To prevent damage to healthy host tissues, the function of the neutrophil is tightly regulated. Neutrophils circulate in an unactivated state and pass continuously through the microvascular circulation. They only enter the tissues when required, a process that involves adhesion to activated endothelium lining the blood vessel, active movement through the endothelial monolayer into the extravascular tissue, and further migration to the site of infection (Zimmerman *et al.* 1997).

At the site of infection neutrophils attempt to phagocytose and destroy bacteria. Their ability to perform this critical function is inhibited by virulence factors such as bacterial capsular polysaccharide and leukocidal toxins. Phagocytosis is also hindered by adverse metabolic states including hypoxia, acidosis, hyperglycemia, and uremia. Successful phagocytosis and killing is stimulated by opsonizing antibody and complement, which bind to the bacterial cell surface and are recognized by a variety of receptors on the neutrophil surface. Reactive oxygen intermediates (free radicals), such as superoxide, the hydroxyl anion, nitric oxide, and peroxynitrite, are produced inside phagocytic vacuoles. These highly reactive molecular species kill bacteria by oxidizing membrane lipids and other structures, destroying their function.

Neutrophils that ingest and kill small numbers of bacteria survive, or die by programmed cell death (apoptosis). They are removed by monocyte–macrophages in a manner that resolves inflammation (Savill and Haslett 1995). If killing is unsuccessful or bacterial toxins are present in sufficient amounts, neutrophils undergo death by necrosis, rupturing to release their tissue-damaging contents and the phagocytosed bacteria, dead or still alive. This event is a potent inducer of further inflammation and the result is an inflammatory lesion at the site of infection with dead and living bacteria, neutrophils, and other host cells; in short, pus develops and an abscess forms. Surgical drainage may be needed to obtain prompt resolution, but the natural history of untreated abscesses includes the potential for spontaneous drainage and cure. Even with deep-seated infections of the musculoskeletal system, resolution may occur by this route. Patients with chronic osteomyelitis frequently describe the extrusion of bony sequestra, which have been separated from underlying healthy bone by the action of neutrophils and osteoclasts. Such bony fragments are expelled through sinus tracts, often with subsequent healing, at least for a time. In the pre-antibiotic era, awaiting the definition and separation of sequestra and aiding their expulsion was the cornerstone of the management of chronic osteomyelitis.

Specific host response

Whereas nonspecific responses generally lead to the clinical appearances and early control of orthopedic infection, specific responses are important in establishing immunity to infection. The role of specific immunity against some of the common musculoskeletal pathogens (e.g. *Staph. aureus*) is not well understood.

Specific immunity is crucially dependent on the recognition of for-

Box 7 Action of neutrophils

- Endothelial cells allow neutrophils to adhere and pass through to tissues
- Neutrophils migrate through extravascular tissue by chemotaxis
- Opsonins and complement on the bacterial surface promote phagocytosis
- Activated neutrophils destroy phagocytosed bacteria using free radicals
- Senescent neutrophils undergo apoptosis and are removed by monocyte–macrophages

eign structures by either immunoglobulin molecules (present on the surface of, and subsequently secreted by, B cells) or another highly variable receptor on the surface of T cells. T-cell activation leads to the proliferation of B and T cells involved in the production of specific antibody and, where relevant, cytotoxic T cells. These events are important in the pathophysiology of infections such as tuberculosis, where chronic inflammation, characterized by the presence of T cells and macrophages, is characteristic.

Interaction between microbial virulence and host response

The clinical presentation of infection is the result of the interaction between the microbial virulence factors and the host responses described above. Which organisms can successfully exploit specific opportunities depends upon the virulence of the pathogen and the overall health of the host. Virulent organisms can attack even apparently normal hosts. For example, primary *Staph. aureus* bacteremia and septic arthritis often have no identifiable predisposing host factor. In contrast, opportunistic pathogens may be unable to cause significant disease unless the host is compromised. Thus, coagulase-negative staphylococci generally cannot cause a wound infection, but will infect a prosthetic joint because of local compromise to host resistance mechanisms.

In the musculoskeletal system, these factors can interact in ways that make it hard to diagnose infection on purely clinical grounds. The musculoskeletal system responds to a variety of insults in relatively limited ways; pain, swelling and loss of function are nonspecific features, and even the addition of redness, warmth, and edema are not diagnostic of infection, merely indicating inflammation.

Two forms of joint-space infection illustrate these points. In native joint infection, the presence of bacteria triggers a host inflammatory response causing pain, loss of movement, an effusion, and a cellular response in the synovial fluid. The patient commonly also develops fever. However, these findings are entirely compatible with non-infective causes of acute arthritis, including gout, pyrophosphate arthropathy, and acute rheumatoid arthritis. In untreated septic arthritis, it appears to be mostly the host response, in the form of chronic inflammatory cells, that destroys the joint surface. Animal models where the inflammatory response is inhibited show less joint damage than controls, whether or not antibiotics are given (Tarkowski and Wagner 1998). However, if antibiotics are witheld, these immuno-suppressed animals die from systemic sepsis.

In prosthetic joint infection (and other forms of foreign body infection including that associated with dead bone), the interaction between host and microbe is particularly intriguing. First, host defenses in the vicinity of foreign materials are greatly impaired, allowing a lower bacterial inoculum to establish infection. This was elegantly

shown by Elek and Conen (1957), who introduced *Staph. aureus* into the skin of guinea pigs (and, later, of medical student volunteers) in the presence or absence of a skin suture. The experiments conclusively showed a dramatic fall in the number of organisms needed to cause infection when the suture was present.

Second, many organisms express cell surface proteins that bind to host proteins. Since these host proteins coat biomaterial surfaces, they can act as a bridge between the biomaterial and the bacterium. *Staph. aureus*, for example, expresses a battery of cellular receptors for extracellular matrix proteins (Foster and Hook 1998). Among these are proteins binding fibrinogen and fibronectin, which appear to be important in adhering to foreign materials (Vaudaux *et al.* 1989). Adherent organisms appear to become resistant to both antibiotic action and host defenses. One reason may be the synthesis of complex polysaccharides, the so-called glycocalyx, in which the organisms live, forming a biofilm (Costerton *et al.* 1999).

These two factors can result in low-virulence organisms being able to establish long-term, often indolent, infection around a foreign body. Because such organisms lack the virulence factors necessary for survival and multiplication in normal tissues, their existence is largely confined to the implant surface and its immediate vicinity, where the host response is impaired. Infections of this sort may be indistinguishable, on gross inspection, from a normal aseptic response to a mechanically loose implant.

The host's inability to clear a device-related infection does not mean that infection is ignored. There is chronic, but relatively ineffective, inflammation. While this may limit bacterial numbers in the tissues, protecting the host from systemic infection, chronic suppuration may lead to sinus formation and to mechanical loosening of the implant. Loosening is thought to be due to the resorption of bone at the interface with the implant, stimulated by inflammatory cytokines (Merkel *et al.* 1999) and possibly by certain bacterial proteins (Meghji *et al.* 1998).

Fundamentals of diagnosis

It is hard for the physician to make a diagnosis that he or she has not already thought of. Given the potentially devastating consequences of misdiagnosing an infection, it is essential that the orthopedic surgeon maintain a high index of suspicion for this possibility. This is easy when there is evidence of acute inflammation (the febrile patient with a wound discharging pus or a red, hot, and painful joint). It is easier to overlook infection when it presents merely as unexplained levels of pain or functional impairment, night pain, early mechanical failure of implants, unexpected nonunion of appropriately stabilized fractures, or postoperative wounds that are merely slow to heal.

Given the overlap between infective and noninfective pathology, it is inevitable that much reliance is placed on diagnostic tests to distinguish the two (Altman 1991). However, all tests generate some erroneous results, giving false positives (positive test result in the absence of true disease) or false negatives (negative test result in the presence of true disease). The performance of a test is commonly described by four parameters.

The **sensitivity** is the proportion of true positives that are test positive. In other words, how good is the test at identifying those with the disease? The **specificity** is the proportion of true negatives that are test negative. In other words, how good is the test at correctly identifying those without the disease? The **positive predictive value** is the proportion of test positives that are true positive and the **negative predictive value** is the proportion of test negatives that are true negative. In general usage, diagnostic tests are used to rule in or rule out a diagnosis, and so the positive and negative predictive values are the most important practical parameters. However, the predictive values of the test vary dramatically with the prevalence of the condition being diagnosed, i.e. the pretest probability. If this is unknown (or cannot be estimated), the predictive values of the test cannot be known either.

This can be illustrated simply by the following scenario. Let us assume that a given diagnostic test for an infection has a sensitivity and a specificity of 90 per cent. Table 1 indicates the distribution of results if 1000 individuals were tested for the presence of infection with a prevalence of infection, in the population, of 50 per cent. Given the stated sensitivity and specificity, of the 500 true positives (i.e. infected persons) in the population, 450 (90 per cent) will have a positive test result, with 50 false negatives. Of the 500 true negatives (uninfected), 450 (90 per cent) will have a negative test result, with 50 false positives. In this case, the positive and the negative predictive values of the test are also 90 per cent and 90 per cent. The test might seem to be performing well.

Tables 2 and 3 show what happens when the prevalence of infection falls, initially to 10 per cent and then to 1 per cent. While the negative predictive value of the test rises to 98.8 per cent (arguably not surprising if the condition is increasingly rare anyway), the posit-

ive predictive value of the test falls dramatically to 50 per cent. Put another way, one could toss a coin to decide whether to believe a positive test result. When the prevalence is lower, at 1 per cent, the negative predictive value rises to 99.9 per cent, but the positive predictive value is 8.3 per cent. Put another way, if the test is used to detect cases and initiate treatment in this population, it will be necessary to treat 11 uninfected persons for every infected individual. This might be considered reasonable for a serious disease and a relatively safe and inexpensive treatment. It would probably not be considered appropriate to guide a decision to perform revision arthroplasty or major bone resection.

An approach that simplifies the diagnostic process is to use an additional parameter that for practical purposes combines sensitivity and specificity, since it is defined as sensitivity divided by (1 − specificity). The **likelihood ratio** compares the likelihood that a positive test result will be found in the true-positive group with the likelihood that it will be found in the true-negative group. The likelihood ratio is a fixed property of the performance of the test, and it can be used (most simply with a nomogram) to relate a pretest probability of disease (based on available epidemiologic data and potentially on prospective natural history studies examining clinical features) to a post-test probability. In our example, the likelihood ratio of the test is always 9. When this is applied to pretest probabilities of infection (based solely on prevalence) of 50 per cent, 10 per cent, and 1 per cent, it gives post-test probabilities of 90 per cent, 50 per cent, and 9 per cent respectively. It is not essential to know the prevalence of a disease, since what is more important for the individual is an estimate of his or her pretest probability of disease. This can be informed by clinical details (ideally obtained from prospective natural history studies) and used with the test result to generate the post-test probability (Halkin et al. 1998).

In practice, not all clinicians are currently applying this approach and some may not yet understand the importance of the issue. To make matters worse, the performance characteristics of many diagnostic tests have not been rigorously defined and validated. For now, the clinician must be aware of the limitations of current diagnostic tests and consider the variability in clinical presentation that differences in microbial and host biology can generate. Isolation of the pneumococcus has little significance from a throat swab, because it is a common colonizing organism, but major significance from a joint aspirate, especially because it would be a very uncommon contaminant. In contrast, a coagulase-negative staphylococcus isolated from a native joint aspirate might well represent a contaminant, because it would be present on the skin through which the aspirate was taken. However, the same organism isolated from a prosthetic joint might represent an infecting pathogen.

In addition to knowing what organisms to expect in which contexts, microbiologists have evolved 'rules of thumb' to help interpret results, few of which have yet been rigorously validated. These

Table 1 Test results for 50 per cent prevalence of infection

	True positive	True negative	Totals
Test positive	450	50	500
Test negative	50	450	500
Totals	500	500	1000

Table 2 Test results for 10 per cent prevalence of infection

	True positive	True negative	Totals
Test positive	90	90	180
Test negative	10	810	820
Totals	100	900	1000

Table 3 Test results for 1 per cent prevalence of infection

	True positive	True negative	Totals
Test positive	9	99	108
Test negative	1	891	892
Totals	10	990	1000

include whether or not organisms are directly visible on a Gram-stained smear of the sample and whether they are isolated from a direct inoculum onto solid media ('direct culture') or are only grown from enrichment media (broth cultures that offer nutritional and osmotic support to organisms that are intrinsically more fastidious in their culture requirements or may have been damaged by antibiotics or the host response). Enrichment cultures are more sensitive, but therefore are more susceptible to contamination and thus are less specific. Solid media require a larger inoculum for convincing growth, while Gram staining is less sensitive still but, with experienced operators, is the most specific. Therefore microbiologists will often consider a single positive direct culture to be meaningful, especially if accompanied by a compatible Gram-stain appearance. In contrast, they will commonly require that more than one enrichment sample yields a similar organism to make a confident statement about the significance of the result, unless the identity of the organism suggests that it is incompatible with contamination or that it cannot be ignored.

Another diagnostic test that appears to be very useful in many situations is histologic examination of involved tissues for the presence of acute inflammatory cells. This has proved especially helpful in prosthetic joint infection, where it correlates well with the isolation of micro-organisms (Pandey *et al.* 1999) and has been used to help define microbiological criteria for diagnosing infection (Atkins *et al.* 1998).

Therefore a recommended approach to diagnosing infection is to begin with clinical suspicion, modifying this on the basis of clinical and epidemiologic features. Noninvasive investigations (such as imaging) must be chosen with some understanding of their sensitivities and specificities. At some point, it is likely that a microbiologic diagnosis will be needed. To avoid culture results such as 'no significant growth' or 'mixed normal flora' it is best to avoid sending superficial swabs. They should be avoided except for seeking methicillin-resistant *Staph. aureus* (**MRSA**) for infection control purposes, because of the problems of colonization and because certain organisms may not survive the transport conditions in the swab. Deeper tissue, either removed by curettage after cleansing and debridement (in an ulcer), or taken as a percutaneous or open biopsy, is of far higher diagnostic value. Sterile aspirates of deep fluid, taken correctly through prepared skin, are useful specimens. Microbiology laboratories recognize this and tend to concentrate efforts on specimens known to be of high quality. Wherever possible, specimens should be sent before antibiotics are commenced. For patients with chronic infections already on treatment, it is generally best (and safe) to stop antibiotics for as long as clinical considerations permit, provided that there is a clearly understood plan for dealing with clinical deterioration.

It is recommended that more than one sample should be sent when infection involves implants or is chronic. Additional samples must be obtained with separate instruments and placed in separate specimen pots to ensure that they are truly independent of one another. Liaison between clinician and laboratory is desirable especially for unusual cases or particularly precious specimens. The specialist in infection can also assist in the choice of empiric antibiotics, the interpretation of the results, and the final choice of treatment. For precision in diagnosis, the physician needs knowledge of sensitivity and specificity of the test(s) against a criterion standard of infection. This, combined with reasonable estimates of pretest probability

Box 10　Fundamentals of diagnosing infection

- Have a high index of suspicion
- The positive predictive value of a test falls with the prevalence of disease
- Gram-stained smears are specific, but not sensitive
- Enrichment cultures are maximally sensitive but have lower specificity
- Antibiotics should be stopped before sampling and multiple samples taken whenever possible
- Histological examination is a valuable adjunct to culture
- Send deep tissue specimens or aspirates, not superficial swabs

(or even rough upper and lower limits), can then be used to generate the post-test probability and to decide upon the treatment plan.

Fundamentals of treatment

Perhaps the most essential question that a clinician must ask when managing infection is: Does the patient need an operation? This is especially the case in orthopedic infection, for the reasons discussed above. Adverse local biology must be corrected if at all possible, with the goal being to drain abscesses, remove dead tissue, stabilize the skeleton, eliminate surgical dead-spaces, and ensure healthy vascularized soft-tissue cover. In this environment, antibiotics can work to maximum effect. Attention must be given to optimizing systemic factors important in wound healing and host defense, such as nutritional state, cardiorespiratory function, diabetic control, uremia and hepatic impairment, and cessation of smoking. Nursing and medical staff must be competent to deal with these issues, while physical and occupational therapy input is important in regaining function. The psychologic state of the patient must be considered, given the chronic nature of some cases and the arduous treatment sometimes necessary.

Antibiotics

Antibiotics have revolutionized the management of all infection, but must not be used as an excuse to avoid surgery when indicated. A comprehensive outline of antibiotic action and mechanisms of resistance is beyond the scope of this chapter. Nevertheless some knowledge assists in understanding 'problem organisms', such as MRSA, and in recognizing the gaps in antibiotic cover inherent in some treatment regimes (Table 4).

A number of cellular targets, against which therapy can be directed, exist in a bacterium. For historical reasons (given the discovery of penicillin that launched antibiotic development) one of the first targets was the bacterial cell wall. In Gram-positive organisms this is a thick structure withstanding an enormously high oncotic pressure (estimated at 1 atm). The wall is composed of chains of sugar residues cross-linked at multiple points by a pentaglycine (i.e. peptide) bridge. Synthesis of this peptidoglycan cell wall depends on a number of enzymes. Because penicillin binds to some of these (whose natural substrates are the sugar intermediates) they are called penicillin-

Table 4 Common bacterial pathogens in orthopedic infection, with their normal biological niches and antibiotic susceptibilities

Organism	Common sites of infection	Normal niches	Antibiotic susceptibilitiesa
Staph. aureus	Native joint Prosthetic joint (acute infection) Bone (acute and chronic) Muscle Skin and soft tissue	Anterior nares Skin, especially if scaling or ulcer	PEN (5%), AUG, METH, CEPH, MERO, ERY, VAN, TEI, CIP, TET, RIF, FUS, LIN, SYN, TRIM
MRSA	Wound, implanted metalware, and prosthetic joints postprocedure	Skin surface (especially wounds and ulcers), nares, throat	VAN, TEI, FUS, RIF, TET, LIN, SYN (resistant to all β-lactams; ERY, CIP, TRIM variable)
Coagulase-negative staphylococci	Implanted metalware and prosthetic joints	Skin surface	VAN, TEI, ERY, FUS, RIF, TET, LIN, SYN, CIP (many strains resistant to PEN, METH, CEPH, ERY, TRIM)
Corynebacteria (diphtheroids)	Implanted metalware and prosthetic joints Rarely, native joint or soft tissue	Skin surface	VAN, TEI, ERY, FUS, RIF, TET, LIN, SYN, CIP (many strains or species resistant to PEN, METH, CEPH)
Propionibacterium acnes	Implanted metalware, particularly spinal instrumentation	Deep dermis (in sebaceous glands)	PEN, AMP, CEPH, VAN, TEI, ERY, FUS, RIF, TET, LIN, SYN (resistance to TET increasing with use for treatment of acne)
β-Hemolytic streptococci	Native joint Prosthetic joint (acute infection) Bone (acute and chronic) Muscle Skin and soft tissue	Skin, throat	PEN, AMP, CEPH, VAN, TEI, ERY, RIF, TRIM, FUS, TET, LIN, SYN (some ERY resistance)
Streptococcus pneumoniae	Native and prosthetic joint (rare)	Throat, respiratory tract	PEN, AMP, CEPH, VAN, TEI, ERY, RIF,TRIM, FUS, TET, LIN, SYN (PEN resistance variably present worldwide)
Enterococcus species	Bone (chronic, open, e.g. diabetic foot ulcer or sinus) Prosthetic joints	Gut, chronic ulcers	AMP, VAN, TRIM, TEI, LIN, SYN, RIF, GENT (GENT resistance variably present; some species AMP resistant)
Bacillus species	Necrotic wounds and muscle	Soil, dirt	PEN (some), CEPH (some), VAN, TEICIP, RIF
Neisseria gonorrhoeae	Joint, tendon sheath	Genital tract, oropharynx and throat	CTX, CIP (many strains PEN resistant)
Haemophilus influenzae	Native joint, bone	Oropharynx, throat and respiratory tract	AUG, CEPH, CIP
Escherichia coli, Proteus species	Native and prosthetic joint, native spine, long bone (chronic, open), metalware	Gut	AMP (few), AUG, CEPH, MERO, TAZO, CIP, TRIM, GENT
Enterobacter species, *Citrobacter* species	Prosthetic joint Fracture fixation metalware and infected non-union	Gut	MERO, CIP, GENT (resistant to AMP, AUG, cephalosporins)
Pseudomonas species	Prosthetic joint Fracture fixation metalware and infected non-union Fibrocartilage (disk space, symphysis pubis, foot puncture wounds)	Water, soil Hospital environment (sinks, soaps) Gut	TAZO, MERO, CEFTAZ, GENT, CIP (resistant to AMP, AUG, cephalosporins)
Anaerobes	Deep wounds	Gut, dental plaque	PEN (especially oral anaerobes), CLINDA, MTZ
Brucella species	Native joint and bone especially spine and sacroiliac joints	Animal reservoir	TET, RIF, CIP, STR
Mycobacterium tuberculosis	Prosthetic joint (rare)	Dormant in human, chronic cavities in lung, chronic infections	INH, RIF, ETH, PYR, STR (multidrug resistance widespread in some areas)

AMP, ampicillin/amoxycillin; AUG, amoxicillin–clavulanic acid (co-amoxiclav or Augmentin); CEFTAZ, ceftazidime; CEPH, cephradine (and usually other cephalosporins); CIP, ciprofloxacin (and usually other fluroquinolones); CLINDA, clindamycin; CTX, ceftriaxone; ERY, erythromycin; ETH, ethambutol; FUS, fusidic acid; GENT, gentamicin and other aminoglycosides; INH, isoniazid; LIN, linezolid; MERO, meropenem (and usually imipenem–cilastin); METH, methicillin (for clinical use, flucloxacillin, cloxacillin, and dicloxacillin); MTZ, metronidazole; PEN, penicillin; PYR, pyrazinamide; RIF, rifampin; STR, streptomycin; SYN, quinupristin–dalfopristin (Synercid); TAZO, piperacillin–tazobactam (Tazocin); TEI, teicoplanin; TET, tetracyclines; TRIM, trimethoprim (and trimethoprim–sulfamethoxazole); VAN, vancomycin.
aHighly variable over time and in different institutions.

Box 11 The role of surgery

- Drainage of abscesses
- Removal of dead tissue
- Stabilization of the skeleton
- Elimination of dead spaces
- Provision of well-vascularized soft-tissue cover
- Antibiotics complement, and do not replace, surgery

binding proteins (**PBPs**). Inhibition of the natural action of PBPs by penicillin affects cell wall synthesis, and cell death, through this and additional pathways, is the usual result (Waxman and Strominger 1983).

The spectacular initial successes of penicillin (compared with the pre-antibiotic era) and the rise of antibiotic resistance led to further developments in the same 'family' of antibiotics—the β-lactams. Modified forms of penicillin and further classes of β-lactam antibiotic, such as the cephalosporins and the carbapenems, were discovered and developed. These have different spectra of activity against bacteria because they target different combinations of PBPs. Some β-lactam structures have been developed to be resistant to penicillinases (e.g. flucloxacillin and cloxacillin which are resistant to the penicillinase of *Staph. aureus*). For others, inhibitors of the bacterial resistance enzyme β-lactamase were developed, restoring the efficacy of the original drug when the two are given in combination (e.g. ampicillin–clavulanate, ampicillin–sulbactam, or piperacillin–tazobactam).

In parallel, drug-discovery programs led to the identification of other classes of antibiotics with different or similar targets. These targets include the following.

- **Protein synthesis** by inhibiting the ribosome: macrolides (e.g. erythromycin), lincosamides (e.g. clindamycin), tetracycline, chloramphenicol, aminoglycosides (e.g. gentamicin), streptogramins (e.g. quinupristin–dalfopristin), rifamycins (e.g. rifampin), and oxazolidinones (e.g. linezolid).

- **Nucleic acid synthesis** by inhibition of folic acid production (sulfonamides and trimethoprim) or by directly affecting DNA replication and supercoiling (quinolones, e.g. ciprofloxacin).

- **Oxidative damage** of multiple intracellular targets by acting as a reducing agent (metronidazole).

- **Cell wall synthesis**, affecting different steps from the β-lactams (glycopeptides, e.g. vancomycin).

Spectra of antibacterial activity vary widely. As a general principle, shaped in part by the evolution of drug resistance, penicillins have activity against Gram-positive and an increasingly limited range of Gram-negative organisms. Cephalosporins have activity against both groups, with successive generations of cephalosporin having more activity against troublesome Gram-negative organisms and a slight reduction in activity against Gram-positive organisms. Carbapenems have very broad spectrum activity against both Gram-positive and Gram-negative organisms, including those expressing extended spectrum β-lactamases that destroy all penicillins and cephalosporins.

Protein synthesis inhibitors are largely useful against Gram-positive organisms, with the important exception of aminoglycosides which remain a mainstay of adjunctive treatment for severe Gram-negative infection. Drugs affecting nucleic acid synthesis are useful against both groups, but resistance evolves relatively easily. Metronidazole has a unique role in the treatment of anaerobic infections, many of which will also respond to penicillins, carbapenems, clindamycin, and some new quinolones. Glycopeptides are only effective against Gram-positive organisms.

It is important in selecting antibiotics to consider the following:

- spectrum of activity against the likely or proven pathogen
- route and frequency of administration
- bioavailability if given by the oral route
- likelihood of side-effects
- patient adherence to the treatment regimen
- cost (but also cost-benefit) of the drug, administration, and any monitoring.

The guiding principle should be to use as narrow a spectrum of antibiotic as is prudent for the organism or infection. This minimizes the ecological impact of the treatment, the potential for certain side-effects (notably *Clostridium difficile* diarrhea), and the development of widespread drug resistance by minimizing the range of organisms exposed to drug. Antibiotics are generally commenced before the causative organism is known, but it is almost always possible (and is good practice in most situations) to obtain a diagnostic sample first (blood culture, aspirate of joint or collection, curettage of ulcer, or biopsy). Empiric therapy needs to take into account the likely pathogens, the prevalence of antibiotic resistance, the severity of the infection, and the possible consequences if the empiric regimen proves to be ineffective. For practical purposes this means that patients with infections that have little potential for rapid progression can be treated with narrow-spectrum agents, with a broadening in coverage if cultures and the clinical course so dictate. Patients with infection that has the potential for rapid local or systemic deterioration should receive broad-spectrum treatment empirically, with a change to narrower-spectrum treatment when culture results allow.

Where bone or orthopedic hardware is involved, especially with a chronic infection, it is highly desirable to take specimens for culture when the patient has been off all antibiotics for at least a few days and preferably more than 2 weeks. This maximizes the chance of isolating all the pathogens from good-quality samples, which is important because antibiotic therapy may need to continue for a prolonged period. A definitive microbiological diagnosis at the outset is exceedingly valuable not only in dictating early treatment but also later, when dealing with side-effects, the patient's requests to stop therapy, and the clinician's uncertainties about the duration of treatment required and the timing of further surgery. It should be stressed that these guidelines do not apply in conditions such as acute osteomyelitis, acute septic arthritis, or spinal epidural abscess. These conditions often have accompanying bacteremia, may cause harm rapidly, and in some cases will respond to medical therapy alone. One or two sets of blood cultures, an aspirate if appropriate, and early empiric antibiotics are the recommended approach if one of these conditions is suspected.

In tandem with the development of antibiotics has been the rise in antibiotic resistance. Microbes can evade the action of antibiotics in a number of ways:

- prevent access of drug by altering uptake systems
- over-express the target so that intracellular concentrations of drug fail to act
- mutate the target with loss of the drug-binding site
- develop novel pathways or functions to bypass those inhibited by the drug
- develop or over-express enzyme systems to destroy the drug
- develop, mutate, or over-express drug export systems.

All these mechanisms are used by various micro-organisms (Cohen and Tartasky 1997). Gram-negative bacteria, such as *Pseudomonas aeruginosa,* have an outer membrane that surrounds the cell wall. Proteins called porins limit the access of many compounds to the cell wall and inner membrane; these porins can be lost by mutation, denying access to particular antibiotics. Protein synthesis inhibitors are vulnerable to mutation of their binding sites on the ribosome, which can become so altered in response to drug pressure that antibiotic-dependent organisms can be generated (although there is no evidence that this extreme is of clinical significance).

Two important antibiotic resistant organisms, MRSA and vancomycin-resistant enterococci (**VRE**), bypass drug action. MRSA expresses the novel penicillin-binding protein PBP2' which, although functional, does not bind β-lactam antibiotics (Utsui and Yokota 1985). VRE makes its cell wall using a quite different synthetic pathway encoded by a substantial number of novel genes that are presumed to have been acquired from a different bacterial species (Gin and Zhanel 1996). Many bacteria express β-lactamases of varying specificities, including the extended-spectrum β-lactamases mentioned above.

While Gram-negative rods were the main concern for antibiotic resistance in the 1970s and 1980s, in the 1990s and at the beginning of the twenty-first century Gram-positive bacteria have re-emerged as the chief resistance problem. Although new antibiotics are under development, with two new drugs active against MRSA and VRE recently licensed (quinupristin–dalfopristin and linezolid), the rise in antibiotic resistance is a major cause for concern. It is for this reason that preventing infection and cross-infection is as important as treating it.

Fundamentals of prevention of infection

Infection

As mentioned, colonization or contamination places organisms in an ideal position to cause infection of surgical wounds or traumatic wounds. Pathogenic bacteria may be present on the skin at the time of incision or may enter the wound on desquamated skin scales (which even a healthy person is continuously shedding). Therefore the prevention of infection requires attention to all aspects of sterile and surgical technique and to the medical state of the patient.

Most postoperative infections start in the operating theatre. Techniques to avoid this include meticulous skin preparation with bactericidal antiseptics, care in hand-washing, gloving, and gowning, keep-

Box 12 Principles of antibiotic use in orthopedics

- Obtain appropriate diagnostic specimens before using antibiotics
- Use narrower-spectrum antibiotics whenever possible
- Use broad-spectrum antibiotics pending culture results when the condition of the patient or the tissues is in jeopardy
- Antibiotics only rarely replace the need for surgery, but are an important adjunct to surgical treatment

ing surgical instruments covered when not in use, operating in laminar air flow when possible, and minimizing operating-room traffic during surgery. Sound surgical technique can also make an important difference, for example reducing trauma to soft tissues by gentle handling, avoiding excessive use of diathermy and suture material, eliminating dead-spaces and hematoma, avoiding excessive tissue tension when closing wounds, and keeping operating time to a minimum.

The natural history of traumatic wounds is a high rate of infection (Gustilo and Anderson 1976; Gustilo *et al.* 1984, 1987), whether of soft tissue or of underlying bone (if fractured). Careful exploration and cleansing of minor wounds and wholesale excision of major wounds (with soft-tissue reconstruction by a plastic surgeon) act to remove necrotic tissue and gross environmental contamination with clothing, plant matter, soil, and grit. These are not only sources of heavy microbial contamination but the foreign materials in question act to potentiate infection, as explained above. This is also the case with fracture-fixation hardware, although the mechanical stability and anatomic reduction conferred by internal fixation may act separately to reduce the risk of infection (Worlock *et al.* 1994).

Outside the operating room, wounds are still at risk of contamination when inspected and dressed. Staff need to pay particular attention to hand-washing, should wear gloves to examine wounds, and should protect wounds from bedding (and vice versa) using sterile drapes. Wounds should generally be left exposed for a minimum period of time while unhealed.

Set against all these considerations, the role of antibiotics is important but limited. Antibiotics will not generally correct for major breaches in sterile technique, but they are an important adjunct to good technique and have been proved, in meta-analyses, to reduce the risk of infection following hip replacement (Glenny and Song 1999) and a number of other procedures. Although prolonged antibiotics given for several days were a part of protocols that improved the management of open fractures (Wilkins and Patzakis 1991), many authorities now prefer to limit antibiotic treatment to the first 24 h, provided that wound debridement and excision take place. There is no evidence that infection rates for other high-risk procedures, such as joint replacement, are lower with prolonged therapy than with treatment for 24 h (Glenny and Song 1999). However, it is important to remember that some antibiotics used in prophylaxis have short half-lives. To ensure adequate levels of antibiotic throughout the operation, it may be necessary, when using some agents (e.g. cefuroxime or cefazolin), to redose with antibiotic intraoperatively if surgery is prolonged beyond 2 to 4 h. Prolonged postoperative antibiotic use increases the selection pressure for resistant bacteria in hospitals and the likelihood of side-effects for the patient.

Antibiotic prophylaxis regimes for elective operations through intact skin must cover aerobic Gram-positive organisms such as *Staph. aureus* and β-hemolytic streptococci. Activity against common aerobic Gram-negative rods is desirable, especially in lower-limb joint replacement. The regime must take into account the prevalence of drug-resistant organisms, in particular MRSA, that might be colonizing the patient. This is especially relevant in patients admitted from long-stay institutions, from hospitals where MRSA is endemic, or when patients have been on antibiotics that might select for resistance. Patients colonized with MRSA should receive appropriate prophylaxis (i.e. adding vancomycin), but the presence of MRSA does not alter the indications for prophylaxis. Regimes following open fractures need to be broader in spectrum in order to cover aerobic Gram-positive and Gram-negative rods and anaerobes. Ideally, prophylaxis for joint replacement should also cover skin commensals, such as coagulase-negative staphylococci. Given the high prevalence of methicillin resistance among hospital strains of these organisms, prophylaxis regimes may need to be adjusted for patients who have been hospitalized prior to joint replacement. Issues such as these should be discussed with the infection control team or an infection specialist, with reference to local antibiotic resistance patterns.

Cross-infection

Antibiotic resistance raises issues of reduced efficacy in treating infection and of increased cost incurred through the use of more expensive alternatives. This is a clinical problem for individual patients, but if resistance becomes widespread or is being transmitted in hospital, it may be disastrous for the institution on quality-assurance, economic, or medico-legal grounds.

Policies to prevent cross-infection rely on an understanding of the key factors involved in transmission. For MRSA, these are direct contact with the skin of an individual who is carrying the organism and, to a lesser extent, acquisition from the environment if it is heavily contaminated, for example with skin scales from another colonized patient with an exfoliating skin condition. Since one cannot know whether a patient is colonized with MRSA before cultures are obtained, universal precautions should be applied to all patients. Key steps in reducing transmission of MRSA are as follows.

- Hand-washing before and after touching all patients.
- The additional use of gloves and aprons if there is close contact with heavily colonized surfaces such as wounds.
- Rigorous attention to standard infection control measures when examining and re-dressing wounds.
- Consideration of decolonization, once colonized patients have a normal integument (i.e. healed skin with no drains, vascular catheters, or urinary catheters).
- Environmental cleaning, especially after MRSA-colonized patients are discharged and before other patients are admitted to the same area.

The following additional measures may be taken in institutions with low endemicity of MRSA that are still mounting control programs.

- Isolation of patients known to be colonized, to reduce the burden of environmental contamination secondary to shedding of skin scales.

- Risk assessment and pre-admission screening for MRSA carriage for all planned admissions.
- Isolation and screening of transfers from high-prevalence wards or institutions.
- Cohorting of bays or wards if numbers of colonized cases exceed the availability of side-rooms.
- Closing wards temporarily if outbreaks cannot be contained or terminated.
- Altering prophylaxis regimes during outbreaks so that even if transmission and colonization cannot be controlled, prophylaxis is appropriate.

It is essential to recognize the distinction between MRSA colonization, which is a problem for the hospital, and MRSA infection, which is a problem for the patient. This distinction and the rationale for control measures, including isolation (which is for the benefit of the institution and other patients, not for the index patient), are not always understood by staff or explained adequately to the patient. It is important that patients are not stigmatized when MRSA colonization or infection is discovered, not least because the majority of cases are hospital acquired. Patients should be reassured that colonization will not prevent planned surgery proceeding, that infection is treatable, and that other aspects of care can still proceed.

The other major area of concern regarding cross-infection, which impacts more directly on health-care providers, is the risk of infection with blood-borne agents. These are predominantly hepatitis B, hepatitis C, and HIV. All may be acquired from needlestick injuries where the health-care worker receives a penetrating wound from a needle or instrument contaminated with blood from an infectious patient. Hepatitis B, a DNA virus, causes acute hepatitis and may be fatal, although fortunately in less than 1 per cent of cases. About 10 per cent of infections result in the carrier state, where the individual remains infectious for over 6 months, and half of these carriers remain surface-antigen-positive for life, placing them at risk of chronic hepatitis, progression to cirrhosis, and liver cancer. A doctor who is hepatitis B surface-antigen (**HBsAg**) positive is not permitted to practise exposure-prone procedures in the United Kingdom. Approximately 30 per cent of needlestick injuries from HbsAg-positive patients will lead to seroconversion. Unless otherwise stated, a needlestick injury refers to a puncture wound with a sharp and contaminated object, most of which are solid needles. Risks are higher if the needle is hollow, rising in proportion to the volume of contaminated blood potentially inoculated. Infection with hepatitis C, an RNA virus, leads to jaundice in only 20 per cent of cases, but 80 per cent of infections become chronic. Chronic infection is also associated with cirrhosis and primary liver cancer. About 3 per cent of needlestick injuries from infected patients lead to seroconversion (Hamid *et al.*1999). Finally, HIV infection leads, after a variable clinically latent period (during which time there are very high levels of circulating virus), to progressively falling CD4 T-cell counts, accompanying impairments of immunity, and AIDS. Seroconversion rates following a needlestick injury from an HIV-positive patient are 0.3 per cent (see Henderson (1995) for excellent review).

The risk of transmission of blood-borne agents can be substantially reduced by adopting standard patterns of behavior that make contact with contaminated blood unlikely even in the event of an accident.

These 'universal precautions' (Centers for Disease Control and Prevention 1988) have been widely adopted and include the following:

- wearing gloves for procedures where there may be contact with body fluids (e.g. venesection or cannulation)
- double gloving for operative procedures
- eye protection where splashes of body fluid are possible
- use of 'blunt needles' for suturing
- avoidance of resheathing of needles
- scrupulous attention to the safe handling and disposal of sharps
- needle-less systems for intravenous infusions
- disposal of blood spillages using hypochlorite solution
- hand-washing
- risk assessment for procedures to identify potential dangers to the operator, assistants, and ancillary staff, including cleaning and portering staff.

Postexposure prophylaxis and immunization

Unfortunately, injuries from sharps during surgical procedures are not uncommon. If the surgeon or another member of the orthopedic team suffers a needlestick injury, the risks of contracting viral infections can be reduced, in the case of hepatitis B and HIV, through immunization or postexposure prophylaxis. In the case of hepatitis B, a recombinant subunit vaccine can elicit high levels of neutralizing antibody (and presumably cytotoxic T cells as well). All health-care workers should receive testing and immunization, if necessary, as a routine part of pre-employment occupational health screening. They should also have periodic checks on antibody titers and booster immunization if required.

Those who experience a needlestick injury need prompt review through the occupational health service. A risk assessment must be carried out, factoring in the nature of the exposure, the immune status of the recipient, and the likelihood that the donor is infectious. Depending upon the result, it may be appropriate for the recipient of the needlestick injury to be offered hepatitis B immune globulin, rapidly followed by an accelerated course of hepatitis B vaccine.

HIV risk also needs to be considered. Following on from the marked success in using anti-retroviral drug monotherapy to effect a 67 per cent reduction in transmission of HIV from a pregnant mother to her newly delivered infant (Connor et al. 1994), there is general agreement that recipients of needlestick injury should be assessed and, if appropriate, offered postexposure prophylaxis. This now takes the form of triple therapy with two nucleoside analogs and a protease inhibitor for 1 month, but it must be noted that a significant number of patients on such drugs experience side-effects of sufficient severity to stop the regimen (Parkin et al. 2000). Postexposure prophylaxis should begin as soon as possible, preferably within 24 h, and not later than 72 h, after the exposure. Of course, the need for postexposure prophylaxis depends upon the status of the 'donor' which in hospital practice can often be determined, although not usually soon enough to inform the initial discussion about prophylaxis. In areas where HIV prevalence is still low, risks associated with a 'blind' needlestick injury, where the donor status cannot be ascertained, are very low even without chemoprophylaxis,

but HIV prevalence may be very high in hospital populations in certain geographic locations.

There is no available postexposure prophylaxis or vaccine against hepatitis C infection, although some authors have advocated prompt use of pooled immunoglobulin after exposure.

It will be evident that universal infection control precautions do not merely minimize risk to health-care workers. They also provide protection for patients against bacterial cross-infection because of the emphasis on risk assessment, hand-washing, and gloving. Worryingly, this has not resulted in universal uptake of precautions or of prompt reporting and assessment following needlestick injuries, possibly because surgeons have an unrealistically low perception of risk (Patterson et al. 1998).

HIV and hepatitis C have focused attention on the risks of acquiring serious infection from blood transfusion, blood product treatment, and organ transplantation. This includes the use of donor bone graft. Given that potential donors are screened, risks of known agents are now minimal. However, there is concern over the new variant of Creutzfeldt–Jakob disease (**nvCJD**), a fatal neurodegenerative condition, which convincingly appears to be caused by the same prion protein that caused the epidemic of bovine spongiform encephalopathy (**BSE**), principally in the United Kingdom (Collinge et al. 1996). The causative agent is an abnormally folded (conformational) variant of a normal host protein. Copies of the abnormal protein accumulate and cannot be degraded by the host. Remarkably, the protein catalyzes the conversion of the normal conformation of the protein to the abnormal one. The BSE epidemic became established because of animal husbandry practices that resulted in the remains of dead cattle being fed to other cattle. Orally ingested prion protein has been shown to be infective in several species. It is assumed, but not proved, that the development of nvCJD is related to the human consumption of contaminated beef. More recently, there have been concerns about potential transmission in white cells, prompting the decision in the United Kingdom to leukocyte-deplete all blood for transfusion (Collinge 1999).

Modeling studies do not yet have the power to estimate the size of the affected human pool. If it becomes clear that large numbers of individuals in the United Kingdom are infected, the inability to destroy the prion by standard autoclaving has major implications for the reuse of surgical instruments and for bone banking. Progress continues on both obtaining more data to predict the size of the human outbreak and developing robust diagnostic tests that could be used to screen bone donors, alongside current screening for the viruses listed above and for syphilis.

Conclusion

Musculoskeletal infections continue to present major management and scientific challenges. They offer paradigms for nonorthopedic conditions (such as prosthetic joint infection as a model for device-related infection), and they illustrate basic principles in the pathogenesis and management of infection.

There are exciting possibilities ahead, including a deeper understanding of the pathogenesis of these infections, with the potential for novel therapies. There are numerous areas, notably pathogenesis, diagnosis, and treatment, requiring further research and a real need to translate research findings into practical improvements in management. Until then, the orthopedic surgeon needs to remain continuously on the alert for infection, asking him- or herself the following questions.

- Does the patient have an infection?
- How will I diagnose it?
- Does the patient understand the condition and its treatment?
- Does the patient need an operation and what will I do?
- Which antibiotics should be used, how, and for how long?
- Does the infection pose a risk to others, including me?
- What help do I need and from whom?
- Was this preventable and what would I do differently next time?

While a strong emphasis on prevention, surveillance, and infection control would be expected to minimize the number of hospital-acquired cases, the very nature of infection as a dynamic and biological entity means that these questions will remain important in orthopedic practice for many years to come. Constant vigilance, surgical courage and determination, and an ability to seek collaborative input will remain key skills in reducing the impact of these serious infections on patient and surgeon alike.

References

Altman, D.G. (1991). Diagnostic tests. In *Practical statistics for medical research*, Vol. 1, pp. 409–19. Chapman & Hall, London.

Atkins, B.L., Athanasou, N., Deeks, J.J., *et al.* (1998). Prospective evaluation of criteria for microbiological diagnosis of prosthetic-joint infection at revision arthroplasty. The OSIRIS Collaborative Study Group. *Journal of Clinical Microbiology*, **36**, 2932–9.

Bassler, B.L. (1999). How bacteria talk to each other: regulation of gene expression by quorum sensing. *Current Opinion in Microbiology*, **2**, 582–7.

Bayer, A.S., Cheng, D., Yeaman, M.R., *et al.* (1998). *In vitro* resistance to thrombin-induced platelet microbicidal protein among clinical bacteremic isolates of *Staphylococcus aureus* correlates with an endovascular infectious source. *Antimicrobial Agents and Chemotherapy*, **42**, 3169–72.

Centers for Disease Control and Prevention (1988). Recommendations for prevention of HIV transmission in health-care settings. *Morbidity and Mortality Weekly Reports*, **36** (Supplement), 1S–19S.

Cerami, A. (1993). Tumor necrosis factor as a mediator of shock, cachexia and inflammation. *Blood Purification*, **11**, 108–17.

Cohen, F.L. and Tartasky, D. (1997). Microbial resistance to drug therapy: a review. *American Journal of Infection Control*, **25**, 51–64.

Collinge, J. (1999). Variant Creutzfeldt–Jakob disease. *Lancet*, **354**, 317–23 .

Collinge, J., Sidle, K.C., Meads, J., Ironside, J., and Hill, A.F. (1996). Molecular analysis of prion strain variation and the aetiology of 'new variant' CJD. *Nature*, **383**, 685–90 .

Connor, E.M., Sperling, R.S., Gelber, R., *et al.* (1994). Reduction of maternal–infant transmission of human immunodeficiency virus type 1 with zidovudine treatment. Pediatric AIDS Clinical Trials Group Protocol 076 Study Group. *New England Journal of Medicine*, **331**, 1173–80 .

Costerton, J.W., Stewart, P.S., and Greenberg, E.P. (1999). Bacterial biofilms: a common cause of persistent infections. *Science*, **284**, 1318–22.

Dinarello, C.A., Gatti, S., and Bartfai, T. (1999). Fever: links with an ancient receptor. *Current Biology*, **9**, R147–50.

Elek, S.D., and Conen, P.E. (1957). The virulence of *Staphylococcus pyogenes* for man: a study of the problems of wound infection. *British Journal of Experimental Pathology*, **38**, 573–86.

Finlay, B.B. and Falkow, S. (1997). Common themes in microbial patho-

genicity revisited. *Microbiology and Molecular Biology Reviews*, **61**, 136–69.

Foster, T.J. and Hook, M. (1998). Surface protein adhesins of *Staphylococcus aureus*. *Trends in Microbiology*, **6**, 484–8.

Ganz, T. and Lehrer, R.I. (1998). Antimicrobial peptides of vertebrates. *Current Opinion in Immunology*, **10**, 41–4.

Gin, A.S. and Zhanel, G.G. (1996). Vancomycin-resistant enterococci. *Annals of Pharmacotherapy*, **30**, 615–24.

Glenny, A. and Song, F. (1999). Antimicrobial prophylaxis in total hip replacement: a systematic review. *Health Technology Assessment*, **3**, 1–57.

Gustilo, R.B. and Anderson, J.T. (1976). Prevention of infection in the treatment of one thousand and twenty-five open fractures of long bones: retrospective and prospective analyses. *Journal of Bone and Joint Surgery, American Volume*, **58**, 453–8.

Gustilo, R.B., Mendoza, R.M., and Williams, D.N. (1984). Problems in the management of type III (severe) open fractures: a new classification of type III open fractures. *Journal of Trauma*, **24**, 742–6.

Gustilo, R.B., Gruninger, R.P., and Davis, T. (1987). Classification of type III (severe) open fractures relative to treatment and results. *Orthopedics*, **10**, 1781–8.

Halkin, A., Reichman, J., Schwaber, M., Paltiel, O., and Brezis, M. (1998). Likelihood ratios: getting diagnostic testing into perspective. *Quarterly Journal of Medicine*, **91**, 247–58.

Hamid, S.S., Farooqui, B., Rizvi, Q., Sultana, T., and Siddiqui, A.A. (1999). Risk of transmission and features of hepatitis C after needlestick injuries. *Infection Control and Hospital Epidemiology*, **20,** 63–4.

Henderson, D.K. (1995). HIV-1 in the health care setting. In *Principles and practice of infectious diseases* (ed. G.L. Mandell, J.E. Bennett, and R. Dolin), pp. 2632–56. Churchill Livingstone, Edinburgh.

Hensel, M., Shea, J.E., Gleeson, C., *et al.* (1995). Simultaneous identification of bacterial virulence genes by negative selection. *Science*, **269**, 400–3.

Hibberd, M.L., Sumiya, M., Summerfield, J.A., Booy, R., and Levin, M. (1999). Association of variants of the gene for mannose-binding lectin with susceptibility to meningococcal disease. Meningococcal Research Group. *Lancet*, **353**, 1049–53.

Holden, I., Swift, I., and Williams, I. (2000). New signal molecules on the quorum-sensing block. *Trends in Microbiology*, **8**, 101–4.

Ji, G., Beavis, R.C., and Novick, R.P. (1995). Cell density control of staphylococcal virulence mediated by an octapeptide pheromone. *Proceedings of the National Academy of Sciences of the United States of America*, **92**, 12 055–9.

Keusch, G.T. (1999). Host responses to infection. In *Infectious diseases* (ed. D. Armstrong and J. Cohen), pp. 2.1–2.20. C.V. Mosby, London.

Kluytmans, J., van Belkum, A., and Verbrugh, H. (1997). Nasal carriage of *Staphylococcus aureus*: epidemiology, underlying mechanisms, and associated risks. *Clinical Microbiology Review*, **10**, 505–20.

Meghji, S., Crean, S.J., Hill, P.A., *et al.* (1998). Surface-associated protein from *Staphylococcus aureus* stimulates osteoclastogenesis: possible role in *S. aureus*-induced bone pathology. *British Journal of Rheumatology*, **37**, 1095–1101.

Merkel, K.D., Erdmann, J.M., McHugh, K.P., *et al.* (1999). Tumor necrosis factor-alpha mediates orthopedic implant osteolysis. *American Journal of Pathology*, **154**, 203–10.

Moxon, E.R., Rainey, P.B., Nowak, M.A., and Lenski, R.E. (1994). Adaptive evolution of highly mutable loci in pathogenic bacteria. *Current Biology*, **4**, 24–33.

Novick, R.P., Ross, H.F., Projan, S.J., *et al.* (1993). Synthesis of staphylococcal virulence factors is controlled by a regulatory RNA molecule. *EMBO Journal*, **12**, 3967–75.

Pandey, R., Drakoulakis, E., and Athanasou, N.A. (1999). An assessment of the histological criteria used to diagnose infection in hip revision arthroplasty tissues. *Journal of Clinical Pathology*, **52**, 118–23.

Parkin, J.M., Murphy, M., Anderson, J., *et al.* (2000). Tolerability and side-effects of post-exposure prophylaxis for HIV infection. *Lancet*, **355**, 722–3.

Patterson, J.M., Novak, C.B., Mackinnon, S.E., and Patterson, G.A. (1998).

Surgeons' concern and practices of protection against bloodborne pathogens. *Annals of Surgery*, **228**, 266–72.

Savill, J. and Haslett, C. (1995). Granulocyte clearance by apoptosis in the resolution of inflammation. *Seminars in Cell Biology*, **6**, 385–93.

Shea, J.E., Hensel, M., Gleeson, C., and Holden, D.W. (1996). Identification of a virulence locus encoding a second type III secretion system in *Salmonella typhimurium*. *Proceedings of the National Academy of Sciences of the United States of America*, **93**, 2593–7.

Slauch, J.M., Mahan, M.J., and Mekalanos, J.J. (1994). *In vivo* expression technology for selection of bacterial genes specifically induced in host tissues. *Methods in Enzymology*, **235**, 481–92.

Strauss, E.J. and Falkow, S. (1997). Microbial pathogenesis: genomics and beyond. *Science*, **276**, 707–12.

Tarkowski, A. and Wagner, H. (1998). Arthritis and sepsis caused by *Staphylococcus aureus*. Can the tissue injury be reduced by modulating the host's immune system? *Molecular Medicine Today*, **4**, 15–18.

Tracey, K.J. and Cerami, A. (1994). Tumor necrosis factor: a pleiotropic cytokine and therapeutic target. *Annual Review of Medicine*, **45**, 491–503.

Tracey, K.J., Fong, Y., Hesse, D.G., *et al.* (1987). Anti-cachectin/TNF monoclonal antibodies prevent septic shock during lethal bacteraemia. *Nature*, **330**, 662–4.

Utsui, Y. and Yokota, T. (1985). Role of an altered penicillin-binding protein in methicillin- and cephem-resistant *Staphylococcus aureus*. *Antimicrobial Agents and Chemotherapy*, **28**, 397–403.

Vaudaux, P., Pittet, D., Haeberli, A., *et al.* (1989). Host factors selectively increase staphylococcal adherence on inserted catheters: a role for fibronectin and fibrinogen or fibrin. *Journal of Infectious Diseases*, **160**, 865–75.

Waxman, D.J. and Strominger, J.L. (1983). Penicillin-binding proteins and the mechanism of action of beta-lactam antibiotics. *Annual Review of Biochemistry*, **52**, 825–69.

Wilkins, J. and Patzakis, M. (1991). Choice and duration of antibiotics in open fractures. *Orthopedic Clinics of North America*, **22**, 433–7.

Worlock, P., Slack, R., Harvey, L., and Mawhinney, R. (1994). The prevention of infection in open fractures: an experimental study of the effect of fracture stability. *Injury*, **25**, 31–8.

Zimmerman, G.A., McIntyre, T.M., and Prescott, S.M. (1997). Adhesion and signaling in vascular cell–cell interactions. *Journal of Clinical Investigation*, **100** (Supplement), S3–5.

1.10 Pain and its control

Henry McQuay

This chapter should act as a signpost. The interested reader is pointed to the best evidence available and to systematic reviews where available, and the efficacy of drugs and other interventions is presented as number needed to treat (**NNT**).

Pain sensation and transmission

The easiest way to think of pain in the nervous system is the idea of pain receptors and nerve cables dedicated to the transmission of pain signals (Fig. 1)—a hard-wired line-labeled system. This view has always had obvious flaws. The return of pain after an initially successful cordotomy, and the phenomenon of phantom limb pain are two examples. In a hard-wired line-labeled system the pain should not recur after the cordotomy and patients should not feel pain in a limb as they did before the accident or amputation. Such flaws mean that the simple view of a 'passive' nervous system does not explain all that we see.

In the peripheral nervous system most of the nociceptive signaling of thermal and mechanical stimuli comes from activation of polymodal nociceptors which are innervated by C-fibers. If tissue is dam-

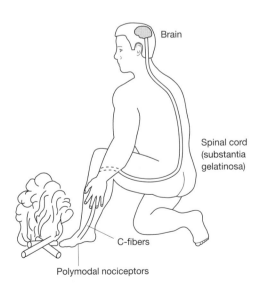

Fig. 1. Simple view of the transmission of pain signals. (After R. Descartes, *L'homme*, 1694.)

aged these fibers also respond to local chemical stimulation and become sensitized to chemical, thermal, and mechanical stimuli. Tissue damage can stimulate the synthesis of arachidonic acid metabolized from adjacent membranes, cleavage of the bradykinin precursor to release active peptide and, via the axon reflex, the release of peptides such as substance P and calcitonin gene-related peptide from the C-fibers. This inflammatory soup, which also contains 5-hydroxy-tryptamine, K^+ ions, and H^+ ions, activates and sensitizes peripheral nerve endings, and causes vasodilatation and plasma extravasation. The net result is swelling, pain, and tenderness, like the contact between warm shower water or clothing and sunburnt skin.

The pharmacology of the dorsal sensory horn of the spinal cord is rich. Transmitters come from afferent fibers, intrinsic neurons, or descending fibers. Most are concentrated in the substantia gelatinosa, one of the densest neuronal areas in the central nervous system, and crucial for the reception and modulation of nociceptive messages from the peripheral fibers. C-fibers terminate in the outer lamina 1 and the underlying substantia gelatinosa, whereas the large tactile fibers terminate in deeper laminas. However, as well as the lamina 1 cells sending long ascending axons to the brain, deep dorsal horn cells also give rise to ascending axons and respond to C-fiber stimulation. The C-fiber input to these deep cells may be relayed via interneurons, or arrive on the dendrites of the cells which pass vertically into the gelatinosa. This, and projection of inhibitory gelatinosa cells towards the deep cells, enables convergence and modulation of the responses of deep cells. Finally, the reason for the good correspondence between the electrophysiology of these cells (behavior, psychophysical studies, and reflex responses to pain) may be that these deep sensory cells both drive the withdrawal reflex and, via ascending projections, are involved in the perception of pain.

At each of these stages the signal can be amplified or damped by endogenous influences, such as mood or endorphins, and exogenous factors, such as drugs or the circumstances of the injury. The classic damping-down scenario is the injured soldier who continues, despite a shattered leg, to escape from the battlefield. Conversely, a stubbed toe when you are tired and miserable is immeasurably more painful than the same injury on a cheerful morning.

For most acute pain the idea of specific cables whose transmission can be blocked is reinforced by the fact that it is possible to operate painlessly on an injured foot by using a local anesthetic block of the foot or a local anesthetic spinal or epidural injection. If or when the operation site becomes the site of chronic pain, the inadequacy of the simple explanation is exposed. Phantom pain needs a more complicated explanation, because the painful foot or hand, the receptors, and the cables are no longer there. The concept of 'pain memory' in the spinal cord and brain has to be invoked.

The idea that the nervous system can change, or is 'plastic', has led to the development of the concept of plasticity, which has had a major impact in both acute and chronic pain (McQuay and Dickenson 1990). The simplest idea is that a memory of a pain is made and stored in the nervous system. Preventing such a memory being laid down led to the idea of pre-empting postoperative pain; any pain after the operation would be easier to treat if the memory had been minimized (McQuay 1995). Long-term sequelae, such as the phantom pain which can occur after amputation, could also be prevented. One issue of importance for treatment is at what level of the nervous system such memories might be stored. If the memory is stored at a 'central' level, for instance in the brain, then attacking the pain in the leg or arm where it originated might not do any good. The memory might be held centrally but require continued input from the periphery to sustain it. Attacking the pain in the leg or arm would then have some logic.

Many treatments or interventions are used to treat both acute pain and chronic pain. Not surprisingly, chronic pain has more twists and turns because its origins may be more complicated and because the nervous system can behave strangely if damaged or continuously bombarded by pain messages. The concept of plasticity has led to some interventions coming into fashion, and to some going out of fashion. Long-term measures, such as cutting the nerves thought to carry a particular pain message, are going out of fashion. The reasoning is that the nervous system will 'rewire'; the pain will re-emerge, and may well be more difficult to manage than it was initially. Better drug control of difficult pain has also reduced the necessity for destructive procedures.

Some definitions

Pain is an unpleasant sensory or emotional experience associated with actual or potential tissue damage, or described in terms of such damage. Chronic pain is that which is still present after 3 months despite sensible treatment. Radicular pain is felt in the distribution of a nerve root, so that pain is felt in an area corresponding to one of the dermatomes down the arm or leg or round the trunk. It is typically caused by compression. Referred pain, or transferred pain, is that which is felt superficially in the dermatome of an affected viscus or other deep structure innervated by that root. An example is pain felt in the left arm because of cardiac disease. Central pain is spontaneous and caused by damage to the central nervous system, often accompanied by dysesthesia. An example is the pain which can occur on the side of the body affected by a stroke—the thalamic or poststroke syndrome. Phantom pain is felt in the missing limb or stump.

Psychological factors

The influence that exogenous factors, such as the circumstances of the trauma, can have on pain has been mentioned. In chronic pain it is sometimes very difficult to disentangle depression from pain. Pain makes depression worse and depression makes pain worse. This pattern is all too familiar to those who manage back pain. The thinking clinician needs to deal with both the pain and the depression.

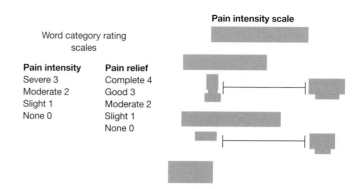

Fig. 2. Categorical and visual analog scales.

Methods of measuring pain

Pain measurement is subjective, and therefore is often thought to be of little value. This is incorrect. If some simple rules are obeyed, pain measurement can be made to work well in research settings and, perhaps even more important, pain can be recorded along with vital signs as part of the normal clinical course.

Research

The same pain scales tend to be used in acute and chronic pain. Proof of their validity dates from 40 years ago (Houde *et al.* 1960). It is especially sensible in chronic pain to use pain scales in conjunction with disability and quality-of-life measures. It makes no sense to invent your own scale. It is far better to use proven tools.

Pain intensity and pain relief can be measured by either word categories or visual analog (100-mm line) scales (Fig. 2).

For rigorous work we use all the scales (Jadad and McQuay 1994). They are clearly not independent, but if a patient gives a silly answer on one scale, out of step with his or her answers on the others, then that is an indication to requestion, thus reducing 'noise'. For chronic work, when patients are recording over long periods, we tend to use diaries with categories, and ask about both pain intensity and pain relief. Another useful scale is the patient's 'global report', sometimes used at the end of the trial period, sometimes serially during the trial. Using the same categories as the pain relief scale, this is a composite view encompassing both pain *per se* and any adverse effects of treatment (Gøtzsche 1990). The clinician's global view is a notorious overestimate and should not be used (Onghena and Van Houdenhove 1992).

Most important and simplest is the idea of including a binary scale because of its clinical relevance. The question is phrased in various forms, around the idea of 'Is your pain at least 50 per cent relieved?', to which the patient answers 'Yes' or 'No'.

Clinical practice

The argument for using pain charts as part of normal practice is to improve the quality of care. It is the fact of a chart rather than the form of the chart which is most important. Examples are the Burford Chart (Burford Nursing Development Unit 1984) or the London Hospital Chart. These should be done together with vital signs, and can then be used for both clinical care and for audit.

Problem areas

Two important groups of patients, children and the unconscious, present particular problems for pain measurement. With unconscious patients there is no alternative to using variations in vital signs, such as blood pressure rise, as a proxy for a report of increased pain. We do not know how well these proxies work. There are special scales for children over 3 years of age (McCrath *et al.* 1993). Below 3 years of age experienced staff interpreting crying and other behavior is the best guide available.

Treatment

This chapter uses systematic reviews when possible to provide the best available evidence for the various interventions used to relieve pain. NNT is used as the measure of clinical significance from quantitative systematic reviews. It shows the effort required to achieve a particular therapeutic target. NNT is treatment specific. It describes the **difference** between active treatment and control. The NNT is given by the equation

$$\text{NNT} = \frac{1}{(\text{IMP}_{act} - \text{TOT}_{act}) - (\text{IMP}_{con} - \text{TOT}_{con})}$$

where IMP_{act} is the number of patients given active treatment achieving the target, TOT_{act} is the total number of patients given the active treatment, IMP_{con} is the number of patients given a control treatment achieving the target, and TOT_{con} is the total number of patients given the control treatment.

An NNT of 1 describes an event which occurs in every patient given the treatment but in no patient in a comparator group. This could be described as the 'perfect' result in, say, a therapeutic trial of an antibiotic compared with placebo. For therapeutic benefit the NNT should be as close as possible to 1; there are few circumstances in which a treatment is close to 100 per cent effective and the control or placebo is completely ineffective, so that NNTs of 2 or 3 often indicate an effective intervention. For unwanted effects, NNT becomes the number needed to harm (**NNH**), which should be as large as possible.

By far the majority of acute pain is managed with analgesics alone. Blocking nerve transmission with continuous epidural local anesthetic is an option after major surgery. Most chronic pain is also managed initially with analgesics, but, by contrast with acute pain, commonly also involves nerve transmission block and alternative methods (Fig. 3). Figure 4 shows a simple plan. As acute pain wanes weaker analgesics are used. If chronic pain increases stronger ones are necessary.

Acute pain

A simple scheme for managing pain after trauma or surgery is shown in Fig. 5.

Low-tech: intermittent opioid injection

Intermittent opioid injection can provide effective relief of acute pain (Gould *et al.* 1992). The main reason that adequate doses are withheld by doctors or nurses is the fear of respiratory depression. Opioids used for people who are not in pain, or in doses larger than

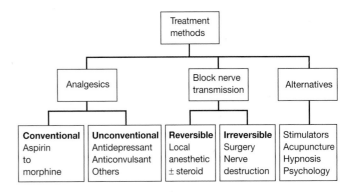

Fig. 3. Treatment methods.

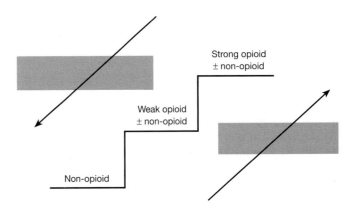

Fig. 4. The pain 'ladder'.

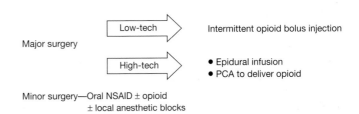

Fig. 5. Overview of acute pain management.

necessary to control the pain, can slow and indeed stop breathing. The principle is that the dose has to be titrated to the effect (Fig. 6). The effect is pain relief. If the dose given has not produced pain relief (the patient is still complaining of pain), and it has all been delivered and absorbed, then it is safe to give another dose. This subsequent dose may be smaller than the first. If it also does not succeed, then the process can be repeated.

There is no compelling evidence that one opioid is better than another, but there is good evidence that pethidine has a specific disadvantage (Szeto *et al.* 1977). Given in multiple doses its metabolite norpethidine can accumulate and act as a central nervous system irritant, ultimately causing convulsions. This is more likely when there is renal dysfunction. This toxic metabolite should preclude using pethidine when multiple injections are likely to be needed. The

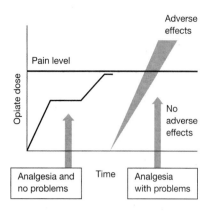

Fig. 6. Principle for safe and effective opiate use.

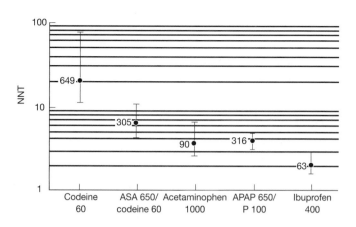

Fig. 7. Relative performances of different analgesics in single dose after surgery. A lower NNT means that the analgesic is more potent. Bars are 95 per cent confidence intervals.

old idea that pethidine is better than other opioids at dealing with colicky pain is no longer tenable (Nagle and McQuay 1990).

Morphine (and its family including heroin and codeine) has an active rather than a toxic metabolite, morphine-6-glucuronide. In renal dysfunction this metabolite can accumulate and, because it is more active than morphine, result in greater effect from a given dose. If, as should be the case, dose is being titrated against effect, this will not matter. Less morphine will be needed. It can be a problem with unconscious patients being dosed by the clock, and whose renal function is compromised (Ball et al. 1985).

We think that there are powerful risk management reasons for using one opioid only, so that everyone is familiar with dosage, effects, and problems. We think that the opioid should be morphine. The importance of good staff education was emphasized by the Cardiff audit where implementing an algorithm for intermittent opioid dosing, together with staff education, had a powerful impact on pain relief and patient satisfaction (Gould et al. 1992). Another advantage of low-tech approaches is the increased risk of adverse events with high-tech approaches (Bates et al. 1995).

High-tech: patient-controlled analgesia

Intermittent opioid injection requires good staffing levels if delays between need and injection are to be minimized. One solution to this logistic problem is to use patient-controlled analgesia (**PCA**). A syringe driver containing opioid is connected to a button and an intravenous line. The patient presses the button and an intravenous dose of opioid is given. This delivers opioid to the same opioid receptors as the intermittent injection, but circumvents any delays. Perhaps not surprisingly there is little difference in outcome between intermittent injection and PCA (Ballantyne et al. 1993). Good risk management with PCA should emphasize the same drug and the same machinery across the clinical service.

High-tech: epidural infusion

Epidural infusion via a catheter can offer continuous relief after trauma or surgery for lower-limb, spinal, abdominal, or chest pain. The current optimal infusate is an opioid–local anesthetic mixture. These two drug classes have a synergistic rather than simply additive effect when used together, so that lower doses of each are required for equivalent analgesia with fewer adverse effects (McQuay 1994).

The risks are those of an epidural (infection, hematoma, abscess),

those of the local anesthetic (cardiac and central nervous system), and those of the opioid ('late' respiratory depression). Wrong doses have been administered (Bates et al. 1995). There is an increased need for urinary catheterization. The risk of persistent neurological sequelae after an epidural is about 1 in 5000 (Kane 1981). Debate continues about whether or not patients with epidural infusions need to be nursed in a high-dependency environment.

Minor surgery (and later after major surgery)

There is an old adage that if patients can swallow it is best to take drugs by mouth. This is very pertinent for pain relief after surgery or trauma. Effective relief can be achieved with oral nonsteroidal anti-inflammatory drugs (**NSAIDs**). There is no sufficient evidence that NSAIDs by injection perform better than the same drug at the same dose given by mouth (Tramèr et al. 1997).

Figure 7 presents the current view of an evolving league table for analgesic performance after surgery. The vertical axis is the NNT for patients to achieve at least 50 per cent relief of pain.

Ibuprofen 400 mg (and other NSAIDs analysed) will produce at least 50 per cent relief of pain for one out of two postoperative patients, acetaminophen (paracetamol) 1 g for one out of four patients. As more data are added the league table should guide prescribing for the postoperative period.

The clear guideline is that the first choice is an oral NSAID. Gastric bleeding is more a problem of chronic use. Acute renal failure can be precipitated in those with pre-existing heart or kidney disease, those on loop diuretics or those who have lost more than 10 per cent of blood volume.

Local anesthetic blocks

There is a necessary distinction between blocks to permit surgery, and blocks combined with a general anesthetic to provide postoperative pain relief. There is clear evidence that blocks can indeed provide good relief in the initial postoperative period (McQuay et al. 1988), and no evidence to suggest that patients with blocks experience rebound, and need more postoperative pain relief. Details of the blocks relevant to orthopedics and trauma can be found elsewhere (Edmonds-Seal et al. 1980; Cousins and Bridenbaugh 1988; Loach

1994). There is strong interest in whether or not there are opioid receptors lurking in the periphery, and whether or not injecting opioid, for instance into the knee joint, can produce effective relief (Stein *et al.* 1991; Kalso *et al.* 1997). The risk of neurological damage is the major drawback (Bridenbaugh 1988). To minimize this risk blocks should not be performed on anesthetized patients.

Acute pain services

One remedy for poor management is the provision of an acute pain service (Royal College of Surgeons of England and College of Anaesthetists 1990). There is dispute about the range of services that should be provided, from a full 'menu' including the high-tech options discussed above (Ready *et al.* 1988) to a service which aims to educate and implement good guidelines for low-tech approaches (Gould *et al.* 1992; Rawal and Berggren 1994). The service can provide a focus for education and a referral service.

Chronic pain

The same analgesics used in acute pain, from NSAIDs through to opioids, are used for the relief of chronic pain. If analgesics relieve the pain to an adequate extent, and with tolerable or controllable adverse effects, then there is little reason to use other interventions. If analgesics are ineffective, other methods have to be considered. If analgesics are effective but cause intolerable or uncontrollable adverse effects, then other methods should be considered. The effectiveness and the adverse effects of analgesics are critical.

It is clear from work with cancer pain that using analgesics according to the World Health Organization (**WHO**) ladder (Fig. 4) can relieve pain for 80 per cent of patients. For most of these the relief will be good, but for a minority it will only be moderate. This presumes that the pain is managed optimally, and we know from audit that this is often not the case. Optimal management requires that the correct drugs are available, and that they are given in the correct dose by the correct route and at the correct time. This needs staff who are well versed in the problems, and who are available to care for the patient. The second problem is the 20 per cent of patients whose pain is not well managed by intelligent use of analgesic guidelines. The other treatment methods in Fig. 3 are necessary to manage those for whom analgesics fail.

Non-opioid analgesics

Oral NSAIDS, combinations, and others

Choosing the best analgesic for long-term use involves the same decisions as in acute pain. Most comparisons are done using single doses, whereas patients with chronic pain take multiple doses. Historically, the efficacy league table for acute pain (Fig. 7) has also proved valid for chronic pain. Despite the fact that the drugs in this category are by far the most widely used, there is remarkably little good evidence about their relative efficacy and adverse effects.

No single-dose trial has shown any efficacy advantage of one NSAID over another (Gøtzsche 1989). This does not fit well with patients' reports on multiple dosing of increased efficacy from NSAIDs with greater anti-inflammatory action. The adverse effect profile may also be different with chronic dosing. The risk of NSAID-induced gastric bleeding is lowest with ibuprofen, and increases with increasing age (Henry *et al.* 1996).

Prophylactic misoprostol should be considered for preventing NSAID-associated gastrointestinal complications in those over 75 years of age, in those with cardiovascular disease, and in those with a history of peptic ulcer or gastrointestinal bleeding (NNTs to prevent one serious gastrointestinal complication in 1 year are 105, 58, 11, and 7 respectively) (Silverstein *et al.* 1995; Shield and Morant 1996).

The efficacy dose–response curve for NSAIDs is flat compared with the dose–response curve for adverse effects such as gastrointestinal symptoms, dizziness, and drowsiness (Eisenberg *et al.* 1994). Therefore increasing the dose to improve analgesia is more likely to increase adverse effects than to improve analgesia.

Centrally acting nonopioids include dipyrone and nefopam. Dipyrone is widely used in certain countries, and is an effective analgesic which can produce blood dyscrasias. The lack of comparative evidence makes it difficult to rank its risk to benefit profile against the other analgesics.

Comparisons NSAIDs alone produced as good analgesia as single or multiple doses of weak opioids alone or in combination with non-opioid analgesics (Eisenberg *et al.* 1994). Adverse effect incidence and patient drop-out rates were the same for multiple doses of NSAIDs or weak opioids in combination with nonopioid analgesics (Eisenberg *et al.* 1994). Conversely, two studies suggest that there is little advantage in osteoarthritis of either NSAIDs over acetaminophen (March *et al.* 1994) or weak opioids in combination with acetaminophen over acetaminophen alone (Kjaersgaard-Andersen *et al.* 1990).

Topical NSAIDs

Many doctors and some pundits (Anonymous 1994) are skeptical about the efficacy of topical NSAIDS. This may not be correct.

Published randomized controlled trials on chronic pain conditions (mainly knee osteoarthritis) studied over 800 subjects treated with topical NSAIDs and 322 subjects who received placebo. The analgesic response for combined placebo treatment was 30 per cent, and for combined topical NSAID preparations it was 63 per cent. For analgesic effects the odds ratio was 3.6 (2.6–4.8) and the NNT was 3.2 (2.6–4.1) (Moore *et al.* 1998).

Opioids

In chronic pain there are two particular problems with opioids (McQuay 1989). The first is that adequate doses are often not available or are not given, primarily because of fear of addiction. The second is that some (rarer) chronic pain states, particularly when the nervous system is damaged, may not respond fully to opioids.

Opioids used for people who are not in pain can induce physical and psychological dependence. This does not happen to patients who receive them for pain relief, for instance after an operation or for severe pain from osteoporotic vertebral collapse. Some governments restrict medical availability on the grounds that if the drugs are available medically this will worsen the wider problem of addiction. There is no evidence for this. The casualties are patients who are deprived of adequate pain relief.

In chronic pain opioids are usually given by mouth. The dose is worked out by titration over a period of days, and then the drug is given regularly without waiting for the pain to return. Initial problems with nausea or dizziness commonly settle. If constipation is likely, laxatives are given.

Patients who cannot swallow can try sublingual, transdermal, or

Table 1 NNT for some analgesic interventions

Condition	Intervention	Outcome	NNT	Reference
Postoperative pain	Ibuprofen 400 mg (good)	> 50% pain relief	2	Moore et al. (1997)
	Acetaminophen 1 g	> 50% pain relief	4	Moore et al. (1997)
	Codeine 60 mg oral (poor)	> 50% pain relief	> 10	Moore and McQuay (1997)
Back pain	Epidural steroid	> 75% relief at 60 days	> 6	Watts and Silagy (1995); McQuay and Moore (1996)
Acute sprains etc.	Topical NSAID (good)	> 50% pain relief	2+	Moore et al. (1998)
Trigeminal neuralgia	Anticonvulsants	> 50% pain relief	2.5	McQuay et al. (1995)
Diabetic neuropathy	Anticonvulsants	> 50% pain relief	2.5	McQuay et al. (1995)
	Topical capsaicin	> 50% pain relief	4.2	Zhang and Li Wan Po (1994)
Diabetic neuropathic pain	Antidepressants	> 50% pain relief	2.5	McQuay et al. (1996)

suppository dosing. Subcutaneous infusion, usually from a small (external) pump is used for terminal patients who cannot manage these other routes. Rarely, the epidural route is used for combination infusion of opioid and local anesthetic.

If pain starts to increase the dose is increased. If sensible dose increases do not produce pain relief, or if increasing the opioid dose provokes intolerable or unmanageable adverse effects, then other methods must be considered, either as well as the opioid or instead of it. A working rule is that if the pain is in a numb area, which is a marker for a damaged nervous system, we would be less confident that opiates would necessarily produce pain relief (Jadad et al. 1992) and the threshold for using other strategies would be lower.

Unconventional analgesics

Unconventional analgesics (McQuay 1988) are drugs which have other indications in other medical settings, and are not normally thought of as analgesics. Treating chronic pain in a tertiary hospital setting, we use these drugs for about one-third of our patients. The hallmark is pain in a numb area—neuropathic pain.

When the patient has symptoms and signs of nervous system damage in the area of their pain we expect the response to conventional analgesics to be reduced. Conventional analgesics have often failed already, which is why the patient has been referred. If not, we try these before embarking on empirical testing to see if any of the unconventional analgesics can provide relief.

Antidepressants

Antidepressants work on the nervous system to relieve depression. We use them in much lower dosage (about half) to relieve pain. Classically they were used to relieve pain that was burning rather than shooting in character, and anticonvulsants were used for shooting pains. Now we tend to use antidepressants as first line for both types of pain, because we have had greater success and because we believe that the antidepressants cause fewer adverse effects (but see Table 1).

We use low doses (median 75 mg amitriptyline at night, maximum 150 mg) compared with those used to control depression. If there is a pain-relieving effect, it occurs well within a week, whereas 10 days is the minimum often quoted for an antidepressant effect. The older (tricyclic) antidepressants seem to be better as analgesics than the selective serotonin reuptake inhibitors. The simplest analogy is that the older drugs are like shotguns, acting on multiple transmit-

ter pathways, whereas the newer ones are more like rifles, designed to be more selective and affect only one pathway.

Anticonvulsants

Anticonvulsants have been used for many years to treat the shooting pains of trigeminal neuralgia and diabetic neuropathy. How they work has never been clear. The pervasive explanation was that they stabilized nerve membranes, preventing them from carrying spurious messages. The current fashionable explanation is that these drugs act as antagonists on the N-methyl-D-aspartate (**NMDA**) mechanism.

Anticonvulsants can provide good relief in neuropathic pain (NNT of 2–3, Table 1) (McQuay et al. 1995). Doses required for analgesic effect are in the anticonvulsant dosing range, and carry a perceived burden of adverse effects. The systematic reviews suggest that there is little difference between the adverse effects of antidepressants and anticonvulsants. Our main use is the traditional role in trigeminal neuralgia and diabetic neuropathy. We also use anticonvulsants in

Table 2 Common nerve blocks

Block	Common indications
Trigger point	Focal pain (e.g. in muscle)
Peripheral	Pain in dermatomal distribution
Intercostal	
Sacral nerves	
Rectus sheath	
Extradural	Unilateral or bilateral pain (lumbosacral, cervical, thoracic, etc.)
	Midline perineal pain
Intrathecal	Unilateral pain (neurolytic injection for pain due to malignancy, limbs, chest, etc.)
	(Midline perineal pain)
Autonomic	
Intravenous regional sympathectomy	Reflex sympathetic dystrophy
Stellate ganglion	Reflex sympathetic dystrophy
	Arm pain
	Brachial plexus nerve compression
Lumbar sympathetic	Reflex sympathetic dystrophy
	Lumbosacral plexus nerve compression
	Vascular insufficiency lower limb
	Perineal pain
Celiac plexus	Abdominal pain

shooting pain which does not respond to antidepressants. Two examples are phantom limb pain and pain in the head and neck due to tumor.

Others

Clonidine and other α_2-adrenergic agonists have analgesic effects in both conventional and neuropathic pain (McQuay 1992). They extend the duration of local anesthetic effect and have a synergistic effect with opioids. Their clinical utility is limited by the adverse effects of sedation and hypotension. In neuropathic pain single doses of clonidine were effective in post-herpetic neuralgia (Max et al. 1988) and in cancer pain (Eisenach et al. 1995). Baclofen is used by intrathecal pump to treat the painful spasms of cerebral palsy. Ketamine and dextromethorphan, both drugs with NMDA antagonist actions, are being used in severe neuropathic pain.

Block nerve transmission

Reversible procedures

Local anesthetics Local anesthetics block nerve conduction reversibly. When the local anesthetic wears off the pain returns. That is the pharmacologically correct statement, but another old saying, that a series of local anesthetic blocks can be used to 'break the cycle' of pain and effect a cure, now has some empirical support (Arner et al. 1990), even if we do not understand the mechanism. Arner and colleagues showed that the duration of pain relief could far outlast the duration of local anesthetic action, and that prolonged relief could result from a series of blocks (Arner et al. 1990). Local anesthetic blocks can thus be diagnostic and therapeutic. Diagnosis of pain, for instance from a 'trapped' lateral cutaneous nerve of the thigh, can be confirmed by local anesthetic block, and a series of blocks may prevent the recurrence of pain.

Pain clinics commonly use such blocks for shoulder pain (suprascapular nerve block) (Emery et al. 1989; van der Heijden 1996), intercostal neuralgia, rectus sheath nerve entrapment, postoperative scar pains, and other peripheral neuralgias (Table 2). What is not clear is the extent to which adding steroid to the local anesthetic makes a difference, either prolonging the duration of effect of a particular procedure or increasing the chance of success of a series of blocks.

Fibromyalgia Similar injections are done for the trigger points of fibromyalgia, but there do not appear to be any controlled comparisons of injections with other treatments.

Intravenous regional sympathectomy Intravenous regional sympathetic blocks (**IRSBs**) are used widely in patients with reflex sympathetic dystrophy. A systematic review of seven randomized controlled trials of IRSBs found that none of the four guanethidine trials showed significant analgesic effect. Two reports, one using ketanserin and one bretylium with 17 patients in total, showed some advantage of IRSBs over controls (Jadad et al. 1995). Adding guanethidine in IRSBs does not appear to be more effective than local anesthetic alone.

Epidural steroids and facet joint blocks Two other common pain clinic procedures (for back pain) are epidural steroid injection and facet nerve blocks. Epidural steroids in back pain have been studied in two systematic reviews (Koes et al. 1995; Watts and Silagy 1995). Overall the combined data showed statistically significant (odds ratios) improvement for both short-term (1 to 60 days) and long-term (12 weeks up to 1 year) treatment. The clinical significance is that the NNT for short-term (1–60 days) greater than 75 per cent pain relief from the 10 trials with short-term outcomes combined, was just under 6, with 95 per cent confidence intervals from 4 to 12 (McQuay and Moore 1996). This means that for six patients treated with epidural steroid one will obtain more than 75 per cent short-term pain relief.

The NNT for long-term improvement (12 weeks up to 1 year) from the five trials combined was about 11, with 95 per cent confidence intervals from 6 to 90. This means that for 11 patients treated with epidural steroid one will obtain more pain relief over this longer-term period. There is still the interesting question of whether local anesthetic alone could achieve these results (breaking the cycle), or whether the steroid is an essential component.

Better results are believed to be achieved the earlier the patient is treated (Benzon 1986), and in patients who have not had back surgery. It may take as long as a week for benefit from the steroid to be felt, and so it is unwise to dismiss the injection as a failure after an hour. If the injection produced incomplete or short-lived relief, then it is worth repeating, and a course of three injections is recommended. No additional benefit accrued from more than three injections (Benzon 1986).

There is considerable current controversy about the potential for epidural steroid to produce long-term neurological sequelae. Intrathecal injection of steroid can produce neurological sequelae. Therefore it is important that intrathecal injection is avoided.

Classically, facet joint injection with local anesthetic and steroid is indicated when pain is worse when sitting, and pain is provoked by lateral rotation and spine extension. Recent studies suggest that whether or not the injection is actually in the facet joint makes little difference (Lilius et al. 1989), and indeed cast some doubt on long-term utility (Carette et al. 1991). Short-lived success (less than 6 weeks) with local anesthetic and steroid is said to be improved by use of cryoanalgesia or radiofrequency blocks to the nerves to the joints.

Irreversible procedures

The destructive procedures are aimed at cutting, burning, or damaging (Table 2) the nerve fibers carrying the pain signals. The flaw in the logic is that the nervous system can all too often rewire, finding a way around the lesion. If that happens, and the pain returns, then it may be even more difficult to manage—severe neuropathic pain can result. In general neurolytic blocks in nonmalignant pain are not recommended, because they do not last for ever, and recurrent pain may be more difficult to manage, and because of the associated morbidity. These neurolytic block procedures do have a place in cancer pain when there is a short (less than 3 month) prognosis, or where alternatives such as painstaking drug control or long-term epidural infusion are not possible. Similar distinction between cancer and noncancer pain holds for celiac plexus block in pancreatic pain. Pain associated with pancreatic cancer responds well to celiac plexus block (Eisenberg et al. 1995), and it may also help those with abdominal or perineal pain from tumor in the pelvis. In chronic pancreatitis results are much less convincing.

The limitation is the potential for motor and sphincter damage. This risk is higher with bilateral and repeat procedures, and the risk is also higher the lower the cord level of the block. Extradural neurolytics have limited efficacy. While claims have been made that the paravertebral approach is preferable, patchy results may be attributed to unpredictable injectate spread. we have found that spinal infusion of a combination of local anesthetic and opioid is superior to neurolytic blocks, providing good analgesia with minimal irreversible morbidity.

Surgery The relevant neurosurgical interventions for orthopedic pain include dorsal column stimulation, rhizotomy, cordotomy, and dorsal root entry zone lesions. The indications are usually nonmalignant neuropathic pain which has failed to respond to pharmacological measures. The difficulties of trials of uncommon surgical procedures are well known. These procedures are usually documented by glowing case series. Longer-term outcomes may not be so good (Abram 1993).

Alternative treatments

Transcutaneous electrical nerve stimulation and acupuncture

The rationale for transcutaneous electrical nerve stimulation (**TENS**) is the gate theory (Melzack and Wall 1965). If the spinal cord is bombarded with impulses from the TENS machine, then it is distracted from transmitting the pathological pain signal. We know from systematic reviews that TENS has limited efficacy in acute (and postoperative) pain, and also in labour pain. As yet there is no systematic review which gathers together the many trials in chronic pain.

Attention to detail makes considerable difference to TENS efficacy in chronic pain (Johnson *et al.* 1992). Patients need to be told that it is useless expecting success unless the machine is connected for at least an hour at a time. They need to be told where to put the electrodes, how to put them on, how to manipulate the stimulus to best advantage, and indeed to turn the machine on.

Three systematic reviews discuss acupuncture in chronic nonmalignant pain (Bhatt Sanders 1985; Patel *et al.* 1989; ter Riet *et al.* 1990). These show that there is an effect, but that in clinical practice it is often short-lived (3 days) and is therefore expensive in time. It is difficult to know the real place of acupuncture, like other complementary interventions, because of the lack of trials comparing complementary with mainstream procedures (a systematic review is given by Puett and Griffin (1994)).

Physiotherapy and variants

Pain clinics keep a very open mind about other interventions. If patients benefit from alternative therapies, we are only too pleased. However, the evidence from back pain suggests that on rigorous outcome measures physiotherapy and other forms of manipulation have only limited success. Such analyses often did not include any measure of quality of life. If they make the patient feel better and they are cheap, then it is a decision for the third-party payer whether or not these physiotherapy manoeuvers should be offered (Brunarski 1984; Ottenbacher and DiFabio 1985; Koes *et al.* 1991; Abenhaim and Bergeron 1992; Anderson *et al.* 1992; Assendelft *et al.* 1992; Shekelle *et al.* 1992; Powell *et al.* 1993).

Behavioral management

Back schools through to behavioral management programs offer a range of help for patients to cope with their (usually back) pain problems. Making decisions about the benefits of psychologically based treatments of medical problems is not easy, and it is especially difficult to compare them with other treatments and to measure relative benefit and cost. Patients whose pain has proved intractable to all reasonable medical and other interventions are chronic consumers of health care—general practitioner or hospital clinic time, analgesic and psychotropic drugs, repeated admissions, and sometimes surgery. If rehabilitation treatment enables these patients to live more satisfying lives with minimum medical help, how can it be most effectively and economically offered?

Randomized comparison of the St Thomas's Hospital 4-week inpatient treatment with 8-week half-day outpatient treatment including fitness training, planned increases in activity, activity scheduling, drug reduction, relaxation, and cognitive therapy as the pain management methods taught by the same staff team (Pither and Nicholas 1991) showed that for every three patients treated as inpatients rather than outpatients, one patient fewer was taking analgesic or psychotropic drugs. For every four patients treated as inpatients rather than outpatients, one patient fewer sought additional medical advice in the year after treatment. For every five patients treated as inpatients rather than outpatients, one patient more had a 10-min walking distance improved by more than 50 per cent. For every six patients treated as inpatients rather than outpatients, one patient fewer was depressed (Bandolier 1995). Systematic reviews include Suls and Fletcher (1985), Mullen *et al.* (1987), Malone *et al.* (1988), Fernandez and Turk (1989), Hyman *et al.* (1989), Cohen *et al.* (1994), Cutler *et al.* (1994), and Gebhardt (1994).

References

Abenhaim, L. and Bergeron, A.M. (1992). Twenty years of randomized clinical trials of manipulative therapy for back pain: a review. *Clinical Investigative Medicine*, **15**, 527–35.

Abram, S.E. (1993). 1992 Bonica Lecture. Advances in chronic pain management since gate control. *Regional Anesthesia*, **18**, 66–81.

Anderson, R., Meeker, W.C., Wirick, B.E., Mootz, R.D., Kirk, D.H., and Adams, A. (1992). A meta-analysis of clinical trials of spinal manipulation. *Journal of Manipulative Physiological Therapy*, **15**, 181–94.

Anonymous (1994). Rational use of NSAIDs for musculoskeletal disorders. *Drug and Therapeutics Bulletin*, **32**, 91–5.

Arner, A., Lindblom, U., Meyerson, B.A., and Molander, C. (1990). Prolonged relief of neuralgia after regional anesthetic blocks. A call for further experimental and systematic clinical studies. *Pain*, **43**, 287–97.

Assendelft, W.J., Koes, B.W., Van der Heijden, G.J., and Bouter, L.M. (1992). The efficacy of chiropractic manipulation for back pain: blinded review of relevant randomized clinical trials. *Journal of Manipulative Physiological Therapy*, **15**, 487–94.

Ball, M., McQuay, H.J., Moore, R.A., Allen, M.C., Fisher, A., and Sear, J. (1985). Renal failure and the use of morphine in intensive care. *Lancet*, **i**, 784–6.

Ballantyne, J.C., Carr, D.B., Chalmers, T.C., Dear, K.B.G., Angelillo, I.F., and Mosteller, F. (1993). Postoperative patient-controlled analgesia: meta-analyses of initial randomised controlled trials. 1. *Clinical Anesthesia*, **5**, 182–93.

Bandolier (1995). http://www.jr2.ox.ac.uk/Bandolier; issue 22.

Bates, D.W., Cullen, D.J., Laird, N., *et al.* (1995). Incidence of adverse drug events and potential adverse drug events. *Journal of the American Medical Association*, **274**, 29–34.

Benzon, H.T. (1986). Epidural steroid injections for low back pain and lumbosacral radiculopathy. *Pain*, **24**, 277–95.

Bhatt Sanders, D. (1985). Acupuncture for rheumatoid arthritis: an analysis of the literature. *Seminars in Arthritis and Rheumatology*, **14**, 225–31.

Bridenbaugh, P.O. (1988). Complications of local anesthetic neural blockade. In *Neural blockade* (ed. M.J. Cousins and P.O. Bridenbaugh), pp. 695–717. Lippincott, Philadelphia, PA.

Brunarski, D.J. (1984). Clinical trials of spinal manipulation: a critical appraisal and review of the literature. *Journal of Manipulative Physiological Therapy*, **7**, 243–9.

Burford Nursing Development Unit (1984). Nurses and pain. *Nursing Times*, **18**, 94.

Carette, S., Marcoux, S., Truchon, R., *et al.* (1991). A controlled trial of corticosteroid injections into facet joints for chronic low back pain. *New England Journal of Medicine*, **325**, 1002–7.

Cohen, J.E., Goel, V., Frank, J.W., Bombardier, C., Peloso, P., and Guillemin, F. (1994). Group education interventions for people with low back pain. An overview of the literature. *Spine*, **19**, 1214–22.

Cousins, M.J. and Bridenbaugh, P.O. (1988). *Neural blockade*. Lippincott, Philadelphia, PA.

Cutler, R.B., Fishbain, D.A., Rosomoff, H.L., Abdel-Moty, E., Khalil, T.M., and Rosomoff, R.S. (1994). Does nonsurgical pain center treatment of chronic pain return patients to work? A review and meta-analysis of the literature. *Spine*, **19**, 643–52.

Edmonds-Seal, J., Paterson, G.M.C., and Loach, A.B. (1980). Local nerve blocks for postoperative analgesia. *Journal of the Royal Society of Medicine*, **73**, 111–14.

Eisenach, J.C., DuPen, S., Dubois, M., Nfiguel, R., and Allin, D. (1995). Epidural clonidine analgesia for intractable cancer pain. The Epidural Clonidine Study Group. *Pain*, **61**, 391–9.

Eisenberg, E., Berkey, C.S., Carr, D.B., Mosteller, F., and Chalmers, T.C. (1994). Efficacy and safety of nonsteroidal anti-inflammatory drugs for cancer pain: a meta-analysis. *Journal of Clinical Oncology*, **12**, 2756–65.

Eisenberg, E., Carr, D.B., and Chalmers, T.C. (1995). Neurolytic celiac plexus block for treatment of cancer pain: a meta-analysis. *Anesthetics and Analgesia*, **80**, 290–5.

Emery, P., Bowman, S., Wedderburn, L., and Grahame, R. (1989). Suprascapular nerve block for chronic shoulder pain in rheumatoid arthritis. *British Medical Journal*, **299**, 1079–80.

Fernandez, E. and Turk, D.C. (1989). The utility of cognitive coping strategies for altering pain perception: a meta analysis. *Pain*, **38**, 123–35.

Gebhardt, W.A. (1994). Effectiveness of training to prevent job-related back pain: a meta-analysis. *British Journal of Clinical Psychology*, **33**, 571–4.

Gøtzsche, P.C. (1989). Patients' preference in indomethacin trials: an overview. *Lancet*, **i**, 88–91.

Gøtzsche, P.C. (1990). Sensitivity of effect variables in rheumatoid arthritis: a meta-analysis of 130 placebo controlled NSAID trials. *Journal of Clinical Epidemiology*, **43**, 1313–18.

Gould, T.H., Crosby, D.L., Harmer, M., *et al.* (1992). Policy for controlling pain after surgery: effect of sequential changes in management. *British Medical Journal*, **305**, 1187–93.

Henry, D., Lim, L.L.-Y., Rodriguez, L.A.G., *et al.* (1996). Variability in risk of gastrointestinal complications with individual non-steroidal anti-inflammatory drugs: results of a collaborative meta-analysis. *British Medical Journal*, **312**, 1563–6.

Houde, R.W., Wallenstein, S.L., and Rogers, A. (1960). Clinical pharmacology of analgesics: a method of assaying analgesic effect. *Clinical Pharmacology and Therapeutics*, **1**, 163–74.

Hyman, R.B., Feldman, H.R., Harris, R.B., Levin, R.F., and Malloy, G.B. (1989). The effects of relaxation training on clinical symptoms: a meta analysis. *Nursing Research*, **38**, 216–20.

Jadad, A.R. and McQuay, H.J. (1994). Pain measurement. In *Outcome measures in trauma* (ed. J. Fairbank, P. Pysent, and A. Carr), p. 1724. Butterworth Heinemann, Oxford.

Jadad, A.R., Carroll, D., Glynn, C.J., Moore, R.A., and McQuay, H.J. (1992).

Morphine responsiveness of chronic pain: double-blind randomised cross-over study with patient-controlled analgesia. *Lancet*, **339**, 1367–71.

Jadad, A.R., Carroll, D., Glynn, C.J., and McQuay, H.J. (1995). Intravenous regional sympathetic blockade for pain relief in reflex sympathetic dystrophy: a systematic review and a randomized, double-blind crossover study. *Journal of Pain and Symptom Management*, **10**, 1320.

Johnson, M.I., Ashton, C.H., and Thompson, J.W. (1992). Long term use of transcutaneous electrical nerve stimulation at Newcastle Pain Relief Clinic. *Journal of the Royal Society of Medicine*, **85**, 267–8.

Kalso, E., Tramer, M., Carroll, D., McQuay, H., and Moore, R.A. (1997). Pain relief from intra-articular morphine after knee surgery: a qualitative systematic review. *Pain*, **71**, 127–34.

Kane, R.E. (1981). Neurologic deficits following epidural or spinal anesthesia. *Anesthesia and Analgesia*, **60**, 150–61.

Kjaersgaard-Andersen, P., Nafei, A., Skov, O., *et al.* (1990). Codeine plus paracetamol versus paracetamol in longer-term treatment of chronic pain due to osteoarthritis of the hip. *Pain*, **43**, 309–18.

Koes, B.W., Assendelft, W.J., van der Heijden, G.J., Bouter, L.M., and Knipschild, P.G. (1991). Spinal manipulation and mobilisation for back and neck pain: a blinded review. *British Medical Journal*, **303**, 1298–303.

Koes, B.W., Scholten, R.P.M., Mens, J.M.A., and Bouter, L.M. (1995). Efficacy of epidural steroid injections for low-back pain and sciatica: a systematic review of randomized clinical trials. *Pain*, **63**, 279–88.

Lilius, G., Laasonen, E.M., Myllynen, P., Harilainen, A., and Grbnlund, G. (1989). Lumbar facet joint syndrome. *Journal of Bone and Joint Surgery*, **71**, 681–4.

Loach, A. (1994). *Orthopaedic anaesthesia*. (2nd edn). Edward Arnold, London.

McGrath, P.J., Ritchie, J.A., and Unruh, A.M. (1993). Paediatric pain. In *Pain management and nursing care* (ed. D. Carroll and D. Bowsher), pp. 100–23. Butterworth Heinemann, Oxford.

McQuay, H.J. (1988). Pharmacological treatment of neuralgic and neuropathic pain. *Cancer Surveys*, **7**, 141–59.

McQuay, H.J. (1989). Opioids in chronic pain. *British Journal of Anaesthesia*, **63**, 213–26.

McQuay, H.J. (1992). Is there a place for alpha 2 adrenergic agonists in the control of pain? In *Toward the use of alpha 2 adrenergic agonists for the treatment of pain* (ed. J.M. Besson and G. Guilbaud), pp. 219–32. Elsevier, Amsterdam.

McQuay, H. (1994). Epidural analgesics. In *Textbook of pain* (ed. P. Wall and R. Melzack), pp. 1025–34. Churchill Livingstone, London.

McQuay, H.J. (1995). Pre-emptive analgesia: a systematic review of clinical studies. *Annals of Medicine*, **27**, 249–58.

McQuay, H.J. and Dickenson, A.H. (1990). Implications of nervous system plasticity for pain management. *Anaesthesia*, **45**, 101–2.

McQuay, H. and Moore, R.A. (1996). Epidural steroids. *Anaesthesia and Intensive Care*, **24**, 284–6.

McQuay, H.J., Carroll, D., and Moore, R.A. (1988). Postoperative orthopaedic pain—the effect of opiate premedication and local anaesthetic blocks. *Pain*, **33**, 291–5.

McQuay, H., Carroll, D., Jadad, A.R., Wiffen, P., and Moore, A. (1995). Anticonvulsant drugs for management of pain: a systematic review. *British Medical Journal*, **311**, 1047–52.

McQuay, H., Nye, B.A., Carroll, D., Wiffen, P.J., Tramèr, M., and Moore, R.A. (1996). A systematic review of antidepressants in neuropathic pain. *Pain*, **68**, 217–27.

Malone, M.D., Strube, M.J., and Scogin, F.R. (1988). Meta analysis of non medical treatments for chronic pain. *Pain*, **34**, 231–44.

March, L., Irwig, L., Schwarz, J., Simpson, J., Chock, C., and Brooks, P. (1994). N of 1 trials comparing a non-steroidal anti-inflammatatory drug with paracetamol in osteoarthritis. *British Medical Journal*, **309**, 1041–6.

Max, M.B., Schafer, S.C., Culnane, M., Dubner, R., and Gracely, R.H. (1988). Association of pain relief with drug side effects in postherpetic neuralgia: a single dose study of clonidine, codeine, ibuprofen, and placebo. *Clinical Pharmacology and Therapeutics*, **43**, 363–71.

Melzack, R. and Wall, P.D. (1965). Pain mechanisms: a new theory. *Science*, **150**, 971–8.

Moore, R.A. and McQuay, H.J. (1997). Single-patient data meta-analysis of 3453 postoperative patients: oral tramadol versus placebo, codeine and combination analgesics. *Pain*, **69**, 287–94.

Moore, R.A., McQuay, H.J., and Gavaghan, D.J. (1997). Deriving dichotomous outcome measures from continuous data in randomised controlled trials of analgesics. *Pain*, **69**, 127–30.

Moore, R.A., Nye, B.A., Carroll, D., Wiffen, P.J., Tramèr, M., and McQuay, H.J. (1998). A systematic review of topically-applied non-steroidal anti-inflammatory drugs. *British Medical Journal*, **316**, 333–8.

Mullen, P.D., Laville, E.A., Biddle, A.K., and Lorig, K. (1987). Efficacy of psychoeducational interventions on pain, depression, and disability in people with arthritis: a meta analysis. *Journal of Rheumatology*, **14** (Supplement), 33–9.

Nagle, C.J. and McQuay, H.J. (1990). Opiate receptors; their role in effect and side-effect. *Current Anaesthesia and Critical Care*, **1**, 247–52.

Onghena, P. and Van Houdenhove, B. (1992). Antidepressant-induced analgesia in chronic non-malignant pain: a meta-analysis of 39 placebo-controlled studies. *Pain*, **49**, 205–19.

Ottenbacher, K. and DiFabio, R.P. (1985). Efficacy of spinal manipulation/mobilization therapy. A meta analysis. *Spine*, **10**, 833–7.

Patel, M., Gutzwiller, F., Paccaud, F., and Marazzi, A. (1989). A meta-analysis of acupuncture for chronic pain. *International Journal of Epidemiology*, **18**, 900–6.

Pither, C.E. and Nicholas, M.K. (1991). Psychological approaches in chronic pain management. *British Medical Journal*, **47**, 743–61.

Powell, F.C., Hanigan, W.C., and Olivero, W.C. (1993). A risk/benefit analysis of spinal manipulation therapy for relief of lumbar or cervical pain. *Neurosurgery*, **33**, 73–8 (discussion 78–9).

Puett, D.W. and Griffin, M.R. (1994). Published trials of nonmedicinal and noninvasive therapies for hip and knee osteoarthritis. *Annals of Internal Medicine*, **121**, 133–40.

Rawal, N. and Berggren, L. (1994). Organization of acute pain services: a low-cost model. *Pain*, **57**, 117–23.

Ready, L.B., Oden, R., Chadwick, H.S., *et al.* (1988). Development of an anaesthesiology based postoperative pain management service. *Anesthesiology*, **68**, 100–6.

Royal College of Surgeons of England and College of Anaesthetists (1990). *Report of the Working Party on Pain after Surgery*. Royal College of Surgeons, London.

Shekelle, P.G., Adams, A.H., Chassin, M.R., Hurwitz, E.L., and Brook, R.H. (1992). Spinal manipulation for low-back pain. *Annals of Internal Medicine*, **117**, 590–8.

Shield, M.J. and Morant, S.V. (1996). Misoprostol in patients taking NSAIDS. *British Medical Journal*, **312**, 846.

Silverstein, F.E., Graham, D.Y., Senior, J.R., *et al.* (1995). Misoprostol reduces serious gastrointestinal complications in patients with rheumatoid arthritis receiving nonsteroidal anti-inflammatory drugs. *American College of Physicians*, **123**, 241–9.

Stein, C., Comisel, K., Haimerl, E., *et al.* (1991). Analgesic effect of intra-articular morphine after arthroscopic surgery. *New England Journal of Medicine*, **325**, 1123–6.

Suls, J. and Fletcher, B. (1985). The relative efficacy of avoidant and non-avoidant coping strategies: a meta analysis. *Health Psychology*, **4**, 249–88.

Szeto, H.H., Inturrisi, C.E., Houde, R., Saal, S., Cheigh, J., and Reidenberg, M. (1977). Accumulation of norperidine, an active metabolite of meperidine, in patients with renal failure or cancer. *Annals of Internal Medicine*, **86**, 738–41.

ter Riet, G., Kleijnen, J., and Knipschild, P. (1990). Acupuncture and chronic pain: a criteria-based meta-analysis. 1. *Clinical Epidemiology*, **43**, 1191–9.

Tramèr, M., Williams, J., Carroll, D., Wiffen, P.J., McQuay, H.J., and Moore, R.A. (1997). Systematic review of direct comparisons of non-steroidal anti-inflammatory drugs given by different routes. *Acta Anaesthesiologica Scandinavica*, **42**, 71–9.

van der Heijden, C.J.M.G. (1996). Steroid injections for shoulder disorders: systematic review of randomised clinical trials. *British Journal of General Practice*, **44**, 309–16.

Watts, R.W. and Silagy, C.A. (1995). A meta-analysis on the efficacy of epidural corticosteroids in the treatment of sciatica. *Anaesthesia and Intensive Care*, **23**, 564–9.

Zhang, W.Y. and Li Wan Po, A. (1994). The effectiveness of topically applied capsaicin. A meta-analysis. *European Journal of Clinical Pharmacology*, **46**, 517–22.

1.11 Biomechanics

A. B. Zavatsky

Introduction

Biomechanics is the application of the principles of mechanics and the techniques of engineering to the study of biologic systems, including the human body. From an early date, one of the major areas of biomechanical study has been the musculoskeletal system or locomotor system. Diagnosis and treatment of disorders and diseases of the musculoskeletal system are the main goals of orthopedics. Practitioners in this field require an understanding of bone, muscle, connective tissue, and nerve. They need to understand how these tissues function and interact on all levels—from genetic and cellular levels to the macroscopic level of the joints and limbs.

There are many reasons why orthopedic surgeons should make an effort to understand the basics of biomechanics. First, the musculoskeletal system is affected not only by genetic and metabolic factors, but also by mechanical factors (Williams *et al.* 1989). This was recognized over a century ago by Wolff (1892), who studied the adaptation of bone to the forces applied to it. The idea that bone perceives and adapts to its functional demands is widely known today as Wolff's law.

Second, many orthopedic surgical procedures are based on simple mechanical principles. For example, a 'closing osteotomy'—an operation which can be used to correct deformity or to reduce pain and disability at an arthritic joint—involves first cutting into two parts one of the bones which meets at the affected joint. A wedge of bone is then removed, followed by realignment and healing of the cut bone ends. The resulting redistribution of load at the joint depends critically on the size and shape of the bone removed, and this should be calculated based on mechanical principles before the procedure is attempted.

Third, the design and application of orthopedic devices and prostheses and of rehabilitation regimes requires a knowledge of the magnitude and frequency of the forces likely to be transmitted by the bones, muscles, and joints during activities of daily living. This also requires an understanding of biomechanics.

Finally, many cases seen by an orthopedic surgeon involve trauma. To understand the mechanisms of traumatic injury, to know how the tissues will react or ultimately fail, and to develop preventative measures requires the assessment of high-speed impact forces, another topic from the realm of mechanics. So, as shown by these examples, a knowledge of basic biomechanics can only be an asset to anyone involved in orthopedics and traumatology.

To cover the range of biomechanical applications in orthopedics would take an entire volume (Nordin and Frankel 1989; Fung 1993; Nigg and Herzog 1994; Simon 1994; Mow and Hayes 1997). Similarly, to explain and illustrate the principles of engineering mechanics (Meriam and Kraige 1993*a,b*) and the techniques of modern engineering would require much space. Indeed, this has been done successfully by others. Instead of duplicating their work, this chapter will explain how loads are transmitted by the bones, muscles, and other soft tissues. In doing so, some basic concepts useful for further study in biomechanics will be introduced.

Loads applied to the body

To find the forces acting in the bones, muscles, and soft tissues of the body, one could attempt to measure them *in vivo*. Direct measurement of forces and strains in living human tissues is not impossible (Komi *et al.* 1987; Beynnon *et al.* 1992), but it is difficult. In addition, ethical considerations mean that most such measurements are done either in animals or *in vitro*. Regardless of which approach is taken, a detailed understanding of the measurement process itself is needed and also a knowledge of the possible physical, biochemical, and physiological interactions of the measurement device with the tissue being measured (Cobbold 1974).

One alternative to direct measurement of forces is the creation and solution of a mathematical model of the system of interest. The particular body or mechanical system to be analyzed is isolated and all the forces or loads which act on it are defined clearly and completely. This isolation of the body of interest is accomplished by means of a 'free-body diagram', which is a diagrammatic representation of the isolated body showing all the forces applied to it by mechanical contact and all body forces, such as those due to gravitational attraction. The construction of the free-body diagram is the single most important step in the solution of problems in mechanics (Meriam and Kraige 1993*a*). Only when a clear free-body diagram has been completed should mathematical relationships between the force quantities be written and solved.

Consider the physical situation in Fig. 1(a), which shows a man carrying a briefcase climbing some stairs. The system of interest is the man, and so he is drawn separately as the first step in constructing a free-body diagram (Fig. 1(b)). Then it is necessary to draw as arrows all the forces acting on the man and to specify their magnitudes, directions, and points of application. In the language of mechanics, these forces are known as vectors. A vector is usually written in boldface type ($\mathbf{F}$) or with an arrow over it ($\vec{F}$).

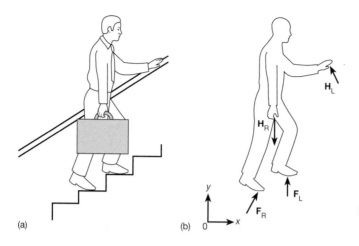

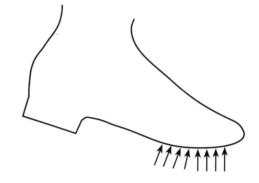

Fig. 2. Distributed forces on the left foot of the man in Fig. 1.

Fig. 1. (a) A man climbing stairs. (b) Free-body diagram of a man climbing stairs, excluding the force of body weight.

Forces may be either concentrated or distributed. When the area over which the force is applied is small compared with the other dimensions of the body, the force may be considered to be concentrated at a point. These are the types of force acting on the man's feet (labeled F_L and F_R in Fig. 1(b)) and on the hand which he rests on the handrail (labeled H_L in Fig. 1(b)). These particular forces are a good example of Newton's third law of mechanics (sometimes known as 'action and reaction'). The man's foot pushes against the stair with a certain force, and the stair pushes back on the foot with a force of the same magnitude and line of action, but in the opposite direction. The forces F_L, F_R, and H_L all have units of newtons (N) in the SI system.

An arrow (labeled H_R) indicating the downward force due to the weight of the briefcase which the man carries in his right hand must also be drawn on the free-body diagram. The force $H_R = m_B g$, where m_B is the mass of the briefcase in kilograms (kg) and g is the acceleration associated with the gravitational force of attraction (9.81 m/s²). Note that 1 N = 1 k m/s². Note also that the force H_R acts downward, towards the center of the Earth.

Distributed forces are applied over an area, or they may be distributed over a volume. The weight of a body or body segment is the force of gravitational attraction distributed over its volume, but this is usually taken as a concentrated force acting through the center of gravity of the body or the relevant body segment. The weight of the man (not included in Fig. 1(b)) is equal to the mass of the man m_M (in kg) times g.

If, instead of the whole man, the bones, muscles, and joints of his feet were of interest, the nonuniform distributed forces (Fig. 2), rather than the concentrated forces F_L and F_R (Fig. 1(b)), would have to be considered. The distributed forces act over the area of contact between the man's feet and the stairs. The parts of these forces perpendicular to the soles of the man's shoes can be thought of as pressures; they have units of force per unit area, namely N/m² or pascals (Pa). Instrumentation has been designed to measure plantar pressure using either shoe insole devices or special plates set in the floor (Lord *et al.* 1986; Alexander *et al.* 1990), but the majority of these devices are limited in that they can only measure pressure in a direction perpendicular to the device itself.

In addition to the forces, pertinent dimensions may also be represented on the free-body diagram. Numerical values for average body segment lengths have been compiled in tables (Winter 1990). The study of such physical measurements of the human body is called anthropometry. In biomechanical studies, a wide variety of physical measurements are required, including not only body segment lengths and masses, centers of mass, and moments of inertia, but also locations of muscle origins and insertions, angles of pull of tendons, and lengths and cross-sectional areas of muscles. In the past, most of these measurements were made on cadavers, but now many subject-specific measurements can be made *in vivo* using plane radiography, CT, or MRI.

It is also usual to indicate a set of co-ordinate axes on the free-body diagram. For simplicity, only two dimensions will be considered in this example, and so in Fig. 1(b) the axes x and y have been added. The x axis points to the right, and the y axis points upward. If a z axis were included, it would point out of the page. The origin O of this global co-ordinate system is fixed on the bottom stair.

Note that each force vector in Fig. 1(b) could instead be drawn as the sum of two perpendicular vectors, one parallel to the x axis and one parallel to the y axis. An example is given in Fig. 3(a), in which $F = F_x + F_y$. The absolute values of the two perpendicular vectors ($|F_x| = F_x$ and $|F_y| = F_y$) are known as the 'components' of the vector F. The graphical construction in Fig. 3(a) is an example of the 'parallelogram law of vector addition', in which the resultant of two vectors is found by drawing each vector to scale and arranging them tip to tail. The resultant then connects the tail of the first vector drawn to the tip of the last vector drawn. The vectors to be added need not necessarily be parallel, nor does it matter in which order they are drawn (Fig. 3(b)).

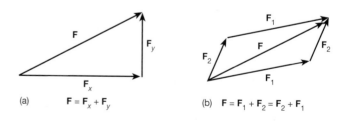

Fig. 3. The parallelogram law of vector addition. (a) Perpendicular forces F_x and F_y add to give F. (b) Forces F_1 and F_2 add to give F_3. Note that the order of addition is not important: $F_1 + F_2 = F_2 + F_1 = F_3$.

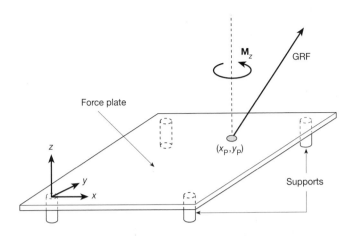

Fig. 4. The force plate. The ground reaction force (**GRF**), the free moment of rotation (**M**$_z$), and the center of pressure (x_p, y_p) are shown. Note that the axis directions differ from those shown in Fig. 1.

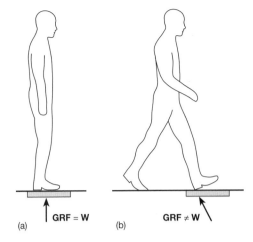

Fig. 5. (a) A static measurement on the force plate. The ground reaction force (**GRF**) equals the man's weight (**W**). (b) A dynamic measurement on the force plate during normal level walking. The ground reaction force (**GRF**) does not equal the man's weight (**W**).

External loads applied to the body can often be measured accurately using force transducers which give an electrical signal proportional to the applied force. Excluding the gravitational force, the most common external force acting on the body is the ground reaction force (**F**$_L$ or **F**$_R$ in Fig. 1(b)) which acts on the foot during standing, walking, or running (Winter 1990). The device used to measure the ground reaction force is called a force plate or force platform and is an important tool in clinical gait analysis (Whittle 1996). Most force plates are rectangular in shape, lie flush with the ground, and are supported below ground level at each corner (Fig. 4). Force transducers are mounted on each support in each axis direction (x, y, z). Summing the x, y, and z components of force measured at each corner gives the x, y, and z components of the ground reaction force. To find the point on the force plate through which the ground reaction force appears to act (the center of pressure x_p, y_p) and what is called the 'free moment of rotation' about a vertical axis (**M**$_z$), a series of equations must be written and solved (Nigg 1994*a*). When a person stands perfectly still with both feet on the force plate, the measured ground reaction force will equal the person's body weight (Fig. 5(a)). When a person walks or runs across the force plate, the force measured no longer equals body weight but is an indication of both the mass and the inertia of the body (Fig. 5(b)). Figures 6(a) to 6(c) show how the components of the ground reaction force change over time during the stance phase of walking. Figure 6(d) shows a normal pattern of ground reaction force vectors as seen in the sagittal plane; this plot is known as a Pedotti diagram or a butterfly diagram. In addition to the force plate, instrumentation has been designed to measure the forces applied to the feet during cycling (Hull and Davis 1981; Newmiller *et al.* 1988; Ruby and Hull 1993).

Statics versus dynamics

Mechanics deals with bodies either in a state of rest or moving under the action of forces. Statics involves a description of the conditions of force that are both necessary and sufficient to maintain a state of equilibrium. When a body is in equilibrium (either stationary or moving at constant velocity, according to Newton's first law of mechanics), the resultant force and resultant moment acting on it are zero ($\Sigma \mathbf{F} = 0$, $\Sigma \mathbf{M} = 0$).

Moment is the term used to describe the tendency of a force to rotate a body about some axis. The magnitude of a moment **M** is proportional to the magnitude of the force **F** which causes it and to the moment arm d, which is the perpendicular distance from the axis about which rotation occurs to the line of action of the force, or $|\mathbf{M}| = |\mathbf{F}|d$, as shown in Fig. 7(a). The moment produced by two equal and opposite but noncollinear forces (**F** and −**F**) a distance d apart is known as a couple **C** with magnitude $|\mathbf{F}|d$ (Fig. 7(b)). Notice that the sum of the two forces is zero since they are equal and opposite. There is no tendency for the forces to translate the body, but they do tend to rotate it. Moments and couples are vectors, and their directions are given by the 'right-hand rule' (Fig. 8).

To check whether the sum of the forces acting on a body is zero, the force vectors must be summed either graphically using the 'parallelogram law' (Fig. 3) or algebraically using the force components. In all but the simplest two-dimensional problems, it is more convenient to add the components. This is especially true if a large number of forces is involved and a computer is used to solve any equations. In two dimensions, to check whether the sum of the moments acting on a body is zero, moments about any point must be summed. Clockwise moments must balance counterclockwise moments. In three dimensions, moments about the x, y, and z axes must be considered.

Dynamics is the study of the motion of bodies under the action of forces. 'Forward dynamics' is the prediction of motion from known forces, while 'inverse dynamics' is the calculation of forces from known motions. Dynamics involves the tendency of unbalanced forces to translate a body and the tendency of unbalanced moments to rotate a body. From Newton's second law, we know that $\Sigma \mathbf{F} = m\mathbf{a}$, or the acceleration of a particle (or of the center of mass of a body) is proportional to the resultant force acting on it and is in the direction of the force. The constant of proportionality is the mass of the particle or body. Note that acceleration, like force, is a vector and has components in the x, y, and z directions. For moments in two

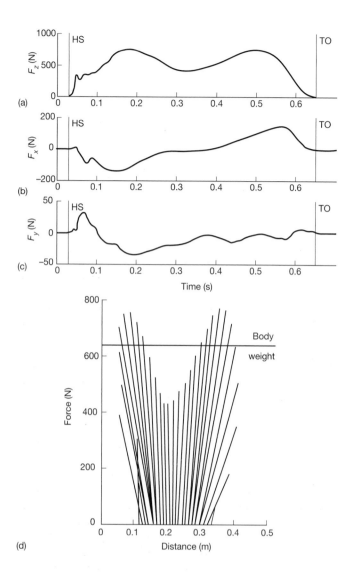

Fig. 6. The ground reaction force during the stance phase of normal gait. (a) The vertical component F_z is positive upward. (b) The fore–aft horizontal component F_x is positive forward. (c) In this case the mediolateral horizontal component F_y is positive laterally. (d) The pattern of ground reaction force vectors as seen in the sagittal plane. HS, heelstrike; TO, toe-off. (Data courtesy of the Oxford Gait Laboratory, Nuffield Orthopaedic Centre NHS Trust, Oxford, UK.)

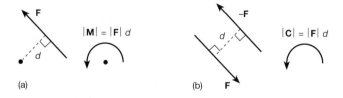

Fig. 7. (a) The moment **M** of force **F** about a point. The length d is the moment arm of the force **F**. (b) Two equal and opposite but noncollinear forces **F** form the couple **C**.

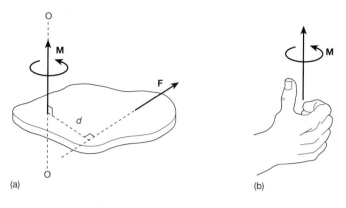

Fig. 8. The 'right-hand rule'. The moment **M** of force **F** about O–O is represented as a vector pointing in the direction of the thumb, with the fingers pointing in the direction of the tendency to rotate. (Adapted from Meriam and Kraige (1993a).)

dimensions, $\Sigma Mz = I\alpha$ where I is the moment of inertia (or tendency of the body to resist rotation) and α is the angular acceleration. The moment of inertia is usually referred to the center of mass of the body or segment. An explanation of how it is calculated and how the moment equation changes for three-dimensional motion is beyond the scope of this chapter (Meriam and Kraige 1993b).

Loads internal to the body

Before finding the forces acting in particular body tissues during activity, it is necessary to quantify the resultant force and moment acting along a limb or at a joint. For static situations, this is relatively easy. A free-body diagram of the body is drawn and an imaginary slice taken through it at the section of interest. This imaginary slice may be through a bone shaft (Fig. 9(a)) or through a joint (Fig. 9(b)). A resultant force **F** and a resultant moment **M** act at this section, and they balance the external loads and segment weights. At a joint, these quantities are sometimes called the 'resultant joint force and moment' or the 'intersegmental force and moment'.

The calculated resultant forces and moments at the sections shown in Fig. 9 do not correspond to actual forces and moments, and they cannot be measured with transducers. They are abstract quantities that are often used not as final results but as inputs to a second step—determination of the distribution of these forces and moments among the structures of the body.

In dynamic situations, the calculation of forces and moments within the body is much more difficult since the accelerations of the various body segments must be taken into account. To do this, the body is usually divided up into segments, and the forces, moments, and accelerations of each segment are considered separately. An example of a two-dimensional link-segment model of the lower limb is shown in Fig. 10. The limb is divided into three segments (thigh, shank, foot), each with its own mass m_i and moment of inertia I_i (Fig. 10(a)). In this simple model, the links are connected by pins. To draw a free-body of each segment, we disconnect the link-segment model at the joints and draw the resultant force and moment at each joint (Fig. 10(c)). On the foot segment, the resultant joint force $\mathbf{R}_a$ at the ankle has two components, R_{x_a} and R_{y_a}. The resultant joint

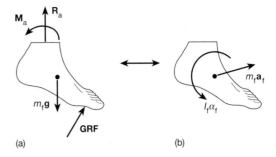

Fig. 11. (a) Free-body diagram and (b) kinetic diagram of the foot during the stance phase of walking.

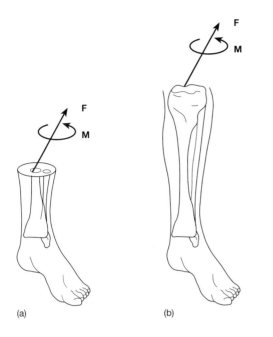

Fig. 9. Resultant force **F** and resultant moment **M** acting at a section (a) through the shank and (b) through the knee. (Adapted from O'Connor (1991).)

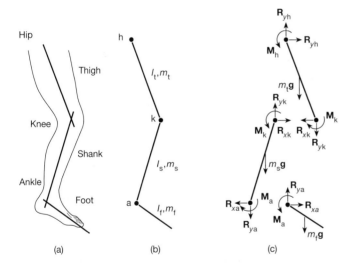

Fig. 10. (a), (b) A sagittal-plane link-segment model of the lower limb. Each link has a mass mi and a moment of inertia li. (c) Free-body diagrams of the three links, each showing the segment weight and the intersegmental forces **F**i and moment **M**i. (Adapted from Winter (1990).)

moment is $\mathbf{M}_a$. On the free-body diagram of the shank segment, $\mathbf{M}_a$ and the components of $\mathbf{R}_a$ are opposite in direction to those drawn on the foot segment. The same is true for the joint reaction force and moment at the knee, as shown on the free-body diagrams of the shank and thigh segments.

In link-segment models of the lower limb, the most distal segment is considered first, followed by the next adjacent segment, moving proximally. Figure 11(a) is a free-body diagram of the foot segment showing all the forces acting on it: the known ground reaction force (**GRF**), the known segment weight ($m_f\mathbf{g}$), and the unknown joint (ankle) reaction force ($\mathbf{R}_a$) and moment ($\mathbf{M}_a$). Figure 11(b) is a 'kinetic diagram' showing the 'inertial forces' $m_i\mathbf{a}_f$ and $I_f\alpha_f$ on the foot. We know from the previous section that, for dynamics in two-dimensions, $\Sigma F = m\mathbf{a}$ and $\Sigma M = I\alpha$, so that the diagrams in Figs 11(a) and 11(b) must be equivalent. When the linear acceleration $\mathbf{a}$ of the center of mass and the angular acceleration α_f of the foot are known, equations to calculate the unknown joint reaction force components (R_{x_a} and R_{y_a}) and the joint reaction moment ($\mathbf{M}_a$) can be written, as will be explained below. Once these are found, the equilibrium of the shank can be considered and, after that, the thigh.

The accelerations needed for a dynamic analysis of a link-segment model can be measured directly using small electronic devices called accelerometers (Morris 1973). These are mounted on or strapped to each segment of interest. Three accelerometers mounted at right angles to each other are needed to measure linear accelerations in three dimensions (a_x, a_y, a_z). To quantify the angular accelerations (α_x, α_y, α_z) of a segment, additional accelerometers must be used. The use of accelerometers in biomedical applications is not widespread, possibly because of problems associated with these measurements (Nigg 1994b), such as how to distinguish between the accelerations of the bone and the surrounding soft tissue and how to separate the measured acceleration into its translational, rotational, and gravitational components.

A second method for finding the accelerations needed for a dynamic analysis of a link-segment model is to measure the sequential positions of each segment and then to differentiate the position data with respect to time, once to obtain segment velocity and twice to obtain segment acceleration. Because measurement errors are magnified in the differentiation process, the position data must first be filtered to remove unwanted noise. Various methods can be used to gather three-dimensional position data. An instrumented spatial linkage (Kinzel *et al.* 1972a, b), a complex version of the conventional electrogoniometer, can be strapped across a joint to measure the relative positions of the two bones. Magnetic tracking systems (An *et al.* 1988) are used to measure the position and orientation of a sensor mounted on a segment relative to a magnetic source. Such systems are accurate and easy to use, but it is important to understand the effects that metal in the experimental environment can have on the measurements.

Optoelectronic motion analysis systems (Fig. 12) are also used to

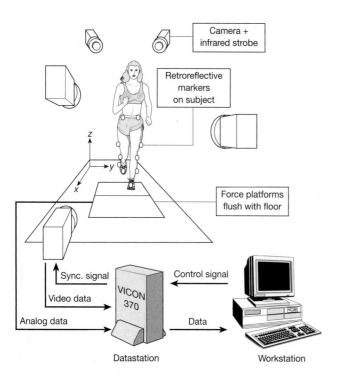

Fig. 12. Schematic diagram of a motion analysis system. (Courtesy of H.S. Gill.)

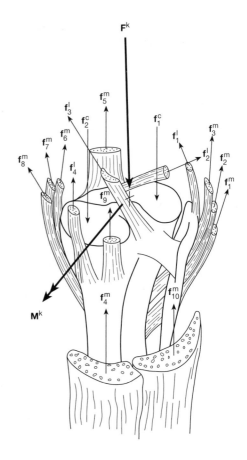

Fig. 13. The indeterminate force system at the knee. (Reproduced from Crowninshield and Brand (1981).)

collect three-dimensional position data. A minimum of three markers are fixed to each body segment of interest, and the changing positions of the markers are recorded by at least two cameras. Some systems use reflective markers, while others use markers containing light-emitting diodes which flash on and off in sequence. Data are analyzed automatically by a computer. A more detailed discussion of motion analysis systems can be found in books on gait analysis (Perry 1992; Winter 1990; Whittle 1996).

The problem of indeterminacy

In mechanics, a system is called 'determinate' if the number of equations describing it is the same as the number of unknown quantities (force, position, etc.) When there are more unknown quantities than there are equations, the system is called 'indeterminate' or 'redundant'. In two dimensions, mechanics provides us with three equations: force equilibrium in the x and y directions (two equations) and moment equilibrium about an axis perpendicular to the plane of interest (one equation). Therefore with three equations, one can solve for three unknown quantities. In three dimensions, there are six equations: force equilibrium in the x, y, and z directions and moment equilibrium about the x, y, and z axes. Therefore in three dimensions, one can solve for six unknown quantities.

The musculoskeletal system is highly indeterminate. Figure 13 shows as an example a sketch of the knee with its known joint force $\mathbf{F}^k$ and joint moment $\mathbf{M}^k$. Also shown on the drawing are all the unknown forces at the knee: muscle forces $\mathbf{f}^m$, ligament forces $\mathbf{f}^l$, and forces $\mathbf{f}^c$ in the articular cartilage which result from contact between

the tibia and the femur. With six equations of equilibrium, it is possible to solve for six unknown quantities. The problem is that there are far more than six unknown forces in Fig. 13—the forces cannot be found using the equations of equilibrium alone. In biomechanics, much effort has gone into trying to solve this 'problem of indeterminacy'. Methods involve either increasing the number of equations or decreasing the number of unknowns.

Structures which carry load

In the fields of orthopedics and traumatology, there is interest in the forces in the bones, muscles, tendons, ligaments, and articular cartilage. These are the tissues which must provide the internal forces and moments discussed above. Muscles produce force and are therefore thought of as 'active' tissues. Bones, tendons, ligaments, and articular cartilage are 'passive' structures, since they take up load only as needed to balance the external, inertial, and muscle forces and moments. Understanding how these tissues produce or carry load can help in calculating the forces within them. For example, knowing that muscles can 'pull' but not 'push', and that ligaments can resist tension but not compression, allows one to reduce the number of unknowns in the indeterminate problem. Theoretical models of the individual tissues can also be formulated. The level of detail required in a model depends, of course, on its final application.

Muscle

As an 'active' tissue, a muscle generates force as a result of neural stimulation. The amount of force that a muscle can produce depends on the lengths and arrangement of its fibers, on its size or physiological cross-sectional area, on its excitability or fiber type, on the contraction velocity and activation level, and on its level of fatigue. Forces produced by the muscles are transmitted by tendons to the skeleton. A muscle that crosses a joint produces a moment about that joint.

It is possible to tell when a muscle is active by detecting with electrodes the electrical signal or electromyogram (**EMG**) associated with its contraction. In most cases in orthopedic biomechanics, electrodes placed on the skin (surface electrodes) are used for this measurement. The EMG is then the sum of the electrical signals from all the motor units within the recording area of the electrode. The raw EMG signal varies in amplitude in a seemingly random way above and below a zero level (Fig. 14). In some cases, it is processed (amplified, filtered, etc.) before use. In order to decide whether a given muscle is 'on' or 'off', the processed EMG signal can be compared qualitatively with the raw EMG of the muscle at rest or quantitatively with the processed EMG recorded during a maximum voluntary isometric contraction. This 'on–off' information is used in biomechanics to reduce the number of unknowns in the indeterminate problem (Morrison 1968). Entire textbooks are devoted to the methods of detecting, processing, and analyzing EMGs (Basmajian and DeLuca 1985; Loeb and Gans 1986).

It is tempting to believe that there is a simple relationship between the amplitude of the EMG signal and the force produced by a muscle. For voluntary isometric contractions only, investigators now report

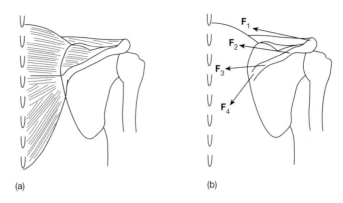

Fig. 15. Representation of muscles with large attachment areas such as the trapezius (a) may need many force vectors (b). (Reproduced from van der Helm and Veenbaas (1991).)

either a linear relationship or a more than linear increase of the EMG signal with force (Basmajian and DeLuca 1985). However, the exact relationship depends on the muscle being studied. Complications arise not only because of the complex relationship between the EMG signal and muscle physiology, but also because the EMG signal recorded for any given muscle is affected by the technical details of the detection procedure and by physiological events occurring in muscles not being monitored (Basmajian and DeLuca 1985). EMG–force relations for dynamically contracting muscles are rare and controversial (Herzog *et al.* 1994).

In many biomechanical models in which a muscle force is unknown, the muscle is represented by a single force vector pointing along the muscle line of action. Many force vectors may be needed for an adequate representation of the mechanical effect of broad pennate muscles with large attachment sites (Fig. 15) (van der Helm and Veenbaas 1991). In simulations in which muscle forces are prescribed, the simplest and most common model of muscle contraction dynamics is the Hill-type model (Fig. 16). The force produced by the contractile process is attributed to the 'contractile element' and depends on the muscle length, the velocity of contraction, and the muscle activation. Hill's equation (Hill 1938) is often modified and used to relate these parameters to muscle force (Zajac 1989). The passive resistance of the muscle to being stretched is represented by a spring, the 'parallel elastic element'. Total muscle force is then the sum of the active and passive elements. Some models include a series elastic element (not shown in Fig. 16) next to the contractile element. The elasticity of the muscle tendon can be included in series with the

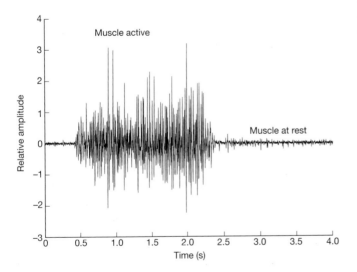

Fig. 14. An EMG signal from the flexor carpi radialis during clenching of the fist in a normal subject. Data collected with a surface electrode and sampled at 4 kHz. Periods of rest and activity are evident. (Data courtesy of S. Taffler, Oxford Orthopaedic Engineering Centre.)

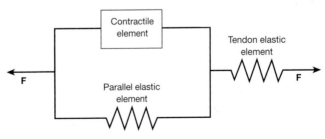

Fig. 16. Hill-type muscle model.

muscle model (Fig. 16). Storage of energy in the elastic elements is thought to be important in activities such as running and jumping (Alexander 1988).

Bone

The mechanical functions of the bones of the skeleton are to support and protect the tissues of the body and to function as a lever system on which the muscles can act. As a result of external forces and muscle forces, bones are subjected to all kinds of loading: tension, compression, bending, shear, torsion, and combinations of these (Fig. 17).

For several reasons, bone is difficult to model using the basic techniques of classical mechanics. Even though many bones appear at first to be either simply tubular or plate-like, on closer inspection their detailed geometry is found to be highly complex. Furthermore, most bones have both cortical and trabecular parts, each made up of different proportions and arrangements of organic and inorganic material. As a result, the ability of bone to resist deformation varies throughout its substance (Keaveny and Hayes 1993).

Since the early 1970s (Brekelmans *et al.* 1972), an advanced computer technique of structural stress analysis called finite-element analysis (**FEA**) has been used in biomechanics to model bone. In FEA, the geometry of the model is defined first. The model is then divided into a number of sections called 'elements', all of which are connected together at points called 'nodes' (Fig. 18). The solution procedure requires that forces be applied to the model only at the nodes. Distributed forces or pressures are divided up amongst relevant nodes, usually automatically by the FEA computer program. In order to prevent rigid body motion, a sufficient number of nodes must be fixed or their displacements limited to, say, translation in one direction only. After the material behavior or stiffness of every element in every direction is defined, the FEA program solves a large number of equations governing force equilibrium at the nodes to find the nodal displacements within the model. From these displacements, strains

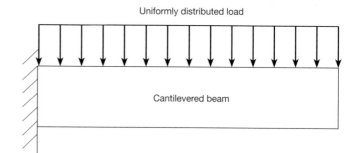

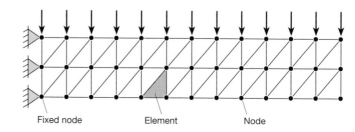

Fig. 18. (a) A uniformly distributed load applied to a cantilevered beam. (b) A simple finite-element model of the beam.

and stresses can be calculated. The amount of computer time needed to solve an FEA problem depends mainly on the number of nodes and the number of ways in which the nodes can move; it can be quite high for three-dimensional models with complex geometries.

During the first decade of FEA use in orthopedic biomechanics, work concentrated on the stress analysis of bones, fracture fixation, and artificial joint design and fixation (Huiskes and Chao 1983). Most of these highly simplified models were of the lower limb, many involving the proximal femur (Fig. 19(a)) and the femoral component of total hip replacement. During this time, most researchers were still learning the capabilities and limitations of FEA in biomechanics. Since then, increased computer capabilities, more sophisticated FEA computer programs, and a better understanding of FEA overall have led to the development of more realistic models of bone (Fig. 19(b)) and bone–implant interactions (Huiskes and Hollister 1993). Iterative procedures are now being used to predict the time-dependent mechanical behavior of bone, to optimize implant design, and to study the relationship between loading and bone shape, bone density, and trabecular architecture. It is also possible to simulate bone growth, maintenance, repair, and remodeling. FEA models of articular cartilage and ligament also now exist. Although FEA is cheap compared with clinical, animal, or laboratory testing methods, the combination of FEA with experimental analyses is many times more powerful than the sum of their individual applications (Huiskes and Hollister 1993).

Articular cartilage

The articulating surfaces of the bones in a synovial joint are covered with a thin layer of connective tissue known as hyaline articular cartilage (a notable exception is the temporomandibular joint in which fibrocartilage covers the bone ends). The mechanical functions of articular cartilage are to transmit compressive forces across the joint,

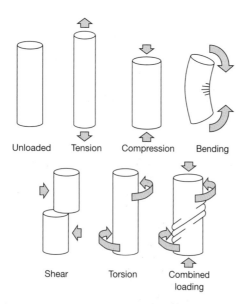

Fig. 17. The types of loads to which bone may be subjected. (Reproduced from Nordin and Frankel (1989).)

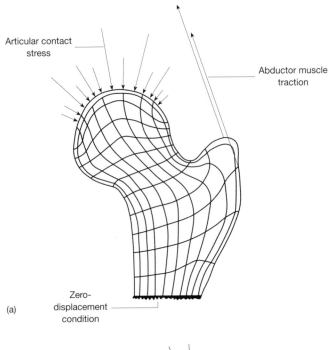

Articular contact stress

Abductor muscle traction

Zero-displacement condition

(a)

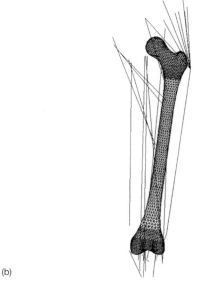

(b)

Fig. 19. (a) Two-dimensional finite-element model of a coronal plane section of a proximal femur. (Reproduced from Brown *et al.* (1980).) (b) Three-dimensional finite-element model of the femur. Lines of action of the major muscle group forces are shown. (Courtesy of K. Polgar, Oxford Orthopaedic Engineering Centre.)

linked to articular cartilage deformation and to its time-dependent responses to loads (Mow 1984). Simple single-phase linear viscoelastic models (see below) can be used to take the time-dependency into account, but for a full representation of fluid flow, cartilage must be modeled as at least a biphasic material, with the solid matrix and the interstitial fluid as the two phases (Torzilli and Mow 1976a,b). A triphasic theory that combines the biphasic theory with an ion phase, representing the cation and anion of a single salt, has since been developed to study the behavior of cartilage under chemical and/or mechanical loads (Lai *et al.* 1991). Both analytical and finite-element methods have been used to find solutions to these mathematical models.

Synovial joints have very low coefficients of friction (order of magnitude 10^{-2}) and experience only minimal amounts of wear, even after many decades of use (Dowson 1990). This is because of the complex lubrication processes involving articular cartilage and synovial fluid. Fluid-film lubrication, in which a thin film of fluid causes surface separation, appears to be the dominant effect. Lubrication occurs by elastohydrodynamic action, in which the bearing surfaces either slide past each other or are squeezed together. The pressure generated in the fluid film supports the load across the joint, but also substantially deforms the articular surfaces and causes fluid to be expelled from the cartilage. Boundary lubrication, in which lubricant is adsorbed on the bearing surfaces, provides additional protection against wear (Mow *et al.* 1989; Dowson 1990).

Ligaments and tendons

Ligaments and tendons are approximately parallel-fibered collagenous tissues that transmit tensile forces across the joints. A ligament connects one bone to another and functions to guide and limit joint movement. A tendon connects a muscle to a bone across a joint, thereby causing joint motion when the muscle contracts. Tendons also store elastic energy.

In models of the musculoskeletal system, ligaments and tendons are often modeled by a small number of tension-only springs (Crowninshield *et al.* 1976). These can be either linear springs, in which the spring force is directly proportional to the amount of stretch, or nonlinear springs, in which the relationship between force and extension is more complicated. It is also possible to model a single ligament as a series of elastic fibers. This gives a better idea of the load distribution across the ligament and of the relationship between ligament structure and function (Zavatsky and O'Connor 1992a,b).

Like articular cartilage, ligaments and tendons contain a high proportion of water and so exhibit time- and history-dependent behavior under load. The quasilinear viscoelastic theory developed by Fung (1993) has been used to model these features of the mechanical behavior of ligaments, tendons, and many other soft tissues. Various extensions to this theory have been proposed, including a finite-element implementation (Puso and Weiss 1998).

Mechanical properties

Almost all work in biomechanics requires some knowledge of the mechanical properties of the tissues of the musculoskeletal system. For instance, when designing a new ligament replacement, it is important to know how much load the natural ligament supports

to distribute the compressive contact force between the bones (by deforming and making the contact area larger), and to allow joint motion with minimal friction and wear (Shrive and Frank 1994).

In some biomechanical models, articular cartilage is considered to be a deformable cushion of linear elastic springs sitting on top of the rigid subchondral bone (An *et al.* 1990). It is also possible to allow for the occurrence of tension, compression, and shear (see Fig. 17) within the depths of the cartilage layer. Such models are useful in certain contexts, but they ignore the fact that fluid flow is intrinsically

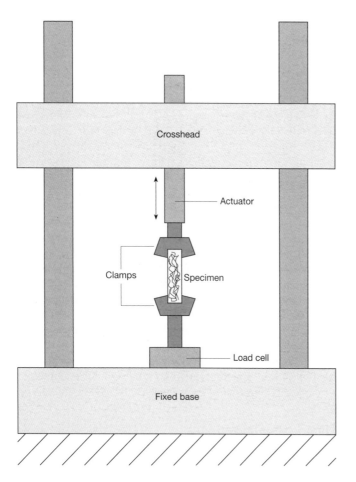

Fig. 20. Schematic diagram of a tensile-testing machine.

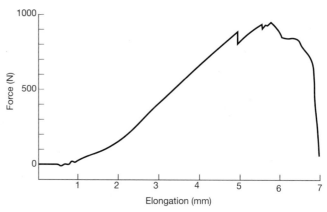

Fig. 21. The force–elongation curve generated from an anterior cruciate ligament tested in tension to failure. (Reproduced from Carlstedt and Nordin (1989), based on data from Noyes (1977).)

before it breaks and how much deformation it undergoes during loading. Another example is the need to know how bone density relates to bone strength, so that various treatments for osteoporosis can be evaluated or compared. Finally, many biomechanical models of the musculoskeletal system require mechanical properties, such as tissue stiffness, as input parameters.

Much information about the mechanical properties of tissues comes from tension and compression tests performed using a tensile-testing machine (Fig. 20). The ends of the tissue specimen are held in special clamps, one attached to the rigid base of the testing machine and the other to a moving actuator (in a hydraulically driven machine) or crosshead (in a screw-driven machine). The movement of the actuator/crosshead up or down is usually controlled electronically, and the load applied to the specimen is measured with a load cell attached to the testing machine. Deformation of the specimen can be measured by tracking the movement of the actuator/crosshead or by attaching an extensometer or strain gage directly to the specimen. In many cases, however, these methods are not accurate enough, and a noncontact optical method must be used. This typically involves recording on high-speed video the positions of reference marks drawn on the specimen before the start of the test (Woo *et al.* 1986). A computer is usually used to set the test parameters (e.g. the testing speed) and to log the force and displacement data.

The output from any tension or compression test is typically a plot of applied load P versus specimen elongation Δl. Figure 21 shows a plot for a tensile test on a ligament. The 'structural properties' of the entire ligament can be found from such a graph. These include the stiffness (slope of the linear part of the curve), energy absorbed (area under the curve), and ultimate (maximum) load and elongation. These values depend, amongst other things, on the geometry of the tissue, such as its cross-sectional area and length, and on the properties of the tissue substance.

To study the 'mechanical properties' of the ligament tissue alone, it is necessary to calculate and plot a graph of stress versus strain. Stress σ is defined as the load P divided by the cross-sectional area A perpendicular to the load: $\sigma = P/A$. Strain ε is defined as the change in specimen length Δl divided by the original length l: $\varepsilon = \Delta l/l$. Mechanical properties such as the elastic modulus (slope of the linear part of the curve), strain energy density (area under the curve), and ultimate (maximum) stress and strain can be found from a graph of σ versus ε (Fig. 22).

Using the tensile-testing machine shown in Fig. 20 it is possible to obtain the mechanical properties in a single direction. This information would be adequate if the material being tested were isotropic, i.e. its mechanical properties were the same in all directions. However, biologic tissues are usually anisotropic, which means that they have oriented structural elements (collagen fibers, trabeculae, osteons, etc.) which lead to very different mechanical properties if the tissue is tested in different directions or if different parts of the tissue are tested (Litsky and Spector 1994). As many as 21 independent quantities (elastic constants) could be required for a full description of the behavior of such materials. Further explanations and details of the structural and mechanical properties of the tissues of the musculoskeletal system are given by Yamada (1970) and by Nordin and Frankel (1989).

It is important to recognize that mechanical measurements on tissues are affected by experimental, biologic, and external factors (Woo *et al.* 1997). Experimental factors include specimen orientation, strain rate, temperature, and tissue hydration. Biologic factors are tissue maturation, age, immobilization, and exercise. Storage by freezing and sterilization are external factors.

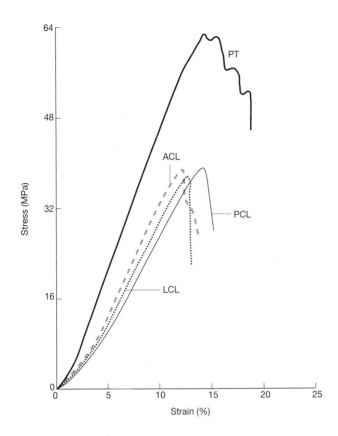

Fig. 22. Typical stress–strain curves for the patellar tendon (PT), anterior cruciate ligament (ACL), posterior cruciate ligament (PCL), and lateral collateral ligament (LCL) fascicle–bone units. Note the much larger elastic modulus and ultimate stress for the PT specimen. (Reproduced from Butler *et al.* (1992).)

Viscoelasticity

In the discussion of the mechanical properties of biologic tissues thus far, time has not been mentioned much. Indeed, the mechanical behavior of engineering materials such as metals and ceramics is usually not time dependent over the range of operating temperatures. In contrast, almost all polymers (plastics) and all biologic materials exhibit time-dependent or viscoelastic properties.

Viscoelasticity is a mechanical behavior involving both fluid-like (viscous) and solid-like (elastic) characteristics. The viscoelastic properties of soft tissues, in particular articular cartilage (Mow *et al.* 1989), have received much attention. The main features of viscoelasticity are shown in Fig. 23. Stress relaxation (Fig. 23(a)) is a decrease in stress in a material subjected to prolonged constant strain. Creep (Fig. 23(b)) is an increase in deformation or strain that occurs when a constant load is applied. Hysteresis (Fig. 23(c)) is a characteristic behavior in which a material property plot follows a closed loop, i.e. the loading and unloading curves are not coincident. Because the area under the curve is related to the strain energy, the hysteresis loop indicates that energy is being dissipated, usually as heat. These features of the behavior of biologic materials are rarely taken into account in models of joints and limbs because the duration of the activity being studied is relatively short, the viscoelastic effects are

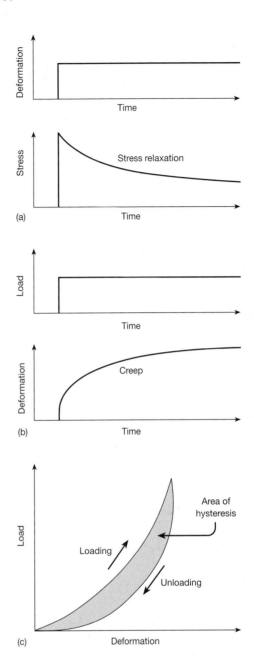

Fig. 23. (a) Stress relaxation; (b) creep; (c) hysteresis.

secondary, or inclusion of such effects would make the models too difficult to solve.

Load transmission across joints

A knowledge of the loads transmitted by the anatomic structures at the joints of the body is necessary for, amongst many other things, the design of joint replacements, an understanding of the mechanical factors which may influence the development of osteoarthritis, and the assessment of the effect of tendon transfer operations in the treatment of cerebral palsy. As explained above and illustrated in Fig. 13, the musculoskeletal system is highly indeterminate, and many methods have been used either to increase the number of equations describing the body in question or to decrease the number of unknowns. Rather than describing the details of various joint models and their solution techniques, in this section we use a simple well-known example to illustrate some important points about the loads across joints.

Consider the situation shown in Fig. 24(a) in which a weight is held in the hand with the elbow joint held fixed at 90° flexion and the forearm parallel to the ground. To find the forces transmitted by the anatomic structures at the elbow joint during this activity, it is

necessary first to draw a free-body diagram of the forearm (Fig. 24(b)) and to calculate the intersegmental force **F** and moment **M** at the elbow. In Fig. 24(b), the weight **W** of the ball and the weight mg of the forearm and hand both act downwards. In this example, it is obvious that the force **F** balances the forces **W** and mg, and so must act upwards, having a vertical component only. In addition, the moment **M** must be counterclockwise to balance the moments of **W** and mg about the center of the elbow joint. Assuming that the arm belongs to a person of height 170 cm and body mass 60 kg, anthropometric tables (Winter 1990) can be used to estimate the length and mass of the forearm and hand ($L = 43$ cm, $m = 1.3$ kg) and the distance of their center of mass from the center of the elbow joint ($a = 29$ cm). The position of the center of mass of the ball from the fingertips is estimated to be $c = 9$ cm.

Solving the equations for static force and moment equilibrium in two dimensions gives **F** = 62.75 N upwards and **M** = 20.70 N m counterclockwise. To distribute **F** and **M** amongst the anatomic structures of the joint, a model of the elbow joint is needed. Figure 24(c) shows a simple model in which it is assumed that the biceps is the only muscle acting. For the elbow position in Fig. 24(a), it is assumed that the line of pull of the biceps is parallel to the humerus and that its insertion is $b = 4$ cm from the center of the elbow joint. It is also assumed that the elbow is a hinge (has a fixed axis of rotation) and that the articular contact force **R** acts vertically at this flexion angle. Using static equilibrium of force and moment in two dimensions (two equations, two unknowns) gives the biceps force **B** = 517 N upwards and the joint reaction force **R** = 454 N downwards.

It is important to note that the magnitudes of both **B** and **R** are larger than the magnitude of the external load **W**. The biceps force **B** is larger because its moment arm b is smaller than the moment arm of the external load ($L-c$). The joint reaction force **R** is larger than **W** because it must balance both **B** and **W**. That the muscle and joint reaction forces are larger than the external loads is true for most joints. Indeed, the joint reaction forces at the hip and knee can be several times body weight. Further details of the elbow problem, together with a summary of joint forces in the upper extremity and the hip joint, are given by An *et al.*(1997).

One further important point to note is that the moment arm of a muscle about a joint may change as the joint flexes. This obviously influences the force that it is necessary for a muscle to provide to balance the moment due to an external load. The changing moment arm of the biceps about the center of the elbow joint is illustrated in Fig. 25.

Conclusions

Much of the progress in the field of biomechanics that has been made over the past half-century has been due to collaborations between scientists, engineers, and clinicians. The scientists and engineers have had to delve into the anatomy and physiology textbooks and the medical literature, while the orthopedic clinicians have had to return to the mathematics and physics that they studied years before. Both sides have benefited, along with many thousands of patients. This chapter has reviewed and explained some of the fundamental concepts and techniques involved in studying the biomechanics of the musculoskeletal system. It is hoped that clinicians have found this

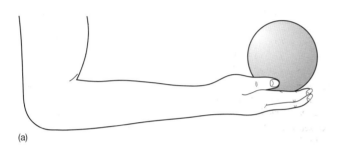

(a)

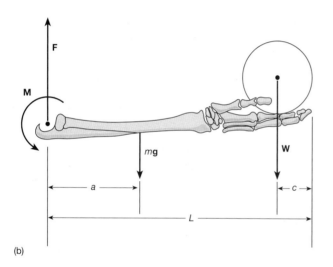

(b)

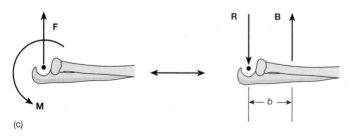

(c)

Fig. 24. (a) A heavy ball is held in the hand with the elbow joint flexed to 90° and the forearm parallel to the ground. (b) A free-body diagram of the situation shown in (a): **W**, weight of the ball; mg, weight of the forearm and hand; **F**, intersegmental force at the elbow joint; **M**, intersegmental moment at the elbow joint. (c) Distribution of **F** and **M** amongst the relevant anatomic structures at the elbow joint: **B**, the biceps muscle force; **R**, the articular contact force. (Reproduced from An *et al.* (1997).)

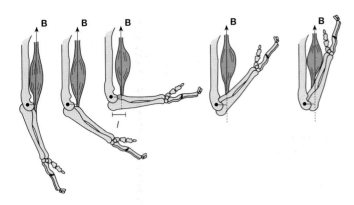

Fig. 25. The biceps (B) at various elbow flexion angles. Note the variations in the moment arm *l* of biceps. (Reproduced from Leveau (1992).)

introduction useful and that they will be encouraged to explore the subject further.

References

Alexander, I.J., Chao, E.Y.S., and Johnson, K.A. (1990). The assessment of dynamic foot-to-ground contact forces and plantar pressure distribution: a review of the evolution of current techniques and clinical applications. *Foot and Ankle*, **11**, 152–67.

Alexander, R.McN. (1988). *Elastic mechanisms in animal movement*. Cambridge University Press.

An, K-N., Jacobsen, M.C., Berglund, L.J., and Chao, E.Y.S. (1988). Application of a magnetic tracking device to kinesiologic studies. *Journal of Biomechanics*, **21**, 613–20.

An, K.-N., Himeno, S., Tsumura, H., *et al.* (1990). Pressure distribution on articular surfaces: application to joint stability and evaluation. *Journal of Biomechanics*, **23**, 1013–20.

An, K.-N., Chao, E.Y.S., and Kaufman, K.R. (1997). Analysis of muscle and joint loads. In *Basic orthopaedic biomechanics* (2nd edn) (ed. V.C. Mow and W.C. Hayes), pp. 1–36. Lippincott–Raven, Philadelphia, PA.

Basmajian, J.V. and De Luca, C.J. (1985). *Muscles alive: their functions revealed by electromyography* (5th edn). Williams and Wilkins, Baltimore, MD.

Beynnon, B., Howe, J.G., Pope, M.H., Johnson, R.J., and Fleming, B.C. (1992) The measurement of anterior cruciate ligament strain *in vivo*. *International Orthopaedics*, **16**, 1–12.

Brekelmans, W.A.M., Poort, H.W., and Slooff, T.J.J.H. (1972). A new method to analyse the mechanical behaviour of skeletal parts. *Acta Orthopaedica Scandinavica*, **43**, 301–17.

Brown, T.D., Way, M.E., and Ferguson, A.B. (1980). Stress transmission anomalies in femoral heads altered by aseptic necrosis. *Journal of Biomechanics*, **13**, 687–99.

Butler, D.L., Kay, M.D., and Stouffer, D.C. (1986). Comparison of material properties in fascicle–bone units from human patellar tendon and knee ligaments. *Journal of Biomechanics*, **19**, 425–32.

Carlstedt, C.A. and Nordin, M. (1989). Biomechanics of ligaments and tendons. In *Basic biomechanics of the musculoskeletal system* (ed. M. Nordin and V.H. Frankel), pp. 59–74. Lea & Febiger, Philadelphia, PA.

Cobbold, R.S.C. (1974). *Transducers for biomedical measurements: principles and applications*. Wiley, New York.

Crowninshield, R.D. and Brand, R.A. (1981). The prediction of forces in joint structures: distribution of intersegmental resultants. *Exercise and Sport Sciences Reviews*, **9**, 159–81.

Crowninshield, R.D., Pope, M.H., and Johnson, R.J. (1976). An analytical model of the knee. *Journal of Biomechanics*, **9**, 397–405.

Dowson, D. (1990). Bio-tribology of natural and replacement synovial joints. In *Biomechanics of diarthrodial joints*, Vol. 2 (ed. V.C. Mow, A. Ratcliffe, and S.L-Y. Woo), pp. 305–45. Springer-Verlag, New York.

Fung, Y.C. (1993). *Biomechanics: mechanical properties of living tissues* (2nd edn). Springer-Verlag, New York.

Herzog, W., Guimaraes, A.C.S., and Zhang, Y.T. (1994). EMG. In *Biomechanics of the musculo-skeletal system* (ed. B.M. Nigg and W. Herzog), pp. 308–36. Wiley, Chichester.

Hill, A.V. (1938). The heat of shortening and the dynamic constants of muscle. *Proceedings of the Royal Society of London*, **126**, 136–95.

Huiskes, R. and Chao, E.Y.S. (1983). A survey of finite element analysis in orthopaedic biomechanics: the first decade. *Journal of Biomechanics*, **16**, 385–409.

Huiskes, R. and Hollister, S.J. (1993). From structure to process, from organ to cell: recent developments of FE-analysis in orthopaedic biomechanics. *Transactions of the ASME: Journal of Biomechanical Engineering*, **115**, 520–7.

Hull, M.L. and Davis, R.R. (1981). Measurement of pedal loading in bicycling. I: Instrumentation. *Journal of Biomechanics*, **14**, 843–56.

Keaveny, T.M. and Hayes, W.C. (1993). A 20-year perspective on the mechanical properties of trabecular bone. *Transactions of the ASME: Journal of Biomechanical Engineering*, **115**, 534–42.

Kinzel, G.L., Hall, A.S., and Hillberry, B.M. (1972a). Measurement of the total motion between two body segments. I: Analytical development. *Journal of Biomechanics*, **5**, 93–105.

Kinzel, G.L., Hillberry, B.M., Hall, A.S., van Sickle, D.C., and Harvey, W.M. (1972b). Measurement of the total motion between two body segments. II: Description of application. *Journal of Biomechanics*, **5**, 283–93.

Komi, P.V., Salonen, M., Jarvinen, M., and Kokko, O. (1987). *In vivo* registration of Achilles tendon forces in man. I. Methodological development. *International Journal of Sports Medicine*, **8** (Supplement 1), 3–8.

Lai, W.M., Hou, J.S., and Mow, V.C. (1991). A triphasic theory for the swelling and deformation behaviors of articular cartilage. *Transactions of the ASME: Journal of Biomechanical Engineering*, **113**, 245–58.

Leveau, B.F. (1992). *Williams and Lissner's biomechanics of human motion* (3rd edn). W.B. Saunders, Philadelphia, PA.

Litsky, A.S. and Spector, M. (1994). Biomaterials. In *Orthopaedic basic science* (ed. S.R. Simon), pp. 447–86. American Academy of Orthopaedic Surgeons, Rosemont, IL.

Loeb, G.E. and Gans, C. (1986). *Electromyography for experimentalists*. University of Chicago Press, Chicago, Illinois.

Lord, M., Reynolds, D.P., and Hughes, J.R. (1986). Foot pressure measurement: a review of clinical findings. *Journal of Biomedical Engineering*, **8**, 283–94.

Meriam, J.L. and Kraige, L.G. (1993a). *Engineering mechanics*. Vol. 1, *Statics* (3rd edn). Wiley, New York.

Meriam, J.L. and Kraige, L.G. (1993b). *Engineering mechanics*. Vol. 2, *Dynamics* (3rd edn). Wiley, New York.

Morris, J. (1973). Accelerometry—a technique for the measurement of human body movements. *Journal of Biomechanics*, **6**, 729–36.

Morrison, J.B. (1968). Bioengineering analysis of force actions transmitted by the knee joint. *Biomedical Engineering*, **3**, 164–70.

Mow, V.C. and Hayes, W.C. (1997). *Basic orthopaedic biomechanics* (2nd edn). Lippincott–Raven, Philadelphia, PA.

Mow, V.C., Holmes, M.H., and Lai, W.M. (1984). Fluid transport and mechanical properties of articular cartilage: a review. *Journal of Biomechanics*, **17**, 377–94.

Mow, V.C., Proctor, C.S., and Kelly, M.A. (1989). Biomechanics of articular cartilage. In *Basic biomechanics of the musculoskeletal system* (2nd edn) (ed. M. Nordin and V.H. Frankel), pp. 31–58. Lea & Febiger, Philadelphia, PA.

Newmiller, J., Hull, M.L., and Zajac, F.E. (1988). A mechanically decoupled two force component bicycle pedal dynamometer. *Journal of Biomechanics*, **21**, 375–86.

Nigg, B.M. (1994*a*). Force. In *Biomechanics of the musculo-skeletal system.* (ed. B.M. Nigg and W. Herzog), pp. 200–24. Wiley, Chichester.

Nigg, B.M. (1994*b*). Acceleration. In *Biomechanics of the musculo-skeletal system* (ed. B.M. Nigg and W. Herzog), pp. 237–53. Wiley, Chichester.

Nigg, B.M. and Herzog, W. (ed.) (1994). *Biomechanics of the musculo-skeletal system.* Wiley, Chichester.

Nordin, M. and Frankel, V.H. (ed.) (1989). *Basic biomechanics of the musculo-skeletal system* (2nd edn.) Lea & Febiger, Philadelphia, PA.

Noyes, F.R. (1977). Functional properties of knee ligament and alterations induced by immobilization. *Clinical Orthopaedics and Related Research*, **123**, 210–42.

O'Connor, J.J. (1991). Load simulation problems in model testing. In *Strain measurement in biomechanics* (ed. A.W. Miles and K.E. Tanner), pp. 14–38. Chapman & Hall, London.

Perry, J. (1992). *Gait analysis: normal and pathological function.* Slack, Thorofare, NJ.

Puso, M.A. and Weiss, J.A. (1998). Finite element implementation of anisotropic quasi-linear viscoelasticity using a discrete spectrum approximation. *Journal of Biomechanical Engineering*, **120**, 62–70.

Ruby, P. and Hull, M.L. (1993). Response of intersegmental knee loads to foot/pedal platform degrees of freedom in cycling. *Journal of Biomechanics*, **26**, 1327–40.

Shrive, N.G. and Frank, C.B. (1994). Articular cartilage. In *Biomechanics of the musculo-skeletal system* (ed. B.M. Nigg and W. Herzog), pp. 79–105. Wiley, Chichester.

Simon, S.R. (ed.) (1994). *Orthopaedic basic science.* American Academy of Orthopaedic Surgeons, Rosemont, IL.

Torzilli, P.A. and Mow, V.C. (1976*a*) On the fundamental fluid transport mechanisms through normal and pathological articular cartilage during function. I: The formulation. *Journal of Biomechanics*, **9**, 541–52

Torzilli, P.A. and Mow, V.C. (1976*b*). On the fundamental fluid transport mechanisms through normal and pathological articular cartilage during function. II: The analysis, solution, and conclusions. *Journal of Biomechanics*, **9**, 587–606.

van der Helm, F.C.T. and Veenbaas, R. (1991). Modelling the mechanical effect of muscles with large attachment sites: application to the shoulder mechanism. *Journal of Biomechanics*, **24**, 1151–63.

Whittle, M.W. (1996). *Gait analysis: an introduction* (2nd edn.) Butterworth Heinemann, Oxford.

Williams, P.L., Warwick, R., Dyson, M., and Bannister, L.H. (1989). *Gray's anatomy* (37th edn). Churchill Livingstone, London.

Winter, D.A. (1990). *Biomechanics and motor control of human movement* (2nd edn). Wiley–Interscience, New York.

Wolff, J. (1892). *The law of bone remodelling.* Trans. P. Macquet and R. Furlong and reprinted by Springer-Verlag, Berlin, 1986.

Woo, S.L.-Y., Orlando, C.A., Camp, J.F., and Akeson, W.H. (1986). Effect of postmortem storage by freezing on ligament behaviour. *Journal of Biomechanics*, **19**, 399–404.

Woo, S.L.-Y., Livesay, G.A., Runco, T.J., and Young, E.P. (1997). Structure and function of ligaments and tendons. In *Basic orthopaedic biomechanics* (2nd edn) (ed. V.C. Mow and W.C. Hayes), pp. 209–52. Lippincott–Raven, Philadelphia, PA.

Yamada, H. (1970). *Strength of biological materials.* Williams and Wilkins, Baltimore, MD.

Zajac, F.E. (1989). Muscle and tendon: properties, models, scaling, and application to biomechanics and motor control. *Critical Reviews in Bioengineering*, **17**, 359–411.

Zavatsky, A.B. and O'Connor, J.J. (1992*a*). A model of human knee ligaments in the sagittal plane. I: Response to passive flexion. *Proceedings of the Institution of Mechanical Engineers, Part H: Journal of Engineering in Medicine*, **206**, 125–34.

Zavatsky, A.B. and O'Connor, J.J. (1992*b*) A model of human knee ligaments in the sagittal plane. II: Fibre recruitment under load. *Proceedings of the Institution of Mechanical Engineers, Part H: Journal of Engineering in Medicine*, **206**, 135–45.

1.12 Locomotion analysis

Richard A. Brand

Introduction

Doctors have used observation of human movement to interpret disease states at least as long as recorded history. The skilled clinician often finds qualitative observational analysis critical to establish the presence of disorders, to distinguish between certain classes of conditions, or to ascertain the severity of disease. The notion of using technology to measure quantitatively and record critical clinical information arose in the nineteenth century. However, despite thousands of studies over more than a hundred years and despite many technical advances, recorded locomotion analysis beyond the observational has never gained widespread clinical use.

Throughout this chapter the term 'observational analysis' is used to refer to those qualitative assessments which a clinician can routinely perform without technology, while the expression 'locomotion analysis' is used specifically to refer to the various means of quantitatively recording and/or assessing locomotion; obviously, these definitions are quite arbitrary.

Although Borelli's landmark static analysis of human and animal bodies *De Motu Animalium* (published in 1680) (Borelli 1989) implies locomotion (Fig. 1), the first scientific work (i.e. systematic exploration of specific questions) on gait came from the Weber brothers in 1836 (Weber and Weber 1836). (They were not, they stated, particularly interested in locomotion *per se*, but rather decided to explore the issues because they wished to work together, and locomotion was an area where an anatomist and a mathematician could both contribute!) Their tools were limited to clocks (which had recently afforded accuracy in the range of fractions of seconds) and rulers. Not surprisingly, their data concentrated on temporal and distance factors of gait (Fig. 2), although they postulated that normal gait minimizes energy expenditure and argued the leg acted as a pendulum during swing (a notion still explored today).

The works of subsequent early investigators remained primarily reports of approaches (Carlet 1872; Marey 1873, 1895) or explorations of specific questions (Braune and Fischer 1885–1901), rather than information obtained for an individual patient. Dercum, a neurologist at the University of Pennsylvania, had seen Muybridge's photographs of human motion, including some of patients with various disorders (Figs 3 and 4), and correctly realized that they might provide a more sensitive analysis than the human eye (Dercum 1888*a*). Collaborating with Muybridge, he commented:

> To show how difficult it is to observe a moving limb, even when the movement is slow, it need only be stated that med-

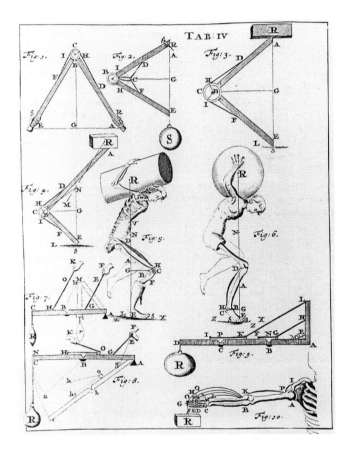

Fig. 1. Borelli used the emerging principles of static analysis to estimate resultant joint forces as well as muscle forces. While he was not the first to recognize the importance of forces in biological function, his prescient insight provided the first quantitative models of biological organisms. When one recalls that Borelli's work preceded the publication of Newton's *Principia Mathematica*, his approaches appear all the more extraordinary.

> ical writers almost without exception describe this gait [locomotor ataxia] erroneously. Almost all lay stress upon rigidity of the leg and insufficient action of the knee-joint. It needs but a hasty examination of the photographs to show how utterly wrong this view is. Every one of the plates reveals the action of the knee joint, and in fact of all of the joints, to be far in excess of the normal. (Dercum 1888*b*)

Mechanik
der
menschlichen
Gehwerkzeuge.

Eine

anatomisch-physiologische Untersuchung

von den Brüdern

Wilhelm Weber

Professor in Göttingen

und

Eduard Weber

Prosector in Leipzig.

Nebst einem Hefte mit 17 Tafeln anatomischer Abbildungen.

Göttingen,

in der Dieterichschen Buchhandlung.

1836.

(a)

Um ein Bild davon zu geben, wie die Zeiträume, wo beide Beine aufstehen, mit denjenigen abwechseln, wo das nicht der Fall ist, wollen wir den Zeitraum, wo ein Bein am Rumpfe hängend in der Luft schwingt, durch eine bogenförmige Linie, den Zeitraum, wo ein Bein auf dem Fussboden steht, durch eine gerade Linie bezeichnen, und durch die obere Reihe von Zeichen die Bewegungen des linken, durch die untere Reihe die des rechten Fusses andeuten, und durch senkrechte Striche die Grenzen der Zeitabschnitte angeben, wo der Körper von beiden oder nur von einem Beine unterstützt wird:

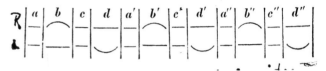

(b)

Fig. 2. The Weber brothers made the first quantitative measurements of locomotion parameters: (a) frontispiece to their seminal work; (b) the relationship of stance and swing phases of gait during level walking, and their overlap. The Weber brothers clearly described the changes in overlap as speed increased.

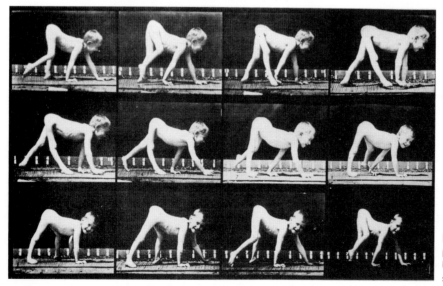

Fig. 3. Muybridge's photographs of a child with a paralytic disorder walking on all fours because of lower-extremity weakness and (in all likelihood) severe hip flexion contractures.

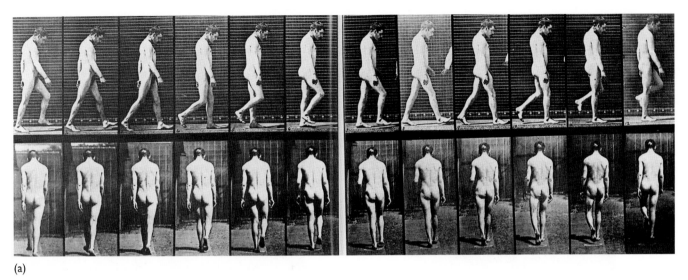

(a)

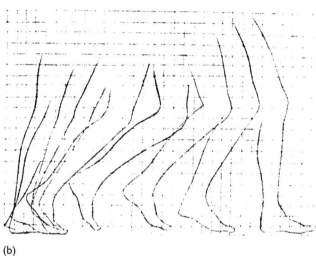

(b)

Fig. 4. Dercum's analysis of Muybridge's photographs of a patient with locomotor ataxia: (a) photograph; (b) Dercum's tracings illustrating knee motion. These recordings disproved the commonly held view of a rigid-knee gait in this disorder.

This seminal study clearly delineated the potential of locomotion analysis of a single patient for purposes of assessment (i.e. a 'clinical' use), as contrasted with exploring some hypothesis (i.e. a 'scientific' use). This chapter focuses on the former, but it is important to keep in mind that some of the criticisms or problems equally apply to the latter. Furthermore, since many authors provide excellent reviews of observational analysis (Steindler 1955; Ducroquet *et al.* 1975; Perry 1992), this chapter will be limited to the use of various recording techniques to provide supplemental information. The fundamental approaches will be reviewed applying those techniques, whilst exploring their capabilities and limitations, providing reasons for the failure of those approaches to achieve widespread clinical use, and criteria required to achieve utility. Current and future technology represents an untapped resource to provide critical clinical information.

The modern concepts of locomotion analysis (i.e. kinematics and kinetics) were established by Braune and Fischer in a series of studies begun in the late 1880s and early 1900s (Braune and Fischer 1885–1901). Extending the static analysis of Borelli, and using Newtonian concepts (and their extrapolations), they realized that one could estimate resultant joint forces and moments by treating limb segments as rigid bodies, then ascertaining their displacement histories

Box 1

- Each limb segment is a rigid body
- Calculate displacement, velocity, and acceleration
- Calculate forces required to produce these
- Redundancy because of indeterminate muscle and ligament forces

(i.e. displacements, velocities, and then accelerations) and inertial properties (i.e. mass and mass distribution). They accomplished this with a five-part procedure:

(1) instrumenting the limb segments with Geisler tubes (Fig. 5(a));

(2) recording displacement histories with four camera views (for three-dimensional analysis) with time-lapse photography (Fig. 5(b));

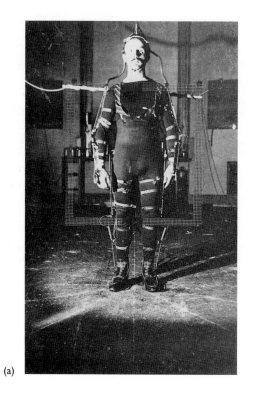

(a)

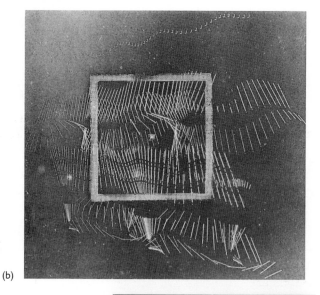

(b)

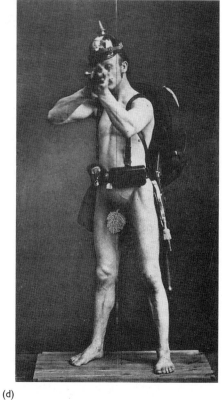

(c)

(d)

(e)

Fig. 5. Critical aspects of the work of Braune and Fischer:
(a) instrumentation of subject's body segments with Geisler tubes;
(b) time-lapse photography from right-oblique camera; (c) displacement
history of body segments as viewed from above; (d) subject with military
gear on a pendulum platform used for ascertaining the overall mass center
of gravity; (e) illustration of intersegmental resultant force and various
muscle forces in one position of the foot during gait.

Box 2

- Clinical tool—prognostic information from one patient
- Scientific tool—statistical information from populations of patients

(3) ascertaining accelerations by transferring the segment displacements to graph paper and graphically differentiating the curves (Fig. 5(c));

(4) estimating segment mass properties using pendulum techniques (Fig. 5(d));

(5) computing intersegmental resultant joint forces using equations of motion (Fig. 5(e)).

They realized that the quantities that they computed did not represent the forces on the articular surfaces, but rather resulted from articular, muscle, and ligament forces. They noted that the problem of computing the articular surfaces was redundant (indeterminant) owing to the fact that there were more unknown muscle, ligament, and articular forces than equations of motions. They extensively discussed, but did not solve the problem (Fig. 5(d)). (Ironically, some contemporary investigators have not recognized the critical distinction between articular forces and intersegmental resultant forces. In a general sense, the two are mathematically linked, but not directly related given that an infinite number of muscle, ligament, and articular force solutions can lead to the same intersegmental result. This error has probably lead to misleading conclusions regarding joint surface responses to forces.) Much of the modern locomotion work described in this chapter builds conceptually on the seminal work of Braune and Fischer.

Locomotion analysis: research versus clinical utility

As implied above, making the distinction between the research and clinical utility of locomotion analysis is critical since such approaches have been very useful to the systematic exploration of well-posed questions, though as yet they have failed to reach widespread clinical utility. The reasons for such divergent applicability arise from distinct requirements of 'clinical' versus 'research' utility.

'Clinical' utility means the study ('testing') of a single patient, and the use of these observations to guide diagnosis, treatment, or prognosis of that patient. Statistical treatment is not generally required, except perhaps to obtain descriptive statistics of multiple trials, or to document that the individual patient's observations fall outside some confidence limits for a 'normal' population.

'Research' or 'scientific' utility means the positing of an explicit hypothesis or question, and the systematic attempts to support or falsify the hypothesis, or unambiguously answer the question. In locomotion analysis, a reasonable number of subjects is required, since all such observations are subject to 'biologic' variability and reproducibility of observations must be ensured. (There are times when very specific questions might be answered by single subject studies.) In addition, we generally perform further statistical treat-

ment to make inferences of the (random or nonrandom) observations based upon limited samples.

Although locomotion analysis has always held great promise to aid the clinician, it has never lived up to its promise. Schwartz and his colleagues recognized that 'Measurement is essential for the interpretation of normal and abnormal phenomena of the human body' and that 'Empiricism fostered by trial and error, must continue to govern the therapy of abnormal function until measurement in some form improves the treatment of disabilities affecting the back and lower extremities' (Schwartz and Heath 1932, 1937; Schwartz et al. 1933, 1934). They described a series of tools to measure certain gait features, but ultimately admitted that 'All methods heretofore developed for recording gait, including those that have been published by others and ourselves, have failed to be of practical clinical value' (Schwartz et al. 1933). By 1937, the group had collected various sorts of recordings in over 2500 patients, but still had not documented clinical usefulness (Schwartz and Heath 1937).

Much more recently, Cappozo (1983) commented on the clinical utility of locomotion analysis following a 3-day conference devoted to the subject: 'From the three-day discussion a state of the art emerged. "A rather disappointing state of the art" was the comment of many observers. It should however be emphasized that the disappointment did not apply to the hardware'. They realized that despite increasing technical sophistication, locomotion analysis had failed to meet its promise.

Means of observation

Concepts of human locomotion analysis arise from the disciplines of kinematics (the branch of mechanics which deals with the motion of bodies) and kinetics (the branch of mechanics which deals with the actions or forces producing motion). Terms specific to the peculiarities of human locomotion (e.g. heel strike) provide a means of communication, although they bear a rather more general connection to well-accepted kinematic concepts. Since the concepts arise from these two disciplines, the means of observation generally include at least some (if not all) elements of motion or force analysis (Table 1). However, the recording of muscle activity (electromyograms) or energy expenditure often provide supplementary (or in some cases critical) information.

Kinematic analysis

Kinematic analysis is the oldest of the approaches, and in its most simple form involves mere observation of movement by the clinician. A skilled clinician can detect many, if not most, of the subtle variations required to make a diagnosis or assessment. For the purposes of this chapter, 'diagnosis' means making a distinction between various disorders which might explain the array of patient symptoms and signs. Conversely, 'assessment' or 'evaluation' refers to the application of a relative (quantitative or semiquantitative) value to an observation, either in relation to a normal population, or the same patient over time. Except in cases where an abnormal movement is so characteristic that it occurs only in a single disorder, locomotion analysis merely allows the clinician to limit the possibilities to one of several disorders. Thus, it does not allow 'diagnosis' in a strict sense. The diagnosis is ordinarily made upon other sorts of observations

Table 1 Tools of locomotion analysis

Kinematics
Still cameras
Movie cameras
Video recorders
Goniometers
Instrumented walkways
Biplanar roentgen stereophotogrammetry
Videofluoroscopy
Optoelectronic systems
Accelerometers
Foot–floor pressures
Foot–shoe pressures

Kinetics
External forces
Force plates
Instrumented transducers
Internal forces
Instrumented implants
Computational models

Electromyography
Surface electrodes
Intramuscular (fine wire or needle) electrodes

Energetics
Oxygen consumption
Computational models of mechanical energy

(e.g. history, neurological examination, laboratory tests, and so on).

The use of recording tools to provide quantitative or semi-quantitative measures often increases the resolution of the observation (i.e. certain observations may be made by a tool which cannot be made even by a skilled clinician), or affords the possibility to compare the observation objectively over time (eliminating the need for precise memory). Furthermore, the use of such tools provides a way to ascertain the average response, which might more accurately reflect the disorder than a potentially atypical response.

Many such tools have been developed (Carlet 1872; Vierordt 1881; Amar 1916, 1920; Schwartz and Heath 1932, 1937; Schwartz et al. 1933, 1934; Cappozzo et al. 1992; Allard et al. 1995). The possibility of capturing movement events increases with the numbers of observation (e.g. frame rate). During the past 20 years, researchers have introduced various techniques, some of which are commercially available. In their simplest form, one merely records patient motion. In their more complicated forms, multiple markers placed upon the body can be tracked by automated or semi-automated (interactive) means, in order to quantify limb segment motion histories.

Parameters of kinematic analysis

At the simplest level, temporal and distance features are recorded as a reflection of a recorded displacement history, for example stride length or cadence in the lower extremity (Gabel et al. 1979), or object-to-nose time of a finger in the upper extremity. With increasing sophistication, it is possible to record analog signals reflecting isolated limb segment motions (e.g. joint angles), three-dimensional reconstructions of segment or total body motions, or even the motions of individual bones. In these latter cases, much information is available to the clinician, but one must select those specific features or parameters of greatest interest. Such parameters include three-dimensional joint motion, joint motion (translational or angular) projected onto some plane (e.g. the sagittal or coronal planes), distance between two critical events, time between two events, limb segment velocities, or limb segment accelerations. Clinically useful observations are ordinarily limited to the more obvious and straightforward features.

Limitations of kinematic analysis

Perhaps the most serious limitation of locomotion analysis relates to inherent biological variability. Movements are never quite identical: they change according to the circumstance and mood of the patient, and they may change over time. Such variability relates to the fact that while the neural system develops limited sorts of strategies for movement, there remain virtually an infinite number of ways to achieve the identical or similar movement. Depending upon the need, one may wish to analyze a single motion, or the means of multiple motions. The infinite number of ways to achieve a given movement (i.e. 'redundancy') relates to mathematical indeterminacy—a state in which there are more unknowns than simultaneous equations and an infinite number of solutions satisfy the equations. About any given joint, there are far more unknown muscle, ligament, capsular, and joint contact forces (or distributions) than equations of motion which those forces must satisfy; therefore a potentially infinite number of combinations of muscle, ligament, capsular, and joint contact forces may satisfy the precise movement.

A second limitation relates to the first, in that some movements will be altered by a particular environment. Laboratory conditions, which are often strange for a patient, limiting in size or shape, or requiring unaccustomed clothing, may result in more or less subtle alterations in movement for physical or psychological reasons. Furthermore, the application of markers, 'umbilical cords', or recording devices may inhibit normal patterns. Many authors conduct and a few have published sensitivity studies (Andriacchi and Strickland 1985; Bell et al. 1990) documenting the range of errors created by these and other sources of error. When interpreting published studies, readers should consider these and additional sources of error or artifact upon the validity of the conclusions.

The measure selected should logically and critically relate to the condition under consideration. For example, measuring knee stance phase flexion–extension in normal level gait will be of little value in a patient with a torn anterior cruciate ligament, since that particular parameter is ordinarily normal (even if another is not) and logically one would not anticipate abnormality.

The measure should clearly distinguish normal and patient populations. For many features, the values for a patient will lie within the considerable normal variability (i.e. confidence intervals) of the measure in a normal population. Furthermore, some parameters (e.g. cadence) vary with age, and many vary with walking velocity (Crowninshield et al. 1978; Winter 1991). Large databases on the normal population are therefore required which afford appropriate matching (Shiavi et al. 1987; Winter 1991). Given the variability of locomotion analysis settings or laboratories, it may be important to insure that local databases are consistent with published databases or even to ascertain an appropriate database for comparison.

For some techniques (e.g. those involving marker or goniometer placement) intratester variability may be an issue. Kerschot et al. (1980) suggested variability of placement of external markers could lead to one standard deviation variability of 2.5° in estimating knee joint flexion extension from interrupted light photography (i.e. potential errors of 5° within two standard deviations). Boone et al. (1978) documented substantial variability (e.g. up to 5° or 6°) differences in the measurement of joint angles between different testers, and somewhat less variability with a given tester measuring the same subject at differing times. They suggested that differences of less than 6° in the upper extremity and 5° in the lower extremity in a given subject over time could not be considered a significant change.

Intermarker distance affects the magnitude of potential errors. In general, errors are unlikely to be more than a few degrees if markers upon which the angles are computed are located over long distances (e.g. estimating knee angles from markers near the hip, at the 'knee center', and at the ankle); however, if markers are located over short distances (e.g. about the foot), the resulting errors might be as much as 10° or 20°. Paradoxically, most sensitivity studies of error have been performed on joints least subject to error.

A reasonable number of trials must be ascertained for each observation. In comparing the reliability of knee joint angles measure by goniometry and interrupted light photography, Kerschot et al. (1980) found that one would need record seven photographic and 20 goniometric gait cycles to achieve one standard deviation of 2°.

More refined techniques generally increase the information available. However, a variety of errors may occur in the various steps required for capturing the additional data, and errors can propagate (Allard et al. 1995). For example, relative motion between the soft tissues and bone during movement inevitably limit reliability, since one is generally interested in the movement of the relatively rigid underlying bones, rather than movement of the soft-tissue envelope (Lafortune and Cavanagh 1985). Markers closest to the bones with a minimum of underlying soft tissue provide the most reliable (i.e. most repeatable) observations, while those held away from the body segment on sticks and/or with substantial underlying soft tissues are the least reliable. Furthermore, if one is interested in movement of the bones, then one must relate external landmarks to bony landmarks, a potential source of substantial error of some centimeters. One potential way to minimize error from marker movement utilizes redundant markers (Kinzel and Gutkowski 1983). To compute full three-dimensional relative motion of two rigid bodies, one must know the displacement histories of a minimum of three landmarks on each rigid body. However, if one uses four, five, six, or more markers on each body segment it is possible to compute the distance between all pairs of markers. Rigidly attached to rigid body, these would always remain the same, but on a body segment such as the thigh, some may move against the overlying soft tissues. If only one or two move relative to the others, a correction can be made for those which move (or move the greatest), and reduce the error of computation of the relative motion of the two limb segments.

In contrast to ascertaining times and distances (which may be more or less directly measured), velocities and accelerations are generally computed using smoothed displacement histories (Woltring 1995). (Accelerations may be directly measured with an accelerometer, but since the accelerations of multiple limb segments are required, this latter method is not generally used for these forms of locomotion analysis.) Many mathematical approaches are available

for such processing, and each includes certain assumptions and potential errors. The choice is somewhat arbitrary, but one must know the specific limitations of whatever technique is chosen, and their potential impact on conclusions.

Other errors include (but are not limited to) calibrating the location of markers, errors in identifying markers, and optical distortion in the recording device. Most investigators will systematically identify and explore such potential problems in their own systems, and in most cases these latter do not incur large errors. In assessing the reliability of the observations, these points should always be considered.

Kinetic analysis

Kinetic analysis involves measurement or calculation of the forces causing observed motions. In clinical terms, this means estimating forces external to the body (e.g. foot–floor forces) or internal forces (e.g. joint or muscle forces). The former require various forms of force transducers (Table 1), while the latter typically require computational models, although internal forces have been measured in humans in a very few specific instances (Kotzar et al. 1991; Bergmann et al. 1993).

Parameters of kinetic analysis

In the simplest cases, forces are directly measured using various transducers (e.g. force plates built into the floor, hand grip strength devices). These devices provide analog or digital records, which can then be analyzed in various ways, most often as peak forces. Accelerations may be ascertained from accelerometers attached to limb segments (Cavagna et al. 1963). While the devices themselves are accurate, they may lead to errors when attached to soft tissues rather than rigidly fixed to bone (Lafortune et al. 1995).

In more complex analyses, it is possible to compute various force parameters using linked-segment mathematical models (including certain assumptions regarding system constraints). Perhaps the most common computes the intersegmental resultant forces and moments (Crowninshield and Brand 1980; Andrews 1995). The intersegmental forces and moments (sometimes termed simply 'joint forces' or 'joint torques') do not represent forces in any actual joint structures, but rather represent the vector sums of all such forces (muscle, ligament, capsule, joint contact forces) acting about a joint. (Although one should distinguish the intersegmental resultant force from the joint contact force, it is important to realize that the joint contact force is ordinarily reported as a single number (magnitude) or vector, and is therefore itself a 'resultant' since that single force is distributed over the articular surface.)

Models computing the intersegmental resultants require estimates of body segment inertial properties and limb motion (segment accelerations) as well as externally measured forces. Computation of both segment inertial properties and accelerations in turn require mathematical models, the latter making assumptions about joint constraints (e.g. hinge joint, ball-and-socket joint). Computation of intersegmental joint forces and moments has become a standard procedure in virtually all gait laboratories, partly owing to marketed software capable of computing these quantities. Linked-segment models also allow the computation of mechanical energy (Elftman 1939; Cavagna et al. 1963; Mansour et al. 1982; Burdett et al. 1983). However, such analyses have rarely been used for clinical purposes.

Considerably more complex modeling procedures are required to estimate forces in actual anatomic structures (Crowninshield and Brand 1981; Zajac and Winters 1990). These latter types of model are generally subject to far more assumptions and limitations than those required for estimating the intersegmental resultants, and accordingly are subject to far greater error and question. For virtually all current clinical uses, one need not consider internal forces other than the rather more simply obtained intersegmental resultant forces and moments.

Limitations of kinetic analysis

Ascertainment of external forces can be accomplished with considerable precision using contemporary devices. One need only be aware of the general accuracy of the device (supplied by the manufacturer, or readily ascertained through calibration procedures if custom made). While accelerometers themselves are reasonably accurate, attachment to the soft tissues may introduce errors (Lafortune et al. 1995).

Conversely, computation of internal forces (i.e. intersegmental resultant forces and moments) is not so straightforward, although 'turn-key' software packages might lead the unsuspecting user to believe they are. As noted above, the following information or data is required: external forces, limb segment accelerations, and body segment inertial properties. Limb segment accelerations normally arise from processing recorded marker displacement data, but a number of steps are required.

Firstly, one must ascertain the 'joint center', not an actual anatomic point, but rather the origin of the required reference frames. Since these are ordinarily anatomically based, the location of specific landmarks must be determined. Obviously, potential errors associated with landmarks (discussed above) apply to these determinations. At the knee, for example, the location of the medial and lateral epicondyle might be determined, then the mid-point of those two locations selected as the 'joint center'. However, the ill-defined nature of the epicondyles and overlying soft tissues may create errors of 1 to 2 cm in locating the 'joint center'. As another example, the 'hip center' may be ascertained by estimating the location of the anterior superior iliac spine and the symphysis pubis, establishing a co-ordinate system from the plane created by those three points, then the hip center location estimated as a percentage of the interanterior superior iliac spine distance from the anterior superior iliac spine and that plane. Such approaches are also subject to errors of several centimeters. Data reported by Andriacchi and Strickland (1985) suggests variability of between 10 and 20 per cent in some joint moment computations assuming errors in estimating hip center location of only 1.6 cm. Precise knowledge of all landmarks is obviously required to record displacement histories of limb segments accurately.

Secondly, a model of the limb is needed. Ordinarily a linked-segment model (Kinzel and Gutkowski 1983) as well as a mathematical technique is used to differentiate the displacement histories to obtain velocities and accelerations (Woltring 1995). Linked-segment models may make a variety of approximations on joint motions, such as a hinge joint at the knee or a ball-and-socket joint at the hip; such assumptions affect model results, although typically not in a major way. The mathematical techniques for smoothing displacement data, and then computing velocities and accelerations can make errors, likely in the range of several to perhaps 10 per cent.

Thirdly, specific inertial properties must be known (e.g. mass center location, mass distribution). Estimates are ordinarily based upon anthropometric measurements on a given patient, then inputting those measurements into anthropometric models from the literature (Dempster 1955; Jensen 1978; Hatze 1979; Jensen and Fletcher 1994). However, both the initial anthropometric measurements and models are subject to certain assumptions and errors likely in the range of 10 to 20 per cent.

All of these uncertainties cause potentially inaccurate computation of the intersegmental joint resultants, and errors may propagate. Unfortunately, such uncertainties are rarely mentioned in current clinically relevant studies or in software documentation. When one interprets the literature on locomotion analysis or the data of a given patient, particularly related to differences of one kinetic parameter relative to a normal database, one must have an appreciation of the potential for these errors: often the uncertainty of the measure exceeds the difference from patient to normal.

Electromyographic analysis

Electromyography (**EMG**) provides a valuable tool for ascertaining temporal activation of a muscle during movement. As a clinical tool, one can determine whether or not a muscle is being activated at an expected ('normal') time and duration. In general, the more cyclic and stereotypical the activity, the greater the potential value for a given subject. For less reproducible activities, it is difficult to distinguish normal from abnormal activation patterns. This situation creates a paradox, since many stereotypical activities occur through 'hard-wired' pattern generators in the central nervous system, and are relatively unaffected by many abnormalities (e.g. level gait in a patient with a tear of the anterior cruciate ligament). Those activities which are most likely to result in abnormal EMG patterns are often those which are not stereotypical and subject to considerable variability. In these cases, distinguishing a normal from an abnormal EMG may be difficult or impossible.

Parameters of EMG analysis

EMG patterns may be analyzed as 'raw' signals, or processed to create 'envelopes' of patterns. All EMG signals are first filtered to exclude motion artifact and eliminate obviously irrelevant signal ('noise'). Typically a 'high-pass filter' eliminates signal below 10 to 20 Hz (the range of signal from motion artifact) and a 'low-pass filter' eliminates signal above 500 to 1000 Hz (the level above which there is no substantial energy content). The resulting raw signals per se may be interpreted only qualitatively, typically determining timing of activation during a cycle of some more or less reproducible activity. Onset of activity is ascertained by presuming some threshold of activity. For clinical purposes, such interpretation often suffices.

However, if one must make a quantitative assessment (e.g Is the signal magnitude greater or lesser after some intervention or is the signal duration different?), then the raw signal may be processed in a variety of ways. Such quantitative assessments are possible only in activities which are reasonably reproducible. Typically this involves rectification (taking the raw signal with its positive and negative voltage signal components and placing all the signal on one side or the other of the zero axis), then smoothing, filtering, or averaging to create an envelope of activity (Hershler and Milner 1978; Shiavi et al. 1983; Winter 1991; Jacobsen *et al.* 1995). The resulting envelopes may then be further processed and analyzed in a variety of ways.

To compare envelope timing and magnitude directly (and quantitatively), both aspects need to be normalized. Timing is normalized by assuming a constant timing for all activity cycles, then mathematically expanding the shorter ones and contracting the longer ones. Signal magnitude may be normalized in a variety of ways: to the maximum signal observed during the test, to the average of all signals, to the maximum voluntary contraction, or to the magnitude during some standard event (i.e. with a fixed joint moment) (Yang and Winter 1984). Each approach has utility in a given situation, and each has certain associated problems.

Once the individual raw signals are processed and normalized, one may then combine any number of curves (typically a given number of cycles from an individual) into an 'ensemble-averaged' curve (Hershler and Milner 1978; Shiavi and Green 1983). The 'average' curve of a number of individuals may then be used to obtain the average of a sample population ('grand ensemble average'). This latter procedure affords the average curve of a normal population (Shiavi *et al.* 1987; Winter 1991), or the average curve for a patient population when answering a specific research question. Alternatively, one may numerically represent a signal using principal component analysis (Wooten *et al.* 1990*a*) or cluster analysis (Wooten *et al.* 1990*b*). The ensemble-averaging approach is far more common, and in clinical practice, one need only the ensemble average of the given patient, plus that for a large, matched normal population.

With the ensemble averages and their variation, it is possible to determine whether various aspects (parameters) of the ensemble from a given patient differ from those of the normal population. Quantities such as the peak magnitudes, or timing to one or two peaks in a cycle, are commonly used. It is also possible to ascertain merely the percentage of time during a given cycle that a muscle is active. This requires the establishment of a threshold of activity. Sometimes this is merely a fixed per cent (e.g. 5 per cent) of the peak; perhaps a more rational approach is to record system noise over some short-time interval (e.g. 10 s) with the subject resting, then process that signal, determine a mean and two or three standard deviations, then presume all signal above those ranges of standard determinations represent 'true' signal, and not noise (Jacobson *et al.* 1995).

Once specific parameters (e.g. peak magnitude, per cent activation time) are ascertained, differences of a given patient from a normal population may be determined using an appropriate statistical test. When examining populations, rather than individual subjects, it is also possible statistically to determine differences between the pattern of entire envelopes. The Kolmogorov–Smirnov test is one such way to examine pattern differences (Hoel 1971; Limbird *et al.* 1988).

Limitations of EMG analysis

EMG signals merely reflect voltage changes within tissues at the site sampled. Obviously those signals arise from electrical discharge throughout the body (and perhaps 'noise' from the environment, such as lighting). In general, electrical discharge from some distant site (e.g. heart muscle activity) is sufficiently small to create no problem in interpretation. However, discharge from adjacent muscles (crosstalk) is often a substantial problem. Surface electrodes are far more subject to this problem since they generally sample larger vol-

umes of tissue. However, intramuscular electrodes are not entirely free from crosstalk, particularly since the location of the electrode is not always well documented (or documentable): if the intramuscular electrode is very near the interface of two muscles, discharge from both will obviously be sampled. Nonetheless, most investigators consider that intramuscular electrodes are essential for distinguishing the activity of two adjacent muscles, particularly those which may act in concert. Crosstalk may be explored by the clinical observer by having the patient perform activities activating a given muscle of interest though not activating adjacent muscles. For example, the popliteus muscle (which cannot be studied by surface electrodes) is activated by active internal rotation of the tibia on the femur with the subject sitting relaxed with the knee at 90°; the overlying gastrocnemius muscles are not activated in this position (Barnett and Richardson 1953). Conversely, when the subject is standing erect and rises onto tiptoes, the gastrocnemius muscles are activated while the popliteus is not. Such tests provide selective activation and insure a signal is activated when appropriate and silent when appropriate, thus confirming proper electrode placement. One then has some confidence that crosstalk will be minimized when studying other activities.

The specific method of hardware or software filtering or smoothing as well as the number of analyzed cycles has a distinct effect on the resulting curves and their statistical analysis. Using a consistent set of data, Gabel and Brand (1994) demonstrated that it was possible to obtain statistically significant or statistically insignificant results merely by altering the processing methods. If considerable smoothing is appropriate for the question asked, then perhaps only three cycles of a reproducible activity from a normal subject may suffice (Arsenault *et al.* 1986). Conversely, smoothing eliminates perhaps biologically important detail from the curves, and if less smoothing is used, up to 20 or more cycles may be necessary (Gabel and Brand 1994).

In determining the percentage of time that a muscle is activated during a given cycle or time of an activity, the per cent activation time will vary depending upon the choice of threshold. That is, a very sensitive threshold will create a greater per cent activation time than a less sensitive threshold. For very repeatable patterns, this will not ordinarily affect the computed activation time substantially, but for nonrepeatable patterns, differing conclusions may result depending upon threshold. As a minimum, it is necessary to be sensitive to this issue, and perhaps explore thresholds in a parametric fashion to ascertain sensitivity to the specific question.

As noted above, quantitatively comparing multiple EMG trials of a given individual to some population average requires normalizing. The signal intimately depends upon electrode placement, thickness of overlying soft tissues, amount of perspiration, cleanliness of the electrodes, and so on. Such variables will result in signals of somewhat differing magnitude even when placing the same electrode at the identical site on different days. Thus, normalization is required even to compare signals between test sessions (intrasubject variability). Perhaps the most common method is to compare signal magnitude of some activity to that recorded in multiple trials of a maximum voluntary contraction of the muscle in question. Even this latter quantity will be somewhat variable, and the number of trials needs to be sufficiently large to be representative, but not conducted in such a way as to introduce fatigue. Normalizing to the maximum voluntary contraction allows comparison of magnitude between various activities in a given individual, but it is important to be cautious in interpreting magnitudes between the same (or differing) activities in multiple individuals since the maximum contraction is variable between individuals. That is, one can compare timing parameters of a given patient to a population norm, but perhaps not magnitude parameters. Alternatively, if one normalizes to some activity which is standardized between all subjects (e.g. the activation of the quadriceps muscles resisting a given torque), then some inferences can be made about relative magnitudes.

When applying statistical tests to biological features, one need always insure coherence of 'statistical' and 'biological' significance: what is statistically significant at some preselected level (e.g. 0.05) may not be biologically or clinically significant and vice versa. Particular care must be taken in interpreting EMG signals with their many layers of processing. The rather sensitive Kolmogorov–Smirnoff test, for example, may show 'statistically significant' (i.e. $p < 0.05$) differences in randomly selected sets of different trials from the same activity of a given subject; such differences can have neither biological nor clinical meaning. However, if care is taken to establish biological or clinical significance at an appropriate level of statistical significance, this is not a problem.

Energy expenditure analysis

For normal subjects, most locomotor functions are metabolically efficient. However, disabled patients often must exert considerable effort. Oxygen consumption allows a reasonably convenient way to assess changes in efficiency over time or occurring as a result of some intervention (Fischer and Gullikson 1978; Brown *et al.* 1980; McBeath *et al.* 1980; DuBow *et al.* 1983; Nowroozi *et al.* 1983; Pinzur *et al.* 1992). The measure is a good one in that it takes into account general or systemic factors such as the cardiopulmonary status of the patient. Furthermore, it relates reasonably well to computed mechanical work (Burdett *et al.* 1983). However, it is sensitive to such factors as walking speed, and patients must be able to reach a steady state for reasonably accurate measurement. Interestingly, the minimum oxygen consumption for a given individual typically occurs at their self-selected walking speed. As a measure for an individual patient, it is rarely useful, although it has been useful to assess various disabilities and the efficacies of various interventions in large groups of patients.

Processing locomotion data

The various locomotion techniques can quickly generate large amounts of data, even for a single patient. Most of the data is continuous, in the form of a time-varying wave (and cyclic for such activities) pattern. For comparison between trials or subjects, many forms of data must be normalized in the time and magnitude domains. While the former is straightforward, the latter is not (see discussion above on EMG). One must then select from among many specific aspects of the patterns which are believed to reflect the disease state in question, then ascertain how they differ from normal. For example, one might select peak magnitudes, timing of peaks, or areas under curves.

Single or even multiple features rarely correlate in any meaningful way with severity of disease, although there may be crude correlations between severity and a parameter such as walking speed. The reason

for this is rather simple: that the impact a disease or treatment has upon a patient arises from a complex compilation of many physical, social, and psychological factors. Any single locomotion measure reflects merely 'the tip of the iceberg'.

Recognizing the problem with single locomotion features, several groups have attempted to incorporate more than one. Chao and his colleagues, in a series of papers, introduced a 'performance index' incorporating many features of an analysis of patients with knee disability. A stepwise discriminate analysis selected and weighted seven gait variables out of a potential 43 to create their index (Chao *et al.* 1980). This procedure generally discriminated between normal and abnormal, although not in all cases. The approach seems intuitively promising, but there remain unsolved problems. Firstly, while the index correlated with a Harris Hip Score (an independent functional scale) when all subjects were considered, the performance index of either the normals or patients alone did not correlate with the hip score; furthermore, it failed to discriminate between the least and most affected patients. Secondly, when they included more additional subjects in a study of 243 patients and considered 54 candidate variables, nine, rather than the original seven, were selected by the stepwise analysis, and the weighting factors changed (Laughman *et al.* 1984). This means the weighting is sensitive to the specific database. If such features were so sensitive, an impractically large database would be needed to ascertain weighting. Thirdly, the weighting coefficients were different for men and women, again demonstrating sensitivity to subgroups. Finally, when the group developed a third performance index for hip disability (Kaufman *et al.* 1987), the weighting factors again changed, illustrating a sensitivity to choice of joint. Mittlmeier *et al.* (1989) reported a seemingly more successful effort to establish a performance index of five parameters of dynamic foot contact pressures. In this case, the index did correlate with an independent clinical rating, but sensitivity to the various features were not explored. Thus, while the approach seems promising, sensitivity of the indices to its individual elements and the database require systematic consideration.

Once the clinician establishes a procedure for selecting and processing locomotion events, there remains the task of statistical analysis. Appropriate tests must be made taking into account normalcy of data, dependence or independence of features. Statistical levels of significance should be established on a rational basis taking into account intra- and intersubject variability, not merely some more or less arbitrary level (e.g. $p = 0.05$); to emphasize a previous point, such statistically significant levels may not be biologically or clinically important and, conversely, statistically insignificant levels may in fact be clinically important.

Requirements for the clinical relevance of locomotion

Given the general failure of locomotion analysis to enter the clinical arena, and all of the cautions noted above, it might be reasonable to ask whether technology can actually achieve clinical utility. The answer is a qualified but definite yes—qualified provided that certain criteria are met.

Doctors order tests for one of five reasons:

- to distinguish between one of several possible disorders explaining some array of symptoms and signs ('diagnosis')
- to select the best among several treatment options
- to screen asymptomatic patients at high risk for developing some problem for which prophylactic or early treatment is critical to long-term outcome
- to predict outcome ('prognosis')
- to determine the severity of disease or injury ('assessment').

From the standpoint of patient care, there are no other reasons for ordering tests; legitimate educational or legal reasons may nonetheless affect a decision to order a test. In fact, decisions over whether or not to treat a patient largely arise from the first three reasons. Knowledge of long-term outcome (prognosis) may affect recommendations for the patient's lifestyle and planning, but less often interventions *per se*. For most medical, administrative (disability ratings), and legal reasons, a clinical assessment is sufficiently precise, and the greater precision of various technical approaches is not required. Disease and injury produce disability as a result of interacting physical and psychological factors, and such factors are more appropriately ascertained by taking a history, observing the overall behavior of the patient, and conducting an appropriate examination, including observations of patient movement when appropriate.

The 'acid tests' of clinical usefulness of any measure are whether that measure predicts a different outcome than would be predicted without the measure, or whether the measure suggests a different treatment than would be recommended without the measure.

Additional criteria arise from problems recognized with various forms of technology. Schwartz *et al.* (1933), recognizing some of these problems, suggested the following criteria for 'any method' of recording gait':

- ease
- rapidity
- economy
- a mechanism which would not change the gait
- constancy of recording (unless the gait were changed)
- measures which when changed in the recording reflected real changes in the gait.

Brand and Crowninshield (1981), unaware of Schwartz's suggestions, proposed several similar criteria. The author would add the following:

- any technique must be accurate and reproducible
- it must not alter the function it intends to measure
- the measure must be stable over time (i.e. not vary during a given day or week or time frame within which a disease does not change)
- the measure must be cost-effective
- the measure must be independent of mood, motivation, and pain
- the measure should clearly distinguish normal from abnormal
- it should not be directly observable by a skilled clinician

- it should be reported in a form analogous to an accepted clinical concept.

This list is not all inclusive; others might propose equally important or more important criteria.

Few would argue with some of these criteria, although a brief amplification of some of the others is appropriate. The first four are not likely to be controversial. However, while most investigators demonstrate reproducibility of the measures, few have demonstrated accuracy by an independent 'gold standard'. For some features (e.g. walking speed) this step is unnecessary, but for others (e.g. joint motion) it may be more important owing to greater measurement errors (Kerschot *et al.* 1980).

There have been few demonstrations of the effect of the measuring system on function, although at least one investigator has documented that intramuscular electrodes do not seriously affect gait. Rather, most investigators assume the laboratory environment and recording apparatus do not affect any measured parameters.

Features substantially dependent upon the patient's mood or motivation are of limited usefulness because they are not reproducible. Locomotion, to a greater or lesser degree, always depends upon the patient's disposition. Patients with chronically painful conditions may be depressed and will not move as well as they might otherwise.

A clinically useful measure should clearly distinguish normal from abnormal. However, many locomotion features (e.g. walking speed) in large populations are defined by Gaussian or non-Gaussian distributions in which data from normal subjects and diseased or injured patients substantially overlap. When this is the case, then a single measure alone may not help in making clinical decisions. Schneider and Chao (1983) reached this conclusion in their study of a variety of parameters of foot–floor reaction force patterns in patients with total knee replacements. Perhaps importantly, they found statistically significant differences with a Fourier analysis of the waveforms. Wong *et al.* (1983) and Wooten *et al.* (1990b) suggested that cluster analysis might more clearly distinguish normal from abnormal gait parameters, while Yamamoto *et al.* (1983) reported principle component analysis techniques based upon 10 gait variables which better distinguished normal from abnormal subjects. Thus, it seems the ability to distinguish normal from abnormal may relate to the procedures for processing the data. Yet many studies fail to address this issue adequately.

The seventh criterion (the measure should be nonobservable) might be more controversial, although it can be effectively argued. In clinical medicine decisions are rarely based upon single observations, but rather an array of observations. In such a situation, semiquantitative information (i.e. an estimate) of each individual observation usually suffices, assuming that observation can be directly made by the clinician. Adding precision or accuracy (by various technical means) rarely adds value. Conversely, many important functions cannot be readily observed (e.g. a patient's blood sugar, or joint moment, or level of muscle activation), yet be critical in making decisions. In such cases, technology to make the measurements proves most useful.

Finally, it is important to formulate features analogous to clinical concepts. Measures not readily contained within the language of clinical medicine will not be readily accepted.

Each of these criteria alone may not prove critical and for a given measure will not likely be equally important. The point is that the likelihood of usefulness and acceptance will increase as more consideration is given to the various criteria.

At the same time, insuring that a gait measure meets all of these criteria will not insure clinical acceptability for decision making. Any measure must be adequately validated and clinical usefulness documented. In this context, 'validated' means the measure correlates well with some more or less independent measure, usually one providing some overall index of function (such as a clinical rating scale). Some years ago my former colleague, Roy Crowninshield, and I went through our files on gait analysis. Among 146 papers, 44 per cent merely described some technique and proposed a potential clinical role, 32 per cent illustrated application with a small number of subjects, 8 per cent proposed a clinical application without illustrative data, and 6 per cent demonstrated an application with a reasonable number of normal subjects or patients. No paper in our files validated the measures!

While clinical rating scales incorporating various features of patient history and examination have been used for decades, few have themselves been validated. (The SF-36 Health Survey represents one such instrument which has been reasonably validated and which has achieved wide use. The SF-36 is perhaps the most widely validated quality-of-life measure (Jaglal *et al.* 2000). it can be used for virtually any medical condition or intervention.) Brand *et al.* (1981) attempted to validate one gait measure (the center of pressure path) against an independent functional rating scale. However, our gait measure correlated neither with the scale nor radiographic changes. Furthermore, the measure failed to distinguish patients clearly from normal subjects. We concluded the center of pressure path had no utility for the intended purpose.

Clinically confirming the utility of locomotion analysis

As noted above, it is important to remember the 'acid tests' of clinical utility.

1. Does the measure (or group of appropriately combined or analyzed features) predict a different outcome than would be predicted without the measure?

2. Does the knowledge of the measure change the clinician's choice of treatment?

A measure which does not meet these tests will never be truly useful nor likely gain wide acceptance.

What strategies, then, can be used to document clinical utility? There are four possible suggestions.

1. Cross-sectional studies of patients in which the clinical evaluation with the measure results in a differently predicted outcome than would be predicted without the measure; such a design might include two clinicians evaluating the same patient.

2. Longitudinal studies which document that the predicted outcome with the new measure is indeed correct.

3. Cross-sectional studies to demonstrate that clinicians recommend differing treatments with and without knowledge of the measure; again, a multiclinician study evaluating the same patients could be considered.

4. Prospective randomized longitudinal trials which document the outcome of treatment (whichever is recommended) is better when the recommendation based upon the new treatment is followed.

In the first and third strategies, one would obviously need two groups of physicians, one with and one without the measure, and both patient and evaluator would need to be blinded with respect to the process of physician decision.

Clinically useful locomotion measures

There are relatively few cases where investigators have addressed clinical utility of locomotion measures in the manner outlined. For illustrative purposes, two such cases are briefly discussed. In both cases, the analysis provided a measure which could not be directly observed by the clinician, and were used to select logically between alternative treatment options, thus meeting the 'acid test'.

It is well known that certain forms of surgery, such as tendon transfers or releases, are not predictable in cerebral palsy. One reason for this is the lack of correlation between presumed muscle strength with voluntary testing and muscle activation during some activities; these patients often do not have sufficient voluntary control to assess muscle strength adequately. In addition, owing to redundancy of muscles, it is difficult to ascertain which muscles are responsible for a given pattern of limb movement. EMGs during gait or upper extremity movements can document which muscles are active at which time and how active they are relative to other muscles, potentially improving our ability to select which patients will benefit from surgery, and which form of surgery is most appropriate. Hoffer and Perry (1983) pioneered the use of EMG for this purpose. For example, when the posterior tibial muscle is active throughout gait, lengthening best corrects equinus induced by that muscle. When the muscle is active only during swing, then tendon transfer is the better procedure. A similar approach has been used in ascertaining the best procedure in the upper extremity (Hoffer 1993; Kozin and Kennan 1993). However, it is important to be aware, that despite the logic and considerable potential of these approaches, utility has not been documented in large series of patients treated with and without the measure.

High tibial osteotomy is frequently performed when only one compartment of the knee joint has deteriorated because of osteoarthrosis. However, the procedure is not very predictable (particularly compared to total knee replacement) and is not performed as often as it might given greater predictability. Prodromos *et al.* (1985) ascertained the preoperative adduction moment correlated with outcome: patients with a low adduction moment did significantly better than those with a high adduction moment at an average follow-up of 3.2 years. In a later study with longer follow-up (3.0–8.9 years) of the same patients, all 14 patients in the low adduction group, but only nine of the 14 in the high adduction group, had good or excellent results (Wang *et al.* 1990). This sort of study indeed fulfils some of the criteria outlined in this chapter, and uses some of the validation strategies.

Summary

It is clear that locomotion analysis has not gained widespread clinical use. Using specific criteria to select a potential tool and measure will help to avoid proposing methods which will likely not gain clinical acceptance, but this alone will not guarantee utility. To insure utility (i.e. to select the best among several treatment options and/or to predict outcome), clinical follow-up studies must be pursued to insure outcomes are actually different with and without the measure or to insure that doctors select different and more appropriate treatments when they have knowledge of the measure than when they do not. However, when the relevant precautions are taken and the appropriate strategies used, locomotion analysis can provide critical information in the evaluation of a given patient.

Further reading

Allard, P., Stokes, I.A.F., and Blanchi, J.-P. (ed.) (1995). *Three-dimensional analysis of human movement.* Human Kinetics, Champaign, IL.

Cappozzo, A., Marchetti, M., and Tosi, V. (1992). *Biolocomotion: a century of research using moving pictures.* Promograph, Rome.

Ducroquet, R., Ducroquet, J., and Ducroquet, P. (1968). *Walking and limping: a study of normal and pathological walking.* Lippincott, Philadelphia, PA.

Groves, R. and Camaione, D.N. (1975). *Concepts in kinesiology.* W.B. Saunders, Philadelphia, PA.

McMahon, T. (1984). *Muscles, reflexes, and locomotion.* Princeton University Press.

Nigg, B.M. and Herzog, W. (ed.) (1994). *Biomechanics of the musculo-skeletal system.* Wiley, New York.

Perry, J. (1992). *Gait analysis: normal and pathological function.* Slack, Thorofare, NJ.

Rose, J. and Gamble, J.G. (1994). *Human walking.* Williams & Wilkins, Baltimore, MD.

Steindler, A. (1955). *Kinesiology of the human body: under normal and pathological conditions.* Thomas, Springfield, IL.

Vaughan, C.L., Murphy, G.N., and du Toit, L.L. (1987). *Biomechanics of human gait: an annotated bibliography* (2nd edn). Human Kinetics, Champaign, IL.

Winter, D.A. (1991). *The biomechanics and motor control of human gait: normal, elderly, and pathological* (2nd edn). University of Waterloo Press.

References

Allard, P., Blanchi, J.-P., and Aïssaoui, R. (1995). Bases of three-dimensional reconstruction. In *Three-dimensional analysis of human movement* (ed. P. Allard, I.A.F. Stokes, and J.-P. Blanchi), pp. 19–40. Human Kinetics, Champaign, IL.

Amar, J. (1916). Trottoir dynamographique. *Comptes Rendus Hebdomadaires des Séances de l'Academie des Sciences*, **163**, 130–2.

Amar, J. (1920). *The human motor.* Routledge, New York.

Andrews, J.G. (1995). Euler's and Lagrange's equations for linked rigid-body models of three-dimensional human motion. In *Three-dimensional analysis of human movement* (ed. P. Allard, I.A.F. Stokes, and J.-P. Blanchi), pp. 145–75. Human Kinetics, Champaign, IL.

Andriacchi, T.P. and Strickland, A.B. (1985). Gait analysis as a tool to assess joint kinetics. In *Biomechanics of normal and pathological human articulating joints* (ed. N. Berme, A.E. Engin, and K.M. Correia da Silva), pp. 83–102. Martinus Nijhoff, Dordrecht.

Arsenault, A.G., Winter, D.A., Marteniuk, R.G., and Hayes, K.C. (1986). How many strides are required for the analysis of electromyographic data in gait? *Scandinavian Journal of Rehabilitation Medicine*, **18**, 133–5.

Barnett, C.H. and Richardson, A.T. (1953). The postural function of the popliteus muscle. *Annals of Physical Medicine*, **1**, 177–9.

Bell, A.L., Pedersen, D.R., and Brand, R.A. (1990). A comparison of the accuracy of several hip joint center location prediction methods. *Journal of Biomechanics*, **23**, 617–21.

Bergmann, G., Graichen, F., and Rohlmann, A. (1993). Hip joint loading during walking and running measured in two patients. *Journal of Biomechanics*, **26**, 969–90.

Boone, D.C., Azen, S.P., Lin, C.-M., Spence, C., Baron, C., and Lee, L. (1978) Reliability of goniometric measurements. *Physical Therapy*, **58**, 1355–60.

Borelli, G.A. (1989). *On the movement of animals* (*De motu animalium*, originally published in 1680), (trans. P. Maquet). Springer-Verlag, Berlin.

Brand, R.A. and Crowninshield, R.D. (1981). Comment on criteria for patient evaluation tools. *Journal of Biomechanics*, **14**, 655.

Brand, R.A., Laaveg, S.J., Crowninshield, R.D., and Ponseti, I.V. (1981). The center of pressure path in treated clubfeet. *Clinical Orthopaedics and Related Research*, **160**, 43–7.

Brand, R.A., Pedersen, D.R., and Friederich, J.A. (1986). The sensitivity of muscle force predictions to changes in physiologic cross-sectional area. *Journal of Biomechanics*, **19**, 589–96.

Braune, W. and Fischer, O. (1895–1901). *Der Gang des Menschen*, Vols I–IV. Teubner, Leipzig.

Brown, M., Hislop, H.J., Waters, R.L., and Porell, D. (1980). Walking efficiency before and after total hip replacement. *Physical Therapy*, **10**, 1259–63.

Burdett, R.G., Skrinar, G.S., and Simon, S.R. (1983). Comparison of mechanical work and metabolic energy consumption during normal gait. *Journal of Orthopaedic Research*, **1**, 63–72.

Cappozzo, A. (1983). Considerations on clinical gait evaluation. *Journal of Biomechanics*, **16**, 302.

Cappozzo, A., Marchetti, M., and Tosi, V. (1992). *Biolocomotion: a century of research using moving pictures.* Promograph, Rome.

Carlet, G. (1872). Sur la locomotion humaine. *Annales des Sciences Naturelles*, Serie 5.

Cavagna, G.A., Saibene, F.P., and Margaria, R. (1963). External work in walking. *Journal of Applied Physiology*, **18**, 1–9.

Chao, E.Y., Laughman, R.K., and Stauffer, R.N. (1980). Biomechanical evaluation of pre- and postoperative total knee replacement patients. *Archives of Orthopaedic and Traumatic Surgery*, **97**, 309–17.

Crowninshield, R.D. and Brand, R.A. (1981). The predictions of forces in joint structures: distribution of intersegmental resultants. In *Exercise and sport science reviews* (ed. D.I. Miller), pp. 159–81. Franklin Institute Press, Seattle, WA.

Crowninshield, R.D., Brand, R.A., and Johnston, R.C. (1978). The effects of walking velocity and age on hip kinematics and kinetics. *Clinical Orthopaedics and Related Research*, **132**, 140–4.

Dempster, W.T. (1955). *Space requirements of the seated operator. WADC Technical Report 55–159.* Wright-Patterson Air Force Base, Dayton, OH.

Dercum, F.X. (1888*a*). A study of some normal and abnormal movements, photographed by Muybridge. In *The Muybridge work at the University of Pennsylvania. The method and the result*, Vol. 9. In *Muybridge's complete human and animal locomotion* (1979). Dover Publications, New York.

Dercum, F.X. (1888*b*). The walk and some of its phases in disease, together with other studies based on the Muybridge investigations. *Transactions of the College of Physicians (Philadelphia)*, **10**, 308–38.

DuBow, L.L., Witt, P.L., Kadaba, M.P., Reyes, R., and Cochran, G.V.B. (1983). Oxygen consumption of elderly persons with bilateral below knee amputations: ambulation by wheelchair propulsion. *Archives of Physical Medicine and Rehabilitation*, **64**, 255–9.

Ducroquet, R., Ducroquet, J., and Ducroquet, P. (1968). *Walking and limping: a study of normal and pathological walking*. Lippincott, Philadelphia, PA.

Elftman, H. (1939). Forces and energy changes in the leg during walking. *American Journal of Physiology*, **125**, 339–56.

Fischer, S.V. and Gullickson, G. (1978). Energy cost of ambulation in health and disability: a literature review. *Archives of Physical Medicine and Rehabilitation*, **59**, 124–33.

Gabel, R.H. and Brand, R.A. (1994). The effects of signal conditioning on the statistical analyses of gait EMG. *Electroencephalography and Clinical Neurophysiology*, **93**, 188–201.

Gabel, R.H., Johnston, R.C., and Brand, R.A. (1979). A gait analyzer/trainer instrumentation system. *Journal of Biomechanics*, **12**, 543–9.

Hatze, H. (1979). *A model for the computational determination of parameter values of anthropomorphic segments*. Tegniese Verslag, Pretoria.

Hershler, C. and Milner, M. (1978). An optimality criterion for processing electromyographic (EMG) signals relating to human locomotion. *IEEE Transactions of Biomedical Engineering*, **5**, 413–20.

Hoel, P.G. (1971). *Introduction to mathematical statistics*. Wiley, San Diego, CA.

Hoffer, M.M. (1993). The use of the pathokinesiology laboratory to select muscles for tendon transfers in the cerebral palsy hand. *Clinical Orthopaedics and Related Research*, **288**, 135–8.

Hoffer, M.M. and Perry, J. (1983). Pathodynamics of gait alterations in cerebral palsy and the significance of kinetic electromyography in evaluating foot and ankle problems. *Foot and Ankle*, **4**, 128–34.

Jacobson, W.C., Gabel, R.H., and Brand, R.A. (1995). Surface versus fine-wire electrode ensemble-averaged signals during gait. *Journal of Electromyography and Kinesiology*, **5**, 37–44.

Jaglal, S., Lakham, Z., and Schatzker, J. (2000). Reliability, validity, and responsiveness of the lower extremity measure for patients with a hip fracture. *Journal of Bone and Joint Surgery, American Volume*, **82A**, 955–62.

Jensen, R.K. (1978). Estimation of the biomechanical properties of three body types using a photogrammetric method. *Journal of Biomechanics*, **11**, 349–58.

Jensen, R.K. and Fletcher, P. (1994). Distribution of mass to the segments of elderly males and females. *Journal of Biomechanics*, **27**, 89–96.

Kaufman, K.R., Chao, E.Y.S., Cahalan, T.D., Askew, L.J., and Bleimeyer, R.R. (1987). Development of a functional performance index for quantitative gait analysis. In *Biomedical sciences instrumentation* (ed. J.D. Enderle), pp. 49–55. Instrument Society of America, Research Triangle Park, NC.

Kerschot, M., Soudan, K., and Van Auderkercke, R. (1980). Objective recording of human gait, a quantitative evaluation of two techniques: electrogoniometry and interrupted light photography. *Acta Orthopaedica Belgica*, **46**, 509–21.

Kinzel, G.L. and Gutkowski, L.J. (1983). Joint models, degrees of freedom, and anatomical motion measurement. *Journal of Biomechanical Engineering*, **105**, 55–62.

Kotzar, G.M., Davy, D.T., Goldberg, V.M., *et al.* (1991). Telemeterized *in vivo* hip joint force data: a report on two patients after total hip surgery. *Journal of Orthopaedic Research*, **9**, 621–33.

Kozin, S.H. and Kennan, M.A.E. (1993). Using dynamic electromyography to guide surgical treatment of the spastic upper extremity in the brain-injured patient. *Clinical Orthopaedics and Related Research*, **288**, 109–21.

Lafortune, M.A. and Cavanagh, P.R. (1985). The measurement of normal knee joint motion during walking using intracortical pins. In *Biomechanical measurement in orthopaedic practice* (ed. M. Whittle and D. Harris). Clarendon Press, Oxford.

Lafortune, M.A., Hennings, W., and Valiant, G.A. (1995). Tibial shock measured with bone and skin mounted transducers. *Journal of Biomechanics*, **28**, 989–93.

Laughman, R.K., Stauffer, R.N., Ilstrup, D.M., and Chao, E.Y.S. (1984). Functional evaluation of total knee replacement. *Journal of Orthopaedic Research*, **2**, 307–13.

Limbird, T.J., Shiavi, R., Frazier, M., and Borra, H. (1988). EMG profiles of knee joint musculature during walking: changes induced by anterior ligament deficiency. *Journal of Orthopaedic Research*, **6**, 630–8.

McBeath, A.A., Bahrke, M.S., and Balke, B. (1980). Walking efficiency before and after total hip replacement as determined by oxygen consumption. *Journal of Bone and Joint Surgery, American Volume*, **62**, 807–10.

Mansour, J.M., Lesh, M.D., Nowak, M.D., and Simon, S.R. (1982). A three dimensional multi-segmental analysis of the energetics of normal and pathological human gait. *Journal of Biomechanics*, **15**, 51–9.

Marey, E.-J. (1873). De la locomotion terrestre: chez les bipèdes et les quadrupèdes. *Journal de l'Anatomie et de la Physiologie Normales et Pathologiques de l'Homme et des Animaux*, **9**, 42–80.

Marey, E.-J. (1895). *Movement*. Heinemann, London.

Mittlmeier, T., Lob, G., Mütschler, W., and Bauer, G. (1989). Assessment of the subtalar joint function after fracture by analysis of the dynamic foot to ground pressure distribution. *Transactions of the Orthopaedic Research Society*, **14**, 248.

Nowroozi, F., Salvanelli, M.L., and Gerber, L.H. (1983). Energy expenditure in hip disarticulation and hemipelvectomy amputees. *Archives of Physical Medicine and Rehabilitation*, **64**, 300–7.

Perry, J. (1992). *Gait analysis: normal and pathological function*. Slack, Thorofare, NJ.

Pinzer, M.S., Gold, J., Schwartz, D., and Gross, N. (1992). Energy demands for walking in dysvascular amputees as related to the level of amputation. *Orthopedics*, **15**, 1033–7.

Prodromos, C.C., Andriacchi, T.P., and Galante, J.O. (1985). A relationship between gait and clinical changes following high tibial osteotomy. *Journal of Bone and Joint Surgery, American Volume*, **67**, 1188–93.

Schneider, E. and Chao, E.Y.S. (1983). Fourier analysis of ground reaction forces in normals and patients with knee joint disease. *Journal of Biomechanics*, **16**, 591–601.

Schwartz, R.P. and Heath, A.L. (1932). The pneumographic method of recording gait. *Journal of Bone and Joint Surgery*, **4**, 783–94.

Schwartz, R.P. and Heath, A.L. (1937). Some factors which influence the balance of the foot in walking: the stance phase of gait. *Journal of Bone and Joint Surgery*, **19**, 431–42.

Schwartz, R.P., Heath, A.L., and Wright, J.N. (1933). Electrobasographic method of gait. *Archives of Surgery*, **27**, 926–34.

Schwartz, R.P., Heath, A.L., Misiek, W., and Wright, J.N. (1934). Kinetics of human gait: the making and interpretation of electrobasographic records of gait. The influence of rate of walking and the height of shoe heel on duration of weight-bearing on the osseous tripod of the respective feet. *Journal of Bone and Joint Surgery*, **16**, 343–50.

Shiavi, R. and Green, N. (1983). Ensemble averaging of locomotor electromyographic patterns using interpolation. *Medical and Biological Engineering and Computation*, **21**, 573–8.

Shiavi, R., Green, N., McFadyen, B., Frazer, M., and Chen, J. (1987). Normative childhood EMG patterns. *Journal of Orthopaedic Research*, **5**, 283–95.

Steindler, A. (1955). *Kinesiology of the human body: under normal and pathological conditions*. Thomas, Springfield, IL.

Vierordt, K.H. (1881). *Das Gehen des Menschen in Gesunden und Kranken Zuständen nach selbstregistrirenden Methoden dargestelt*. Laupp, Tubingen.

Wang, J.-W., Kuo, K.N., Andriacchi, T.P., and Galante, J.O. (1990). The influence of walking mechanics and time on the results of proximal tibial osteotomy. *Journal of Bone and Joint Surgery, American Volume*, **72**, 905–9.

Weber, W. and Weber, E. (1836). *Mechanik der Menschlichen Gehwerkzeuge*, Dieterichshen, Buchhandlung, Gottingen.

Winter, D.A. (1991). *The biomechanics and motor control of human gait: normal, elderly, and pathological* (2nd edn). University of Waterloo Press.

Woltring, H.G. (1995). Smoothing and differentiation techniques applied to 3-D. In *Three-dimensional analysis of human movement* (ed. P. Allard, I.A.F. Stokes, and J.-P. Blanchi), pp. 79–99. Human Kinetics, Champaign, IL.

Wong, M.A., Simon, S., and Olsen, R.A. (1983). Statistical analysis of gait patterns of persons with cerebral palsy. *Statistics in Medicine*, **2**, 345–54.

Wooten, M.E., Kadaba, M.P., and Cochran, G.V.B. (1990*a*). Dynamic electromyography. I. Numerical representation using principal component analysis. *Journal of Orthopaedic Research*, **8**, 247–58.

Wooten, M.E., Kadaba, M.P., and Cochran, G.V.B. (1990*b*). Dynamic electromyography. II. Normal patterns during gait. *Journal of Orthopaedic Research*, **8**, 259–65.

Yamamoto, S., Suto, Y., Kawamura, H., Hashizume, T., and Kakurai, S. (1983). Quantitative gait evaluation of hip diseases using principal component analysis. *Journal of Biomechanics*, **16**, 717–26.

Yang, J.F. and Winter, D.A. (1984). Electromyographic amplitude normalization methods: improving their sensitivity as diagnostic tools in gait analysis. *Archives of Physical Medicine and Rehabilitation*, **65**, 517–21.

Zajac, F. and Winters, J.M. (1990). Modeling musculoskeletal movement systems: joint and body-segment dynamics, musculotendinous actuation, and neuromuscular control. In *Multiple muscle systems: biomechanics and movement organization* (ed. J.M. Winters and S.L.-Y. Woo), pp. 121–48. Springer-Verlag, New York.

1.13 Imaging

Eric A. Brandser and Georges Y. El-Khoury

Introduction

Medical imaging is exceedingly important for the management of patients with orthopedic problems. Imaging is crucial to diagnosis and staging of many illnesses, and is often an extension of the history and physical examination. Imaging is also important for following patients over time, documenting favorable outcome or complications.

Box 1 Imaging modalities

- Plain radiography
- Conventional tomography
- CT
- MRI
- Ultrasound
- Nuclear medicine
- Arthography etc.

There are a number of imaging modalities available to the practicing orthopedist, including plain radiography, conventional tomography, CT, MRI, ultrasound, nuclear medicine studies, and studies where iodinated contrast is injected such as arthrography. Each modality has advantages and disadvantages. They can also complement each other and may have an appropriate order in which they are best performed to maximize diagnostic information while minimizing risk and cost.

Plain radiography

Plain radiography as we know it is changing and, like the rest of the field of medical imaging, the change is accelerating. This change is the result of advances in computers, picture archiving and communication systems, teleradiography, and digital display of images. However, in most units the hard film copy of radiographic images is and will continue to be, for the foreseeable future, the primary means for storing and viewing radiographic images. Regardless of the image medium, all radiographic images are produced by exposing the patient to X-rays.

X-rays, which are a form of radiation belonging to the electromag-netic spectrum, were discovered by Wilhelm Conrad Roentgen in 1895. Diagnostically useful X-rays are able to traverse the patient and transmit diagnostic information. When these X-rays are captured by the appropriate receptor, an image is formed which can be recorded on a film or displayed on a television screen for viewing by physicians. The plain radiographic examination is the best and most available imaging study for the initial evaluation of patients with musculoskeletal problems. Generally, plain radiography should precede any complex imaging studies such as CT or MRI; interpretation of these complex studies should not be undertaken without the plain radiographic examination being available for comparison.

Box 2 Principles of radiology in clinical practice

- Whatever the imaging medium, all radiographic images involve exposing the patients to X-rays
- Plain radiography should normally precede special investigation to assist interpretation

Understanding the physical principles of X-ray generation, X-ray interaction with living tissue, and image formation is key to obtaining high-quality diagnostic examinations. When these principles are effectively utilized, radiation exposure to patients and medical staff is kept to a minimum.

X-rays used in medical imaging are either generated in X-ray tubes or emitted from radioactive isotopes. Those generated in X-ray tubes are used in radiography, fluoroscopy, conventional tomography, and CT. X-rays emitted from radioactive isotopes are used in nuclear

Box 3 Radiological principles of creating an image

- The smaller the anode, the sharper the image
- Only large anodes can withstand heavy exposures
- Short exposures minimize blurring from patient movement
- The quantity of X-rays is proportional to the current (mA)
- The operating property of the X-rays is determined by the voltage (kV_p)

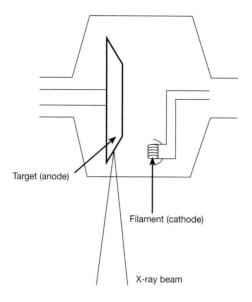

Fig. 1. Diagram of X-ray tube. Rotation of the anode increases the heat capacity of the tube and allows more X-rays to be generated.

medicine and are called γ-rays. In the X-ray tube (Fig. 1), X-rays are generated when a fast stream of electrons is suddenly stopped by the target or anode (positive terminal). The electrons originate on the negative terminal of the tube which is also known as the cathode or filament. The area of the target bombarded by electrons is known as the focal spot. In clinical practice, radiography of bones and joints is best performed with a small focal spot, preferably 1 mm or less. A small focal spot produces sharper images and better trabecular detail. The ability of the X-ray tube to achieve high X-ray outputs is limited by the heat generated at the target or anode. The only disadvantage of a small focal spot is in its inability to withstand large exposures, such as for thick body parts like the lumbar spine or pelvis; the significant heat focused on a small area can cause the target to melt. A large focal spot allows greater heat loading and therefore less damage to the target. To increase the heat capacity of the X-ray tube, the rotating anode was developed (Fig. 1). The target rotates, and the heat is spread over the entire disc, increasing heat capacity. Both the filament and the target are made of tungsten which has a very high melting point. Patient motion also reduces clarity; this can be minimized by making short exposures as well as asking the patient to remain perfectly still during the exposure.

The quantity of X-rays emitted from the X-ray tube is proportional

Box 4 Techniques for reducing dose and improving image in radiography

- Filters remove X-ray wavelengths which are not useful, thus reducing dose
- Grids reduce blurring from scattering
- Decreasing field size reduces scatter and overall dose
- Rare-earth-intensifying scan reduces X-ray dose required for good image

to the number of electrons flowing from the filament (cathode) to the target (anode); this is measured in milliamperes (mA) and is preselected by the technologist. The quality, or penetrating properties, of the X-ray beam is determined by the energy of the electrons striking the target. This is determined by the kilovoltage setting (kV_p). Typically, a spectrum of X-rays of different wavelengths (polychromatic) or energies emerge from the X-ray tube with each exposure. The very low energy X-rays are not diagnostically useful and increase radiation dose to the patient because they are absorbed by the tissues. Modern X-ray tube casings are designed with filters to remove the low energy radiation from the X-ray beam. Filtration is an essential technique utilized to change the composition and improve the quality of the X-rays beam. It increases the ratio of X-rays in the beam which are useful for imaging compared to those which only increase the patient's dose of radiation. High-energy X-rays pass through the patient, carrying information, and are therefore diagnostically useful. Aluminum (1–3 mm thick) is the most commonly used general purpose filter.

Primary X-rays travel in a straight line from the tube to the receptor. X-rays that interact with the tissues can be deflected from the primary X-ray beam, giving rise to scattered radiation. Although high energy diagnostic X-rays are generally favored because less radiation is absorbed by the patient, they generate significant scatter radiation which results in foggy images and diminished tissue contrast on radiographs. Without scatter control, the information content of X-ray images is severely compromised. To control scatter and improve image quality, radiographic grids are employed. The use of a fixed or a reciprocating (motorized) grid are the most commonly applied techniques for controlling scatter in medical radiography. Grids are made of very thin lead strips separated by X-ray-transparent spacers. The degree of scatter is proportional to the thickness of the structure being radiographed as well as the field size. Thicker body parts produce much more scatter than thinner parts. Larger field size results in more scatter and less tissue contrast on images. Limiting the field size, or restricting the size of the beam to the area of interest achieves two very important objectives: it reduces scatter and cuts radiation to the patient.

Between 80 and 95 per cent of the scattered X-rays are absorbed by the grid, which is placed between the patient and image receptor. Thin body parts, such as hands, feet, and cervical spine, produce little scatter and therefore can be radiographed without grids. One caveat regarding the use of grids relates to the fact that some grids are focused and proper alignment and distance of the grid from the X-ray tube should always be maintained otherwise the image quality deteriorates very rapidly. This could become a serious problem in examinations performed in bed or in the operating room using portable X-ray machines and grid cassettes.

Variations in tissue composition give rise to differences in how much of the primary X-ray beam is transmitted through the patient. The term for how much of the primary beam is stopped is called attenuation. Structures that stop much of the primary beam have high attenuation. Bone has high beam attenuation, whereas inflated lung has low beam attenuation, and appears dark on a radiograph, while bones appear white on the radiograph. Fat attenuates X-rays more than air while water and soft tissues attenuate it more than fat but less than bone. These variations in the ability of the different tissues to attenuate the X-ray beam form the basis for tissue contrast on radiographic images.

In conventional radiography, in contradistinction to digital radiography, the receptor is the film cassette which consists of the film and two intensifying screen, one on each side of the film. The function of the intensifying screens is to convert the X-rays into visible light which in turn exposes the film. Where more X-rays pass through the patient and reach the intensifying screen, more visible light is generated by the screens which darkens the radiographic film. The efficiency of the intensifying screen in converting X-rays to visible light is important in reducing the radiation dose to the patient. State-of-the-art radiography relies almost exclusively on the use of rare earth screen systems which are more efficient than the old calcium tungstate screens. There are specialized extremity cassettes used for thin parts, and these contain a single intensifying screen as well as special film with photosensitive emulsion on one side only. This system is frequently used in orthopedic work; it produces high detail images. However, a much higher radiation dose is required.

Digital radiography

The radiographic film has multiple functions: it serves as the X-ray detector (in combination with the screens), it displays the images for the physician to see on viewboxes, and it serves as part of the patient's medical records as an image archive. However, film does not perform all these functions equally well. A major problem with film as an X-ray detector in orthopedics is related to the limited and non-linear exposure latitude which places a critical dependency on proper radiographic technique. The wide variation in extremity thickness may result in underexposure in one part and overexposure in another on the same radiograph. An alternative to the conventional radiographic film is the digital image or radiograph which is a quantized representation of the spatial modulation of the X-ray beam after it passes through the patient. In digital radiography, the conventional screen-film system is replaced with a storage phosphor plate which is two to four times more efficient than the fastest rare earth screen film combination. A laser image reader extracts the latent image from the phosphor plate and the data is handled by an image processor. Interactive workstations are connected to the image processor thus replacing the light boxes for viewing images. Images can be manipulated to improve density and contrast, they can be enlarged or minimized; images can also be transmitted from station to station. The dose to the patient is reduced because the storage phosphor is more sensitive than the screen-film system; repeat exposures due to technical errors are also eliminated because the image contrast and density can be manipulated at the workstation.

Box 5 Digital radiography

- Dosage is reduced
- Not so dependent on radiographer expertise
- Image can be manipulated electronically
- Stored on computer memory
- Cost is high but falling
- Quality was low but is rising

The data required for digital representation may be considerable, but computer memory is progressively becoming cheaper. A conservative estimate for a single 14 inch × 17 inch image is about 40 megabytes, compared with only 16 megabytes for a 30-image set from a CT study. Digital radiography is particularly suited for evaluation of musculoskeletal trauma, soft-tissue abnormalities, scoliosis, and other spinal problems. The limitation of digital radiography at this point includes high cost, restricted patient throughput, and increased perception of image noise. In spite of these limitations, computed radiography is a new alternative to screen-film radiography without significant differences in diagnostic quality. Digital radiography is effectively replacing conventional film radiography at many institutions around the world.

Radiographic techniques

For most orthopedic problems, two orthogonal radiographic views of the structure under investigation are considered a basic requirement. Depending on the anatomic region, additional views are often needed. In the trauma setting, two orthogonal views may be difficult to obtain in the shoulder because of pain and splinting; a transscapular view can be substituted for the axillary view. For subtle undisplaced fractures of the radial head, oblique views can be very helpful. When a nondisplaced fracture of the scaphoid is suspected it is advantageous to put the long axis of the scaphoid parallel to the film (Fig. 2). Small avulsion fractures at the dorsum of the triquetrum are best detected on mildly pronated lateral views of the wrist (Fig. 3). The pisiform, pisitriquetral joint, and the hook of the hamate are best visualized on mildly supinated lateral views as well as carpal tunnel views (Fig. 4).

For the assessment of displaced pelvic fractures, pelvic inlet and outlet views in addition to an anteroposterior (**AP**) view of the pelvis are quite helpful. Judet views are recommended for acetabular fractures, and are important for correct classification of fracture type. Hip fractures are best evaluated with AP and cross-table lateral views. In the setting of slipped capital femoral epiphysis, some pediatric orthopedists advise against frog-leg lateral views of the hip because of the stress on the femoral head in the abducted and externally rotated position, possibly aggravating the slip. Therefore, AP views of the pelvis and cross-table lateral views of the hips are the favored examination for evaluating the patient with suspected slipped capital femoral epiphysis. When subtle undisplaced fractures of the tibial plateau are suspected, right and left oblique views may be added to the standard AP and lateral views. Standing AP views of the knees are recommended for patients with osteoarthritis, to demonstrate the extent of articular cartilage loss (Fig. 5). Many authorities believe that radiography for ankle injuries is overutilized, and several criteria have been suggested to limit unnecessary examinations; the Ottawa criteria are probably the best known and are applied by our emergency physicians (Stiell *et al.* 1994).

It is not necessary for orthopedic surgeons to know all the appropriate views that can be used. X-ray departments will arrange for appropriate views, provided that the diagnosis under consideration is clearly stated in the request form.

Neck pain can be initially evaluated with an AP and lateral views of the cervical spine. The American College of Radiology has developed appropriateness criteria for the use of imaging studies in the trauma

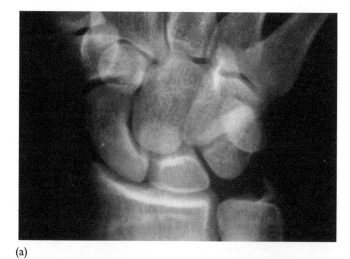

(a)

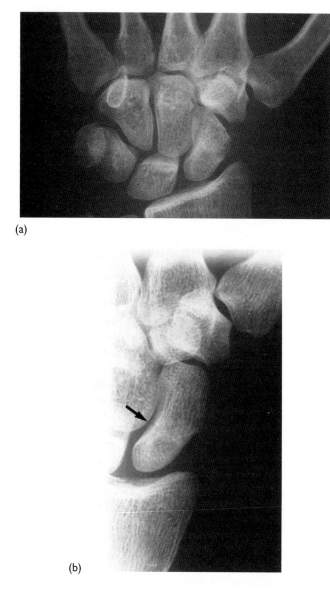

(a)

(b)

(b)

Fig. 2. Scaphoid view demonstrating a subtle fracture. (a) The routine PA view of the wrist was unremarkable and showed no fractures. (b) The scaphoid view, obtained by placing the hand and wrist in ulnar deviation along with 15° of cephalad angulation of the X-ray tube, shows a subtle non-displaced fracture (arrow).

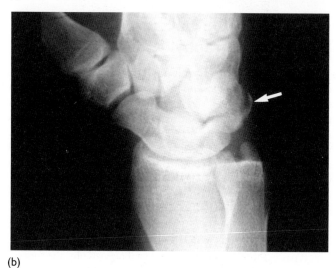

Fig. 3. Avulsion fracture of the triquetrum demonstrated on mildly pronated lateral view of the wrist. (a) PA view of the wrist shows no abnormalities of the triquetrum. (b) Mildly pronated lateral view clearly demonstrates the avulsion fracture of the dorsum of the triquetrum (arrow).

setting (American College of Radiology 1995). Six clinical scenarios cover the vast majority of patient presentations. The criteria vary depending on the symptoms and signs of the patient at the time of admission to the emergency department. The basic examination for the injured neck consists of AP, lateral, and open-mouth views; oblique views, CT, or MRI may be added depending on the patient's condition. AP and lateral views of the thoracic spine are sufficient for most clinical investigations. If the upper thoracic spine or lower cervical spine is obscured by the shoulders, a swimmer's view is usually quite helpful. For the lumbar spine, AP and lateral views are typically sufficient. Occasionally, oblique views are used to look for defects in the pars interarticularis, but these oblique views add signi-

ficant radiation dose to the patient, increase the cost of the examination, and should not be used routinely.

Conventional tomography

Conventional tomography (also known as body section radiography) has been mostly replaced by CT. However, in places where CT is not available, conventional tomography is still an excellent and affordable substitute. Conventional tomography is effective in solving some diagnostic orthopedic problems because of the high radiographic tissue contrast of bone. On a plain radiograph, bony structures are superimposed over each other. Conventional tomography is capable of blurring superimposed structures and bringing into focus structures of interest. There are a wide variety of tomographic units, but they

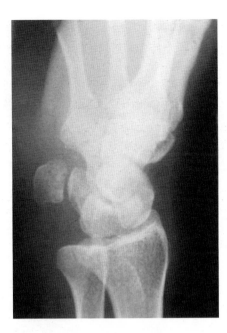

Fig. 4. Mildly supinated lateral view of the wrist demonstrates a pisiform fracture which was difficult to see on routine views.

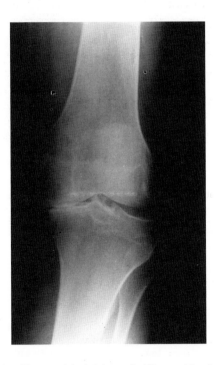

Fig. 5. Standing AP view of the left knee of a 70-year-old male showing marked narrowing of the joint space medially indicating almost total loss of cartilage. Varus deformity of the knee and mild lateral subluxation of the tibia are also present.

all share the same principle components of an X-ray tube and film cassette connected to a rigid arm. When the X-ray tube moves in one direction, the film moves in the opposite direction around a fulcrum or focal plane. The amplitude (distance) of tube travel is measured

Box 6 Conventional tomography

As the exposure is taking place:

- the X-ray tube moves one way
- the film moves in the other direction
- only the plane of interest stays in focus
- other structures are blurred out
- the radiation dose is higher than with CT

in degrees and is referred to as the tomographic angle. The plane of interest within the patient is positioned at the level of the fulcrum and is the only plane that stays in sharp focus. Structures above or below the fulcrum are blurred.

Radiation protection

A discussion of the biological effects of ionizing radiation is beyond the scope of this chapter; however, exposure of patients to medical X-rays continues to command increased attention by society and public health officials (Hendee 1991). If basic principles of radiation protection are adhered to, the same level of diagnostic information can be achieved with minimal risk to patients and health workers. With any radiographic study, one should try to maximize the distance between the patient and the radiation source, maximize filtration of the X-ray beam, and use the fastest film-screen speed feasible. Gonadal shielding and appropriate collimation should always be attempted. Exposure time should be kept to a minimum. Appropriate personnel radiation-monitoring devices should be worn by health professionals whenever there is a possibility of exposure to radiation.

Nuclear medicine

Radionuclide scintigraphy continues to be an integral part of the diagnostic work-up in patients with musculoskeletal disease. It has a high sensitivity in detecting early bone and joint disease; it surveys the entire skeleton quickly and at reasonable cost. However, a major

Box 7 Radiation protection

- Always consider carefully the need for a radiograph
- Maximize distance between X-ray source and patient
- Maximize beam filtration
- Use fastest film possible
- Minimize exposure time
- Shutter down the field
- Use gonadal shields
- Train staff in proper radiation protection
- Monitor staff radiation levels

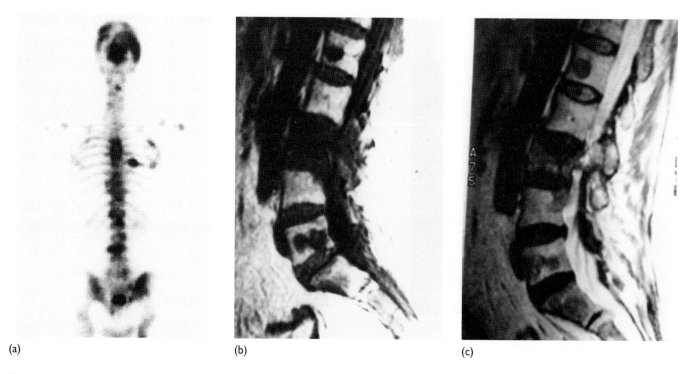

(a)   (b)   (c)

Fig. 6. 51-year-old female with breast cancer and bony metastasis. (a) Posterior view from a [^{99}Tc^m]MDP bone scan showing multiple areas of increased radiotracer uptake in the skull, spine, pelvis, shoulders, and ribs. Note the lack of soft tissue and renal activity due to 'sink' phenomenon of metastases. (b) T_1-weighted and (c) T_2-weighted sagittal images depict the metastatic deposits and encroachment on the thecal sac.

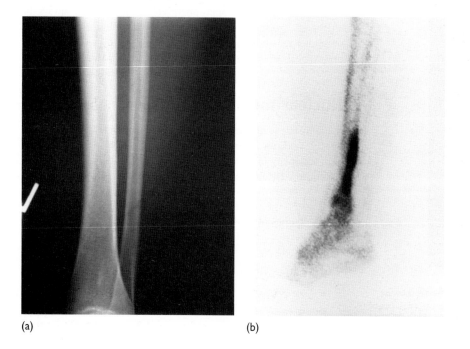

(a)   (b)

Fig. 7. Bone scans are more sensitive than plain radiographs in detecting stress fractures. (a) Lateral plain radiograph of the left tibia is normal. (b) [^{99}Tc^m]MDP bone scan clearly shows marked increase in radiotracer uptake where patient is symptomatic. Patient responded well to reduced athletic activity.

limitation of bone scintigraphy is its lack of specificity; any condition that influences osteoblastic activity or blood flow to the bone can result in an abnormal bone scan. Bone scintigraphy is most widely used in the detection and follow-up of metastatic bone disease (Fig. 6), early detection of stress fractures (Fig. 7), and in the search for an osteoid osteoma. Its role in musculoskeletal infections, and staging of primary malignant neoplasm of bone has for the most part been replaced by MRI.

The most commonly used radiopharmaceutical in bone scintigraphy is technetium-labeled methylene diphosphonate ([**99Tcm]MDP**). The physical properties of technetium-99m make it a very attractive scanning agent. It has a half-life of 6 h, emits a 140-keV photon, and is readily available. The radiopharmaceutical is injected intravenously; it is rapidly taken up by bone and scanning usually begins 2 to 3 h after the injection. The tracer is excreted by the kidney, and by 24 h, 50 to 60 per cent of the injected dose is eliminated in the urine. The radiation dose to bladder wall and pelvic organs depends on the frequency of voiding; consumption of liquids and frequent voiding should be encouraged after the examination. Bone scintigraphy should be avoided in pregnant and lactating patients.

The exact mechanism of how [^{99}Tc^m]MDP localizes in bone is not well understood, but it is felt that this compound adsorbs primarily to the mineral phase of bone, with little binding to the organic phase. In the growing skeleton, the epiphyseal and apophyseal growth centers normally show increased radiotracer compared to the rest of the skeleton.

The spine is the most common site for skeletal metastasis, and except for few limitations radionuclide bone scintigraphy is the primary imaging examination used to detect and follow metastatic bone disease. It has been repeatedly shown to be more sensitive than plain radiography. The tracer does not localize mainly in the cancerous tissue but in the bone which surrounds and reacts to the metastatic tissue. Very aggressive lytic metastasis may show cold or photopenic areas on bone scan, because surrounding bone fails to react to it. Multiple myeloma can frequently present with photopenic lesions or even a negative bone scan (Woolfenden *et al.* 1980; Ludwig *et al.* 1992). Bone scans are also insensitive for the detection of skeletal

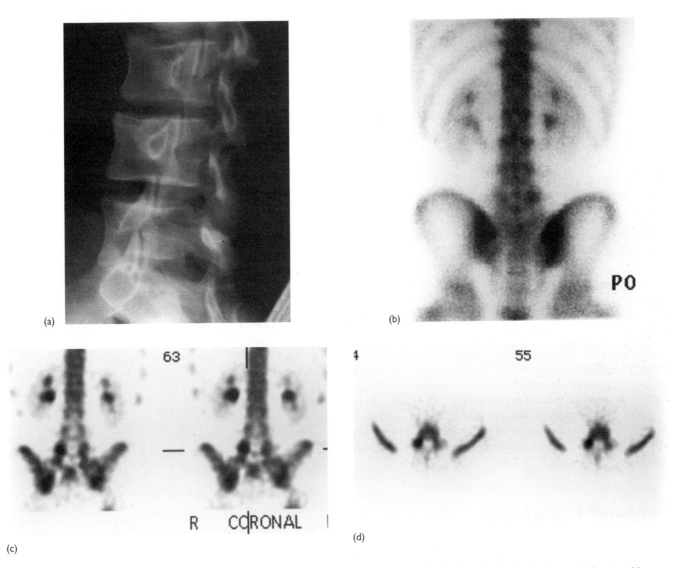

Fig. 8. SPECT imaging of the spine in suspected acute or subacute spondylolysis. This 16-year-old boy had low back pain of a few weeks duration. (a) Oblique radiograph of the lower lumbar spine is inconclusive. (b) A planar [^{99}Tc^m]MDP scan suggests abnormal increased activity at L5 on the right. SPECT images in the (c) coronal and (d) axial planes show a definite increase in radiotracer uptake in the region of the right pars interarticularis of L5.

lesions due to Langerhans' cell histiocytosis (histiocytosis X); therefore radiographic bone surveys are recommended for patients with this disease.

Bone metastases are very uncommon at initial presentation in patients with primary malignant bone tumors and therefore radionuclide bone scintigraphy is not indicated. Bone scintigraphy was shown not to be useful in differentiating between benign and malignant bone lesions or in reliably defining the local extent of malignant tumors. While bone scanning is not indicated for most primary bone tumors, evaluation of patients with osteosarcoma is probably an exception. This is because, although the yield for metastasis at the time of diagnosis is small, the presence of a metastasis would substantially affect patient management (Goldstein *et al.* 1980; Holder 1990). During follow-up of treated patients with osteosarcoma, a small percentage may develop asymptomatic osseous metastasis prior to lung metastasis; therefore routine bone scans are recommended by some authors (Goldstein *et al.* 1980; Holder 1990).

Stress fractures

A bone scan is a very sensitive technique for the detection of stress fractures. A bone scan can be positive 1 or 2 weeks before the radiographic appearance of a stress fracture.

Osteoid osteoma

Osteoid osteoma can be difficult to detect, particularly if it occurs intracapsularly, where the bone and periosteal reaction to the nidus is limited, or if the nidus is located in the posterior elements of a vertebra where the anatomy is fairly complex. SPECT imaging is especially helpful in detecting osteoid osteomas of the spine. SPECT is a technique where tomographic images are generated from data acquired by a special rotating camera system. The images can be reconstructed in any plane, and the main advantage of SPECT imaging is to increase conspicuity of lesions that would be masked by overlying normal activity. One such example is spondylolysis (Fig. 8).

Computed tomography

CT is fundamentally different from conventional tomography or radiography, which are modalities that involve directing an X-ray beam through the patient, and detecting the transmitted rays with film. A CT scanner is a machine where an X-ray source and a set of X-ray detectors are positioned opposite each other within the gantry

of the scanner. The detectors are connected electronically to one or more microcomputers which are also connected to a display and control terminal.

During the acquisition of a CT image, the X-ray tube and the detector array rotate around the patient while the X-ray tube generates an X-ray beam that is directed through the patient to the detector array. The detectors measure the amount of radiation transmitted through the patient. Each detector continuously records the amount of X-ray transmission. Since some structures in the body attenuate more X-rays than others, differing amounts of radiation will be transmitted through to the detector array depending upon what structures are being imaged.

Each image generated by the CT scanner is made up of many tiny boxes called pixels, short for 'picture elements'. The spatial resolution of the image is, in part, determined by the size of the pixels. Each pixel in the image is assigned a value, called the CT number, based on the calculated attenuation of X-rays in that region of the patient compared to a standard attenuation of water, which is arbitrarily assigned a CT number of zero. CT numbers larger than zero are represented by lighter shades of gray on the image, and numbers less than zero are represented by darker shades of gray. That is why lung parenchyma, which is mostly air and has a very low CT number is blacker than bone, which has a higher CT number. An image can now be acquired in seconds (and in some cases, fractions of a second).

After an image is acquired, the CT numbers can be displayed with many different windows and levels. For example, to demonstrate soft tissues, the display is set to optimize visualization of different densities of soft-tissue structures such as fat, muscle, and water. However, a display optimized for soft tissues leaves the bones nearly completely white, obscuring any subtle changes in density. Therefore, to display the architecture of bones, a CT display with a higher level and wider window is used.

Advantages

There are several advantages to CT over conventional tomography for evaluating orthopedic patients. While CT has intrinsically less spatial resolution than conventional radiography or tomography, the significant increase in contrast resolution provides better evaluation of bones and adjacent soft tissues. Another advantage of CT is that if overlapping axial images are obtained of an area of interest, multiplanar reconstructions can be performed in virtually any plane. This technique is especially important with spiral CT (discussed below).

Disadvantages

While CT is a powerful modality, there are several disadvantages to this technique. If a given scanner does not have multiplanar reconstructive capability, scanning is often limited to the axial plane. This can be problematic when attempting to image fractures or abnormalities that are parallel to the scanning gantry. For example, a chance fracture of the lumbar spine or a dens fracture in the cervical spine can be entirely missed on axial CT images because of volume averaging and the fact that the fracture runs in a plane parallel to the gantry. This fracture will be detected if multiplanar reconstructions are performed (Fig. 9). CT uses ionizing radiation to obtain images, and this is a disadvantage when the modality is compared with ultrasound or MRI, which do not use ionizing radiation. Cost is a relative disadvantage, as CT is more expensive than plain radiography, conventional tomography, or ultrasound; however, it is less expensive than MRI. Another limitation of CT is that in patients who have had prior orthopedic instrumentation, extensive artifacts from the metal can hamper the diagnostic utility of CT scans.

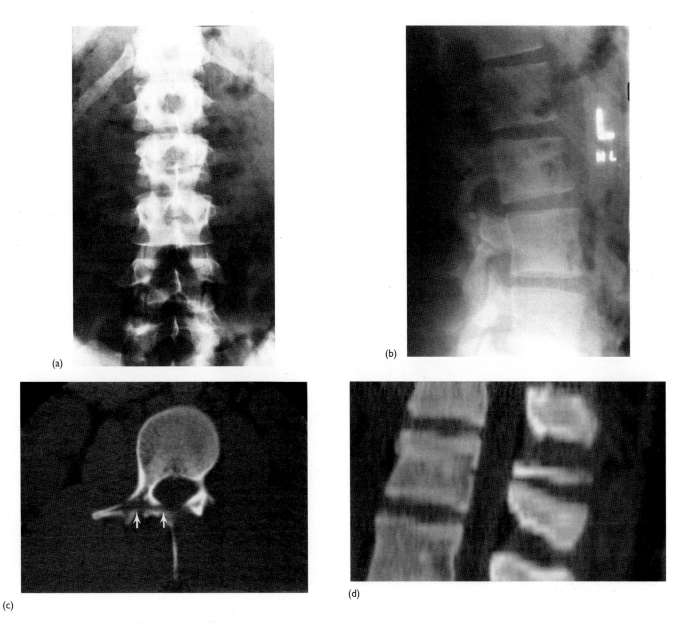

(a)

(b)

(c)

(d)

Fig. 9. Chance fracture of L2 in a 17-year-old male involved in a motor vehicle accident. Such a fracture may be difficult to appreciate on axial CT section. (a) AP and (b) lateral views of the lumbar spine show the fracture traversing the body, pedicles and splitting the spinous process. (c) The fracture is very subtle on an axial section through L2 (arrows), because the plane of section passes through the plane of the fracture. (d) Midline sagittal reconstruction clearly depicts the fracture.

Spiral CT

Newer technology for CT acquisition has been developed and has several names including spiral, helical, and volumetric CT. With

spiral CT, the patient continuously moves into the gantry while the X-ray tube and detectors continuously rotate without interruption. This generates a continuous data set of transmitted X-ray information over a volume of the patient. The computer then reconstructs individual slices from this helical volume data set and displays them in the same manner as conventional CT.

There are several advantages to spiral CT over conventional CT. Once the volume data set is acquired, the computer can reconstruct an infinite number of closely spaced overlapping images, without increasing patient radiation dose. Spiral CT is much faster than conventional CT. The speed of acquisition not only increases the throughput of the patient, but also minimizes the chance of patient motion during the study.

Box 10 Spiral CT

- Infinite number of overlapping images are possible
- Faster than conventional CT
- Reduces patient movement blurring

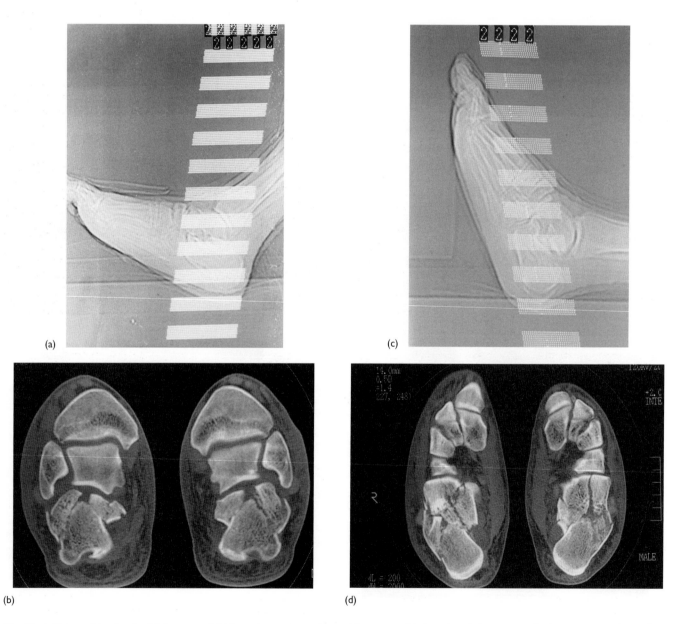

(a)

(c)

(b)

(d)

Fig. 10. A 56-year-old male who fell from a roof. (a) Lateral scout image shows oblique coronal orientation of slices, perpendicular to posterior facet of subtalar joint. (b) CT slice delineates the posterior facet to advantage in this patient with bilateral calcaneal fractures. Articular gaps and step-off is easily demonstrated with this plane of section. (c) Lateral scout image showing orientation of longitudinal scan. (d) Images obtained in the longitudinal orientation better demonstrate extension of fractures in an AP dimension, and are the best way to evaluate the calcaneocuboid joint.

Indications

CT is very useful for demonstrating fractures, especially when there is intra-articular extension or when anatomy is complex and plain films do not convey enough information to the treating orthopedist. An example is fracture of the calcaneus, where involvement of the posterior subtalar joint is common but difficult to assess by plain radiographs. In this setting, images are obtained both perpendicular to the posterior facet of the subtalar joint and parallel to the long axis of the calcaneus (Fig. 10).

In the setting of acetabular trauma, CT is an adjunct to plain films for categorization of fracture type, and is very helpful for preoperative planning in those patients needing open reduction and internal fixation. CT is superior to plain film for detecting intra-articular fracture fragments, and shows impaction of the posterior articular surface of the acetabulum more clearly. CT alone is not sufficient for characterizing fracture type, but should be interpreted in conjunction with the AP and Judet oblique films.

CT is a useful tool for evaluating patients with known scaphoid fracture, and when delayed or non-union is suspected. Images are acquired along both the sagittal and coronal long axes of the scaphoid (Fig. 11). When detecting motion across the fracture is important, images can be obtained along the sagittal long axis with the patient in both ulnar and radial deviation of the wrist. Radial deviation accentuates any humpback deformity, whereas the images obtained with ulnar deviation tend to minimize the deformity.

CT is a useful modality for evaluating certain patients with suspected or known bone neoplasms. In a patient with suspected osteoid osteoma, CT may show the nidus and surrounding sclerotic bone better than plain film and MRI (Fig. 12) and is more scientific than bone scan. However, for most bone neoplasms, once a diagnosis is suggested by plain radiographs, MRI is often more useful than CT.

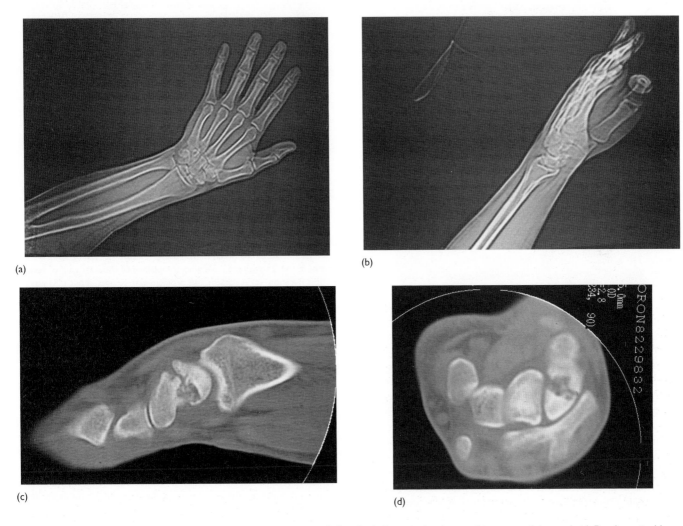

(a)

(b)

(c)

(d)

Fig. 11. Optimal positioning for CT of the scaphoid. Images are acquired along both the sagittal and coronal long axes of the scaphoid. For the sagittal long axis view, the patient is placed prone on the table with arm overhead and elbow flexed approximately 45°. The wrist is placed in ulnar deviation with the volar surface of the hand resting on the table. (a) Scout image from a CT study showing correct position of the wrist for the sagittal long axis study. For the coronal long axis view, the patient remains prone with the arm abducted and elbow flexed approximately 45° and the wrist in supination. The palm faces the top of the head. (b) Scout image demonstrating proper position for the coronal long axis view. (c) Sagittal long axis image from a 22-year-old male with nonunion showing fracture line with resorption along fracture, and apex dorsal angulation. (d) Coronal long axis view demonstrates fracture, resorption, angulation, and sclerosis of the proximal pole.

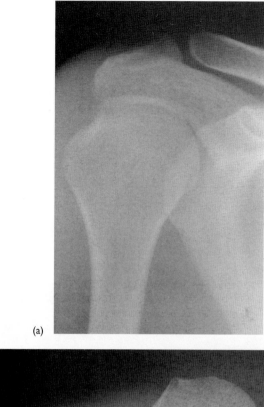

(a)

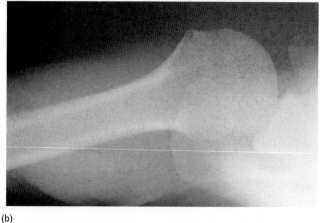

(b)

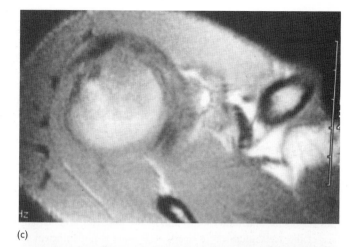

(c)

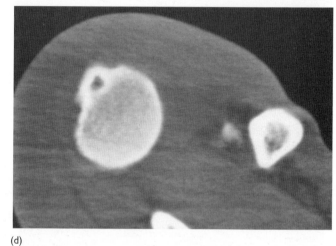

(d)

Fig. 12. MRI is frequently unhelpful in detecting the nidus in osteoid osteoma and occasionally can be confusing. (a), (b) Plain radiographs were normal in this 23-year-old male who complained of shoulder pain of several months duration. (c) A rotator cuff problem was suspected but MRI was not very helpful except for showing some marrow edema in the humeral head. (d) Thin-section CT clearly depicts the nidus and mild bony reaction.

Both CT and MRI can be helpful in atypical stress fractures where longitudinal fractures or diffuse uptake at bone scan makes the diagnosis difficult (Fig. 13). CT is also useful for detecting insufficiency fractures of the sacrum. Plain films are insensitive due to overlying bowel gas and osteopenia. Bone scan can make the diagnosis, but occasionally is not specific enough to differentiate insufficiency fracture from other etiologies such as metastasis. In this setting, CT is very specific (Fig. 14).

CT can be performed along with other procedures such as arthrography, or to guide needle placement during percutaneous biopsies. For example, CT arthrography of the shoulder is performed to detect tears of the anterior glenoid labrum. CT arthrography can be used to demonstrate radiolucent intra-articular bodies in patients with synovial chondromatosis and to evaluate whether an osteochondral defect has intact overlying cartilage. CT is commonly used to guide deep biopsies, especially of the spine. Exact needle position is easily demonstrated, and needles can be placed safely within a vertebra via a transpedicular or extrapedicular approach. In the thoracic spine, a costotransverse approach is also used to place a needle within a vertebral body.

Magnetic resonance imaging

MRI is a powerful tool for the evaluation of many orthopedic diseases. It is now the primary imaging technique for internal derangement of the knee, disk disease, muscle and tendon injuries, early detection of osteonecrosis, and evaluation and staging of many soft-tissue and bone neoplasms. MRI is fundamentally different from radiographic techniques, and a basic understanding of its physical principles, terminology, indications, contraindications, and future trends is essential for the practicing orthopedist.

Physical principles

The basic principle of clinical MRI is that hydrogen atoms in the body have an unpaired proton and exhibit a spin; this results in a

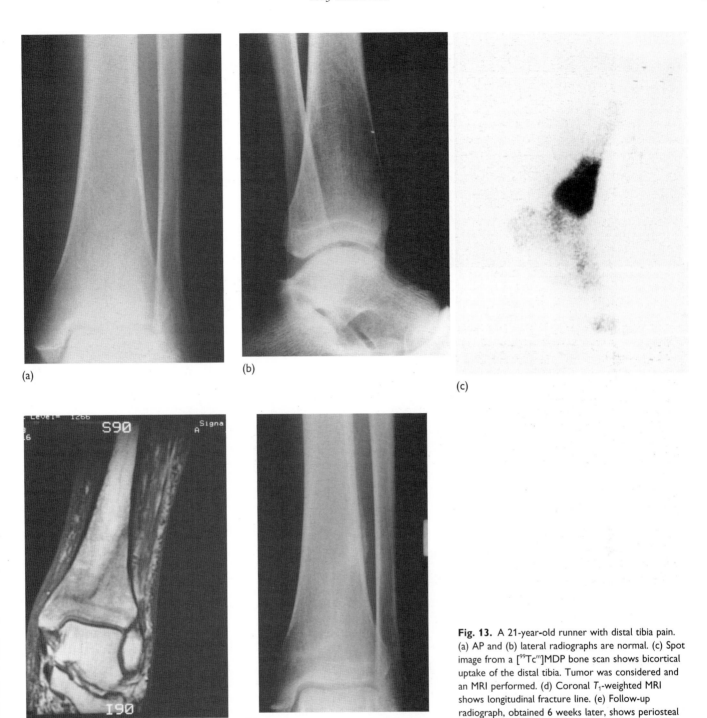

Fig. 13. A 21-year-old runner with distal tibia pain. (a) AP and (b) lateral radiographs are normal. (c) Spot image from a [^{99}Tc^m]MDP bone scan shows bicortical uptake of the distal tibia. Tumor was considered and an MRI performed. (d) Coronal T_1-weighted MRI shows longitudinal fracture line. (e) Follow-up radiograph, obtained 6 weeks later, shows periosteal reaction of healing stress fracture.

small magnetic moment and therefore will react to external magnetic fields. Any nucleus with an unpaired proton or neutron (^{1}H, ^{31}P, ^{23}Na) has a magnetic moment and could be used for MRI, but ^{1}H is the most abundant element in the body and so is easiest to image. Outside an external magnetic field, the spins of the many hydrogen atoms are oriented in a random fashion. However, when a subject is placed in a strong magnetic field, some of the protons align with the magnetic field. This process occurs over a short period of time, and eventually an equilibrium state is reached between protons aligned with and against the magnetic field.

Once at equilibrium, the protons not only have a spin, but they also precess around the axis of the magnetic field, analogous to the wobble of a spinning top (Fig. 15). The frequency of precession is proportional to the strength of the external magnetic field and to a constant specific to each proton. Hydrogen atoms in different tissues (fat versus muscle) will have different constants and precess at different frequencies.

The equilibrium of spin alignment can be disturbed by applying a radiofrequency pulse at the frequency of precession; when this occurs, some of the protons are tipped out of alignment with the

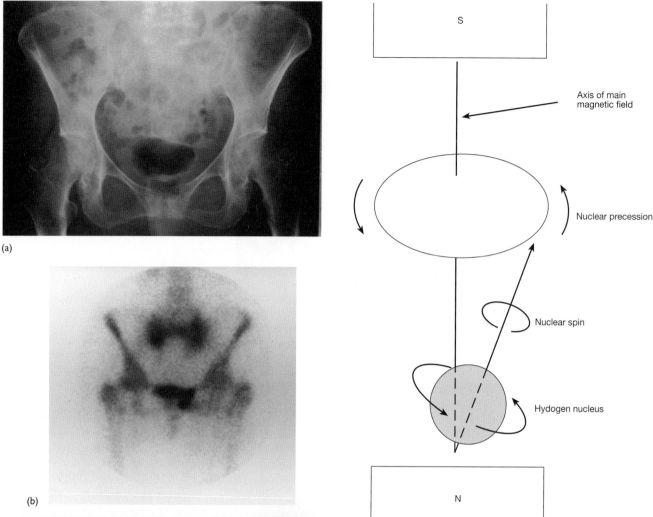

(a)

(b)

(c)

Fig. 14. Sacral insufficiency fracture in a 69-year-old female. (a) AP radiograph is suboptimal for evaluating sacrum due to overlying bowel gas and osteopenia. (b) Anterior view bone scan image shows increased uptake in both sacral ala and on both sides of the symphysis pubis. The pattern of uptake in the sacrum resembles the 'H' logo on a Honda automobile, and is called the 'Honda sign'. Insufficiency fracture was considered likely, but a history of breast carcinoma prompted CT scanning. (c) Axial CT scan shows bilateral sacral ala fractures (arrows).

Fig. 15. Diagram of a hydrogen proton in an external magnetic field. Note that the nucleus has spin as well as precession around the main direction of the external magnetic field.

main magnetic field. As the protons come back into alignment, they emit electromagnetic radiation in the radiofrequency spectrum that is collected and turned into magnetic resonance images.

An MRI image is made up of little squares called pixels. These pixels are generated by dividing the x and y axes of the image into columns and rows. If one adds the thickness of the image in space, then the term 'voxel' is used. As outlined above, after hydrogen protons are excited into the transverse plane by a radiofrequency pulse, they undergo relaxation and emit radio signals. The process of image generation takes these signals and relates them finally into the signal intensities present in each pixel of a given image.

Definitions

Resonance

As mentioned above, the frequency of precession is directly proportional to the strength of the external magnet. The external magnetic

Box 11 How MRI works

- Hydrogen atoms align themselves in a magnetic field because of their charge
- They then precess (wobble) at a frequency characteristic of the tissue
- A radiofrequency pulse disturbs this precession
- As they return to normal a radio signal is emitted
- The radio signals are collected and converted into a magnetic resonance image

field is set at a gradient where field strength gradually decreases across the scanned part, so that each slice or position is encoded with a known frequency of precession. Resonance is the process of synchronizing the radiofrequency pulse emitted by the transmitter with the precessing frequency of the nuclei in the sample for energy transfer to occur.

T_1 relaxation time

Also called longitudinal relaxation or spin–lattice relaxation time, T_1 relaxation time is a tissue-specific time constant. It is the time required for 63 per cent of the deflected nuclei to realign with the external magnetic field and return to equilibrium state, after the termination of a 90° radiofrequency. T_1 images depict anatomy well: fat is white, water is black.

T_2 relaxation time

Also called transverse relaxation time or spin–spin relaxation time, this is a tissue-specific time constant describing the rate at which nuclei lose their phase coherence after being tipped from equilibrium. Immediately after a radiofrequency pulse, the deflected nuclei are in phase with each other and emitted signal is maximal. With T_2 relaxation, the phase coherence decreases and the signal becomes weaker. This occurs at an exponential rate with a time constant T_2. For most clinically used pulse sequences, a 'refocusing' 180° pulse is used to rephase the nuclei before signal collection. T_2 images show pathology well. Fat is black, water white.

T_1 and T_2 relaxation following the 90° radiofrequency pulse occur simultaneously. However, the T_2 decay occurs much more rapidly than T_1 relaxation. For most soft tissues, the range of T_1 relaxation time is 220 to 3000 ms; T_2 relaxation time varies from 55 to 200 ms.

Pulse sequences

A pulse sequence is a precisely defined pattern of radiofrequency pulses and listening intervals. The most commonly used pulse

Box 12 Signals measured in MRI

- T_1 relaxation depicts anatomy
- T_2 relaxation demonstrates pathology
- In T_2 images water is white, fat is black
- In T_1 images water is black, fat is white

sequences in the study of the musculoskeletal system is the spin–echo sequence. It consists of a 90° pulse followed by a pause, after which a 180° pulse is applied. Then after an additional pause, the receiver coil is set to listen to a signal (echo) emitted from the tissues; after a longer pause, the cycle is repeated (Fig. 16).

After the initial 90° pulse sequence, a period of time elapses before the tissue emits a signal that is collected by the MRI unit to generate images. This time period is called the 'time to echo' (**TE**). The period of time between two pulse sequences, or the time between two 90° radiofrequency pulses is called the 'time of repetition' (**TR**). Different tissues will have different signal intensities depending upon what values of TR and TE are selected.

A spin–echo sequence can be T_1 weighted, accentuating the T_1 properties of tissue, or T_2 weighted, accentuating the T_2 properties of the tissue. T_1-weighted sequences have an echo time (TE) less than or equal to 40 ms and a repetition time (TR) less than or equal to 800 ms. T_2-weighted sequences have a TE greater than or equal to 80 ms and a TR greater than or equal to 1500 ms. 'Proton density' weighted images are generated when the TR is long, minimizing T_1 effects, and the TE is short, minimizing the T_2 effects. As a result, the main determinant of signal intensity in such a sequence is proton density. In general, T_1-weighted sequences depict anatomy better and T_2-weighted images show pathology to advantage.

On T_1-weighted images, tissues with a short T_1 have high signal intensity and are bright. An example of a substance with a short T_1 is fat. Tissue with long T_1, such as cerebrospinal fluid, have low signal intensity. On T_2-weighted sequences, tissues with a short T_2 have low signal intensity. Examples include tendon and ligament. Tissues with a long T_2, such as cerebrospinal fluid, are bright on T_2-weighted sequences. Inflamed, edematous tissue has more extracellular water than normal and will therefore be lower in signal intensity on T_1-weighted images and will be higher in signal on T_2-weighted images than normal tissue. Most tumors appear relatively dark on T_1-weighted images, less than fat and similar to muscle. On T_2-weighted images, most tumors show increased intensity, but not usually as bright as cerebrospinal fluid.

Fast imaging

Conventional spin–echo images are the mainstay of MRI, but the T_2-weighted images take a long time to acquire and are susceptible to motion artifacts. Other pulse sequences have been developed that generate images in much less time; one such sequence is called fast spin–echo. This sequence reduces time by acquiring more than one line from the image at a time. Imaging times can be cut significantly because up to 32 lines of the image can be acquired in a single repetition. There are advantages and disadvantages to the fast spin–echo sequences. Besides reducing time of acquisition, fast spin–echo images have less distortion of the image when hardware or metal is present in the scanned area. One disadvantage to fast spin–echo sequences is that edema is harder to detect than with spin–echo images. Spin–echo T_2-weighted images have traditionally been used to detect edema that is often present as a sign of many pathologic processes. These T_2-weighted sequences are sensitive for detecting edema because signal intensity of fat is low and signal intensity of water is high on T_2-weighted images. However, with fast spin–echo T_2-weighted images, the signal from fat is not suppressed and edema can be masked. To overcome this limitation, methods to suppress the signal from fat are often employed.

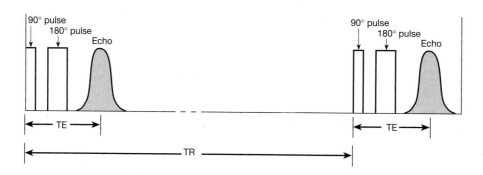

Fig. 16. Spin–echo pulse sequence. It consists of a 90° pulse followed by a pause, after which a 180° pulse is applied. Then after an additional pause, the receiver coil is set to listen to a signal (echo) emitted from the tissues; after a longer pause, the cycle is repeated.

Fat suppression

The two currently used methods of suppressing fat signal are frequency selective chemical presaturation and inversion recovery. Chemical presaturation is a technique that is applied to other sequences such as fast spin–echo, whereas inversion recovery is a pulse sequence itself, and cannot be combined with other sequences. When using chemical presaturation, the machine takes advantage of the fact that the hydrogen protons in fat have a slightly faster precessional rate than water hydrogen protons. By placing a very selective radiofrequency pulse that only deflects fat hydrogens immediately before the main pulse sequence, signals from fat can be nullified, and signals from all other tissues unaffected. This is usually used with fast spin–echo T_2-weighted sequences to increase the conspicuity of edema or fluid. Chemical saturation can also be used with T_1-weighted images after the administration of contrast. Increases in signal from contrast accumulation are more conspicuous when surrounding fat (bright on T_1-weighted images) is dark.

Inversion recovery sequences can effectively decrease signals from fat, but they have the disadvantage of a long TR, and take a relatively long time to acquire. Newer inversion recovery pulse sequences include a fast inversion recovery sequence, which still suppresses fat signal and is very sensitive for edema, but is acquired rapidly, similar to fast spin–echo (Fig. 17). One important point is that if fat suppression is desired for images obtained following contrast administration, chemical saturation should be used and inversion recovery avoided. Inversion recovery will suppress the signal changes caused by the contrast, whereas chemical saturation will not.

Contrast agents

Several contrast agents have been approved for clinical use by the Food and Drug Administration; all are based on gadolinium chelates. Gadolinium is a transition element which has paramagnetic activity. Paramagnetic atoms possess unpaired electrons in their outer shells, thus creating their own small local magnetic field. Paramagnetic agents act by shortening both the T_1 and T_2 relaxation times of nearby hydrogen nuclei. The T_1 shortening produces a higher (brighter) signal on T_1-weighted images. Following an intravenous administration, a contrast agent is distributed in a complex manner but enhancement of tissues is roughly proportional to blood flow to the tissue. The increased concentration on contrast in areas with increased blood flow results in increased signal on T_1-weighted

images. Therefore, following contrast administration, T_1-weighted sequences are typically obtained and compared with T_1-weighted images before contrast.

Contrast is most commonly used as an intravenous agent, but can also be instilled into joints, resulting in an MR arthrogram. This has been applied to the shoulder for improving the characterization and detection of labral abnormalities and in the knee for evaluating osteochondral fragments and postoperative menisci.

Clinical applications

MRI has been used to evaluate numerous orthopedic conditions; a thorough discussion of each indication is beyond the scope of this chapter. However, a brief review of the most common indications for orthopedic MRI is presented.

Knee

MRI is a commonly used modality to diagnose internal knee derangement. MRI has almost completely replaced arthrography for diagnosing internal derangement of the knee. It is an effective modality for diagnosing tears of the anterior cruciate ligament.

MRI is also accurate for detection of meniscal tears. Normal menisci have low signal intensity on all pulse sequences, and tears are seen as linear increased signal that contacts a surface of the meniscus on two consecutive images. Another sign of meniscal tears is abnormal contour of the meniscus, with truncation being a sign of a displaced fragment (Fig. 18). Following partial meniscectomy, retears are difficult to diagnose by MRI. Intra-articular contrast is a method to improve the characterization of the postoperative meniscus.

Diagnosing anterior cruciate ligament tear by MRI can be done by detecting abnormalities of the ligament itself, such as increased signal within the ligament, or by detecting secondary signs that the anterior cruciate ligament is torn. Primary signs include abnormal increased signal of the anterior cruciate ligament, either diffuse or focal, and abnormal orientation of the ligament; that is, when the ligament fails to run parallel to the intercondylar line of Blumensaat. Secondary signs can be used to diagnose anterior cruciate ligament tears. Secondary signs demonstrate laxity of the knee or denote a prior severe injury. Signs of prior injury include bone contusions, medial collateral ligament injury, and hemarthrosis, and signs of abnormal laxity of the knee include anterior translation of the tibia, abnormal posterior position of the posterior horn of the lateral meniscus, and abnor-

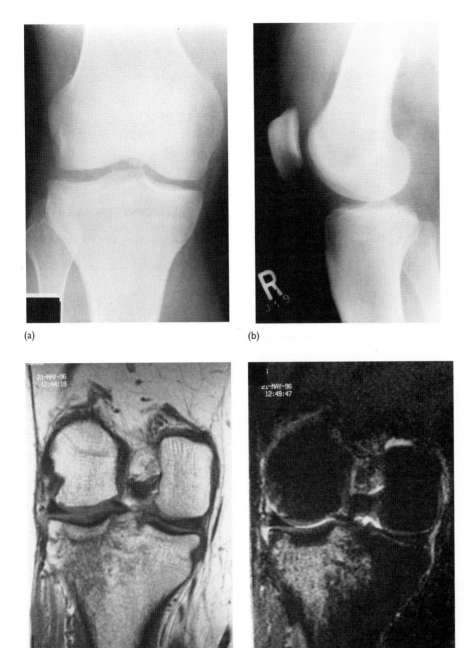

(a)

(b)

(c)

(d)

Fig. 17. Lateral tibial plateau fracture in a 39-year-old patient involved in a motor vehicle accident with persistent right knee pain. (a) AP radiograph shows no abnormality. (b) Lateral radiograph is notable for a joint effusion, but no fracture is seen. (c) Coronal T_1-weighted MRI image shows decreased signal in the bone under the lateral tibial plateau. (d) Coronal inversion recovery sequence shows the increased signal within the posterolateral tibial plateau. Note also the slight central depression of the lateral plateau articular surface.

mal orientation of the posterior cruciate ligament such as hyper-buckling.

Posterior cruciate ligament tears are less common than anterior, and can also be diagnosed by MRI. Any increase in signal is abnormal (Sonin *et al.* 1995). Conversely, the anterior cruciate ligament often has some strands of increased signal within it, and this can be problematic for detecting subtle anterior cruciate ligament tears, and decreases the accuracy of MRI for evaluating partial anterior cruciate ligament tears. Medial collateral ligament injuries are well demonstrated by MRI, and coronal plane images are optimal for evaluating the medial collateral ligament. Normally, the medial collateral ligament is seen as a moderately robust low intensity structure arising from the femoral epicondyle and extending beyond the knee joint to

insert on the tibia. With injury, abnormal signals are seen both deep and superficial to the medial collateral ligament, and if the ligament is focally disrupted or not visualized at all, then complete tear is diagnosed.

While knee MRI is usually performed to evaluate possible internal derangement of the knee, other clinical questions are often solved by MRI. For example, in a patient with persistent pain following trauma in whom plain films are negative, MRI can show contusions or occult fractures (Fig. 19).

MRI can be used to evaluate patients with suspected injury to the patellar ligament (Fig. 20). The normal patellar ligament has uniformly low signal intensity on T_1-weighted, T_2-weighted, and proton density images. In patellar tendinitis or partial tearing, the ligament

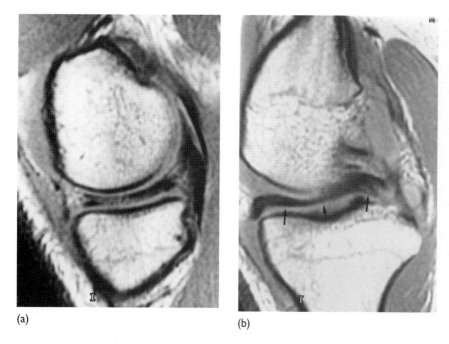

(a)   (b)

Fig. 18. Bucket-handle tear of the medial meniscus. An 18-year-old male involved in a football injury with significant knee pain and locking. (a) Oblique sagittal proton density weighted sequence of the peripheral medial meniscus shows that the meniscus is thinner than normal and does not have the normal rectangular appearance of the peripheral meniscus. (b) Centrally, an abnormal band of dark signal intensity is present, due to the flipped bucket-handle fragment of the medial meniscus (arrows).

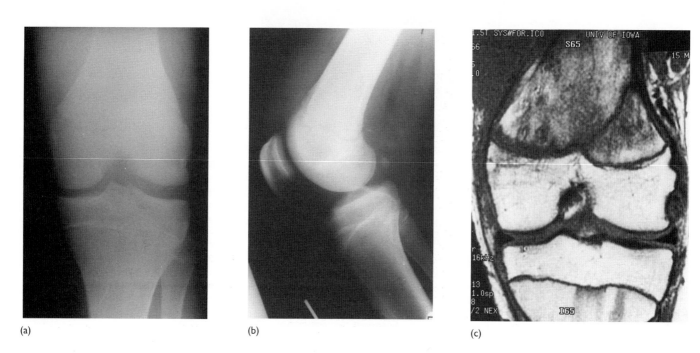

(a)   (b)   (c)

Fig. 19. Occult fracture detected by MRI in a 15-year-old football player following left knee injury. Plain (a) AP and (b) lateral radiographs shows a joint effusion, but no fractures are detected. (c) Coronal T_1-weighted image of the knee reveals a Salter–Harris type II fracture involving the distal femur.

may show increased signal intensity on T_1-weighted, T_2-weighted, and proton density images; it also shows increased AP diameter proximally and the margins of the affected ligament become indistinct, especially posterior to the thickened segment (El-Khoury *et al.* 1992).

One artifact that commonly occurs with musculoskeletal MRI is the magic-angle phenomenon (Fig. 21). This artifact occurs when a tendon is oriented approximately 55° out of the main magnetic field. When in this orientation, tendons have falsely increased signal

intensity. This effect occurs with pulse sequences that have a short TE, such as T_1-weighted or proton density sequences. The artifact does not occur with longer TEs, such as T_2-weighted images. Many tendons can be affected by the magic-angle phenomenon. The supraspinatus tendon, just proximal to its insertion on the greater tuberosity, commonly shows this artifact. This is why rotator cuff tears should not be diagnosed from the short TE pulse sequences. Other tendons that commonly show magic-angle effects are the patellar

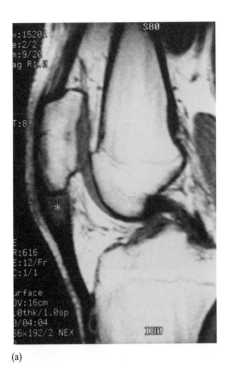

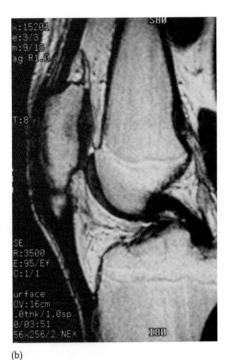

(a)

(b)

Fig. 20. A 21-year-old patient with anterior knee pain. (a) T_1-weighted image shows AP thickening of the proximal patellar ligament (asterisk) with increased signal and adjacent low signal within the prepatellar fat. (b) T_2-weighted image shows increase in signal within the proximal ligament, due to edema.

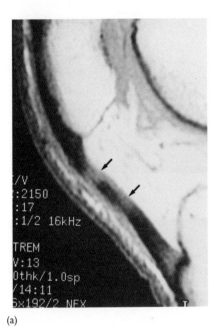

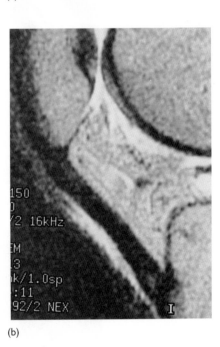

(a)

(b)

Fig. 21. Magic-angle artifact. (a) Proton-density-weighted image of the patella shows patchy increased signal of the patellar ligament (arrows). The patient had no symptoms at this location. (b) T_2-weighted image shows normal signal intensity of the tendon, separating this artifact from patellar tendonitis.

ligament, the foot flexor tendons such as flexor hallucis longus, and occasionally the peroneal tendons. If increased signal is seen on a short TE sequence, it is important to confirm the abnormality on a long TE sequence.

Shoulder

Tendon degeneration or tendinopathy and partial tears are demonstrated by MRI as areas of increased signals on the T_2-weighted images that does not completely span the thickness of the tendon. A complete tear of the rotator cuff will have full thickness increased signal on T_2-weighted spin–echo sequences (Fig. 22). Many imaging

centers use oblique planes to image the rotator cuff, including sequences that are both parallel and perpendicular to the long axis of the supraspinatus tendon. Fat suppression and magnetic resonance arthrography will increase the conspicuity of cuff abnormalities (Fig. 23).

Foot

Many disorders of the foot and ankle can be evaluated by MRI. For the Achilles tendon, axial and sagittal planes are sufficient for evaluation (Fig. 24). However, the other tendons that cross the ankle joint do not run in a straight course, but curve around the ankle and

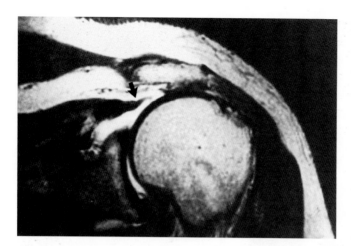

Fig. 22. Large full-thickness rotator cuff tear with retraction. A 67-year-old male with long-standing shoulder pain and clinical question of rotator cuff tear. Oblique coronal T_2-weighted sequence shows that the rotator cuff has torn completely and is retracted (arrow). The humeral head is high riding with associated irregularity of the undersurface of the acromium. These findings are consistent with a long-standing rotator cuff tear.

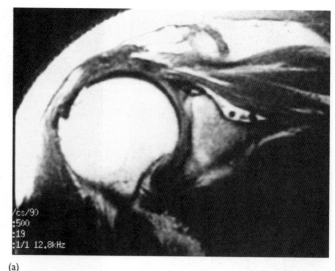

(a)

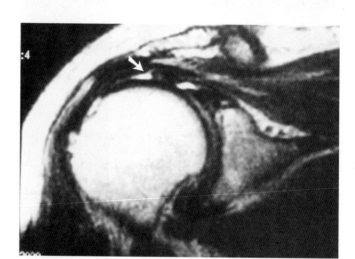

(b)

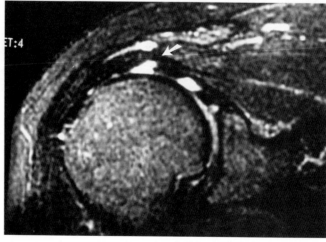

(c)

hindfoot roughly parallel to the posterior facet of the subtalar joint. Therefore, in order to image these tendons in cross-section, oblique imaging planes should be used. When studying the foot flexors and extensors, sagittal sequences are followed by oblique coronal sequences that are perpendicular to the posterior facet of the subtalar joint (Fig. 25). Three-dimensional gradient echo acquisitions allow multiplanar reformatted images, and this is very useful when demonstrating tendons that follow a complex or oblique course.

Spine

MRI has proven itself as an excellent method to depict the anatomy of the entire spine, including direct visualization of the vertebra, intervertebral disks, ligaments, cord, and surrounding cerebrospinal fluid. From an orthopedic standpoint, MRI is very useful for evaluating patients with possible disk disease, metastatic disease, congenital anomalies, and trauma.

MRI is very sensitive for detecting abnormal signal and morphology of intervertebral disks. Normally the disk is lower in signal intensity than vertebral bone marrow on T_1-weighted images, and higher in signal on T_2-weighted images. With disk degeneration, signal remains low on the T_2-weighted images. Morphological abnor-

Fig. 23. Partial thickness rotator cuff tear. A 59-year-old male with right shoulder pain and clinical question of rotator cuff tear. (a) Oblique coronal T_1-weighted sequence shows diffuse increase in signal intensity throughout the supraspinatus tendon. Tendon pathology cannot be separated from magic-angle artifact. (b) T_2-weighted oblique coronal image shows increased signal along the articular surface of the supraspinatus tendon which does not extend completely through the tendon (arrow), and is diagnostic of a partial thickness rotator cuff tear. (c) A fat-suppressed oblique coronal T_2-weighted sequence better demonstrates the partial thickness tear (arrow). With fat suppression, fluid is much more conspicuous than with fast spin–echo T_2-weighted sequences that do not employ fat suppression.

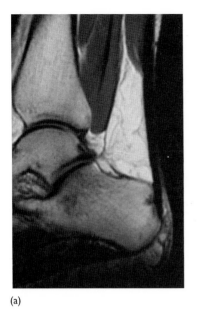

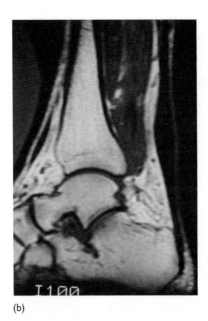

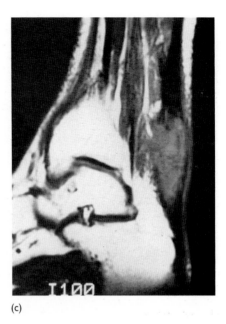

(a)   (b)   (c)

Fig. 24. Spectrum of injuries to the Achilles tendon. (a) Sagittal T_1-weighted image shows normal Achilles tendon. Note that the tendon shows no focal enlargement and has uniform low signal intensity. (b) Tendinosis or partial tearing is demonstrated by fusiform swelling of the tendon. This appearance is also seen following repair of complete tears. (c) With complete tendon tear, an area of discontinuity and abnormal signal is present, usually between 4 and 10 cm from the insertion of the tendon.

malities have been given many names, including disk bulges, herniations, extrusions, migrated free fragments, etc.

While MRI is very sensitive for detecting abnormal disks, care must be taken when interpreting the study to correlate with the patient's symptoms. In an asymptomatic population, 38 per cent of patients had disk abnormalities at more than one level by MRI criteria (Jensen *et al.* 1994). MRI with contrast enhancement is the best technique to study individuals with the failed back syndrome, and differentiating recurrent disc herniation from epidural scarring following surgery.

For evaluating patients with suspected metastases to the spine, MRI is the procedure of choice. It shows the extent of bony involvement, degree of compression of the cord, and extraspinal extension of the tumor. It is more specific than bone scan for characterizing metastatic deposits, and the entire spine can be surveyed in the right clinical setting. Metastases replace the normal fatty bone marrow and therefore appear as focal low signal areas on T_1-weighted images. MRI is also helpful for distinguishing benign from metastatic etiologies of compression fractures. If a part of the affected vertebral body marrow is intact, then the fracture is likely benign. Metastatic compression fractures typically show diffuse complete replacement of the marrow signal. One caveat to this rule is in the setting of acute compressions. The edema associated with acute compression fracture leads to diffuse replacement of the marrow signal, and resembles metastatic deposit. In this setting, the best approach is to repeat the MRI in 6 weeks if the clinical suspicion for metastatic disease is low, or to biopsy the collapsed vertebra in the setting of higher suspicion.

Patients with vertebral osteomyelitis can be a diagnostic challenge. Patients usually present with back pain, and the working diagnosis is disk-related disease. The typical plain radiographic features of adjacent vertebral endplate destruction with loss of intervertebral disk height may lag for several weeks. Often, the white blood cell count

and erythrocyte sedimentation rates are non-specific, and no fever is present. In this setting, MRI is a very sensitive method to detect vertebral osteomyelitis and diskitis. The classic findings are adjacent vertebra with abnormal replacement of marrow signal with edema, low signal on T_1-weighted and high signal on T_2-weighted images. The intervertebral disk usually shows increased signal on T_2-weighted images as well.

Neoplasms

MRI has been extensively used to evaluate patients with soft-tissue and bone neoplasms. For most tumors, there are no tissue-specific features that allow definitive diagnosis. Notable exceptions include lipoma and soft-tissue hemangioma. The MRI appearance of a benign lipoma is characteristic, and fatty tumors can easily be demonstrated by MRI. However, differentiating the low grade liposarcoma from a benign lipoma with some internal septations can be quite difficult. It is generally agreed that interpretation of MRIs on patients with suspected bone tumors should not be done without the plain films at hand. Use of intravenous contrast is also controversial.

The main use of MRI in the evaluation of patients with tumors is staging and postoperative follow-up. MRI is superior to plain film for detecting the extent of disease for surgical planning. It can be difficult to separate precisely peritumoral edema from actual tumor, but many surgeons resect beyond the margin of edema when attempting wide excision. When evaluating a patient with primary bone malignancy, it is important to scan the entire extremity involved to detect any occult skip metastases. For the postoperative patient, MRI can be used to detect recurrent disease. However, hematoma or seroma in the surgical bed are often present and can make exclusion of recurrent or residual tumor difficult. Follow-up scans will typically show stable or decreasing size of seromas and hematoma whereas tumors generally increase in size.

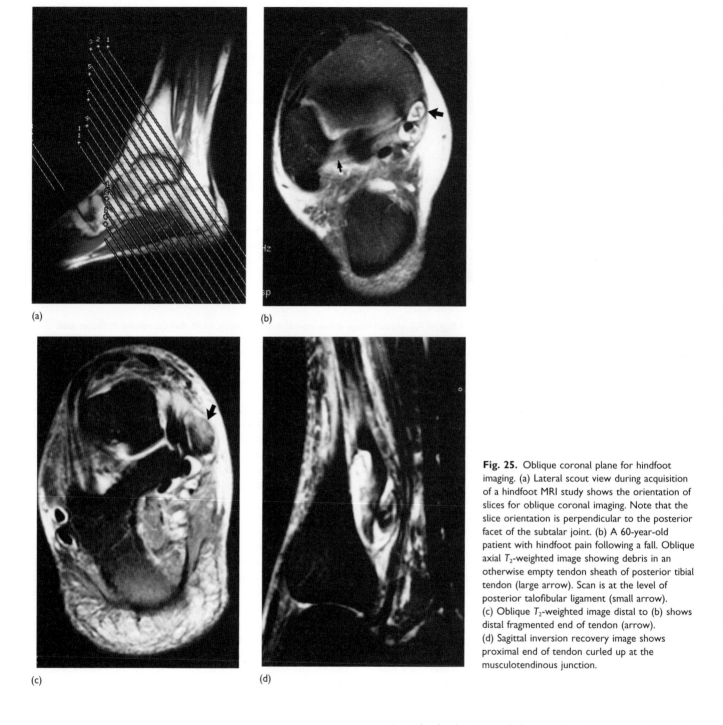

(a)

(b)

(c)

(d)

Fig. 25. Oblique coronal plane for hindfoot imaging. (a) Lateral scout view during acquisition of a hindfoot MRI study shows the orientation of slices for oblique coronal imaging. Note that the slice orientation is perpendicular to the posterior facet of the subtalar joint. (b) A 60-year-old patient with hindfoot pain following a fall. Oblique axial T_2-weighted image showing debris in an otherwise empty tendon sheath of posterior tibial tendon (large arrow). Scan is at the level of posterior talofibular ligament (small arrow). (c) Oblique T_2-weighted image distal to (b) shows distal fragmented end of tendon (arrow). (d) Sagittal inversion recovery image shows proximal end of tendon curled up at the musculotendinous junction.

Ultrasound

Orthopedic ultrasound is an underused modality in the United States, whereas there is significant experience in Europe. Several features make ultrasound an attractive diagnostic modality. Ultrasound generates images with high frequency sound waves, in the order of 3 to 12 MHz, and no ionizing radiation is used. Ultrasound machines are fairly portable, and can be set up in the orthopedic clinic, making availability of ultrasound similar to plain films. Another significant advantage is that it can be used for dynamic assessment of tendon motion. The disadvantages of ultrasound are that it is labor intensive from the physician standpoint, it is operator dependent and there is a learning curve for proficient interpretation, field of view is limited, and tissue characterization is limited when compared to other modalities such as MRI.

The main indications for ultrasound in orthopedic practice include evaluation of developmental dysplasia of the hip, detecting fluid collections, evaluation of tendons, especially the rotator cuff and tendons about the hindfoot, and the detection of deep venous thrombosis in the postoperative patient.

Box 13 Ultrasound

Advantages

- Portable
- No ionizing radiation
- Can do dynamic studies

Disadvantages

- Labor intensive
- Operator dependent
- Limited field of view
- Tissue characterization limited

Conclusion

Diagnostic imaging has expanded considerably from the plain film, and many imaging options are available to the practicing orthopedist. Each modality has its own advantages and disadvantages, and an advantage for evaluating one problem can be a disadvantage for another. Therefore, a good understanding of the various available modalities allows the referring orthopedist to maximize diagnostic efficiency, yielding cost-effective, accurate, and rapid diagnosis for their clinical patients.

References

American College of Radiology (1995). Cervical Spine Trauma, Expert Panel on Musculoskeletal Imaging. In *ACR appropriateness criteria for imaging and treatment decisions*, p. MS2. American College of Radiology, Reston, Vancouver.

El-Khoury, G.Y., Wira, R.L., Berbaum, K.S., Pope, T.L. Jr, and Monu, J.U.V. (1992). MR imaging of patellar tendinitis. *Radiology*, **184**, 849–54.

Goldstein, H., McNeil, B.J., Zufall, E., Jaffe, N., and Treves, S. (1980). Changing indications for bone scintigraphy in patients with osteosarcoma. *Radiology*, **135**, 177–80.

Hendee, W.R. (1991). Personal and public perceptions of radiation risks. *RadioGraphics*, **11**, 1109–19.

Holder, L.E. (1990). Clinical radionuclide bone imaging. *Radiology*, **176**, 607–14.

Jensen, M.C., Brant-Zawadzki, M.N., Obuchowski, N., Modic, M.T., Malkasian, D., and Ross, J.S. (1994). Magnetic resonance imaging of the lumbar spine in people without back pain. *New England Journal of Medicine*, **331**, 69–73.

Ludwig, H., Kumpan, W., and Sinzinger H. (1992). Radiography and bone scintigraphy in multiple myeloma: a comparative analysis. *British Journal of Radiology*, **55**, 173–81.

Sonin, A.H., Fitzgerald, S.W., Hoff, F.L., Friedman, H., and Bresler, M.E. (1995). MR imaging of the posterior cruciate ligament: normal, abnormal and associated injury patterns. *RadioGraphics*, **15**, 551–61.

Stiell, I.G., McKnight, R.D., Greenberg, G.H., *et al.* (1994). Implementation of the Ottawa ankle rules. *Journal of the American Medical Association*, **271**, 827–32.

Woolfenden, J.M., Pitt, M.J., Durie, B.G.M., and Moon, T.E. (1980). Comparison of bone scintigraphy and radiography in multiple myeloma. *Radiology*, **134**, 723–8.

INDEX

Page numbers in **bold** refer to major sections of the text

Page numbers in *italics* refer to pages on which figures and tables may be found

vs denotes differential diagnosis or comparison

Since the major subjects of this book are orthopedics and trauma, entries have been kept to a minimum under these keywords, and readers are advised to seek more specific references

Indexing style/conventions used

Alphabetical order. This index is in letter-by-letter order, whereby hyphens, en–rules and spaces within index headings are ignored in the alphabetization. Terms in brackets, prepositions and '*vs*' are excluded from initial alphabetization.

Cross-references. Cross-reference terms in *italics* are either general cross-references, or refer to subentry terms within the same main entry (the main entry term is not repeated) i.e. they are not main entry terms.

Abbreviations used in subentries (without explanation):

BCG Bacille Calmette–Guérin

nvCJD new variant Creutzfeldt–Jakob disease

CT Computed tomography

MRC Medical Research Council

MRI Magnetic resonance imaging

SPECT Single photon emission computed tomography

UHMWPE ultra-high molecular-weight polyethylene

D

dacarbazine 291
Dacron 1674
dactinomycin
  extra-abdominal desmoid tumors 206
  Wilms' tumor 362
dactylitis 398
  tuberculous 1543
Dall–Miles plate 1100
dancers
  ankle arthritis 1219
  flexor hallucis longus tendon dysfunction 1304–5
dapsone 1374
Darrach resectional arthroplasty 842–3, 859, 1939, 1940
data
  analysis 15–17
  bimodal *16*
  collection 20–1
  interval 15
  nominal 15
  normally distributed 15
  ordinal 15
  types 14, 15
databases
  general hospital discharge 1585
  outcome assessment 1584–5
  review 31
d'Aubigne–Postel hip score 2196
deafness 1343, 1347
Deane knee prosthesis *1142*
debridement
  bone defects 2404
  bone infection 2395, 2399
  childhood fractures 2637–8
  childhood osteomyelitis 2421
  tibial open fractures 2734
decision analysis 21–2, 28, 1586
  patient perceptions 27
decision-making 19
  avoiding decisions that can cause harm 27
  clinical intuition 28
  group approach 28
  hip arthroplasty 29
  inconsistency 27
  individual approach 28
  maximum expected utility analysis 26
  surgical intervention 29
decision tree 24
  expected utility 25
  options 26
  outcomes 26
  outcome worth 24
decision under certainty 23–4
decompression sickness
  avascular necrosis 973, 974
  osteonecrosis 728, 1160
    femoral head 981
    knee 1164
deductive reasoning 19
deep vein thrombosis 1598–9
  acetabular fractures 2198
  anatomy 1598
  classification 1598
  clinical evaluation 1598
  complications 1599
  femoral shaft fracture 2250
  high tibial osteotomy 1121
  immobility 1598
  incidence 1598
  investigations 1598
  management 1598–9
  prophylaxis 29, 1599
  pulmonary embolism relationship 395
  spinal cord injuries 2148
  spinal deformity surgery 572
  stasis 1598

tibial plateau fractures 2290
total knee replacement 1139
ultrasound 476
venographic 1038
defensins 403
deflazacort 1330
Dega pelvic osteotomy 2473
degenerative change
  adult scoliosis 616
  vs alkaptonuria 1361
  arthritis 175
  glenohumeral joint 2040
  intervertebral disk 552–3, 558, 2063, 2065
  loose bodies in elbow joint 804, 806
  neuropathies 1478
  patellectomy 1125, 1126
  radiographic evaluation of cervical spine 487–9
  scoliosis 616, 619, 621
  spondylarthrosis 1366
  spondylolisthesis 528, 544–5, 634
  thoracic spine *498–502, 503*, 504
  triangular fibrocartilage 840–1
Déjrine–Sottas disease 1477
Delpech's law 2577
deltoid ligament 1307
  ankle fracture 2327
  sprains 1308–9
deltoid muscle 2002, 2013
  abduction contracture 757
  atrophy 660, 678–9
  detached *679*
  dysfunction 738
  obstetric brachial plexus palsy 2773
  paralysis 895, 1853
    poliomyelitis 1527
  shoulder girdle inspection 685
  splitting *679*
  strengthening 713
  wasting 661
  weakness 659
denervation, surgical 800
Denham pin 1612
Denis–Browne bar 2591
dens 2083, 2088–90
  blood supply 2095
dental treatment, antibiotic prophylaxis 1797
dentine 60
  inherited disorders 1318
dentinogenesis imperfecta 60, 1318
Denys–Drash syndrome 361
Depo-Medrol 124
depression
  low back pain 520
  pain 416, 518, 520
  spinal cord injuries 2150–1
  whiplash injury 2117
de Quervain syndrome 815, 820, 888–9
  extensor pollicis brevis subcompartment 887
  operative release 889
  splintage 888
  steroid injection 888
Dercum FX 439, 441
dermadesis 1563
dermal sinus 2532
dermatomes 582
  chart *508*
  testing in cervical spine trauma 2070, 2085
dermatomycosis 944
dermatomyositis 1394–5, *1474*
  calcinosis 1363
  heterotopic calcinosis 1382
  vs osteomalacia 1337
  tendon rupture 892
dermoid tumor 2533, 2534
  low back pain 548
desensitization exercises 1851
desferrioxamine 400

desmin
  leiomyosarcoma 311
  malignant peripheral nerve sheath tumor 317
  rhabdomyosarcoma 324
desmoid tumors 101, 102
  extra-abdominal **204–7**
    adjuvant treatment 207
    amputation 207
    anatomic distribution 204, *205*
    chemotherapy 206–7
    clinical features 204–5
    hormonal relationship 204, 207
    imaging 205
    metachronous disease 206
    pain 205
    pathology 205
    recurrence 205, 206, 207
    resection margin 206
    surgical resection 207
    treatment 205–6
    vs fibrosarcoma 308
  intra-abdominal 204
desmoplastic fibroma 286, 307
desmopressin 1457
detection bias 1586
developing countries, tuberculosis 1532, 1545, 1554
developmental anomalies
  foot 2583–4
  knee 1156–7
    osteoarthritis 1412
  kyphosis 629–30
  Ollier's disease 190
  osteoarthritis 1411–12
  see also congenital anomalies; hip dysplasia, developmental
Dewar and Harris procedure 753–4
dexamethasone
  multiple myeloma 271
  spinal vasogenic edema reduction 357
dextromethorphan 421
Deyerle screws 2219
diabetes, maternal 550
diabetes mellitus
  amputation 1496
  back pain 510
  Candida albicans infection 944
  Dupuytren's disease 878
  epidemiology 1251–2
  frozen shoulder 745, 746
  gout 1379
  hand abscess *934, 936*
  hand infections 934, 1828
  hip disorders 957
  injury and soft-tissue coverage 1652
  neuropathic joint destruction 800
  pathophysiology 1252–4
  peripheral neuropathy 1252
  protective sensation loss 1252
  pulp infections 1829
  sensory neuropathy 1252
  trigger finger 889
diabetic foot 1251–61
  abscess formation 1257
  Akin osteotomy 1261
  amputation 1252
  ankle 1255
  autonomic neuropathy 1253
  brace *1260*
  Charcot joint 1253, *1254*
  clinical examination 1254–5
  gangrene 1257, 1258
  hallux valgus 1261
  hyperglycemia 1257
  imaging 1255, 1257
  insensate 1252
  ischemia 1255
  malperforan ulcerations 1253, 1255, 1258
  motor dysfunction 1252–3

patella (*continued*)
  lateral facet 1173
    chondromalacia 1176
  maltracking of component 1142
  metal-backed components 1143
  nerve plexus 1125
  ossification center 1166, 1174
  osteochondrosis dissecans 1176
  polyethylene cemented components 1143
  postoperative mobilization 1206
  preparation for knee replacement 1131
  Q angle 1168, 1169
  resurfacing 1176–7, 2438
  revision 1147
    failed 1151
  stability 2753, 2754
  stabilizers 1168
  subluxation 1168–9
  taping 1170
  tendon shortening 1144
  tracking 1144, 1168, 1169, 1170
  transverse separation 2728
  vascular circle 1125
patellar entrapment syndrome 1206
patellar ligament
  load 1125
  MRI diagnosis of injuries 471–2
  tenotomy 2482
patellar retinaculum release 2574
patellar tendon 1168, 2265
  allograft 1195
  attachment 1145–6
  autografts 2760–1
  avulsion 1151
  bone-block graft 1199–206
  detachment 1169
  graft 1194–5, 1196–7, 1208
    harvesting 1200–1
  implant attachment 93
  peritendonitis 1175
  reattachment 2269, 2270
  repair 1150
  rupture 1787–8
  stress–strain curve *435*
  stretching 1206
  tendonitis 1175
patellectomy 1125–6, 1174, 2271
  anterior knee pain syndrome 1125, 1126
  comminuted fracture 2258
  complete 2728
  degenerative disease 1125, 1126
  history 1125
  indications 1125
  osteochondritis dissecans 1176
  partial 2269, 2271, 2728
  technique 1126
  total 2269, 2271
patellofemoral dysfunction 1140
patellofemoral joint 1166–77
  arthritis 1176–7
  biomechanics 1167–8
  dislocation 1168–9, 2273
  instability 1168–9
  osteoarthritis 2272
  pain 1176, 1199, 1472, 2539
  reaction force 1168
  stabilization 1167
patellofemoral ligament 2273
patello–femoral–quadriceps mechanism 2753
patellomeniscal ligament 2753
pathogenesis 401–4
pathogens, genome sequences 402
pathognomic findings 20, 21–2
patient-controlled analgesia (PCA) 418
patients
  adolescent and lumbar disk herniations 529
  management tools 12
  unconscious 417

young
  biopsy technique 98
  expandable endoprostheses 233
  massive prostheses 90–1, 93
  osteofibrous dysplasia 223
  osteosarcoma surgery 231–2, 234
  see also age of patient/aging
Patte test 666
Pauwel fracture classification 1578, 2217
Pavlik harness 2544, 2545
  congenital knee dislocation 2574
Pavlov ratio 2103, 2105
Pax-1 gene expression 584
PC-10 antibody 188
PCA Uni knee prosthesis 1214
pectoralis major muscle 2002
  rupture 1788
  transfer 2488, *2489*
    to biceps tendon 896, *897*2769
    to scapula 755–6, 895
pectoralis minor muscle 2038, 2043
  avulsion 2044
  transfer to scapula 755
pectus excavatum 1483
  neurofibromatosis 1492
pedestrian injury triad *366*
pedorthic treatment 1272
Pedotti diagram 427
Pelite foot orthosis inserts 1263
Pellegrini–Stieda disease 1158–9
pelvic brim 2172, *2173*
  access 2194
pelvic fixation 607
pelvic obliquity 605
  Duchenne muscular dystrophy 606
  poliomyelitis 1529, 1530–1
  spinal dysraphism 1476
pelvic osteotomy 8, 955
  acetabular rim syndrome 960
pelvic replacements 91–4
pelvic ring
  anatomy 2155–6
  disruption 2156
  lumbar spine connection 2156
pelvic ring fractures
  abdominal injury 2157, 2162
  acetabular fractures 2158
  angiography 2160, 2161, 2162
  associated conditions 2156–7, 2162, 2165
  avulsion 2155
  bed rest 2165–6
  bleeding 2160–2
  bucket-handle lateral compression injury 2158
  children 2714, 2715–16
  classification 2157–8, 2165
    outcome 2168
  complications 2167, 2169–70
  compression 2165
  CT scanning 2159, 2160
  external fixation 2160–1, 2166, 2167
    intermittent 2169
    pin insertion sites 2166
  fracture–dislocation 2155
  functional outcome 2167
  genitourinary injury 2157, 2162, 2170
  hematuria 2160
  high-energy trauma 2155
  iliac wing 2165, 2166–7
  implant placement 2167
  incidence 2155
  internal fixation 2166–7, 2169
  investigations 2158–60
  limb-length discrepancy 2168–9
  malunion 2169–70
  management 2160, 2165–70
  mechanisms 2165
  mobilization 2161, 2165–6
  mortality 2162, 2163

  natural history 2168–9
  neurologic injury 2157, 2159, 2169, 2170
  nonunion 2168–9, 2170
  open 2162–3
  open reduction 2169
  pain 2161, 2168
  pelvic sling 2166
  plate fixation 2166
  posterior injury 2165
  prevalence 2155
  radiography 2159
  reduction 2167, 2169
  retrograde urethrocystogram 2160
  rotationally deformed 2168
  sacroiliac joint 2165, 2166–7
  sacrum 2165, 2167
  screws 2166
  SF-36 score 2167–8
  skeletal traction 2166
  soft-tissue damage 2156
  stable 2166
  surgical approach 2166–7
  surgical result measurement 2167–8
  treatment algorithm *2163*
  ultrasonography 2160
  undisplaced 2168
  unstable *2163*, 2170
    internal fixation 2169
  urethra 2170
  urinary bladder 2170
  vertical instability 2168
  vertical shear 2158, 2165
  wound debridement/irrigation 2163
pelvic sling 2166
pelvic veins 2156
pelvis 947–1105
  antishock clamp 2161
  bony 2155–6
  chondrosarcoma *246*
    of bone *244*
    central 239
    dedifferentiated 246
  chordoma *295*
  distraction 1543
  Ewing sarcoma *257*, 258, 262
  fractures 1606, 1610
    bleeding 1608
    children 2713–18
    displaced 457
    external fixation 1608, 1609, 1610, 1723
    sacral plexus injury 1857
    sciatic nerve injury 1857
    stress 1761
    tibial plafond fractures 2311
    vascular injury 1597
  fusion 2469
  injury 1606
  irradiation 961
  levels 564–5
  ligaments 2155–6
  metastatic bone disease due to carcinoma 349–51
  obliquity 967
    cerebral palsy 1475
  osteosarcoma 234, *236*
  osteosclerotic myeloma 273, *274*
  osteotomy 955, 960, 1531, 2473
  periacetabular region resection 91
  stability 2155
  subacute osteomyelitis 1426
  tilt 2605
  tumors 91–4
  unstable 1608, 1609
Pemberton osteotomy *2483*
D-penicillamine 1283, 1374
penicillin 408
  allergy 1796, 1797
  bite infections 1830
  childhood gonococcal arthritis 2425

popliteal angle 2455
  measurement 1475
popliteal artery
  injury 1666
  repair with reversed interposition vein graft *1678*
  shunt 1672
  tibial plateau fractures 2281
  trifurcation 2731, 2741
popliteal cysts 1155
popliteal varix 1159
popliteal vein repair *1678*
popliteal vessels
  injury in children 2727
  injury in total knee replacement 1137–8
  supracondylar fractures of femur 2254
porins 409
Porphyromonas, bites 940
positive predictive value 22–3, 405
postconcussive syndrome 389
postexposure prophylaxis 411
postherpetic neuralgia 421
postphlebitic limb 395
postpolio syndrome 1269, 1476–7
  ankle–foot orthosis 1274
  arthrodesis of foot/ankle 1274
  foot disorders 1273–4
  walking aids 1274
poststroke syndrome 416
postural deformity in adult scoliosis 616
postural round back 629–30
  imaging 629, 630
  treatment 629–30
power analysis 6–7, 13–14
power grasp 849
practice parameters 32
precision pinch 848
prediction rules 28
Predictive Salvage Index (PSI) 1683, *1684*, 1685
predictive value of positive test 22–3
prednisolone
  connective tissue disease 1392, 1394, 1399
  dermatomyositis 1394
  hemophilic synovitis 1462
  polymyalgia rheumatica 1396
  polymyositis 1394
  rheumatoid arthritis 1375
  systemic vasculitis 1395, 1398, 1399
prednisone
  multiple myeloma 271
  non-Hodgkin lymphoma 280
pregnancy
  avascular necrosis 973
  back pain 510
    chronic 550
  disk prolapse 549–50
  idiopathic scoliosis 576
  osteochondroma 181
  osteoporosis 1330, *1331*
    transient 956
  smoking 2618
  twin 2584
prenatal diagnosis, genetic conditions of skeleton 67,
    68, 69
pressure analysis 1283
pressure sores 2148
prevention 4
prevertebral shadow 2105
Prevotella, bites 940
PRICE mnemonic 1781
primitive neuroectodermal tumors 256
  children 2534
  vs neuroblastoma 359
  vs non-Hodgkin lymphoma 276
principle component analysis 449
prion diseases 411
probability *(p)* 13
  estimating 24
  odds ratio 23

pretest 405, 406
  tests 22
  utility 26
probability theory 20
probenecid 1380
procoagulants, activated 1598
profilometry 1092
profunda femoris, perforating branches 995
progestins 344
progestogen 1328
progressive osseous heteroplasia 1367–8
progress zone 80
prolactin 1330
proliferating cell nuclear antigen 317
pronator compression test 906
pronator quadratus muscle 1958, 2683
  grafts 1902
pronator syndrome 848, 905–6
pronator teres muscle 2678, 2683
  transfer 1854
Propionibacterium
  implants for spinal deformities 573
  prosthetic joint infection 1450
Propionibacterium acnes 407
  scoliosis surgery 579
  septic hip arthroplasty 1078
proprioception 387–8
proptosis 1397–8
prospective studies 5–6
prostaglandin(s)
  osteoid osteoma 151–2
  pulmonary dysfunction 1649
  unicameral bone cyst 121
prostaglandin D$_2$ 1094
prostaglandin E$_2$
  giant cell tumour of bone 162
  infection 402–3
  membrane from bone–cement interface 1086
  metastatic bone disease due to carcinoma 341
  osteoclasts 1093
  osteolysis 1093, 1094
  pain generation 558
  polyethylene 1086
prostate cancer
  metastases 103
  metastatic bone disease due to carcinoma 344
  stromal bone 1768
prosthesis 432
  congenital limb deficiency 2617
  elbow level deficiency 2620
  failure management 93
  femur 2623, *2624*
  hand deformities 2499–500
  humerus deficiency 2620
  infection 404, 406, 1443–53
    amputation 1452
    antibiotics 1446, 1451, 1452–3
    classification 1446–7
    clinical presentation 1447
    debridement 1451
    diagnosis 1447–8
    exchange arthroplasty 1451–2
    excision arthroplasty 1452
    foreign material 1444
    fusion 1452
    Gram stain 1449
    hematogenous 1446
    host factors 1444
    imaging 1448–9
    implant factors 1444
    incidence 1444
    intraoperative cultures 1449–50
    intraoperative investigations 1449
    joint aspiration 1449, *1450*
    mechanisms 1444–5
    microbiology 1445
    micro-organisms 1444–5
    operative factors 1444

  operatively-acquired 1445–6
  polymorphonuclear leukocytes 1449
  postoperative investigations 1449–50
  preoperative investigations 1448–9
  prevention 1445–6
  retention 1451
  risk factors 1444
  treatment 1450–3
  intertrochanteric pathologic lesions 351, 352
  ischial bearing extension 2623, *2624*
  leg 2621, *2622*
  limb-deficient child 2619, 2621
    transverse upper-limb 2619–20
  metastatic bone disease due to carcinoma 346, 347
  see also acetabular component of hip prosthesis;
      amputation, prostheses; hip, prosthesis;
      implants; implants, extendible; knee, prosthesis
proteins
  intraneural accretion 1252
  noncollagen 1318, *1319*
protein synthesis inhibitors 408
proteoglycans 77
  articular cartilage 379, 380
  tendons 381
Proteus
  prosthetic joint infection 1445
  pyogenic spinal infection 650
Proteus mirabilis
  cephalosporins 1795
  postoperative infections 1791
prothrombin complex concentrates 1464
proton-pump inhibitors 1394
protrusio acetabulae 956, 961, 962–4
  anatomy 962–3
  bone grafts 963–4
  classification 963
  clinical evaluation 963
  imaging 996
  incidence 962
  management 963
  rheumatoid arthritis 968–9
  severity grades 962
  total hip replacement in rheumatoid arthritis 972
  tuberculosis 1539
proximal interphalangeal joint (PIP) 2504
  dislocations in children 2704
  symphalyngism 2509
proximal myopathy 1334
Prunus spinosa (blackthorn) 887
pseudachondroplasia 37, *51*
  features *1322*
pseudarthrosis
  adult scoliosis surgery 621
  back pain 510, 516
  bone graft union rates 1103
  Boyd classification 1488–90
  clavicle 62, 698, 2615
  congenital 2526
    child 2611–16
    clavicle 698, 2615
    femur 2616
    forearm 2615
    tibia 2611–15
  external fixation 1719
  femur 62, 2616
  fibula 1490
  irradiated spine 633
  neurofibromatosis 1485, 1488–92
    free vascularized bone grafts 1491–2
    management 1491–2
    surgical procedures 1491–2
  neurofibromatosis type 1 1481, 1483
  post-traumatic 2493
  radiotherapy for tumors 624
  radius 1491
  rheumatoid arthritis 493
  scoliosis surgery 579
  spinal fusion failure 573, 579, 581